a LANGE medical book

Basic & Clinical
Immunology

eighth edition

Edited by

Daniel P. Stites, MD
Professor and Chairman
Department of Laboratory Medicine
University of California, San Francisco

Abba I. Terr, MD
Clinical Professor of Medicine
Stanford University School of Medicine
Stanford, California

Tristram G. Parslow, MD, PhD
Associate Professor of Pathology
and of Microbiology and Immunology
University of California, San Francisco

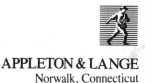

APPLETON & LANGE
Norwalk, Connecticut

Copyright © 1994 by Appleton & Lange
Paramount Publishing Business and Professional Group
Copyright © 1991 by Appleton & Lange
Copyright © 1987, 1984, 1982, 1980, 1978, 1976 by Lange Medical Publications

94 95 96 97 98 / 10 9 8 7 6 5 4 3 2 1

Prentice Hall International (UK) Limited, *London*
Prentice Hall of Australia Pty. Limited, *Sydney*
Prentice Hall Canada, Inc., *Toronto*
Prentice Hall Hispanoamericana, S.A., *Mexico*
Prentice Hall of India Private Limited, *New Delhi*
Prentice Hall of Japan, Inc., *Tokyo*
Simon & Schuster Asia Pte. Ltd., *Singapore*
Editora Prentice Hall do Brasil Ltd., *Rio de Janeiro*
Prentice Hall, *Englewood Cliffs, New Jersey*

ISBN: 0835-0561-9
ISSN: 0891-2076

Acquisitions Editor: Martin Wonsiewicz
Production Editor: Jennifer Sinsavich

PRINTED IN THE UNITED STATES OF AMERICA

ISBN   0-8385-0561-9

Table of Contents

Preface . . . . **xix**

History of Immunology **1**

David W. Talmage, MD

The Origin of Immunology 1
Cellular Versus Humoral Immunity 2
The Period of Serology 2
The Rebirth of Cellular Immunology 2
The Advent of Molecular Immunology 3

Immunogenetics & Genetic Engineering 3
Immunology Time Line 3
Nobel Prize Winners in Immunology 4
Summary 5

SECTION I BASIC IMMUNOLOGY

1. The Phagocytes: Neutrophils & Macrophages **9**

Tristram G. Parslow, MD, PhD

Ontogeny of Blood Cells 9
Neutrophils 10

Mononuclear Phagocytes: The Monocyte-
   Macrophage System 17

2. Lymphocytes & Lymphoid Tissue **22**

Tristram G. Parslow, MD, PhD

B Cells 24
T Cells 26
Requirements for Activation of B or
   T Lymphocytes 30

Lymphoid Organs 31
Lymphocyte Circulation & Homing 38

3. The Immune Response **40**

Joel W. Goodman, PhD

Clonal Organization & Dynamics of Lymphocyte
   Populations 40
The Immune Response 42
Antigen Processing & Presentation 42
Mechanisms of Antigen Elimination 46
Inflammation 47

Localization of Immune Responses 47
Quantitative & Kinetic Aspects of Immune
   Responses 48
Programmed Cell Death in the Immune
   System 49

4. Immunogens & Antigens **50**

Joel W. Goodman, PhD

Immunogens 50
Adjuvants 51
B Cell Antigens & B-Cell Epitopes 52
Conformational & Linear Epitopes 53
Haptens 54

T Cell Antigens, T Cell Epitopes,
   & Immunogenicity 55
Thymus-Independent Antigens 56
Vaccines 56

5. Antigen Presentation & the Major Histocompatibility Complex **58**

Joel W. Goodman, PhD

Human Leukocyte Antigens 58
Genetic Organization of the MHC 58
Antigen Presentation by Class I & Class II MHC
   Proteins 61

Antigen-Presenting Cells 62
MHC & Immune Responsiveness 64
MHC & Disease 64

6. Immunoglobulin Proteins 66
Joel W. Goodman, PhD, & Tristram G. Parslow, MD, PhD

Organization & Diversity of Immunoglobulin
    Proteins 66
Classification of Immunoglobulins & Their
    Constituent Chains 68
Carbohydrate Moieties of Immunoglobulins 72
Biologic Activities of Immunoglobulins 73

Fc Receptors 74
Immunoglobulin Variable Regions 74
The 3-Dimensional Structure of
    Immunoglobulins 77
Immunoglobulin Gene Superfamily 78

7. Immunoglobulin Genes, B Cells, & the Humoral Immune Response 80
Tristram G. Parslow, MD, PhD

Immunoglobulin Genes Are Formed Through
    DNA Rearrangement in B Cells 80
Immunoglobulin Gene Rearrangements & Early
    B Cell Ontogeny 84

Maturation & Release of Virgin B
    Lymphocytes 86

8. T Lymphocytes & Natural Killer Cells 94
John B. Imboden, Jr., MD

T Cell Antigen Receptor 94
Accessory Molecules & TCR Coreceptors 97
T Cell Subsets & Heterogeneity 99

T Cell Ontogeny 101
Natural Killer Cells 102

9. Cytokines 105
Joost J. Oppenheim, MD, Francis W. Ruscetti, PhD & Connie Faltynek, PhD

Interleukin-1 & Tumor Necrosis Factor 105
Interleukin-2 112
Interleukin-6 & Related Cytokines 113
The Interferons 114
Interleukin-4 & Interleukin-13 116
Interleukin-5 117
Interleukin-7 117
Interleukin-9 117

Interleukin-10 117
Interleukin-12 117
Transforming Growth Factor ß 117
Interleukin-8 & the Chemokine Family of
    Cytokines 118
Hematopoietic Colony-Stimulating Factors 120
Cytokine Receptor Families 121
Overview & Prospects 121

10. Complement & Kinin 124
Michael M. Frank, MD

The Complement System 124
Functions of Complement 124
Pathways of Complement Activation 124
Nomenclature 124
The Classic Complement Pathway 125
The Classic Pathway C5 Convertase 127
The Alternate Complement Pathway 128
The Late Components C5–9 & the Membrane
    Attack Complex 128
Control Mechanisms 129
Genetic Considerations 131
Biologic Consequences of Complement
    Activation in Inflammation 131

Complement Receptors & Related Membrane
    Proteins 132
The Kinin Cascade 133
Proteins of the Kinin Cascade 133
Steps in Kinin Activation 133
Amplification & Regulation of Kinin
    Generation 134
Plasma Inhibitors of Kinin Generation 134
Low-Molecular-Weight Kininogen & Tissue
    Kallikrens 134
Functions of Kinins in Disease 135

11. Inflammation 137
Abba I. Terr, MD

Inflammatory Cells 138
Mediators of Inflammation 142

Types of Immunologically Mediated
    Inflammatory Responses 145

SECTION II IMMUNOLOGIC LABORATORY TESTS

12. Clinical Laboratory Methods for Detection of Antigens & Antibodies **151**
R. P. Channing Rodgers, MD

Methods & Interpretation 152
Applications: Serum Immunoglobulin Levels in Health & Disease 155
Electrophoresis & Immunoelectrophoresis 156
Zone Electrophoresis 157
Immunoelectrophoresis 158
Electroimmunodiffusion 164
Immunochemical & Physicochemical Methods 166
Chromatography 166
Serum Viscosity 168
Cryoglobulins 168
Pyroglobulins 169
Detection of Immune Complexes 169
Nephelometry 170
Binder-Ligand Assays 170
Radioimmunoassay 171
Types of Analytic Methods 173
Comparing Analytic Performance of Different Methods 175

Glossary of Assay Terminology 176
Immunohistochemical Techniques 178
Immunofluorescence 178
Other Immunohistochemical Techniques 183
Agglutination 184
Agglutination Techniques 184
Hemagglutination Inhibition 185
Clinically Applicable Tests that Involve Agglutination Reactions 185
Complement Assays 186
Hemolytic Assays 187
Measurement of Individual Complement Components 188
Monoclonal Antibodies 189
Technique of Monoclonal Antibody Production 190
Comparative Sensitivity of Quantitative Immunoassays 191
Predictive Value Theory 191

13. Clinical Laboratory Methods for Detection of Cellular Immunity **195**
Daniel P. Stites, MD

Delayed Hypersensitivity Skin Tests 195
Assays for Human Lymphocytes & Monocytes 197
T Lymphocyte Assays 198
B Lymphocyte Assay 200
Flow Cytometry 202
Lymphocyte Activation 203
Methods & Interpretations 205
Mixed Lymphocyte Culture & Cell-Mediated Lympholysis 208

Clinical Application of T & B Cell Assays 209
Natural Killer Cells 209
Monocyte-Macrophage Assays 209
Neutrophil Function 209
Tests for Motility 210
Tests for Recognition & Adhesion 211
Tests for Ingestion 211
Tests for Degranulation 211
Tests for Intracellular Killing 212

14. Molecular Genetic Techniques for Clinical Analysis of the Immune System **216**
Tristram G. Parslow, MD, PhD

Nucleic Acid Probes 216
Hybridization Assays 217
Southern Blot 218
Gene Rearrangement Assay for Lymphocyte Clonality 220

In Situ Hybridization 221
Target Amplification Techniques: Polymerase Chain Reaction 221
Methods of Analyzing RNA 223
Overview & Prospects 224

15. Blood Banking & Immunohematology **226**
Elizabeth Donegan, MD & Edith L. Bossom, AB, MT (ASCP), SBB

Blood Groups 226
Erythrocyte Antigens 226
Methods for Detection of Antigen & Antibodies to Erythrocytes 229

Transfusion Reactions 230
Rh Isoimmunization 233
Blood Component Therapy 234

16. **Histocompatibility Testing** **237**
Beth W. Colombe, PhD

Histocompatibility Testing & Transplantation 237
Rationale for Tissue Typing for
   Transplantation 237
Antibodies to Detect Sensitization to HLA
   Antigens 240
Serologic Methods in Histocompatibility
   Testing 240
Tissue Typing by the Lymphocytotoxicity
   Test 240
Tissue-Typing Reagents: HLA Alloantisera 242

Monoclonal Antibodies to HLA Antigens 242
Specificity of HLA Antibodies: Private &
   Public 242
Tissue Typing for Class II HLA Antigens by
   Serologic Methods 243
Cross-Matching 244
Cellular Assays for Histocompatibility 246
Histocompatibility Testing by Molecular-Biologic
   Methods 248

17. **Laboratory Evaluation of Immune Competence** **256**
Daniel P. Stites, MD

Utility of Laboratory Tests 256
Variability of Tests 256
Limitations of Testing 257
Clinical Utility of Testing 257
Specific Testing for Immune Competence 257

T Cells 258
B Cells 259
NK Cells 261
Complement 261
Phagocytic Cells 261

SECTION III CLINICAL IMMUNOLOGY _____

18. **Mechanisms of Immunodeficiency** **263**
Arthur J. Ammann, MD

19. **Antibody (B Cell) Immunodeficiency Disorders** **266**
Arthur J. Ammann, MD

X-Linked Infantile Hypogammaglobulinemia 266
Transient Hypogammaglobulinemia of
   Infancy 270
Common, Variable Unclassifiable
   Immunodeficiency 271

Immunodeficiency With Hyper-IgM 273
Selective IgA Deficiency 273
Selective IgM Deficiency 276
Selective Deficiency of IgG Subclasses 276
X-Linked Lymphoproliferative Syndrome 277

20. **T Cell Immunodeficiency Disorders** **279**
Arthur J. Ammann, MD

Congenital Thymic Aplasia 279
Chronic Mucocutaneous Candidiasis 282

Immunodeficiency Associated With Natural
   Killer Cell Deficiency 284

21. **Combined Antibody (B Cell) & Cellular (T Cell) Immunodeficiency Disorders** **286**
Arthur J. Ammann, MD

Severe Combined Immunodeficiency Disease 286
T Cell Membrane Signaling & Cytokine
   Defects 288
Cellular Immunodeficiency With Abnormal
   Immunoglobulin Synthesis 289
Immunodeficiency With
   Ataxia-Telangiectasia 290
Immunodeficiency With Thrombocytopenia,
   Eczema, & Recurrent Infection 292

Immunodeficiency With Thymoma 293
Immunodeficiency With Short-Limbed
   Dwarfism 294
Immunodeficiency With Enzyme Deficiency 295
Graft-Versus-Host Disease 297
Immunodeficiency With Cell Membrane
   Abnormalities 298

22. **Phagocytic Dysfunction Diseases** **303**
Arthur J. Ammann, MD

Chronic Granulomatous Disease 303
Glucose-6-Phosphate Dehydrogenase
   Deficiency 305
Myeloperoxidase Deficiency 306
Alkaline Phosphatase Deficiency 306
Chédiak-Higashi Syndrome 306

Job's Syndrome 306
Tuftsin Deficiency 306
Elevated IgE, Defective Chemotaxis, Eczema, &
   Recurrent Infection 307
Leukocyte Movement Disorders 307
Miscellaneous Phagocytic Disorders 307

23. **Complement Deficiencies** **309**
Michael M. Frank, MD

Alternate-Pathway Components Deficiencies 309
Classic-Pathway Component Deficiencies 309
C3 & Terminal-Component Deficiencies 310
Complement Deficiencies & Autoimmunity 311

Complement Regulatory Factor Deficiencies 311
Hereditary Angioedema 311
Complement Receptor Deficiencies 312
Complement Allotype Variants 312

24. **Mechanisms of Hypersensitivity** **314**
Abba I. Terr, MD

Definitions 314
Prevalence 314
Allergens 314
Susceptibility to Allergy 314
Mechanisms & Classification of Allergic
    Disease 315
The IgE/Mast Cell/Mediator Pathway 315
The IgE or IgM/Complement/Neutrophil
    Pathway 317

The Effector T Lymphocyte/Lymphokine
    Pathway 317
Clinical Evaluation 317
General Considerations 317
History 317
Physical Examination 318
Laboratory Testing 318

25. **The Atopic Diseases** **327**
Abba I. Terr, MD

General Considerations 327
Atopic Allergens 329
Allergic Rhinitis 332

Asthma 335
Atopic Dermatitis 341
Allergic Gastroenteropathy 343

26. **Anaphylaxis & Urticaria** **347**
Abba I. Terr, MD

Anaphylaxis 347

Urticaria & Angioedema 354

27. **Immune-Complex Allergic Diseases** **357**
Abba I. Terr, MD

The Arthus Reaction 357
Serum Sickness 358

Allergic Bronchopulmonary Aspergillosis 359

28. **Cell-Mediated Hypersensitivity Diseases** **363**
Abba I. Terr, MD

Allergic Contact Dermatitis 363
Photoallergic Contact Dermatitis 365

Hypersensitivity Pneumonitis 366

29. **Drug Allergy** **371**
H. James Wedner, MD

Immunologic Basis of Drug Allergy 371
Diagnosis of Drug Allergy 374
Treatment of Drug Allergy 375
Penicillin Allergy 375

Sulfonamide Allergy 377
Insulin Allergy 378
Pseudoallergic Reactions 379
Conclusions 379

30. **Mechanisms of Disordered Immune Regulation** **380**
Alfred D. Steinberg, MD

Disease Mechanisms 380
Lessons from Experimental Animals 383

Conclusions 385

31. **Rheumatic Diseases** **387**
Kenneth H. Fye, MD & Kenneth E. Sack, MD

Systemic Lupus Erythematous 387
Rheumatoid Arthritis 392
Juvenile Arthritis 397
Sjögren's Syndrome 399

Progressive Systemic Sclerosis 401
Polymyositis-Dermatomyositis 404
Ankylosing Spondylitis 406
Reiter's Syndrome 407

Psoriatic Arthritis 408
Relapsing Polychondritis 408
Relapsing Panniculitis 408

Hereditary Complement Deficiencies & Collagen
    Vascular Diseases 409
Hypogammaglobulinemia & Arhtritis 409

32. Endocrine Diseases 412
James R. Baker, Jr. MD

Mechanisms of Development of Autoimmune
    Endocrine Disease 412
Organ-Specific Autoantibodies 412
Thyroid Autoimmune Diseases 413
Chronic Thyroiditis 413
Transient Thyroiditis Syndromes 415
Graves' Disease 417

Disorders of the Endocrine Pancreas 419
Insulin-Dependent Diabetes Mellitus 419
Adrenal Insuffiency 421
Lymphocytic Adenohypophysitis 421
Premature Ovarian Failure 422
Idiopathic Hypoparathyroidism 422
Autoimmune Polyglandular Syndromes 422

33. Hematologic Diseases 425
John Vivian Wells, MD, FRACP, FRCPA & James P. Isbister, FRACP, FRCPA

Leukocyte Disorders 425
Leukopenia 425
Erythrocyte Disorders 427
Immune Hemolytic Anemias 427
Paroxysmal Nocturnal Hemoglobinuria 433
Aplastic Anemia & Related Disorders 433
Platelet Disorders 434

Idiopathic Thrombocytopenic Purpura 435
Drug-Induced Immune Thrombocytopenias 438
Posttransfusion Purpura 438
Coagulation Disorders 438
Hemophilia & Von Willebrand's Disease 438
Circulating Inhibitors of Coagulation 439

34. Cardiac & Vascular Diseases 442
Thomas R. Cupps, MD

Cardiac Diseases 442
Pericardial Diseases 442
Myocardial Diseases 442
Endomyocardial Diseases 443
Vascular Diseases: The Vasculitides
Small-Vessel Vasculitis 444
Syndromes Associated With Small-Vessel
    Vasculitis 445

Systemic Necrotizing Vasculitis 447
Wegener's Granulomatosis 450
Takayasu Arteritis 453
Thromboangiitis Obliterans 455
Other Vasculitic Syndromes 455

35. Gastrointestinal, Hepatobiliary, & Orodental Diseases 457
Stephen P. James, MD, Warren Strober, MD & John S. Greenspan, BDS, PhD, FRCPath

Gastrointestinal Diseases 457
Gluten-Sensitive Enteropathy 457
Non-Gluten Hypersensitivity 459
Crohn's Disease 459
Ulcerative Colitis 461
Alpha Heavy-Chain Disease 462
Pernicious Anemia 462
Whipple's Disease 463
Hepatobiliary Diseases 463
Hepatitis A 464
Hepatitis B 464

Hepatitis D 466
Hepatitis C 466
Hepatitis E 467
Autoimmune Chronic Active Hepatitis 467
Primary Biliary Cirrhosis 468
Orodental Diseases 470
Local Oral Diseases Involving Immunologic
    Mechanisms 471
Recurrent Aphthous Ulceration 474
Acquired Immunodeficiency Syndrome 475
Oral Candidiasis 476

36. Renal Diseases 478
Curtis B. Wilson, MD, Winson W. Tang, MD, Lili Feng, MD, Yiyang Xia, MD & David M. Ward, MB, ChB, FRCP

Anti-Glomerular Basement Membrane Antibody-
    Induced Glomerulonephritis 479
Immune Complex Glomerulonephritis 481
Tubulointerstitial Nephritis 487

Minimal-Change Nephropathy 489
Focal Glomerulosclerosis 489
Vasculitis 489

37. Dermatologic Diseases 492
Sanford M. Goldstein, MD & Bruce U. Wintroub, MD

Bullous Pemphigoid 492
Herpes Gestationis 495
Dermatitis Herpetiformis 497
Epidermolysis Bullosa Acquisita 499

Pemphigus Vulgaris & Pemphigus Foliaceus 500
Linear IgA Bullous Dermatosis 503
Discoid Lupus Erythematous 504

38. Neurologic Diseases 507
Hillel S. Pantich, MD & Paul S. Fishman, MD, PhD

Demyelinating Diseases 507
Acute Disseminated Encephalomyelitis 507
Multiple Sclerosis 508
Acute Inflammatory Demyelinating
    Polyneuropathy 511
Chronic Demyelinating Polyneuropathies 513
Disorders of Neuromuscular Transmission 513
Myasthenia Gravis 513
Myasthenic Syndrome 515

Immunologic Abnormalities in Other Neurologic
    Diseases 515
Paraneoplastic Cerebellar Degeneration 515
Amyotrophic Lateral Sclerosis 516
Alzheimer's Disease 517
Slow & Latent Virus Infections of the Nervous
    System 517
Progressive Multifocal Leukoencephalopathy 517

39. Eye Diseases 520
Mitchell H. Friedlaender, MD & G. Richard O'Connor, MD

Antibody-Mediated Diseases 520
Vernal Conjuctivitis & Atopic
    Keratoconjuctivitis 520
Rheumatoid Diseases Affecting the Eye 521
Other Antibody-Mediated Diseases 523
Cell-Mediated Diseases 523

Ocular Sarcoidosis 523
Sympathetic Ophthalmia & Vogt-Koyanagi-
    Harada Syndrome 524
Other Cell-Mediated Diseases 525
Corneal Graft Reactions 526

40. Respiratory Diseases 528
John F. Fieselmann, MD & Hal B. Richerson, MD

Drug-Induced Respiratory Diseases 528
Eosinophilic Pneumonias 530
Occupational & Environmental Lung
    Diseases 533
Sarcoidosis 533
Idiopathic Pulmonary Fibrosis 534
Goodpasture's Syndrome 536

Pulmonary Vasculitis Syndromes 537
Pulmonary Manifestations of
    Immunodeficiency 537
Lung Transplantation 538
Adult Respiratory Distress Syndrome 538
Allergic Asthma 539
Allergic Bronchopulmonary Aspergillosis 539

41. The Mucosal Immune System 541
Warren Strober, MD & Stephen P. James, MD

Functions 541
Anatomy 541
Immunoglobulin A 544
Production of Other Immunoglobulins in the
    Mucosa 548

Regulation of IgA Synthesis at Mucosal Sites 548
Oral Unresponsiveness 549
Mucosal Homing 549
Breast Milk Immunology 550
Summary 550

42. Reproduction & the Immune System 552
Karen Palmore Beckerman, MD

Reproductive Tract Anatomy & Immunity 552
Mucosal Immunity 553
Defense Against Pathogens Versus Tolerance of
    Sperm "Invasion" 554
The Testis & The Ovary 554
Fertilization, Implantation, & the Immune
    Response to Fetal Tissues 554
Implantation 555
Trophoblast Invasion of Maternal Tissues 555
The Placenta as an Immune Organ 557
Immunity in Pregnancy 558

Background: Altered Susceptibility to Infection in
    Pregnancy 558
Proposed Mechanisms of Altered Immunity in
    Pregnancy 558
Infertility & Spontaneous Abortion 559
Recurrent Spontaneous Abortion 561
Isoimmunization 561
Historical Background 562
Pathophysiology of Isoimmune Hydrops 562
ABO Incompatibility 562
Anti-Rh Ig Prophylaxis 563

Management of the Isoimmunized Pregnancy 564
Heterosexual Transmission of HIV 565
HIV Infection & the Reproductive System 565

Neonatal Alloimmune Thrombocytopenia 565
Perinatal Transmission of HIV 566
Conclusion 567

43. **Mechanisms of Tumor Immunology** **569**
Philip D. Greenberg, MD

Development of Tumors 569
Antigens on Tumor Cells 570
Immunologic Effector Mechanisms Potentially
    Operative Against Tumor Cells 572

Potential Mechanisms by Which Tumor Cells
    May Escape from an Immune Response 574
Immunotherapy 575

44. **Cancer in the Immunocompromised Host** **578**
John L. Ziegler, MD

Immune Surveillance 578
Immunocompromise & Cancer 579
Congenital Immunodeficiency & Neoplasia 580
Cancer in Organ Transplant Recipients 581
Cancer in Patients With Autoimmune
    Disorders 582

Second Tumors in Cancer Patients 582
Human Immunodeficiency Virus Infection & the
    Development of Cancer 583
Conclusions 586

45. **Neoplasms of the Immune System** **588**
John W. Parker, MD & Robert J. Lukes, MD

Classification 588
General Considerations 588
Immunologic Features 589
DNA Analysis 592
Cytogenetics 596
Molecular Genetics 599
Therapy 600
Lymphocytic Neoplasms of B Cell Origin 601
Acute Lymphocytic Leukemia 602
Small Lymphocytic Lymphomas
    & Leukemias 603
Prolymphocytic Leukemia 604
Follicular Center Cell Lymphomas 604
Immunoblastic Sarcoma of the B Cell Type 605
Hairy Cell Leukemia 606
Plasmacytoid Lymphocytic Lymphoma 606
Plasm Cell Neoplasms & Dyscrasias 607
Multiple Myeloma 607
Solitary Plasmacytoma 608
Amyloidosis 608
Heavy-Chain Diseases 608
Benign Monoclonal Gammopathy 609
Cryoglobulinemia 609

Benign Hypergammaglobulinemia Purpura 610
Lymphocytic Neoplasms of T Cell Origin 610
Acute Lymphocytic Leukemia of T Cell
    Type 610
Convoluted T Cell Lymphoma 612
Small T Lymphocyte Neoplasms 612
Peripheral T Cell Lymphomas 613
Lymphoepithelioid Lymphocytic Lymphoma of
    T Cell Type 613
Cutaneous T Cell Lymphomas 613
Hodgkin's Disease 614
Neoplasms of the Mononuclear Phagocyte
    System 616
Histiocytic Medullary Reticulosis 616
Other Malignant Histiocytoses 616
Acute Myelomonocytic Leukemia 617
Acute Monocytic Leukemia 617
Interrelation of Granulocytic & Lymphocytic
    Leukemias 617
Natural Killer Cell/Large Granular Lymphocyte
    Leukemia 617
Benign Condition Mimicking or Associated With
    Neoplasms of the Immune System 618

46. **Mechanisms of Immunity to Infection** **622**
John Mills, MD & David J. Drutz, MD

Nonimmunologic Defenses Against Infection 622
Immunologic Defenses Against Infection 624

Immunopathology of Infection 625

47. **Bacterial Diseases** **627**
John L. Ryan, PhD, MD

Serodiagnosis 627
Exotoxins & Endotoxins 627
Toxogenic Bacterial Diseases 628

Encapsulated Bacteria 631
Intracellular Bacterial Pathogens 633
Conclusions 635

48. Viral Infections **637**

John Mills, MD

Influenza Virus 637
Respiratory Syncytial Virus 639
Measles Virus 641
Hepatitis B Virus 642

Hepatitis A Virus 645
Rabies Virus 646
Poliovirus 646

49. Fungal Diseases **649**

David J. Drutz, MD

Systemic Invasive Mycoses: Primary
  Pathogens 654
Blastomycosis 654
Coccidiomycosis 654
Histoplasmosis 657
Paracoccidioidomycosis 658

Systemic Invasive Mycoses: Opportunistic
  Pathogens 659
Cryptococcosis 660
Aspergillosis 661
Mucormycosis 662
Pneumocytosis 663

50. Parasitic Diseases **666**

James McKerrow, PhD, MD & Donald Heyneman, PhD

Immune Response to Protozoa 666
Malaria 666
Toxoplasmosis 668
Leishmaniasis 669
African Trypanosomiasis 671

Immune Response to Helminths 673
Trematodes 673
Cestodes 675
Nematodes 676

51. Spirochetal Diseases **680**

Charles S. Pavia, PhD & David J. Drutz, MD

Syphilis 680
Nonvenereal Treponematoses 684
Lyme Disease 684

Relapsing-Fever Borreliosis 686
Leptospirosis 687

52. Virus Infections of the Immune System **689**

Suzanne Crowe, MBBS, FRACP & John Mills, MD

Human Immunodeficiency Virus 689
Cytomegalovirus 700
Epstein-Barr Virus 701

Human T Cell Leukemia Virus Types I & II 703
Human Herpesvirus Type 6 705

53. Opportunistic Infections in the Immunocompromised Host **706**

Lowell S. Young, MD

Host Defects Predisposing to Infection 706
Approach to the Immunocompromised
  Patient 706
Disease Associations 707
Appropriate Diagnosis 708

Diagnostic Tests 708
Treatment 709
Reversal of Underlying Immunologic Defects 709
Prophylaxis 709

SECTION IV IMMUNOLOGIC THERAPY

54. Immunologic Therapy **711**

Abba I. Terr, MD

Modulation of the Immune Response 712
Antigen-Specific Therapy 712

Antigen-Nonspecific Therapy 713
Modulation of the Inflammatory Response 715

55. Immunization 717

Moses Grossman, MD

Historical Overview 717
Types of Immunization 717
Active Immunization 717
Passive Immunization 727
Combined Passive-Active Immunization 734
Clinical Indications for Immunization 734
Herd Immunity 734
Antigenic Shift & Antigenic Variation 734

Specific Diseases 735
Age at Immunization 735
Simultaneous Immunization with Multiple
   Antigens 736
Immunization for Foreign Travel 737
Vaccines for Special Populations 737
Vaccines Currently in Development 737
HIV Infection 738

56. Allergy Desensitization 739

Abba I. Terr, MD

Methods 739
Immunologic Effects 741
Adverse Effects 741

Indications 742
Monitoring Desensitization 742
Desensitization With Modified Allergens 743

57. Clinical Transplantation 744

Marvin R. Garovoy, MD, Peter Stock, MD, Ginny Bumgardner, MD, PhD,
Fraser Keith, MD & Charles Linker, MD

Kidney Transplantation 744
ABO Testing 744
Liver Transplantation 749
Pancreas Transplantation 752
Heart Transplantation 754

Combined Heart-Lung & Lung
   Transplantation 756
Bone Marrow Transplantation 758
Bone Transplantation 761
Future of Transplantation 762

58. Immunosuppressive Therapy 765

Alan Winkelstein, MD

Corticosteroids 765
Cytotoxic Drugs 768
Cyclosporin 775
FK-506 776

Plasmapheresis 777
Intravenous Gamma Globulin 777
Antilymphocyte Antibodies 778
Monoclonal Antibodies 778

59. Immunomodulators 781

Lawrence R. Hennessey, MD & James R. Baker, Jr, MD

Compounds Derived from Bacteria 781
Compounds Derived from Eukaryotic
   Organisms 782

Biochemical Agents 784

60. Anti-Inflammatory Drugs 786

James S. Goodwin, MD

Corticosteroids 786
Aspirin & Other Nonsteroidal Anti-Inflammatory
   Drugs 789
Colchicine 791

Gold, D-Penicillamine, & Antimalarials 791
Drugs That Suppress Immediate-Hypersensitivity
   Reactions 792

Appendices 795
Glossary of Terms Commonly Used in Immunology 797
Acronyms & Abbreviations Commonly Used in Immunology 812
The CD Classification of Hematopoietic Cell Surface Markers 817
Glossary of Symbols Used In Illustrations 819
Index 821

The Authors

Arthur J. Ammann, MD
Director, Ariel Project for the Prevention of HIV Transmission from Mother to Infant; Chairman, Health Advisory Board Pediatric AIDS Foundation; Adjunct Professor, Pediatric Immunology, University of California, San Francisco.

James R. Baker, Jr., MD
Associate Professor, Internal Medicine and Pathology, University of Michigan, Ann Arbor.

Karen Palmore Beckerman, MD
Assistant Professor, University of California, San Francisco; Acting Chief of Obstetrics, San Francisco General Hospital.

Edith Bossom, AB, MT, (ASCP) SBB
Former Supervisor, Blood Bank, University of California, San Francisco.

Ginny L. Bumgardner, MD, PhD
Assistant Professor of Surgery, Division of Transplantation, Ohio State University College of Medicine, Columbus, Ohio

Beth W. Colombe, PhD
Associate Director, Immunogenetics and Transplantation Laboratory, Department of Surgery, University of California, San Francisco.

Suzanne Crowe, MBBS, FRACP
Head, AIDS Pathogenesis Research Unit, MacFarlane Burnet Centre and Staff Physician, Fairfield Hospital, Melbourne, Australia.

Thomas R. Cupps, MD
Associate Professor of Medicine, Department of Medicine, Division of Rheumatology, Immunology, and Allergy, Georgetown University Medical Center, Washington, DC.

Elizabeth Donegan, MD
Associate Professor of Clinical Laboratory Medicine, Pathology, Microbiology, and Immunology, University of California, San Francisco.

David J. Drutz, MD
Clinical Professor of Medicine, Seton Hall University, School of Graduate Medicine; Adjunct Professor of Microbiology and Immunology, Temple University Medical School, Philadelphia.

Connie R. Faltynek, PhD
Principal Research Investigator, Sterling Winthrop Pharmaceutical Research Division, Collegeville, Pennsylvania.

Lili Feng, MD
Assistant Member, Department of Immunology, The Scripps Research Institute, La Jolla, California.

John F. Fieselmann, MD
Assistant Professor, Division of Pulmonary Diseases, Department of Internal Medicine, University of Iowa Hospitals, Iowa City.

Paul S. Fishman, MD, PhD
Associate Professor of Neurology, University of Maryland School of Medicine; Staff Neurologist, Veterans Affairs Medical Center, Baltimore, Maryland.

Michael M. Frank, MD
Professor and Chairman, Department of Pediatrics, Duke University Medical Center, Durham, North Carolina.

Mitchell H. Friedlaender, MD
Director of Cornea and Refractive Surgery, Division of Ophthalmology, The Scripps Clinic and Research Foundation, La Jolla, California.

Kenneth H. Fye, MD
Clinical Professor of Medicine, Department of Medicine, University of California, San Francisco.

Marvin Garovoy, MD
Director, Immunogenetics and Transplantation Laboratory, Department of Surgery, University of California, San Francisco.

Sanford M. Goldstein, MD
Assistant Professor, Department of Dermatology, University of California, San Francisco.

Joel W. Goodman, PhD
Professor, Department of Microbiology and Immunology, University of California, San Francisco.

James S. Goodwin, MD
George and Cynthia Mitchell Distinguished Professor, Director, Division of Geriatric Medicine, Department of Internal Medicine, University of Texas Medical Branch, Galveston.

Philip D. Greenberg, MD
Professor of Medicine and Immunology, University of Washington,; Member, Fred Hutchinson Cancer Research Center, Seattle, Washington.

John S. Greenspan, BDS, PhD, FRCPath
Professor of Oral Pathology and Chair, Department of Stomatology, School of Dentistry, Professor of Pathology, School of Medicine, University of California, San Francisco.

Moses Grossman, MD
Professor Emeritus, Department of Pediatrics, University of California, San Francisco.

Lawrence R. Hennessey, MD
Fellow in Allergy and Immunology, University of Michigan Medical Center, Ann Arbor.

Donald Heyneman, PhD
Professor Emeritus, Department of Parasitology, University of California, San Francisco.

John B. Imboden, Jr., MD
Associate Professor, Department of Medicine, Veterans Administration Medical Center, University of California, San Francisco.

James P. Isbister, FRACP, FRCPA
Head, Department of Hematology, Royal North Shore Hospital of Sydney, St. Leonards, New South Wales, Australia.

Stephen P. James, MD
Division of Gastroenterology, University of Maryland Hospital, Baltimore.

Fraser Keith, MD
Professor of Surgery, Division of Cardiothoracic Surgery, Department of Surgery, University of California, San Francisco.

Charles Linker, MD
Associate Clinical Professor of Medicine, Division of Hematology/Oncology, University of California, San Francisco.

Robert J. Lukes, MD
Professor Emeritus, Department of Pathology, University of Southern California, San Francisco.

James H. McKerrow, PhD, MD
Professor, Departments of Pathology and Pharmaceutical Chemistry, Veterans Administration Medical Center, San Francisco, California.

John Mills, MD
Director, Macfarlane Burnet Centre for Medical Research, Fairfield, Australia.

G. Richard O'Connor, MD
Professor Emeritus, Department of Ophthalmology, University of California, San Francisco.

Joost J. Oppenheim, MD
Chief, Laboratory of Molecular Immunoregulation, National Cancer Institute, Frederick, Maryland.

Hillel S. Panitch, MD
Professor of Neurology, University of Maryland School of Medicine; Clinical Investigator, Research Service, Veterans Affairs Medical Center, Baltimore.

John W. Parker, MD
Professor of Pathology and Vice Chairman, Department of Pathology; Director, University of Southern California Clinical Laboratories, University of Southern California School of Medicine, Los Angeles.

Charles S. Pavia, PhD
Director, NYCOM Immunodiagnostic Laboratory, Old Westbury, New York; Associate Professor of Medicine and Microbiology, New York Medical College, Valhalla, New York.

Hal B. Richerson, MD
Professor of Internal Medicine, University of Iowa College of Medicine, Iowa City.

R. P. Channing Rodgers, MD
National Library of Medicine, National Institutes of Health, Bethesda, Maryland.

Francis W. Ruscetti, PhD
Chief, Laboratory of Leukocyte Biology, MRMP, DCT, NCI-FCRDC Frederick, Maryland.

John L. Ryan, PhD, MD
Executive Director, Clinical Infectious Diseases, Merck Research Laboratories; Clinical Associate Professor Department of Medicine, University of Pennsylvania, Philadelphia.

Kenneth E. Sack, MD
Clinical Professor of Medicine, Department of Medicine, University of California, San Francisco.

Alfred D. Steinberg, MD
Principal Scientist, The MITRE Corporation, McLean, Virginia.

Peter Stock, MD
Transplantation Service, University of California, San Francisco.

Warren Strober, MD
Chief, Division of Immunology and Rheumatology, Department of Medicine, Stanford University School of Medicine, Stanford, California.

David W. Talmage, MD
Distinguished Professor, University of Colorado, Health Sciences Center, Denver.

Winson W. Tang, MD
Research Associate, Department of Immunology, The Scripps Research Institute, La Jolla, California.

David M. Ward, MB, ChB, FRCP
Professor of Clinical Medicine, Chief of Clinical Nephrology, Director of Dialysis and Pheresis Programs, University of California, San Diego.

Stephen Wasserman, MD
The Helen M. Ranney Professor of Medicine; Chairman, Department of Medicine, University of California, San Diego.

H. James Wedner, MD
Department of Allergy and Immunology, Washington University School of Medicine, St. Louis.

John Vivian Wells, MD, FRACP, FRCPA, FACP
Senior Staff Specialist in Clinical Immunology, Kolling Institute, Royal North Shore Hospital, St. Leonards, Australia.

Curtis B. Wilson, MD
Member, Department of Immunology, The Scripps Research Institute, La Jolla, California.

Alan Winkelstein, MD
Professor of Medicine, University of Pittsburgh School of Medicine; Medical Director and Vice President, Central Blood Bank, Pittsburgh.

Bruce U. Wintroub, MD
Professor and Chairman, Department of Dermatology, University of California, San Francisco.

Yiyang Xia, MD
Research Associate, Department of Immunology, The Scripps Research Institute, La Jolla, California.

Lowell S. Young, MD
Director, Kuzell Institute, San Francisco, California.

John L. Ziegler, MD
Professor of Medicine, University of California, San Francisco.

Preface

The 8th edition of *Basic and Clinical Immunology* continues the tradition of a popular textbook for health care students and practitioners. The book is an attempt at a comprehensive and comprehensible treatise on immunology, which began with the first edition in 1976.

The key features of the 8th edition are as follows:

- The first section of the book, Basic Immunology, has been extensively revised under the expert guidance of our new editor, Dr. Tristram Parslow. The number of authors has been reduced for increased consistency and to focus on essential concepts.
- As before, the subject matter of the book is restricted to human immunology. Nevertheless, the results of critical experiments with certain animal models are included whenever they help to explain human diseases.
- Numerous illustrations simplify the identification of cells and their chemical products and receptors using a uniform set of symbols throughout the book. A glossary of these symbols is provided at the end of the book for easy reference.
- The sections and chapters of the book are organized to emphasize normal immunologic function and disease processes.
- It is recognized that immunology is not an easy subject, both because of its intrinsic complexity and because of the vast array of information currently available. The authors—all experts in their particular fields—have made every effort to write in a readable style without sacrificing essential details.

The book is divided into four sections, including Basic, Laboratory, and Clinical Immunology, as in previous editions, and a new fourth section, Immunotherapy. This section describes the drugs and other forms of therapy used to treat immunologic diseases. It also deals with the ways in which the immune system is manipulated for treatment of other diseases through immunization, immune suppression, and immune modulation.

Section I, Basic Immunology (Chapters 1–11), which introduces the science of immunology, has been reorganized and extensively rewritten. Our goal in this section is to provide a comprehensive overview of basic immunobiology that could serve either as a textbook for introductory courses or as a concise, state-of-the-art review for practicing physicians and scientists from immunology and other fields. We have tried to make the presentation lucid and accessible for beginning students, emphasizing major concepts while incorporating the latest experimental findings and theories throughout. The most important themes are presented at an increasing level of detail in successive chapters, and references to pertinent articles are provided at the end of each chapter for those who wish to explore further.

Section II, Immunologic Laboratory Tests, is extensively updated with new methods and techniques that are rapidly being added to aid in clinical diagnosis. A new chapter, entitled "Molecular Genetic Techniques for Clinical Analysis of the Immune System," describes the key molecular biological methods that are rapidly becoming standard in clinical laboratories. Histocompatibility testing is treated in a separate chapter. A chapter on the assessment of immune competence through laboratory testing provides a critical overview of the efficient use and avoidance of misuse of the enormous number and variety of tests now available.

Section III, Clinical Immunology, is subdivided into 5 categories. Two of these—

Immunodeficiency Diseases and Allergic Diseases—expand these important subjects, which were treated as individual chapters in previous editions. The large number of diseases characterized by a variety of immunologic abnormalities, autoimmunity, and disordered immune regulation in which the underlying cause is unknown are again grouped together. As in previous editions, these fascinating diseases are discussed in separate chapters based on the organ or body system involved. A fourth category covers neoplasms of the immune system and neoplasms that arise in patients with diseased immune systems. The fifth category, infections, makes a full circle from the origin of immunology, which concerned protection against infectious diseases, to a central concern of viral infections of the immune system itself, including acquired immune deficiency syndrome (AIDS).

The Clinical Immunology subsections each begin with a brief introductory chapter that is both an overview and an essay on the subject of the chapters that follow. The editors hope that this feature will serve as a conceptual framework for the details that must be learned by beginning and advanced students of immunology.

ACKNOWLEDGMENTS

The editors are deeply grateful to Martin Wonsiewicz for his expertise and advice during the preparation of this 8th edition. The meticulous editing skills of Yvonne Strong and the artistic drawings of Linda Harris helped to make this an informative and understandable text on a difficult subject. Special thanks are due Drs. D. Bainton, A. De-Franco, J. Edman, and Z. Werb for their insightful reviews of several new chapters. Finally, the authors and editors are indebted to the editorial staff of Appleton & Lange, particularly Lee Jackson, for their efforts and patience.

Recommendations about diagnosis and treatment of disease are based on the best scientific and clinical information currently available. They are intended, however, as guidance to the clinician and not necessarily as recommendations for specific cases. Furthermore, we recognize that we may have overlooked errors despite our best efforts. We would be grateful if our readers would point these out so that they may be corrected in the next edition.

San Francisco
October 1993

Daniel P. Stites, MD
Abba I. Terr, MD
Tristram G. Parslow, MD, PhD

History of Immunology

David W. Talmage, MD

THE ORIGIN OF IMMUNOLOGY

Immunology began as a branch of microbiology; it grew out of the study of infectious diseases and the body's responses to them. The concepts of contagion and the germ theory of disease are attributed to Girolamo Fracastoro, a colleague of Copernicus at the University of Padua, who wrote in 1546 that "Contagion is an infection that passes from one thing to another . . . The infection is precisely similar in both the carrier and the receiver of the contagion . . . The term is more correctly used when infection originates in very small imperceptible particles." Fracastoro's conclusions were remarkable because they were contrary to the philosophy of his time in that he postulated the existence of germs that were too small to be seen. He was a practical physician who gave more credence to his own observations than to traditional beliefs.

It was more than 2 centuries later that another physician, Edward Jenner, extended the concept of contagion to a study of the immunity produced in the host. This was the beginning of immunology. Jenner, a country doctor in Gloucestershire, England, noted in 1798 that a pustular disease of the hooves of horses called "the grease" was frequently carried by farm workers to the nipples of cows, where it was picked up by milkmaids. "Inflamed spots now begin to appear on the hands of the domestics employed in milking, and sometimes on the wrists . . . but what renders the Cowpox virus so extremely singular, is, that the person who has been thus affected is for ever after secure from the infection of Small Pox; neither exposure to the variolous effluvia, nor the insertion of the matter into the skin, producing this distemper."

Jenner was unclear about the nature of the infectious agent of cowpox and its relation to smallpox, but he reported 16 cases of resistance to smallpox in farm workers who had recovered from cowpox. He described how he deliberately inserted matter "taken from a sore on the hand of a dairymaid, on the 14th of May, 1796, into the arm of the boy by means of two superficial incisions, barely penetrating the cutis, each about half an inch long." Two months later, Jenner inoculated the same 8-year-old boy with matter from a smallpox patient, a dangerous but accepted procedure called **variolation.** However, the boy developed only a small sore at the site of inoculation. His exposure to the mild disease cowpox had made him immune to the deadly disease smallpox. In this manner Jenner began the science of immunology, the study of the body's response to foreign substances.

Immunology has always been dependent on technology, particularly lens-making and microscopy. Eyeglasses were introduced into Europe in the 14th century, (perhaps by Marco Polo), and telescopes were used by Galileo in 1609 to discover the moons of Jupiter. However, useful microscopes were not available until the middle of the 19th century. After that, progress in microbiology was rapid. In 1850, Davaine reported that he could see anthrax bacilli in the blood of infected sheep. In 1858, Wallace and Darwin jointly submitted reports proposing evolution through natural selection, and in the same year, Pasteur demonstrated to the French wine industry that fermentation was due to a living microorganism. In 1864, Pasteur disproved the theory of spontaneous generation; in 1867, Lister introduced aseptic surgery; and in 1871, DNA was discovered by Miescher. Anthrax was first transmitted from in vitro culture to animals by Koch in 1876, thus fulfilling **Koch's postulates,** which he had said were required to prove that the bacteria caused the disease. Between 1879 and 1881, Pasteur developed the first 3 attenuated vaccines (after cowpox); these were for chicken cholera, anthrax, and rabies.

Bacteriology and histology were recognized as established scientific fields during this period. The gonococcus, the first human pathogen, was isolated in 1879 by Neisser, and 10 other pathogens were isolated in the next decade. Of particular importance to immunology was the isolation of the diphtheria bacillus by Klebs and Loeffler in 1883; this led to the production of the first defined antigen, diphtheria toxin, by Roux and Yersin in 1888. In that same year, the first antibodies, serum bactericidins, were reported by Nuttall, and Pasteur recognized that nonliving substances as well as living organisms could induce immunity. This led to the discovery of antitoxins by von Behring and Kitasato in 1890 and later to the development of toxoids for diphtheria and tetanus.

CELLULAR VERSUS HUMORAL IMMUNITY

In 1883, Metchnikoff observed the phagocytosis of fungal spores by leukocytes and advanced the idea that immunity was due primarily to white blood cells. This provoked an intense controversy with the advocates of **humoral immunity.** The discovery of complement in 1894 by Bordet and **precipitins** in 1897 by Kraus appeared to favor the humoral side of the controversy. Ehrlich's side chain theory, proposed in 1898, was an attempt to harmonize the 2 views. According to Ehrlich, cells possessed on their surfaces a wide variety of side chains (we would call them antigen receptors) that were used to bring nutrients into the cell. When toxic substances blocked one of these side chains through an accidental affinity, the cell responded by making large numbers of that particular side chain, some of which spilled out into the blood and functioned as circulating antibodies.

In 1903, Sir Almoth Wright reported that antibodies could aid in the process of phagocytosis, thus effectively settling the controversy over cellular versus humoral community. Wright called these antibodies "opsonins." This followed the practice of labeling antibodies according to their observed action, eg, agglutinins, precipitins, hemolysins, and bactericidins.

It was gradually realized that antibodies could have deleterious as well as beneficial effects and could produce hypersensitivity. The term "anaphylaxis" was coined by Richet and Portier in 1902 to denote the frequently lethal state of shock induced by a second injection of antigen. The term "allergy" was introduced by von Pirquet in 1906 to denote the positive reaction to a scratch test with tuberculin in individuals infected with tuberculosis.

THE PERIOD OF SEROLOGY

Blood group antigens and their corresponding agglutinins were discovered by Landsteiner in 1900. This led to the ability to give blood transfusions without provoking reactions. Landsteiner was a dominant figure in immunology for 40 years, developing the concept of the antigenic determinant and demonstrating the exquisite specificity of antibodies for chemi-

cally defined haptens, a term he applied to simple chemicals that could bind to antibodies but were by themselves incapable of stimulating antibody formation. Landsteiner rejected Ehrlich's side chain theory because he was able to make antibodies against a seemingly infinite number of different substances, synthetic as well as natural.

In 1901, Bordet and Gengou introduced the complement fixation test, which became a standard diagnostic test in the hospital laboratory. The word "immunology" first appeared in the *Index Medicus* in 1910, and the *Journal of Immunology* began publication in 1916. The first 30 years of the Journal were devoted almost exclusively to a study of serologic reactions.

Landsteiner's book, *The Specificity of Serological Reactions,* was published in German in 1933 and in English in 1936. Marrack's text, *The Chemistry of Antigens and Antibodies,* was published in 1935. Antibodies were viewed as being formed directly on antigens, which functioned as templates, in a theory published by Breinl and Haurowitz in 1930. In 1939, Tiselius and Kabat showed that antibodies were gamma globulins, and in 1940, Pauling proposed the variable-folding theory of antibody formation. According to Pauling's theory, gamma globulin peptides are folded into a complementary configuration in the presence of antigen. This fit the "Unitarian" view of antibodies generally accepted at that time, which held that all antibodies were the same except for their specificity.

Immunochemistry was a natural outgrowth of this chemical approach to immunology. The quantitative precipitin test was developed by Heidelberger, Kendall, and Kabat and was used to study the structure of polysaccharide antigens.

THE REBIRTH OF CELLULAR IMMUNOLOGY

Two events of 1941–1942 heralded the rediscovery of the cell by immunologists. Coons demonstrated the presence of antigens and antibodies inside cells by the new technique of **immunofluorescence,** and Chase and Landsteiner reported that delayed hypersensitivity could be transferred by cells but not by serum. The very next year (1943), Avery, MacCleod, and McCarty reported that DNA was responsible for the transfer of hereditary traits in bacteria.

In 1945, Owen discovered blood chimeras in cattle twins, and in 1948, Fagraeus showed that antibodies were made in plasma cells. In 1949, Burnet and Fenner published their adaptive enzyme theory of antibody formation, which again established immunology as a biologic science. They also proposed the "self-marker" concept, which was the first formal explanation of self tolerance.

In 1953, Billingham, Brent, and Medawar demonstrated acquired immunologic tolerance in bone marrow chimeras in mice injected with allogeneic bone marrow at or before birth. In that same year, Watson and Crick described the double helix of DNA. The close association in the development of immunology and molecular biology is illustrated by these 2 discoveries. Two years later, Jerne proposed his natural selection theory of antibody formation, in which randomly diversified gamma globulin molecules were thought to replicate after binding to injected antigen. Jerne's theory explained the known facts of immunology of that time, such as immunologic memory and the logarithmic rate of rise of antibody. However, this theory was incompatible with the new concepts of cellular and molecular biology. Within 2 years, 2 new theories of antibody production were proposed, the first by Talmage and the second by Burnet. Both theories substituted randomly diversified cells for randomly diversified gamma globulin molecules and proposed that the interaction of antigen with receptors on the cell surface stimulated antibody production and the replication of the selected cell.

After more than 30 years, the cell selection theory and the name given to it by Burnet—**clonal selection**—have become part of the established dogma of immunology. This theory has been confirmed by numerous experiments and was popularized in 1975 by the development of Köhler and Milstein of the technique of producing monoclonal antibodies.

Cellular immunology reached its zenith in 1966 with the discovery by Claman, Chaperon, and Triplett of the presence and cooperation of **B cells** and **T cells.** Since that time, the study of the development, specificity, and activation of B cells and T cells has occupied the energy of a great many immunologists.

THE ADVENT
OF MOLECULAR IMMUNOLOGY

By 1959, the field of protein chemistry had reached the point at which it was possible to analyze the structure of the antibody molecule in detail. In that same year, the 3 fragments of immunoglobulins, 2 Fab's and one Fc, were separated by Porter, and the heavy and light chains were separated by Edelman. The discovery of common and variable regions by Putnam and by Hilschmann and Craig came in 1965. Edelman et al reported the first complete amino acid sequence of an immunoglobulin molecule in 1969.

The 1960s and 1970s saw similar advances in the identification, separation, and characterization of other molecules important to the immune system, such as complement components, interleukins, and cell receptors. These studies were greatly enhanced by the application of monoclonal antibody technology, which allowed sensitive and specific identification and isolation of many such molecules.

The first monoclonal antibody identifying a T cell subset (OKT4, now called CD4) was described by Kung et al in 1979. The elusive T cell receptor was finally isolated in 1982–1983 by Allison et al and Haskins et al. The steps required for antigen processing and presentation and the chemical reactions required for lymphocyte activation by antigen were also elucidated.

IMMUNOGENETICS
& GENETIC ENGINEERING

The major histocompatibility antigens were discovered by Gorer in 1936, but it was not until 1968 that McDevitt and Tyan showed that immune response genes were linked to the genes of the major histocompatibility complex. Six years later, Doherty and Zinkernagel reported that the recognition of antigen by T cells was restricted by major histocompatibility complex molecules. During this time, the technology of recombinant DNA was developed. This led to the demonstration of immunoglobulin gene rearrangement by Tonegawa et al in 1978 and the production of transgenic mice by Gordon et al in 1980. The identification of genes for the T cell receptor by Davis et al came in 1984.

IMMUNOLOGY TIME LINE

1798   Edward Jenner
        Cowpox vaccination.

1880   Louis Pasteur
        Attenuated vaccines.

1883   Elie I. I. Metchnikoff
        Phagocytic theory.

1888   P. P. Emile Roux and A. E. J. Yersin
        Bacterial toxins.

1888   George H. F. Nuttall
        Bactericidal antibodies.

1890   Robert Koch
        Hypersensitivity.

1890   Emil A. von Behring and Shibasaburo Kitasato
        Diphtheria antitoxin.

1894   Jules J. B. V. Bordet
        Complement.

1897   Rudolf Kraus
        Precipitins.

1898   Paul Ehrlich
        Side chain theory.

1900   Karl Landsteiner
        Blood group antigens and antibodies.

1902   Charles R. Richet and Paul J. Portier
        Anaphylaxis.

1903   Almoth E. Wright
        Opsonins.

1905   Clemens P. von Pirquet and Bela Schick
        Serum sickness.

1906   Clemens P. von Pirquet
        Allergy.

1930   Friedrich Breinl and Felix Haurowitz
        Template theory.

1939   Arne Wilhelm Tiselius and Elvin A. Kabat
        Identity of antibodies with gamma globulins.

1941   Albert H. Coons et al
        Immunofluorescence.

1942   Karl Landsteiner and Merrill W. Chase
        Transfer of delayed-type hypersensitivity with cells.

1945   Ray D. Owen
        Chimeras in bovine twins.

1948   Astrid E. Fagraeus
        Antibodies in plasma cells.

1949   F. Macfarlane Burnet and Frank Fenner
        Adaptive enzyme theory.

1953   Rupert E. Billingham, Leslie Brent, and Peter B. Medawar
        Bone marrow chimeras in mice.

1955   Niels K. Jerne
        Natural selection theory.

1957   David W. Talmage and F. Macfarlane Burnet
        Cell selection theories.

1959   Rodney R. Porter and Gerald M. Edelman
        Structure of antibodies.

1966   Henry N. Claman et al
        Cooperation of T and B cells.

1968   Hugh O. McDevitt and Marvin L. Tyan
        Linkage of immune response genes to major histocompatibility complex genes.

1974   Peter C. Doherty and Rolf M. Zinkernagel
        T cell restriction.

1975   Cesar Milstein and Georges J. F. Kohler
        Monoclonal antibodies.

1978   Susumu Tonegawa
        Immunoglobulin gene rearrangement.

1979   Patrick Kung, Gideon Goldstein, Ellis Reinherz, and Stuart Schlossman
        Monoclonal antibody to CD4 marker on T cells.

1980   Jon W. Gordon et al
        Transgenic mice.

1983   James Allison, Kathryn Haskins et al
        T cell receptor isolation.

1984   Mark Davis et al
        T cell receptor genes.

NOBEL PRIZE WINNERS IN IMMUNOLOGY

1901   EMIL ADOLF VON BEHRING for his work on serum therapy, especially application against diphtheria.

1905   ROBERT KOCH for his investigations and discoveries in relation to tuberculosis.

1908   PAUL EHRLICH and ELIE METCHNIKOFF for their work on immunity.

1913   CHARLES ROBERT RICHET for his work on anaphylaxis.

1919   JULES BORDET for his discoveries relating to immunity, particularly complement.

1928   CHARLES JULES HENRI NICOLLE for his work on typhus.

1930   KARL LANDSTEINER for his discovery of human blood groups.

1960   FRANK MACFARLANE BURNET and PETER BRIAN MEDAWAR for their discovery of acquired immunologic tolerance.

1972   GERALD MAURICE EDELMAN and

RODNEY ROBERT PORTER for their discoveries concerning the chemical structure of antibodies.

1977   ROSALYN YALOW for the development of radioimmunoassays of peptide hormones.

1980   BARUJ BENACERRAF, JEAN DAUSSET, and GEORGE DAVIS SNELL for their discoveries concerning genetically determined structures on the cell surface that regulate immunologic reactions.

1984   NEILS K. JERNE, GEORGES F. KÖHLER, and CESAR MILSTEIN for theories concerning the specificity in development and control of the immune system and the discovery of the principle for production of monoclonal antibodies.

1987   SUSUMU TONEGAWA for his discovery of the genetic principle for generation of antibody diversity.

1990   JOSEPH E. MURRAY and E. DONNALL THOMAS for their work on human organ and cell transplantation.

SUMMARY

Immunology began as a study of the response of the whole animal to infection. Over the years, it has become progressively more basic, passing through phases of emphasis on serology, cellular immunology, molecular immunology, and immunogenetics. At the same time, immunology has grown to encompass many fields such as allergy, clinical immunology, immunochemistry, immunopathology, immunopharmacology, tumor immunology, and transplantation. Thus, it has always provided an excellent mix of fundamental and applied science.

Immunology has always depended upon and stimulated the application of technology, such as the use of microscopy, electrophoresis, radiolabeling, immunofluorescence, recombinant DNA, and transgenic mice. In general, immunology has not become an inbred discipline but has maintained close associations with many other fields of medical science. From a base in microbiology, immunologists have spread out into all of the basic and clinical departments.

REFERENCES

Alexander HL: The history of allergy. In: *Immunological Diseases.* Samter M (editor). Little Brown, 1965.

Allison JP, McIntyre BW, Bloch D: Tumor specific antigen of murine T-lymphoma defined with monoclonal antibody. *J Immunol.* 1982;**129**:2293.

Billingham RE, Brent L, Medawar PB: Actively acquired tolerance of foreign cells. *Nature* 1953;172:603.

Bordet J: *Traite de L'Immunité dans les Maladies infectieuses,* 2nd ed. Masson, 1937.

Brack C, et al: A complete immunoglobulin gene is created by somatic recombination. *Cell* 1978;**15**:1.

Burnet FM: A modification of Jerne's theory of antibody production using the concept of clonal selection. *Aust J Sci* 1957;**20**:67.

Burnet FM, Fenner F: *The Production of Antibodies.* Macmillan (Melbourne), 1949.

Claman HN, Chaperon EA, Triplett RF: Thymus-marrow cell combination. Synergism in antibody production. *Proc Soc Exp Biol Med* 1966;**122**:1167.

Coons AH et al: Immunological properties of an antibody containing a fluorescent group. *Proc Soc Exp Biol Med* 1941;**47**:200.

Doherty PC, Zinkernagel RM: T-cell mediated immunopathology in viral infections. *Transplant Rev* 1974; **19**:89.

Dubos R: *The Unseen World.* Rockefeller Univ Press, 1962.

Edelman GM: Dissociation of gamma globulin. *J Am Chem Soc* 1959;**81**:3155.

Ehrlich P: On immunity with special reference to cell life. *Proc R Soc London Ser B* 1900;**66**:424.

Fagraeus A: The plasma cellular reaction and its relation to the formation of antibodies in vitro. *J Immunol* 1948; **58**:1.

Foster WD: *A History of Medical Bacteriology and Immunology.* Heineman, 1970.

Gay FP: Immunology, a medical science developed through animal experimentation. *J Am Med Assoc* 1911; **56**:578.

Gordon JW et al: Genetic transformation of mouse embryos by microinjection of purified DNA. *Proc Natl Acad Sci USA* 1980;**77**:7380.

Haskins K et al: The major histocompatibility complex restricted antigen receptor on T cells. I. Isolation with a monoclonal antibody. *J Exp Med* 1983;**157**:1149.

Hedrick SM et al: Isolation of cDNA clones encoding T cell-specific membrane-associated proteins. *Nature* 1984; **308**:149.

Jerne NK: The natural selection theory of antibody formation. *Proc Natl Acad Sci USA* 1955;**41**:849.

Köhler G, Milstein C: Continuous culture of fused cells secreting antibody of predefined specificity. *Nature* 1975; **256**:495.

Kung PC et al: Monoclonal antibodies defining distinctive human T cell antigens. *Science* 1979;**206:**347.

Landsteiner K: *The Specificity of Serological Reactions.* Thomas, 1936; reissued by Dover, 1962.

Landsteiner K, Chase MW: Experiments on transfer of cutaneous sensitivity to simple compounds. *Proc Soc Exp Biol Med* 1942;**49:**688.

McDevitt HO, Tyan ML: Transfer of response by spleen cells and linkage to the major histocompatibility (H-2) locus. *J Exp Med* 1968;**128:**1.

Parrish HJ: *A History of Immunization.* E & S Livingstone, 1965.

Parrish HJ: *Victory with Vaccines.* E & S Livingstone, 1968.

Pauling L: A theory of the structure and process of formation of antibodies. *J Am Chem Soc* 1940;**62:**2643.

Porter RR: The hydrolysis of rabbit gamma globulin and antibodies with crystalline papain. *Biochem J* 1959; **73:**119.

Talmage DW: Allergy and immunology. *Annu Rev Med* 1957;**8:**239.

Talmage DW: A century of progress: Beyond molecular immunology. *J Immunol* 1988;**141(Suppl):**S5.

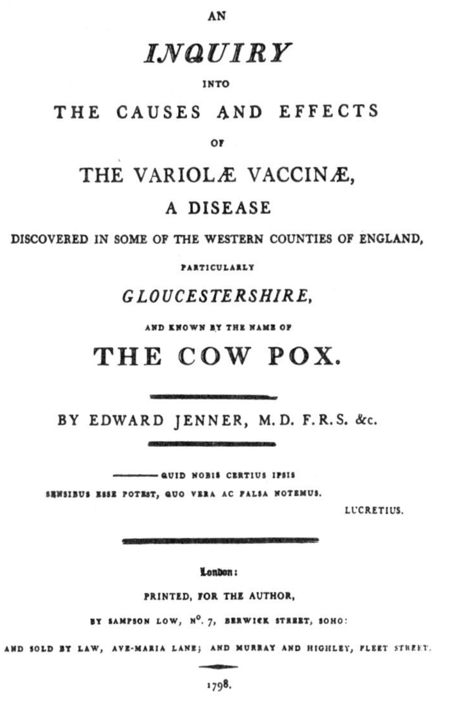

AN
INQUIRY
INTO

THE CAUSES AND EFFECTS

OF

THE VARIOLÆ VACCINÆ,

A DISEASE

DISCOVERED IN SOME OF THE WESTERN COUNTIES OF ENGLAND,

PARTICULARLY

GLOUCESTERSHIRE,

AND KNOWN BY THE NAME OF

THE COW POX.

BY EDWARD JENNER, M.D. F.R.S. &c.

———— QUID NOBIS CERTIUS IPSIS
SENSIBUS ESSE POTEST, QUO VERA AC FALSA NOTEMUS.
LUCRETIUS.

London:

PRINTED, FOR THE AUTHOR,

BY SAMPSON LOW, Nº. 7, BERWICK STREET, SOHO:

AND SOLD BY LAW, AVE-MARIA LANE; AND MURRAY AND HIGHLEY, FLEET STREET.

1798.

Figure I. Face plate from first edition (1798) of Jenner's inquiry into the Causes and Effects of . . . the Cow Pox

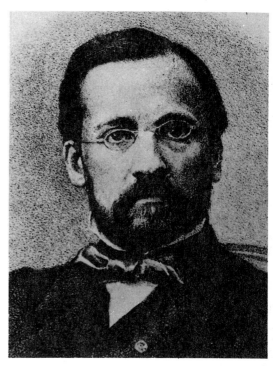

Figure 2. Louis Pasteur (1822–1895). (Courtesy of the Museum of the Pasteur Institute, Paris.)

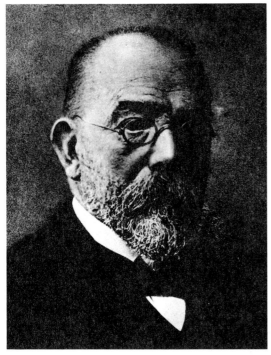

Figure 3. Robert Koch (1843–1910). (Courtesy of the Museum of the Pasteur Institute, Paris.)

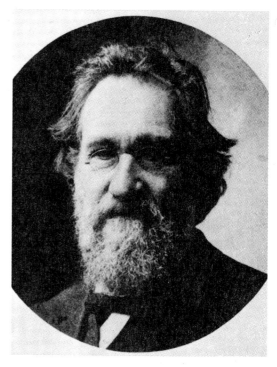

Figure 4. Elie Metchnikoff (1845–1916). (Courtesy of the Rare Book Library, the University of Texas Medical Branch, Galveston.)

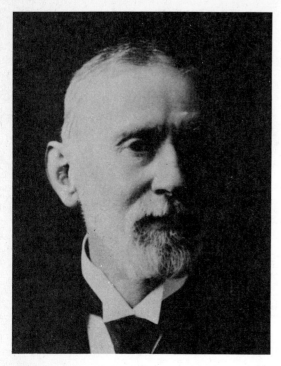

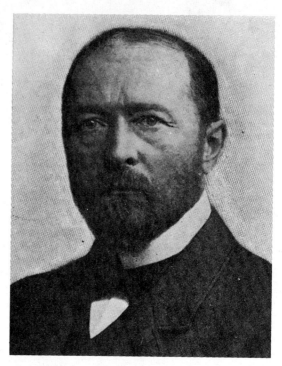

Figure 5. Paul Ehrlich (1854–1915). (Courtesy of the Museum of the Pasteur Institute, Paris.)

Figure 6. Emil von Behring (1854–1917). (Courtesy of the Museum of the Pasteur Institute, Paris.)

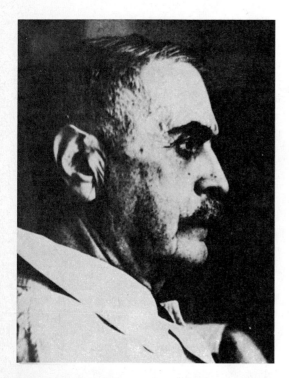

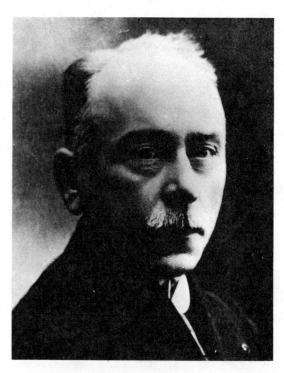

Figure 7. Karl Landsteiner (1868–1943). (Courtesy of the Museum of the Pasteur Institute, Paris.)

Figure 8. Jules Bordet (1870–1961). (Courtesy of the Museum of the Pasteur Institute, Paris.)

Section I.
Basic Immunology

The Phagocytes: Neutrophils & Macrophages

1

Tristram G. Parslow, MD, PhD

The human body has many ways to protect itself. Some are simply physical barriers, like the skin's tough, outer keratin layer that shields the living cells beneath it from a hostile environment. Others are potent biochemical substances that offer relatively nonspecific protection against a broad range of microorganisms. For example, tears and many other bodily secretions contain the enzyme **lysozyme,** which acts to digest and weaken the protective walls surrounding bacterial cells. A more elaborate chemical barrier is provided by the group of blood proteins that together make up the **complement** pathway (see Chapter 10); these proteins mediate a cascade of enzymatic reactions that can be triggered by molecular features on the surfaces of some microorganisms and that may ultimately lead to lysis or enhanced phagocytosis of the foreign invader. During serious infections, the body also produces increased amounts of a different group of serum proteins known as the **acute-phase proteins,** some of which have antimicrobial effects. For example, the **C-reactive protein** binds to the so-called C protein on the surfaces of pneumococci and thus promotes their destruction by the complement cascade.

But by far the most complex, dynamic, and effective defense strategies are carried out by specialized cells that travel through the body to search out and destroy microorganisms and other foreign substances. In human beings, 3 major groups of cells provide this type of defense (Table 1–1). Two of these—the **neutrophils** and the **monocyte-macrophage** series—are phagocytic cells, which act primarily by engulfing and digesting bacteria, cellular debris, and other particulate matter. The third group, which comprises the **lymphocytes** and their relatives, has little phagocytic capacity but instead participates in a host of other protective reactions that are known collectively as **immune responses.** Both phagocytes and lymphocytes are essential for health; they often act in concert and are to a great extent dependent on one another for maximal effectiveness. However, it is useful to begin by focusing on the properties and limitations of phagocytic cells as guardians of the body and to consider why these cells alone cannot provide a sufficient defense against many types of pathogenic agents.

ONTOGENY OF BLOOD CELLS

Neutrophils, monocytes, and lymphocytes each spend a portion of their lives circulating in the blood. Like all other blood cells, they arise from a common stem cell precursor through a process called **hematopoiesis.** Hematopoietic activity begins in mesenchyme surrounding the yolk sac during early embryogenesis but soon moves to the fetal liver and spleen, which serve as the principal sites of hematopoiesis until the fourth or fifth month of gestation. Thereafter, the process shifts increasingly to the bone marrow, where it continues throughout life. In the adult, hematopoiesis is confined largely to marrow of the spinal column, proximal femurs and humeri, iliac bones, ribs, and sternum. Hematopoiesis in the liver and spleen subsides to undetectable levels by puberty, although it can resume at any time in response to abnormal demand.

The physical characteristics of **hematopoietic stem cells** are not yet fully known, since techniques for purifying these cells have only recently been developed. They are thought to constitute approximately 0.01% of all cells in the bone marrow and are defined by their ability not only to regenerate themselves through mitotic division but also to produce differentiated progeny of all red and white blood cell types. The pathways by which these progeny cells

Table 1–1. Properties of the 3 major human cell lineages involved in host defense.[1]

	Neutrophils	Monocyte-Macrophages	Lymphocytes[2]
Primary effector function	Phagocytosis	Phagocytosis	Varies
Cytoplasmic granules	Many	Moderate	No
Can synthesize new membrane or secretory proteins	No	Yes	Yes
Terminally differentiated	Yes	Usually	No
Principal normal location	Blood, marrow	All tissues	Lymphoid tissues
Immunoregulatory cytokine production	No[3]	Yes	Yes
Antigen presentation[4]	No	Yes	Yes

[1]The properties as listed apply to the mature cells of each lineage.
[2]Several distinct subtypes of lymphocytes have been described, and their functional properties differ widely (see Chapter 2). Properties shown are those of B and T lymphocytes.
[3]Except certain chemokines (see Chapter 9).
[4]To helper T lymphocytes (see Chapter 5).

differentiate are outlined in Fig 1–1. In general, individual cells can become irreversibly committed to any one of 3 main alternative differentiation pathways that yield erythrocytes, lymphocytes, or myeloid cells. Both neutrophils and monocytes are products of the myeloid lineage, as are megakaryocytes (the cells that produce platelets), mast cells, eosinophils, and basophils. The last 3 cell types are involved in certain specialized types of immune reactions and are discussed in Chapter 11. Neutrophils, eosinophils, and basophils are sometimes referred to as **granulocytes**.

The growth and maturation of cells within each lineage is precisely controlled by hormonal factors that are present in the marrow microenvironment. Some of the most important of these regulatory factors belong to 2 diverse families of polypeptide hormones known as the **interleukins** and the **colony-stimulating factors** (see Chapter 9). Myeloid differentiation depends particularly on 2 such factors, known as interleukin-3 (**IL-3**) and granulocyte-monocyte colony-stimulating factor (**GM-CSF**), which enhance the production and maturation of all myeloid cell types. In the late stages of the myeloid pathway, 2 other factors, called granulocyte colony stimulating factor (G-CSF) and monocyte colony-stimulating factor (M-CSF), act to favor selective outgrowth of

neutrophils or monocytes, respectively. Direct cell-to-cell contacts with marrow stromal elements, extracellular matrix components, and other hematopoietic cells also play a critical although poorly understood role in regulating hematopoiesis.

NEUTROPHILS

Neutrophils make up an army of more or less identical circulating phagocytes that are poised to respond quickly and in vast numbers wherever tissue injury has occurred. The mature cells, which are also known as segmented neutrophils (segs) or polymorphonuclear leukocytes (polys, or PMNs), can easily be identified under the light microscope by their characteristic multilobed nucleus and by the abundant storage granules in their cytoplasm (Fig 1–2). The granules are specialized lysosomes—membrane-bounded vesicles containing digestive enzymes and other proteins that can be used to break down particles that have been engulfed by the cell. Most neutrophil granules are of 2 types, called **azurophilic granules** and **specific granules,** respectively, each containing a particular assortment of proteins (Table 1–2). Immature neutrophil precursors have a well-developed rough endoplasmic reticulum and Golgi apparatus that enable them to synthesize the granules, but these organelles disappear or are greatly diminished as the cells mature, leaving the fully mature neutrophil unable to produce new secretory or membrane proteins. Whereas the immature forms replicate briskly, a mature neutrophil is **terminally differentiated**—that is, it lacks the ability to replicate by cell division.

Neutrophils grow to full maturity in the bone marrow and are usually retained in the marrow for an additional 5 days as part of a large reserve pool. They are then released into the bloodstream, where they normally constitute one-half to two-thirds of all circulating white blood cells. An adult has approximately 50 billion neutrophils in the circulation at all times, each of which is terminally differentiated and is programmed to die after a lifespan of only 1 or 2 days. Thus, the marrow must produce vast numbers of neutrophils each day to maintain a stable circulating population. To meet this demand, roughly 60% of all marrow hematopoietic activity is devoted to neutrophil production, compared with only 20–30% devoted to erythrocyte formation.

Tissue Invasion by Neutrophils

Once released from the marrow, neutrophils normally circulate continuously in the blood throughout their brief lives. If their journey carries them into a site of injury or infection, however, the cells will rapidly adhere to the endothelial lining of local blood vessels, migrate through the vessel walls, and invade the affected tissues, where they may accumulate in vast numbers. This response is directed in large part

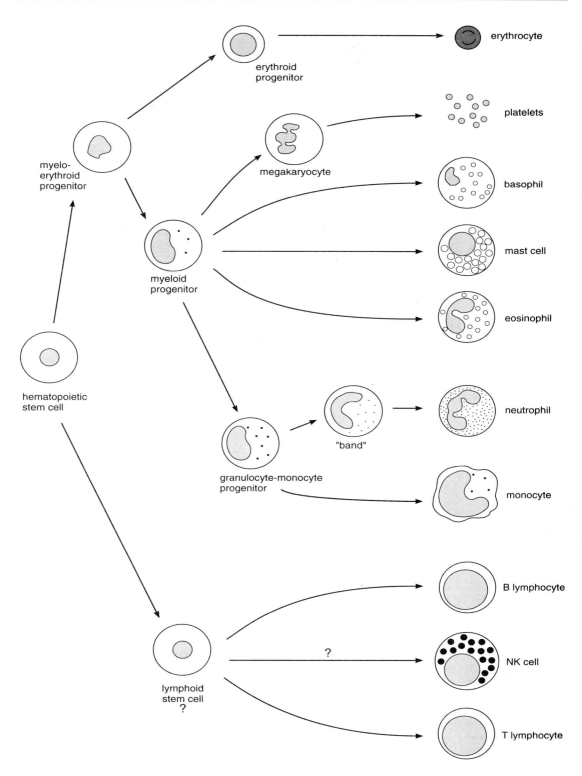

Figure 1–1. Schematic overview of hematopoiesis, emphasizing the erythroid, myeloid, and lymphoid pathways. This highly simplified depiction omits many recognized intermediate cell types in each pathway. All of the cells shown here arise in the bone marrow except T lymphocytes, which develop from marrow-derived progenitors that migrate to the thymus (see Chapter 2). A common lymphoid stem cell is believed to exist but has not yet been isolated. The histogenesis of natural killer (NK) cells is unknown.

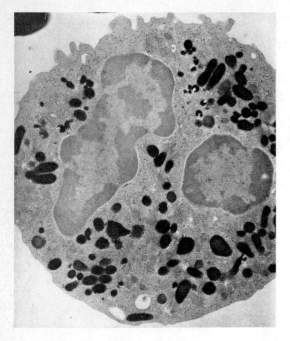

Figure 1–2. Electron micrograph of a human neutrophil. The single elongated nucleus is constricted at multiple sites to form segments, only two of which appear in this section. The cytoplasm contains numerous storage granules that differ in appearance and enzyme content; the peroxidase-containing (azurophilic) granules are stained darkly in this preparation. Note the absence of rough endoplasmic reticulum. The cell is 14 μm in diameter. (Courtesy of Dorothy F. Bainton.)

Table 1–2. Some contents of neutrophil granules.[1]

	Azurophilic Granules	**Specific Granules**
Microbicidal proteins	Defensins Myeloperoxidase Lysozyme	Lysozyme NADPH oxidases
Proteases	Elastase Cathepsin G Azurocidin Collagenase	Collagenase Gelatinase Plasminogen activator
Acid hydrolases	Cathepsins B and D β-Glucuronidase β-Glycerophosphatase N-Acetyl-β-glucosaminidase N-Acetyl-β-galactosaminidase α-Mannosidase Acid phosphatase Ribo- and deoxyribonucleases Lipases	
Other proteins		Lactoferrin Histaminase Vitamin B_{12}-binding protein Membrane receptors for N-formylated oligopeptides Complement (C3b, C5a) Fibrinogen Fibronectin Laminin Vitronectin

[1]Modified and reproduced, with permission, from Bainton D: Developmental biology of neutrophils and eosinophils. Page 303 in: *Inflammation: Basic Principles and Clinical Correlations*, 2nd ed. Gallin JI, Goldstein IM, Snyderman R (editors). Raven Press, New York, 1992.

by biochemical substances, known as **neutrophil chemotactic factors** (Table 1–3), that are released from damaged or infected tissues and are detected by receptors on the neutrophil surface membrane. In general, these chemotactic factors are substances that signify the presence of an injury rather than its exact cause. Many are host-derived molecules that are produced either directly as a result of tissue damage or indirectly by the host response to it. They include fragments of fibrin or collagen (as might be generated in a wound), soluble factors released by activated platelets or mast cells, and certain by-products of the complement protein cascade. Other neutrophil chemoattractants are unique products of bacterial metabolism, the most notable of which are peptides containing **N-formylmethionine** residues. This modified amino acid is present at the amino termini of proteins from most types of bacteria but is not found in proteins of human origin; it therefore serves as a telltale sign that bacteria are present within a host tissue.

Every neutrophil carries many different surface receptors, each one specific for a different type of chemoattractant. When even a nanomolar amount of a chemotactic factor diffuses from an injured tissue

into the blood, it can be detected by neutrophils as they pass through the local circulation. The neutrophils respond by associating tightly with the inner vessel wall, in a phenomenon known as **margination.** This takes place most commonly in postcapillary venules—small, thin-walled vessels in which blood flows relatively slowly—and results from changes not only in the neutrophil but also in the local endothelial cells. Margination occurs in 2 phases (Fig 1–3). The first phase is mediated primarily by oligosaccharide-binding membrane proteins called **selectins.** One of these, called **L-selectin,** is constitutively expressed on neutrophils, and its binding activity appears to increase after exposure to chemotactic factors. Two others, called **P-selectin** and **E-selectin,** appear on the surfaces of endothelial cells only after these cells have been "activated" by exposure to bacterial cell wall components, activated thrombin, or other factors that indicate nearby tissue injury (Table 1–4). These selectins on the neutrophil and endothelial surfaces allow each cell type to bind

Table 1–3. Major neutrophil chemotactic factors.

Endogenous
  Fibrin fragments
  Collagen fragments
  Complement derivatives (especially C5a)
  Chemokines, especially IL-8
  Platelet-activating factor (PAF)
  Leukotriene B_4 (LTB_4)
  Prostaglandin D_2 (PGD_2)
Exogenous
  N-formylated oligopeptides
    (ie, N-formylmethionyl or N-formylnorleucyl)

Table 1–4. Factors that induce expression of surface adhesion proteins on endothelial cells.

Adhesion Protein	Kinetics[1]	Major Inducers
P-selectin	Rapid (min)	Thrombin Histamine Complement derivatives Peroxide
E-selectin	Slow (h)	Interleukin-1 Tumor necrosis factor Bacterial endotoxin (LPS)[2]
ICAM-1	Slow (h)	Interleukin-1 Tumor necrosis factor Interferon γ

[1]Endothelial cells constitutively harbor P-selectin on the membranes of intracytoplasmic granules called Weibel-Palade bodies, from which it can be translocated rapidly onto the cell surface. Induction of E-selectin or ICAM-1 requires new mRNA and protein synthesis and is correspondingly slower.
[2]LPS, lipopolysaccharide.

particular oligosaccharide residues (and certain other ligands) on the surface of the other. Selectin-mediated binding is relatively weak, however, so that the neutrophil may initially continue to roll or skip a short distance along the vessel wall under the force of the flowing blood.

Contact with the endothelium, together with the influence of chemotactic factors, rapidly induces the transition into the second phase of margination, in which proteins called **integrins** appear on the neutrophil surface (Fig 1–3). The integrins can be expressed very quickly because neutrophils, which lack the ability to synthesize membrane proteins de novo, carry presynthesized integrins on the membranes of small vesicles in their cytoplasm; when a neutrophil

is appropriately simulated, these organelles quickly fuse with the plasma membrane, so that the adhesion proteins are transferred to the cell surface. Each integrin binds tightly to a particular endothelial cell surface protein; for example, the integrins known as **Mac-1** and leukocyte functional antigen type 1 (**LFA-1**) each bind an endothelial adhesion protein called intercellular adhesion molecule type 1

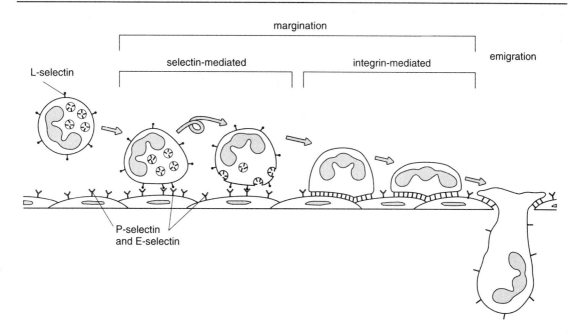

Figure 1–3. Neutrophil margination and emigration. The initial weak binding is mediated by selectins on the neutrophil and on activated endothelial cells. On contact with the endothelium, L-selectin is rapidly shed from the neutrophil surface, and presynthesized integrins (including Mac-1 and LFA-1) are translocated from cytoplasmic storage granules onto the neutrophil plasma membrane. The integrins mediate tight binding to the endothelial surface and later facilitate emigration and migration through the adjacent tissue. The emigrating neutrophil passes between endothelial cells, with their active collaboration.

(**ICAM-1**). This strong, integrin-mediated binding prevents further movement of the neutrophil and causes it to flatten out against the endothelial surface.

Once attached, neutrophils actively insinuate themselves between endothelial cells to migrate out of the venule and into the adjacent tissue in a process termed **emigration.** The neutrophils then travel by ameboid motion up the concentration gradient of chemotactic factors until they arrive at the focus of injury or infection. Emigration and chemotaxis are facilitated in part by integrins on the neutrophil surface that bind to fibronectin and other components of the extracellular matrix.

Phagocytosis & Microbicidal Activity of Neutrophils

On arrival at an injured site, neutrophils immediately begin the process of engulfing any bacteria, cel-

lular debris, or foreign particulate matter in the area. The mechanisms by which these cells are able to recognize such a wide range of target particles are not fully understood. Some types of targets, such as unencapsulated bacteria, carbon particles, or polystyrene beads, are probably recognized by virtue of nonspecific surface properties such as hydrophobicity. Others may fortuitously carry particular oligosaccharides or other chemical moieties that are recognized by receptors on the neutrophil surface. Submicroscopic particles that bind an individual receptor may be taken into the cell through receptor-mediated endocytosis, but larger (diameter, >100 nm), multivalent particles, such as bacteria, are thought to be engulfed through a progressive "zippering" process as increasingly large numbers of receptors on the cell surface membrane come into contact with the particle surface (Fig 1–4).

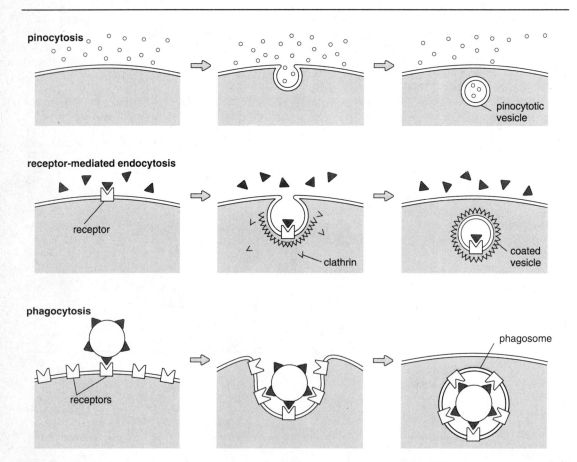

Figure 1–4. Three major pathways for bringing extracellular materials into a cell. Pinocytosis ("cell drinking") occurs through formation of minute surface vesicles filled with unmodified extracellular fluid. Receptor-mediated endocytosis is triggered by the binding of a soluble ligand to one or more specific surface receptors; the resulting polymerization of clathrin protein on the cytoplasmic aspect of the plasma membrane leads to invagination of the receptor and formation of a coated pit. Phagocytosis occurs when multiple surface receptors sequentially engage the surface of a target particle, usually >100 μm in diameter. Pinocytotic and coated vesicles, like phagosomes, are lined by a single lipid bilayer derived from the plasma membrane.

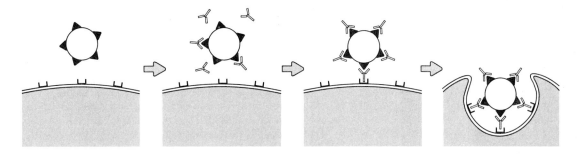

Figure 1–5. Opsonization. The opsonin protein (in this case, an immunoglobulin) binds to the surface of a particle, enabling the particle to be recognized by opsonin-specific receptors on the phagocyte surface.

Many types of particles, including most species of encapsulated bacteria, do not interact effectively with any cellular receptor and hence cannot be phagocytized directly. However, phagocytosis of such particles can occur when their surfaces are coated with certain host-derived proteins. Proteins that have this ability to enhance phagocytosis are known as **opsonins.** Many different human proteins function as opsonins, but by far the most important are the complement derivatives and a group of proteins called **immunoglobulins** that are secreted by some cells of the lymphocyte lineage (see Chapters 2 and 6). Opsonization occurs because the phagocyte carries surface receptors for the opsonin protein: when such a protein coats a target particle, it allows receptor-mediated engulfment (Fig 1–5). The opsonizing effect of immunoglobulins, for example, is mediated through immunoglobulin receptors, called **Fc receptors,** on the phagocyte surface. Similarly, some products of the complement pathway act as very potent opsonins because the phagocytes express surface **complement receptors.**

Particles that have been engulfed by a neutrophil are initially contained within membrane-bounded vacuoles called **phagosomes.** Seconds after engulfment, storage granules in the neutrophil cytoplasm begin to fuse with each phagosome, emptying their contents into its lumen (Fig 1–6). This process is known as **degranulation.** The neutrophil granules contain an extensive array of enzymes and other substances that can kill and degrade bacteria or dissolve other phagocytized materials (Table 1–2). Among the most abundant are a class of small (roughly 30 amino acids long) antimicrobial peptides called **defensins,** which kill by permeabilizing bacterial or fungal cell membranes and which constitute 30–50% of total granule protein. Other granule contents include the bactericidal enzyme **lysozyme,** numerous proteases, and **lactoferrin,** a protein that inhibits bacterial growth by chelating iron. The cell also acidifies the phagosome by actively pumping hydrogen ions into its interior; this not only promotes hydrolysis of the target directly but also enhances the activities of many granular enzymes.

In addition, a family of potent **NADPH-dependent oxidases** attached to the granule membranes project into the lumen of the phagocytic vacuole after degranulation. These oxidases act to convert molecular oxygen into highly reactive singlet oxygen, which spontaneously dismutates to form hydrogen peroxide (Table 1–5). In the presence of the abundant granular enzyme **myeloperoxidase** (which accounts for 5% of

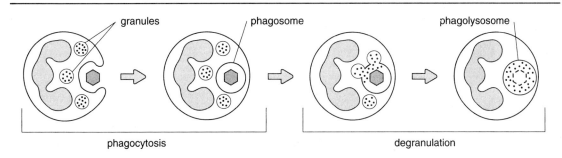

Figure 1–6. Engulfment and digestion of a target by a neutrophil. In the process of degranulation, multiple types of cytoplasmic granules may fuse with the phagosome, disgorging their contents into its lumen to inactivate and degrade the target particle.

Table 1–5. The major oxidative microbicidal pathway in neutrophils.[1]

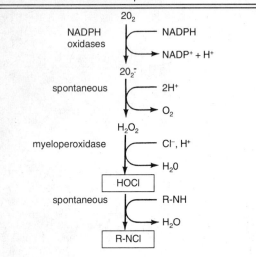

[1]Hypochlorous acid (HOCl) and organic chloramines (R-NCl) probably account for most of the target oxidization that takes place in vivo. The superoxide (O_2^-)and hydrogen peroxide (H_2O_2) intermediates in this pathway are also strong oxidizing agents but probably proceed along the pathway too quickly to play a major direct role in attacking target particles. "R-NH" denotes any organic primary or secondary amine.

the dry weight of a neutrophil), this hydrogen peroxide combines with chloride ions to form hypochlorous acid (HOCl), a potent oxidizing agent that is the active ingredient of household bleach. The hypochlorous acid is consumed almost instantaneously as it oxidizes amines, thiols, nucleic acids, proteins, and other biomolecules in the target particle, but a substantial portion reacts to form organic chloramines (R-NCl), a less powerful but much longer-lived class of oxidizing agents. Together, these oxidative pathways provide some of the most important antimicrobial effects of the neutrophil. Their vigorous action is manifested by a pronounced, transient increase in overall oxygen consumption by the neutrophil (called a **respiratory burst** or **metabolic burst**) that occurs immediately after phagocytosis and can persist for as long as 3 hours.

Neutrophils in Host Defense

The types of injuries that attract neutrophils into a tissue are nearly always accompanied by the local release of cellular chemical mediators which produce swelling, redness, heat, and pain at the involved site (see Chapter 11). These local effects, combined with an infiltration of neutrophils, constitute the pattern of host response known as **acute inflammation.** The first wave of invading neutrophils can be detected as early as 30 minutes after an acute injury; the cells generally accumulate to significant levels within 8–12 hours and will continue to arrive in increasing

numbers until the production of chemotactic signals subsides. Since neutrophils cannot replicate and since they survive for only a short time, many die at the site of inflammation and must be replaced by new cells from the circulation. In severe acute infections or other periods of high demand, the rate at which neutrophils are produced and released from storage in the bone marrow often increases dramatically, so that the blood neutrophil concentration rises severalfold. This greatly increases the number of cells available for delivery to the injured site. If marrow output is especially great, immature neutrophils that have unsegmented, rod-shaped nuclei (and hence are called **bands**) may also be released into the bloodstream. When the demand eventually wanes, the peripheral neutrophil concentration gradually returns to normal over a period of days or weeks.

If a localized response is prolonged or intense, enzymes released from dying neutrophils may liquefy nearby host cells and foreign material alike to form a viscous semifluid residue called **pus**—another hallmark of acute inflammation. Granule contents can also escape accidentally from living neutrophils during the course of phagocytosis, since degranulation often begins before a target particle has been completely engulfed (Fig 1–7). An extreme example of this occurs when neutrophils confront a target (such as a splinter) that is too large to engulf: in such a case, the cells attach themselves to the target and discharge granule contents (primarily from the specific granules) onto its surface, in a process called **extracellular degranulation.** Although beneficial in some cases, extracellular release of granule contents carries the risk of serious damage to host tissues and plays a prominent role in the pathogenesis of several human diseases, including gout, some forms of glomerulonephritis, and autoimmune arthritis.

The neutrophilic phagocyte system has many advantageous properties. First, neutrophils are attracted by a limited number of stimuli, which generally signal the presence of tissue injury no matter what its cause. This ensures that the cells can respond to many different types of injuries, including those that the host has never encountered before. Thus, acute trauma, foreign bodies, thermal or chemical burns, bacterial infections, and many other types of injuries can each provoke an intense neutrophil response. In addition, because large numbers of neutrophils are continually present in the blood and because nearly all of them respond to the same set of chemotactic stimuli, vast numbers of the cells can be mobilized without delay. Moreover, neutrophils are highly effective at killing certain bacteria, and their ability to digest cellular debris and exogenous particulate matter provides an important first step in the healing process.

Nevertheless, a defense system based solely on neutrophils would have some very significant limitations. In particular, these cells are completely unable

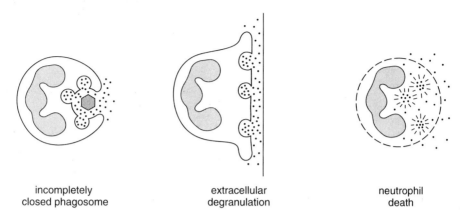

incompletely
closed phagosome

extracellular
degranulation

neutrophil
death

Figure 1–7. Some means by which the contents of neutrophil granules may be released into the extracellular milieu. Extracellular degranulation (also called "frustrated phagocytosis") occurs when the cell encounters a target that is too large to engulf. Neutrophil death, and the inadvertent release of granule contents from incompletely closed phagosomes, are common during intense or prolonged neutrophil reactions.

to recognize many types of potentially injurious agents and so do not respond to them until tissue damage has occurred. For example, neutrophils cannot detect or eradicate most types of proteinaceous toxins or individual viral particles circulating in the blood, since these generally do not bind to any neutrophil surface receptor. When neutrophils are called into action, they have only a limited repertoire of possible responses, consisting mainly of phagocytosis and the intracellular or extracellular discharge of their granule contents. Finally, the neutrophil system by itself has almost no ability to modify its responses on the basis of past exposure. Left on its own, this system of phagocytes would respond (or fail to respond) in the same stereotypical manner to a given pathogen no matter how many times it had encountered that same pathogen before.

MONONUCLEAR PHAGOCYTES: THE MONOCYTE-MACROPHAGE SYSTEM

Nearly all tissues, organs, and serosal cavities harbor a population of resident phagocytes. Most contain only a diffuse scattering of individual phagocytic cells that remain inconspicuous under normal conditions and are very similar to one another in appearance and function. In some tissues, however, phagocytes are especially abundant or have distinctive morphologic features and are known by specific names: examples include the Kupffer cells that line sinusoids of the liver (and account for nearly 10% of total liver mass), osteoclasts in bone, and microglial cells of the brain (Table 1–6). Regardless of their location or appearance, all of these tissue-associated phagocytes belong to a single lineage known as the

mononuclear phagocyte system and are derived from a circulating white blood cell called the monocyte.

Monocytes are relatively large (12–20 μm in diameter) cells with kidney-shaped nuclei, loose nuclear chromatin, and fairly abundant cytoplasm that is well stocked with the types of organelles needed to synthesize secretory and membrane proteins (Fig 1–8). They also contain a substantial supply of cytoplasmic **lysosomes,** which contain most of the same enzymatic constituents found in neutrophil azurophilic granules; however, lysosomes in monocytes are less numerous than the granules in neutrophils and are not readily seen under the light microscope. Monocytes are not very abundant in the peripheral circulation, accounting for only 1–6% of all nucleated blood cells. They are produced in the bone marrow and are then released into the blood,

Table 1–6. Cells of the monocyte-macrophage lineage.

Tissue	Cell Type Designation
Blood	Monocytes
Bone marrow	Monocytes and monocyte precursors (monoblasts, promonocytes)
Any solid tissue	Resident macrophages (histiocytes)
Skin	Langerhans cells
Liver	Kupffer cells
Lung	Alveolar macrophages
Bone	Osteoclasts
Synovium	Type A synovial cells
Central nervous system	Microglia
Pleural cavity	Pleural macrophages
Peritoneal cavity	Peritoneal macrophages
Chronic inflammatory exudate	Exudate macrophages
Granuloma	Epithelioid cells, multinucleated giant cells

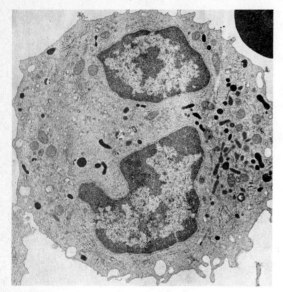

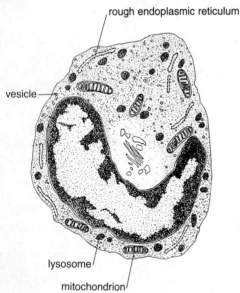

Figure 1–8. Electron micrograph (top) and diagram (bottom) of a human monocyte. Cytoplasmic granules (lysosomes) are present but are much less numerous than in neutrophils. However, the cell retains the abundant Golgi apparatus and rough endoplasmic reticulum needed to synthesize additional granules or secretory proteins as needed. The cell is 12–20 μm in diameter. (Courtesy of Dorothy F. Bainton.)

where they circulate for only about 1 day before settling into a permanent site of residence in a tissue. Once settled in this manner, the cells are called tissue **macrophages,** or **histiocytes.** The criteria by which the cells select their tissue residence is presently unknown. Those that enter some tissues (such as the liver or brain) subsequently undergo changes in mor-

phology or function, presumably in response to factors in the local microenvironment.

Macrophage Activation & Phagocytic Responses

A tissue macrophage lives for approximately 2–4 months. During this time, some macrophages remain immobile while others wander incessantly by ameboid motion. In either case, the cell continually samples its surrounding environment by pinocytosis (Fig 1–4) and through an extensive array of receptors on its surface (Table 1–7). Whenever it encounters certain stimuli, the macrophage undergoes a process known as **activation,** in which it rapidly increases its metabolic rate, motility, and phagocytic activity. Activated macrophages are somewhat larger than their inactive counterparts, owing mainly to an increase in cytoplasmic volume, and are much more efficient at killing bacteria and other pathogens. The range of stimuli that can activate macrophages is very large: direct contact with certain microorganisms or inert particles, with bacterially derived endotoxin or host tissue breakdown products, or with protein components of the complement or blood coagulation systems can each lead to activation. Activation can also be enhanced by certain polypeptide hormones (notably one known as **interferon γ [IFN γ]**) that may be secreted by nearby lymphocytes (see Chapter 9).

Activated macrophages are avid phagocytes that

Table 1–7. Ligands bound by macrophage surface receptors[1]

Opsonins
    Complement components (C3 and C4 products)
    Immunoglobulins (especially IgG; via Fc receptors)
    Carbohydrates and carbohydrate-binding proteins (mannose-, fucose-, galactose-, and N-acetylglucosamine-containing oligosaccharides)
Chemotactic factors
    N-formyl oligopeptides
    Complement components (C5a)
    Thrombin
    Fibrin
Growth factors and cytokines
    Colony-stimulating factors (GM-CSF, M-CSF)
    Interleukins (IL-1, IL-3, IL-6, IL-10)
    Interferons (IFN α, IFN β, IFN γ)
    Tumor necrosis factors (TNF)
    Transforming growth factor β (TGFβ)
Hormones and other mediators
    Insulin
    Histamine
    Epinephrine
    Calcitonin
    Parathyroid hormone
    Somatomedins
Miscellaneous
    Transferrin
    Lactoferrin
    Modified low-density lipoproteins
    Fibronectin

[1]Modified and reproduced, with permission, from Klein J: *Immunology,* Blackwell Scientific, Boston, 1990.

engulf whatever foreign particles or cellular debris they encounter. They move somewhat less rapidly than neutrophils but have the advantage of being much longer-lived. They also are larger and hence can engulf larger targets, including entire senescent or damaged host cells. Like neutrophils, macrophages recognize some target particles directly by their surface properties. However, the cells also express receptors for complement components, immunoglobulins, and other opsonins, and a coating of such opsonins is essential for phagocytosis of many types of particles. Engulfment occurs through the zippering process described earlier (Fig 1–4) and encloses the target particle in a phagosome; cytoplasmic lysosomes then fuse with the phagosome, disgorging their contents into its lumen.

In comparison with the action of neutrophils, macrophage phagocytosis tends to be a slower, less dramatic process: the metabolic burst that occurs after engulfment is less pronounced, and engulfed matter tends to be broken down gradually and relentlessly over time. This is in part a reflection of the limited number of lysosomes that are available in the macrophage at a given moment. However, unlike neutrophils, macrophages retain all of the organelles needed to synthesize secretory proteins and so can produce new lysosomes as needed. Ultimately, the offending particles are usually completely annihilated. For example, red blood cells that leak from a damaged vessel to form a bruise are soon engulfed by tissue macrophages and broken down into their component molecules. Most engulfed bacteria meet the same fate. Other materials may resist degradation but still remain sequestered within the macrophage and so are prevented from contacting the surrounding tissue. For example, large numbers of inhaled carbon particles often persist for years within macrophages in the lungs of cigarette smokers.

Macrophage Secretory Activity

Activated macrophages not only function as phagocytes but also specifically secrete an enormous variety of biologically active substances into the surrounding tissues. More than 100 secretory products of macrophages have been identified so far, a partial list of which is presented in Table 1–8. Certain of these can be secreted individually in response to specific stimuli, whereas others are released in combination as part of a more generalized response. Some products, such as lysozyme, complement components, and hydrogen peroxide, have antimicrobial activity. Others, such as elastases and collagenases, act to liquefy the extracellular matrix; this facilitates cellular migration and helps clear the way for the healing process. Macrophages also secrete numerous **cytokines,** which influence the growth and activities of other cell types (see Chapter 9). These include colony-stimulating factors (which promote hematopoietic cell growth), fibroblast growth factors, prosta-

Table 1–8. Secretory products of macrophages.

Enzymes
Lysozyme
Acid hydrolases (proteases, nucleases, glycosidases, phosphatases, lipases, etc)
Elastase
Collagenase
Plasminogen activator
Angiotensin-converting enzyme

Mediators
Interferons (IFN α, IFN β)
Colony-stimulating factors (GM-CSF, M-CSF, G-CSF, and others)
Interleukins (IL-1, IL-6, IL-8, IL-10, IL-12)
Chemokines
Tumor necrosis factor α
Platelet-derived growth factor
Platelet-activating factor (PAF)
Transforming growth factor β (TGFβ)
Angiogenesis factors
Nitric oxide
Arachidonate derivatives (prostaglandins, leukotrienes)

Complement components
C1–C9
Properdin
Factors B, D, I, and H

Coagulation factors
Factors V, VII, IX, and X
Prothrombin
Thromboplastin

Reactive oxygen species
Hydrogen peroxide
Superoxide anion
Singlet oxygen
Hydroxyl radicals

Miscellaneous
Glutathione
Nucleosides (adenosine, thymidine, guanosine, etc)

glandins, and chemoattractant peptides (chemokines) that draw lymphocytes and other blood cells into the vicinity.

Macrophages in Host Defense

Most macrophages are thought to be terminally differentiated, although some appear capable of limited replication within tissues. Some of the factors secreted by activated macrophages attract other nearby macrophages and blood monocytes, but the relatively slow movement and small numbers of such cells limit the speed of their response. Generally, 7–10 days must pass before significant numbers of macrophages arrive at an injured site. In most cases, there is little or no accompanying increase in marrow production or blood concentration of these cells.

Eventually, large numbers of macrophages may congregate around targets that are large, numerous, or resistant to digestion. Such macrophage aggregates are called **granulomas** (Fig 1–9) and may contain subpopulations of lymphocytes, fibroblasts, or other cell types. Macrophages in such lesions are often called **epithelioid cells,** since they tend to interdigitate closely with one another through complex

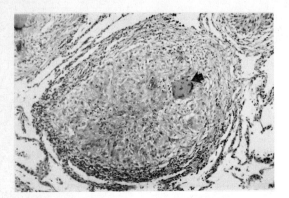

Figure 1–9. A granuloma—a distinctive pattern of macrophage reaction against foreign material. This photomicrograph shows a single, roughly spherical granuloma, 1–2 mm in diameter, in the lung. It is composed almost entirely of epithelioid macrophages, with a thin, surrounding rim of fibroblasts and normal lung tissue. At one site, several individual macrophages have fused to form a multinucleated giant cell (arrow). Granulomas often contain other types of inflammatory cells (especially lymphocytes) in addition to macrophages. (Courtesy of Martha Warnock)

surface folds and microvilli and so form a continuous sheet of cells that resembles an epithelium. This interdigitation serves to entrap material within the granuloma. Individual macrophages may also fuse to form large **multinucleated giant cells,** which are able to engulf correspondingly larger targets such as splinters, multicellular parasites, and surgical suture material.

Viewed in isolation, macrophages suffer from many of the same limitations that were described above for neutrophils. They are a fairly homogeneous group of phagocytic cells that recognize a fixed number of potential targets. They are, moreover, less numerous, slower to respond, and less effective than neutrophils at killing most bacteria. However, there is an additional facet of their biology that places macrophages among the most important components of the immune system: unlike neutrophils, macrophages are able to control the actions of lymphocytes—a far more abundant and versatile population of defensive cells. Macrophages affect lymphocyte responses in at least 2 major ways. First, activated macrophages secrete potent immunoregulatory peptides, such as tumor necrosis factor and IL-1, that control lymphocyte proliferation, differentiation, and effector function. Second, activated macrophages also are among the most important types of **antigen-presenting cells,** ie, cells that process and display foreign substances in a form that can be recognized and responded to by lymphocytes. Through these 2 types of regulatory interactions with lymphocytes, macrophages play a crucial role in initiating and coordinating nearly all types of immune responses. The mechanisms and consequences of these interactions will be explored in detail in subsequent chapters.

REFERENCES

Hematopoiesis

Clark SC, Kamen R: The human hematopoietic colony-stimulating factors. *Science* 1987;**236:**1229.

Dexter TM, Spooncer E: Growth and differentiation in the hemopoietic system. *Annu Rev Cell Biol* 1987;**3:**423.

Dorshkind K: Regulation of hemopoiesis by bone marrow stromal cells and their products. *Annu Rev Immunol* 1990;**8:**111.

Sachs L: The molecular control of blood cell development. *Science* 1987;**238:**1374.

Phagocytosis and Endocytosis

van Oss DJ: Phagocytosis: An overview. *Methods Enzymol* 1986;**132:**3.

Goldstein JL et al: Receptor-mediated endocytosis. *Annu Rev Cell Biol* 1985;**1:**1.

Target Recognition and Antimicrobial Effector Mechanisms

Babior BM: The respiratory burst oxidase. *Trends Biochem Sci* 1987;**12:**241.

Lehrer RI et al: Defensins: Antimicrobial and cytotoxic peptides of mammalian cells. *Annu Rev Immunol* 1993;**11:**105.

Retrosen D, Gallin JI: Disorders of phagocyte function. *Annu Rev Immunol* 1987;**5:**127.

Snyderman R, Pike MC: Chemoattractant receptors on phagocytic cells. Annu Rev Immunol 1984;**2:**257.

Weiss SJ: Tissue destruction by neutrophils. *N Engl J Med* 1989;**320:**365.

Neutrophils

Lehrer RI et al: Neutrophils and host defense. *Ann Intern Med* 1988;**109:**127.

Malech HL, Gallin JI: Neutrophils in human diseases. *N Engl J Med* 1987;**317:**687.

Monocyte-Macrophages

Adams DO, Hamilton TA: The cell biology of macrophage activation. *Annu Rev Immunol* 1984;**2:**283.

Hamilton TA, Adams DO: Molecular mechanisms of signal transduction in macrophages. *Immunol Today* 1987;**8:**151.

Endothelial Cells

Jaffe EA: Cell biology of endothelial cells. *Hum Pathol* 1987;**18:**234.

Pober JS, Cotran RS: Cytokines and endothelial cell biology. *Phys Rev* 1990;**70:**427.

**Adhesion Proteins
and Leukocyte-Endothelial Interactions**

Bevilacqua MP: Endothelial-leukocyte adhesion molecules. *Annu Rev Immunol* 1993;**11:**767.

Hynes RO: Integrins: Versatility, modulation, and signaling in cell adhesion. *Cell* 1992;**69:**11.

Lasky LA: Selectins: Interpreters of cell-specific carbohydrate information during inflammation. *Science* 1992;**258:**964.

Ruoslahti E: Integrins. *J Clin Invest* 1991;**87:**1.

Lymphocytes & Lymphoid Tissues

Tristram G. Parslow, MD, PhD

The normal adult human body contains on the order of a trillion (10^{12}) lymphocytes, most of which appear virtually identical to one another when examined by conventional histologic techniques. The typical lymphocyte is a small, round, or club- shaped cell, 5–12 μm in diameter, with a roughly spherical nucleus, densely compacted nuclear chromatin, and cytoplasm so scanty as to be scarcely detectable under the light microscope. The cytoplasm contains scattered mitochondria and free ribosomes but lacks any distinctive organelles (Fig 2–1). Despite this uniform appearance, several very different types of lymphocytes can be distinguished on the basis of their functional properties and by the specific proteins they express. The most fundamental distinction is the division of these cells into 2 major lineages known as T (thymus-derived) cells and B (bone-marrow-derived) cells.

The relative proportions of T and B cells vary among tissues (Table 2–1); in peripheral blood, they account for about 75 and 10% of all lymphocytes, respectively. The remaining 15% of peripheral blood lymphocytes belong to a separate and rather enigmatic lineage known as natural killer (NK) cells, which differ from other lymphocytes in many significant respects and have some unusual properties that will be described later in this book (see Chapter 8). The present chapter focuses exclusively on T and B cells, which are the cells involved in most types of immune responses.

T and B lineage cells both arise from a subset of hematopoietic stem cells in the bone marrow or fetal liver that become committed to the lymphoid* pathway of development (Fig 2–2). There is considerable

evidence for the existence of a committed marrow progenitor, called the **lymphoid stem cell,** that serves as a common precursor for both T and B cells; however, such cells have not yet been purified or characterized definitively. The progeny of these putative stem cells follow divergent pathways to mature into either B or T lymphocytes. Human B lymphocyte development takes place entirely within the bone marrow. T cells, on the other hand, develop from immature precursors that leave the marrow and travel through the bloodstream to the thymus, where they proliferate and differentiate into mature T lymphocytes.

The thymus and bone marrow are sometimes referred to as **primary lymphoid organs** because they provide unique microenvironments that are essential for **lymphopoiesis**—the initial production of lymphocytes from uncommitted progenitor cells. Together, the thymus and marrow produce approximately 10^9 mature lymphocytes each day, which are then released into the circulation. Lymphopoietic activity is controlled in part by soluble factors elaborated within these organs. For example, growth of early lymphoid progenitors requires at least 2 cytokines, called interleukin-3 (**IL-3**) and stem cell factor (**SCF**), found in both the thymic and marrow microenvironments. In addition, the thymus produces a number of hormones that selectively promote later stages of T cell development. Lymphopoiesis also depends on direct contact of the lymphoid precursor cells with marrow and thymic stromal elements, with the extracellular matrix, and with one another. In general, lymphocytes are produced and released by the marrow and thymus at a more or less constant rate, irrespective of whether the cells are needed for an immune response at the moment. T lymphopoiesis in the thymus continues until about the time of puberty, at which time the organ normally involutes, but B cells continue to be produced by the marrow throughout life.

Mature lymphocytes that emerge from the thymus or bone marrow are in a quiescent **"resting"** state:

---

*The word "lymphocyte" refers to cells at a specific stage in the T- or B-cell lineage. The term "lymphoid" is used to denote the entire lineages (encompassing cells at all developmental stages), or tissues in which cells from these lineages normally predominate.

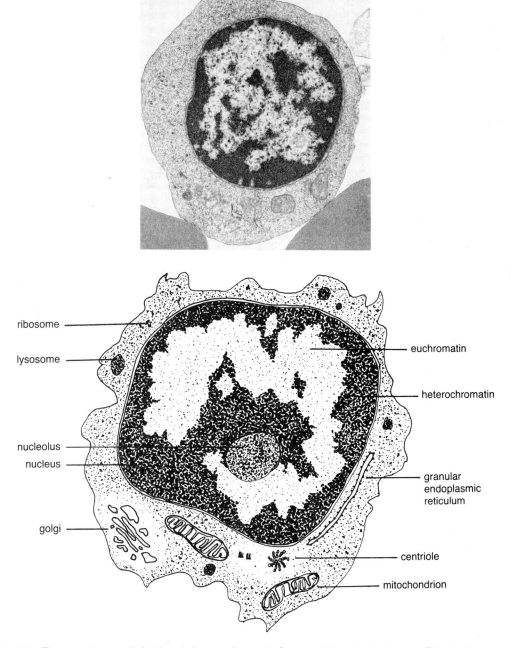

ribosome

lysosome

euchromatin

heterochromatin

nucleolus

nucleus

granular
endoplasmic
reticulum

golgi

centriole

mitochondrion

Figure 2–1. Electron micrograph (top) and diagram (bottom) of a normal human lymphocyte. This slightly tangential section exaggerates the amount of cytoplasm present: in most resting lymphocytes, the nucleus accounts for 90% of total cell volume. Note the dense nuclear chromatin and the bland cytoplasm, which lacks any obvious secretory organelles. (Courtesy of Imok Cha and Noel Weidner.)

they are mitotically inactive (that is, they are in the G_0 phase of the cell cycle) and, although they are potentially capable of undergoing cell division and of carrying out immunologic functions, they have not yet been stimulated to do either. When dispersed into the bloodstream, these so-called "naive" or **"virgin"** lymphocytes migrate efficiently into various **secondary** (or **peripheral**) **lymphoid organs,** such as the spleen, lymph nodes, or tonsils. The function of the secondary lymphoid organs is to maximize encoun-

Table 2–1. Proportions of lymphoid cell types in normal human tissues.

Tissue	Approximate % of[1]:		
	T Cells	B Cells	NK Cells
Peripheral blood	70–80	10–15	10–15
Bone marrow	5–10	80–90	5–10
Thymus	99	<1	<1
Lymph node	70–80	20–30	<1
Spleen	30–40	50–60	1–5

[1]Includes cells at all recognizable stages of development in each lineage.

ters between lymphocytes and foreign substances, and it is from these sites that most immune responses are launched.

Most virgin lymphocytes have an inherently short life span and are programmed to die within a few days after leaving the marrow or thymus. However, if such a cell receives signals that indicate the presence of a specific foreign substance or pathogen, it may respond through a phenomenon known as **activation,** in the course of which it may undergo several successive rounds of cell division over a period of several days (Fig 2–3). Some of the resulting progeny cells then revert to the resting state to become **memory lymphocytes**—cells that resemble the virgin T or B lymphocyte from which they are derived but which can survive for many years. Such memory lymphocytes make up a large proportion of the cells in the

immune system of an adult, and, like virgin lymphocytes, are constantly poised to undergo further cycles of activation and cell division. Thus, one consequence of activating a virgin lymphocyte is that some of its progeny become long-term constituents of the host immune system. The other progeny of an activated virgin lymphocyte differentiate into **effector cells,** which survive for only a few days but, during that time, carry out specific defensive activities against the foreign invader.

Lymphocyte proliferation can thus take place in 2 very different contexts. The first (lymphopoiesis) is confined to the thymus and marrow and results in the de novo production of short-lived, quiescent virgin lymphocytes that are then released into the periphery. This occurs autonomously at a rate dictated by the marrow and thymus themselves. The second form of replication takes place in peripheral tissues and occurs only when lymphocytes become activated as part of an immune response. This stimulus-dependent proliferation gives rise to long-lived memory cells and also to short-lived effector cells that actively carry out specific immune functions. The nature of these latter functions depends on the lymphocyte lineage from which the effector cells arose.

B CELLS

The defining feature of cells in the B cell lineage is their ability to synthesize proteins called **immuno-**

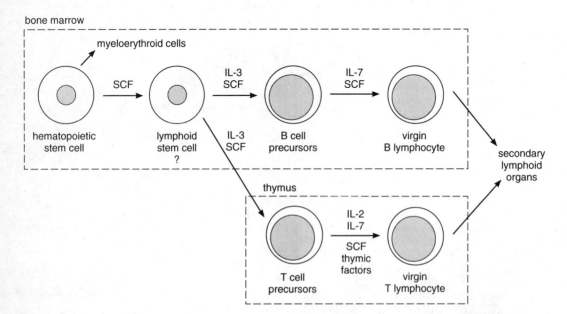

Figure 2–2. Schematic overview of lymphocyte development (lymphopoiesis). In this simplified diagram, most intermediate stages are omitted. The characteristics of cells that migrate to the thymus are unknown. A few of the regulatory molecules needed for proliferation at particular stages of development are indicated. SCF, stem cell factor.

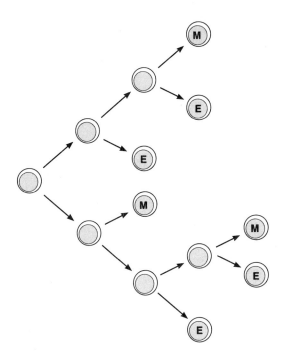

Figure 2–3. Lymphocyte activation leads to both cell division and differentiation. At each cell division, individual cells can cease dividing and differentiate into memory (M) or effector (E) cells. In this example, a single activated lymphocyte gives rise to 4 effector and 3 memory cells after 4 cycles of division.

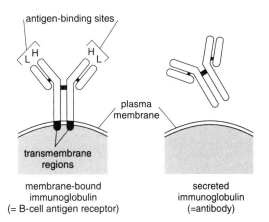

Figure 2–4. Membrane-bound and secreted forms of an immunoglobulin protein. This diagram depicts one of the many types of immunoglobulins, each of which is composed of paired light-chain (L) and heavy-chain (H) polypeptides. The amino termini of the L and H chains are juxtaposed to form the binding site for an antigen. A hydrophobic region (shaded) at the carboxy termini of the heavy chains anchors the membrane-bound protein onto the cell surface. When this region is absent, the immunoglobulin is secreted from the cell.

globulins (Fig 2–4). No other cell expresses these proteins. The immunoglobulins are an extremely diverse family of proteins, each made up of 2 related types of polypeptides called **heavy chains** and **light chains.** Each immunoglobulin binds specifically and with high affinity to its own particular small molecular ligand, which may be any of a vast number of chemical determinants found in proteins, carbohydrates, lipids, or other macromolecules. The molecular determinants bound by various immunoglobulin proteins can be referred to collectively as **antigens**— an important term that is considered more thoroughly in Chapter 4.

Mature B cells can express immunoglobulin in 2 different forms that each serve unique functions (Fig 2–5). In resting (virgin or memory) B lymphocytes, immunoglobulins are expressed only on the cell surface, where they serve as membrane-bound receptors for specific antigens. Each resting lymphocyte may express tens of thousands of membrane immunoglobulins on its surface. By contrast, the effector cells of the B lineage (called **plasma cells**) are uniquely specialized to secrete large amounts of immunoglobulin proteins into their surrounding milieu. Secreted immunoglobulins retain the ability to recognize and bind their specific ligands and are often referred to as

antibodies; they normally circulate at a serum concentration of 7–26 g/L in an adult and so account for about 25% of total serum protein. Binding of an antibody to its target antigen can have a variety of effects that are beneficial to the host. For example, antibody binding may sequester and inactivate a toxic protein in the blood or may block receptors on a viral particle that would otherwise enable the virus to adhere to host cells. Many secreted immunoglobulins also are potent opsonins, in that they promote phagocytosis of bacteria or other targets to which they bind. The properties of immunoglobulins are discussed in much

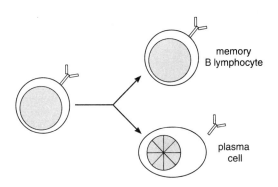

Figure 2–5. The progeny of an activated B lymphocyte can differentiate into either memory B lymphocytes or antibody-secreting plasma cells.

more detail in Chapter 6. For the present, it is enough to say that these binding proteins not only serve as surface receptors for foreign substances but also can be released to search out and bind their targets at a considerable distance from the cell.

When an activated B lymphocyte divides, some of its progeny become memory B cells, while the remainder differentiate into plasma cells. Plasma cells are oval or egg-shaped and have abundant cytoplasm and eccentrically placed round nuclei (Fig 2–6). Clumps of dark-staining chromatin are often distributed around the inner aspect of the nuclear membrane in plasma cells, giving the nuclei a characteristic "pinwheel" or "clock face" appearance under the light microscope. The protein-secretory organelles are well represented, including a large paranuclear Golgi apparatus and abundant rough endoplasmic reticulum. Immunoglobulins usually are not present on the surface of a plasma cell but are produced in copious amounts in the cytoplasm and are then secreted into the extracellular space. Plasma cells have a relatively short lifespan (on the order of days to a few weeks) and are terminally differentiated. Unless new plasma cells are continually produced, the existing ones soon die out and immunoglobulins are no longer secreted. Thus, activation of B cells typically results in a transient wave of proliferation, followed by a burst of antibody secretion that increases and then subsides over several days or a few weeks.

The main function of B-lineage cells is to secrete antibodies into the blood and other body fluids and hence to make these fluids inhospitable to foreign invaders. They are the principal cell type involved in **humoral immunity**—that is, in protective effects that are mediated through tissue fluids. However, B cells also play 2 additional roles in the immune system. First, they can function as **antigen-presenting cells,** by processing and displaying foreign substances in a manner that can be recognized by T lymphocytes. Second, activated B cells can secrete certain **lymphokines** and other factors that influence the growth and activities of other immunologically important cells. These last 2 functions are discussed in more detail in later chapters.

T CELLS

T lymphocytes do not express immunoglobulins but, instead, detect the presence of foreign substances by way of surface proteins called **T cell receptors.** These receptors form a heterogeneous class of membrane proteins, which, on most T cells, are made up of a pair of transmembrane polypeptides known as the α and β chains. T cell receptors are closely related to immunoglobulins in evolution and share with them a number of structural and functional properties (see Chapter 8), including the ability to detect specific small molecular ligands called **antigens.** Unlike im-

munoglobulins, however, T cell receptor proteins are never secreted, and, as a result, T cells lack the ability to strike their targets at long distance. Instead, they exert their protective effects either through direct contact with a target or by influencing the activity of other immune cells. Together with macrophages, T cells are the primary cell type involved in a category of immune responses called **cell-mediated immunity.**

Unlike B cells, T cells can detect foreign substances only in specific contexts. In particular, T lymphocytes will recognize a foreign protein only if it is first cleaved into small peptides, which are then displayed on the surface of a second host cell, called an **antigen-presenting cell.** Virtually all types of host cells can present antigens under some conditions, but certain cell types are specially adapted for this purpose and are particularly important in controlling T cell activity. These specialized antigen-presenting cells include macrophages and B lymphocytes, as well as other cell types that we will encounter later. Presentation depends in part on specific proteins, called **major histocompatibility complex (MHC)** proteins, on the surface of the presenting cells. Foreign peptides are attached noncovalently onto the MHC proteins for display, and it is the combination of peptide and MHC protein that can be recognized by a T cell receptor. Thus, T lymphocytes must directly touch the surfaces of other cells to detect antigens as well as to produce most of their immunologic effects.

Mature, functional T lymphocytes express a number of characteristic surface proteins in addition to T cell receptors (Table 2–2). Many of these proteins are referred to by the initials **CD** (which stands for "**cluster of differentiation**") followed by a unique identifying number. This system of nomenclature was originally developed for membrane proteins or protein complexes that could be identified by their physical properties (such as molecular weight) or their interactions with specific antibodies but whose biological functions had not yet been determined. It is most often used for proteins that are expressed on lymphocytes and other hematopoietic cells, although several of the proteins that carry CD designations are also expressed on one or more nonhematopoietic cell types. Proteins that have been named in this manner are listed in the Appendix, along with a brief summary of their properties and the cell types on which each is expressed. We will encounter several of these proteins repeatedly, since they are very useful for distinguishing among different types of cells and often participate directly in immune cell functions.

For example, surface T cell receptors are always expressed in conjunction with 5 other transmembrane surface polypeptides that are known collectively as the **CD3 complex.** These CD3 proteins are physically associated with the T cell receptors through noncovalent attachments; they serve to transmit signals from

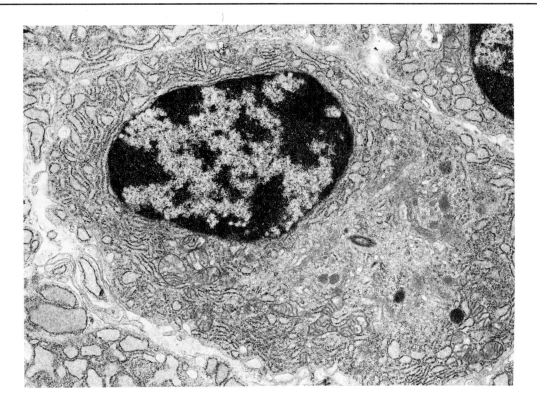

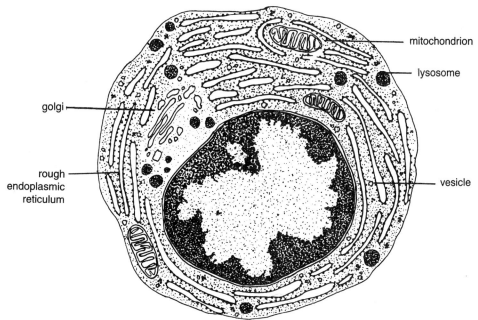

Figure 2–6. Electron micrograph (top) and diagram (bottom) of a plasma cell, the effector cell of the B lymphoid lineage. The abundant rough endoplasmic reticulum and Golgi complex in the cytoplasm allow these cells to synthesize large amounts of immunoglobulins in a form that is then secreted from the cell. (Courtesy of DF Bainton.)

Table 2–2. Some important surface molecules on T lymphocytes.

Marker	Major Function or Significance
T cell receptor	Antigen binding.
CD3 complex	Signal transduction from T cell receptor; lineage-specific marker.
CD2, CD5, CD7	Lineage-specific markers.
CD4	Subset-specific marker (mainly on helper cells); interaction with class II MHC proteins.
CD8	Subset-specific marker (mainly on cytotoxic cells); interaction with class I MHC proteins.
IL-2 receptor Class II MHC proteins Transferrin receptor CD25, CD29, CD54, CD69 CD40 ligand (CD40L)	Activation-specific markers
IL-1 receptor IL-6 receptor TNFα receptor	Other cytokine receptors
Fc receptors	Immunoglobulin binding
LFA-1, ICAM-1	Cell-cell adhesion molecules

Table 2–3. Major T-cell subsets found in blood and peripheral tissues.

Surface Phenotype	Predominant Function	Proportion of Total Blood T Lymphocytes	T Cell Receptor Type
CD4+CD8−	Helper	70%	α/β
CD4−CD8+	Cytotoxic	25%	α/β, rarely γ/δ
CD4−CD8−	Cytotoxic	4%	γ/δ
CD4+CD8+	?	1%	α/β

the receptors into the cytoplasm and must be present for the receptors to be transported onto the cell surface. Because the CD3 proteins are expressed almost exclusively by T-lineage cells and are easier to detect and much less structurally diverse than the receptors themselves, their presence is commonly used to identify T lymphocytes in extrathymic tissues. However, surface expression of the receptor-CD3 complex occurs relatively late in T cell ontogeny. Two other proteins, called **CD2** and **CD7,** appear at an earlier stage of T cell development in the thymus, continue to be displayed on the surfaces of virtually all T-lineage cells and are almost never found on other cell types. CD2 and CD7 therefore serve as very useful general markers for recognizing all cells in this lineage.

Nearly all mature T lymphocytes that are found in peripheral blood and secondary lymphoid organs are CD2+CD3+CD7+—that is, they each express CD2, CD3, and CD7 on their surface. However, the class of CD2+CD3+CD7+ T lymphocytes as a whole is actually made up of distinct subpopulations that have very different immunologic functions and express their own distinctive surface markers. These subpopulations are often referred to as **T cell subsets** (Table 2–3). The 2 most important T cell subsets can be distinguished by 2 additional surface proteins known as CD4 and CD8. Mature, functional T lymphocytes almost always express only one of these 2 proteins, and this correlates with important differences in cell function (Fig 2–7). Most T lymphocytes that express surface **CD8** protein have **cytotoxic** ac-

tivity—the ability to kill cells that have foreign macromolecules on their surfaces. Cytotoxic T lymphocytes (**Tc cells** or **CTLs**) are extremely important in the defense against viral infections: host cells that are infected by a virus can often be identified by the presence of viral peptides on their surfaces, and killing these cells is essential to eradicate the disease. In contrast, T lymphocytes that express **CD4** protein generally are not cytotoxic but instead function as **helper T cells** (**TH cells**) which promote proliferation, maturation, and immunologic function of other cell types. For example, specific lymphokines secreted by

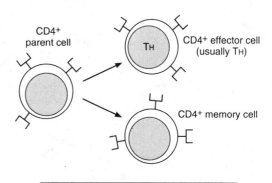

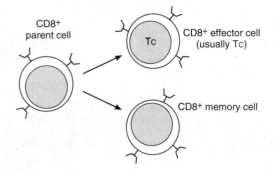

Figure 2–7. The progeny of activated T lymphocytes retain the surface phenotype (CD4+ or CD8+) of their parents.

helper T cells are very important in controlling the activities of B cells and of cytotoxic T cells.

Altogether, roughly 70% of T cells in human blood or secondary lymphoid tissues are CD4+CD8– (also called CD4 cells), whereas 25% are CD4–CD8+ (or simply CD8 cells). Cells with either of these phenotypes are often referred to as **single-positive** lymphocytes and are the cells most commonly involved in immune responses. Approximately 4% of T cells outside the thymus are CD4–CD8– **double-negative** lymphocytes; nearly all of these express an alternative form of T cell receptor composed of polypeptides called γ and δ (see Chapter 8). The remaining 1% of extrathymic T cells are **double-positive** CD4+CD8+ cells, whose function is unknown.

The correlation of CD4 or CD8 with TH and TC cell function, respectively, is strong but not absolute: a few CD8 cells have helper activity, and a few CD4 cells are cytotoxic. Expression of CD4 or CD8 actually correlates most closely with the type of MHC protein that a T cell can recognize, as will be described in Chapters 3 and 5.

Virgin and memory T lymphocytes ordinarily remain in the resting state, and in this state they do not exhibit significant helper or cytotoxic activity. When activated, however, these cells can undergo several rounds of mitotic division to produce multiple daughter cells. Some of these daughter cells return directly to the resting state as memory cells, but others become effector cells that actively express helper or cytotoxic activity. The daughter cells resemble their parents: activated CD4+ cells can produce only CD4+ daughter cells, whereas activated CD8+ cells yield only CD8+ progeny. The effector cells of the T lineage tend to have slightly more cytoplasm and

looser chromatin than their resting counterparts but cannot reliably be distinguished from them under the light microscope. However, the effector cells display several types of surface proteins (such as CD25, CD29, transferrin receptors, and a group of MHC proteins known as class II MHC proteins) that are not found on resting T cells, and they also express increased amounts of some constitutive T cell markers (such as CD2). When the activating stimuli are withdrawn, cytotoxic or helper activity gradually subsides over a period of several days as the effector cells either die or revert to the resting state.

AN OVERVIEW OF LYMPHOCYTE ACTIVATION

The term **"lymphocyte activation"** denotes an ordered series of events through which a resting lymphocyte is stimulated to divide and produce progeny, some of which become effector cells (Fig 2–8). The full response thus includes both the induction of cell proliferation (**mitogenesis**) and the expression of immunologic functions. Lymphocytes become activated when specific ligands bind to receptors on their surfaces. The ligands required are different for T cells and B cells (see below), but the response itself is similar in many respects for all types of lymphocytes.

The earliest event known to take place when a T or B cell binds ligands that cause activation is a marked increase in activity of cytoplasmic **protein tyrosine kinases (PTKs)**—proteins that have the ability to catalyze the phosphorylation of tyrosine residues in other proteins. This increase occurs within seconds and reflects the functional activation of a variety of

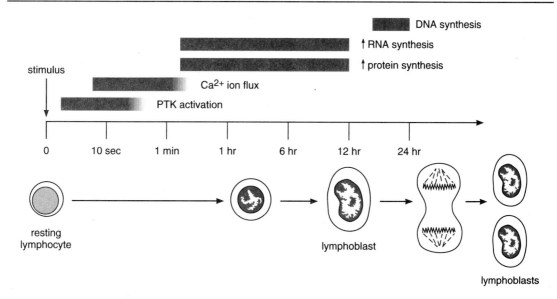

Figure 2–8. Major biochemical and morphologic events in lymphocyte activation. PTK, protein tyrosine kinase.

different PTKs. Phosphorylation is a common mechanism of regulating protein function; indeed, many of the PTKs must themselves be phosphorylated before they can become active. Several important types of lymphocyte surface receptors (including membrane immunoglobulin and T cell receptor proteins) are physically linked to specific cytoplasmic PTK proteins, which become active when the receptor binds its target ligand. These receptor-associated PTKs, in turn, may then activate other types of PTKs through phosphorylation, so that almost immediately a host of different PTKs are recruited into the response. By phosphorylating still other types of substrates, such as proteins that control cytoskeletal organization, expression of specific genes, and entry into the cell cycle, these newly activated PTKs appear to be either directly or indirectly responsible for triggering all subsequent events in lymphocyte activation. At present, however, the functions of most individual PTKs are uncertain.

One almost immediate effect of the PTK cascade is to activate the enzymatic breakdown of a specific class of phospholipids (called phosphatidylinositides) within the cell. The products of this hydrolysis include 2 small organic molecules, **diacylglycerol (DAG)** and **inositol 1,4,5-trisphosphate (IP₃)**, which are released into the cytoplasm and serve as second messengers to trigger additional changes in cellular physiology. Among the most notable changes is a rapid, marked increase in the concentration of **intracellular free calcium ions,** which flood into the cytosol from organellar storage pools and from the extracellular medium, reaching maximal concentrations within 1 minute after contact with the activating stimulus. Like PTK activation, these rapid calcium fluxes are thought to be critical for initiating the subsequent events in activation.

Within the first hour after stimulation, the rates of oxidative metabolism and of overall protein and RNA synthesis in the lymphocyte rise. The chromatin begins to decondense as previously silent genes are transcribed and the cell prepares to undergo mitosis. After 2–4 hours, specific proteins that are thought to regulate cell proliferation, such as the product of the proto-oncogene **c-*myc*,** become detectable in the nucleus. In parallel with these biochemical events, the morphology of the cell changes in a process known as **blast transformation**: its overall diameter increases to 15–30 μm as both its nucleus and cytoplasmic enlarge; the nuclear chromatin becomes loose and pale-staining; and the cell acquires a prominent nucleolus (reflecting a high rate of RNA synthesis). Within 8–12 hours, the changes are sufficiently marked that the cell can be recognized under the light microscope as a **lymphoblast**—a lymphocyte poised to begin mitosis. DNA synthesis takes place at around 18–24 hours after stimulation. The first cell division occurs 2–4 hours later and, depending on the conditions, can be repeated 5 or more times in succession, at intervals as

brief as 6 hours. The effector cells produced as a result of each division mature completely within a few days and express the immune functions typical of their lineage for several days thereafter.

REQUIREMENTS FOR ACTIVATION OF B OR T LYMPHOCYTES

What are the stimuli that can lead to lymphocyte activation in vivo? Certainly, the most important are the innumerable foreign **antigens** that are recognized and bound by membrane immunoglobulins or T cell receptor proteins. A few types of antigens are in themselves sufficient to activate B cells—these are usually highly polymeric proteins or polysaccharides that are able to interact simultaneously with many immunoglobulin proteins on the surface of a single cell. Such multivalent antigens act to **cross-link** the immunoglobulins to one another, so that eventually a great many immunoglobulins are gathered at one pole of the cell surface at the point of contact with antigen—a phenomenon known as **capping** (Fig 2–9A). This dense local aggregation of immunoglobulins, each of which is bound to antigen, transmits a very effective signal and is enough to trigger B cell activation.

Activation can also be induced under artificial conditions by cross-linking other types of surface molecules (Table 2–4). Among the agents used for this purpose are certain lectins (sometimes called **mitogens**), which can activate T and/or B cells by cross-linking surface glycoproteins. Similar results can be obtained by using multivalent antibody complexes to cross-link some T cell surface proteins (such as CD3) that are able to transmit signals to the cytoplasm. Alternatively, lymphocytes can be activated pharmacologically by being treated with agents that directly in-

Table 2–4. Mitogens and other conditions used to activate lymphocytes in vitro.

Mitogen or Condition	Specificity
Lectins	
Concanavalin A	T cells
Helix pomatia lectin	T cells
Phytohemagglutinin	T cells; few B cells
Pokeweed mitogen	T and B cells
Wheat germ agglutinin	T cells
Artificial cross-linking of specific surface proteins	
Immunoglobulins	B cells
T cell surface markers (eg, CD3)	T cells
Pharmacologic agents	
Phorbol myristyl acetate plus calcium ionophore (eg, ionomycin)	T and B cells

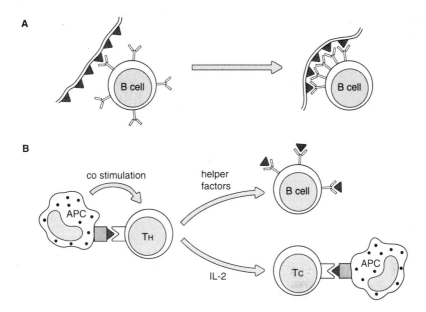

Figure 2–9. General requirements for lymphocyte activation. **A:** Some highly polymeric antigens that cross-link multiple antigen receptors are sufficient to activate B cells. **B:** Activation by a monomeric antigen requires additional stimuli supplied by another cell type. Costimulators from the antigen-presenting cell (APC) are necessary to activate a TH cell, which in turn provides helper factors for B cells and/or interleukin-2 (IL-2) for Tc cells.

duce calcium fluxes and other important signaling events, thereby bypassing the surface receptors entirely. Such potent artificial activators are often used in clinical testing to study lymphocyte responses in vitro.

The majority of antigens encountered in nature, however, are not polymeric and so do not cross-link receptors. Even when many copies of such an antigen bind individual immunoglobulins on a B cell, they generate only an incomplete signal, which fails to activate the cell. B cells can be activated by these more common antigens only if they are simultaneously stimulated by a nearby activated helper T lymphocyte. This stimulation may be delivered by lymphokines secreted from the T cell, but is transmitted most efficiently through direct contact of the B cell with T cell surface proteins. In either case, the helper-cell-derived proteins (which will be referred to in this book as **helper factors**) interact with non-immunoglobulin receptors on the B cell to generate a second signal. The combined effects of the helper factors and the bound antigen then act synergistically to cause B cell activation.

In a similar manner, T lymphocyte responses to most antigens also require 2 types of stimuli simultaneously. The first is provided by the antigen, which, if appropriately displayed by MHC proteins on an antigen-presenting cell, can be recognized and bound by T cell receptors. When it binds an antigen-MHC complex, the T cell receptor sends a signal to the cell interior, but this signal alone is usually not enough to

cause activation. For helper T cells, full activation also requires contact with other specific ligands, known as **costimulators,** that are expressed on the surface of the antigen-presenting cell. Activation of a cytotoxic T cell, on the other hand, generally requires **IL-2,** a cytokine secreted by activated helper T cells.

In summary, it is important to recognize that activation of a lymphocyte is controlled not only by antigen binding but also by interactions with other cells (Fig 2–9B): all T cells must cooperate with antigen-presenting cells, whereas B cells and cytotoxic T cells depend on helper T lymphocytes. These interactions either require direct surface-to-surface contact or are mediated by highly labile cytokines that act only over extremely short distances. Owing to this interdependence among cell types, lymphocyte activation occurs most commonly and efficiently in the secondary lymphoid organs, where lymphocytes, antigens, and antigen-presenting cells encounter one another at close quarters.

LYMPHOID ORGANS

Lymphocytes are normally present in the blood at a concentration of approximately 2500 cells/mm^3 and so account for roughly one-third of all peripheral white blood cells. Each individual lymphocyte, however, spends most of its life within solid tissues, entering the circulation only periodically to migrate from one resting place to another. Indeed, at any given moment, no more than 1% of the total lymphocyte population can be found in the blood. Most of the remaining cells are contained in specialized lymphoid organs such as the lymph nodes, thymus, tonsils, Peyer's patches, and white pulp of the spleen, where they carry out most of their functions.

Lymph Nodes & Lymphatic Circulation

Driven by the hydrostatic pressure within capillary lumens, water and low-molecular-weight solutes from the blood plasma continually leach out through blood vessel walls and into the lower-pressure interstitial space. This slow leakage occurs in all solid organs and is the source of the nutrient-rich **interstitial fluid** that permeates every available niche in the tissues and bathes each individual cell. Most of this fluid returns directly to the bloodstream through the walls of nearby venules, but a substantial amount (totaling approximately 120 ml/h in an adult at rest) does not. Instead, this portion of the interstitial fluid flows through the tissues at an almost imperceptible rate and is eventually collected in a branching network of flaccid, thin-walled channels known as primary lymphatic vessels. These vessels ramify throughout almost all organs of the body (except the brain, eyeballs, marrow cavities, cartilage, and placenta) but are often difficult to discern in tissue sections, since they collapse easily and are delimited only by a single delicate layer of lymphatic endothelial cells. Once the fluid enters these vessels, it is known as **lymph.** Flowing slowly along the primary lymphatics, the lymph empties into progressively larger-caliber lymphatic vessels, which ultimately converge and drain their contents into the right and left subclavian veins in the thorax (Fig 2–10). Thus, the lymphatic vasculature serves as a slow-flowing, low-pressure drainage system that collects a small proportion of the interstitial fluid from throughout the body and returns it to the bloodstream.

During its passage along the lymphatic vessels, the lymph flows through a series of bean-shaped organs called **lymph nodes,** which range from as little as 1 mm to about 25 mm in diameter. Nodes are distributed along the entire length of the lymphatic vasculature, tend to increase in size toward the venous end of the system, and often occur in chains or clusters that receive flow exclusively from a particular organ or region of the body (Fig 2–10). Especially prominent clusters of lymph nodes can be found in the neck and axillae (draining the head and arms), in the inguinal and paravertebral regions (draining the legs and pelvis), and the root of the mesentery (draining the gut).

In its simplest form, a lymph node can be viewed as a localized dilatation of the lymphatic vessel, filled with dense aggregates of lymphocytes and macrophages that cling to a loose meshwork of connective tissue fibers called **reticulin** fibers. The reticulin mesh is produced by specialized fibroblasts known as **reticular cells,** small numbers of which are also pres-

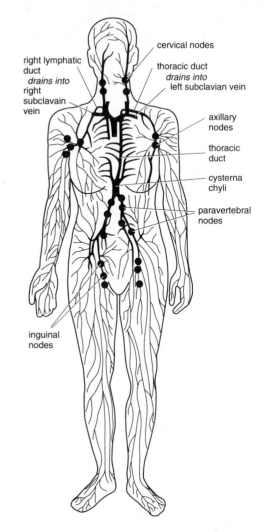

Figure 2–10. Lymphatic vascular system. Lymphatic vessels draining the right arm and right side of the head and neck converge to form the right lymphatic duct; the thoracic duct receives lymph from the remainder of the body. Only a few major collections of lymph nodes are depicted.

ent in the node. The node functions as a physical and biologic filter: as lymph fluid percolates through its internal lattice of cells, the macrophages and lymphocytes survey the fluid for any bacteria, viruses, or foreign macromolecules that may have been carried along with it from the tissues.

Larger nodes show an organized internal structure, which is schematized in Fig 2–11. The entire node is surrounded by a fibrous capsule. Lymph flows into the node along several **afferent lymphatic vessels** on one surface of the node and enters a narrow **subcapsular sinus** that is lined primarily by macrophages. The lymph then percolates sequentially through two more or less distinct regions of predom-

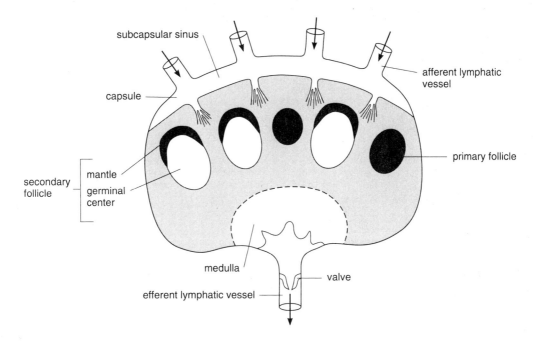

Figure 2–11. Idealized structure of a lymph node. Lymph enters via afferent vessels, passes through the cortex (shaded) and medulla, and exits via a single efferent vessel. Large lymphatic vessels often contain valves that prevent backward flow of the lymph.

inantly lymphoid tissue, called the **cortex** and the **medulla,** and finally exits through an **efferent lymphatic vessel** on the opposite side, at a region known as the hilus. Each node also receives a rich supply of blood that enters via an arteriole at the hilus, flows through a dense bed of capillaries and venules in the cortex and medulla, and then returns to the hilus to drain out through small veins.

The lymph node cortex usually contains several discrete spherical or ovoid cellular aggregates called **lymphoid follicles** (Fig 2–11). These follicles are composed mainly of memory B lymphocytes, a smaller number of T cells (virtually all of which are helper cells), and a specialized type of supporting cell called the **follicular dendritic cell.** The latter cells are so named because they are found only in lymphoid follicles and exhibit many long, delicate cytoplasmic processes that radiate out like tentacles to encircle each follicular lymphocyte. The origin and function of follicular dendritic cells are poorly understood, but they appear to be responsible for assembling memory B cells into follicles and regulating their subsequent activities.

Lymphoid follicles are labile structures that can disappear and re-form at different sites over time and can enlarge in response to infections or other immune challenges. They are of 2 types (Fig 2–12). **Primary follicles** contain predominantly mature, resting B cells; since these have dense nuclei and little cytoplasm, a primary follicle appears as a relatively dark-staining mass on conventional histologic preparations. **Secondary follicles,** on the other hand, appear as a pale-staining sphere known as the **germinal center,** with a cap (or **mantle**) of more darkly staining mature B lymphocytes overlying it on the afferent side of the node. The pale staining of the germinal center reflects the fact that, in this portion of the follicle, most of the lymphocytes are in various stages of activation and blast transformation and hence have more cytoplasm and looser chromatin than do resting lymphocytes. Numerous individual macrophages are also present in the germinal center, and occasional plasma cells may be seen.

Secondary follicles are not present at birth, and they form only after repeated exposure to substances that provoke an immune response. Although their physiology is not well understood, the presence of secondary follicles clearly denotes an ongoing B cell immune response. Secondary follicles are thought to arise when a few helper T cells become activated in response to an antigen, migrate into a primary follicle, and in turn help activate the resident B cells. The B cells then replicate to generate secretory plasma cells, which may remain in the germinal center or migrate to the medulla of the node; the antibodies that these cells secrete are carried away by the lymph flow and into the bloodstream. Proliferating B cells in a germinal center also undergo a process called **affinity maturation,** in which the B cells that respond most vigorously to the antigen are allowed to prolif-

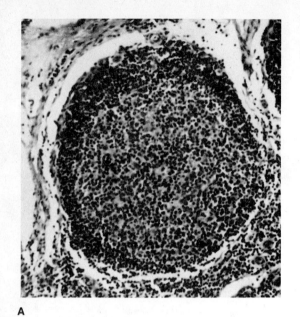

Figure 2–12. Structures of lymphoid follicles. ***A***: A secondary follicle in the cortex of a lymph node, from a hematoxylin-eosin–stained section. Note the round, pale-staining germinal center and darker, overlying cap (mantle). Because follicles are often cut tangentially in standard tissue sections, the mantle is sometimes erroneously thought to completely encircle the germinal center. (Contributed by Brian Herndier.) ***B***: At the top are photomicrographs of a primary (left) and a secondary (right) follicle from a hematoxylin-eosin–stained section of a lymph node. The diagrams below schematically depict the relationship between a follicular dendritic cell (white with shaded nucleus) and the surrounding lymphoid cells in a primary follicle (left) and a germinal center (right). The relatively pale staining properties of the germinal center result mainly from the abundant cytoplasm and large, pale-staining nuclei of the B cell blasts it contains. (Contributed by Roger Warnke.)

A

primary

secondary

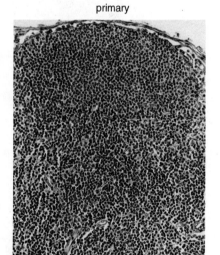

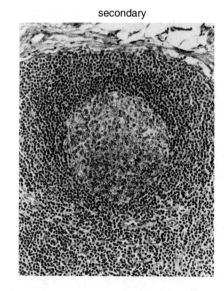

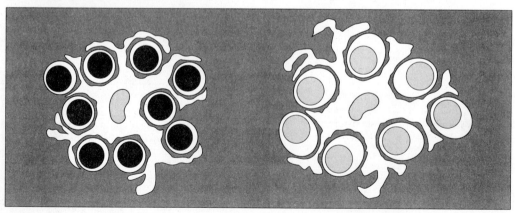

primary follicle

germinal center
of secondary follicle

B

erate while others selectively die (see Chapter 7). The phagocytosed remains of B cells that have died in this process can be seen within the macrophages of a germinal center.

The regions of lymph node cortex lying outside the follicles are populated primarily by T cells, about two-thirds of which are helper cells. T cells are especially abundant in the ill-demarcated region of cortex known as the **paracortex,** which lies between the lymphoid follicles and the medulla. Here, as in the T cell-rich zones of all secondary lymphoid organs, the T cells are accompanied by a smaller population of supporting cells, called **interdigitating cells,** that have antigen-presenting activity. The **medulla** usually is less densely cellular than the cortex, and often contains a scattering of plasma cells along with mature B and T lymphocytes and macrophages.

The lymph that flows into a node may carry with it microorganisms or other foreign matter from the tissues. When such a substance enters a lymph node, some of the lymphocytes and macrophages in the node may respond by activation. As a result, some of the resident lymphocytes begin to proliferate, inflammatory mediators are released locally, blood flow to the node increases markedly, and the normal, slow lymphocyte emigration from the node ceases entirely. If these responses are sufficiently pronounced, the node may become noticeably enlarged—a condition known as **lymphadenopathy.** Rapid enlargement of a lymph node can occur, for example, when an infection develops in the region it drains. Swelling usually decreases when the infection ends, although repeated bouts of swelling can lead to permanent enlargement and induration by scarring the interior of a node.

Spleen

The spleen (Fig 2–13) filters blood much as the lymph nodes filter lymph. Located just below the diaphragm on the left side of the abdomen, the spleen weighs approximately 150 g in an adult and is enclosed in a thin and rather fragile connective-tissue capsule. Blood enters by way of the splenic artery at the hilum and passes into a branching network of progressively smaller arterioles that radiate throughout the organ. Each arteriole is encased in a cylindrical cuff of lymphoid tissue that consists mainly of mature T cells and is called the **periarteriolar lymphoid sheath.** Primary and secondary lymphoid follicles protrude at intervals from the sheath; these are identical to the follicles found in other lymphoid tissues and are composed mainly of B cells. The arterioles, sheaths, follicles, and a small amount of associated connective tissue are together called the splenic **white pulp,** which is visible as a delicate latticework

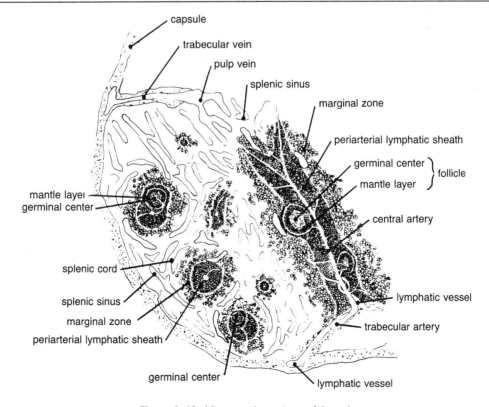

Figure 2–13. Microscopic anatomy of the spleen.

on the cut surface of the organ. Blood flows from the arterioles into the **red pulp**—a spongy, blood-filled network of reticular cells and macrophage-lined vascular sinusoids that makes up the bulk of the spleen—and then exits by way of the splenic vein.

During the course of each day, approximately half the total blood volume passes through the spleen, where lymphocytes and macrophages survey it continually for evidence of infectious agents or other contaminants. The spleen thus serves as a critical line of defense against blood-borne pathogens. Splenic macrophages also have the important function of recognizing and eliminating any abnormal, damaged, or senescent red or white cells from the blood. Surgical removal of the spleen (most often performed because it has been lacerated by trauma) is usually well tolerated in an adult but causes a persistent rise in the percentage of malformed circulating erythrocytes and a modestly increased risk of sepsis due to diplococci or other pyogenic bacteria.

Tonsils, Peyer's Patches, & Other Subepithelial Lymphoid Organs

Vast numbers of individual T and B lymphocytes, macrophages, and plasma cells lie just below the mucosal epithelia in many regions of the alimentary, genitourinary, and respiratory tracts. Especially dense populations of such cells can normally be found around bronchial lumens or in the lamina propria and submucosa of the large and small intestines, where they are well situated to detect any foreign substances that contact these body surfaces. In most areas, the cells form a diffuse, disorganized mass, punctuated only occasionally by isolated lymphoid follicles.

At other sites, the cells are organized into discrete, stable anatomic structures. For example, **tonsils** are nodular aggregates of macrophages and lymphoid tissue located immediately beneath the stratified squamous epithelium of the nasopharynx and soft palate. Tonsils lack a capsule and afferent lymphatic vessels but have many of the other constituents of a lymph node, including lymphoid follicles; their function is to detect and respond to pathogens in the respiratory and alimentary secretions. The overlying epithelium plunges downward into the substance of a tonsil to form deep crypts whose contents are continually monitored by the tonsillar cells. Similar unencapsulated lymphoid nodules, called **Peyer's patches,** are present in the ileal submucosa of the small bowel, where they serve to detect substances that diffuse across the intestinal epithelium (Fig 2–14). Together, all of the organized and diffuse lymphoid tissues found in submucosal regions of the body can be viewed as a single functional unit, called the **mucosa-associated lymphoid tissue (MALT),** which will be discussed in Chapter 41. One important function of these tissues is to secrete antibodies across the mucosal surface as a defense against external pathogens.

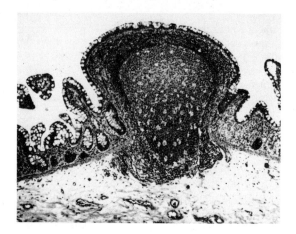

Figure 2–14. Microscopic anatomy of a Peyer's patch, a secondary lymphoid follicle beneath the mucosal epithelium of the small intestine. (Contributed by Linda Ferrell.)

The skin, too, is an important site of immune surveillance. Small populations of lymphocytes are constantly present in the dermis and epidermis, although they usually are inconspicuous and do not normally form lymphoid follicles. In addition, the epidermis contains a resident subpopulation of antigen-presenting cells, called **Langerhans cells,** each of which sends out a network of dendritic branches that intertwine between epidermal epithelial cells over a relatively large area. These Langerhans cells account for about 5% of all epidermal cells. When it encounters foreign substances, a Langerhans cell secretes cytokines that attract additional lymphocytes from the nearby circulation and it also presents the foreign substances on its surface to help initiate an immune response. Macrophages in the dermis play a similar role as antigen-presenting sentinels.

Thymus

Unlike the other lymphoid organs described above, the thymus is involved in lymphocyte production and maturation rather than in immune surveillance per se. It is the primary site at which T lymphocytes differentiate and become functionally competent. The organ itself arises during embryogenesis as 2 endodermal buds from the third pharyngeal pouches; these invade downward into the superior mediastinum and then fuse to form a solid, V-shaped epithelial mass. During the third month of gestation, this mass becomes colonized by primitive, marrow-derived lymphoid stem cells that are carried to it by way of the blood. It is not yet clear whether these migrating stem cells are already committed to T cell differentiation or become committed only after entering the thymus. The epithelial component of the thymus is made up of sheets and islands of squamous cells that elaborate a variety of small peptide hormones, the best characterized of which are thymulin, thymopoietin, thymic humoral factor, and several forms of thymosin. These hormones have been proposed to play a role in attracting T cell precursors from the blood and also to promote their subsequent maturation within the thymus. Once inside the organ, T cells pack themselves densely into the interstices between epithelial cells, stretching them apart until the epithelium comes to resemble a loose network of stellate cells that cling to one another via desmosomes. In this microenvironment, T cells proliferate briskly, giving the thymus one of the highest rates of cell division in the body.

The fully developed thymus is composed of 2 lobes, each comprising multiple lobules (Fig 2–15). Lymphocytes are packed more densely toward the periphery of each lobule than near its center, and this gives rise to the appearance of an outer cortex and inner medulla, although there is no sharp anatomic border between these 2 zones. In some areas of the medulla, the epithelium forms small keratized whorls, called **Hassell's corpuscles,** whose significance is unknown. Apart form the epithelial cells and a few macrophages and other supporting elements, virtually all cells in the thymus are T cells. T lymphocytes residing in the thymus are often called **thymocytes.** Of these, a minor proportion (approximately 10%) are CD4–CD8– cells. Unlike the rare double-negative T cells found outside the thymus, these are somewhat enlarged, have a high rate of mi-

totic activity, and are presumed to be primitive T cell precursors. A second subpopulation (15% of thymic T cells) consists of single-positive thymocytes that express only CD4 or CD8 alone and are nearly indistinguishable from the mature T lymphocytes found elsewhere throughout the body. Such single-positive cells are most abundant in the thymic medulla and are thought to be fully mature virgin T lymphocytes that are preparing to leave the organ.

The vast majority of lymphoid cells in the thymus, however, are small T cells that express both CD4 and CD8 proteins together on their surfaces. These double-positive thymocytes account for roughly 75% of all thymic T cells. They are not immunologically functional and are thought to represent a transient intermediate stage in T cell development. Amazingly, nearly all of these double-positive thymocytes (at least 99%) die without ever leaving the thymus: the thymic cortex is studded with individual dying thymocytes, and phagocytosed debris from the dead thymocytes can be seen within cortical macrophages and epithelial cells. Thus, the thymus is a site for both prolific replication and wholesale slaughter of T cells. As discussed in later chapters, the T cell deaths that occur in the thymus are part of a rigorous **selection** process that is essential for creating a functioning immune system.

The developmental relationships among the various classes of thymocytes are outlined in Fig 2–16. Blood-borne lymphocyte progenitors enter the thy-

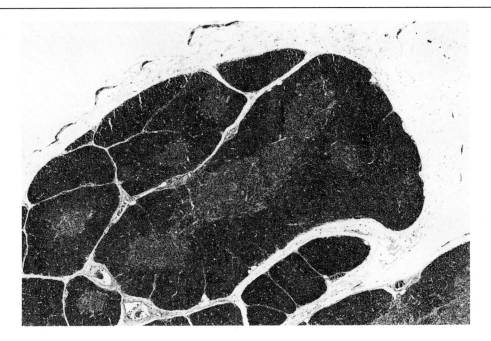

Figure 2–15. Microscopic anatomy of the thymus. This photomicrograph shows a portion of a thymic lobule from a hematoxylin-eosin–stained section, illustrating the dense outer cortex and pale inner medulla. (Contributed by Gordon Honda.)

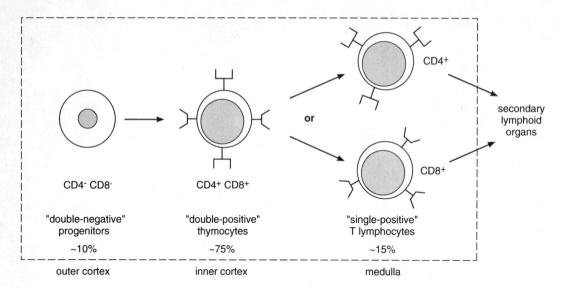

Figure 2–16. Model for intrathymic T cell maturation. Developing thymocytes pass through 3 successive stages of differentiation as they migrate from the outer cortex to the medulla and then exit the thymus. Some identifiable intermediate stages have been omitted. The sequence depicted applies to most T cells that express α/β T cell receptors. For details, see Chapter 8.

mus and form a pool of replicating cells located mainly near the periphery of the cortex; it is not known whether this replicating pool is stable or must continually be replenished with new marrow precursors. The progeny of the replicating cells appear first as double-negative thymocytes and then progress to the double-positive stage in which they express T cell receptors along with both CD4 and CD8 on their surfaces. Each individual thymocyte then selectively and permanently shuts off expression of either CD4 or CD8 (apparently choosing between these 2 markers at random), and so becomes a single-positive thymocyte. This differentiation process is plainly arduous, since fewer than 1% of the cells produced in the thymus are able to complete it. Although the factors that determine which thymocytes will survive are not entirely known, the selection process depends in part on specific interactions with thymic macrophages or epithelial cells, at least some of which are mediated through the T cell receptor (see Chapter 8). The small percentage of single-positive cells that survive ultimately leave the thymus as mature T lymphocytes. There is a general tendency for the cells to migrate from the cortex toward the medulla as they differentiate, though this may not be true of all thymocytes.

The thymus is relatively large and highly active at birth, weighing an average of 22 g. It continues to enlarge for several years, although at a lower rate than the rest of the body, and reaches its peak weight (around 35 g) at puberty. Thereafter, it begins to involute as the lymphoid components recede and are replaced by fatty connective tissue. Little more than 6 g of thymic tissue (most of it epithelial) persists into adulthood. This normal regression probably signifies that the thymus produces enough virgin T lymphocytes early in life to seed the entire immune system and that it is then no longer necessary. Consistent with this view, removal of the thymus at any time after birth generally does not cause significant immunologic abnormalities. However, complete congenital absence of the thymus results in the absence of T lymphocytes and produces profound, life-threatening immunodeficiency.

LYMPHOCYTE CIRCULATION & HOMING

Lymphocytes are migratory cells: their tissue distribution is determined by the rates at which they enter and exit particular sites, as well as by local replication. Individual lymphocytes in a lymph node, for example, do not remain there permanently but instead detach themselves periodically from the reticulin matrix and exit through efferent vessels, carried along by the lymph flow. They eventually are carried into the bloodstream and so enter the general circulation, which disperses them throughout the body. Similarly, lymphocytes continually exit from other secondary lymphoid organs through the lymph vessels or, in the case of splenic lymphocytes, by passing directly into the blood. Through this means, a small proportion of the lymphocyte population is constantly in motion, shuttling through other organs and surveying the body for foci of infection or contamination.

Lymphocytes in the blood are attracted back into

solid tissues by way of specialized blood vessels known as **high endothelial venules.** Such vessels are a modified form of postcapillary venules, which are found in all lymphoid organs; they can be recognized under the light microscope by the cuboid shape of the endothelial cells that line them. Some lymphocytes passing through these venules tend to bind tightly to the specialized endothelium and then infiltrate between endothelial cells and out into the tissue. Binding occurs because proteins known as **homing receptors** on the lymphocyte surface have a strong affinity for determinants, called **vascular addressins,** on the high endothelium. High endothelial cells in different target organs, such as lymph nodes or Peyer's patches, express addressins that are characteristic of that organ and are recognized by a specific type of homing receptor. Thus, when a circulating lymphocyte expresses a particular homing receptor, it will tend to bind and infiltrate a specific tissue or organ. Homing to lymph nodes, for example, results from an interaction between **L-selectin** on the surface of some lymphocytes and a glycoprotein addressin (CD34) on the endothelium. Lymphocytes bearing surface **CD29,** on the other hand, bind preferentially

to the surface integrin VCAM-1 on the high endothelium of Peyer's patches. Lymphocytes also carry other types of surface adhesion proteins that serve to strengthen the interaction with endothelium but do so in a non-tissue-specific fashion.

High endothelial venules are a constant feature of lymphoid organs but may also appear transiently at any site in the body where an immune response is occurring. They arise by differentiation of pre-existing capillaries in response to a lymphokine called gamma interferon (IFN γ) that is elaborated locally by activated helper T cells. These vessels then serve as a portal for circulating lymphocytes to enter the site and join in an immune response. By this means, lymphocytes and other reactive cells can accumulate wherever they are needed in the body. If a response is sufficiently intense and prolonged, the assembled lymphocytes, plasma cells, and antigen-presenting cells may arrange themselves spatially in a manner that resembles a permanent lymphoid organ, complete with secondary lymphoid follicles. Such reactive, and usually temporary, encampments are sometimes referred to as **tertiary lymphoid organs.**

REFERENCES

Ontogeny & Subtypes of T and B Lymphoid Cells

Adkins B et al: Early events in T-cell maturation. *Annu Rev Immunol* 1987;**5**:325.

Ikuta K et al: Lymphocyte development from stem cells. *Annu Rev Immunol* 1992;**10**:759.

Kincade PW et al: Cells and molecules that regulate B lymphoiesis in bone marrow. *Annu Rev Immunol* 1989;**7**:111.

Podack ER, Kupfer A: T cell effector functions: Mechanisms for delivery of cytotoxicity and help. *Annu Rev Cell Biol* 1991;**7**:479.

Vitetta ES et al: Memory B and T cells. *Annu Rev Immunol* 1991;**9**:193.

Secondary Lymphoid Organs

Bohnsack JF, Brown EJ: The role of the spleen in resistance to infection. *Annu Rev Med* 1986;**37**:49.

Bos JD, Kapsenberg ML: The skin immune system: Its cellular constituents and their interactions. *Immunol Today* 1986;**7**:235.

Szakal AK et al: Microanatomy of lymphoid tissue during humoral immune responses: Structure-function relationships. *Annu Rev Immunol* 1989;**7**:91.

Lymphocyte Activation

Clark EA, Lane PJL: Regulation of human B-cell activation and adhesion. *Annu Rev Immunol* 1991; **9**:97.

Crabtree GR: Contingent genetic regulatory events in T lymphocyte activation. *Science* 1989;**243**;355.

DeFranco AL: Molecular aspects of B-lymphocyte activation. *Annu Rev Cell Biol* 1987;**3**:143.

Parker DC: T cell-dependent B-cell activation. *Annu Rev Immunol* 1993;**11**:331.

Ullman K et al: Transmission of signals from T lymphocyte antigen receptor to the genes responsible for cell proliferation and immune function. *Annu Rev Immunol* 1990;**8**:421.

Lymphocyte Recirculation & Homing

Picker LJ, Butcher EC: Physiological and molecular mechanisms of lymphocyte homing. *Annu Rev Immunol* 1992;**10**:561.

Springer TA: Adhesion receptors in the immune system. *Nature* 1990;**346**:425.

Yednock TA, Rosen SD: Lymphocyte homing. *Adv Immunol* 1989;**44**:313.

3

The Immune Response

Joel W. Goodman, PhD

The immune system has at least 3 major functional properties that distinguish it from all of the body's other defenses. The first is its extreme **specificity**— the ability to recognize and distinguish among a vast number of different target molecules and to respond (or not respond) to each of these individually. Second, the immune system **discriminates between self and nonself,** so that it normally coexists peacefully with all of the innumerable proteins and other organic materials that make up the host but responds vigorously against foreign substances, including cells or tissues from other people. Third, the immune system has **memory,** ie, the ability to be molded by its experiences so that subsequent encounters with a particular foreign pathogen provoke more rapid and more vigorous responses than occurred at the initial encounter.

These properties of the immune system seemed impenetrable mysteries only a few decades ago, but in recent years they have begun to yield to research. A great deal is now understood about the mechanisms that give rise to immunologic specificity and memory, and the processes underlying self-nonself discrimination are beginning to be unraveled as well. What has emerged is the realization that the lymphocyte population in each person constitutes an extraordinarily interactive network of mobile cells that are almost as diverse as the foreign substances they respond to and that their diversity is the result of molecular genetic processes that may well be unique to these cells. Moreover, it is now recognized that each person's immune system is continually evolving in response to its environment and experience as the individual cells communicate and cooperate with one another to control their own proliferation, differentiation, and immunologic functions.

The interplay of molecular and cellular events that takes place during even the simplest immune response is dauntingly complex, and many aspects of immune system function are still incompletely understood. As a result, the subject can be especially bewildering and intimidating to the uninitiated. The goal of this chapter is therefore to present an introduction to the subject by describing the organization of lymphocyte populations and the essential elements of an immune response in a stepwise and simplified fashion. Each of these topics will then be addressed more rigorously and in much greater detail in subsequent chapters of this book.

CLONAL ORGANIZATION & DYNAMICS OF LYMPHOCYTE POPULATIONS

Virgin lymphocytes are continually released from the primary lymphoid organs into the periphery, each carrying surface receptors that enable it to bind substances called **antigens.** Antigen-binding in B cells is mediated by surface immunoglobulin proteins, whereas in T cells it is mediated by T cell receptors. The sequences of these 2 types of proteins are extremely diverse, so that as a group they can bind an enormous variety of antigens (see Chapters 6 and 7). Antigen-binding, when accompanied by other stimuli, can lead to activation of a T or B cell. Virgin lymphocytes that fail to become activated die within a few days after entering the periphery, but those that become activated survive and proliferate, yielding daughter cells that may then undergo further cycles of activation and proliferation.

All of the progeny cells derived from any single virgin lymphocyte constitute a lymphocyte **clone.** Some members of each clone differentiate into effector cells, whereas the remainder are memory cells; however, apart from this, all cells within a clone are identical to one another in nearly all respects, reflecting their common ancestry. For example, B cell clones contain only B cells, and each T cell clone is made up entirely of either CD4+ or CD8+ cells.

A fundamental property of lymphocytes is that all of the immunoglobulin or T cell receptor proteins expressed by cells in a given clone are identical. Although each individual lymphocyte typically has thousands of such proteins on its surface, all of these have precisely the same amino acid sequence and are identical to those expressed by all other cells in the same clone. Since the sequence of an immunoglobulin or T cell receptor protein determines which antigens it will bind, it follows that any single lymphocyte can recognize and respond to only a very small subset of the total universe of possible antigens. This same antigen specificity, moreover, is shared by all other cells in the clone (with the exception of occasional somatic mutants, discussed in Chapter 7). Thus, each lymphocyte or clone of lymphocytes has a uniquely restricted specificity for antigens—a phenomenon known as **clonal restriction.** The immune system as a whole is able to recognize many different antigens because it is made up of a vast number of different lymphocyte clones, each of which has very limited antigen specificity.

The antigen specificity of each virgin lymphocyte is determined through an essentially random genetic process during the early stages of its development and is permanently fixed by the time the cell enters the periphery (see Chapter 7). It has been estimated that the lymphopoietic system is able to produce lymphocytes with approximately 10^8 alternative antigen specificities, and this range of possible specificities is known collectively as the **primary lymphocyte repertoire.** Roughly 10^9 virgin lymphocytes enter the periphery each day, so that at least a few with any given specificity are likely to be present at all times. Whenever any one of these encounters its specific antigen under conditions that favor activation, it can give rise to multiple daughter cells, some of which

are long-lived memory cells. With each successive exposure to the same antigen, the antigen-specific clone expands further and so comes to represent an increasing proportion of the total lymphocyte population (Fig 3–1). In this manner, exposure to an antigen selectively promotes the growth of any clones that recognize it without affecting other cells in the population—a phenomenon known as **clonal selection.** On the other hand, if no further contact with an antigen occurs, the specific memory cells will tend to die out, though this usually occurs over a period of years or decades. Thus, the lymphocyte population is continually evolving over time as individual clones expand or subside, depending on the specific antigens to which the host is exposed.

The antigen specificity of a given clone applies not only to its ability to recognize antigens but also to its effector functions. For example, cytotoxic effector T cells generally will attack a target cell only if it bears the particular surface antigen recognized by their T cell receptors; hence, the sequence of the T cell receptor defines not only the antigen that can activate the T cell clone but also the targets it will attack. Similarly, the antibodies secreted by a B cell clone have exactly the same binding specificity as the surface immunoglobulins expressed on that clone. Clonal restriction thus ensures that the immune response mounted by a lymphocyte clone is directed with a high degree of specificity against the antigen that induced its activation. The speed and intensity of response to a given antigen is determined largely by clonal selection: the larger the specific clone, the more lymphocytes are available that can recognize the antigen and can participate in the immune response.

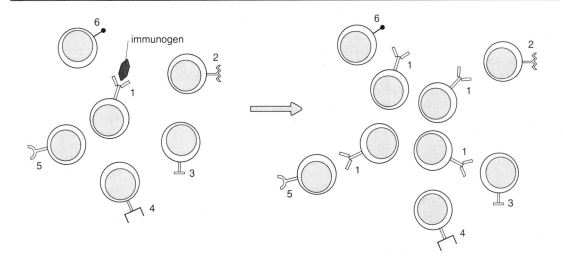

Figure 3–1. Clonal selection of lymphocytes by a specific immunogen. The unimmunized lymphocyte population (**left**) is composed of cells from many different clones, each with its own antigen specificity, indicated here by the distinctive shapes of the surface antigen receptors. Contact with an immunogen leads to selective proliferation (positive selection) of any clone or clones that can recognize that specific immunogen (**right**).

The principles of clonal restriction and clonal selection were first postulated by Burnet, Jerne, Talmadge, and others in the 1950s and still rank among the most important conceptual insights in the history of immunology. Clonal restriction is the primary basis for the extreme specificity of immune responses: each clone of lymphocytes can respond only to the limited set of antigens recognized by its unique immunoglobulin or T cell receptor proteins and, when activated, carries out effector functions that are specifically directed against that same antigen. Clonal selection, on the other hand, is principally responsible for the phenomenon of immunologic memory: exposure to an antigen sculpts and hones the lymphocyte population so that it can respond more quickly and more vigorously the next time the same antigen is encountered.

THE IMMUNE RESPONSE

Every **immune response** is a complex and intricately regulated sequence of events involving several cell types. It is triggered when an antigen enters the body and encounters a specialized class of cells called antigen-presenting cells (APCs). These APCs capture a minute amount of the antigen and display it in a form that can be recognized by antigen-specific helper T lymphocytes. The helper T cells become activated and, in turn, promote the activation of other classes of lymphocytes, such as B cells or cytotoxic T cells. The activated lymphocytes then proliferate and carry out their specific effector functions, which, in most cases, successfully inactivate or eliminate the antigen. At each stage in this process, the lymphocytes and APCs communicate with one another through direct contact or by secreting regulatory cytokines. They also may interact simultaneously with other cell types or with components of the complement, kinin, or fibrinolytic systems, resulting in phagocyte activation, blood clotting, or the initiation of wound healing. Immune responses may be either localized or systemic but are nearly always highly specific, focusing their full force against the antigen while causing little or no damage to normal host tissues. The responses are also precisely controlled and normally terminate soon after the inciting antigen is eliminated.

Fig 3–2 provides a schematic overview of the sequence of events that take place during a prototypical immune response. The following sections will describe each step of this response in turn.

Immunogens & Antigens

Immunologists often use the term **antigen** when referring to the agent that triggers an immune response. Strictly speaking, however, this term actually refers to the ability of a molecule to be recognized by an immunoglobulin or T cell receptor and hence to serve as the target of a response. For reasons that will be explained in Chapter 4, not all antigens are capable of inducing immune responses. Instead, a molecule or collection of molecules that can induce an immune response in a particular host is most properly referred to as an **immunogen.** Typical immunogens include pathogenic microorganisms (such as viruses, bacteria, or parasites), foreign tissue grafts, or otherwise innocuous environmental substances such as the proteins in pollen, grasses, or food.

Proteins are, in general, the most potent immunogens. Other classes of molecules, such as lipids, carbohydrates, or nucleic acids, most commonly become the targets of immune responses when they are linked to an immunogenic protein (as in lipoproteins, glycoproteins, or nucleoprotein complexes). Many of the immunogens encountered in nature are actually composites of several different immunogenic substances. A single bacterium, for example, is made up of a multitude of proteins and other molecules that may each elicit a specific immune response. In the prototypic immune response depicted in Fig 3–2, the immunogen is a virus that, like most viruses, contains several immunogenic proteins.

ANTIGEN PROCESSING & PRESENTATION

Responses to most proteinaceous immunogens can begin only after the immunogen has been captured, processed, and presented by an APC (Fig 3–2). The reason for this is that T cells only recognize immunogens that are bound to **major histocompatibility complex (MHC)** proteins on the surfaces of other cells (see Chapter 5). There are 2 different classes of MHC proteins, each of which is recognized by one of the 2 major subsets of T lymphocytes. **Class I MHC** proteins are expressed by virtually all somatic cell types and are used to present substances to **CD8** T cells, most of which are cytotoxic. Therefore, almost any cell can present antigens to cytotoxic T cells and thus serve as the target of a cytotoxic response. **Class II MHC** proteins, on the other hand, are expressed only by macrophages and a few other cell types and are necessary for antigen presentation to **CD4** T cells—the subset that includes most helper cells. Since helper-cell activation is necessary for virtually all immune responses, the class II-bearing APCs play a pivotal role in controlling such responses. In fact, unless otherwise stated, the term "antigen-presenting cell" usually refers only to these specialized cells that bear class II MHC proteins.

Exogenous immunogens can be captured in a variety of ways. The APC depicted in Fig 3–2 is a macrophage, ie, a voracious phagocyte that can readily capture particulate immunogens. Other types of APCs have less phagocytic capacity and tend to rely instead on receptor-mediated endocytosis or on pinocytosis

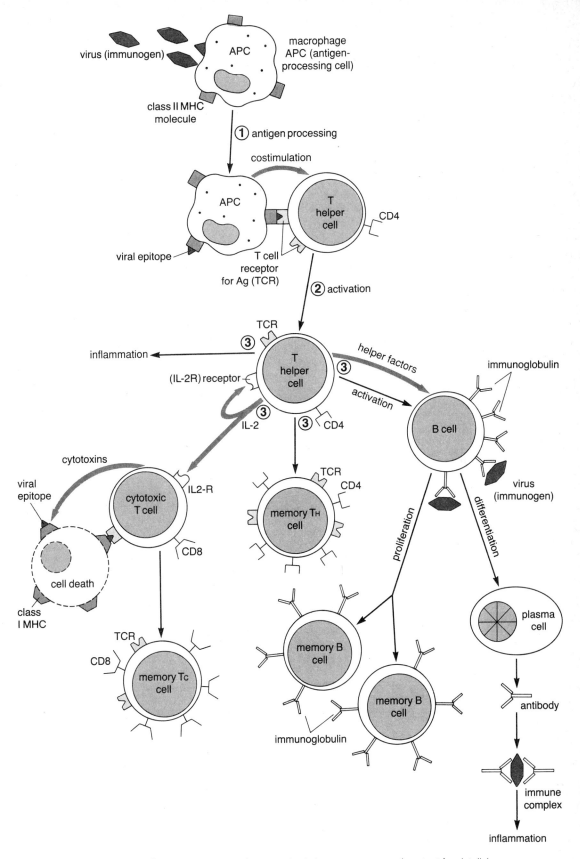

Figure 3–2. Sequence of events in a prototypic immune response (see text for details).

43

(see Chapter 1)—pathways that are also used quite effectively by macrophages. By using these three pathways, APCs can capture a very broad range of different immunogenic substances, and most APCs exhibit little or no antigen specificity. Indeed, a given APC may present several different antigens simultaneously, one on each of its many surface MHC proteins. The capture mechanisms are relatively inefficient, however, so that relatively high local concentrations of an exogenous immunogen are required for optimal activity of most APCs.

Exogenous immunogens that are captured by an APC become enclosed within membrane-lined vesicles in its cytoplasm and, within these vesicles, undergo a series of alterations called **antigen processing** (Fig 3–3). The full range of chemical modifications that can occur during processing is not known; it probably depends on the chemical nature of the immunogen. Processing of most, if not all, proteinaceous immunogens appears to involve denaturation and partial proteolytic digestion, so that the immunogen is cleaved into short peptides. A limited number of the resulting peptides then associate noncovalently with class II MHC proteins and are transported to the APC surface, where they can be detected by helper T cells. This process is called **antigen presentation.** A CD4 helper T lymphocyte that comes into direct contact with an APC may become activated, but it will do so only if it expresses a T cell receptor protein that can recognize and bind the particular peptide-MHC complex presented by the APC.

Activation of Helper T Lymphocytes

Helper T (TH) cells are the principal orchestrators of the immune response because they are needed for activation of the 2 other lymphoid effector cell types: cytotoxic T (T_C) cells and antibody-secreting plasma cells. TH cell activation occurs early in an immune response (Fig 3–2) and requires at least 2 signals. One signal is provided by binding of the T cell antigen receptor to the antigenic peptide-MHC complex on the APC surface and is transmitted through the CD3 protein complex (see Chapter 8). The second, **costimulatory** signal also requires contact with the APC and is thought to result from binding of a separate signal-transmitting protein on the T cell surface with a specific ligand on the APC. One interaction that is known to generate such a costimulatory signal is the binding of a T cell surface protein designated **CD28** to any one of a small family of APC surface proteins designated **B7** (see Chapter 8). Other surface protein pairs may also mediate costimulation.

Together, the 2 signals induce the helper T cell to begin secreting a cytokine known as interleukin-2 (**IL-2**) and also to begin expressing specific high-affinity **IL-2 receptors** on its surface (Fig 3–4). IL-2 is a highly potent mitogenic factor for T lymphocytes and is essential for the proliferative response of activated T cells. The IL-2 protein has a very short half-life outside the cell and so acts only over extremely short distances. In fact, IL-2 is thought to exert its greatest effects on the cell from which it is secreted—a phenomenon known as an **autocrine effect.** Even if a T cell has received both activation signals from contact with an APC, it will not begin to proliferate in the absence of IL-2 activity or if its own surface IL-2 receptors are blocked. The IL-2 secreted by an activated TH cell can also act on cells in the immediate vicinity, in a so-called **paracrine effect;** this is especially important for activating Tc cells, which generally do not produce enough IL-2 to stimulate their

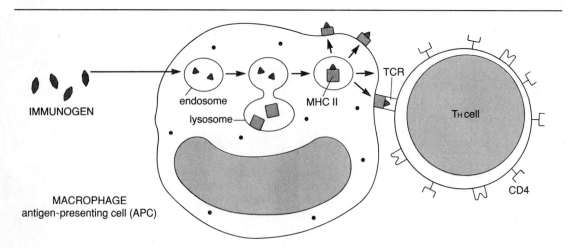

Figure 3–3. Capture, processing, and presentation of antigen by an APC. The immunogen is captured by phagocytosis, receptor-mediated endocytosis, or pinocytosis and is broken down into fragments. Some fragments (antigens) become associated with class II MHC proteins and are transported to the cell surface, where they can be recognized by CD4 T cells. TCR, T cell receptor.

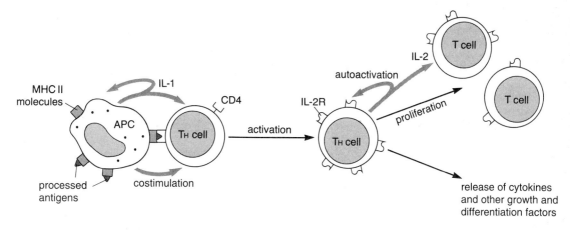

Figure 3–4. TH cell activation. The APC presents an antigen in the context of class II MHC to the TH cell and also provides a costimulatory signal. The 2 signals lead to activation of the TH cell. The APC also releases IL-1, which acts on both the APC and the TH cell to promote activation. Activation leads to IL-2 receptor expression and IL-2 secretion by the TH cell, resulting in autocrine growth stimulation.

own proliferation (see below). In addition to IL-2, activated TH cells secrete other cytokines that promote the growth, differentiation, and functions of B cells, macrophages, and other cell types (see Chapter 9).

The contact between an APC and an antigen-specific TH cell also has effects on the APC. One of most important is that the APC may begin to release a cytokine called interleukin-1 (**IL-1**). This cytokine appears to act primarily in an autocrine manner on the APC itself: it increases surface expression of class II MHC proteins and of various adhesion molecules and thereby strengthens binding of the TH cell and enhances antigen presentation (Fig 3–4). At the same time, IL-1 functions in a paracrine manner on the TH cell to promote IL-2 secretion and IL-2 receptor expression, and thus it potentiates the TH proliferative

response. Macrophages produce relatively large amounts of IL-1 and smaller amounts of 2 additional cytokines—tumor necrosis factor (**TNF**) and interleukin-6 (**IL-6**)—that can mimic or synergize with IL-1 activity (see Chapter 9). Other types of APCs produce the same cytokines, although in various proportions. The signal for their secretion appears to be transmitted to the APC at least in part by the class II MHC protein when it binds an appropriate T cell. Thus, TH cell contact with an APC leads to bidirectional signaling events that enhance the immunologic functions of both cells.

Activation of B Cells & Cytotoxic T Cells

While the TH cells are being activated as described above, some B cells may also have been engaging the

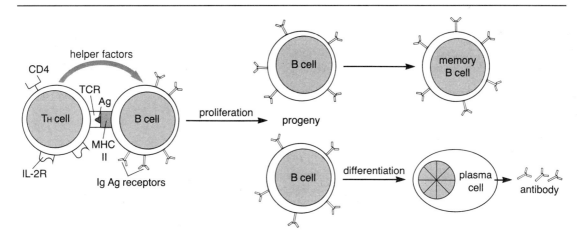

Figure 3–5. B cell activation. Antigen-binding to the surface immunoglobulins, coupled with soluble or contact-mediated helper factors from an activated TH cell, lead to proliferation and differentiation. Cytokines involved in TH cell help include IL-2, IL-4, and IL-6.

immunogen through their antigen receptors, which are membrane-bound forms of the antibodies they will later secrete (see Chapters 6 and 7). Unlike T cells, B cells recognize an immunogen in its free, un-processed form (Fig 3–2). Specific antigen-binding provides one type of signal that can lead to B cell activation. A second type is provided by activated TH cells in the form of soluble cytokines termed helper cell factors (Fig 3–5). The best characterized TH-de-rived cytokines involved in B-cell activation are IL-2 and 2 other interleukins designated IL-4 and IL-6, each of which has a very short radius of activity. TH cells also promote B cell activation through direct contact, since some surface proteins on activated TH cells also can act as helper factors. In fact, contact with an activated TH cell may be sufficient to activate a resting B cell even though its surface immunoglob-ulins have not engaged an antigen; this is known as **bystander** B cell activation. However, the combina-tion of antigen-binding and helper factors yields the strongest mitogenic signals, so that over time anti-gen-specific clones quickly outgrow any activated bystanders. Some cells in the activated clone differ-entiate into plasma cells that secrete antibodies spe-cific for the immunogen.

Tc lymphocytes function to eradicate cells that ex-press foreign antigens on their surfaces, such as virus-infected host cells (Fig 3–6). Most Tc cells ex-press CD8 rather than CD4 and hence recognize anti-gens in association with class I rather than class II MHC proteins. When a somatic cell is infected by a virus, some immunogenic viral proteins may undergo processing within the cell, and the resulting peptides may then appear as surface complexes with class I MHC molecules. These peptide-MHC complexes may then be recognized by the T cell receptor of an antigen-specific clone, providing one of 2 signals necessary for Tc cell activation. This first signal alone induces high-affinity IL-2 receptors on the Tc cell. The second signal is furnished by IL-2 secreted from a nearby activated TH lymphocyte. On receiving both signals, the activated Tc cell acquires cytotoxic

activity, enabling it to kill the cell to which it is bound, as well as any other cells bearing the same peptide-MHC class I complexes. In some cases, kill-ing occurs because the Tc releases specific toxins onto the target cell; in others, the Tc induces the tar-get cell to commit suicide (see below). The activated Tc cell also proliferates, giving rise to additional Tc cells with the same antigen specificity.

MECHANISMS OF ANTIGEN ELIMINATION

The ultimate function of the immune system is to seek out and destroy foreign substances in the body. Depending in part on the nature of the foreign sub-stance, this can be accomplished in several ways. One, described in the preceding section, is the direct **cytotoxic** killing of antigen-bearing target cells by activated Tc cells (Fig 3–6). Most other immunologic effector mechanisms require antibodies; the most im-portant of these are listed below.

Toxin Neutralization
Antibodies specific for bacterial toxins or the venom of insects or snakes bind these antigenic pro-teins and, in many cases, directly inactivate them by steric effects. In addition, formation of an antigen-an-tibody complex promotes the capture and phagocyto-sis of these toxins by macrophages and other phago-cytes (see the section on opsonization, below). Because of their effectiveness, preformed antibodies against toxins or venom are often injected prophylac-tically or therapeutically as a means of protecting unimmunized individuals who have recently been, or are at risk of being, exposed to specific toxins.

Virus Neutralization
Antibodies specific for proteins on the surface of a virus may block the attachment of the virus to target cells, particularly if the antibodies bind at or close to the site of cell binding on the virus. This provides a

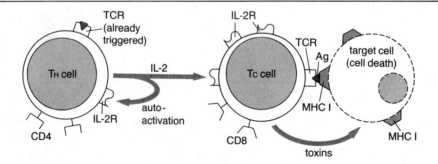

Figure 3–6. Tc cell activation requires contact with specific antigen in the context of a class I MHC molecule on the surface of a target cell. It also requires IL-2 from a nearby activated TH cell. The activated Tc cell kills the target cell either by secreting cytotoxins (as shown) or by inducing it to commit suicide.

means by which preexisting antibodies can protect against new viral infections. Once viral infection has become established, however, neutralization is often less important than the cytotoxic action of Tc cells for eradicating the infection.

Opsonization & Phagocyte Activation

Antibodies that coat bacteria or other particulate antigens can function as **opsonins** to promote phagocytosis. This occurs because macrophages and other phagocytes carry surface **Fc receptors** that facilitate engulfment of antibody-coated particles (see Chapters 1 and 6). Thus, just as macrophages control lymphocyte function through their role as APCs, B lymphocytes regulate macrophage function by directing these phagocytes to specific antigenic targets through the process of opsonization.

Immune responses also affect phagocyte functions in other ways. For example, IL-1 stimulates macrophages to express surface receptors for gamma interferon (**IFNγ**), a cytokine released from activated Tн cells that is a potent macrophage activator. The resulting activation increases the phagocytic activity of the macrophage and may cause it to secrete numerous other cytokines and mediators (see Chapter 1). Activated lymphocytes also produce IL-2, IL-3, and IL-4, as well as colony-stimulating factors (see Chapter 9), which regulate macrophage growth and function.

Activation of Complement

Certain types of antibodies can activate the **complement pathway** when they are complexed with an antigen (see Chapters 6 and 10). If the antibody is bound to the surface of a cell, such as a bacterium, the cascade of complement enzyme reactions may lead to lysis of the cell, providing an important means of killing foreign invaders. Some products of the complement cascade also act as opsonins when bound to an antigen-antibody complex, whereas others are chemoattractive for neutrophils. Still others cause the release of inflammatory mediators such as histamine from mast cells and basophils (see Chapter 11).

Antibody-Dependent Cell-Mediated Cytotoxicity (ADCC)

One major class of antibodies, called IgG (see Chapter 6), binds to Fc receptors on the surfaces of natural killer (NK) cells and certain other cell types and enables them to carry out a form of antigen-specific cell killing called **antibody-dependent cell-mediated cytotoxicity (ADCC).** The IgG antibodies bound on the surface of the cell enable it to bind specifically to antigen-bearing target cells, which might be bacteria or multicellular parasites, and to kill the target cell with cytotoxins. The antibodies are said to "arm" the cells to perform ADCC, and they are absolutely required for such killing; this fact distinguishes ADCC from Tc-mediated cytotoxicity, which occurs independently of antibodies.

INFLAMMATION

Although lymphocytes and APCs are the key cells in all immune responses, other types of cells may be recruited into the response. For example, cytokines or other products released by activated lymphocytes and macrophages may chemoattract neutrophils or eosinophils, stimulate proliferation of fibroblasts and endothelial cells, or cause mast cells and basophils (see Chapter 11) to discharge other bioactive substances into the local tissues. These agents, as well as products of the complement cascade, may lead directly or indirectly to increased local vascular perfusion, capillary permeability, accumulation of extravascular fluid, and pain. In some instances, other enzymatic pathways such as the kinin, clotting, and fibrinolytic systems may also become activated (see Chapters 10 and 11).

The entire, integrated host reaction—encompassing the immune response along with all of its associated secondary phenomena—is called **inflammation.** Soluble factors that trigger the various secondary aspects of inflammation are known collectively as **inflammatory mediators** and are said to be **proinflammatory.** The cells involved (including lymphocytes, neutrophils, mast cells, and many others) are often referred to as **inflammatory cells.** Different features of inflammation predominate in different settings, giving rise to several distinct categories of inflammatory reactions (see Chapter 11). Most aspects of inflammation are potentially beneficial since they help to defend the host against toxins, pathogens, or other injurious substances. However, excessive or inappropriate inflammatory reactions can lead to discomfort, disability, and even death. For this reason, drugs and other therapeutic measures that suppress inflammation play an important role in contemporary medical practice.

LOCALIZATION OF IMMUNE RESPONSES

The initial response to an immunogen depends partially on its route of entry into the body. Most immunogens enter via one of 3 routes. Those that enter through the bloodstream are most likely to be detected by macrophages and other APCs in the spleen, which then becomes the principal site of the immune response. By contrast, immunogens that enter the skin and subcutaneous connective tissues are usually detected by resident APCs, such as epidermal Langerhans cells or dermal macrophages, and, in addition, may be carried via the lymphatic circulation into regional lymph nodes; the immune response then begins both at the site of contact and in the affected nodes. Alternatively, an immunogen may enter the body by traversing mucosal surfaces of the respiratory or gastrointestinal tract; in this case, it immediately encounters the submucosal lymphoid tissues, which launch a response that is directed both locally and into the adjacent lumen from which the immunogen came (see Chapters 2 and 41).

Regardless of the site at which a response begins, there is always some trafficking of lymphocytes to other sites via the blood and lymphatic vessels, so that the entire immune system can eventually be recruited into the response if the immunogen is especially abundant, widely disseminated, or resistant to immune elimination. Some types of APCs are likewise capable of migrating through the blood or lymphatics (see Chapter 5), carrying immunogens along with them into distant lymphoid organs.

QUANTITATIVE & KINETIC ASPECTS OF IMMUNE RESPONSES

The quantitative aspects of immune function have been studied most extensively for B cells, since B cell activity can easily be monitored by the concentrations of specific antibodies in the serum—an area of investigation known as **serology.** The general conclusions of such studies, however, are thought to be applicable to T cell responses as well.

At any given moment, active T and B effector cells account for roughly 1% of the total lymphoid population in a normal host. These belong to many different clones (the exact number is unknown and no doubt varies widely), most of which are probably involved in ongoing, low-level immune responses against the many antigens encountered in everyday life. As a result, the serum of a normal, healthy adult contains innumerable different types of antibody molecules. Each is present in only minute amounts, but altogether they account for roughly 20% of total serum protein. Each of these circulating antibodies provides a low level of protection against its specific antigen.

When a person or animal is exposed to significant amounts of an antigen and mounts a B cell response, the concentration of serum antibodies against that antigen generally rises. Serum from such an immunized individual is often called a **specific antiserum.** It is important to remember, however, that even in the serum of highly immunized individuals, antibodies against a given antigen make up only a small fraction of the total and that antibodies with many other specificities are also present.

An individual's first encounter with a particular immunogen is called a **priming event** and leads to a relatively weak, short-lived response designated the **primary immune response.** This is divisible into several phases (Fig 3–7). The **lag** or **latent phase** is the time between the initial exposure to an immunogen and the detection of antibodies in the circulation, which averages about 1 week in humans. During this period, activation of TH and B cells is taking place. The **exponential phase** is marked by a rapid increase in the quantity of circulating antibodies and reflects the increasing numbers of secretory plasma cells. After an interval during which the antibody level remains relatively constant because secretion and degradation are occurring at approximately equal rates (the **steady-state** or **plateau phase**), the antibody level gradually declines (**declining phase**) as synthesis of new antibody wanes. The decline indicates that new plasma cells are no longer being produced and that existing plasma cells are dying or ceasing antibody production; this generally signifies that the immunogen has been eradicated. Thus, the duration of a humoral immune response is limited

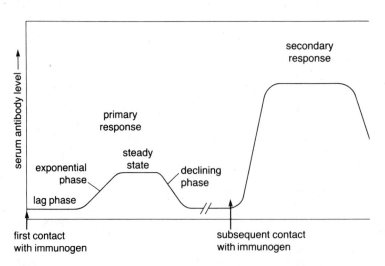

Figure 3–7. Primary and secondary immune responses (see text for details).

primarily by the duration of the antigenic stimulus and by the relatively short life spans of the plasma cells involved in the response.

Subsequent encounters with the same immunogen lead to responses that are qualitatively similar to the primary response but manifest marked quantitative differences (Fig 3–7). In such a **secondary** or **anamnestic immune response,** the lag period is shortened and antibody levels rise more rapidly to a much higher steady-state level, thereafter remaining in the serum at detectable levels for much longer periods. The large numbers of antigen-specific memory T and B cells generated during the primary response are responsible for the rapid kinetics and the greater intensity and duration of secondary responses.

PROGRAMMED CELL DEATH IN THE IMMUNE SYSTEM

Antigen-dependent proliferation of a lymphocyte clone is an example of **positive selection;** ie, the antigen promotes growth of the cells on which it acts. Under some conditions, however, contact with antigens or other stimuli results in **negative selection** of a responsive clone, meaning that cells in the clone selectively die. Negative selection of lymphocytes is a common event and is essential to the ability of the immune system to discriminate self from nonself. In particular, most virgin T or B cells whose antigen receptors recognize components found in normal host tissues are thought to be selectively killed before they leave the bone marrow or thymus, as a means of protecting the host against attack by these potentially **autoreactive** (ie, self-reactive) cells. This may account for the observation that at least 99% of developing thymocytes die within the thymus (see Chapter 1). Thus, the clonal composition of the immune system is shaped not only by positive clonal selection but also by the active elimination of potentially deleterious clones.

The mechanisms responsible for such physiologic or **programmed cell death** are not fully known and probably are numerous. Lymphocyte death in many settings occurs not because the cell has been killed but, rather, because it has been instructed to commit suicide. A lymphocyte undergoing such suicide actively degrades its own chromosomal DNA, inspissates its nucleus and cytoplasm, and then breaks itself down into small fragments that can readily be ingested by macrophages. Such ritualized cell suicide, called **apoptosis,** is common among normal thymocytes, bone marrow progenitors, and germinal-center B cells (see Chapter 2), as well as in lymphoid cells that have been deprived of essential growth factors or exposed to steroids, ionizing radiation, or other toxic agents. Nonlymphoid cell types can also undergo apoptosis; indeed Tc cells sometimes kill by inducing apoptosis of the target cell.

The importance of negative selection is illustrated by the **follicular lymphomas**—a common cancer of B cells in humans (see Chapters 7 and 45). A major factor in pathogenesis of this disease is a cellular protein called **Bcl-2,** which acts through an unknown mechanism to block many forms of programmed cell death. The normal function of Bcl-2 is unknown, but it has been proposed to be involved in regulating cellular life spans. In follicular lymphoma, a clone of B cells arises that expresses abnormally high levels of Bcl-2 protein and hence is resistant to killing; as a result, these cells accumulate in abnormally large numbers and eventually evolve into a cancer. This implies that a high, controlled rate of programmed lymphocyte death normally benefits the host by restricting the growth of individual clones and of the lymphoid population as a whole, providing a counterforce against stimuli that might otherwise drive excessive lymphocyte proliferation.

REFERENCES

Brodsky FM, Guagliardi LE: The cell biology of antigen processing and presentation. *Annu Rev Immunol* 1991;**9:**707.

Burnet FM: A modification of Jerne's theory of antibody production using the concept of clonal selection. **Aust J Sci** 1957;**20:**67.

Cohen JJ et al: Apoptosis and programmed cell death in immunity. *Annu Rev Immunol* 1992;**10:**267.

Gray D: Immunological memory. *Annu Rev Immunol* 1993;**11:**49.

Green DR et al: Activation-induced apoptosis in lymphoid systems. *Semin Immunol* 1992;**4:**379.

Parker DC: T cell-dependent B-cell activation. *Annu Rev Immunol* 1993;**11:**331.

Podack ER, Kupfer A: T cell effector functions: Mechanisms for delivery of cytotoxicity and help. *Annu Rev Cell Biol* 1991;**7:**479.

Vitetta ES et al: Cellular interactions in the humoral immune response. *Adv Immunol* 1989;**45:**1.

von Boehmer H, Kisielow P: Self-nonself discrimination by T cells. *Science* 1990;**248:**1369.

4

Immunogens & Antigens

Joel W. Goodman, PhD

A great many foreign substances evoke immune responses when they enter the body. The response may involve exclusively the humoral or the cellular limb of the immune system but most commonly involves both. Any substance that is capable of inducing an immune response is called an **immunogen** and is said to be **immunogenic.** As a rule, immune responses are carried out only by T and/or B cell clones which produce immunoglobulin or T cell receptor proteins that recognize the immunogen. Substances that are recognized by a particular immunoglobulin or T cell receptor, and so can serve as the target of an immune response, are called **antigens** and are said to be **antigenic.** Thus, all immunogens are also antigens (Fig 4–1).

Many immunogens, including all microbial pathogens, are complex assemblages containing several different types of molecules, not all of which are antigenic. For example, the response to an enveloped virus is usually directed against protein components of the viral particle but not against the lipids that make up much of the viral envelope. Even when a single pure protein serves as an immunogen, the response is usually directed against only a few discrete clusters of amino acid residues within the larger polypeptide. The specific set of chemical features that is recognized by a given antibody or T cell receptor is called an **epitope,** or antigenic determinant. In other words, an epitope is the specific site to which a particular immunoglobulin or T cell receptor binds. It follows that every immunogen must contain one or more epitopes which enable it to serve as an antigen. However, not all antigens or epitopes are immunogenic—in other words, not every chemical substance that can be bound by an immunoglobulin is, in itself, capable of inducing an immune response. This chapter will explore the properties that enable a substance to serve as the stimulus for, or the target of, an immunologic attack.

IMMUNOGENS

The ability to evoke an immune response depends not only on the physicochemical nature of a substance itself but also on other factors, such as the mode of immunization, the characteristics of the organism being immunized, and the sensitivity of the methods used to detect the response. The factors that confer immunogenicity on molecules are complex and incompletely understood, but it is known that certain conditions must be satisfied for a molecule to be immunogenic.

A. Chemical Composition: Large, macromolecular proteins are, in general, the most potent immunogens. Polysaccharides, short polypeptides, and some synthetic organic polymers (eg, polyvinylpyrrolidone) can also be immunogenic under certain circumstances. Pure lipids and nucleic acids have not been shown to be immunogenic, although antibodies that react with them can be elicited by immunization with nucleoprotein or lipoprotein complexes; this is probably the mechanism of origin of the anti-DNA antibodies found in the serum of many patients with **systemic lupus erythematosus** (see Chapter 31). Thus, lipids and nucleic acids are examples of molecules that are antigenic but not immunogenic.

B. Molecular Size: Extremely small molecules such as amino acids or monosaccharides are usually not immunogenic, implying that a certain minimum size is necessary for immunogenicity. However, there is no fixed threshold mass below which all substances are inert and above which all are active, but, rather, there is a gradient of immunogenicity with molecular size. A few substances with molecular weights below 1000 have proven to be immunogenic, but as a rule molecules with molecular weights below 10,000 are only weakly immunogenic or not immunogenic at all. The most potent immunogens are proteins with molecular weights greater than 100,000.

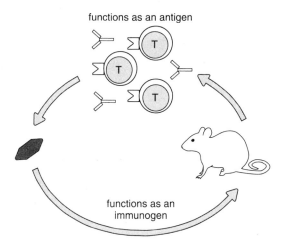

functions as an antigen

functions as an
immunogen

Figure 4–1. Immunogens and antigens. A substance is referred to as an immunogen to indicate that it induces an immune response and is referred to as an antigen to indicate that it serves as the target of the response.

C. Chemical Complexity: A molecule must possess a certain degree of chemical complexity to be immunogenic. This principle is most clearly illustrated by synthetic polypeptides. Homopolymers of a single amino acid are poor immunogens regardless of size, whereas copolymers of 2 or—even better—3 amino acids are often quite active. Once again, it is difficult to define a discrete threshold, but the general rule is that immunogenicity increases with structural complexity. Aromatic amino acids contribute more to immunogenicity than do nonaromatic residues: thus, simple random polypeptides that contain tyrosine are better immunogens than are comparable polypeptides without tyrosine, and immunogenicity of such polymers is directly proportionate to their tyrosine contents. Attachment of tyrosine chains to the weakly immunogenic protein gelatin (which contains few aromatic amino acids) markedly enhances its immunogenicity.

D. Genetic Constitution of the Host Animal: The ability to respond to a particular immunogen is genetically predetermined. For example, pure polysaccharides are immunogenic when injected into mice or humans but not when injected into guinea pigs or rabbits. Much information about the genetics of immune responsiveness has accrued from studies with inbred strains of animals. As one of many examples, some strains of guinea pig produce a vigorous antibody response against the simple polypeptide poly-L-lysine, whereas other strains give no detectable response; crossbreeding studies among these strains indicate that the ability to respond to poly-L-lysine is inherited as an autosomal dominant trait. Many analogous phenomena have been described in humans. Selective responsiveness of this type reflects

a number of hereditary factors, the best understood of which include (1) the repertoires of different immunoglobulins and T cell receptor proteins that an individual is able to produce (see Chapters 7 and 8) and (2) the ability of antigen-presenting cells to present specific types of molecules to T lymphocytes (see Chapter 5).

E. Foreignness: The immune system normally discriminates between self and nonself, so that only molecules that are foreign to the host are immunogenic. Hence, albumin isolated from the serum of a rabbit and injected back into the same or another rabbit will not yield an immune response—every rabbit is **tolerant** to this endogenous protein. Yet the same protein, if injected into other vertebrate species, is likely to evoke substantial antibody responses, depending on the dose of antigen and the route and frequency of injection. The mechanisms that enable an animal to discriminate self from nonself are as yet incompletely understood, but some of the processes that contribute to this discrimination will be considered in Chapters 7 and 8.

F. Method of Administration: Whether a substance will evoke an immune response also depends on the dose and mode of administration. A quantity of substance that has no effect when injected intravenously may evoke a copious antibody response when injected subcutaneously, particularly if it is accompanied by an adjuvant (see below). The threshold dose required for a response under particular conditions varies among immunogens. In general, once the threshold dose is exceeded, increasing doses lead to increasing, although less than proportionate, responses. However, excessive doses may not only fail to induce a response but also establish a state of specific unresponsiveness, or tolerance, to subsequent exposures—a phenomenon that is sometimes referred to as **high-zone tolerance.**

ADJUVANTS

The response to an immunogen is often enhanced if it is administered as a mixture with substances called **adjuvants.** Adjuvants function in one or more of the following ways: (1) by prolonging retention of the immunogen, (2) by increasing the effective size of the immunogen, or (3) by stimulating the local influx of macrophages and/or other immune cell types to the injection site and promoting their subsequent activities.

A number of adjuvants have been used in experimental animals, the most potent being **complete Freund's adjuvant** (CFA), a water-in-oil emulsion containing killed mycobacteria. CFA appears to work by providing a depot for the immunogen and by stimulating macrophages and certain lymphocytes, but its very strong inflammatory effects preclude its use in humans. The most widely used adjuvant for humans is **alum precipitate,** a suspension of aluminum hydroxide onto which the immunogen is adsorbed. This adjuvant increases the effective particle size of the immunogen and so promotes its ingestion and presentation by macrophages (see Chapter 5). It further increases the antigen-presenting activity of the macrophages by potentiating the secretion of interleukin-1 (IL-1). **Muramyl dipeptide,** a glycosylated protein fragment derived from mycobacterial cell walls, has also been found to possess adjuvant activity.

B CELL ANTIGENS
& B CELL EPITOPES

Large molecules are the strongest immunogens and are usually correspondingly strong antigens. However, only restricted portions of these molecules are recognized and bound by any given antibody or T cell receptor. Such binding sites on an antigen are called **epitopes,** or antigenic determinants. A single antigenic molecule may contain several distinct epitopes, and most large antigens do (Fig 4–2). For any given antigen in a particular individual, the regions that are recognized by immunoglobulins (called **B cell epitopes**) are often different from those that are recognized by T cell receptors (called **T cell epitopes**). The concept of T cell epitopes is somewhat complicated in that T cells recognize their

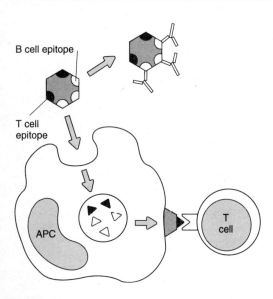

B cell epitope

T cell epitope

APC

T cell

Figure 4–2. Most large antigens contain multiple epitopes. B cell epitopes (white) are regions that can be bound by immunoglobulin proteins. T cell epitopes (black) are recognized by T lymphocytes only after being processed and presented in association with an MHC protein on the surface on an antigen-presenting cell (APC).

epitopes only in association with major histocompatibility complex (MHC) molecules on cell surfaces. In contrast, epitope recognition by an antibody is a relatively straightforward bimolecular interaction that occurs in solution and is correspondingly easier both to study experimentally and to understand. Therefore, B cell antigens and epitopes are discussed first.

The number of separate epitopes on an antigenic molecule generally is proportionate to its size and chemical complexity. One way to estimate how many B cell epitopes are present on a given antigen is to determine the number of antibody molecules that can bind to each molecule of antigen under saturating conditions. By using this approach, it has been estimated, for example, that hen egg albumin (MW 42,000) has about 5 B cell epitopes, whereas thyroglobulin (MW 700,000) has about 40. This approach provides only minimal estimates, since steric hindrance may prevent simultaneous occupation of all epitopes by bound antibodies. Moreover, these numbers are somewhat misleading, since different regions of an antigen can be utilized preferentially as epitopes by different individuals or different animal species or even by a single individual at different times. In fact, the weight of evidence currently suggests that virtually any region on the exposed surface of a protein has the potential to serve as a B cell epitope.

Size & Location of B Cell Epitopes

The antigen-binding site on any single immunoglobulin molecule has a fixed size (see Chapter 5), and this, in turn, dictates the maximum spatial dimensions of its epitope. Studies with homopolymers of sugars or amino acids, either alone or conjugated to immunogenic proteins, indicate that a single epitope can encompass as few as 3–6 amino acid or sugar residues. On the other hand, x-ray crystallographic studies of individual antibodies bound to complex, native proteins have revealed contacts involving nearly 20 amino acid residues on the antigen simultaneously. Thus, a reasonable rule of thumb may be that B cell epitopes on polypeptides generally encompass about 3–20 amino acid residues.

Antibody responses against native, folded proteins are almost always directed against residues on the protein surface, since it is these residues that are exposed and accessible for binding. This principle has been demonstrated most vividly by immunizing animals with synthetic polypeptides comprising an invariant backbone decorated with numerous side branches composed of alanine (A), tyrosine (Y), and glutamate (E) (Fig 4–3). When the branches were synthesized so that all alanines were clustered at the outer termini, with tyrosine and glutamate nearer the backbone, most of the antibodies produced were alanine-specific. Conversely, when the alanines were situated near the backbone and the tyrosines and glutamates were exposed, tyrosine- and glutamate-spe-

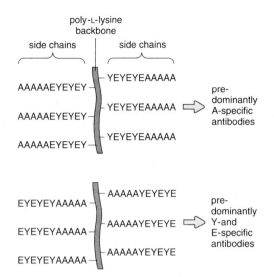

Figure 4–3. The most exposed residues on an antigen are most likely to function as B cell epitopes. In this schematic representation of an experiment by Sela and colleagues (*Science* 1969;**166:**1365), animals were immunized with synthetic polypeptides consisting of a poly-L-lysine backbone with side chains composed of alanine (A), tyrosine (Y), and glutamate (E) residues. The residues that were located at the most exposed termini of the side chains served as the preferred (immunodominant) B cell epitopes.

cific antibodies were obtained. In each instance, the most exposed region served as the dominant epitope of the antigen. In similar fashion, antibodies directed against complex, branched polysaccharides, such as those found on many glycoproteins, react most often with the terminal carbohydrate residues.

B cell epitopes on native globular proteins have a disproportionate tendency to be made up of polar (as opposed to hydrophobic) amino acids residues, since polar residues are much more frequently found on the external surface than in the hydrophobic interiors of such proteins. This correlation has some value in predicting the locations of epitopes on proteins: the greater the average polarity of a polypeptide region, the higher the likelihood that it will be antigenic.

Conformational & Linear Epitopes

The residues that make up a B cell epitope must all lie within a very limited 3-dimensional space in order to make simultaneous contact with an antibody molecule. In many instances, all of the amino acid or sugar residues that form a given epitope are positioned sequentially in the linear sequence of a protein or polysaccharide antigen. Because these residues are covalently linked to one another and can-

not move far apart, epitopes of this type are not affected by heat denaturation or other treatments that alter the 3-dimensional structure of a protein. Such epitopes are called **linear** (or **sequential**) **epitopes** (Fig 4–4).

Other B cell epitopes, by contrast, form only when the critical residues are brought together in space through folding of the polypeptide or polysaccharide chain into its normal 3-dimensional conformation. Epitopes of this type are called **conformational epitopes,** and, by definition, are lost if the antigen is denatured and fails to refold properly. Many conformational epitopes are made up of residues located at 2 or more discontinuous sites along the linear sequence of an antigen, as depicted in Fig 4–4. However, this is not always the case. For example, repeating polymers of the tripeptide tyrosine-alanine-glutamine form α-helices in solution and can evoke specific antibodies. Individual tripeptides with this sequence, by contrast, do not have an ordered conformation and will not bind to antibodies prepared against the helical polymer, even though they can be recognized by specific antibodies prepared in other ways. Thus, the α-helical form of this simple, continuous peptide sequence can function as a conformational epitope.

Antibodies that recognize conformational epitopes are often used to study changes that occur in the 3-dimensional structures of proteins during physiologic processes. For example, antibodies have been described that can discriminate between the oxygenated and nonoxygenated forms of hemoglobin by detecting small differences in alignment of the globin subunits. There are many other examples of such conformation-specific antibody binding.

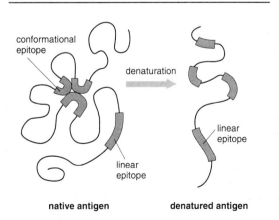

Figure 4–4. Conformational and linear epitopes in a polypeptide antigen. After denaturation, the conformational epitope can no longer be recognized by antibodies but the linear epitope is unaffected.

Immunodominance

Large antigens usually contain numerous epitopes. In a given individual, and under a given set of circumstances, however, only one or a few of these may serve as the primary target of an immune response. In a B cell response, for example, one epitope might evoke antibodies in larger quantities and with higher binding affinities than do the other available epitopes. Such a preferred epitope is said to be **immunodominant.** The same term can also be applied to individual residues within any single epitope that contribute disproportionately to interactions with the antibody. For example, when an antibody recognizes a sequence at the end of a polymer, the terminal residue of this sequence is almost invariably the most critical for binding and hence is immunodominant. The other residues in such a terminal epitope generally exhibit decreasing degrees of immunodominance with increasing distance from the terminus.

HAPTENS

Much of our understanding of antigen-antibody interactions comes from studies of small molecules that are not immunogenic but can be bound by antibodies of appropriate specificity. Molecules with these characteristics were first uncovered in the early 20th century by the pioneering experiments of Landsteiner, who was studying the immunologic properties of certain small aromatic amines (Fig 4–5). These compounds in free form cannot induce antibody responses. However, Landsteiner found that when they were coupled covalently to immunogenic proteins which were then injected into animals, the resulting immune responses included antibodies that were capable of binding the free aromatic amine. This demonstrated that a nonimmunogenic molecule could become the target of an antibody response when attached to an immunogenic protein. Landsteiner named substances that had this property **haptens,** from the Greek word *haptien* ("to fasten"). The proteins or other immunogens onto which haptens are

fastened for such experiments are called **carriers.** In some instances, the hapten alone constitutes the entire epitope for an antibody. More typically, however, the hapten simply serves as one of the residues that contribute to the epitope, together with amino acid residues from the carrier.

Most small, nonimmunogenic compounds will behave as haptens if coupled to an appropriate carrier. This has practical importance, since it provides a simple way of obtaining antibodies directed against virtually any small molecule, regardless of its inherent immunogenicity. Even antibodies that are specific for particular metal ions have been obtained in this manner.

Just as importantly, the discovery that antibodies could be raised against small, chemically defined haptens provided an experimental system which could be used to determine precisely which chemical features of an epitope are responsible for its interaction with antibodies. Taking this approach, Landsteiner and others were able to demonstrate that antibodies raised against a particular hapten would also bind other, chemically similar molecules. In general, the more structurally similar a compound was to the original hapten, the more likely it was to bind the antihapten antibody (Table 4–1). Through studies of these simple model epitopes, it soon became clear that an antibody not only recognizes specific chemical features (such as the polarity, hydrophobicity, or ionic charge) of its epitope but also recognizes the overall shape of the epitope in 3-dimensional space. This then led to the more general realization that antibodies bind to their epitopes because the 2 mole-

Table 4–1. Effect of variations in epitope structure on the strength of binding by anti-hapten antibodies.[1]

	ortho	meta	para
R = sulfonate	+	+++	±
R = arsonate	–	+	–
R = carboxylate	–	±	–

[1]In this typical experiment, an antiserum raised against the hapten *m*-aminobenzene sulfonate (R = sulfonate, in the *meta* position) was tested for its ability to bind this or various structurally related compounds. Binding affinity was graded from absent (–) to very strong (+++). Sulfonate and arsonate are both tetrahedral and negatively charged, but arsonate is the bulkier of the two owing to the larger size of the arsenic atom as well as the presence of additional hydrogen atoms. Carboxylate is also negatively charged but is planar rather than tetrahedral. (Based on data from Landsteiner K, van der Scheer J: On cross reactions of immune sera to azoproteins. *J Exp Med* 1936;**63**:325.)

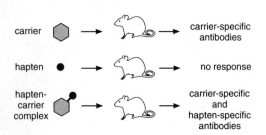

Figure 4–5. Haptens are substances that are antigenic but not immunogenic.

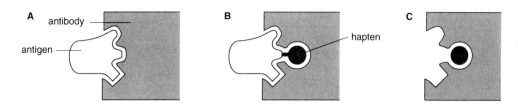

Figure 4–6. Schematic illustration of the complementarity between a B cell epitope and the antigen-binding site on an antibody protein. Antibodies raised against **(A)** an antigen or **(B)** a hapten-carrier complex are fully complementary to their cognate epitopes. **(C):** An antibody whose epitope includes a hapten will also bind the isolated hapten, although it usually has lower affinity for the free hapten than for the hapten-carrier complex. Note that binding of the hapten interferes with binding of the hapten-carrier complex; this fact is often used as a basis for demonstrating low-affinity hapten binding by hapten-specific antibodies.

cules are spatially and chemically **complementary** to one another: the antigen-binding residues in an antibody protein form a 3-dimensional surface that is precisely complementary to its epitope, so that epitope and antibody fit together in a "lock-and-key" relationship (Fig 4–6). The more perfectly an epitope matches the chemical and spatial contours of an antibody, the more tightly it will be bound. This complementarity between immunoglobulins and their epitopes is an extremely important concept to understand, since it is the mechanism by which the humoral immune system recognizes and distinguishes among antigenic molecules.

The binding of an antibody to a hapten or antigen other than the one that induced its formation is called a **cross-reaction.** Cross-reacting antigens generally have some, but not all, of the features responsible for the strong binding of an antibody to its homologous (or **cognate**) antigen. Although the antigen-binding sites on most antibodies are somewhat flexible and can compensate for minor variations in epitope structure, antibodies generally have a lower affinity for a cross-reacting antigen than for their cognate antigen. If any of the individual residues that make up an epitope is absent, this also reduces overall complementarity and results in a lower binding affinity. As a result, although many antibodies raised against a specific hapten-carrier complex will bind to either the free hapten or the free carrier, they tend to have significantly lower affinity for these individual components than for the complete complex (Fig 4–6.)

T CELL ANTIGENS, T CELL EPITOPES, & IMMUNOGENICITY

Epitope recognition by a T cell receptor (TCR) occurs through complementary interactions that are, in most respects, identical to those described above. Unlike an antibody, however, a TCR does not bind free antigens but instead recognizes its epitope as part of a complex with MHC proteins on the surface of an antigen-presenting cell (APC). Both the epitope and the MHC molecule contribute to the complementarity required for effective TCR binding (see Chapter 5). Before being presented by an APC, most proteinaceous antigens must undergo processing, in the course of which the antigen is degraded into peptides that then can serve as T cell epitopes. Because they recognize only processed antigens, T cells show no preference for epitopes that lie on the surfaces (as opposed to the interior) of globular proteins and rarely recognize specific conformational features of the native antigen. Moreover, APCs often present only a few of the peptides that can be obtained from an antigen (see Chapter 5) and thereby tend to limit the number that can serve as T cell epitopes. Nevertheless, some large proteins have been found to contain as many as 50 separate T cell epitopes, and T cells show the same exquisite specificity as antibodies in recognizing their cognate antigens.

Studies with small, well-defined antigens have shown that humoral and cell-mediated immune responses can be directed against different regions of a single molecule. For example, the human hormone glucagon, which is only 29 amino acids long, contains separate B cell and T cell epitopic regions: when mice are immunized with human glucagon, they produce antibodies only against the amino-terminal part of the molecule, whereas their T cells respond only to the carboxy-terminal portion. Similarly, the small organoarsenate molecule L-tyrosine-p-azobenzenearsonate (ABA-Tyr), with a molecular weight of only 409, induces cellular immunity but little or no antibody production in a variety of animal species. When animals are immunized with a hapten covalently attached to ABA-Tyr, they respond with hapten-specific antibodies and ABA-Tyr-specific T cells.

T cell epitopes not only serve as the targets for cytotoxic T cell responses but also are essential for nearly all B cell responses. This is because T cell epitopes are needed to activate helper T lymphocytes, which, in turn, are required for B cell responses against nearly all antigens. Thus, as a rule, a molecule must contain at least one T cell epitope in order to be immunogenic. Molecules that contain only B cell epitopes (such as haptens or the amino-terminal portion of human glucagon) may serve very well as targets for antibody responses but are unable to induce such responses themselves.

THYMUS-INDEPENDENT ANTIGENS

A few types of molecules have been reported to induce antibody responses without the apparent participation of T lymphocytes. Most such **thymus-independent antigens** are polymers composed of many repeating chemical units, and they may activate B lymphocytes directly by cross-linking specific B cell surface receptors (see Chapter 2). Certain lectins, some polymeric proteins, and many polysaccharides have been reported to be thymus-independent antigens. Recent careful analysis of the responses to such antigens indicates that many, if not all, do require some degree of T cell help, although significantly less than that required by conventional **thymus-dependent antigens.** It may therefore be more accurate to view them as thymus-efficient, rather than thymus-independent.

One striking property of the responses to thymus-independent antigens is that no apparent **memory** is engendered: even after repeated exposures, the antibody responses are quantitatively modest, occur after a relatively long lag period, and in all other respects resemble primary humoral responses. (In particular, the antibodies produced are nearly all of the IgM class; see Chapter 6). This implies that clonal expansion of antigen-specific helper T cells is required for many of the characteristic features of secondary antibody responses and that an immunogen must contain at least one T cell epitope in order to induce functional immunologic memory.

VACCINES

A **vaccine** is a nonpathogenic immunogen that, when inoculated into a host, induces protective immunity against a specific pathogen. Most human vaccines that are currently in use are prepared from bacteria or viruses that either have been **killed** (with heat or chemical treatments) or are **attenuated** (that is, have been selected for the lack of certain characteristics that are necessary to cause disease).

Two promising new approaches to vaccine development have emerged in the modern era of biomedical technology. One is based on the use of recombinant DNA techniques, which make it possible to create laboratory bacteria, yeasts, or cultured cells that produce any desired protein in virtually unlimited quantities. By using this approach, vaccines can be prepared that contain only a single immunogenic surface protein from the pathogen of interest. For example, a **recombinant vaccine** containing the major surface protein of the hepatitis B virus has recently been approved for clinical use.

The other approach relies on the chemical synthesis of short peptides that correspond to known B cell epitope sequences of proteins from the infectious organism. These short (usually 6–15-amino-acid) polypeptide epitopes may be linked to immunogenic carriers to create **synthetic vaccines.** This approach is predicated on the assumption that the isolated epitopes will act as haptens to induce antibodies, which will then recognize the same epitopes in the native pathogen. Indeed, it has been shown that antibodies raised against isolated surface epitopes do react with native proteins, although the affinities of binding are usually lower than with the peptides themselves.

One major caveat to using B cell epitopes as vaccines, however, is that immunologic memory induced by hapten-carrier complexes is directed mainly against the carrier, which bears the T cell epitopes. Thus, an encounter with the native pathogen after immunization with such a vaccine would elicit little or no secondary response. Although protective antibody titers might be obtainable even without memory, this does represent a serious potential limitation for this type of vaccine. One possible way around this dilemma would be to design synthetic vaccines that incorporate both T cell and B cell epitopes derived from the pathogen in question. An experimental vaccine against the malaria parasite *Plasmodium falciparum* was created through this approach and was found to induce not only high-titer antibody responses but also specific memory in immunized animals. Although this vaccine technology is still in its infancy, it may offer a simple and flexible approach to prophylaxis against many human and animal pathogens.

REFERENCES

Benjamin DC et al: The antigenic structure of proteins: A reappraisal. *Annu Rev Immunol* 1984;**2:**67.

Good MF et al: The T cell response to the malaria cir-

cumsporozoite protein: An immunological approach to vaccine development. *Annu Rev Immunol* 1988;**6:**663.

Goodman JW: Antigenic determinants and antibody combining sites. Page 127 in: *The Antigens.* Vol 3. Sela M (editor). Academic Press, 1975.

Goodman JW: Modeling determinants for recognition by B cells and T cells. *Prog Allergy* 1989;**56**:1.

Goodman JW, Sercarz EE: The complexity of structures involved in T cell activation. *Annu Rev Immunol* 1983; **1**:465.

Landsteiner K: *The Specificity of Serological Reactions.* Harvard Univ Press, 1945.

Livingston AM, Fathman CG: The structure of T cell epitopes. *Annu Rev Immunol* 1987;**5**:477.

Milch DR: Synthetic T and B cell recognition sites: Implications for vaccine development. *Adv Immunol* 1989; **45**:195.

Reichlin M: Amino acid substitution and the antigenicity of globular proteins. *Adv Immunol* 1975;**20**:71.

Sela M: Antigenicity: Some molecular aspects. *Science* 1969;**166**:1365.

Zanetti ME et al: The immunology of new generation vaccines. *Immunol Today* 1987;**8**:18.

5

Antigen Presentation & the Major Histocompatibility Complex

Joel W. Goodman, PhD

Immune responses to essentially all protein antigens require initial processing and presentation of the antigen to T cells by accessory antigen-presenting cells (APCs). The reason for this requirement is that T cells recognize foreign antigens only when they are first broken down into short peptides, which are then displayed in association with **major histocompatibility complex (MHC)** proteins on cell surfaces. The role of APCs is thus to offer antigenic peptides complexed with MHC molecules to the available repertoire of T cells. The critical point is that MHC molecules are obligatory components of the antigen complex recognized by T cells. Indeed, the ability of T cells to recognize specific features of the MHC proteins is critical for their survival in the thymus and for the ability of the immune system to discriminate self from nonself (see Chapter 8). Because the MHC plays such a central role in the immune response, an understanding of its genetic organization and molecular structure is absolutely essential. This chapter will consider the features of MHC genes and proteins and their role in antigen presentation to T cells.

HUMAN LEUKOCYTE ANTIGENS (HLA)

The human MHC is also known as the HLA complex—an appellation that derives from the recognition in the 1950s that many people, particularly those who had received multiple blood transfusions or had been pregnant several times, had antibodies in their serum that reacted with the leukocytes of other members of the population. The antigens involved were termed **human leukocyte antigens (HLA).** It was quickly realized that they played a central role in the success or failure of organ transplants, and this, in turn, provided an impetus for detailed investigation of the HLA complex. Interest in the MHC increased still further as its central role in the regulation of im-

mune responses, and its association with particular diseases, became apparent in the 1970s.

HLA and the genes that encode them are subdivided into 3 types (called classes I, II, and III) on the basis of their molecular structure. Class I and II molecules are structurally similar cell surface glycoproteins that are involved in antigen presentation to T cells. Class III comprises an assortment of proteins, including several components of the complement system, that are structurally unrelated to classes I and II and are grouped with them solely because they are situated in the same chromosomal region. Class III proteins are not relevant to antigen presentation and are not considered further in this chapter.

HLA **class I antigens** are expressed on all somatic cells, whereas **class II antigens** are found on relatively few cell types (see below). The 2 HLA classes service different T cell subsets. Class II proteins are required for the presentation of antigen to CD4 (usually helper) T cells, which are therefore said to be **class II restricted,** whereas CD8 (usually cytotoxic) T cells respond only to antigens associated with class I molecules and are said to be **class I restricted.** Thus, the 2 classes of HLA molecules are distinguishable on the basis of their cell type distribution and their function in antigen presentation.

GENETIC ORGANIZATION OF THE MHC

The human MHC (HLA complex) spans approximately 3.5×10^6 bp on the short arm of chromosome 6 (Fig 5–1). It is divisible into 3 separate regions, which contain the class I, class II, and class III genes. There are 3 genes within the class I region, designated the **HLA-A, -B, and -C loci.** Similarly, there are 3 class II genes, known as the **HLA-DP, -DQ, and -DR loci.** Each of these genes exists in multiple different allelic forms—that is, a given copy of chromosome 6 can contain any one of many alternative

58

The HLA Complex

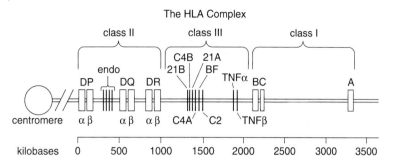

Figure 5–1. Organization of the HLA complex on the short arm of human chromosome 6. Regions encoding the 3 classes of MHC proteins are indicated by braces. Endo denotes a cluster of genes within the class II region that encode proteasome components and peptide-transport proteins required for processing endogenous antigens (see text). Class III proteins are unrelated to class I and II and are not involved in antigen presentation. Among proteins encoded in the class III region are tumor necrosis factors α and β, and complement factors C2, C4, B, and F.

versions of each gene that yield proteins with distinct sequences. For example, at least 24 different alleles of HLA-A and 50 alleles of HLA-B have been identified in the human population, and the actual number of functionally distinct alleles may be substantially higher. Indeed, the HLA complex is the most polymorphic genetic system known.

Each person inherits 2 copies of chromosome 6 and thus can express up to 6 different class I and 6 different class II proteins (ie, the products of 2 different alleles at each locus). Because of the extreme polymorphism of these loci, the probability that any 2 individuals will express identical sets of HLA proteins is very low. This, together with the fact that HLA antigens are highly immunogenic, presents a major problem in matching donors and recipients for organ transplantation (see Chapter 16).

Class I HLA Proteins

Each class I protein is expressed on the cell surface as a dimer composed of 2 noncovalently linked polypeptide chains: a polymorphic heavy or **α chain** (MW 43,000) encoded by genes at the A, B, and C loci in the HLA complex on chromosome 6, and a smaller (MW 12,000) nonpolymorphic polypeptide called **β$_2$-microglobulin (β$_2$m)** encoded by a single gene on chromosome 15. Each of these dimeric molecules is anchored to the cell membrane by the C-terminal region of the α chain, as depicted schematically in Fig 5–2. The extracellular region of the α chain is divided into 3 discrete folded domains (called α1, α2, and α3), each of which is structurally similar to immunoglobulin proteins (see Chapter 6). Almost all the polymorphic amino acid residues are in the α1 and α2 domains. The nonpolymorphic β$_2$m also has an immunoglobulinlike domain and is associated with the nonpolymorphic α3 domain of the heavy chain (Fig 5–2). Although B$_2$m is not directly involved in the antigen presentation function of class I proteins, it is thought to facilitate the transport of

the newly synthesized proteins from the endoplasmic reticulum to the cell surface and probably serves to stabilize their structure.

X-ray diffraction analysis of crystallized class I protein has revealed its 3-dimensional structure, in-

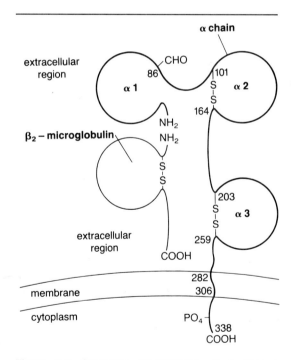

Figure 5–2. Schematic representation of a class I HLA protein. The molecule consists of an MW 44,000 polymorphic transmembrane polypeptide (α chain) noncovalently associated with an MW 12,000 nonpolymorphic polypeptide (β$_2$-microglobulin). The 3 extracellular domains of the α chain are designated α1, α2, and α3. The binding site for immunogenic peptides (T cell determinants) is formed by the cleft between the α1 and α2 domains.

cluding the site at which peptides are bound for presentation to CD8 T cells. Most of the molecule has a β-pleated sheet structure, but the α1 and α2 domains each contain an α-helix (Fig 5–3). These 2 helices are adjacent and roughly parallel to one another and together form the walls of a groove in the distal surface of the molecule, which serves as the **peptide-binding site** (Fig 5–4). A β-pleated sheet contributed by portions of both the α1 and α2 domains serves as the floor of the site. Most of the polymorphic residues of the class I molecule are located in the walls and floor of the groove and thus have the effect of conferring slightly different contours to the binding site in different allelic forms of the protein. Peptides bind noncovalently within the groove in an extended, rodlike conformation.

Each allelic form of a class I protein has its own specificity for peptide binding, which is determined by the sequences of the walls and floor of the peptide-binding site. It should be emphasized that although peptide binding by class I proteins is somewhat selective, it is not as highly specific as the binding of antigen by antibody, so each class I protein can bind a fairly wide range of peptides. Consequently, even the limited number of different class I proteins (no more than 6) expressed by each individual possesses a diverse peptide-binding capacity, sufficient to enable a normal individual to mount class I restricted responses to most antigens. Since a single cell may express on the order of 10^6 class I proteins on its surface, each cell has the potential to present many alternative peptides simultaneously.

The peptides bound by class I proteins are remarkably uniform in size, with most of those characterized thus far being 8–10 amino acids long. High-resolution x-ray diffraction imaging of such peptides nestled within the class I binding site has shown that amino acid residues in the site interact mainly with the backbone of the peptide, leaving its side chains free to interact with the T cell antigen receptor. The binding groove is constricted at both ends by nonpolymorphic HLA residues that bind the amino and carboxyl termini of the peptide backbone, and these tend to limit the size of peptides that can be accommodated in the site. The fact that a class I protein mainly recognizes the uniform backbones of peptides accounts for its relative peptide-binding degeneracy. In contrast, the highly specific T cell receptor interacts with the side chains, which vary from one peptide to another.

Class II HLA Proteins

The **class II proteins,** HLA-DP, -DQ, and -DR, are also each composed of 2 noncovalently associated polypeptides, but, unlike the class I molecules, both chains are encoded by polymorphic genes located within the HLA complex (Fig 5–1). Each class II protein consists of an **α chain** (MW 34,000) and a **β chain** (MW 29,000), which are both anchored in the cell membrane and have 2 extracellular immunoglobulinlike domains apiece (Fig 5–5). Polymorphism of class II molecules is confined to the N-terminal domain of each chain, which are designated the α1 and β1 domains.

X-ray crystallography has shown that the α1 and β1 domains in a class II molecule come together to form a **peptide-binding site,** which is very similar to that found in a class I protein. The class II α1 and β1 domains each contain a helical segment and β-sheet structures that form one wall and half the floor, respectively, of a peptide-binding cleft on the protein surface (Fig 5–6). As with class I, essentially all the polymorphism of class II molecules is localized to the walls and floor of this cleft, resulting in a distinctively contoured site for each allelic variant. The peptide-binding characteristics of class II molecules are generally analogous to those of class I, in that pep-

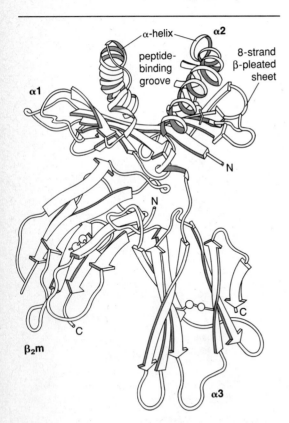

Figure 5–3. Diagrammatic structure of a class I HLA molecule (side view). In this ribbon diagram of the polypeptide backbone, the polypeptides are oriented as in Fig 3–2, but only the extracellular region is depicted. The peptide-binding site is a cleft (or groove) formed by 8 strands of β-pleated sheet and a pair of α-helices from the α1 and α2 domains. The β-sheet structure forms the floor and the two α helices the walls of the cleft. β-strands are depicted as broad arrows and α-helices as narrow coils. (Modified and reproduced, with permission, from Bjorkman PJ et al: Structure of the human class I histocompatibility antigen HLA-A2. *Nature* 1987;**329**:506.)

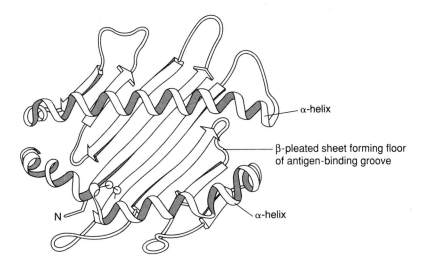

Figure 5–4. Peptide-binding site of a class I HLA molecule, viewed along an axis perpendicular to the cell surface. Eight strands of β-pleated sheet contributed by the α1 and α2 domains forms the floor of the site, and 2 α-helices, one from each of the 2 domains, form the walls. The groove accommodates peptides 8–9 amino acid residues long, leaving them partially accessible for interaction with the T cell antigen receptor. (Modified and reproduced, with permission, from Bjorkman PJ et al: Structure of the human class I histocompatibility antigen HLA-A2. *Nature* 1987;**329:**506.

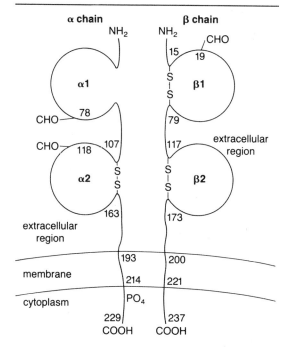

Figure 5–5. Schematic representation of a class II HLA molecule. The molecule consists of an MW 34,000 polypeptide (α chain) noncovalently associated with an MW 29,000 polypeptide (β-chain).

tides are bound in an extended conformation through noncovalent contacts that mostly involve the backbone, rather than the side chains, of the peptide. Hence, each class II protein has degenerate specificity (ie, can bind a fairly wide range of peptides). The binding cleft in class II proteins is open at both ends and preferentially binds somewhat longer peptides (10–18 amino acids) than those bound by class I (8–10 amino acids). The result is that class II-restricted CD4 T lymphocytes are presented with larger peptide determinants than are class I-restricted CD8 T cells, although the same antigen receptors are used by both T cell subsets. The immunologic significance of this difference is unknown.

ANTIGEN PRESENTATION BY CLASS I & CLASS II MHC PROTEINS

Class I and class II MHC proteins have considerable structural homology and similar peptide-binding sites, but they function differently in antigen presentation. One important difference is that they present immunogenic peptides to different T cell types: class I presents to CD8 T cells and class II to CD4 T cells. Another key difference is that the 2 classes of MHC proteins associate with peptides that have been produced through different processing pathways within the cell. Class I molecules bind peptides derived from **endogenously** synthesized proteins (eg, viral proteins in virus-infected cells), whereas class II molecules bind peptides derived from **exogenous** proteins (ie, those in the external medium) that have been in-

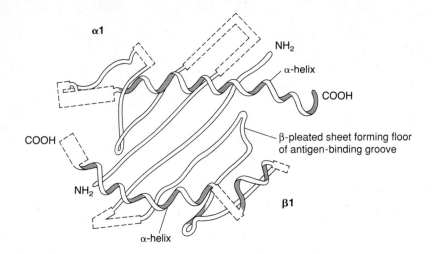

Figure 5–6. Structure of the peptide-binding site of a class II HLA molecule, viewed as in Fig 5–4. The binding site is similar to that of class I molecules, except that it is formed by the α1 and β1 domains of the class II molecule and is relatively open at both ends to accommodate longer peptides. (Modified and reproduced, with permission, from Brown JH et al: Three-dimensional structure of the human class II histocompatibility antigen HLA-DR1. *Nature* 1993;**364:**33.)

ternalized by APCs. This dichotomy ensures that cells which harbor intracellular infectious agents are recognized and attacked by class I-restricted cytotoxic T cells, whereas class II-restricted helper T cells respond to the universe of soluble antigens, providing activating signals for antibody production by B lymphocytes. The difference in antigen presentation pathway appears to be related to the requirements for assembly and transport to the cell surface of class I and class II proteins, as will be described in the following section.

Assembly & Transport of Peptide-MHC Complexes

MHC molecules, like other membrane proteins, are synthesized by polyribosomes in association with the rough endoplasmic reticulum (RER). When first synthesized, they are anchored in the RER membrane and project into its lumen. Class I MHC molecules bind peptides while still in the RER. Recent experimental findings suggest that the binding of a peptide by a class I α chain induces a conformational change which facilitates association with β_2 and that this, in turn, promotes transport of the class I molecule from the RER to the cell surface (Fig 5–7). The peptides that associate with class I molecules are derived from partial proteolytic digestion of endogenously synthesized proteins in the cytoplasm. This digestion appears to be carried out at least in part by proteases that reside in large (26S) multienzyme cytoplasmic complexes known as **proteasomes.** Some of the resulting peptides are then actively pumped from the cytoplasm into the RER lumen in an ATP-dependent manner by specialized **peptide-transporter proteins.** Two such proteins, called the transporters of antigenic peptides 1 and 2 (**TAP1** and **TAP2**), have been

characterized thus far; each is an integral RER membrane protein containing multiple transmembrane regions and an ATP-binding domain. TAP1, TAP2, and at least two components of the proteasome are encoded by a cluster of genes within the class II MHC locus (see Fig 5–1); each can occur in several alternative allelic forms which may have different substrate specificities. The proteolytic and peptide-transport mechanisms each act most efficiently on only a subset of peptides, and this presumably influences which peptides can be presented by class I MHC.

In contrast, class II molecules must be transported from the RER to an endosomal compartment before they bind peptides (Fig 5–7). While in the RER, newly synthesized class II molecules associate with another protein called the **invariant chain (Ii);** this protein is believed to obstruct the class II peptide-binding site sterically, preventing interaction of the site with any endogenous peptides in the RER lumen. The complex of class II protein and bound invariant chain is then transported via membrane vesicles to an endosomal compartment, where it encounters peptides derived from endocytosed, exogenous proteins. Here, the invariant chain is dissociated and degraded, permitting binding of the exogenous peptides to the now unoccupied peptide-binding groove. The resulting peptide-protein complex is then translocated onto the cell surface.

Thus, class I and class II proteins travel different routes and encounter antigen in different cellular compartments. This difference in routing is believed to determine the source of peptide that becomes associated with each class: either endogenously synthesized and transported to the endoplasmic reticulum (endogenous pathway; class I) or endocytosed and

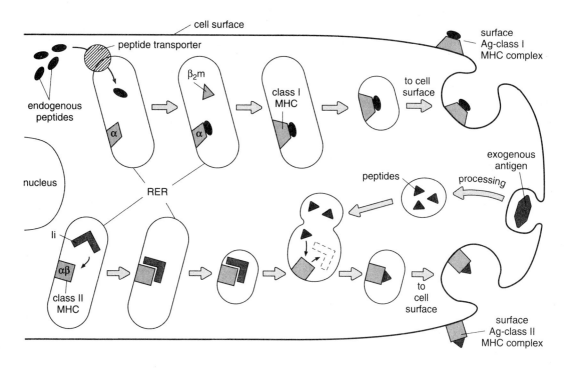

Figure 5–7. The pathways of assembly and transport for antigen-MHC complexes containing class I (top) and class II (bottom) HLA molecules. MHC polypeptides of both classes are initially expressed in the rough endoplasmic reticulum (RER). Class I proteins sequentially bind endogenous peptides and β_2-microglobulin (β_2m) in the RER lumen and are then transported to the cell surface. Class II proteins associate with invariant chain (Ii) in the RER and so are prevented from binding endogenous peptides; they are translocated instead to an endosomal compartment, where Ii dissociates and is replaced by exogenous peptides.

degraded in an endosomal compartment (exogenous pathway; class II).

ANTIGEN-PRESENTING CELLS

Virtually all somatic cells express class I proteins and therefore can present endogenous antigens to CD8 T cells. They do so, for example, when infected with a virus, and usually are killed by the lymphocyte as a result. In contrast, only a few cell types express class II proteins; such cells are uniquely able to present exogenous antigens to CD4 helper T cells, and so are important for nearly all immune responses. It is to these latter cell types that the term "antigen-presenting cell" usually refers. The major types of antigen presenting cells are discussed below.

Macrophages

Most types of macrophages express class II proteins constitutively, and the level of class II expression is increased when the macrophage is activated. Macrophages are widely distributed in lymphoid and nonlymphoid tissues and, because of their prodigious phagocytic capacity (see Chapter 1), are especially important for presenting antigens from particulate immunogens such as bacteria.

B Lymphocytes

Although they lack significant phagocytic activity, B cells are able to capture, process, and present small molecular antigens to helper T cells. They are especially effective in presenting the antigens that bind specifically to their surface immunoglobulins. Antigen presentation by B cells and its importance for humoral immunity are considered in detail in Chapter 7.

Dendritic Cells

Cells in this category are known by a variety of names depending on their location in the body but are thought to represent different forms of a single cell type. All have in common an unusual, spidery shape imparted by their many long cytoplasmic processes. They are found as a diffuse, minor population in all surface epithelia and many solid organs but can also migrate through the blood and lymph. Members of this group include epidermal **Langerhans cells**, the "veiled" cells of lymph, **blood dendritic cells** (which make up less than 0.1% of all nucleated blood cells), and the **interdigitating cells** that are found throughout the T cell zones of lymphoid organs. All are derived from a common marrow precursor, although not from monocytes. These cells have little phagocytic capacity but express abundant class II protein and are highly efficient at capturing and presenting antigens. Being motile, they may also travel through the body in search of rare T cells with appropriate antigen specificity. Dendritic cells appear to be particularly important in initiating primary immune responses and responses against antigens that contact the body surface. For example, when an immunogen is applied to the skin, some Langerhans cells migrate from the site into dermal lymphatics and are carried to the T cell zones of regional lymph nodes, carrying processed antigens with them for presentation.

Despite the unfortunate similarity in names and morphology, follicular dendritic cells (FDCs) are *not* related to the dendritic cells described above, and are not considered to be APCs. FDCs are found only in primary and secondary lymphoid follicles (in fact, they may be responsible for assembling these follicles), and, although their origin remains obscure, they are not descendants of any marrow precursor. They are not appreciably phagocytic, and they do not express class II MHC protein. Possible functions of FDCs are discussed in Chapter 7.

MHC & IMMUNE RESPONSIVENESS

The ability to mount immune responses to particular antigens is strongly influenced by the MHC. This influence has been demonstrated clearly in experimental studies with inbred strains of mice, which are homozygous at each MHC locus and consequently express a more limited set of MHC molecules than do outbred animals. Fortunately, we are able to manipulate mice experimentally, which has made demonstration of the influence of the MHC on immune responsiveness relatively straightforward. For example, certain strains of mice fail to express one of the class II loci because of a gene deletion at that locus; such mice do not respond to pigeon cytochrome *c*, which is a strong antigen in most other mouse strains. When the missing class II gene is artificially reintroduced into these mice, they express the corresponding class II protein and gain the ability to respond to pigeon cytochrome *c*. Since only the class II gene was introduced into these mice, it would appear that it was solely responsible for the observed effect on immune responsiveness.

The foregoing experiment illustrates the importance of the MHC for **determinant selection**—the multistage process by which each individual's immune system selects the specific immunogens (and the specific epitopes from within complex immunogens) to which it will respond. The influence of the MHC on determinant selection stems from the fact that any given allelic form of an MHC protein is able to bind only a finite range of peptides. Thus, an individual with a particular subset of class II genes may lack a class II molecule capable of binding peptides from a particular foreign protein, so that no part of the protein can be presented to helper T cells. In such a case, no immune response could occur. Deficiencies of this type in determinant selection are sometimes readily apparent in inbred homozygous animals because their repertoire of MHC proteins is relatively limited. Humans (being outbred) are much more genetically diverse and so are less likely to manifest major gaps in determinant selection. Even if such gaps occur in humans, the extreme polymorphism of the MHC helps to ensure that at least some members of the population will be able to respond against almost any potential pathogen. This is clearly advantageous and provides a teleological explanation for why polymorphism has been preserved in the MHC system.

MHC & DISEASE

Certain human diseases occur more frequently among individuals who carry particular MHC alleles. These diseases include the susceptibility to certain infectious agents, as well as to a number of **autoimmune disorders** (that is, disorders that are thought to involve an inappropriate immune attack against host tissues; see Chapter 30). In each instance, the association with MHC is statistically significant but not absolute: it appears likely that other genes apart from the MHC, as well as unknown environmental factors, also play roles in these diseases, making it very difficult to unravel the story completely. For example, the strongest HLA-disease association found thus far (Table 5–1) is that of **ankylosing spondylitis,** a degenerative disease of the spine whose cause is un-

Table 5–1. Some MHC-associated disorders in the US Caucasian population.

Disorder	HLA Allele	Relative Risk[1]
Ankylosing spondylitis	B27	80
Juvenile rheumatoid arthritis	Dw14	47
	Dw4	26
Reiter's syndrome	B27	40
Insulin-dependent diabetes mellitus	DQw8	32
Acute anterior uveitis	B27	8
Sjögren's syndrome	DR3	6
Graves' disease	DR3	4
Systemic lupus erythematosus	DR2	3

[1]Chance that a person who is heterozygous for the indicated allele will develop the disease, expressed as a multiple of the risk in the population that does not carry this allele.

known. About 90% of Caucasian patients with this disease express a particular HLA-B allele designated HLA-B27, compared with only 9% of the control Caucasian population. The association in the American black population is much lower, with only about 48% of patients expressing HLA-B27, and this argues strongly that the B27 allele is not obligatory for development of ankylosing spondylitis.

The role played by the MHC in HLA-associated diseases is thought to reflect, at least in part, determinant selection. For example, the tissue destruction in ankylosing spondylitis appears to result from a cell-mediated autoimmune reaction against an unknown antigen in vertebral tissues. If peptides from this presumed antigen bind more avidly to B27 than to other class I proteins, it would be expected that individuals expressing B27 would be more likely to develop class I-restricted immunity to that antigen and concomitant disease. Conversely, HLA-associated susceptibility to infectious disease could be due to an inability of the particular HLA protein to associate effectively

with processed antigens from the pathogen, thereby limiting the capacity of the individual to mount an immune response against it.

Although the role of determinant selection in HLA-associated disease remains unproven, there is evidence in animal populations that reduced MHC polymorphism may predispose a population to infectious disease. Reduced polymorphism arises within a shrinking population from limited breeding stock and reflects the limited number of MHC alleles within the population. Numerous studies suggest that reduced polymorphism limits the range of antigens to which a population can respond, as would be predicted by determinant selection. Such findings again underscore the survival value to a species of extreme MHC polymorphism: although there may be individuals within a species that are unable to respond to a given pathogen because they lack the appropriate MHC alleles, polymorphism ensures that at least some individuals will be able to respond and that the species as a whole will survive.

REFERENCES

Bjorkman P, Parham P: Structure, function and diversity of class I major histocompatibility complex molecules. *Annu Rev Biochem* 1990;**59**:253.

Brodsky F, Guagliardi L: The cell biology of antigen processing and presentation. *Annu Rev Immunol* 1991;**9**:707.

Brown JH et al: Three-dimensional structure of the human class II histocompatibility antigen HLA-DR1. *Nature* 1993;**364**:33.

Germain RN, Margulies DH: The biochemistry and cell biology of antigen processing and presentation. *Annu Rev Immunol* 1993;**11**:403.

Kappes D, Strominger J: Human class II major histocompatibility complex genes and proteins. *Annu Rev Biochem* 1988;**57**:991.

Klein J: *Natural History of the Major Histocompatibility Complex*. John Wiley & Sons, 1986.

Matsumura M et al: Emerging principles for the recognition of peptide antigens by MHC class I molecules. *Science* 1992;**257**:927.

Neefjes JJ et al: Selective and ATP-dependent translocation of peptides by the MHC-encoded transporter. *Science* 1993;**261**:769.

Steinman RM: The dendritic cell system and its role in immunogenicity. *Annu Rev Immunol* 1991;**9**:271.

6

Immunoglobulin Proteins

Joel W. Goodman, PhD, & Tristram G. Parslow, MD, PhD

Immunoglobulin proteins are the critical ingredients at every stage of a humoral immune response. When expressed on the surfaces of resting B lymphocytes, they serve as receptors that can detect and distinguish among the vast array of potential antigens present in the environment. On binding their cognate antigens, surface immunoglobulins can initiate a cascade of molecular signaling events that may culminate in B cell activation, clonal proliferation, and the generation of plasma cells. The immunoglobulins that are secreted as a result then function as **antibodies,** traveling through the tissue fluids to seek out and bind to the specific antigenic molecules that triggered their production.

The two hallmarks of immunoglobulins as antigen-binding proteins are the **specificity** of each for a particular antigenic structure and their **diversity** as a group. In addition to antigen binding, however, immunoglobulins possess **secondary biologic activities** that are critical for host defense. These include, for example, the abilities to function as opsonins, to activate the complement cascade, and to cross the placental barrier. Immunoglobulin proteins are heterogeneous with respect to these latter activities, which are determined by structural features independent of those that dictate antigen specificity. In this chapter, we will consider how the structures of immunoglobulins account for their specificity, diversity, and secondary biologic activities.

ORGANIZATION & DIVERSITY OF IMMUNOGLOBULIN PROTEINS

The immunoglobulins are an enormous family of glycoproteins that are composed of 82–96% polypeptide and 4–18% carbohydrate by weight. Almost all of the biologic properties of immunoglobulins derive from the structure of their polypeptide components. Antibodies are bifunctional molecules in that they bind specifically to antigens and also initiate a variety of secondary phenomena—such as complement activation, opsonization, or signal transduction—that are unrelated to their antigen-binding specificity. As discussed below, these 2 independent aspects of immunoglobulin function reside in separate regions of each protein.

The sheer diversity of immunoglobulins was for a long time a major barrier to understanding their structures. A serum specimen from a normal person contains a tremendous number of different antibody molecules, each of which is present in only minute amounts and (owing to its unique structure) has its own distinctive set of physical properties such as molecular weight and isoelectric point. When a serum specimen is fractionated by electrophoresis, for example, the immunoglobulins are found to migrate as a broad band (called the **gamma globulin** fraction) that reflects the presence of innumerable different proteins, each with slighly different electrophoretic properties. This extreme diversity made it virtually impossible to isolate sufficient amounts of any single antibody protein from a normal donor to permit a thorough biochemical analysis.

Two major discoveries during the 1950s and 1960s finally opened up the field of immunoglobulin protein chemistry. The first was the finding that enzymes and reducing agents could be used to digest or dissociate immunoglobulins into smaller components. This revealed that diversity was confined largely to specific regions of the immunoglobulin molecules; other regions were much more uniform and could be isolated in pure form, making them accessible for structural analysis. The second breakthrough came with the realization that patients who had certain types of B lymphoid cancers (such as **multiple myeloma**) contained in their blood and urine large amounts of a single, homogeneous type of immunoglobulin protein secreted by the malignant B cell clone. Purification and characterization of such **myeloma proteins** made it possible to study individual antibodies and permitted (by 1969) the determination

66

of the first complete amino acid sequence of an immunoglobulin. The development, in 1975, of laboratory methods for immortalizing individual clones of antibody-secreting cells gave birth to **monoclonal antibody** technology (see Chapter 12) and made it possible to obtain homogeneous antibodies of virtually any specificity in unlimited quantities. At about the same time, the isolation and characterization of immunoglobulin genes (see Chapter 7) revolutionized the study of this protein family by making it relatively easy to isolate, analyze, and even design immunoglobulin proteins of all types. Information gleaned from all these approaches forms the basis for our current detailed understanding of immunoglobulin protein structure.

The 4-Chain Basic Unit

Every immunoglobulin molecule is made up of 2 different types of polypeptides. The larger of these, called **heavy (H) chains,** are roughly twice as large as the smaller **light (L) chains.** Every immunoglobulin contains equal numbers of heavy- and light-chain polypeptides and can be represented by the general formula $(H_2L_2)_n$. The chains are held together by noncovalent forces and also by covalent interchain disulfide bridges to form a bilaterally symmetrical structure as depicted in Fig 6–1. All normal immunoglobulins conform to this basic structure, although some, as we shall see, are composed of more than one of these 4-chain basic units.

The heavy and light polypeptide chains are both composed of a number of folded globular **domains,** each of which is 100–110 amino acids long and contains a single intrachain disulfide bond (Fig 6–1). Although the amino acid sequences of the individual domains vary, they fold into very similar 3-dimensional conformations (a roughly cylindric assembly of β-strands known as the **immunoglobulin barrel**), owing in part to the fairly constant location of the intrachain disulfide. Light chains always contain 2 of these domains, whereas heavy chains contain either 4 or 5.

All of the light chains and all of the heavy chains in any single immunoglobulin protein are identical. When different immunoglobulins are compared, however, the sequences of these chains vary widely.

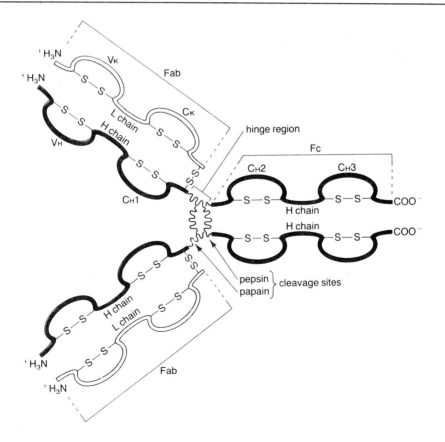

Figure 6–1. Schematic model of an IgG1 (κ) human antibody molecule showing the basic 4-chain structure and domains (V_H, C_H1, etc). Sites of enzymatic cleavage by pepsin and papain are shown.

In both heavy and light chains, this variability is confined largely to the N-terminal domain, whereas the sequences of the other domains remain relatively constant. For this reason, the N-terminal domain in a heavy- or light-chain polypeptide is called the **variable region,** abbreviated V_H or V_L, respectively. The other domains are collectively termed the **constant region,** abbreviated C_H or C_L. Light-chain polypeptides contain only a single C_L domain but heavy-chain C_H regions comprise 3 or more domains, which are numbered sequentially (C_H1, C_H2, etc) beginning with the domain closest to V_H.

Within an immunoglobulin unit, the heavy and light chains are aligned in parallel, as shown in Fig. 6–1. Each V_H domain is always positioned directly adjacent to a V_L domain and this pair of domains together forms a single **antigen-binding site.** Each basic 4-chain unit thus contains 2 separate but identical antigen-binding sites and so is said to be **divalent**. The antigen-specificity of a given protein is determined by the combined sequences of its V_H and V_L domains and for this reason varies widely among immunoglobulins. Each C_H1 domain interacts closely with the C_L domain, and in most types of immunoglobulins the 2 are linked covalently by one or more disulfide bridges. Each of the remaining C_H domains is aligned with its counterpart on the opposite heavy chain and may be linked to it by disulfide bonds. Overall, the protein has a T- or Y-shaped configuration when viewed schematically. The region at the base of each arm in the T or Y, located between the C_H1 and C_H2 domains, is called the **hinge region;** in most immunoglobulins, it has a loose secondary structure that confers flexibility, enabling the 2 arms to move relatively freely with respect to each other.

Enzymatic Digestion Products of Immunoglobulins

Immunoglobulins are rather resistant to proteolytic digestion but are most susceptible to cleavage near the hinge region (Fig 6–1), which usually lies adjacent to the site of interchain disulfides linking the 2 heavy chains together. The enzyme **papain** happens to cleave this region on the N-terminal side of the inter-heavy-chain disulfides and so splits an immunoglobulin into 3 fragments of roughly similar size. Two of these are identical to one another, and each consists of an entire light chain along with the V_H and C_H1 domains of one heavy chain; these fragments thus contain the antigen-binding sites of the protein and so are called **Fab fragments** (ie, antigen-binding fragments). Each Fab fragment is **monovalent** with respect to antigen-binding activity. The third fragment comprises the carboxy-terminal portions of both heavy chains held together by disulfides. The structure of this third fragment is identical for many different immunoglobulin molecules, so that fragments of this type can often be crystallized even if they are derived from a heterogeneous antibody population. Hence, this third fragment is designated the crystallizable or **Fc fragment.** Most of the secondary biologic properties of immunoglobulins (such as the ability to activate complement) are determined by sequences in the Fc region of the protein. This is also the region that is recognized by the **Fc receptors** found on many types of cells.

A somewhat different pattern of cleavage occurs with the enzyme pepsin, which cleaves on the carboxy-terminal side of the inter-heavy-chain disulfides. This yields a single large fragment called an **F(ab)$'_2$** fragment, which roughly corresponds to 2 disulfide-linked Fab fragments and has divalent antigen-binding activity. The Fc region, on the other hand, is extensively degraded by pepsin and usually does not survive as an intact fragment.

Characterization of these proteolytic fragments in the 1960s was an important step toward understanding antibody structure, because it provided the first evidence that the antigen-binding and secondary functions of antibodies reside in separate regions of the protein. Such fragments are still used today when it is necessary to dissociate different aspects of antibody function for diagnostic or research purposes.

CLASSIFICATION OF IMMUNOGLOBULINS & THEIR CONSTITUENT CHAINS

Immunoglobulins are composed of heavy and light chains. The N-terminal domain (V region) in both types of chains is highly variable and mediates antigen-binding. The remaining portion (C region) of each chain, by comparison, is far less variable. Nevertheless, every normal person produces several alternative forms of heavy and light chains that each have distinctly different C-region amino acid sequences (Table 6–1). These alternative forms of the immunoglobulin chains can be distinguished from one another by their physical properties (such as molecular weight) or serologically by using antibodies (usually obtained from animals that have been immunized with human Fc fragments) that recognize specific features in the various human C regions. Whereas these normal variations in sequence of the light-chain C region have no impact on immunoglobulin function, those in the heavy-chain C region significantly affect the secondary biologic properties of immunoglobulins.

Light Chain Types & Subtypes

All light chains have protein molecular weights of approximately 23,000 but can be classified into 2 distinct **types,** called **kappa** (κ) and **lambda** (λ), on the basis of their C_L-region sequences. There are no

Table 6–1. Properties of human immunoglobulin chains and related polypeptides.

Chain	H Chains					L Chains		Secretory Component	J Chain
	γ	α	μ	δ	ε	κ	λ	SC	J
Classes in which chain occurs	IgG	IgA	IgM	IgD	IgE	All classes	All classes	IgA	IgA, IgM
Subclasses or subtypes	1,2,3,4	1,2	...	...	...	...	1,2,3,4,5,6	...	...
Molecular weight (approximate)	50,000[1]	55,000	70,000	62,000	70,000	23,000	23,000	70,000	15,000
V region subgroups	$V_H I$–$V_H IV$					$V_\kappa I$–$V_\kappa IV$	$V_\lambda I$–$V_\lambda IV$		
Carbohydrate (average percentage)	4	10	15	18	18	0	0	16	8
Number of oligosaccharides (average)	1	2 or 3	5	?	5	0	0	?	1

[1]60,000 for γ3.

known functional differences between these 2 types, and each can associate with any of the various classes of heavy chains. Nevertheless, expression of 2 distinct light-chain types is common among mammalian species. Indeed, the amino acid sequence similarities between human and mouse kappa chains are much greater than those between the kappa and lambda chains within each species—a finding that supports the conclusion that the 2 light-chain types arise from 2 genes that separated from one another during evolution prior to the divergence of mammalian species.

The C regions of all κ light chains produced by an individual are essentially identical. In contrast, one individual person may express as many as 6 slightly different forms of the λ C region. These various **subtypes** of λ differ from one another only slightly in C-region amino acid sequence and are functionally identical, although each is encoded by a separate chromosomal locus.

A given immunoglobulin molecule always contains exclusively κ or one of the λ chains, never a mixture. Similarly, any given B lineage cell produces only one type of light chain. When the entire population of immunoglobulins (or of B lineage cells) in an individual is considered, the proportion of κ to λ chains that are produced varies from species to species; in humans, the ratio is about 2:1.

Heavy-Chain Classes & Subclasses

Humans express 5 different **classes** (or **isotypes**) of immunoglobulin heavy chains, which differ considerably in their C_H-region sequences and in their physical and biologic properties. All of the heavy chains in any given immunoglobulin molecule are identical. The 5 classes of heavy chains are designated μ, δ, γ, α, and ε, and immunoglobulins that contain these heavy chains are designated the IgM, IgD, IgG, IgA, and IgE classes, respectively. The γ and α classes are further divided into **subclasses** (γ1, γ2, γ3, γ4, α1, and α2) on the basis of relatively minor differences in C_H sequence and function; the corresponding immuno-

globulin subclasses are denoted IgG1, IgG2, etc. Heavy chains representing the various subclasses within a class are much more similar to one another than to the other classes. Normal individuals express all 9 classes and subclasses, because each is encoded by a separate genetic locus and is inherited independently.

The heavy-chain polypeptides range in molecular weight from about 50,000 to 70,000. The μ and ε chains are made up of 5 globular domains apiece (one V_H and 4 C_H), whereas γ and α chains each contain only 4 domains. The δ chain has an intermediate molecular mass attributable to an extended hinge region. The γ3 chain also has an extended hinge that consists of about 60 amino acid residues; of these, 14 are cysteines, which accounts for the large number of inter-heavy-chain disulfide bonds in IgG3 (see below). In some mammalian species, the charge characteristics of the various IgG subclasses differ sufficiently to permit their separation by electrophoretic techniques, but this is not true of humans.

Composition of Immunoglobulin Classes & Subclasses

The class of the H chain determines the class of the immunoglobulin. Thus, there are 5 classes of immunoglobulins: **IgG, IgA, IgM, IgD,** and **IgE.** A given molecule in any of these classes may contain either κ or λ light chains. For example, 2 γ chains (of any of the 4 subclasses) combined with either 2 κ or 2 λ L chains constitute an IgG molecule—the most abundant class of immunoglobulins in sera from adults. Similarly, 2 μ chains together with 2 L chains form an IgM monomer unit of the type found on the surfaces of many B cells. The secreted form of IgM, however, is a pentameric macroglobulin that consists of 5 of these basic 4-chain units along with an additional polypeptide called **J chain** (Fig 6–2). Each IgM pentamer contains 10 identical antigen-binding sites and so has **polyvalent** binding activity. IgA accounts for only about 10–15% of serum immunoglobulin but is the predominant class of antibody found in body se-

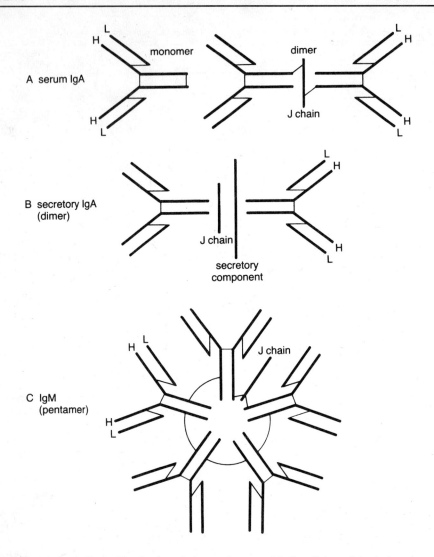

Figure 6–2. Highly schematic illustration of polymeric human immunoglobulins. Polypeptide chains are represented by thick lines; disulfide bonds linking different polypeptide chains are represented by thin lines.

cretions. The membrane-bound form of IgA is a single 4-chain unit, but the secreted form can polymerize to form polyvalent assemblages comprising 2–5 of these basic units along with J chain and (in secreted IgA) yet another polypeptide called **secretory component** (Fig 6–2). The properties of the individual chains are summarized in Table 6–1, and those of the immunoglobulin classes are compared in Table 6–2.

One noteworthy structural difference between the immunoglobulin classes or subclasses lies in the number and arrangement of interchain disulfide bridges within each 4-chain unit (Fig 6–3). In IgA2, for example, the L chains are covalently linked to each other rather than to the H chains, so that L-H binding is entirely due to noncovalent forces. In other subclasses, the L-H bond may be situated either close to the junction of the V_H and C_H1 domains (as in IgG2 or IgA1) or, alternatively, near the junction between C_H1 and C_H2 (as in IgG1).

Membrane & Secreted Immunoglobulins

Immunoglobulins of all classes can exist in either membrane-bound or secreted forms. The membrane forms always exist as individual 4-chain units, and their heavy chains contain an additional carboxy-terminal sequence of approximately 40 amino acid residues. This sequence consists of a highly acidic region of 12–14 residues, followed by a strikingly hydrophobic sequence of about 26 residues. The hydrophobic por-

Table 6–2. Properties of human immunoglobulins.

	IgG	IgA	IgM	IgD	IgE
H chain class	γ	α	μ	δ	ϵ
H chain subclasses	$\gamma1, \gamma2, \gamma3, \gamma4$	$\alpha1, \alpha2$			
L chain type	κ and λ	κ and λ	κ and λ	κ and λ	κ and λ
Molecular formula	$\gamma_2 L_2$	$\alpha_2 L_2$[1] or $(\alpha_2 L_2)_2 SC^2 J^3$	$(\alpha_2 L_2)_5 J^3$	$\delta_2 L_2$	$\epsilon_2 L_2$
Sedimentation coefficient (S)	6–7	7	19	7–8	8
Molecular weight (approximate)	150,000	160,000[1] or 400,000[4]	900,000	180,000	190,000
Electrophoretic mobility (average)	γ	Fast γ to β	Fast γ to β	Fast γ	Fast γ
Complement fixation (classic)	+	0	++++	0	0
Serum concentration (approximate; mg/dL)	1000	200	120	3	0.05
Serum half-life (days)	23	6	5	3	2
Placental transfer	+	0	0	0	0
Mast cell or basophil degranulation	?	0	0	0	++++
Bacterial lysis	+	+	+++	?	?
Antiviral activity	+	+++	+	?	?

[1]For monomeric serum IgA.   [3]J chain.
[2]Secretory component.   [4]For secretory IgA.

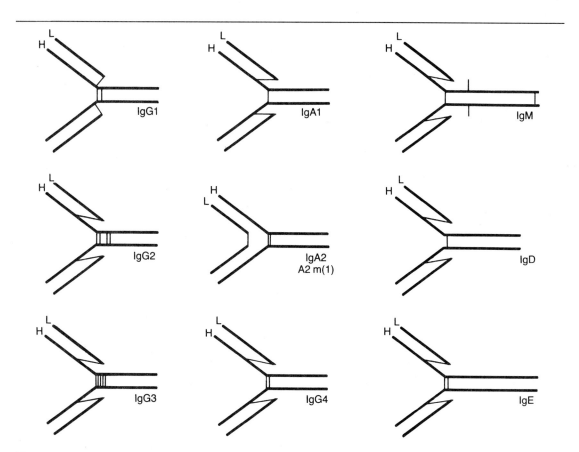

Figure 6–3. Distribution of interchain disulfide bonds in various human immunoglobulin classes and subclasses. H chains are represented by long thick lines and L chains by short thick lines. Disulfide bonds are represented by thin lines. The number of inter-heavy-chain disulfide bonds in IgG3 may be as large as 14.

tion is the **transmembrane** component that anchors the heavy chain (and, hence, the entire 4-chain unit) into the cell membrane. It is similar in hydrophobicity and length to known transmembrane segments of other proteins, and it satisfies the requirements for the formation of a membrane-spanning α-helix. Whereas the acidic portion of the membrane segment shows little amino acid sequence conservation among heavy-chain classes, the hydrophobic sequences of μ and γ chains show substantially greater homology to each other than do the C-region domains of those classes. This is puzzling, because transmembrane segments of other proteins seem to have little in common aside from length and hydrophobicity.

Secreted immunoglobulins lack the terminal transmembrane segment as a result of alternative RNA splicing (see Chapter 7). In its place, the secreted forms of μ and α (but not of the other classes) contain short terminal sequences, called **tail pieces,** that mediate polymerization of 4-chain units and also serve as contact sites for the J chain.

Allotypic (Allelic) Forms of Heavy & Light Chains

The heavy-chain classes and subclasses and the light-chain types and subtypes are each encoded by separate genetic loci, so that all are normally present in a single haploid genome. Some of these individual loci, however, exist in more than one form within the population; the alternative forms (**alleles**) generally differ from one another by only one or, at most, a few amino acid substitutions. Such minor alternative forms at a given immunoglobulin locus are called **allotypes.** In humans, allotypes have been found for γ, α and ε H chains and for κ L chains. Thus far, allotypic forms of λ L chains or of μ and δ H chains have not been observed.

Allotypic variation has no effect on immunoglobulin function and is primarily of interest because the variant C-region sequences can be immunogenic in some circumstances. For example, during the course of pregnancy mothers may become immunized against paternal allotypic determinants expressed on fetal immunoglobulins. Alternatively, immunization may result from blood transfusions. In addition, patients with rheumatoid arthritis can develop "**rheumatoid factors**"—antibodies that are directed against normal IgG—which occasionally recognize allotypic determinants.

J Chain & Secretory Component

As noted above, the secreted forms of IgM and IgA generally exist as polymers of the basic 4-chain unit that include a single additional polypeptide called **J chain.** J chain is a small (MW 15,000) acidic protein that is structurally unrelated to heavy and light chains but is synthesized by all plasma cells that secrete polymeric immunoglobulins. In these polymeric as-

semblies, J chain is disulfide-bonded to the penultimate cysteine residue in the tail piece of the α or μ chains. Its function seems to be to facilitate proper polymerization, although whether it is required for polymerization remains controversial.

Secretory component is a single polypeptide with a molecular weight of approximately 70,000. It is associated only with IgA and is found almost exclusively in body secretions. The carbohydrate content of secretory component is high but not precisely known. Its amino acid sequence is invariant and shows no appreciable resemblance to J chain or to any of the immunoglobulin polypeptides. Secretory component can exist either in free form or bound to IgA molecules; the latter interaction is usually noncovalent, but disulfide bonds have been implicated in a small proportion of human IgA. Free secretory component can even be observed in secretions from individuals who lack measurable IgA in their serum or secretions.

Secretory component is synthesized not by lymphocytes but, rather, by mucosal epithelial cells that overlie Peyer's patches and other submucosal lymphoid tissues. Such epithelial cells take up IgA that is secreted from the lymphoid cells beneath them, associate it with secretory component, and transport the resulting complex across the epithelial barrier into secretions. The exact function of secretory component is unknown, but it is presumed to facilitate transepithelial passage of IgA.

CARBOHYDRATE MOIETIES OF IMMUNOGLOBULINS

Significant amounts of carbohydrate are present in all immunoglobulins in the form of simple or complex side chains covalently bonded to amino acids of the polypeptide chains (Table 6–1). The function of these carbohydrate moieties is poorly understood. They may play important roles in the secretion of immunoglobulins by plasma cells and in the biologic functions associated with the C_H regions.

In general, carbohydrate is found only in secretory component, J chain, and the C regions of H chains; it is not found in L chains or in V_H regions. Exceptions to these rules have occasionally been observed. Surveys of a limited number of pure immunoglobulins indicate that IgM and IgE bear an average of 5 oligosaccharides each; IgG, one oligosaccharide; and IgA, 2 or 3 oligosaccharides. This agrees with the overall carbohydrate content of immunoglobulins, which is highest for IgM, IgD, and IgE, followed by IgA and then by IgG (Table 6–1). Nevertheless, it is clear that immunoglobulins of a given class (or even different molecules of a single myeloma protein) can differ considerably with respect to carbohydrate content. Secretory component is more heavily glycosylated than immunoglobulin chains; this accounts for the higher carbohydrate content of secretory IgA than of serum IgA.

The carbohydrate chains of immunoglobulins are in most cases attached by means of an N-glycosidic linkage between an N-acetylglucosamine residue in the carbohydrate and an asparagine residue of the polypeptide. However, other linkages have also been observed, including occasional O-glycosidic linkages between an amino sugar of an oligosaccharide and a serine or threonine residue in the polypeptide chain.

BIOLOGIC ACTIVITIES OF IMMUNOGLOBULINS

As previously noted, immunoglobulins are bifunctional molecules that bind antigens and, in addition, initiate other biologic processes that are independent of antibody specificity. These 2 kinds of activities are each localized to a particular part of the protein: antigen-binding to the combined V_H and V_L domains and the other activities to the C_H domains (particularly those of the Fc segment). These latter activities, some of which are summarized in Table 6–2, are considered in this section.

Immunoglobulin G (IgG)

IgG accounts for approximately 75% of the total serum immunoglobulin in normal adults and is the most abundant antibody produced during secondary humoral immune responses in the blood. Within the IgG class, the relative concentrations of the 4 subclasses are approximately as follows: IgG1, 60–70%; IgG2, 14–20%; IgG3, 4–8%; and IgG4, 2–6% (Table 6–3). These values vary somewhat among individuals; it appears that the propensity to produce IgG antibodies of one subclass or another is at least partly an inherited trait.

IgG is the only class of immunoglobulin that can cross the placenta in humans, and it is responsible for protection of the newborn during the first months of life (see Chapter 42). The subclasses are not equal with respect to this property, IgG2 being transferred less efficiently than the others. The adaptive or biologic value of this inequality, if any, is obscure.

Antigen-bound IgG is also capable of fixing (that is, binding and activating) serum complement, and

Table 6–3. Properties of human IgG subclasses.

	IgG1	IgG2	IgG3	IgG4
Abundance (% of total IgG)	70	20	6	4
Half-life in serum (days)	23	23	7	23
Placental passage	+++	+	+++	+++
Complement fixation	+	+	+++	–
Binding to Fc receptors	+++	+	+++	–

once again the subclasses do so with unequal efficiency (IgG3 > IgG1 > IgG2 > IgG4). IgG4 is completely unable to fix complement by the classic pathway, which requires binding of a protein called **C1q**, but may be active in the alternative pathway (see Chapter 10). The C1q binding site on the other IgG proteins appears to reside in the C_H2 domain.

Macrophages and certain other cell types express surface receptors that bind the Fc regions of IgG molecules. These interact principally with C_H3 domains and bind IgG1 and IgG3 with much higher affinity than they bind the other subclasses. The properties of these receptors are considered in a later section.

Immunoglobulin A (IgA)

IgA is the predominant immunoglobulin produced by B cells in Peyer's patches, tonsils, and other submucosal lymphoid tissues. Therefore, although it accounts for only 10–15% of serum immunoglobulin, it is by far the most abundant antibody class found in saliva, tears, intestinal mucus, bronchial secretions, milk, prostatic fluid, and other secretions. On B cell surfaces, IgA exists as a monomer (MW 160,000) comprising only one 4-chain unit. In the blood or in secretions, it multimerizes to form disulfide-linked polymers of up to 5 such units that are associated with one molecule each of J chain and (in secretions) secretory component. The predominant secreted forms of IgA are dimers and trimers (Fig 6–2). The 2 subclasses, IgA1 and IgA2, are expressed at a 5:1 ratio in the blood and have similar properties. Specific Fc receptors for IgA have been observed but are not well characterized.

Immunoglobulin M (IgM)

IgM constitutes approximately 10% of normal serum immunoglobulins and is normally secreted as a J-chain-containing pentamer with a molecular weight of approximately 900,000. IgM antibody predominates in early primary immune responses to most antigens, although it tends to become less abundant subsequently. It is the class most frequently found as "natural" antibodies against such antigens as the blood group determinants (see Chapter 5). IgM (often accompanied by IgD) is the most common immunoglobulin expressed on the surfaces of B cells, particularly virgin B lymphocytes. IgM is also the most efficient complement-fixing immunoglobulin: a single molecule of antigen-bound IgM suffices to initiate the complement cascade. Fc receptors specific for IgM exist but have not been well characterized.

Immunoglobulin D (IgD)

The IgD molecule is a monomeric 4-chain unit with a molecular weight of approximately 180,000. Although IgD is commonly found on the surfaces of B lymphocytes that also bear surface IgM, it is rarely secreted in significant amounts and only traces of it are normally found in the blood. In cells that coexpress IgD and IgM, both classes of heavy chains are produced by alternative splicing of a single RNA (see Chapter 7) and have identical antigen specificity. The IgD on these cells can bind antigen and transmit signals to the cell interior, with consequences that appear identical to those produced by IgM. When such B cells become activated, surface IgD expression ceases.

The physiologic function of IgD is unknown. It is relatively labile to degradation by heat or proteolytic enzymes. There are isolated reports of IgD with antibody activity toward insulin, penicillin, milk proteins, diphtheria toxoid, nuclear components, or thyroid antigens. Its presence on many mature virgin lymphocytes has suggested an as yet unproven role in B cell differentiation or tolerance.

Immunoglobulin E (IgE)

Although it normally represents only a minute fraction (0.004%) of all serum antibodies, IgE is extremely important from the clinical standpoint because of its central involvement in **allergic disorders.** Two specialized types of inflammatory cells that are involved in allergic responses—the **mast cell** and the **basophil**—carry a unique, high-affinity Fc receptor that is specific for IgE antibodies. Thus, despite the very low concentration of IgE in body fluids (roughly 10^{-7} M), the surfaces of these cells are constantly decorated with IgE antibodies, adsorbed from the blood, that serve as antigen receptors. When its passively bound IgE molecules contact an antigen, the mast cell or basophil releases inflammatory mediator substances that produce many of the acute manifestations of allergic disease (see Chapters 11 and 24). Elevated levels of serum IgE may also signify infection by **helminths** or certain other types of multicellular **parasites** (see Chapter 50). Like IgG and IgD, IgE exists only in monomeric form.

Fc RECEPTORS

Many cell types that cannot synthesize immunoglobulins are able to adsorb circulating antibodies onto their surfaces by way of **Fc receptors.** Receptors for each of the heavy-chain classes have been observed, but only those for γ and ε have been characterized at the molecular level. Humans express 3 different Fcγ and 2 different Fcε receptors, each of which has a characteristic tissue distribution and biologic properties (Table 6–4). In general, the high-affinity receptors of each type (designated FcγRI and FcεRI, respectively) are most likely to bind immunoglobulins under normal conditions and so produce the most notable biologic effects.

The physiologic functions of Fc receptors differ among cell types. Binding of secreted IgG molecules onto Fcγ receptors on macrophages or natural killer cells serves to "arm" these cells to carry out **antibody-dependent cell-mediated cytotoxicity (ADCC)** (see Chapter 3). Fc receptors also facilitate phagocytosis of antibody-coated particles through the phenomenon of **opsonization** and are important for triggering chemotaxis and **degranulation** in neutrophils and other phagocytes. Binding of antigens to the FcεRI-associated IgE on a basophil or mast cell provides the signal for degranulation and can lead to allergic symptoms. In contrast, Fc receptors on B lymphoid cells enable these cells to sense local antibody concentrations, providing an important feedback pathway that limits further antibody production.

IMMUNOGLOBULIN VARIABLE REGIONS

The V regions, which coincide with the N-terminal domains of light and heavy chains, mediate antigen binding and are by far the most heterogeneous portions of these proteins. Indeed, no 2 human myeloma proteins from different patients have ever been found

Table 6–4. Properties of human Fc receptors.

	Associated Markers[1]	Affinity (K_d)	Relative Subclass Preference	Cell Type Distribution
IgG receptors				
FcγRI	CD64	10^{-8}M	IgG1 = IgG3 > IgG4	Monocytes, macrophages
FcγRII	CD32	10^{-7}M	IgG1 = IgG3 > IgG2	Monocytes, macrophages, neutrophils, eosinophils, B lymphocytes
FcγRIII	CD16	10^{-6}M	IgG1 = IgG3	Macrophages, neutrophils, eosinophils, NK cells[2]
IgE receptors				
FcεRI	—	10^{-9}M	—	Mast cells, basophils
FcεRII	CD23	10^{-7}M	—	Eosinophils, monocytes, macrophages, platelets, some T and B cells

[1]CD designations generally apply to only one polypeptide chain of these multichain receptors.
[2]NK, natural killer (see Chapter 8).

to have identical V-region sequences. However, some clear patterns can be discerned. V_H regions show significantly more resemblance to one another than to V_L regions, while V_κ and V_λ sequences each have characteristic features that distinguish them from each other and from V_H. Thus, V_H, V_κ, and V_λ sequences can be recognized as separate groups that each associate with their own characteristic constant regions. There is never any mixing: a given V_H sequence, for example, may be found on heavy chains of any class (μ, δ, γ, α, or ε) but is never found on a light chain.

Framework & Hypervariable Regions

Variable regions within any single group are not uniformly variable across their entire 110-amino-acid spans. Instead, they consist of relatively invariant stretches (called **framework regions**) of 15–30 amino acids separated by shorter regions of extreme variability (called **hypervariable regions**) that are each 9–12 amino acids long. V_H and V_L regions each contain 3 hypervariable regions, whose approximate locations are depicted in Fig 6–4. Antigen-binding is mediated by noncovalent interactions that primarily involve amino acids in the hypervariable regions of each chain; hence, the sequences of these regions are the primary determinants of antigen specificity. Hypervariable regions are also called **complementarity-**

determining regions (CDRs) and within each chain are designated CDR1, CDR2, and CDR3, beginning with the one nearest the amino terminus. CDR3 is usually the longest and most variable of the three, since specialized genetic mechanisms act to increase sequence diversity in this region (see Chapter 7).

V-Region Subgroups

When sequences of many variable regions from any one type of chain (V_H, V_κ, or V_λ) are compared, they are found to form subgroups that are more similar to one another than to the remaining V regions in the group. For example, human V_κ regions have been classified into 4 **subgroups,** and similar subgroups exist for the V_H and V_λ regions. The subgroups differ from one another principally in the length and position of amino acid insertions and deletions within their framework regions.

Idiotypes

The term **idiotype** refers to the unique V-region amino acid sequences of the homogeneous immunoglobulin molecules produced by a single B cell clone. Thus, there are as many idiotypes as there are B cell clones (perhaps about 10^8 in an adult).

The concept of idiotype (which means "self type") was first derived from experiments in which inbred

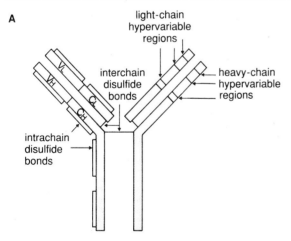

A

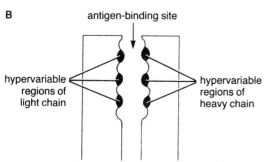

B

Figure 6–4. A: Schematic depiction of an IgG molecule showing the approximate locations of the hypervariable regions (also called complementarity-determining regions [CDRs]) in the heavy and light chains. Each CDR is roughly 9–12 residues long and is centered around residues 30–33, 56, or 94–98 of the polypeptide chain. **B:** Schematic depiction of how the 3 CDRs in each heavy- and light-chain pair might form an antigen-binding site.

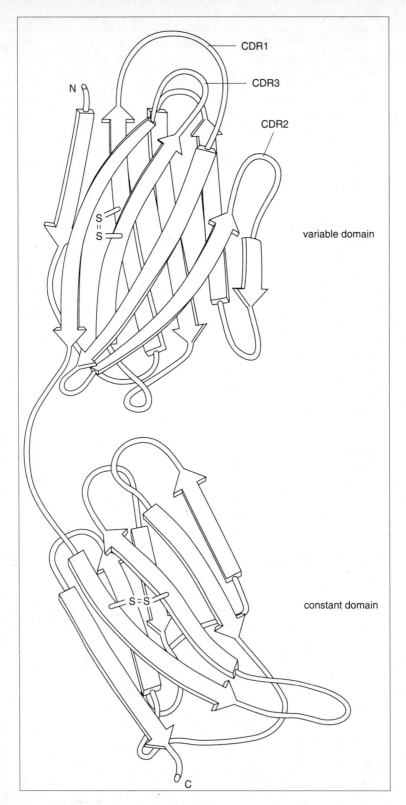

Figure 6–5. Three-dimensional structure of a light chain. In this ribbon diagram tracing the polypeptide backbone, β-strands are shown as wide ribbons, other regions as narrow strings. Each of the 2 globular domains consists of a barrel-shaped assembly of 7–9 antiparallel β-strands. The three hypervariable regions (CDR1, CDR2, and CDR3) are flexible loops that project outward from the amino-terminal end of the V_L domain.

animals were inoculated with purified antibody proteins that had been raised against a particular antigen in genetically identical animals. The inoculated animals mounted an antibody response against the injected immunoglobulin, implying that some sequences within it were recognized as foreign, but these antibodies would not react with other immunoglobulins from the same strain of animal. The antiserum produced in such a response was called an **anti-idiotype** antiserum. It was soon observed that the reaction between an anti-hapten antibody and its corresponding anti-idiotypic antiserum could, in some cases, be inhibited by the hapten, indicating that the idiotypic determinants were close to or within the antigen-binding site. It is now known that anti-idiotype antibodies specifically recognize sequences in the hypervariable regions of the target antibody, which are unique to that antibody and determine its antigen specificity. Thus, in current usage, the term "idiotype" refers to the global characteristics of the antigen-binding site in a given immunoglobulin, which are determined by the hypervariable sequences of its particular V_H and V_L domains.

THE 3-DIMENSIONAL STRUCTURE OF IMMUNOGLOBULINS

The complete 3-dimensional structures of several immunoglobulin molecules have been deduced from x-ray crystallographic studies. Such studies provide conclusive evidence that all of the individual globular domains in heavy and light chains share a common folded structure, despite the considerable differences in their amino acid sequences. Each domain is folded into a rigid, roughly cylindric scaffold made up of 7–9 strands of antiparallel β-sheet that are aligned like the staves of a barrel (Fig 6–5). In V_H and V_L domains, the 3 hypervariable sequences each occupy a position between individual β-strands and form relatively flexible loops that project outward from one "rim" of the barrel to participate in antigen-binding. A single antigen-binding site is formed by the apposition of 6 hypervariable loops: 3 from V_H and 3 from V_L.

Complete crystallographic structures have been obtained for only a few antibodies or Fab fragments complexed with their target antigens or with haptens. These structures confirm the expectation that antigen-binding is carried out mainly by residues in the hypervariable regions (especially CDR3) but demonstrate that nearby residues in the framework regions can also participate in binding. In general, haptens tend to bind by nestling into small (10–15-Å) crevices in the antigen-binding site, whereas macromolecular antigens interact over larger regions on the surface of the site. For example, 16 separate residues in lysozyme were found to interact with nearly 20 residues spread over a 20- by 30-Å surface formed by the six CDR loops of one anti-lysozyme Fab fragment.

Structural studies also reveal the strong tendency of immunoglobulin domains to adhere to one another laterally through noncovalent (especially hydrophobic) bonding (Fig 6–6). Thus, pairs of heavy and light chains are held together side by side not only by disulfide bonds but also by extensive noncovalent interactions between the C_H1 and C_L domains. Simi-

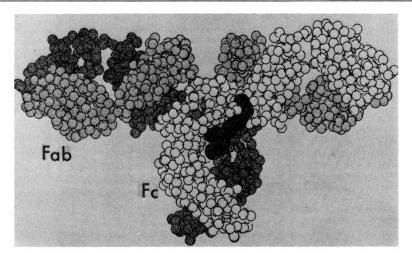

Figure 6–6. Three-dimensional structure of an immunoglobulin molecule. (Reproduced, with permission, from Silverton EW, Navia MA, Davies DR: Three-dimensional structure of an intact human immunoglobulin. *Proc Natl Acad Sci USA* 1977;**74:**5140.)

larly, the heavy chains within each 4-chain unit adhere to one another in part through strong hydrophobic contacts between C_H3 domains. These interdomain interactions are mediated by hydrophobic residues that occupy one lateral face of the barrel and that tend to be relatively conserved among all immunoglobulin domains.

IMMUNOGLOBULIN GENE SUPERFAMILY

The repetitive domain structure of immunoglobulin polypeptides reflects the manner in which their genes evolved. It is thought that the common ancestor of all immunoglobulin proteins was a single primordial exon that encoded a single copy of the barrellike polypeptide domain. In light of the tendency of modern immunoglobulin domains to adhere to one another noncovalently, it could be speculated that the protein product of this exon originally served to mediate some advantageous protein-protein interaction in—or, perhaps, surface interactions among—the ancestral cells that expressed it. Over evolutionary time, this unique primordial exon appears to have been reduplicated many times at the DNA level, so that additional copies were produced at both nearby and distant chromosomal locations. The sequences of these individual copies then diverged as a result of random mutations and natural selection. Every modern immunoglobulin light chain can thus be viewed as a tandemly duplicated descendent of the primordial domain, whereas heavy chains each represent tandem arrays of 4 or 5 such domains.

The descendants of this hypothetic primordial domain have been found not only in immunoglobulins but also in many other types of proteins (Table 6–5). Although their sequences have diverged greatly, the single or multiple immunoglobulinlike domains in

Table 6–5. The immunoglobulin gene superfamily.[1]

Immunoglobulin heavy and light chains
T cell receptor α, β, γ, and δ chains
CD3 complex γ, δ, and ε chains
Major histocompatibility complex proteins, class I and class II, and β$_2$-microglobulin
T cell differentiation antigens CD2, CD7, CD4, and CD8
Other CD proteins: CD1, CD5, CD16, CD19, CD22, CD28, CD54, CD56, and CD58
Adhesion proteins: VCAM-1, ICAM-1, ICAM-2, LFA-3, and N-CAM
Cytokine receptors for IL-1, IL-6, M-CSF, G-CSF, stem-cell factor (SCF), and platelet-derived growth factor (PDGF)
Poly-Ig receptor
Thy-1
Carcinoembryonic antigen

[1]VCAM-1, vascular cell adhesion molecule type 1; ICAM-1 and -2, intercellular adhesion molecule types 1 and 2; LFA-3, leukocyte functional antigen type 3; N-CAM, neural cell adhesion molecule. ICAM-1 and LFA-3 are also designated CD54 and CD58, respectively.

each of these proteins can be recognized by their size and 3-dimensional shape, by the characteristic position of the intrachain disulfide bond, and by a few other conserved features. In recognition of their common ancestry, these proteins (or their corresponding genes) are known collectively as the **immunoglobulin gene superfamily.** Most, but not all, are integral membrane proteins. In any given member of this family, the immunoglobulinlike domains may be found in association with other, unrelated types of domains that confer specialized activities, such as transmembrane signaling. Members of this superfamily are found at widely scattered chromosomal locations, are expressed in diverse cell types, and subserve many different functions, but in each case the immunoglobulinlike sequences appear to retain their ancestral function of interacting with other immunoglobulinlike domains in the same or other proteins.

REFERENCES

Early Studies of Immunoglobulin Protein Chemistry

Hilschmann N, Craig LC: Amino acid sequence studies with Bence Jones protein. *Proc Natl Acad Sci USA* 1965;**53**:1403.

Porter RR: Structural studies of immunoglobulins. *Science* 1973;**180**:713.

Wu TT, Kabat EA: An analysis of the variable regions of Bence Jones proteins and myeloma light chains and their implications for antibody complementarity. *J Exp Med* 1970;**132**:211.

Immunoglobulin Chains & Related Polypeptides

Kehry M et al: The immunoglobulin μ chains of membrane-bound and secreted IgM molecules differ in their C-terminal segments. *Cell* 1980;**21**:393.

Koshland ME: The coming of age of the immunoglobulin J chain. *Annu Rev Immunol* 1985;**3**:425.

Natvig JB, Kunkel HG: Immunoglobulins: Classes, subclasses, genetic variants, and idiotypes. *Adv Immunol* 1973;**16**:1.

Biologic Properties of Immunoglobulins

Blattner FR, Tucker PW: The molecular biology of immunoglobulin D. *Nature* 1984;**307**:417.

Spiegelberg HL: Biological activities of immunoglobulins of different classes and subclasses. *Adv Immunol* 1974;**19**:259.

Antibody Structure

Alzari PN et al: Three-dimensional structure of antibodies. *Annu Rev Immunol* 1988;**6:**555.

Amit AG et al: Three-dimensional structure of an antigen-antibody complex at 2.8 Å resolution. *Science* 1986;**233:**747.

Colman PM: Structure of antibody-antigen complexes: implications for immune recognition. *Adv Immunol* 1988;**43:**99.

Davie JM et al: Structural correlates of idiotypes. *Annu Rev Immunol* 1986;**4:**147.

Davies DR, Padlan EA: Antibody-antigen complexes. *Annu Rev Biochem* 1990;**59:**439.

Fc Receptors

Ravetch JV, Kinet J-P: Fc receptors. *Annu Rev Immunol* 1991;**9:**457.

Immunoglobulin Gene Superfamily

Hunkapiller T, Hood L: Diversity of the immunoglobulin gene superfamily. *Adv Immunol* 1989;**44:**1.

Williams AF, Barclay AN: The immunoglobulin superfamily—domains for cell surface recognition. *Annu Rev Immunol* 1988;**6:**381.

7

Immunoglobulin Genes, B Cells, and the Humoral Immune Response

Tristram G. Parslow, MD, PhD

To contend with the almost unlimited variety of antigens that it may encounter, the human immune system is able to produce an estimated 10^8 different antibody molecules, each with a unique specificity for antigen. How can so many different antibody proteins be encoded in the genes of every human being? As discussed in this chapter, the source of this diversity of antibodies lies in the structure of the immunoglobulin genes and in the remarkable ability of B cells to create and modify these genes by rearranging their own chromosomal DNA. The properties of immunoglobulin genes, in turn, provide a basis for understanding many aspects of B cell differentiation and of the humoral immune response. Although the antigen specificity of each B cell is determined randomly early in its life by the structure of its immunoglobulin genes, its survival, proliferation, and secretory activity are all ultimately governed by the antigens it encounters.

IMMUNOGLOBULIN GENES ARE FORMED THROUGH DNA REARRANGEMENT IN B CELLS

The antigen specificity of an antibody is determined by amino acid sequences within its paired heavy- and light-chain variable domains, which together form the antigen-binding site (see Chapter 6). To produce antibodies with many different specificities, the immune system must have the genetic capability to produce a very large number of different variable-domain sequences. The sequence of the constant region, on the other hand, is generally the same for all heavy or light chains of a given immunoglobulin class and has no effect on an antigen specificity. In fact, the entire family of immunoglobulin proteins consists of a relatively small number of different constant-region domains linked in various combinations with an almost unlimited assortment of variable-region sequences. In 1965, Dreyer and Bennett

first recognized that these interchangeable combinations of protein domains must be the result of an active reshuffling of gene fragments that took place within the B cell chromosomes. This was a revolutionary insight, because it implied that a cell could efficiently manipulate its chromosomes to change the structure of genes that it had inherited. And yet this proved to be only a part of the story: nearly a decade later, Tonegawa made the remarkable discovery that the inherited chromosomes contain no immunoglobulin genes at all but only the building blocks from which these genes can be assembled. Since that time, studies by many investigators have revealed in detail the extraordinary process through which a B cell precursor assembles an immunoglobulin gene.

As with most human genes, the information that codes for an immunoglobulin protein is dispersed along the DNA strand in multiple coding segments (**exons**) that are separated by regions of noncoding DNA (**introns**); after the gene is transcribed into RNA, introns are removed from the transcript and the exons are joined by RNA splicing. Unlike nearly all other genes, however, the immunoglobulin DNA sequences that are found in germ cells or other non-lymphoid cell types do not exist as intact, functional genes. This is because the exons that code for variable domains are normally broken up along the chromosome into still smaller gene segments; these segments each lack some of the features needed for proper RNA splicing and so cannot function individually as exons. Before a developing B cell can begin to synthesize immunoglobulin, it must first fuse 2 or 3 of these gene segments to assemble a complete variable-region exon. This fusion of gene segments is achieved through a highly specialized process that requires cutting, rearrangement, and rejoining of the chromosomal DNA strands. Only developing lymphocytes possess the enzymatic machinery that is needed to carry out this process of immunoglobulin gene rearrangement.

Light-Chain Genes

The kappa (κ) light chain genes are simplest and will be considered first. All of the genetic information needed to produce κ chains lies within a single locus on chromosome 2 (Fig 7–1). The constant domain of the protein (amino acids 109–214) is encoded by an exon called $C_κ$ and only one copy of this exon is found on the chromosome. The sequence encoding any given variable domain, however, is contained in 2 separate gene segments called the variable ($V_κ$) and joining ($J_κ$) segments. The $V_κ$ segment encodes approximately the first 95 amino acids of the variable domain; the shorter $J_κ$ segment codes for the remaining 13 (amino acids 96–108). In contrast to the single $C_κ$ exon, multiple $V_κ$ and $J_κ$ segments are present, each with a somewhat different DNA sequence. The 5 $J_κ$ segments are clustered near the $C_κ$ exon, while at least 100 different $V_κ$ segments lie scattered over a region that spans more than $2 × 10^6$ bp of DNA (roughly 1% of the length of chromosome 2). This wide separation between $V_κ$ and $J_κ$ segments is found in the DNA of all nonlymphoid cells. When an immature hematopoietic cell becomes committed to the B lymphocyte lineage, however, it selects one Vκ and one Jκ segment and fuses these. This process of **V/J joining** is accomplished by highly precise enzymatic manipulation of specific sites in the chromosomal DNA. In some instances, this involves precise deletion of all the DNA that normally separates the $V_κ$ and $J_κ$ segments; in others, the 2 segments are brought together by inverting a portion of the chromosomal strand with no overall loss of DNA (Fig 7–2). The result in either case is that the $V_κ$ and $J_κ$ segments become permanently and covalently joined to one another, side by side on the rearranged chromosome, to form a single continuous exon. Transcription can then begin at one end of the $V_κ$ segment and pass through both the fused $V_κ/J_κ$ exon and the nearby $C_κ$ exon. When transcribed together, these 2 exons contain all of the information needed to synthesize a particular κ protein.

The organization of the κ genes thus accounts for the unusual properties of this light-chain protein family. Since there is only one $C_κ$ exon, all κ proteins must have identical constant-region sequences. On the other hand, because the cell can choose from among many alternative $V_κ$ and $J_κ$ segments and can join these together in various combinations, a large number of different variable-domain sequences can result. For example, 100 $V_κ$ and 5 $J_κ$ segments could in theory give rise to $(100 × 5 =)$ 500 different variable domains. This reshuffling process, known as **combinatorial joining,** is the most important source of light-chain protein diversity.

Lambda (λ) light chains arise from a similar gene complex on chromosome 22. Joining of $V_λ$ and $J_λ$ segments occurs in a manner identical to that of the κ segments. A given chromosome 22, however, may contain up to 6 slightly different copies of the $C_λ$ exon (corresponding to various subtypes of λ protein), each with a nearby $J_λ$ segment. A $V_λ$ segment (of which there are approximately 100) may fuse to any of these alternative $J_λ$ segments, and the resulting $V_λ/J_λ$ exon can then be transcribed together with the adjacent $C_λ$ exon. The B cell selects only one of the available $J_λ$ segments for V/J joining and, in so doing, determines which $C_λ$ subtype will be expressed (Fig 7–3).

Heavy-Chain Genes

All immunoglobulin heavy chains are derived from a single region on chromosome 14 (Fig 7–4). Each heavy chain constant region is encoded by a cluster of several short exons. The μ constant region, for example, is divided among 5 exons known collectively as the Cμ sequence. Constant-region (C_H) sequences for each of the 9 heavy-chain isotypes are arrayed in tandem along the chromosome in the following order: $C_μ$, $C_δ$, $C_{γ3}$, $C_{γ1}$, $C_{α1}$, $C_{γ2}$, $C_{γ4}$, $C_ε$, $C_{α2}$; only a single copy of each is present. The 6 J_H segments and at least 100 (perhaps as many as 1000) V_H segments are arranged in a manner analogous to those of the κ gene. In contrast to the light-chain genes, however, a third type of gene segment, called the diversity (D_H) segment, must also be used in forming a heavy-chain variable region. Several of these D_H segments (the exact number is unknown), each coding for 2 or 3 amino acids, lie between the J_H and V_H segments on the unrearranged chromosome. In assembling the heavy-chain gene, a B cell must

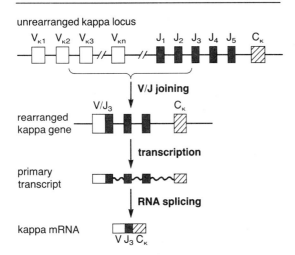

Figure 7–1. Assembly and expression of the κ light-chain locus. A DNA rearrangement event fuses one V segment (in this example, $V_κ2$) to one J segment ($J_κ3$) to form a single exon. The V/J exon is then transcribed together with the unique $C_κ$ exon, and the transcript is spliced to form mature κ mRNA. Note that any unrearranged J segments on the primary transcript are removed as part of the intron during RNA splicing.

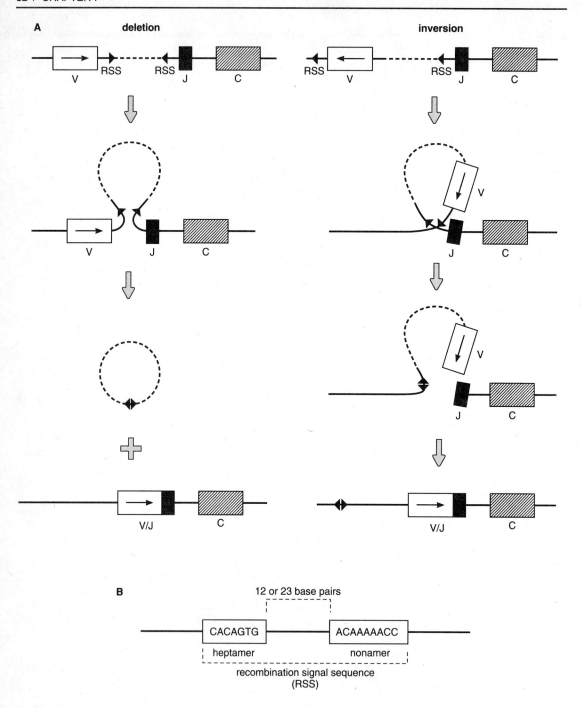

Figure 7–2. Mechanism of immunoglobulin κ gene rearrangement. **A:** Site-specific cleavage and religation of the chromosomal DNA is guided by a pair of recombination signal sequences (RSS) flanking V and J gene segments. The chromosome segment undergoes either deletion (left) or inversion (right), depending on the original orientation of the V segment with respect to the J and C segments. If deletion occurs, the DNA that originally separated V and J is released as a covalently closed circle and subsequently is degraded. **B:** The RSS, consisting of a pair of short DNA sequences (heptamer and nonamer) separated by either 12 or 23 bp of DNA, marks all sites of recombinase action in both heavy- and light-chain genes.

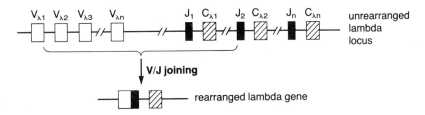

Figure 7–3. Assembly of a λ light-chain gene. An individual λ locus contains up to 6 alternative C_λ exons, each with nearby J_λ segment. In this example, DNA rearrangement fuses $V_{\lambda 1}$ with $J_{\lambda 2}$; the resulting gene will produce light chains that contain $C_{\lambda 2}$.

complete 2 DNA rearrangement events, first bringing together one D_H and one J_H segment, and subsequently linking these to a V_H segment. This sequence is termed **V/D/J joining.**

Use of the D_H segment greatly increases the amount of heavy-chain diversity that can be produced. For example, 100 V_H, 10 D_H, and 6 J_H segments could give rise to ($100 \times 10 \times 6$ =) 6000 different heavy-chain variable domains, and these, when combined with 500 κ-chain variable domains, could form (500×6000 =) 3 million different antigen-binding sites! Even with a relatively small number of gene segments, then, the immune system can generate enormous antibody diversity through combinatorial joining.

Additional diversity of heavy-chain variable-regions arises because the V/D/J rearrangement process is somewhat imprecise, so that the site at which one segment fuses with another can vary by a few nucleotides. As a result, the DNA coding sequence that remains at the junction between any 2 segments can also vary. Moreover, during assembly of a heavy-chain gene (but not one of light-chain genes), a few nucleotides of random sequence (called **N regions**) are often inserted at the points of joining between the V, D, and J segments; these insertions are known to be

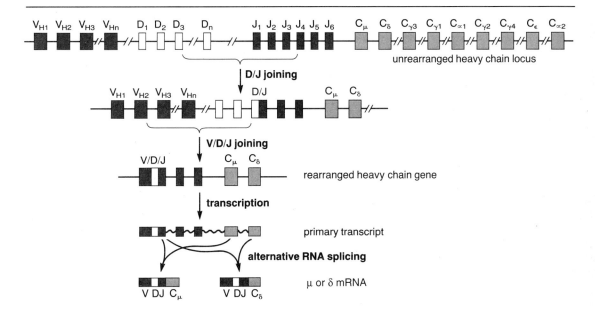

Figure 7–4. Rearrangement and expression of the heavy-chain locus. Unlike the light-chain genes, assembly of a heavy-chain V region exon requires 2 sequential DNA rearrangement events involving 3 different types of gene segments. The D_H and J_H segments are joined first and are then fused to a V_H segment. Nine alternative C region sequences are present; of these, however, only C_μ and C_δ are initially transcribed. The primary transcript can be spliced in either of 2 ways to generate mRNAs that encode μ or δ heavy chains with identical V domains. This diagram is highly schematic: each C_H sequence is actually composed of multiple exons whose aggregate length is more than 3 times longer than that of the V/D/J exon.

produced by **terminal deoxynucleotidyltransferase (TdT),** a nuclear enzyme that is expressed in immature lymphocytes. The variations in gene sequence that result from **imprecise joining** or from the insertion of N regions contribute substantially to overall antibody diversity. Moreover, these processes selectively affect the sequences that code for the third **hypervariable region (CDR3)** of the heavy- or light-chain variable domain (see Chapter 6); hence, the diversity they engender has a disproportionately strong effect on antigen specificity. At the same time, however, these processes greatly increase the risk that 2 segments may be joined in an improper translational reading frame, resulting in a nonfunctional gene. In practice, such unsuccessful rearrangements occur frequently and generally cannot be reversed or repaired; they represent a cost paid by the immune system in exchange for greater potential gene diversity.

In general, only the C_H region located immediately downstream of the V/D/J exon can be expressed. Because the V/D/J exon is originally assembled at a site adjacent to the C_μ locus, the gene always produces μ heavy chains when it is first rearranged. For this reason, virgin B lymphocytes always express IgM on their surfaces. Expression of one of the other C_H regions can occur only after a cell becomes activated in the periphery, as described below. One important exception to this rule is the C_δ sequence, which lies very near the C_μ region and is often transcribed along with the V/D/J and C_μ exons. This produces RNA that can be spliced to yield either μ or δ mRNA (Fig 7–4) and so enables the cell to simultaneously express IgM and IgD antibodies that have identical variable-domain sequences. Such coexpression of IgM and IgD on the surface membrane is a common phenotype of mature B lymphocytes.

Molecular Basis of V/(D)/J Rearrangement

Active gene rearrangements of the type that produce V/(D)/J joining (that is, either V/J or V/D/J joining) were first thought to be a unique property of the immunoglobulin genes. Subsequently, however, identical rearrangements were found to be involved in producing the genes that encode T lymphocyte antigen receptors, which are similar to immunoglobulins in many respects (see Chapter 8). Rearrangement of both the immunoglobulin and T cell antigen receptor gene families is carried out by the same molecular machinery: a presumably complex system of enzymes and other proteins that are known collectively as the **V/(D)/J recombinase.** This term must be used loosely, however, since none of the proteins that carry out lymphocyte gene rearrangements has yet been identified with certainty. It appears that at least some of the steps in recognizing, cleaving, and religating the various gene segments may be carried out by cellular enzymes that are also involved in more common types of DNA repair. In addition, 2 recently identified proteins known as **RAG-1** and **RAG-2** (the products of recombination-activating genes 1 and 2, respectively) have been found to act together to stimulate V/(D)/J recombination. It is not yet known whether the RAG-1 and RAG-2 proteins participate directly in recombination or simply regulate the expression of recombinase components.

The V/(D)/J recombinase is known to identify potential rearrangement sites on the chromosome by the presence of a pair of short DNA sequences (7 and 9 bp long) that together form the **recombination signal sequence** (Fig 7–2B). These sequences are found immediately adjacent to each unrearranged V, D, or J segment; their relative positions and orientations guide the recombinase to ensure that segments are joined in the proper order and alignment to produce a functional exon.

V/(D)/J recombinase activity appears to be unique to B and T lymphoid cells: no other cell type has yet been proven to manipulate its chromosomes in this manner. Moreover, recombinase activity is present only during the early phases of lymphoid development that take place within the lymphopoietic organs. By the time a virgin B cell emerges from the marrow, it has rearranged both its heavy- and light-chain genes and has forever lost the ability to perform further V/(D)/J rearrangements. The orderly manner in which the recombinase carries out its task defines the stages of B cell ontogeny.

IMMUNOGLOBULIN GENE REARRANGEMENTS & EARLY B CELL ONTOGENY

The DNA rearrangements that assemble immunoglobulin genes occur in a strict developmental sequence (Fig 7–5). The first rearrangements take place in a population of mitotically active bone marrow cells, sometimes referred to as **pro-B cells,** which are perhaps the most primitive recognizable cells in the B lineage. These cells are not well characterized but are known to display surface CD10 and CD19, as well as the nuclear proteins TdT, RAG-1, and RAG-2 (Fig 7–6).

The first rearrangement that occurs in a pro-B cell is the joining of D_H and J_H segments in the heavy-chain genes. This occurs on both copies of chromosome 14. The cell then attempts to join a V_H segment to the fused D_H/J_H segment on one of its 2 chromosomes. If this first attempt yields a functional gene, the cell (for reasons discussed below) carries out no further rearrangements of its other heavy-chain locus. If, on the other hand, the first rearrangement fails, a second attempt at V/D/J assembly is made with the other chromosome 14. Because of the error-prone nature of V/D/J joining, about 50% of pro-B cells fail at both tries to produce a functional heavy-chain gene;

pro-B cell

pre-B cell

early
B lymphocyte

1) express TdT
2) assemble one functional heavy chain gene
3) express cytoplasmic μ chains
4) stop heavy chain rearrangements
5) stop TdT expression

1) assemble one functional light chain gene
2) express surface heavy (μ ± δ) and light chains
3) stop all rearrangements

Figure 7–5. Major genetic events in early B cell ontogeny. Listed are the sequences of events that occur in progressing from each stage of development to the next. Note that the ability to perform V/(D)/J rearrangements is lost by the time the cell becomes an early B lymphocyte.

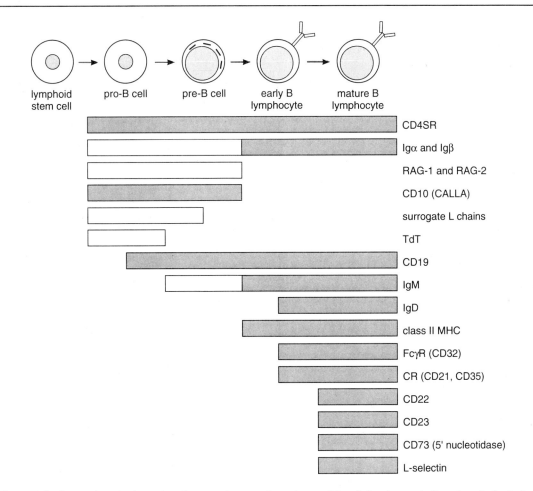

lymphoid stem cell   pro-B cell   pre-B cell   early B lymphocyte   mature B lymphocyte

CD4SR

Igα and Igβ

RAG-1 and RAG-2

CD10 (CALLA)

surrogate L chains

TdT

CD19

IgM

IgD

class II MHC

FcγR (CD32)

CR (CD21, CD35)

CD22

CD23

CD73 (5' nucleotidase)

L-selectin

Figure 7–6. Expression of selected marker proteins at various stages of B cell development. Open bars indicate that a protein is expressed only within the cytoplasm of a cell; stippled bars indicate surface expression.

unable to proceed further through the maturation pathway, these cells simply die in the marrow.

Successful V/D/J rearrangement on either chromosome allows the cell to immediately begin synthesizing heavy-chain proteins. The heavy chains produced at this stage are all of the μ isotype and have a short hydrophobic region at their carboxy termini that causes them to integrate into cellular membranes. This membrane-associated form of μ protein is called μ_m. Heavy chains generally cannot be transported to the cell surface unless they are complexed with light chains; therefore, most of the μ_m initially remains within the rough endoplasmic reticulum. However, a few of the heavy chains associate with proteins of a different type, known as **surrogate light chains,** to form a complex that is displayed transiently on the surface membranes of these immature cells. The surrogate light chains are not true immunoglobulin proteins: they are expressed only in primitive B cell precursors, are derived from genes that do not undergo somatic rearrangement, and have no role in immune responses per se. Nevertheless, they are thought to be essential for regulating early B cell development. When the μ_m and surrogate light chain proteins reach the cell surface, they are believed to transmit a signal back into the cell, perhaps after contacting some unknown ligand. In effect, this signal notifies the cell that it has produced a functional heavy-chain protein. In response, the cell permanently halts any further rearrangements of its heavy-chain genes and stops expressing TdT. It also ceases to express surrogate light chains, so that the temporary signaling complex disappears from the cell surface. These events mark the transition into the next phase of ontogeny, known as the pre-B stage.

Pre-B cells are defined as cells that do not yet express immunoglobulin light chains but contain μ_m heavy chains in their cytoplasm (Figs 7–5 and 7–6). They are found almost exclusively in the marrow and represent a transient phase in B cell development that lasts for about 2 days. On entering this phase, the cells cease dividing and will not resume mitosis until they have become fully mature and encountered antigen in the periphery. The most important event taking place in pre-B cells is the rearrangement of light-chain genes, which usually begins only after heavy-chain rearrangements have ceased. Because TdT no longer is expressed, no N-region nucleotides are inserted as the light-chain genes rearrange. V/J joining is attempted on each chromosome 2 or 22 in succession, until a functional κ or λ gene is produced. As soon as either type of light-chain protein appears, it associates with the existing heavy chains and the resulting 4-chain units are transported to the cell surface as monomeric membrane IgM. At that moment, the cell enters the B lymphocyte stage of development and permanently loses the ability to perform additional V/J rearrangements, presumably because RAG-1, RAG-2, and other essential components of the recombinase are lost or inactivated. It seems likely that the signal to shut off the recombinase is sent by the IgM molecules themselves when they first reach the cell surface.

As outlined above, the successful assembly of a single heavy- or light-chain gene prevents all other genes of that type from undergoing rearrangement in the same cell. Consequently, only one heavy-chain and one light-chain gene can give rise to protein in any individual B lymphocyte—a phenomenon termed **allelic and isotypic exclusion.** If the lymphocyte subsequently divides in the periphery, chromosomes bearing the active rearranged genes will be passed on to its progeny and the daughter cells will continue to express these genes without performing further V/J or V/D/J rearrangements. For this reason, all of the immunoglobulin molecules produced by a given B lymphocyte and its progeny have identical antigen specificity and light-chain type (κ or λ). This is the molecular basis of the phenomenon known as **clonal restriction** (see Chapter 3). The diversity of antibody molecules produced by the immune system as a whole reflects the fact that innumerable B cell precursors each rearrange their genes independently and in different combinations, resulting in a large assortment of clones that each possess a unique specificity for antigen.

MATURATION & RELEASE OF VIRGIN B LYMPHOCYTES

The moment it begins to express surface IgM, a cell is considered to have become a B lymphocyte. Nevertheless, it is not yet ready to exit the bone marrow or to participate in immune responses. Instead, such **early B lymphocytes** remain in the marrow for another 1–3 days, during which time they acquire additional surface molecules that distinguish them as **mature B lymphocytes** (Fig 7–6). One such marker is surface **IgD,** which, as noted previously, is produced by alternative splicing of some of the RNA transcripts arising from the rearranged heavy-chain gene; the IgM and IgD on any individual lymphocyte both incorporate the same light chains and have identical antigen specificity. Other surface markers that appear on mature B lymphocytes include complement receptors; a membrane-anchored enzyme called **5′ nucleotidase (CD73),** whose function is unknown; the lectinlike oligosaccharide-binding protein **CD23;** and the adhesion proteins LFA-1, ICAM-1, and **CD22.** Individual cells also begin to express surface homing receptors, such as **L-selectin,** which will target them to lymph nodes or other peripheral sites. At about the same time, the cells acquire **class II MHC** proteins, which enable them to present antigens to helper T cells, and they also begin surface expression of **CD40,** a protein involved in receiving T cell help (see below). With the acquisition of these various accessory molecules, the mature lymphocytes become competent for immunologic function. They are then released from the marrow to disseminate through the bloodstream and colonize secondary lymphoid organs.

The developmental pathway outlined above is typical of the B cell population as a whole but does not apply strictly to all of its cells. Individual B-lineage cells may differ significantly in the types and amounts of surface markers they express or the sequence in which these markers are acquired. Thus far, however, it has not proven fruitful to distinguish any specific subsets of B lymphocytes. One possible exception is the small, enigmatic subpopulation of B cells that express surface CD5, a protein of unknown function that is also expressed on most T lymphocytes. These **CD5 B cells** are long-lived cells that are found principally in the peritoneal cavity and appear to be derived from precursor cells that are present in infant but not adult bone marrow. They are disproportionately more likely than other B cells to produce autoreactive immunoglobulins (ie, antibodies that recognize determinants in host tissues). Remarkably, the malignant cells in nearly all cases of human B cell **chronic lymphocytic leukemia** carry the CD5 marker. No unique immunologic function has yet been assigned to CD5 B cells, however, and it is not clear whether they represent a truly distinct developmental lineage.

Virgin B lymphocytes are continually produced in the bone marrow, independently of exogenous antigens. The marrow of an adult releases approximately 10^9 virgin B cells into the circulation each day regardless of the immunologic history of the individual. The vast repertoire of variable regions expressed by these cells is also unaffected by prior antigen exposure, being determined by the more or less random joining of V, D, and J gene segments into various combinations. As a result, no more than about one in 100,000 newly minted B cells is capable of recognizing any individual epitope. Moreover, although they can home efficiently into lymphoid tissues or sites of ongoing inflammation, virgin B cells are mitotically and immunologically inert and have very limited life spans. Nearly all will die within a few days unless they are roused from their quiescent state. Only those that become activated will survive.

B Lymphocyte Activation

Surface immunoglobulin is anchored in the membrane by a short, hydrophobic tail at the carboxyl terminus of the heavy chain. Since the tail projects only a few amino acids into the cytoplasm, an immunoglobulin alone cannot transmit signals across the membrane. Instead, membrane immunoglobulins of all types must associate with two other proteins, called **Ig-α** and **Ig-β**, to form a functional signaling complex (Fig 7–7). Ig-α and Ig-β are transmembrane glycoproteins, each of which includes a large

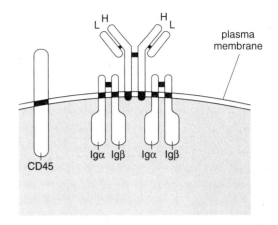

Figure 7–7. Antigen-receptor transmembrane signaling complex on mature B cells. Ig-α and Ig-β are disulfide-linked to one another but associate noncovalently with membrane immunoglobulins through their transmembrane and extracellular domains. The CD45 isoform CD45R is not physically linked with the antigen-receptor complex but may modulate its effects.

cytoplasmic domain resembling those of the CD3 proteins of T cells. Like the CD3 complex, Ig-α and Ig-β are thought to link the surface immunoglobulin with cytoplasmic protein tyrosine kinases (PTKs), which become functionally activated upon antigen binding.

With the exception of highly polymeric substances that act as T-independent antigens (see Chapter 4), most antigens are not sufficient by themselves to activate B cells. Antigen binding alone produces some changes (such as IL-2 receptor induction) that make the cell more receptive to other stimuli, but full activation under ordinary conditions requires help from activated CD4+ T cells. This help can come in the form of secreted cytokines—notably IL-2, IL-4, IL-6, and IL-10—which act only over extremely short distances from the helper cell. Although these cytokines are effective in combination, none is necessary or sufficient to mediate T cell help. On the other hand, direct contact with an activated CD4+ cell can produce a powerful helper effect even in the absence of cytokine secretion. Indeed, such contact can even activate B cells that have not bound antigen (the so-called **bystander** effect), although a combination of antigen binding and contact help yields the strongest proliferative responses. Contact-mediated help results from specific interactions between membrane proteins on the Tн and B cell surfaces. The best-characterized interaction of this type occurs between the B cell protein **CD40** and a protein called **CD40 ligand** (or **CD40L**) which appears on Tн cells only after they become activated. Binding of CD40 to CD40L appears to be an extremely important and effective mechanism of delivering T cell help in vivo. An inherited defect in CD40L causes a form of congenital immunodeficiency known as **hyper-IgM syndrome,** in which humoral immunity is impaired owing to a deficiency of T cell help.

In cells that coexpress surface IgM and IgD, both are capable of antigen-binding and signal transduction, and they produce identical effects. Certain accessory molecules on the B cell (such as CD22, complement receptors, and class II MHC proteins) can send signals that augment activation when they bind their cognate ligands. In contrast, activation tends to be suppressed by the binding of antigen-antibody complexes (especially those containing IgG) to B cell surface **Fc receptors;** this provides a negative feedback mechanism that may be important for terminating B cell responses once saturating amounts of antibody have been produced.

Another surface protein that may modulate activation is **CD45,** a membrane-spanning glycoprotein whose cytoplasmic domain has **protein tyrosine phosphatase** activity (ie, the ability to dephosphorylate tyrosines in other proteins). CD45 is found on all hematopoietic cells, but its molecular weight varies considerably among cell types owing to differences in the size of the extracellular domain that result from alternative mRNA splicing. B lymphocytes express the largest (MW 220,000) isoform of CD45, designated **CD45R.** Although its precise role is unknown, CD45R may function to prevent unwanted PTK activation in resting B cells or may transmit a signal that inhibits activation when it contacts some unknown ligand.

B Lymphocytes as Antigen-Presenting Cells

The encounter between a B cell and its cognate antigen occurs most often in a lymphoid organ (where the cells are most abundant) but may also take place in the bloodstream or in an inflamed tissue. A soluble protein antigen may bind directly to the cell surface immunoglobulin, but this interaction alone is not sufficient to activate the cell. Instead, the B lymphocyte must first function as an antigen-presenting cell to obtain help from nearby CD4+ T cells.

Human B lymphocytes constitutively express surface class II MHC proteins and so can present antigens to helper T cells without prior activation. Although a B cell could, in principle, present any antigen, it is exceptionally efficient at presenting antigens that bind to its surface immunoglobulins. This is because the immunoglobulin acts as a high-affinity receptor, enabling the B cell to capture concentrations of its cognate antigen several orders of magnitude lower than those needed to engage the low-affinity, broad-specificity receptors on other types of antigen-presenting cells. The bound antigen is taken into the B cell by receptor-mediated (in this case, immunoglobulin-mediated) endocytosis to be processed, and the resulting peptides are then displayed on the B-cell surface, where they may be recognized by T cells that have the appropriate antigen and MHC specificities (Fig 7–8). Note that, if the antigen is a complex protein, the B cell may produce and display from it many different processed peptides that can serve as T cell epitopes; these may or may not correspond to the B cell epitope originally recognized by the immunoglobulin. If this sequence of events leads to helper T cell activation, the presenting B cell is also likely to become activated, since it not only is receiving signals from the bound antigen but also is already in direct contact with the helper cell (Fig 7–8). Activated B cells express surface **B7** proteins, which are T cell costimulators, and they may also secrete **IL-6** and **TNFα**, which (like IL-1) increase the efficiency of Tн cell activation.

Although they offer unique advantages, B cells also have important limitations as antigen-presenting cells. They are not always present in large numbers at most sites in the body, and, because they have little phagocytic capacity, they are unable to process many types of particulate antigens. Most importantly, in an unimmunized person, B cells specific for any given antigen are exceedingly rare. Consequently, other types of antigen-presenting cells usually play the dominant role in initiating primary humoral responses. B cells then become increasingly important in this capacity at each subsequent encounter with antigen.

Immunoglobulin Secretion

When a B cell becomes activated and divides, its daughter cells do not regain the capacity for V/(D)/J rearrangement but, rather, continue to express the rearranged genes they inherited from their clonal forebears. Some undergo further differentiation to become **plasma cells,** which secrete large amounts of immunoglobulin derived from the same genes. Many of the cells that commit to becoming plasma cells migrate to the bone marrow in order to do so. As a result, the marrow contains the great majority of the

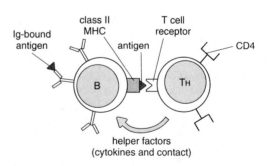

Figure 7–8. Antigen presentation by a B lymphocyte to a CD4+ T lymphocyte. Presentation does not require, but is likely to result in, activation of the B cell. Ig, immunoglobulin.

body's plasma cells and is the main source of circulating antibodies, especially during secondary immune responses. Plasma cells cannot replicate, and they survive for only a few days; hence, humoral responses wane quickly after an antigenic challenge subsides. At its peak, however, a plasma cell may secrete thousands of antibody molecules per minute.

The shift from producing membrane-bound to secreted immunoglobulin reflects a subtle change in the structure of the heavy-chain mRNA (Fig 7–4). The short hydrophobic tail that anchors a heavy-chain protein onto the cell membrane is encoded by the final 2 exons of every C_H region; when a B lymphocyte matures into a plasma cell, it produces an alternative form of heavy-chain mRNA that lacks these final exons and so encodes a heavy-chain protein that can be secreted from the cell (see Fig 2–4). For μ chains, this slightly truncated mRNA is designated μ_s. Clones that coexpress surface IgM and IgD almost always secrete only IgM (in pentameric form, complexed with J chains); IgD is rarely secreted, and, indeed, its function is unknown.

Memory B Lymphocytes

Most cells within a proliferating clone that do not differentiate into plasma cells instead revert to the resting state to become memory B lymphocytes. Many of these memory cells ultimately take up residence within lymphoid follicles, where they survive for years; if subsequently activated, they undergo further cycles of replication to produce still more memory and effector cells. In general, the progeny at each stage continue to express the same immunoglobulin genes as their parents. However, 2 specialized types of genetic processes occur at high frequency whenever memory B cells proliferate in the periphery. These processes, known as class switching and somatic hypermutation, further diversify the immunoglobulin genes expressed by some of the replicating cells and permanently alter the characteristics of their progeny. In the following sections, we will consider each of these phenomena in turn.

Heavy-Chain Class Switch

As a B cell clone proliferates, individual daughter cells often appear that express a heavy-chain class (such as γ or α) which differs from that of the founder (Fig 7–9A). This phenomenon is called **class switching** or isotype switching. It results from a specialized type of DNA rearrangement in the expressed heavy-chain gene, whereby a new C_H region is moved to a position adjacent to the existing V/D/J exon by deletion of all intervening C_H sequences on the chromosome (Fig 7–9B). Although class switching bears some resemblance to V/(D)/J joining, the 2 processes are believed to occur through entirely different enzymatic pathways. In particular, switching occurs in mature B cells that can no longer carry out V/(D)/J joining, and it occurs at chromosomal sites (called

switch regions) that are located several hundred bases away from the V/D/J and C_H exons themselves. Because class switching occurs by deleting one or more C_H regions, it is normally irreversible. Switching does not change the structure of the V/D/J exon and so does not affect antigen specificity.

Through the process of class switching, a preassembled V/D/J exon that was originally linked to C_μ can become associated with any of the other heavy-chain constant-region sequences. By this means, the effector function of an antibody (such as its ability to activate complement or to cross the placental barrier) can be changed without altering its specificity for antigen. The choice of a new C_H isotype is strongly influenced by lymphokines and other factors acting on the B cell. For example, the microenvironment found in Peyer's patches favors switching to $C_{\alpha 1}$, resulting in the production of IgA. Similarly, exposure to IL-4 promotes switching to C_ε. If a cell that has switched continues to divide, its progeny (both memory and plasma cells) will also express the new heavy-chain isotype. As a rule, subclones expressing non-μ isotypes become increasingly prevalent during clonal B cell proliferation, and their isotype distribution increasingly reflects the peripheral tissue in which the proliferation has occurred: memory cells in subepithelial regions most commonly express IgA, whereas IgM- and IgG-expressing memory cells predominate elsewhere.

Somatic Hypermutation

Fully assembled V/J and V/D/J exons in lymphocytes have been found to undergo point mutation at an unusually high rate during the course of an immune response. This phenomenon, termed **somatic hypermutation,** occurs mainly when memory B cells replicate within the germinal centers of secondary lymphoid follicles. Its mechanism is unknown but appears quite specific, since adjacent regions on the chromosome (including the C_H or C_L exon) are not affected. Although the mutations are presumably introduced into the variable-region exon at random, they can have the effect of either increasing or decreasing the affinity of the resulting immunoglobulin for its target antigen. Individual cells that express higher-affinity mutants are likely to be more effective at antigen presentation and also to receive stronger mitogenic signals through their surface immunoglobulins; they therefore gain a growth advantage. At the same time, unknown processes operating within the germinal center act to selectively eliminate cells that bear lower-affinity immunoglobulins, so that subclones expressing high-affinity mutants soon come to predominate. This selection process is thought to account for a phenomenon known as **affinity maturation,** ie, the observation that antibodies produced later in an immune response tend to have higher affinity for the target antigen than do those produced earlier.

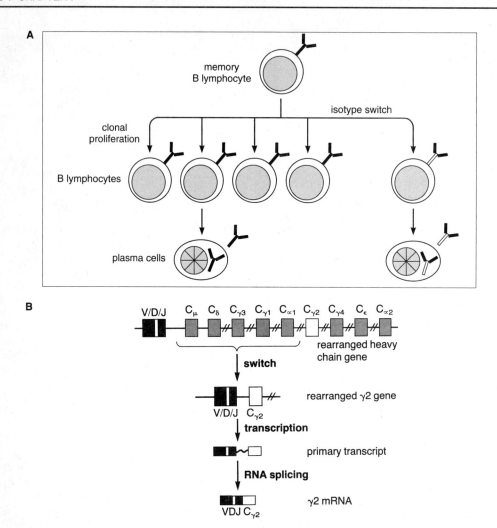

Figure 7–9. Heavy-chain class switch. **A:** During clonal proliferation of an activated memory B cell, some daughter cells may arise that express a different heavy-chain isotype and pass this trait on to their progeny. **B:** Class switching takes place when a fully assembled heavy-chain locus undergoes an additional DNA rearrangement event that places a new C_H sequence adjacent to the V/D/J exon. This occurs by deletion of the intervening C_H exons and is carried out by an enzymatic pathway distinct from that of V/D/J rearrangement. In the example shown, the gene switches to the C 2 isotype.

Primary & Secondary Humoral Responses

Of necessity, the properties of a primary humoral immune response (ie, the antibody response that occurs the first time an individual encounters a given antigen) reflect the properties of virgin lymphocytes (Table 7–1). Because B cells with the appropriate specificity are rare in unimmunized hosts, most of the antigen must be processed by low-affinity accessory cells and presented to antigen-specific helper T cells, which are also correspondingly rare. The helper cells must then contact and activate the B cells, which must in turn proliferate and differentiate into plasma cells in sufficient numbers to be effective. These factors account for the lag time (typically 5–10 days) re-

quired to reach peak serum antibody concentrations in a primary response and for the relatively low concentrations achieved. The antibodies are predominantly IgM—the type secreted by most direct progeny of virgin B cells—and have, on average, low antigen affinities. Indeed, a relatively large percentage of the antibodies are likely to come from "by-stander" B cells, ie, cells that were incidentally activated by a nearby active helper cell but whose immunoglobulins may have little or no affinity for the antigen in question.

Subsequent responses, by contrast, are increasingly dominated by antigen-specific memory cells, whose sheer numbers enhance both the speed and in-

Table 7–1. Comparison of primary and secondary humoral immune responses.

	Primary Response	Secondary Responses
Antigen presentation	Mainly by non-B cells	B lymphocytes increasingly important
Antigen concentration needed to induce response	Relatively high	Relatively low
Antibody response		
Lag phase	5–10 days	2–5 days
Peak concentration	Relatively low	Relatively high
Class(es)	Mostly IgM	Other classes (IgG, IgA, etc) often predominate, in tissue-specific manner
Average antigen affinity	Relatively low	Relatively high
Nonspecific antibodies	Abundant	Relatively rare

tensity of the response (Table 7–1). In a highly immunized lymph node, as many as one in a few hundred B cells may be specific for the target antigen. Memory B cells may serve as the principal antigen-presenting cells in secondary responses and so enable helper T cells to become activated at very low concentrations of antigen. In the process, the B cells themselves are ideally positioned for activation, since they are stimulated strongly both by the bound antigen and by direct contact with the helper cells (Fig 7–8). The responding B cells are more likely to express high-affinity antibodies that enable them to survive selection in the germinal center, and, although some produce IgM, a substantial number arise from class-switched subclones that instead secrete IgG, IgA, or IgE. These latter isotypes therefore tend to predominate in secondary responses, depending on the site at which the response occurs: secondary responses in the blood are predominantly IgG, whereas those at mucosal surfaces are mainly IgA.

The **follicular dendritic cells** (FDCs) found in all lymphoid follicles probably play an important role in controlling humoral responses. FDCs express abundant surface Fc receptors and are therefore very efficient at capturing antigen-antibody complexes. In the presence of preformed antibodies, FDCs can trap antigens within lymphoid follicles and so help potentiate secondary responses. Once displayed on the FDC surface, antigens may persist for weeks or even months, suggesting a possible role for these cells in maintaining immunologic **memory**.

B Cell Tolerance

The random assembly of V, D, and J segments during lymphopoiesis inevitably produces some B cell clones whose immunoglobulins recognize "self" determinants on normal host cells or tissues. Because such autoreactive immunoglobulins are potentially deleterious to the host, stringent measures are needed to ensure that they will not be secreted. In most cases, these measures operate successfully: the immune system remains specifically **tolerant** toward the many self determinants to which it is continually exposed. Recent experimental work has begun to shed light on the mechanisms by which immunologic tolerance is established and maintained. Although it is too soon to generalize extensively from these initial findings, some important aspects of B cell tolerance have already emerged.

In principle, B cell tolerance could be achieved either by eliminating any cells that express an autoreactive antibody (**clonal deletion**) or by permitting such cells to survive in a functionally inactive state (**clonal anergy**). It appears that the body uses both these approaches. Clonal deletion is thought to take place among early B lymphocytes in the marrow, perhaps at the moment when they first begin to express complete immunoglobulins on their surfaces. There is evidence that contact of surface immunoglobulins with a self antigen at this stage transmits a signal that arrests further development of the early B cell and that the arrested cell subsequently dies. It is not yet known whether deletion can also take place at other body sites and at later stages of B cell development. By contrast, several distinct forms of clonal anergy have been observed among mature B cells in the periphery. In some cases, the affected cells fail to express surface immunoglobulins, although they may retain the ability to secrete immunoglobulins if artificially activated. In other cases, autoreactive immunoglobulins continue to be expressed on the cell surface but fail to transmit an effective signal to the cell upon binding the cognate antigen. Still other B lymphocytes appear to be functionally inactive only because the corresponding helper T cells are absent or anergic (see Chapter 8). Indeed, it has been proposed that contact of surface immunoglobulins with a cognate antigen in the absence of appropriate T-cell help may be a crucial factor in initiating many different forms of B cell anergy. It remains to be determined precisely what roles clonal anergy and deletion each play in maintaining self tolerance and how these processes come to be circumvented in autoimmune diseases.

Immunoglobulin Gene Rearrangements and B Cell Malignancy

Apart from their role in generating antibody diversity, immunoglobulin gene rearrangements are gaining increasing importance in clinical diagnosis and research. Rearrangement of these genes can be detected in biopsy or blood specimens by using a technique known as the Southern blot, and their presence provides a highly sensitive and specific means of di-

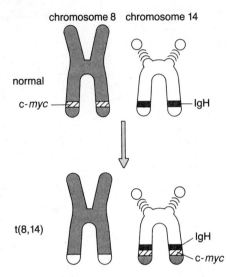

chromosome 8   chromosome 14

normal

c-*myc*

IgH

t(8,14)

IgH

c-*myc*

Figure 7–10. The t(8,14) chromosomal anomaly of Burkitt's lymphoma. A reciprocal translocation of genetic material exchanges the distal ends of the long arms of chromosomes 8 and 14. This transposes the c-*myc* proto-oncogene from chromosome 8 into the active immuno-globulin heavy-chain locus on chromosome 14 and contributes to the development of a malignancy.

agnosing lymphoid cancers (see Chapter 14). Perhaps more importantly, errors in immunoglobulin gene re-arrangement are now thought to contribute to the genesis of several major types of leukemia and lymphoma. For example, the cells of **Burkitt's lymphoma,** a B lymphocytic malignancy, usually contain a specific chromosomal abnormality called **t(8,14),** in which a portion of chromosome 8 has been translocated onto chromosome 14 (Fig 7–10). In this translocation, breakage of chromosome 14 occurs within the immunoglobulin heavy-chain locus, while the breakpoint on chromosome 8 coincides with a cellular proto-oncogene known as **c-*myc*.** As a result, the c-*myc* gene is moved to a position directly adja-cent to the heavy-chain gene. It is thought that this proximity to the transcriptionally active heavy-chain locus alters the expression of the proto-oncogene and that this, along with other damage to c-*myc* that can occur during translocation, contributes to malig-nant transformation. Less commonly, the cells of Burkitt's lymphoma may lack t(8,14), and instead exhibit a closely related anomaly in which the c-*myc* locus is translocated into the κ or λ light-chain gene on chromosome 2 or 22, producing the same effects.

A similar type of chromosomal anomaly, desig-nated **t(14,18),** is observed in at least 90% of cases of **follicular lymphoma,** the most common human B cell malignancy. In this translocation, the gene on chromosome 18 that encodes the cytoplasmic mem-brane protein **Bcl-2** is moved to a position immedi-ately adjacent to the heavy-chain locus on chromo-some 14. B cells carrying the t(14,18) anomaly express unusually high levels of structurally normal Bcl-2 protein and hence are resistant to being killed by many of the physiologic processes that normally induce apoptosis (see Chapter 3). As a result, they tend to accumulate in great numbers and evolve into a malignancy (see Chapter 45). In both t(14,18) and Burkitt's anomalies, the chromosomal breakpoint in affected immunoglobulin loci occurs directly beside a J segment; this strongly implies that each of these translocations results in part from an error in immu-noglobulin gene rearrangement.

REFERENCES

Immunoglobulin Gene Organization & Rearrangements

Dreyer WJ, Bennett JC: The molecular basis of antibody formations: A paradox. *Proc Natl Acad Sci USA* 1965;**54**:864.

Honjo T et al (eds.): *Immunoglobulin Genes.* Academic Press, 1989.

Tonegawa S: Somatic generation of antibody diversity. *Nature* 1983;**302**:575.

V/(D)/J Recombinase

Akira SJ, Okazaki K, Sakano H: Two pairs of recombi-nation signals are sufficient to cause immunoglobulin V-(D)-J joining. *Science* 1987;**238**:1134.

Gellert M: Molecular analysis of V(D)J recombination. *Annu Rev Genet* 1992;**26**:425.

Lewis S, Gellert M: The mechanism of antigen receptor gene assembly. *Cell* 1989;**59**:585.

Schatz D et al: V(D)J recombination: Molecular biology and regulation. *Annu Rev Immunol* 1992; **10**:359.

Other Sources of Antibody Diversity

French DL et al: The role of somatic hypermutation in the generation of antibody diversity. *Science* 1989;**244**:1152.

Komori T et al: Lack of N regions in antigen receptor variable region genes of Tdt-deficient lymphocytes. *Science* 1993;**261**:1171.

Max EE et al: Variation in the crossover point of kappa immunoglobulin gene V-J recombination: Evidence from a cryptic gene. *Cell* 1980;**21**:793.

Heavy-Chain Class Switching & Immunoglobulin Secretion

Cebra JJ, Komisar JL, Schweitzer PA: C_H isotype "switching" during normal B-lymphocyte develop-ment. *Annu Rev Immunol* 1984;**2**:493.

Early P et al: Two mRNAs can be produced from a single immunoglobulin μ gene by alternative RNA process-ing pathways. *Cell* 1979;**20**:313.

Finkelman FD et al: Lymphokine control of in vivo immunoglobulin isotype selection. *Annu Rev Immunol* 1990;**8:**303.

Harriman W et al: Immunoglobulin class-switch recombinations. *Annu Rev Immunol* 1993;**11:**385.

B Cell Surface Receptors & Signaling

Gordon J, Guy GR: The molecules controlling B lymphocytes. *Immunol Today* 1987;**8:**339.

Nossal GJV: Immunologic tolerance and the collaboration between antigen and lymphokines in lymphocyte signaling. *Science* 1989;**245:**145.

Reth M: Antigen receptors on B lymphocytes. *Annu Rev Immunol* 1992;**10:**97.

Venkitaraman A et al: The B-cell antigen receptor of the five immunoglobulin gene classes. *Nature* 1991; **352:**777.

Zola H: The surface antigens of human B lymphocytes. *Immunol Today* 1987;**8:**308.

B Cell Ontogeny, Tolerance, & the Humoral Immune Response

Clark EA, Lane PJL: Regulation of human B-cell activation and adhesion. *Annu Rev Immunol* 1991;**9:**97.

Goodnow CC: Transgenic mice and analysis of B cell tolerance. *Annu Rev Immunol* 1992;**10:**489.

Goodnow CC et al: The need for central and peripheral tolerance in the B repertoire. *Science* 1990;**248;**1373.

Hayakawa K, Hardy RR: Normal, autoimmune, and malignant CD5+B cells: The Ly-1 B lineage. *Annu Rev Immunol* 1988;**6:**197.

Kincade PW et al: Cells and molecules that regulate B lymphopoiesis in bone marrow. *Annu Rev Immunol* 1989;**7:**111.

Rolink A, Melchers F: Molecular and cellular origins of B lymphocyte diversity. *Cell* 1991;**66:**1081.

Schwartz RH: Acquisition of immunological self-tolerance. *Cell* 1989;**57:**1073.

Vitetta ES et al: Cellular interactions in the humoral immune response. *Adv Immunol* 1989;**45:**1.

Chromosomal Translocations in Lymphoid Neoplasia

Croce CM, Nowell PC: Molecular basis of human B cell neoplasia. *Blood* 1985;**65:**1.

Korsmeyer SJ: Chromosomal translocations in lymphoid malignancies reveal novel protooncogenes. *Annu Rev Immunol* 1992;**10:**785.

T Lymphocytes & Natural Killer Cells

John B. Imboden, MD

The success of the specific immune system depends on the remarkable ability of thymus-derived (T) lymphocytes to recognize and discriminate among a wide range of different foreign antigens. Antigen recognition activates T cells to perform their effector functions leading, for example, to the production of lymphokines that promote humoral and cellular immune responses to the antigen. This chapter will emphasize the cellular and molecular interactions involved in the T cell response to antigen. It also will review T cell development and the mechanisms by which the normal T cell system distinguishes between foreign and self antigens, thereby avoiding autoimmunity.

T CELL ANTIGEN RECEPTOR

Structure of the T Cell Receptor

T lymphocytes do not "see" soluble antigens but, rather, recognize antigen in the form of peptide fragments that are bound to class I and class II molecules of the major histocompatibility complex (MHC) locus. The **T cell receptor** for antigen (**TCR**) is a complex of at least 8 polypeptide chains (Fig 8–1). Two of these (the α and β chains) form a disulfide-linked dimer that recognizes antigenic peptides bound to MHC molecules and therefore is the actual ligand-binding structure within the TCR. The TCR α and β chains are similar in many respects to immunoglobulin proteins. The amino-terminal regions of the α and β chains are highly polymorphic, so that within the entire T cell population there are a large number of different TCR α/β dimers, each capable of recognizing a particular combination of antigenic peptide and MHC. The TCRs on individual T cells contain only a single type of α/β dimer; therefore, individual T cells respond only to a specific combination of antigen and MHC.

The α/β dimer is associated with a complex of pro-

teins designated **CD3.** The CD3 chains are not polymorphic and range in size from 16 to 28 kDa. They are involved in signal transduction and thus allow the TCR to convert the recognition of antigen/MHC into intracellular signals for activation. Compared with TCR α and β, whose intracellular regions are only several amino acids in length, the CD3 chains have large cytoplasmic domains, ranging from 45–55 amino acids for CD3 ϵ, δ, and γ to 113 amino acids for CD3ζ.

TCR α & β Genes & Generation of TCR Diversity

To generate the diversity of TCRs required to recognize a wide spectrum of antigenic determinants, the TCR α and β genes use a combinatorial strategy of **DNA rearrangement** similar to that of the immunoglobulin genes (see Chapter 7). The germline TCR β gene contains 20–30 V (variable), 2 D (diversity), and 13 J (joining) gene segments (Fig 8–2). When the TCR β gene rearranges early in T cell ontogeny, one of the V_β region segments becomes linked to one of the D_β regions and to one of the J_β segments to form a single exon. After transcription, RNA splicing fuses this V/D/J exon to the single C_β (constant) region exon to form a TCR β mRNA that encodes a functional protein. The potential diversity generated by this **combinatorial joining** is equal to the number of possible V segments multiplied by the number of D segments and by the number J segments. Similarly, in the TCR α locus, there are approximately 100 V segments and 50 J segments (but no D segments). To form a functional TCR α chain gene, a V_α segment joins to a J_α segment.

Although both TCR and immunoglobulin genes undergo V/(D)/J recombination, there are several interesting differences in the mechanisms used by these 2 gene families to generate diversity. Relative to the immunoglobulin genes, which have 250–1000 V regions, the TCR genes have a more limited array of V

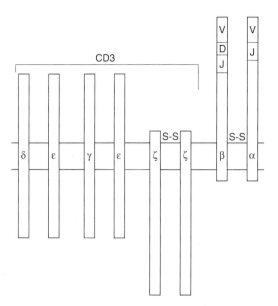

Figure 8–1. T cell antigen receptor. The TCR is a complex of 8 transmembrane proteins. The α and β chains form a disulfide-linked (S–S) dimer that is responsible for the recognition of antigenic peptides bound to class I and class II MHC molecules. The amino-terminal regions of the α and β chains, which are formed through rearrangements of V, D, and J segments, are highly polymorphic. The α/β dimer is noncovalently associated with the CD3 complex, which converts the recognition of antigen into transmembrane signals. The CD3 polypeptides are not polymorphic and have larger cytoplasmic domains than TCR α and β do. The CD3 complex consists of 3 sets of dimers. There are 2 CD3 ε chains, one paired with CD3γ and the other with CD3δ. The ζ chain exists either as a disulfide-linked ζ-ζ homodimer (as shown here) or as a heterodimer with either η (an alternatively spliced form of ζ) or the γ chain of the high-affinity Fcε receptor (not to be confused with CD3γ). The functional importance of this variation in the ζ dimer is not understood.

segments. Moreover, the TCR α gene does not take maximal advantage of its available V-region repertoire, since it actually uses only a fraction of its 100 V-region segments. Compared with the immunoglobulins, therefore, the TCR chains have restricted V-region diversity, which limits the diversity that can be generated through combinatorial mechanisms alone. As in immunoglobulin genes, diversity is further enhanced by **imprecise joining** of the gene segments and by the insertion of non-germline-encoded nucleotides (**N regions**) between segments during the rearrangement process. These mechanisms each enhance **junctional diversity,** ie, the diversity of sequences at the junctions between V_α and J_α, and between V_β, D_β, and J_β segments. N-region insertion is carried out by the enzyme **terminal deoxynucleotidyltransferase**

(TdT), which is expressed in the nuclei of immature T cells at the stage when V/(D)/J recombination occurs. Unlike immunoglobulin genes, however, TCR genes do not undergo somatic hypermutation.

TCR Recognition of Antigen

For T cells to respond to an antigen, the antigen must first be processed into peptides, which in turn bind to the groove on the "top" of class I or II MHC molecules (see Chapter 5). The resulting complex of peptide and MHC molecule forms the ligand for the TCR. It is likely, but not yet formally proven, that contacts with both the peptide and the MHC molecule are critical for TCR binding. It is important to emphasize a further constraint on TCR recognition: the T cell system is heavily biased toward recognizing peptides bound to **self** MHC molecules, ie, the specific subset of MHC alleles that are expressed by the individual host. Thus, for example, T cells from an HLA B27[+] individual will recognize an antigenic peptide in the context of B27 but may not respond to the same peptide bound to other HLA B molecules. This **restriction** to self MHC molecules occurs because, during T cell development, there is **positive selection** for T cells whose TCRs have the potential to recognize peptides presented by self MHC.

It is not known precisely how the TCR interacts with the peptide-MHC complex. The x-ray crystallographic structures of peptide-class I MHC complexes have been solved, but we do not yet have crystallographic structures of TCR-peptide-MHC complexes or even of isolated TCR α/β dimers. However, from the MHC structure and structural studies of antibody-antigen complexes, it has been possible to generate a plausible model for the interaction of the TCR with its ligand. In this model, the V segments of the TCR α and β chains contact the α-helices that form the sides of the peptide groove of the MHC molecule (see Chapter 5), while the junctional regions (the V_α/J_α and $V_\beta/D_\beta/J_\beta$ joints) contact the peptide itself (Fig 8–3). One appealing feature of this model is that the regions of maximal diversity in the TCR chains form the contact sites for the antigenic peptide. Junctional diversity, therefore, may allow the TCR repertoire to recognize a wide array of antigenic peptides.

Interaction of the TCR with Superantigens

Superantigens are a class of bacterial toxins and retroviral proteins that have the remarkable ability to bind both class II MHC molecules and the TCR β chain. In so doing, they act as a "clamp" between the TCR and class II molecules, providing signals to the T cell. It is important to grasp the differences between classic antigenic peptides and superantigens. Superantigens are not processed, and they interact with the MHC molecule outside of the peptide-binding groove. On the T cell side, superantigens bind to V_β segments only, without regard to the D and J regions

A α gene locus

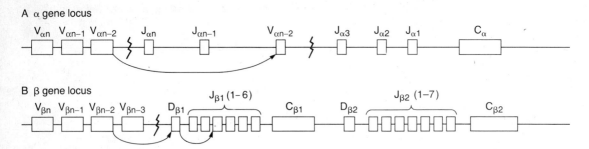

B β gene locus

Figure 8–2. Rearrangement of the TCR α and β genes. The TCR α gene locus contains multiple V and J segments, only some of which are shown here. Similarly, the TCR β gene locus contains multiple V, D, and J segments. During T cell ontogeny, the TCR genes rearrange (arrows), so that one of the V_α segments pairs with a J_α segment and a V_β segment pairs with a D_β and J_β segment. The two C (constant) segments in the β gene are very similar, and differential use of $C_\beta 1$ and $C_\beta 2$ does not contribute to TCR diversity.

or the TCR α chain (Fig 8–4). Superantigens differ in the V_β segments that they can bind, with any given superantigen binding only one or a few V_β segments. Individual superantigens, therefore, activate only T cells whose TCRs contain particular V_β segments.

Because superantigens recognize only the V_β segment but not the other components of the TCR α/β dimer, a superantigen has the capability of activating 1–10% of peripheral T cells. This is orders of magnitude more than even the most potent conventional antigen. Exposure to a superantigen, therefore, can lead

to massive T cell activation, and the ensuing lymphokine release accounts for many of the manifestations of acute exposure to bacterial toxins that have superantigen capabilities. This probably explains the clinical features of **toxic shock syndrome,** which can be induced by the *Staphylococcus aureus* toxin TSST-1, a superantigen that activates human T cells expressing $V_\beta 2$. In the acute phase of toxic shock syndrome there is marked and selective proliferation of T cells that bear $V_\beta 2$: in one reported case, 70% of peripheral T cells were $V_\beta 2^+$ in the acute phase of the disease.

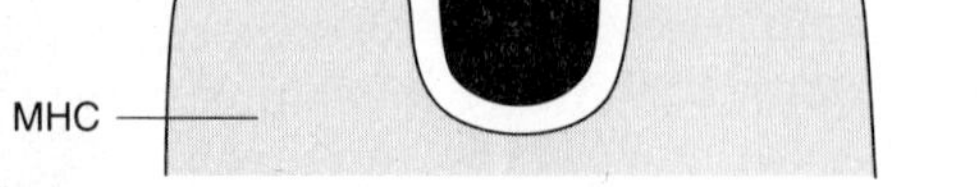

Signal Transduction by the TCR

The recognition of appropriately presented antigen is one of the most important stimuli that can activate T cells to proliferate and to perform their effector functions. Activation of helper T cells, for example, leads to the production of lymphokines that promote cellular and humoral immune responses, whereas ac-

Figure 8–3. Model for the recognition of antigen-MHC by the TCR. The antigenic peptide is shown in black. The J_α and J_β regions are crosshatched, and the D_β region is stippled. Computer modeling suggests that the V_α and V_β regions of the TCR may contact the α-helices that form the sides of the peptide-binding groove of MHC molecules, while the V_α/J_α and $V_\beta/D_\beta/J_\beta$ joints interact with the antigenic peptide itself. This model has considerable appeal, because the most highly variable regions of the TCR, generated through junctional diversity, contact the antigen. Junctional diversity, therefore, may greatly increase the range of peptides recognized by the T cell system.

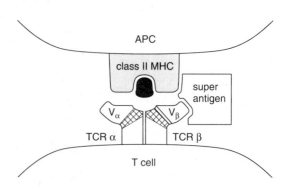

Figure 8–4. Model of the interactions between the TCR, class II MHC molecule, and a superantigen. The superantigen interacts with the MHC molecule outside the peptide groove and binds only to the V_β segment of the TCR.

tivation of cytotoxic T cells results in the lysis of the antigen-bearing cells. Each of these T cell responses depends on the ability of the TCR to generate intracellular signals for activation. The earliest known TCR-induced signal, which occurs within 5 seconds of stimulation, is the induction of **protein tyrosine kinase (PTK)** activity. Because none of the known components of the TCR has intrinsic kinase activity, it is likely that the TCR couples to nonreceptor, cytoplasmic PTK. Three PTKs have been implicated in TCR signaling: p59*fyn*, p56*lck*, and ZAP70 (Fig 8–5). **p59*fyn*** associates with the cytoplasmic domains

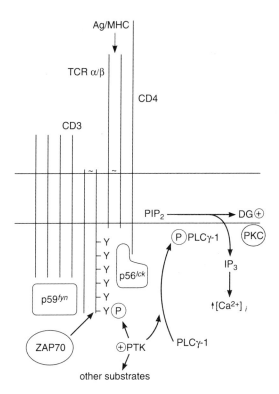

Figure 8–5. Scheme of the early events in transmembrane signaling by the TCR. The CD3 components of the TCR are associated with the protein tyrosine kinase (PTK) p59*fyn*, and the CD4 coreceptor is associated with the PTK p56*lck*. Stimulation of the TCR by antigen plus MHC leads to an increase in PTK activity. The initial PTK activation probably involves a combination of p59*fyn* and p56*lck*. One substrate is the CD3 ζ chain, which, when tyrosine phosphorylated, binds a third PTK, ZAP70. The TCR-activated PTKs phosphorylate a variety of intracellular molecules, including phospholipase Cγ-1 (PLCγ-1). Tyrosine phosphorylation (P) activates PLCγ-1, which then hydrolyzes its substrate, the membrane phospholipid phosphatidylinositol bisphosphate (PIP$_2$), releasing diacylglycerol (DG) and inositol trisphosphate (IP$_3$). DG activates protein kinase C (PKC), a family of serine/threonine kinases, while IP$_3$ triggers an increase in the concentration of cytoplasmic free Ca^{2+} ([Ca^{2+}]$_i$).

of CD3 ε, γ, ζ, and η. As discussed below, **p56*lck*** binds to the cytoplasmic domains of CD4 or CD8 and may be brought into proximity of the TCR through the interactions of CD4 or CD8 with the TCR. **ZAP70** associates with CD3 ζ following TCR stimulation; tyrosine phosphorylation of ζ appears to be the signal for ZAP70 binding.

TCR-mediated PTK activation leads to the tyrosine phosphorylation of a number of intracellular proteins. It is likely that this phosphorylation regulates the activities of key enzymes and signaling molecules, thereby allowing the TCR to transduce signals for activation. One known substrate for a TCR-activated PTK is **phospholipase C-γ1 (PLC-γ1)**, an enzyme that, when active, hydrolyzes **phosphatidylinositol bisphosphate (PIP$_2$),** a membrane phospholipid. Tyrosine phosphorylation activates PLC-γ1, and the ensuing breakdown of PIP$_2$ generates two second messengers: **diacylglycerol and inositol $_{1,4,5}$-trisphosphate (IP$_3$).** Diacylglycerol activates the **protein kinase C** family of serine/threonine protein kinases. IP$_3$ binds to a channel-like intracellular receptor, stimulating the release of Ca^{2+} from internal stores into the cytoplasm. In T cells, an IP$_3$ receptor also has been found in the plasma membrane, indicating that IP$_3$ may promote increases in the concentration of cytoplasmic free calcium ([Ca^{2+}]$_i$) by stimulating Ca^{2+} influx as well as intracellular Ca^{2+} release. Elevations in [Ca^{2+}]$_i$ and in protein kinase C activity function synergistically and appear to be important mediators for many subsequent events in T cell responses, including the production of interleukin-2 (**IL-2**) and the triggering of cytolytic activity. One consequence of the increase in [Ca^{2+}]$_i$ is the activation of **calcineurin,** a Ca^{2+}-dependent serine phosphatase that plays a key role in the activation of the IL-2 gene. Calcineurin is the target of **cyclosporin** and **FK506**, 2 immunosuppressive drugs that block TCR-mediated induction of IL-2. These drugs are widely used in clinical transplantation to prevent graft rejection.

ACCESSORY MOLECULES & TCR CORECEPTORS

Interactions Between T Cells & Antigen-Presenting Cells

When a T cell encounters an antigen-presenting cell (APC), the outcome is determined in part by the specificity of its TCR and in part by **costimulatory** signals it receives through other receptors. Activation occurs only if the TCR recognizes its particular antigen-MHC combination, and signals transmitted from the TCR alone are sufficient to cause certain biochemical changes in a T cell. However, the T cell response is also influenced by a number of non-TCR proteins on its surface that recognize specific ligands on the APC. These so-called **accessory receptors** subserve 2 general functions: (a) to enhance adhesion between the T cell and the APC, and (b) to transduce signals across the plasma membrane.

It is likely that the initial interaction between a T cell and an APC is independent of the TCR. The affinity of the TCR for its ligand (antigen-MHC) appears to be low and may not be sufficiently strong to give stable binding to another cell, particularly if relatively small numbers of MHC molecules bear the specific peptide of interest. The initial binding thus appears to depend primarily on other T cell molecules that bind ligands on the APC surface. An example of such an **adhesion molecule** is **CD2,** which binds a widely expressed cell surface molecule designated **LFA-3.** The binding of CD2 to LFA-3, and of other adhesion molecules to their ligands, results initially in a relatively nonspecific adhesion of the T cell onto the APC, which allows the T cell to survey the surface of the APC for the appropriate combination of antigenic peptide and MHC molecule. If the TCR recognizes its antigen, then TCR-mediated signals lead to changes that further stabilize the interaction between the T cell and the APC. For example, these signals lead to increased expression of CD2 and also modify the T cell surface adhesion molecule **LFA-1** so that there is an increase in the affinity of LFA-1 for its ligand on the APC.

Other types of accessory molecules, including Fc receptors, complement receptors, and mitogen receptors, can all contribute to the signaling events that activate T cells. A detailed survey of these signaling molecules is beyond the scope of this chapter. Instead, we will restrict our comments to the CD4 and CD8 "coreceptors" and to CD45 and CD28.

CD4 & CD8 Coreceptors

The expression of CD4 and CD8 divides mature T cells into 2 mutually exclusive subsets: those that recognize antigen in the context of class II MHC molecules (CD4+ cells) and those that recognize antigen bound to class I molecules (CD8+ cells). **CD4** binds directly to class II MHC molecules, probably at a site within these proteins that is located near the membrane surface and is not directly involved in peptide binding. **CD8,** on the other hand, binds to class I MHC molecules. It is possible, therefore, that CD4 and CD8 interact with the same MHC molecule as the TCR during T cell activation (Fig 8–6). There is considerable evidence to support this notion and to suggest that CD4 and CD8 are in close proximity to the TCR, functioning as **coreceptors.** This approximation of the TCR and CD4/CD8 has important consequences for signaling, because the cytoplasmic domains of CD4 and CD8 are noncovalently associated with the PTK p56^{lck}. CD4 and CD8, therefore, may serve to bring p56^{lck} into proximity with the TCR complex, allowing this kinase to participate in the signaling response to antigen recognition. A number of experiments indicate that the TCR-CD4 (or TCR-

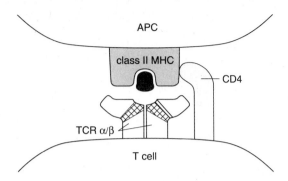

Figure 8–6. Model of the recognition by the TCR and CD4 coreceptor of an antigenic peptide bound to a class II MHC molecule. CD4 binds to the same MHC molecule as the TCR but interacts with a membrane-proximal region that is not directly involved in peptide binding. One consequence of this coreceptor function of CD4 is to bring p56^{lck} into proximity with the TCR.

CD8) supercomplex is far more effective in transducing signals for activation than is the TCR alone.

CD45—a Tyrosine Phosphatase Required for TCR Signaling

CD45 is a large (180 to 220 kDa) cell surface molecule that is expressed by all leukocytes, including all T lymphocytes. Signal transduction by the TCR requires the coexpression of CD45, whose cytoplasmic domain has **tyrosine phosphatase** activity. T cells that lack CD45 cannot respond to antigen, even though they express normal levels of the TCR. It appears that CD45 is required for functional coupling of the TCR and its PTKs. An attractive hypothesis is that the CD45 phosphatase removes tyrosine phosphorylations that inhibit signaling. A likely target of such inhibitory phosphorylation is the PTK p56^{lck}. Phosphorylation of p56^{lck} on a carboxy-terminal tyrosine (Tyr-505) decreases its kinase activity. By dephosphorylating Tyr-505, CD45 may allow this PTK to be activated during antigen recognition.

CD45 protein can exist in several distinct **isoforms** that differ in the structures of their extracellular domains as a result of alternative RNA splicing. Some T cells express a 205- to 220-kDa isoform designated **CD45RA,** whereas others express a 180-kDa isoform called **CD45RO.** At one time it appeared that the CD45RO isoform might be a marker for memory T cells, but current evidence suggests instead that it signifies recent activation: soon after a T cell is activated, splicing of its CD45 mRNA changes so that CD45RO is expressed in place of CD45RA; however, this change persists for only a few weeks and the cell subsequently reverts to CD45RA expression. It is not known what role, if any, this transient alteration plays in modulating T cell activation.

CD28, the 2-Signal Model of T Cell Activation, & Anergy

Several years ago an interesting in vitro phenomenon was observed: if a T cell clone is stimulated by a chemically modified APC, the T cell is not activated but instead becomes **anergic**—ie, it enters the state of **anergy,** in which it remains viable but is refractory to stimulation by antigen. This observation suggests that anergy might be induced whenever the signals delivered by a TCR are not accompanied by a particular costimulus, which chemically modified APCs are unable to deliver. In other words, normal T cell activation requires the delivery to the cell of both the TCR signals and a second signal generated by accessory molecules. In the absence of the second signal, TCR stimulation induces a state of anergy. The nature of this costimulus has been the subject of considerable interest. It appears that, at least in certain circumstances, the costimulus can be delivered through the T cell surface molecule designated **CD28.** The ligands for CD28 are proteins in the **B7** family of cell surface molecules found on activated B cells, macrophages, and other APCs. At least three B7 proteins have been identified which share approximately 25% sequence identity; their individual roles in costimulation have not been determined. The idea is that the signals resulting from the CD28-B7 interaction provide the necessary costimulus that permits TCR-mediated signaling to result in activation rather than anergy (Fig 8–7). This model suggests that CD28 may provide a means of manipulating the immune response to specific antigens. Recent studies support this notion. For example, blockade of B7 (which prevents CD28 from binding) results in prolongation of allograft survival in experimental animals. Nevertheless, certain types of T cell immune responses can occur in the absence of CD28, suggesting that alternative pathways of costimulation may also exist.

T CELL SUBSETS & HETEROGENEITY

The T cell population is heterogenous with respect to both functional capabilities and cell surface phenotype. Broadly speaking, T cells are divided into helper T cells (TH cells) which promote cell-mediated and antibody responses, and cytotoxic T cells (Tc cells), which lyse antigen-bearing target cells. Some of the phenotypic and functional characteristics of T cell subsets result from commitments made during T cell ontogeny and are stable over the life span of the mature T cell. The decision to become a CD4+ T cell or a CD8+ T cell, for example, appears to be irreversible. CD4+CD8– T cells do not convert to CD4– CD8+ T cells and vice versa. Mature T cells, however, are capable of further differentiation. T cell activation, for example, induces the appearance of a variety of new cell surface molecules. Certain of these, such as the receptor for IL-2, are only transiently expressed and thus can be used as markers to detect recently activated T cells. T cell activation also induces long-lasting changes: once activated, a T cell does not appear to revert completely to its original

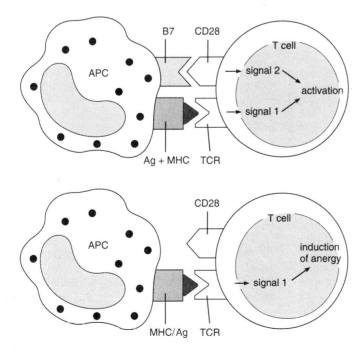

Figure 8–7. The 2-signal model of T cell activation. Activation of T cells is thought to require TCR-derived signals (signal 1) and a costimulus (signal 2). At least under certain conditions, CD28 delivers signal 2. The ligand for CD28, B7, is expressed on APCs. In the absence of the costimulus, the unopposed TCR signals cause the T cell to enter a state of unresponsiveness known as anergy.

state. Differentiation following activation is responsible for another major dichotomy in the T cell population: virgin versus memory T cells.

Helper T Cells

Helper T cells were so named because they provide signals that augment cell-mediated immune responses and that are necessary for B cells to differentiate into antibody-producing cells. When activated, helper T cells produce soluble lymphokines that can regulate the activities of T cells, B cells, monocytes, and other cells of the immune system. T cell help for B cell differentiation also involves direct binding of the helper T cell to the B cell. This cell-cell interaction leads to direct stimulation of CD40 and other receptors on the B cell and also results in exposure of the B cell to high local concentrations of lymphokines. Helper T cells usually express CD4 and thus most often respond to "professional" APCs, which are the only cells that normally express class II MHC molecules (see Chapter 5). It should be emphasized, however, that expression of CD4 correlates better with restriction by MHC class II molecules than with helper function. Thus, some CD4+ T cells have cytolytic activity. Similarly, some CD8+ T cells function as helper cells.

Heterogeneity of Helper T Cells: TH0, TH1, & TH2 Cells

On the basis of the array of lymphokines they produce, T cell clones can be placed into one of 3 categories: TH1, TH2, and TH0. **TH1** clones produce **IL-2** and gamma interferon (**IFN γ**) but not IL-4 or IL-5. **TH2** clones, on the other hand, produce **IL-4** and **IL-5** but not IL-2 or IFN γ. TH0 clones combine the lymphokine profiles of TH1 and TH2 cells. Broadly speaking, the lymphokines produced by TH1 cells promote cell-mediated immune responses, augment IgM and IgG2 synthesis by B cells, and activate macrophages. The TH2-derived lymphokines, on the other hand, lead to enhanced IgG1 and IgE responses and to increased numbers of local and/or circulating eosinophils (**eosinophilia**).

Until recently, the physiological significance of TH1 and TH2 cells remained uncertain, and it was not known whether TH1 and TH2 cells actually developed in vivo. It is now clear, however, that certain human immune responses are dominated by one of these 2 subsets of helper T cell. Such polarized responses have been most clearly identified following parasitic infections. Infection by **helminths,** for example, leads to a predominantly TH2 response. The resulting production of IL-4 and IL-5 is probably responsible for the elevated IgE levels and eosinophilia, respectively, that are characteristic of helminthic infections. Conversely, in most mouse strains, the protozoan intracellular parasite **Leishmania major** elicits a TH1 response. These animals develop a brisk cell-mediated reaction and clear the infection. Certain mouse

strains, however, develop a response to *L major* that is dominated by TH2 cells; this leads to a vigorous antibody response, but no cell-mediated reaction, against the protozoan. In the latter strains, the parasite evades the immune response, disseminates, and eventually kills the host.

It is not precisely clear why certain immune responses are dominated by either TH1 or TH2 cells and why others (perhaps the majority) fail to polarize into one of these 2 types. It appears likely that TH0, TH1, and TH2 cells derive from precursor T cells that, depending on environmental influences, can differentiate into any one of these TH subtypes. Recent evidence indicates that the lymphokine interleukin-12 (**IL-12**) can selectively promote the production of TH1 cells. Conversely, the development of a polarized TH2 response appears to be promoted by IL-4 but inhibited by IFN γ.

Cytotoxic T Cells

Cytotoxic T lymphocytes (also called TC cells or CTLs) respond to antigen recognition by lysing the antigen-bearing cell. TC cells are usually CD8+ and recognize antigen in the context of class I MHC molecules. As in other interactions between lymphocytes and APCs, the initial contact between a TC cell and its target is mediated primarily by adhesion molecules on the surfaces of the two cells. If specific binding then occurs between the TCR and peptide-MHC complexes, signals are transmitted that lead to increased expression of adhesion proteins by both cells. As a result, the cells bind more strongly to one another over a larger area of their surfaces and often interdigitate their membranes. The TC cell then kills the target through one of at least two distinct mechanisms. One mechanism ("murder") involves the synthesis and directed extracellular release of cytotoxic proteins onto the target cell. Toxic proteins that can be secreted by TC cells include **perforin** (previously known as cytolysin) and a family of at least 4 serine proteases, called **granzymes,** that are evolutionarily related to complement component C9 (see Chapter 10). Together, these proteins produce 10–20-nm pores in the target cell membrane, and so kill the cell by osmotic lysis. Alternatively, cytotoxic cells can stimulate some target cells, through mechanisms that are not yet understood, to undergo **apoptosis** or programmed cell death ("induced suicide"). These two alternative pathways of killing may not be mutually exclusive. After killing, the activated TC cell disengages from its target but is not inactivated, and so can kill again.

Cytotoxic lymphocytes play a prominent role in host defense against infection by viruses and other intracellular parasites, because proteins encoded by these pathogens enter the endogenous pathway for antigen presentation (see Chapter 5) and therefore are expressed on the surface of the infected cell as a complex with class I MHC proteins. TC cells are also important in allograft rejection and contribute to the pathogenesis of some autoimmune diseases. The ability of Tc lymphocytes to lyse cancer cells that express tumor-specific antigens is well documented, but this phenomenon is variable and of uncertain relevance to cancer immunity ("immunosurveillance") in vivo.

Suppressor T Cells

There is a large literature describing T cells that appear to terminate, or suppress, immune responses. At present, however, the significance, and even the existence, of these **suppressor T cells** is in doubt. One difficulty has been the inability to firmly establish the cellular and molecular basis for suppression or to identify specific surface markers that characterize a subset of T cells with suppressor activity. It should also be pointed out that certain phenomena which were previously attributed to suppressor T cells may instead reflect helper T cell heterogeneity and the pleiotropic effects of lymphokines. TH1 cells, for example, provide help for cell-mediated reactions, in large part because of their ability to produce IFN γ. As noted above, IFN γ inhibits Th2 cells and thus would diminish IgG1 responses; an experimental system that looked at IgG1 responses, therefore, would consider TH1 cells to be suppressors.

γ/δ T Cells

Members of a small subset (<5%) of mature T cells do not express a TCR α/β dimer. These cells instead have a second form of the TCR that is composed of a CD3 complex together with a dimer of polypeptides designated γ and δ. The TCR γ and δ genes are highly homologous to the TCR α and β genes and, as is the case with α and β, are assembled through rearrangements of germline V and J segments (for TCR γ) or of V, D, and J segments (for TCR δ). Interestingly, the TCR δ gene lies within the TCR α locus.

The physiologic roles of γ/δ T cells remain uncertain. These cells can be either CD4−CD8− or CD4−CD8+. They have cytotoxic activity and can produce lymphokines. It appears likely that they recognize antigen, but relatively little is known about their specificities or MHC restriction. They appear to be the predominant T cell type in certain epithelial tissues, such as the skin.

T CELL ONTOGENY

Stages of Thymocyte Development

T cells develop from bone marrow-derived progenitor cells that undergo maturation in the thymus (Fig 8–8). Early in development, thymocytes express several cell surface molecules (such as CD2 and CD7) that are characteristic of the T cell lineage, but they lack many others, including CD4 and CD8, and thus are known as **double-negative thymocytes.** Rearrangement of the TCR genes begins in the double-

negative stage. Cells that are destined to become α/β T cells rearrange first the TCR β gene and then the TCR α gene. If rearrangements lead to the formation of functional TCR α and β proteins that can form a dimer, the α/β dimer and CD3 molecules are coexpressed at low levels on the cell surface. At this point in development, the thymocytes begin to express both CD4 and CD8 and so become **double-positive thymocytes.** With further maturation into T cells, the level of TCR expression increases and the cells lose expression of either CD4 or CD8, becoming **single-positive thymocytes.** At this stage, thymocytes have acquired the phenotype of mature peripheral T cells and soon exit the thymus.

Interestingly, the first T cells to mature during fetal development are γ/δ T cells. The development of these early γ/δ T cells is highly regulated: they appear in successive waves, with each wave characterized by the use of particular V_γ segments. By contrast, γ/δ T cells that are produced after the time of birth no longer exhibit this coordinated pattern of V_γ expression, whose significance is unknown.

Negative Selection of Thymocytes

A remarkable feature of the T cell system is its ability to distinguish foreign antigens, which elicit an immune response, from self antigens, which do not. One mechanism of self tolerance (but not the only one) is to **delete** T cells whose TCRs recognize self antigens in combination with self MHC molecules. Deletion of autoreactive thymocytes occurs in the double-positive stage. At this point in ontogeny, stimulation of the TCR triggers apoptosis. Presentation of self antigens in the thymus, therefore, induces programmed cell death of CD4+CD8+ thymocytes whose TCRs recognize the self antigens—a phenomenon known as **negative selection.**

Positive Selection of Thymocytes

In addition to the deletion of autoreactive thymocytes, the T cell development process selects for T cells whose TCRs are able to recognize foreign antigens bound to self MHC molecules. The molecular basis for this phenomenon, known as **positive selection,** is obscure. Positive selection accomplishes 2 remarkably difficult feats. First, it occurs in the absence of the foreign antigen and therefore is not the result of a simple TCR recognition event. Second, it selects T cells whose TCRs recognize self MHC molecules yet are not autoreactive.

Self Tolerance

Deletion of autoreactive thymocytes is a major mechanism for avoiding a T cell response to self, but it is not the only one. The deletional mechanism is not completely effective, and some autoreactive T cells escape from the thymus. This may suggest that certain self antigens are not presented in the thymus and therefore cannot induce the deletion of their cognate

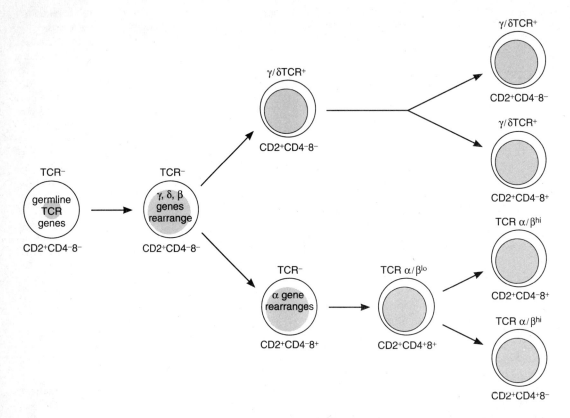

Figure 8–8. Stages in thymocyte development. Progenitor cells migrate from the bone marrow to the thymus. At the earliest stages of development, they express several T cell surface molecules, such as CD2, but still have germline configurations of their TCR genes. Thymocytes destined to become α/β T cells pass through a critical CD4⁺CD8⁺ phase during which autoreactive T cells are deleted.

T cells. In several experimental animal models, mature peripheral T cells whose TCRs can react to autoantigens are rendered anergic (ie, the autoreactive T cells are still present but are unable to respond to the self antigen). The molecular basis of this anergy is unknown.

It seems probable that there are mechanisms for self tolerance in addition to deletion and anergy. It is possible that certain self antigens are sequestered from the immune system. Although MHC molecules do not distinguish between peptides derived from foreign and self proteins, certain self antigens might not be presented to the immune system because they never encounter class II molecules. Recall that only class II molecules can present antigen to the pivotal CD4+ T cells and that class II molecules are very limited in their tissue expression (they are normally found only on professional APCs). Another potential mechanism for tolerance is suppression. As discussed above, there is little hard evidence for the existence of suppressor T cells. Currently suppression remains an intriguing, but not firmly established, means of regulating an immune response to self.

NATURAL KILLER (NK) CELLS

Natural killer cells (**NK cells**) make up a discrete lymphocyte lineage that is distinct from T cells and B cells. NK cells are large lymphocytes that contain cytoplasmic granules and were defined initially by their ability to kill certain tumor cells and virus-infected cells in vitro. The precise physiologic roles of NK cells remain to be defined. They appear to be involved in host defense against certain viral infections and, possibly, against malignancies. NK cells also can be stimulated to produce a variety of cytokines and may have complex regulatory roles.

Development & Tissue Distribution of NK Cells

Like T and B lymphocytes, NK cells derive from a bone marrow precursor, but, apart from this, little is known about their ontogeny. The requirements for development of the NK cell lineage are clearly distinct from those of T cells and B cells. For example, children with severe combined immunodeficiency may lack T cells and B cells but have normal NK cells. Conversely, a few patients have been identified in whom NK cells are absent but T and B cell development is normal.

NK cells make up about 15% of peripheral blood lymphocytes and 3–4% of splenic lymphocytes. Appreciable numbers of NK cells are also found in the lung interstitium, the intestinal mucosa, and the liver. Unlike T cells, they are rare in the thymus and lymph nodes and are not usually found in thoracic duct lymph.

Natural Killing

Several features distinguish natural killing from killing mediated by antigen-specific cytolytic T cells. Lysis of tumor target cells by NK cells does not require the expression of MHC molecules on the surface of a target cell and therefore cannot be triggered through a conventional TCR that recognizes a specific combination of antigenic peptide and MHC protein. Moreover, NK cell activity against tumor targets is spontaneous: it is readily apparent in individuals who have not previously been exposed to the target cell. A cytolytic T cell response, in contrast, requires prior sensitization.

The cell surface receptors that NK cells use to recognize and respond to tumor target cells have not been well defined and remain an area of intense investigation. One attractive model is that NK cells express 2 types of receptors: one that triggers cytolytic activity, and a second that inhibits killing. According to this model, NK cells will lyse a target cell only if the target expresses ligands for the stimulatory receptors and lacks ligands for the inhibitory receptors.

Little is known about the identity of the stimulatory NK receptors or the nature of their ligands on target cells. There has been progress, however, in understanding inhibition of natural killing. In the mouse, a cell surface molecule designated **Ly-49,** whose expression is restricted largely to NK cells, appears to function as an inhibitory receptor. Ly-49 interacts with certain class I MHC molecules and, as a result of this interaction, prevents the NK cell from killing its target. Disruption of the Ly-49/MHC interaction (by the addition of monoclonal antibodies to either component) enables NK cells to lyse formerly resistant targets. Conversely, expression of a class I MHC molecule thought to be a ligand for Ly-49 renders formerly susceptible targets resistant. The Ly-49 inhibitory signals, therefore, are dominant over stimulatory signals. These properties of Ly-49 offer a possible explanation for the long-standing observation that expression of class I MHC molecules on target cells correlates inversely with susceptibility to killing by NK cells. Ly-49 is a member of a family of closely related molecules, raising the possibilities that individual NK cells express multiple family members and that differential expression of members of the Ly-49 family define NK cell subsets with differing spectra of susceptible targets.

Although most studies of NK activity have examined the killing of tumor cells in vitro, it is quite clear that NK cells can kill certain tumors in vivo as well. By implication, NK cells might play a key role in host defense against malignancies, but this point has been difficult to establish experimentally. The roles that NK cells play in immune surveillance against tumors and in host defense against established malignancies remain uncertain.

Lymphokine-Activated Killing

Exposure to certain lymphokines, particularly **IL-2,** activates NK cells to kill a broader spectrum of tumor targets than can be killed by untreated NK cells. Indeed, NK cells are the primary source of **lymphokine-activated killer (LAK)** cells, which are generated when human peripheral blood mononuclear cells are cultured in IL-2 and which have been proposed as a potential biologic agent for antineoplastic therapy.

Distinctions between NK Cells and T Cells

Cytolytic T cells also can be stimulated by IL-2 to acquire LAK activity. This initially led to some confusion regarding discrimination between NK cells and T cells, particularly in the activated state. These cell populations, however, are distinct. Unlike T cells, NK cells do not productively rearrange their TCR genes and do not express a cell surface TCR-CD3 complex. Moreover, most NK cells express **CD16** (a low-affinity Fc receptor that binds IgG in immune complexes) and **CD56,** whereas these molecules generally are not found on T cells. Thus, analysis of the expression of CD3, CD16, and CD56 helps to distinguish NK cells (which are always CD3– and usually CD16+CD56+) from T cells (which are always CD3+ and usually CD16–CD56–).

Antibody-Dependent Cell-Mediated Cytotoxicity

In addition to their ability to mediate natural killing, NK cells can kill antibody-coated cells. This antibody-dependent cell-mediated cytotoxicity (**ADCC**) activity requires the binding of the Fc region of the antibody to the NK cell surface Fc receptor, **CD16,** which in turn activates the cytolytic apparatus of the NK cell.

Cytokine Production by NK Cells

Stimulation of NK cells either with IL-2 or with CD16 ligands leads to the production of IFN γ, TNFα, granulocyte-macrophage colony-stimulating factor (GM-CSF), and colony-stimulating factor-1. The ability to produce cytokines implies that NK cells are likely to have regulatory roles and that the functions of NK cells are not limited to their cytolytic activity. Indeed, NK cells can modulate hematopoiesis and may play a major role in regulating extramedullary hematopoiesis. They also appear capable of modulating B cell responses.

Roles of NK Cells in Host Defenses against Microbial Agents

Despite the attention given to the tumoricidal capacities of NK cells, it is by no means certain that the major physiologic function of NK cells is related to their ability to kill tumor cells. In humans, recurrent viral infections, particularly with varicella-zoster virus, cytomegalovirus, and Epstein-Barr virus, dominate the clinical manifestations of a selective deficiency in NK cells. This experiment of nature suggests that a major role of NK cells is to defend against viral infections, a conclusion that is further supported by animal studies. The latter also implicate NK cells in host responses to certain bacterial and parasitic infections. NK cells may therefore help protect against a range of infectious agents, possibly by acting as a front line of defense that is operative before a specific response can be mounted by the T cell and B cell systems.

REFERENCES

T Cell Receptor

Appleby MW et al: Defective T cell receptor signaling in mice lacking the thymic isoform of p59^{fyn}. *Cell* 1992;**70:**741.

Davis MM, Bjorkman PJ: T-cell antigen receptor genes and T-cell recognition. *Nature* 1988;**334:**395.

Marrack P, Kappler J: The staphylococcal enterotoxins and their relatives. *Science* 1990;**248:**705.

Matsui K et al: Low affinity interaction of peptide-MHC complexes with T cell receptors. *Science* 1991; **254:**1788.

Schreiber SL, Crabtree GR: The mechanism of action of cyclosporin and FK506. *Immunol Today* 1992; **13:**136.

Accessory Molecules

Harding FA et al: CD28-mediated signalling co-stimulates murine T cells and prevents induction of anergy in T-cell clones. *Nature* 1992;**356:**607.

Janeway CA: The T cell receptor as a multicomponent signaling machine: CD4/CD8 coreceptors and CD45 in T cell activation. *Annu. Rev. Immunol.* 1992;**10:**645.

Jenkins MK et al: CD28 delivers a costimulatory signal involved in antigen-specific IL-2 production by human T cells. *J Immunol* 1991;**147:**2461.

Rudd CE et al: The CD4 receptor is complexed in detergent lysates to a protein-tyrosine kinase (pp58) from human T lymphocytes. *Proc Natl Acad Sci USA* 1988;**85:**5190.

Veillette A et al: The CD4 and CD8 T cell surface molecules are associated with the internal membrane tyrosine-protein kinase P56^{lck}. *Cell* 1988;**55:**301.

T Cell Heterogeneity

Havran WL, Allison JP: The immunobiology of T cells with invariant γδ antigen receptors. *Annu Rev. Immunol.* 1991;**9:**679.

Mosmann TR, Coffman RL: Th1 and Th2 cells: different patterns of lymphokine secretion lead to different functional properties. *Annu Rev Immunol* 1989; **7:**145.

Vitetta ES et al: Memory B and T cells. *Annu Rev Immunol* 1991;**9:**193.

T Cell Ontogeny

Kappler JW et al: T cell tolerance by clonal deletion in the thymus. *Cell* 1987;**49:**273.

von Boehmer H: Developmental biology of T cells in T cell receptor transgenic mice. *Annu Rev Immunol* 1990;**8:**531.

Natural Killer Cells

Trinchieri G. Biology of natural killer cells. *Adv Immunol* 1989;**47:**187.

Cytokines

9

Joost J. Oppenheim, MD, Francis W. Ruscetti, PhD, & Connie Faltynek, PhD

Many critical interactions among cells of the immune system are controlled by soluble mediators called **cytokines.** Over the past 3 decades, much has been learned about the molecular nature and biologic effects of these important regulatory molecules. The cytokines are a diverse group of intercellular signaling proteins that regulate not only local and systemic immune and inflammatory responses but also wound healing, hematopoiesis, and many other biologic processes.

Over 100 structurally dissimilar and genetically unrelated cytokines have been identified to date. Most are peptides or glycoproteins with molecular weights (MW) of between 6000 and 60,000. They are extremely potent compounds that act at concentrations of 10^{-10}–10^{-15} M by binding to specific surface receptors on target cells. Unlike endocrine hormones, they are not produced by specialized glands but, rather, by a variety of different tissues and individual cells. Cytokines produced by lymphocytes are also known as **lymphokines,** whereas those produced by monocytes or macrophages are called **monokines.** Only a few cytokines—such as transforming growth factor β (TGFβ), erythropoietin (Epo), stem cell factor (SCF), and monocyte colony-stimulating factor (M-CSF)—are normally present in detectable amounts in the blood and are able to influence distant target cells. Most other cytokines act only locally over extremely short distances, in either a **paracrine** manner (ie, on adjacent cells) or an **autocrine** manner (ie, on the producing cell itself).

Each cytokine is secreted by particular cell types in response to specific stimuli and produces a characteristic constellation of effects on the growth, mobility, differentiation, or function of its target cells. They may be secreted individually or as part of a coordinated response along with other, unrelated cytokines. Their activities often overlap considerably, and, indeed, one cytokine may induce the secretion of other cytokines or mediators, producing a cascade of biologic effects.

This chapter will focus primarily on the cytokines and cytokine receptors that participate in immune and inflammatory responses (Table 9–1). We will first consider IL–1, IL–2, and IL–6, tumor necrosis factor (TNF), and the interferons (IFN) as prototypes and then summarize the essential properties of other cytokines. Cytokines can now be produced in unlimited quantities by using recombinant DNA techniques, and so many are being tested as potential therapeutic agents; we will briefly summarize the clinical experience with them to date. For more information, readers are referred to the cited texts, monographs, and reviews.

INTERLEUKIN-1 (IL-1) & TUMOR NECROSIS FACTOR (TNF)

IL-1 and TNF are structurally unrelated cytokines that bind to different cellular receptors, yet their spectra of biologic effects so resemble one another that these 2 cytokines are almost interchangeable (Fig 9–1; Table 9–2). Their importance in immune responses stems in large part from their ability to enhance the activation of helper T lymphocytes by antigen-presenting cells (APCs). IL-1 and TNF are each secreted by APCs on contact with an antigen- and MHC-specific helper T cell, and they can provide a **costimulatory** signal that promotes T cell activation (see Chapter 3). This appears to occur primarily through autocrine effects on the APC itself: by inducing expression of various adhesion molecules, IFN γ receptors, and class II major histocompatibility complex (MHC) proteins on the surface of an APC, IL-1 and TNF increase the efficiency with which it can bind and activate T cells. In addition, IL-1 and TNF act in a paracrine fashion on the T cell, augmenting IL-2 secretion, expression of surface receptors for IL-2 and IFN γ, and all subsequent events leading to clonal proliferation. Through their ability to potentiate helper cell activation, IL-1 and TNF can promote nearly all types of humoral and cellular immune re-

Table 9–1. Major properties of human interleukins and other immunoregulatory cytokines.

	Earlier Terms	Principal Cell Source	Principal Effects[1]
Interleukins			
IL-1 α and β	Lymphocyte-activating factor, B cell activating factor, hematopoietin	Macrophages, other APCs, other somatic cells	Costimulation of APCs and T cells B cell proliferation and Ig production Acute-phase response of liver (see Table 9–3) Phagocyte activation Inflammation and fever Hematopoiesis
IL-2	T cell growth factor	Activated TH1 cells, TC cells, NK cells	Proliferation of activated T cells NK and TC cell functions B cell proliferation and IgG2 expression
IL-3	Multi-colony-stimulating factor	T lymphocytes	Growth of early hematopoietic progenitors
IL-4	B cell growth factor I, B cell stimulatory factor I	TH2 cells, mast cells	B cell proliferation, IgE expression, and class II MHC expression TH2- and TC-cell proliferation and functions Eosinophil and mast cell growth and function Inhibition of monokine production
IL-5		TH2 cells, mast cells	Eosinophil growth and function
IL-6	IFN-β2, hepatocyte-stimulating factor, hybridoma growth factor	Activated TH2 cells, APCs, other somatic cells	Synergistic effects with IL-1 or TNF to costimulate T cells Acute-phase response of liver (see Table 9–3) B-cell proliferation and Ig production Thrombopoiesis (see Table 9–4)
IL-7		Thymic and marrow stromal cells	T and B lymphopoiesis TC cell functions
IL-8		Macrophages, other somatic cells	Chemoattractant for neutrophils and T cells (see Table 9–5)
IL-9		Cultured T cells	Some hematopoietic and thymopoietic effects
IL-10	Cytokine synthesis inhibitory factor	Activated TH2, CD8 T, and B lymphocytes, macrophages	Inhibition of cytokine production by TH1 cells, NK cells, and APCs Promotion of B cell proliferation and antibody responses Suppression of cellular immunity Mast cell growth
IL-11		Stromal cells	Synergistic effects on hematopoiesis and thrombopoiesis
IL-12	Cytotoxic lymphocyte maturation factor, NK cell stimulatory factor	B cells, macrophages	Proliferation and function of activated TC and NK cells IFN γ production TH1 cell induction; suppresses TH2 cell functions Promotion of cell-mediated immune responses
IL-13		TH2 cells	IL-4-like effects
Other cytokines			
TNFα	Cachectin	Activated macrophages, other somatic cells	IL-1-like effects (see Table 9–2) Vascular thrombosis and tumor necrosis
TNFβ	Lymphotoxin	Activated TH1 cells	IL-1-like effects (see Table 9–2) Vascular thrombosis and tumor necrosis

(*continued*)

Table 9–1. Major properties of human interleukins and other immunoregulatory cytokines. (continued)

	Earlier Terms	Principal Cell Source	Principal Effects[1]
Other cytokines (cont'd.)			
INF α and β	Leukocyte interferons, type I interferons	Macrophages; neutrophils, other somatic cells	Antiviral effects Induction of class I MHC on all somatic cells Activation of macrophages and NK cells
INF γ	Immune interferon, type II interferon	Activated TH1 and NK cells	Induction of class I MHC on all somatic cells Induction of class II MHC on APCs and somatic cells Activation of macrophages, neutrophils, and NK cells Promotion of cell-mediated immunity (inhibits TH2 cells) Induction of high endothelial venules Antiviral effects
TGFβ		Activated T lymphocytes, platelets, macrophages, other somatic cells	Anti-inflammatory (suppression of cytokine production and class II MHC expression) Anti-proliferative for macrophages and lymphocytes Promotion of B-cell expression of IgA Promotion of fibroblast proliferation and wound healing

[1]All of the listed processes are enhanced unless otherwise indicated.

sponses. In this regard, both cytokines often act together with IL-6, with which they produce synergistic effects.

IL-1 and TNF also act directly on many other types of immune and inflammatory cells (Fig 9–1A). For example, they can directly promote growth and differentiation of B cells—particularly during the transitions from pre-B cells into mature B lymphocytes and from lymphocytes into plasma cells. They also can activate neutrophils and macrophages, stimulate hematopoiesis, and induce expression of numerous other cytokines and inflammatory mediators. Moreover, both IL-1 and TNF produce a broad range of effects on nonhematopoietic cell types (Fig 9–1B), which will be discussed below.

Interleukin-1

IL-1 can be produced by virtually all nucleated cell types, including all members of the monocyte-macrophage lineage, B lymphocytes, natural killer (NK) cells, T lymphocyte clones grown in cell culture, keratinocytes, dendritic cells, astrocytes, fibroblasts, neutrophils, endothelial cells, and smooth muscle cells. Like all other species examined to date, humans express 2 distinct molecular forms of IL-1, called **IL-1α** and **IL-1β**. These are peptides, 159 and 153 amino acids long, respectively, that are encoded by separate genes and share only 26% amino acid sequence similarity. Nevertheless, the potency and biologic activi-

ties of IL-1α and IL-1β are virtually identical, and they bind with about the same affinity to the same cell surface receptors. Many cell types express both IL-1 genes, but their relative levels of expression can vary widely. For example, human monocytes produce predominantly IL-1β, whereas keratinocytes produce mainly IL-1α. The biologic significance of this disparity is unknown. A few cell types can also express a third gene that codes for a protein known as **IL-1 receptor antagonist (IL-1RA),** which is biologically inactive but competes for binding of IL-1 receptors and so is a competitive inhibitor of IL-1α and IL-1β.

IL-1α and IL-1β are initially synthesized as propeptides (MW 31,000), which are then processed enzymatically, either at or beyond the outer cell membrane, to yield the mature cytokines (MW 17,000). The IL-1α propeptide is biologically active, but the IL-1β precursor is not. Although IL-1 generally acts as a soluble extracellular protein, biologically active IL-1α (but not IL-1β) has also been detected on the surfaces of cells and may thus participate in interactions that require cell-to-cell contact.

A few tissues express IL-1 constitutively; for example, the skin contains significant amounts of IL-1, as do amniotic fluid, sweat, and urine. In contrast, macrophages and most other cell types produce IL-1 only in response to external stimuli, such as bacterial **lipopolysaccharide (LPS),** urate or silicate particles, or the **adjuvants** aluminum hydroxide and muramyl

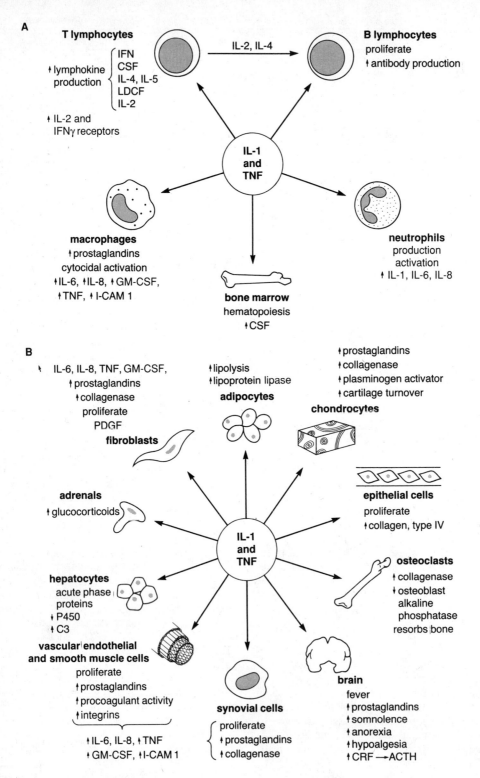

Figure 9–1. Actions of IL-1 and TNF on hematopoietic and lymphoid tissues **(A)** and nonlymphoid cells and tissues **(B).** Activities of the two individual cytokines differ in some respects, as detailed in Table 9–2.

Table 9–2. Target cells and actions of IL-1 and TNF.

Target Cells or Tissues	Effects	IL-1	TNF
T lymphocytes	Costimulate T cell activation Induce IL-2 receptors Induce lymphokine production	+ + +	+ + +
B lymphocytes	Promote proliferation Enhance immunoglobulin expression	+ +	+ +
Monocytes and macrophages	Chemoattract Activate to cytotoxic state Induce production of prostaglandins, IL-1, IL-6, GM-CSF, and chemokines	− + +	± + +
Neutrophils	Activate to produce cytokines	+	+
Endothelial and vascular smooth muscle cells	Increase adhesiveness for leukocytes (ICAM-1) Induce procoagulant activity, cytokine production, and class I MHC Induce mitogenesis and angiogenesis	+ + +	+ + +
Hematopoietic cells	Inhibit some precursor growth and differentiation Stimulate precursor cells	− +	+ −
Hepatocytes	Induce some acute-phase proteins Decrease cytochrome P-450 Increase plasma Cu; decrease plasma Fe and Zn	+ + +	+ + +
Neuroendocrine cells	Stimulate glucocorticoid secretion Induce fever Induce somnolence and anorexia	+ + +	+ + +
Osteoblasts	Decrease alkaline phosphatase	+	+
Osteoclasts	Increase bone resorption and collagenase	+	+
Chondrocytes	Increase cartilage turnover	+	+
Fibroblasts and synovial cells	Induce collagenase, chemokines, other cytokines	+	+
Adipocytes	Decrease lipoprotein lipase Increase lipolysis	+ +	+ +
Epithelial cells	Induce proliferation Increase type IV collagen secretion	+ +	ND[1] ND
Pancreatic β cells	Modulate insulin secretion	+	−
Dendritic cells	Enhance ability to activate T cells	+	ND
Tumor cells	Cytostatic and cytolytic effects	+	+

[1]ND, no data available.

dipeptide (see Chapter 4). It is thought that, during the process of antigen presentation, IL-1 production by the presenting cell is initially triggered by contact with the T cell and may then be increased further in response to TNF, colony-stimulating factor (CSF), or IL-2 released from the T cell when it becomes activated. Prostaglandins, a class of small molecules that are important mediators of inflammation (see Chapter 10), can also regulate IL-1 expression; for example, IL-1 production by macrophages is enhanced by leukotrienes but is suppressed by products of the cyclooxygenase pathway such as prostaglandin E_2. Increased circulating levels of IL-1 are also observed during the luteal phase of the menstrual cycle and during strenuous exercise.

IL-1 Receptors & Signal Transduction

IL-1α and IL-1β bind to high-affinity receptors (K d ≈ 10^{-10} M) found on all their target cells. The numbers of receptors range from 50 or fewer on T lymphocytes to several thousand on fibroblasts. Two distinct receptors have been cloned, both of which are transmembrane glycoproteins that bind IL-1α and IL-1β equally. These receptors share only 28% sequence similarity but have comparable 3-dimensional structures that each include 3 extracellular immunoglobulinlike domains. The type 1 receptor (**IL-1RI**) is 517 amino acids long, has a 217-amino-acid cytoplasmic tail, and transmits signals into the cytoplasm when it binds IL-1; it appears responsible for signaling in all IL-1-responsive cells. The type II receptor (**IL-1RII**), in contrast, has only a 29-amino-acid intracytoplasmic tail and cannot transduce signals. The extracellular domain of IL-1RII is released in soluble form at sites of local inflammation and into the serum during times of systemic inflammation. This soluble IL-1RII is produced in relatively large amounts, binds IL-1β much more strongly than it binds IL-1α or IL-1RA, and is proposed to function as an endogenous inhibitor of IL-1β at inflammatory sites.

Receptors for IL-1 are expressed constitutively on responsive cells, but their level of expression is modulated by a variety of agents. For example, IL-1 itself, as well as GM-CSF, G-CSF, and corticosteroids each increase the expression of IL-1 receptors and enhance IL-1 responsiveness of bone marrow cells. TFFβ decreases IL-1 receptor expression.

The mechanism of signal transduction by IL-1 is still controversial. After IL-1 binds, the receptor-cytokine complex is immediately internalized and subsequently degraded, and it must then be replaced by newly synthesized receptors. IL-1 binding to only 5–10% of the IL-1RI molecules on a cell (ie, occupancy of fewer than 5–200 receptors/cell) appears sufficient to trigger cellular responses. The earliest events observed after binding include phosphorylation of serine and threonine residues on a number of cytoplasmic proteins. Some of the phosphorylated proteins directly or indirectly activate specific transcription factors, which in turn bind to chromosomal DNA containing IL-1 responsive genes, leading to activation or inhibition of those genes.

Tumor Necrosis Factor

Human TNF exists in 2 distinct forms called TNFα and TNFβ. **TNFα** was first described as an activity in the serum of lipopolysaccharide (LPS)-treated animals that was capable of inducing hemorrhagic necrosis of certain tumors. It later was discovered independently as **cachectin,** a circulating mediator of the wasting syndrome associated with certain parasitic diseases. TNFα is produced predominantly by activated macrophages and less so by other cell types. **TNFβ,** which is primarily a product of activated T lymphocytes, has also been called **lymphotoxin.** TNFα and TNFβ both bind to the same receptors on target cells and consequently have the same biologic activities. As noted above, these activities extensively overlap those of IL-1.

The degree of similarity between TNFα and TNFβ is only 28% at the amino acid level. They are encoded by 2 separate genes that are both located within the MHC complex on chromosome 6; hence, they are sometimes referred to as class III MHC proteins, although they have no structural resemblance to class I or class II MHC molecules. Both are synthesized as propeptides and are processed intracellularly to yield the mature forms, which are 157 and 171 amino acids long, respectively. It has been proposed that an active membrane-bound form of TNFα may exist that can mediate tumor cell killing through direct contact.

TNF Receptors & Signal Transduction

Two types of high-affinity receptors for TNFα and TNFβ have been identified. The MW 75,000 (type II) receptor binds TNFα and TNFβ with about 10-fold higher affinity ($K_d = 5 \times 10^{-11}$ M) than does the MW 55,000 (type I) receptor. Each TNF receptor has a large extracellular binding domain, a hydrophobic transmembrane region, and an intracellular signal-transducing tail. TNF binds to these receptors as a trimer, with each trimer binding simultaneously to 2 or 3 of either the type I or type II receptors. This ligand-mediated cross-linking of the receptors is thought to initiate signal transduction, resulting in a cascade of protein phosphorylation and gene activation very similar to that produced by IL-1. The 2 types of TNF receptor are thought to elicit distinct responses: the type I receptor reportedly promotes cytotoxic activity and fibroblast proliferation, whereas the type II receptor promotes T lymphocyte proliferation.

Like the IL-1 receptors, TNF receptors are internalized after ligand binding and are modulated by a variety of regulatory factors. For example, IL-2 increases expression of both types of TNF receptors, whereas IFN γ selectively induces type II. Activated cells shed TNF receptors from the cell surface, and this may serve to antagonize TNF activity during inflammatory responses.

Nonimmunologic Effects of IL-1 & TNF

TNF appears primarily responsible for a laboratory phenomenon known as the localized **hemorrhagic Schwartzman reaction,** in which 2 successive injections of bacterial LPS given 24 hours apart into the same solid tissue site produce localized coagulation, hemorrhage, and tissue necrosis. This occurs because LPS-induced secretion of TNF by macrophages can stimulate endothelial cells to produce prostaglandins, IL-6, and a protein called procoagulant factor (or tissue factor III), which can initiate the clotting cascade. These local coagulation and inflammatory effects block the blood supply and may account for the ability of TNF to cause infarcts and hemorrhagic necrosis of tumors, the property that led to its initial discovery. There is also a systemic form of the Schwartzman reaction, in which 2 doses of LPS given intravenously induce **disseminated intravascular coagulation—**widespread thrombosis that obstructs capillaries, depletes the supply of coagulation factors, and may lead to hemorrhages, shock, and death. This systemic reaction is thought to mimic certain effects of severe bacterial sepsis and is mediated, at least in part, by TNF. Repeated injections of IL-1 can also yield local Schwartzman reactions, and low doses of IL-1 act synergistically with TNF to mimic the fatal systemic effects of **septic shock.**

TNF and IL-1 are among the most important inducers of the **acute-phase response,** in which hepatocytes produce increased amounts of certain plasma proteins that are thought to be of value in nonspecific host defense against infections (Table 9–3). Their effect in this regard is less pronounced than that of IL-6 (see below).

Both IL-1 and TNF can activate endothelial cells

Table 9–3. Plasma proteins of the acute-phase response.[1]

Inducible by IL-1, IL-6, or TNF
Complement factor C3
Haptoglobin
C-reactive protein
α_1-Acid glycoprotein
Factor B
Serum amyloid proteins A and P
Regulated only by IL-6
Albumin[1]
Prealbumin[1]
Fibrinogen
Hemopexin
Cysteine proteinase inhibitor
α_1-Antichymotrypsin
α_2-Macroglobulin

[1]Hepatocyte synthesis and plasma concentration of each of the listed proteins are increased during the acute-phase response, except those of albumin and prealbumin, which are decreased.

and thus promote neutrophil migration into an inflamed site. They induce the production of endothelial growth factors and have angiogenic activity. Acting alone or synergistically, they can induce a number of effects that are mediated through the hypothalamus: they are **endogenous pyrogens** (ie, they induce **fever**) and directly induce the secretion of corticotropin-releasing factor, which stimulates the release of adrenocorticotropic hormone from the pituitary and thus induces **glucocorticoid** production by the adrenals. The latter effect results in negative feedback, since glucocorticoids suppress the production of both IL-1 and TNF.

Both IL-1 and TNF stimulate alkaline phosphatase activity in osteoblasts, bone resorption by osteoclasts, cartilage turnover by chondrocytes, and proliferation by fibroblasts and synovial cells. Increased levels of IL-1 and TNF are found in inflammatory joint fluids and may contribute to the fibrosis and thickening of **arthritic joints.** Preliminary reports suggest that administration of IL-1RA and TNF antagonists can ameliorate the symptoms and signs of rheumatoid arthritis.

IL-1 synergizes with CSFs to stimulate proliferation and differentiation of early hematopoietic progenitors of the marrow. In addition, IL-1 induces bone marrow stromal cells to produce a number of the hematopoietic CSFs, as well as receptors for G-CSF and SCF. TNF also actively induces CSF production by bone marrow stromal cells and macrophages but directly inhibits rather than promotes stem cell proliferation. Both TNF and IL-1 enhance production and release of neutrophils from the marrow. IL-1 and, to a lesser extent, TNF can protect against the marrow-suppressive effects of radiation if given 1 day prior to exposure.

IL-1 stimulates epithelial cell proliferation and function, including the production of basement membrane collagen; the effect of TNF on epithelial cells is

unknown. IL-1, but not TNF, selectively affects pancreatic β cells and causes changes in plasma insulin levels. Both TNF and IL-1 exhibit indirect antiviral effects that are mediated in part by the induction of IFN β. TNF and IL-1 can kill or inhibit the growth of many tumor cells in vitro, although TNF is effective against a wider variety of cell types and kills them more rapidly than does IL-1. The **cachexia** (ie, wasting) induced by TNF is probably related to its ability to increase lipoprotein lipase activity and hence deplete fat cells. IL-1 is also reported to have this capability, but to a significantly lesser degree.

Overall, the considerable overlap in the biologic activities of IL-1 and TNF is probably advantageous in that it provides alternative pathways for mobilizing host reactions in emergencies. Moreover, IL-1 and TNF regulate one another, and their ability to synergize enables them to achieve maximal effects at suboptimal concentrations. This is economical, results in enormous amplification of host reactions, and increases the efficiency of the host defense system.

IL-1, TNF, & Their Inhibitors as Therapeutic Agents

Both IL-1 and TNF have been investigated as possible therapeutic agents, with emphasis on their immunostimulatory and antineoplastic activities. Neither has yet proven useful in practice, however, largely because of their numerous side effects. The pharmacologic properties of TNF and IL-1 at high concentrations are similar, although TNF causes more vascular occlusion, tumor necrosis, and capillary leakage, whereas IL-1 (owing to its more potent hematopoietic effects) provides greater protection against lethal doses of radiation and against bone marrow suppression caused by cancer chemotherapeutic agents.

Antagonists of IL-1 and TNF are of considerable therapeutic interest as a means of ameliorating chronic inflammatory diseases. IL-1 and TNF activities can potentially be inhibited by factors that affect their synthesis, release, receptor binding, or signal transduction. Potent nonspecific antagonism to both these cytokines is exhibited by TGFβ and by corticosteroids. In addition to reducing IL-1 production, TGFβ inhibits IL-1RI expression and induces the production of IL-1RA—it is a "triple threat!" Corticosteroids not only reduce the production of IL-1 and TNF but also increase expression of IL-1RII, which can further inhibit IL-1 effects. Inhibitors of the lipoxygenase pathway likewise reduce the amount of IL-1 released, whereas leukotrienes appear to increase it (see Chapter 11). β-Melanocyte-stimulating factor has been reported to inhibit IL-1 activity through an unknown mechanism.

IL-1RA can competitively inhibit IL-1 binding to its receptor; however, it must be present in substantial (at least 100-fold) molar excess over IL-1 to yield effective competition. Moreover, IL-1RA is unable to prevent activation of helper T cells by APCs, presumably because alternative pathways of costimulation are available. The shed extracytoplasmic domain of IL-1RII can selectively bind and inhibit IL-1β and probably plays a significant antagonistic role in vivo. Interestingly, certain poxviruses have also been found to encode soluble IL-1β-binding proteins that are secreted from infected cells and may tend to suppress antiviral immune responses.

INTERLEUKIN-2

IL-2 is an autocrine and paracrine growth factor that is secreted by activated T lymphocytes and is essential for clonal T cell proliferation. It was first discovered in 1976 by virtue of its ability to enhance mitogenesis of human T lymphocytes and to support continuous growth of normal T cells in culture. The discovery of IL-2 (then called **T cell growth factor**) was a major advance in immunology, because it made it possible for the first time to propagate and study individual clones of normal T cells that maintained their immunologic properties. Its essential role in T cell proliferation, together with its effects on cytokine production and on the functional properties of B cells, macrophages, and NK cells, places IL-2 among the most critical immunoregulatory cytokines.

The IL-2 molecule is an MW 15,400 polypeptide, 133 amino acids long, that is encoded by a single gene on human chromosome 4. It can be glycosylated to various degrees to produce higher-molecular weight species, although the glycosyl side chains are not necessary for function. Its amino acid sequence bears no similarity to that of any other known cytokine, but x-ray crystallographic analysis indicates that it has a 3-dimensional structure resembling those of IL-4 and granulocyte-macrophage CSF (GM-CSF). IL-2 is a globular protein composed of 4 α-helices that are arranged to form hydrophobic planar faces around a very hydrophobic core. This configuration is maintained in part by the single intrachain disulfide bond, which is essential for biologic activity.

Resting T lymphocytes do not synthesize or secrete IL-2 protein but can be induced to do both by appropriate combinations of antigen and costimulatory factors (see Chapter 8) or by exposure to polyclonal mitogens (see Chapter 2). Studies of isolated T cell subtypes indicate that antigen-induced IL-2 production occurs mainly in CD4 helper T cells. However, CD8 lymphocytes and some NK cells also can be induced to secrete IL-2 under certain conditions. When normal human lymphocytes are exposed to a T cell mitogen, IL-2 mRNA expression becomes detectable after 4 hours, reaches peak concentration at 12 hours, and thereafter declines rapidly. The abrupt disappearance of the mRNA reflects not only the cessation of IL-2 gene transcription but also the instability of IL-2

mRNA, which has a half-life of less than 30 min. Synthesis and release of IL-2 protein follow a similar time course, resulting in a transient burst of secretion that quickly subsides. Because IL-2 has a very short half-life in the circulation, it acts only on the cell that secreted it or on cells in the immediate vicinity.

IL-2 Receptors & Signal Transduction

The high-affinity IL-2 receptor **(IL-2R)** is not expressed on resting T cells but is induced to maximal levels within 2–3 days after the cells become activated. Expression then declines to undetectable levels by 6–10 days after activation. The decline in receptor expression occurs regardless of whether IL-2 is present, indicating that it is autonomously regulated. This ensures that, within a few days after activation, the T cell will become refractory to IL-2, so that clonal proliferation will cease. If such a cell is then reactivated, IL-2R reappears on the cell surface and IL-2-dependent proliferation resumes until the receptors again disappear 4–7 days later. The transient nature of IL-2R expression helps to maintain the cyclical, self-limiting pattern of normal T cell growth in vivo. In contrast, T cells that have been transformed by **human T cell leukemia virus type I (HTLV-I),** the agent of **adult T cell leukemia** syndrome, constitutively express IL-2R. This is thought to be important for the mechanism of cellular transformation by HTLV-I.

The high-affinity IL-2R found on activated T lymphocytes is composed of 3 different polypeptides designated α, β, and γ. All 3 are integral membrane proteins that associate noncovalently with one another. Each can bind IL-2 independently with low affinity, but the 3 in combination yield a high-affinity binding site. The α chain (MW 55,000) has only 13 cytoplasmic amino acids and has no signaling activity; it is the protein recognized by an antibody, called **anti-Tac,** which is widely used to detect IL-2R for diagnosis or research. The β and γ chains (MW 75,000 and 64,000, respectively) have larger cytoplasmic domains (286 and 86 residues, respectively), which can work together cooperatively to transmit signals. IL-2 binding is followed almost immediately by the onset of protein tyrosine kinase (PTK) activity in the cytoplasm. Since none of the IL-2R chains has intrinsic kinase activity, the receptor is presumably linked directly or indirectly with cytoplasmic PTKs whose identity is unknown.

Effects of IL-2 on T Lymphocytes

When exposed to appropriate activating stimuli, resting CD4 T lymphocytes begin to express both IL-2 and surface IL-2R and shortly thereafter begin to proliferate. Interference with either the IL-2 or its receptor (for example, by treatment with specific antibodies) blocks the proliferative response. CD8 T cells are generally unable to produce adequate amounts of IL-2 and so require exogenous IL-2 from helper cells in order to proliferate. Because of its effect on lymphocyte proliferation, IL-2 can be used to establish proliferating clones of normal human CD4 or CD8 T cells in vitro, provided the cells are also continually exposed to mitogens or other activating stimuli that can maintain IL-2 receptor expression.

The addition of IL-2 to activated normal human lymphocytes directly promotes several other cellular functions as well as proliferation. For example, IL-2-stimulated T cells exhibit enhanced cytotoxicity and produce lymphokines such as IFN γ, TNFβ, and TGFβ; B cell growth factors such as IL-4 and IL-6; and hematopoietic growth factors such as IL-3, IL-5, and GM-CSF. The congenital inability to produce IL-2 does not appear to affect thymic anatomy or T cell development in mice but does result in a potentially fatal deficiency of cytotoxic T cell function. Some forms of T cell **anergy** are associated with a selective inability of individual clones to produce IL-2. The immunosuppressive drugs **cyclosporin A** and **FK506** act in part by blocking the induction of IL-2 and IL-2R in helper T lymphocytes.

IL-2 Effects on Non-T Cells

NK cells are unique among lymphoid cells in that they constitutively express IL-2R and thus are always IL-2-responsive. Because they express only the β and γ chains, unstimulated NK cells bind IL-2 with relatively low affinity and proliferate only in response to correspondingly higher IL-2 concentrations. Once stimulated by IL-2, however, NK cells begin to express the Il-2Rα chain and so acquire high-affinity receptors. IL-2-stimulated NK cells have enhanced cytolytic activity and secrete numerous cytokines, including several (IFN γ, GM-CSF, and TNFα) that are potent activators of macrophages. IL-2 also induces **lymphokine-activated killer (LAK)** activity, which is predominantly due to NK cells.

Activated or transformed **B lymphocytes** express high-affinity IL-2R at approximately 30% the density found on activated T cells. IL-2 enhances proliferation and antibody secretion by normal B cells, although at concentrations 2–3-fold higher than are required to obtain T cell responses. It also influences the **heavy-chain class switch,** biasing B cells toward expression of IgG2 antibodies.

Human monocytes and **macrophages** constitutively express low levels of IL-2Rβ chain, but inducibly express high-affinity receptors containing all 3 chains on exposure to IL-2, IFN γ, or other activating agents. Continued exposure of an activated macrophage to IL-2 enhances its microbicidal and cytotoxic activities and promotes secretion of hydrogen peroxide, TNFα, and IL-6. Recent reports indicate that IL-2 can activate **neutrophils** as well.

IL-2 & Related Molecules as Therapeutic Agents

Administration of IL-2 to normal or immunodefi-cient mice has been shown to enhance immune responses, particularly those mediated by cytotoxic T lymphocytes or NK cells. Its potential use in humans, unfortunately, is limited by severe toxic side effects that occur at pharmacologic IL-2 dosages. One of the most important of these is the **"vascular leak syndrome,"** characterized by the accumulation of edema fluid in the pleural cavities, peritoneum, and other extravascular spaces; this may result from the ability of IL-2 to induce other cytokines that activate endothelial cells. IL-2 treatment can also lead to elevated serum cortisol levels, with consequent immunosuppressive effects. High-dose IL-2 has been tested as an immunostimulatory agent in the treatment of a variety of cancers and has produced partial remissions in some patients with **renal cell carcinoma** or metastatic **melanoma.** It has also been tested at low doses as a treatment for the T cell anergy that occurs in patients with **lepromatous leprosy;** although some clinical benefit was observed, the anergy persisted, and the beneficial effects appear to have been attributable to activation of macrophages and NK cells.

Efforts have also been made to suppress immune responses by preventing interaction of IL-2 with its cellular receptor. Animal studies suggest that treatment with anti-IL-2R antibodies which interfere with this interaction may prolong the survival of tissue allografts and may induce long-term tolerance to the graft. In addition, fusion proteins made by linking IL-2 covalently to toxins (such as diphtheria toxin) are being explored as selective poisons that could be used to eradicate cells bearing surface IL-2R. Such fusion proteins are highly efficacious in vitro and may prove useful in treating **adult T cell leukemia** and other IL-2R-expressing cancers (see Chapter 45).

INTERLEUKIN-6 (IL-6) & RELATED CYTOKINES

IL-6 is a cytokine with multiple biologic activities on a variety of cells (Table 9–4). Its major activities include synergizing with IL-1 and TNF to **costimulate** immune responses; inducing the **acute-phase response** in liver cells; enhancing B cell replication, differentiation, and immunoglobulin production; costimulating hematopoiesis and thrombopoiesis; and supporting the growth of transformed hepatocyte and myeloma cell lines in tissue culture. IL-6 was initially called interferon-β2 (IFN β2) because it appeared to exhibit antiviral activity and to cross-react with some antisera to IFN β (see below). However, subsequent studies show that IL-6 itself has no antiviral activity, though it acts to induce small amounts of interferon.

The gene for IL-6 is located on human chromosome 7. The reported MW of IL-6 ranges between 22,000 and 30,000, owing to variations in the degree of glycosylation and phosphorylation of the single polypeptide. IL-6 can be produced by many cell

Table 9–4. The human IL-6 family of cytokines.

	IL-6	IL-11	LIF	OSM	CNTF
Predominant cell sources	Activated TH2 cells Macrophages Endothelial cells Fibroblasts	Stromal cells	T cells Macrophages Fibroblasts	Macrophages T cells	Glial cells
Unique effects	T cell costimulator Coinduces cachexia Induces glucocorticoids Increases bone resorption Promotes keratinocyte growth			Promotes smooth muscle and fibroblast growth	Enhances survival of ciliary neurons
Shared effects[1]	Acute-phase response	+	+	+	+
	B cell and plasma cell growth, Ig production	+	–	–	–
	Hematopoiesis	+	+	+	–
	Leukemic cell growth	?	+	+	–
	Neurotrophic activity	?	+	+	+
	Endothelial cell growth	?	+	+	–

[1]Ability to induce or enhance the indicated processes.

types, including activated T and B lymphocytes, monocytes, endothelial cells, epithelial cells, and fibroblasts. Its expression is induced by a variety of stimuli, including TNF, IL-1, platelet-derived growth factor, and any factors that activate T lymphocytes.

The IL-6 Receptor Family

High-affinity receptors for IL-6, with a K_d of 10^{-10}–10^{-12} M, are expressed by a variety of cell types, including macrophages and myelomonocytic cell lines, hepatocytes, resting T cells, activated or Epstein-Barr virus-infected B cells, and plasma cells. Each target cell expresses 10^2–10^4 IL-6 receptors. The receptor consists of 2 glycoprotein chains; the MW 80,000 **IL-6Rα** chain lacks a cytoplasmic domain and binds IL-6 with low affinity; and the resulting complex of IL-6Rα and IL-6 is then bound with high affinity by the MW 130,000 **IL-6Rβ** chain, which transduces a signal into the cytoplasm.

Over the past few years, the Il-6Rβ chain has also been found to form part of the receptors for 4 structurally unrelated cytokines: interleukin-11 (**IL-11**), leukocyte inhibitory factor (**LIF**), oncostatin M (**OSM**), and ciliary neurotrophic factor (**CNTF**). Each of these cytokines has its own specific receptor containing a unique α chain that mediates ligand binding. The IL-6Rβ chain functions as a common signal-transducing portion in each of these receptors; this may account for the reported overlap in the biologic activities of these structurally dissimilar cytokines.

Activities of the IL-6 Cytokine Family

IL-6 has certain biologic activities that are not exhibited by other known members of the family (Table 9–4), although further study may yet uncover new family members which share these capabilities. Alone among these cytokines, IL-6 acts as a co-stimulant that synergistically augments the mitogenic effects of IL-1 and TNF on helper T cells. This effect

is in part (but not entirely) due to its ability to increase IL-2 receptor expression. IL-6 is also very effective in enhancing TNF- or IL-1-induced cachexia and glucocorticoid synthesis and is able independently to stimulate osteoclast activity and keratinocyte growth. It does not activate expression of any other known cytokines and has relatively little autonomous effect on immune cells at physiologic concentrations. This suggests that its main immunologic function is to potentiate the effects of other cytokines.

IL-6 is the most important inducer of the hepatic **acute-phase response** (Table 9–3), although IL-11, LIF, and OSM share this activity, as do IL-1 and TNF. The capacities of IL-6 to stimulate growth of lymphoid cell lines and to promote immunoglobulin synthesis are shared by IL-11. Since malignant B cells of multiple myeloma both produce and respond to IL-6, it may act as an autocrine growth factor for these cells. IL-11 has stimulatory effects on hematopoiesis, as do IL-6 and LIF. The leukemic-cell inhibitory and myelocytopoietic activities of LIF are also exhibited by OSM and IL-6. OSM was initially discovered as an inhibitor of melanoma cell growth. CNTF promotes survival of ciliary neurons by preventing apoptosis. Most effects of CNTF are neuron-specific, because the distribution of CNTF receptor appears limited to neural tissues. IL-6 and LIF also have some trophic effects on neural cells.

THE INTERFERONS (IFNs)

In 1957, it was discovered that cells exposed to inactivated viruses produce at least one soluble factor that can "interfere" with viral replication when applied to newly infected cells. The factor was named **interferon.** It has since been shown that the interferons consist of a large family of secretory proteins that have in common not only their antiviral activity but also the ability to inhibit proliferation of vertebrate cells and to modulate immune responses. Interferons do not exert their antiviral effects by acting on viral particles but, rather, by inducing an antiviral state within the host cell that makes it inhospitable to viral replication. This, as well as the antiproliferative and immunomodulatory effects of interferons, reflects their ability to regulate specific gene expression and metabolic activity in their target cells.

Many different types of proteins can induce an antiviral state in vertebrate cells and therefore are, by definition, interferons. Their molecular and biologic properties differ so widely that it is useful to classify the interferons into distinct types. Classifications can be drawn on the basis of amino acid sequence, cell of origin, stimulus for induction, or other criteria. It is most important, however, to recognize that one interferon, called IFN γ, differs in nearly all significant respects from the others. In particular, although IFN γ has the antiviral activity typical of all interferons, this is far outweighed by its importance as an immunoregulatory molecule. For this reason, we will first consider the predominantly antiviral (type I) interferons as a group and then examine the unique properties of the only immune (type II) interferon, IFN γ.

The Antiviral IFNs (IFN α, IFN β, & IFN ω)

Most cell types can synthesize **type I IFNs** and will do so in response to infection by viruses, bacteria, or protozoa or when exposed to certain cytokines (Fig 9–2). These IFNs can also be induced artificially by treating cells with double-stranded RNA molecules, which presumably mimic the genomes of certain RNA viruses. One inducer of type I IFN that is used frequently for research is **poly(I:C)**—a heteroduplex of polyinosinate and polycytodinate RNA chains. Type I IFNs are not normally found in tissues or serum but appear rapidly during viral infections.

There are 3 major forms of type I IFN, called IFN α, IFN β, and IFN ω. **IFNα** is the primary IFN produced by **leukocytes** and consists of proteins (MW 18,000–20,000) encoded by a family of at least 18 closely related genes, of which 14 are functional. The amino acid sequences of these various IFN α proteins are approximately 90% identical to one another. **Fibroblasts** and most other nonleukocytic cells primarily express **IFN β**, a protein that is only about 30% identical to IFN α. Small amounts of IFN β are also expressed by leukocytes. There are 6 **IFN ω** genes, of which only one is functional; it resembles the IFN α genes and is primarily expressed by leukocytes.

All 3 forms of type I IFN bind to a single receptor, which is expressed on nearly all cell types. The molecular characteristics of the receptor are not yet fully known. Binding of a type I IFN to this receptor induces or increases expression of at least 30 different gene products in the target cell (Fig 9–2). Among the proteins whose expression is increased are the **class I MHC** molecules, which function to present endogenous antigens to CD8 T cells. Induction of class I MHC enhances the ability of a virally infected cell to

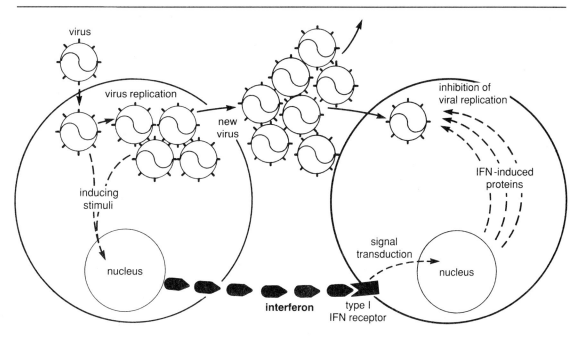

Figure 9–2. Schematic representation of the induction and activity of a type I interferon.

present viral antigens and so to be killed by cytotoxic T cells. IFN-inducible proteins include a specific protein kinase and 2′–5′-oligoadenylate (2–5A) synthetase. The latter 2 enzymes both require the presence of double-stranded RNA for activity. When activated, the protein kinase phosphorylates a component of the cellular translational machinery (called eukaryotic initiation factor 2 [eIF2], and thereby inhibits protein synthesis. The 2–5A synthetase produces short chains of adenylate residues joined by 2′–5′ phosphodiester bonds; these bind and activate a cellular endoribonuclease that specifically degrades single-stranded RNA. These enzymes, together with other IFN-inducible proteins, combine to yield a relatively nonspecific inhibition of gene expression that is particularly potent against viruses.

In addition to inhibiting viral replication, type I IFNs can modulate specific cellular functions. They are able to arrest the growth of (but generally do not kill) many types of cells in culture, including transformed cell lines. They also may either inhibit or promote cellular differentiation, depending on the cell type and the timing and dosage of IFN.

Immune IFN (IFN γ)

IFN γ (also called type II IFN or immune IFN) differs in virtually all respects from the type I IFNs. There is only a single active form of IFN γ protein—a homodimer of MW 18,000 polypeptides that can be glycosylated to various degrees. It arises from a single gene and shows no appreciable resemblance to the other IFNs. The receptor to which it binds is likewise unrelated to the receptor for type I IFN. Although IFN γ has some antiviral activity (which led to its discovery and is the source of its name), it is much less active in this regard than the type I IFNs. Moreover, IFN γ expression is not inducible by infection or by double-stranded RNA. It is therefore best regarded as an entirely distinct immunoregulatory cytokine.

IFN γ is a lymphokine that is secreted by nearly all CD8 T cells, by some CD4 T cells (particularly those of the TH1 subset [see Chapter 8]), and to a minor degree by NK cells. Each of these cell types secretes IFN γ only when activated, usually as part of an immune response.

Nearly all cell types express receptors for IFN γ and respond to this cytokine by increasing surface expression of class I MHC proteins. As a result, virtually any cell in the vicinity of an IFN γ-secreting lymphocyte becomes more efficient at presenting endogenous antigens and hence a better target for cytotoxic killing if it harbors an intracellular pathogen. Unlike the type I IFNs, IFN γ also increases the expression of class II MHC proteins on class II-bearing cells and so promotes antigen presentation to CD4 T lymphocytes as well. It also induces de novo expression of class II MHC proteins on venular endothelial cells and on some other epithelial and connective-tissue cells that do not otherwise express them,

thus recruiting these cell types to function as APCs at sites of intense immune activity.

IFN γ is also the most potent known activator of macrophages. Exposure to IFN γ greatly enhances the microbicidal (and, to a lesser degree, cytotoxic) activity of macrophages and induces them to secrete monokines such as IL-1, IL-6, IL-8, and TNF α. It also activates neutrophils, NK cells, and vascular endothelial cells. In the presence of IFN γ, venular endothelial cells become more adhesive for neutrophils (see Chapter 1) and may differentiate to form high endothelial venules, which attract lymphocytes from the circulation (see Chapter 2).

Although IFN γ tends to promote the differentiation of B cells and CD8 T cells into immunologically active effector cells, it does not promote lymphocyte proliferation and may, in fact, suppress it to some degree. IFN γ enhances the activity of TH1 cells and therefore augments cell-mediated immunity, but it inhibits the proliferation of TH2 cells and thus tends to suppress humoral immunity. It not only decreases the production of IL-4 by TH2 cells but also potently inhibits the effects of IL-4 on B cells, particularly inhibiting IgE production.

INTERLEUKIN-4 & INTERLEUKIN-13

IL-4 is an MW 15,000–20,000 glycoprotein secreted by activated CD4 T cells of the TH2 subset and by mast cells. It was initially identified as a helper factor for B-cell proliferation, and so was called B cell growth factor I (BCGF-I). It is mitogenic for activated B cells, although its effect is usually less pronounced than that of IL-2 and always requires other activating stimuli. IL-4 was also previously called B cell stimulatory factor I (BSF-I) because of its ability to induce class II MHC expression on resting B cells. IL-4 is a major regulator of the heavy-chain class switch, since it promotes switching to immunoglobulin E (IgE). It also induces expression of the low-affinity Fcε receptor. Thus, IL-4 acts on B cells at many stages.

IL-4 also appears to promote the induction of TH2 cells, which control (among other things) the proliferation and activities of eosinophils and mast cells. The indirect effect of IL-4 on these cells, coupled with its direct effect on IgE production, suggests a central role in allergic diseases. In contrast, IL-4 suppresses the induction and function of TH1 cells, which control many facets of cellular immunity, suggesting that IL-4 may have clinical utility in the treatment of T cell-mediated autoimmunity and graft-versus-host disease.

In addition to the above effects, IL-4 promotes cytotoxic T cell activity, enhances IL-3-mediated mast cell growth, acts synergistically with CSFs to enhance the growth of various hematopoietic cells, and induces the adhesion molecule VCAM-1 on endothelial cells. It also has multiple effects on macrophages: it can activate macrophage cytocidal functions and increase macrophage expression of class II MHC proteins. However, it inhibits the release of proinflammatory cytokines, such as IL-1, IL-6, IL-8, and TNF α, from activated monocytes. IL-4 has also exhibited some antitumor activity, especially when injected locally, and is currently undergoing clinical trials in this regard.

A newly characterized lymphokine, **IL-13,** was recently found to have many properties overlapping those of IL-4. It is a TH2 cell product that enhances the production of IgE and suppresses the production of monokines.

INTERLEUKIN-5

IL-5 is a disulfide-linked homodimeric glycoprotein with an MW of 40,000–50,000. It was originally described as a growth factor for murine B cells but does not have significant stimulatory activity on human B cells. The major function of IL-5 in humans is to stimulate the production of **eosinophils.** IL-5 not only increases the numbers of eosinophils but also has been reported to increase their function. In vivo studies have clearly demonstrated that IL-5 is the major cytokine regulating eosinophilia during helminth infections and allergic diseases. Human IL-5 also enhances the activities of basophils by priming them to release mediators such as histamine and leukotrienes in response to other signals.

INTERLEUKIN-7

IL-7 is an MW 25,000 glycoprotein secreted by bone marrow stromal cells that functions as a **growth factor** for both T and B cell precursors. Together with SCF, it provides a powerful mitogenic stimulus to thymocytes and pre-B cells. It is thought to provide the signal that initiates rearrangement of T cell receptor genes during fetal thymocyte development. It induces IL-2 receptor expression, but most of its proliferative effect occurs independently of IL-2. Mature human peripheral blood T lymphocytes do not respond significantly to IL-7 unless costimulated or previously activated. IL-7 administration results in pronounced leukocytosis in normal mice and hastens recovery of leukocytes in mice made leukopenic by sublethal irradiation or cytotoxic agents; the majority of its pharmacologic effect in vivo is on B-lineage cells, with a more modest increase observed in T lymphocytes.

IL-7 enhances the function of mature, activated lymphocytic cells, particularly those with cytotoxic activity. It can also induce **lymphokine-activated killer (LAK)** activity, but to a substantially lesser degree than IL-2. At high concentrations, IL-7 also in-creases macrophage cytotoxic activity and induces cytokine secretion by monocytes.

INTERLEUKIN-9

IL-9 is a heavily glycosylated polypeptide lymphokine with an apparent MW of 30,000–40,000. It is secreted by some cultured T cells and has growth-promoting effects on several hematopoietic cell types in vitro. Its physiologic role has not been firmly established.

INTERLEUKIN-10

IL-10 is an MW 18,000 protein produced by TH2 cells, CD8 T cells, monocytes, keratinocytes, and activated B cells. It was originally called **cytokine synthesis inhibitory factor** because of its ability to inhibit cytokine production by activated T lymphocytes. In particular, IL-10 inhibits the production of cytokines such as IL-2 and IFN γ by TH1 cells, and therefore tips the regulatory balance in favor of humoral immune responses. IL-10 also inhibits cytokine production by NK cells and macrophages. Indeed, the suppression of TH1 activity appears to be an indirect effect resulting from direct impairment of the accessory-cell functions of macrophages and dendritic cells. IL-10 also has a direct stimulatory effect on B cells and promotes antibody production.

INTERLEUKIN-12

IL-12 is a structurally unique heterodimer composed of distinct MW 35,000 and 40,000 disulfide-linked subunits. It was originally called cytotoxic lymphocyte maturation factor (CLMF) or NK cell stimulatory factor (NKSF). IL-12 is produced predominantly by B cells and macrophages. It promotes the proliferation of activated T lymphocytes and NK cells, enhances the lytic activity of NK and LAK cells, and is the most potent inducer of IFN γ production by resting or activated T and NK cells. In addition, it selectively promotes the differentiation of TH1 lymphocytes and thus promotes cell-mediated immunity, but it suppresses TH2-dependent functions such as the production of IL-4, IL-10, and IgE antibodies. IL-12 also induces the production of GM-CSF, TNF, IL-6, and, to a small extent, IL-2. It synergizes with IL-2 in promoting cytotoxic T cell responses.

TRANSFORMING GROWTH FACTOR β

TGFβ was initially discovered as a growth factor for fibroblasts that promoted wound healing. However, it also has considerable antiproliferative activity and acts as a negative regulator of immunity and hematopoiesis (Fig 9–3). TGFβ is produced by many cell types, including activated macrophages and T lymphocytes. Humans express at least 3 forms of TGFβ, called TGFβ-1, -2, and -3. These are the products of separate genes, but they all bind to the same 5 types of high-affinity cell surface receptors. TGFβ receptors are expressed in widely different numbers by many cell types. Type I and II receptors transduce signals, whereas the function of type III, IV, and V receptors is not yet clear.

TGFβ has antiproliferative effects on a wide variety of cell types, including macrophages, endothelial cells, and T and B lymphocytes (Fig 9–3). It also suppresses the production of most lymphokines and monokines and reduces the cellular expression of class II MHC proteins and of IL-1 receptors. TGFβ at 10^{-10}–10^{-12} M blocks the proliferative effects of IL-2 on T and B cells and of IL-1 on thymocytes. In addition, TGFβ inhibits T cell-dependent antibody production, mixed-leukocyte reactions, and the in vitro generation of cytotoxic T cells. It also inhibits the

induction of NK cell activities and of LAK cells by IL-2. Thus, TGFβ is unique in that it can act as a negative-feedback regulator that dampens immunologically mediated reactions.

TGFβ also has some activities that tend to potentiate inflammation. It is chemoattractive for neutrophils and monocytes, and it stimulates monocyte expression of adhesion proteins. In humans, TGFβ promotes switching of B cells to the IgA antibody class. These effects may account for the observation that instilling TGFβ into inflamed joints exacerbates the inflammation.

INTERLEUKIN-8 & THE CHEMOKINE FAMILY OF CYTOKINES

Over the past 8 years, a new family of cytokines has been characterized whose members have **chemoattractant** activity for leukocytes and fibroblasts (Table 9–5). These **chemokines** range in MW from 8000 to 11,000, share 20–50% amino acid

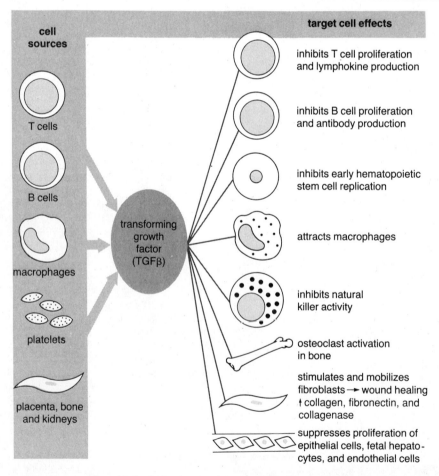

Figure 9–3. Cell sources and target cell effects of TGFβ.

Table 9–5. The human chemokines.

	Predominant Cell Source	Chemoattracted Cells	Other Activities[1]
α subfamily[2]			
IL-8	Monocytes, neutrophils, NK cells, somatic cells	Neutrophils, T lymphocytes, basophils	Neutrophil activation, neutrophil degranulation, acute inflammation
GRO	Monocytes, endothelial cells, fibroblasts	Neutrophils	Neutrophil degranulation, fibroblast growth, melanoma cell growth
ENA-78	Epithelial cells	Neutrophils	Neutrophil activation
CTAP III/βTG	Platelets, monocytes	Fibroblasts	Fibroblast activation
NAP-2	Platelets	Neutrophils	Neutrophil activation
PF-4[3]	Platelets	Fibroblasts	Endothelial adhesiveness, inhibition of angiogenesis
IP-10	Monocytes, endothelial cells, fibroblasts, keratinocytes	Monocytes, activated T cells	Integrin expression by T cells, chronic inflammation
β subfamily[2]			
MCP-1	Monocytes, endothelial cells, fibroblasts, keratinocytes	Monocytes, basophils, mast cells	Macrophage activation, macrophage secretory activity, chronic inflammation, basophil degranulation (histamine release)
RANTES	T lymphocytes, platelets	Monocytes, T lymphocytes, basophils, eosinophils, mast cells	Macrophage activation, integrin expression by T cells, chronic inflammation, basophil degranulation (histamine release)
MIP-1α	T lymphocytes, monocytes	Monocytes, T lymphocytes	Integrin expression by T cells (especially CD8 T cells), inhibition of marrow stem cell growth
MIP-1β	T lymphocytes, monocytes	Monocytes, T lymphocytes	Integrin expression by T cells (especially CD4 T cells)
I-309	Cultured T cells	Monocytes	Macrophage activation

[1]All of the listed processes are enhanced unless otherwise indicated.
[2]Members of the α subfamily are encoded on chromosome 4; β subfamily members are encoded on chromosome 17.
[3]PF-4, platelet factor 4.

sequence similarity with one another, bind to structurally analogous receptors, and are active at concentrations of 10^{-8}–10^{-11} M. Chemokines act predominantly to influence the functions, rather than the growth, of target cells.

Each chemokine is produced by particular cell types and is chemoattractive for specific types of leukocytes or fibroblasts (Table 9–5). Chemokines can be classified into an α subgroup, whose members are encoded by a cluster of genes on chromosome 4, and a β subgroup, whose genes are clustered on chromosome 17. No uniform system of nomenclature has yet been adopted for these proteins, and they carry names that focus upon a variety of different attributes. One **(IL-8)** is an interleukin.

Agents that induce expression of the chemokines include a battery of macrophage activators, polyclonal mitogens and antigens that activate T cells, and inducers of platelet aggregation. In addition, a number of proinflammatory cytokines, such as IL-11, IL-2, IFN γ, TNFα, and platelet-derived growth factor (PDGF), are potent inducers of various chemokines. The chemokines, by contrast, have little or no ability to induce other types of cytokines.

Two distinct but related chemokine receptors have been identified to date. One binds only IL-8, but the second can also bind at least 3 other chemokines. Such promiscuity at the receptor level probably accounts for the overlapping biologic activities of the chemokines. The IL-8 receptors are 70% identical to each other and belong to the **rhodopsin** receptor family, members of which characteristically consist of polypeptides that contain 7 transmembrane regions. Neutrophils and basophils each express several thousand of these receptors per cell.

As a group, the chemokines appear capable of selectively attracting fibroblasts and every type of inflammatory cell to an inflamed site. Their contribution to physiologic immune reactions is still incompletely defined. Local injection of IL-8 or some other chemokines results in rapid accumulation of neutrophils (2–3 hours). IL-8 is found in the blood of patients with systemic inflammatory reactions and severe trauma and can readily be detected at inflammatory sites, in synovial fluid in rheumatoid arthritis, in extracts of psoriatic skin, and in the circulation of patients in septic shock. Thus, IL-8 is implicated as a major participant in acute inflammatory reactions. Single injections of some of the β chemokines induce primarily monocytic or lymphocytic infiltrates, suggesting a role in chronic inflammation, whereas others attract eosinophils and stimulate basophil degranulation and so might play a role in allergy and in the host response to parasites.

HEMATOPOIETIC COLONY-STIMULATING FACTORS

CSFs are cytokines that stimulate individual pluripotent stem cells or their committed progeny (found mainly in the bone marrow in adults) to produce large numbers of erythrocytes, platelets, neutrophils, monocytes, eosinophils, and basophils. Each CSF acts on cells with particular developmental capabilities and is named according to the predominant cell types whose production it induces in in vitro stem cell cultures (Table 9–6). Thus, granulocyte-monocyte CSF (**GM-CSF**) stimulates production of granulocytes and mononuclear phagocytes; granulocyte CSF (**G-CSF**) yields granulocytes; monocyte CSF (**M-CSF**) yields monocytes; and erythropoietin (**Epo**) stimulates production of erythrocytes. Interleukin-3 (**IL-3**), also known as multi-CSF, stimulates pluripotent stem cells to produce all types of hematopoietic cells. In addition to maintaining homeostasis under normal conditions, these cytokines marshall bone marrow responses to environmental stresses, such as infection or trauma. In vivo administration of CSFs can also yield effects that extend beyond their in vitro activities, presumably because CSFs can induce other cytokines or their receptors, and directly influence the functions of some mature leukocytes.

The various CSFs are unrelated to one another structurally and bind to distinct cell surface receptors. Nevertheless, many have overlapping functions and induce quite similar biologic effects. This is particularly true of CSFs that influence granulocyte and

macrophage production (Table 9–6). The biologic significance of this redundancy is not clear. Some cytokines (eg, IL-1, IL-6, and IL-11) have little or no independent effect on hematopoiesis but act synergistically with others that do. The recently discovered SCF is the most potent of these synergistic CSFs: it interacts with many other cytokines to promote growth of myeloerythroid and lymphoid progenitors and hence increases the production of all blood cells.

Hematopoiesis is controlled by at least 30 known cytokines. Some of these—such as SCF, M-CSF, and Epo—are present at all times, whereas others are produced in response to specific stimuli. For example, IL-2, IL-3, IL-4, and IL-5 are expressed by T cells only when these cells become activated. Similarly, fibroblasts and endothelial cells secrete G-CSF and GM-CSF only when stimulated by IL-1, TNFα, or other products of activated macrophages. Some of the regulatory interactions occur within a single cell type; for example, activated macrophages can secrete M-CSF and GM-CSF, which promote macrophage production.

Many aspects of hematopoiesis and its control are incompletely understood. At any given moment, the majority of pluripotent stem cells are thought to be in a resting, nonmitotic state (ie, in the G_0 phase of the cell cycle). Their entry into the mitotic cycle can be induced by SCF, IL-11, IL-6, and IL-1. Other factors, such as TGFβ, IFN γ, MIP-1α, and TNFα, cause cycling stem cells to revert to the resting state. It is not clear how the progeny of stem cells become committed to a particular cell lineage or how CSFs might influence this process. Most evidence is compatible with the view that commitment occurs randomly but that the committed cells subsequently survive only if the appropriate CSFs are present. According to this model, IL-3 is required to support growth of the most primitive progenitors; GM-CSF supports early multilineage precursors; and Epo, G-CSF, M-CSF, IL-5, or IL-7 is required for survival of cells committed to specific lineages.

Several of the CSFs profoundly affect cells that participate in immunity and inflammation. Macrophages produced in the presence of GM-CSF alone have better APC activity and, when activated, have greater cytotoxic activity than those produced by M-CSF. In contrast, M-CSF-treated macrophages are less functionally active, in part because M-CSF reduces MHC protein expression and stimulates production of IL-1RA. GM-CSF and TNFα are essential for the generation of **dendritic cells** from their marrow-derived precursor forms, and the local release of these cytokines by activated macrophages, neutrophils, and keratinocytes in the course of an immune response is thought to stimulate circulating dendritic-cell progenitors to differentiate into functional APCs. Both cytokines also potentiate the activity of mature dendritic cells.

Many CSFs are currently being tested for possible

Table 9–6. Human hematopoietic growth factors.

	Predominant Cell Source	Cells Whose Production is Enhanced
SCF	Fibroblasts, hepatocytes, endothelial cells, epithelial cells, stromal cells	All hematopoietic cell types, gonadal cells, melanocytes
IL-3	T lymphocytes	Neutrophils, monocytes, eosinophils, erythrocytes, megakaryocytes
GM-CSF	T lymphocytes, monocytes, fibroblasts, endothelial cells	Neutrophils, monocytes, eosinophils, erythrocytes, megakaryocytes, dendritic cells
G-CSF	Monocytes, fibroblasts	Neutrophils
M-CSF	Monocytes, lymphocytes, fibroblasts, endothelial cells, epithelial cells	Monocytes, placental trophoblast cells
Epo	Kidney cells	Erythrocytes

clinical use. GM-CSF and G-CSF may prove to be of value in preventing the therapy-induced granulocytopenia that is the major cause of death among cancer patients undergoing chemotherapy or radiation therapy. These 2 cytokines may also have protective activity against bacterial septicemia. A combination of SCF and IL-11 shows promise for preventing thrombocytopenia in several therapeutic settings. In contrast to many of the other cytokines, CSFs appear to produce relatively few toxic side effects.

CYTOKINE RECEPTOR FAMILIES

The characterization of many cytokine receptors and their corresponding genes has revealed that most belong to larger multigene families (Table 9–7). The members of each family share distinctive structural features and are thought to be evolutionarily related. For example, the receptors for IL-1, M-CSF, SCF, G-CSF, and IL-6 each contain an immunoglobulinlike domain in their extracellular regions and thus belong to the **immunoglobulin gene superfamily** (see Chapter 6).

The TNF receptors, on the other hand, are members of a family of receptors that each contain 4 cysteine-rich regions in their extracellular domains. This family also includes the receptors for **nerve growth factor** and for a protein called **fas antigen,** as well as 3 T-cell surface proteins (ligands) that are specifically bound by CD27, CD30, and CD40, respectively. The **CD27** and **CD30** ligands transmit costimulatory signals to a T cell when bound by CD27 or CD30 on an APC. CD40 ligand is **(CD40L)** recognized by CD40 on B cell surfaces, and this interaction transmits an activating signal to the B cells. The interaction between fas antigen and its receptor induces apoptosis in the fas-bearing cell.

Many of the remaining cytokines belong to a newly described group called the cytokine receptor or **hematopoietin receptor family.** This family includes the receptors for IL-2, IL-3, IL-4, IL-5, IL-6, IL-7, IL-9, GM-CSF, G-CSF, Epo, LIF, growth hormone, and prolactin. Members of this receptor family can be recognized by a distinctive set of 4 spaced cysteines in their extracellular domains, as well as by a conserved sequence motif (Trp-Ser-X-Trp-Ser) located near the external membrane surface. It has been proposed that receptor dimerization is a required common mechanism for signal transduction by receptors of this family. The dimers can be either homodimers, as in IL-4 receptors, or more complex heterodimers, as in the IL-6 receptor and some of the other members of this family.

The divisions among families are not mutually exclusive, and some receptors can be assigned to multiple families. For example, the IL-6 receptor belongs to both the hematopoietin receptor and immunoglobulin superfamilies and also is the prototype of a third family (called the IL-6 receptor family) whose members all share a common β subunit that mediates transmembrane signal transduction.

OVERVIEW & PROSPECTS

The cytokines as a group serve as crucial intercellular signaling molecules that are responsible for the multidirectional communication among immune and inflammatory cells engaged in host defense, as well

Table 9–7. Cytokine receptor families.

	Distinguishing Features	Ligands of Member Receptors
Hematopoietin (cytokine receptor) family	Trp-Ser-X-Trp-Ser motif; 4 extracellular Cys residues.	IL-2, IL-3, IL-4, IL-5, IL-6, IL-7, IL-9, GM-CSF, G-CSF, Epo, LIF, growth hormone, prolactin
Immunoglobulin superfamily	Ig-like extracellular domain.	IL-1, IL-6, M-CSF, G-CSF, SCF
TNF family	4 Cys-rich extracellular regions.	TNF, CD27, CD30, CD40, fas antigen, nerve growth factor
IL-3 family	Common β subunit.	IL-3, IL-5, GM-CSF
IL-6 family	Common β subunit.	IL-6, IL-11, LIF, OSM, CNTF
IL-8 family	Rhodopsin-like proteins with 7 transmembrane domains.	IL-8, GRO, PF4, βTG, IP-10, RANTES, MIP-1α and β, MCP-1, C5a, substance P, vasoactive intestinal polypeptide, platelet-activating factor
Tyrosine kinase family	Intrinsic Tyr kinase activity in cytoplasmic domain.	M-CSF, SCF, platelet-derived growth factor, fibroblast growth factor
TGFβ family	Intrinsic Thr/Ser kinase activity in cytoplasmic domain.	TGFβ, inhibins, activins, Mullerian inhibiting substance, bone morphogenetic protein
IFN family	Type I (for IFN α, β, and ω), type II (for IFN γ)	IFNα, β, ω, and γ, IL-10

as among other somatic cells in the connective tissues, skin, nervous system, and other organs. Cytokines regulate one another's production and activities through competition, synergism, and mutual induction, producing a complex network of cytokine cascades and regulatory circuits with positive or negative feedback effects. In addition, other types of biologic mediators, such as corticosteroids and prostaglandins, have agonistic or antagonistic effects on some cytokine activities. The biologic responses to cytokines can also be regulated through effects on the specific cytokine receptors expressed by responsive cells, and these receptors may provide a useful therapeutic target for modulating cytokine activity.

It has recently become clear that some viruses encode cytokinelike proteins that probably play an important role in the viral life cycles. For example, Epstein-Barr virus produces an IL-10-like activ-

ity. Other viruses, such as the poxviruses, encode cytokine-binding proteins whose structures sometimes resemble those of the corresponding cellular receptors and that are able to sequester the active cytokines in vivo. It has been speculated that these so-called "virokines" or "viroceptors" are descended from cellular proteins whose genes were usurped by the viruses to enable them to interfere with host defenses.

Owing to the complexity of cytokine interactions, the therapeutic use of these agents is still in its infancy. Nevertheless, some disease states have already been shown to respond to IFN or to IL-2. Specific agonists and antagonists of the cytokines and their receptors can be expected to play an important role in future therapy of inflammatory, infectious, autoimmune, and neoplastic diseases.

REFERENCES

General

Arai K et al: Cytokines: Coordinators of immune and inflammatory responses. *Annu Rev Biochem* 1990; **59:**783.

Balkwill FR: *Cytokines in Cancer Therapy.* Oxford Univ Press, 1989.

Durum SK, Oppenheim JJ: Proinflammatory cytokines and immunity. In: *Fundamental Immunology,* 3rd ed. Paul WE (editor). Raven Press, 1993.

Howard M et al: T cell derived cytokines and their receptors. In: *Fundamental Immunology,* 3rd ed. Paul WE (editor). Raven Press, 1993.

Oppenheim JJ, Rossio J, Gearing A (editors): *Clinical Applications of Cytokines.* Oxford Univ Press, 1993.

Thompson A (editor): *Cytokine Handbook.* 2nd ed. Academic Press, 1993.

Interleukin-1

Dinarello CA: Biology of interleukin-1. *FASEB J* 1988;**2:**108.

Dinarello CA: IL-1 and IL-1 antagonism. *Blood* 1991; **77:**1627.

Dinarello CA, Thompson RC: Blocking IL-1: IL-1RA in vivo and in vitro. *Immunol Today* 1991;**12:**404.

Neta R, Oppenheim JJ: IL-1: Can we exploit Jekyll and subjugate Hyde? *Biol Ther Cancer Updates* 1992; **2:**1.

Neta R, et al: Relationship of TNF to interleukins. In: *TNF: Structure, Function, and Mechanisms of Action.* Vilcek J, Aggarwal B, (editors): Marcel Dekker, 1992.

Tumor Necrosis Factor

Beutler B (editor): *Tumor Necrosis Factors: The Molecules and Their Emerging Role in Medicine.* Raven Press, 1992.

Beutler B, Cerami A: The biology of cachectin/TNF—a primary mediator of host response. *Annu Rev Immunol* 1989;**7:**625.

Old LJ: Tumor necrosis factor (TNF). *Science* 1985;**230:**630.

Vilcek J, Aggarwal B (editors): *TNF: Structure, Function, and Mechanisms of Action.* Marcel Dekker, 1992.

IL-6 Family

Grove RI et al: Oncostatin M is a mitogen for rabbit vascular smooth muscle cells. *Proc Natl Acad Sci USA* 1993;**90:**823.

Ip NY et al: CNTF and LIF act on neuronal cells via shared signalling pathways that involve the IL-6 signal transducing component gp130. *Cell* 1992; **69:**1121.

Metcalf D: Leukemia inhibitory factor—a puzzling polyfunctional regulator. *Growth Factors* 1992;**7:**169.

Paul SR, Schendel P: The cloning and biological characterization of recombinant human interleukin 11. *Int Cell Cloning* 1992;**10:**135.

Interferons

Pestka S et al: Interferons and their actions. *Annu Rev Biochem* 1987;**56:**727.

Sen GC, Lengyel P: The interferon system. A bird's eye view of its biochemistry. *J Biol Chem* 1992; **267:**5017.

Williams BRG: Signal transduction and transcriptional regulation of interferon-α-stimulated genes. *J Interferon Res* 1991;**11:**207.

Lymphokines

Moore KW et al: IL-10. *Annu Rev Immunol* 1993; **11:**165.

Mosmann TR, Moore KW: The role of IL-10 in cross-regulation of T_H1 and T_H2 responses. *Immunol Today* 1991;**12:**A49.

Ruscetti FW: Interleukin-2. In *Immunophysiology.* Oppenheim J, Shevach E (editors). Oxford Univ Press, 1990.

Schwartz RH: Costimulation of T lymphocytes: Role of CD28 in interleukin-2 production and immunotherapy. *Cell* 1992;**71:**1065.

Smith KA: Low-dose IL-2 immunotherapy. *Blood* 1993;**81:**1402.

Interleukins-4, -5, & -7

Henney CS: Interleukin-7: Effects on early events in lymphopoiesis. *Immunol Today* 1989;**10:**170.

Paul WE: Interleukin-4: A prototypic immunoregulatory lymphokine. *Blood* 1991;**77:**1859.

Sanderson CF: Interleukin-5, eosinophils, and disease. *Blood* 1992;**79:**3101.

Hematopoietic Cytokines

Gearing A et al: Elevated levels of GM-CSF and IL-1 in the serum, peritoneal, and pleural cavities of GM-CSF transgenic mice. *J Exp Med* 1992;**175:**877.

Metcalf D: Control of granulocytes and macrophages: Molecular, cellular, and clinical aspects. *Science* 1991;**254:**529.

Moore MAS et al: Cytokine networks involved in hemopoietic stem cell proliferation and differentiation. *CIBA Symp* 1990;**148:**43.

Schrader JW: Biological effects of myeloid growth factors. *Bailliere's Clin Haematol* 1992;**5:**509.

Zsebo KM et al: Radioprotection of mice by recombinant rat stem cell factor. *Proc Natl Acad Sci USA* 1992;**89:**9464.

Chemokines

Kuna P et al: Monocyte chemotactic and activating factor is a potent histamine-releasing factor for human basophils. *J Exp Med* 1992;**175:**489.

Oppenheim JJ et al: Properties of the novel proinflammatory supergene intercrine cytokine family. *Annu Rev Immunol* 1991;**9:**617.

Schall TJ: Biology of the RANTES/SIS cytokine family. *Cytokine* 1991;**3:**165.

Growth Factors

Kovacs EJ: Fibrogenic cytokines: The role of immune mediators in the development of scar tissue. *Immunol Today* 1991;**12:**17.

Piez KA, Sporn MB: TGFβ's: Chemistry, biology, and therapeutics. *Ann NY Acad Sci* 1990;**593:**379.

Shull NM, et al: Targeted disruption of mouse TFGβ1 gene results in multifocal inflammatory disease. *Nature* 1992;**359:**693.

Sporn MB, Roberts AB: TGFβ: Problems and prospects. *Cell Regul* 1990;**1:**875.

Wahl SM: Transforming growth factor beta (TGFβ) in inflammation: A cause and a cure. *J Clin Immunol* 1992;**12:**61.

Cytokine Receptors

Honda M et al: Human soluble IL-6 receptor: Its detection and enhanced release by HIV infection. *J Immunol* 1992;**148:**2175.

Layton MJ et al: A major binding protein for LIF in normal mouse serum: Identification as a soluble form of the cellular receptor. *Proc Natl Acad Sci USA* 1992;**89:**8616.

Lee J et al: Characterization of two high affinity human IL 8 receptors. *J Biol Chem* 1992;**267:**M283.

Massague J: Receptors for the TGFβ family. *Cell* 1992;**69:**1067.

Miyajima A et al: Common subunits of cytokine receptors and the functional redundancy of cytokines. *Trends Biochem Sci* 1992;**17:**378.

Smith CA et al: A receptor for TNF defines an unusual family of cellular and viral proteins. *Science* 1990;**248:**1019.

Taga T, Kishimoto T: Cytokine receptors and signal transduction. *FASEB J* 1992;**6:**3387.

Waldmann TR: The multi-subunit IL-2 receptor. *Annu Rev Biochem* 1989;**58:**875.

10

Complement & Kinin

Michael M. Frank, MD

Complement activation, kinin generation, blood coagulation, and fibrinolysis are physiologic processes that occur through sequential cascadelike activation of enzymes normally present in their inactive forms in plasma. Although they are 4 distinct systems and perform different functions, they interact with one another and with various cell membrane proteins. The first two—complement and kinin—are the subjects of this chapter because of their involvement in immunologic effector responses.

THE COMPLEMENT SYSTEM

Complement is a collective term used to designate a group of plasma and cell membrane proteins that play a key role in the host defense process. Table 10–1 lists the major proteins, their molecular weights, and their serum concentrations.

FUNCTIONS OF COMPLEMENT

This complex system, which now numbers more than 25 proteins, acts in at least 3 major ways. The first and best-known function of the system is to cause **lysis** of cells, bacteria, and enveloped viruses. The second is to mediate the process of **opsonization,** in which foreign cells, bacteria, viruses, fungi, etc, are prepared for phagocytosis. This process involves the coating of the foreign particle with specific complement protein fragments that can be recognized by receptors for these fragments on phagocytic cells (see Chapter 1).

The third function of the complement proteins is the generation of peptide fragments that regulate features of the inflammatory and immune responses. These proteins play a role in vasodilatation at the site

of inflammation, in adherence of phagocytes to blood vessel endothelium, in egress of the phagocytes from the vessel, in directed migration of phagocytic cells into areas of inflammation, and, ultimately, in clearing infectious agents from the body.

PATHWAYS OF COMPLEMENT ACTIVATION

Most of the early-acting proteins of the complement cascade are present in the circulation in an inactive form. The proteins undergo sequential **activation** to ultimately cause their biologic effects.

Two major pathways of complement activation operate in plasma. A general scheme of the system is shown in Fig. 10–1. The first complement activation pathway to be discovered is termed the **classic complement pathway.** Under normal physiologic conditions, activation of this pathway is initiated by antigen-antibody complexes. The second pathway, known as the **alternative complement pathway,** was discovered more recently, although phylogenetically it probably is the older activation pathway. It does not have an absolute requirement for antibody for activation. Both pathways function through the interaction of proteins termed **components.** Both proceed by means of sequential activation and assembly of a series of components, leading to the formation of a complex enzyme capable of binding and cleaving a key component, C3, which is common to both pathways. Thereafter, the 2 pathways proceed together through binding of the terminal components to form a membrane attack complex, which ultimately causes cell lysis.

NOMENCLATURE

The proteins of the classic pathway and the terminal components are designated by numbers following the letter C. Proteins of the alternative pathway are

Table 10–1. Molecular weights and serum concentrations of complement components.

	Molecular Weight	Serum Concentration (μg/mL)
Classic pathway component		
C1q	410,000	70
C1r	85,000	34
C1s	85,000	31
C2	102,000	25
C3	190,000	1200
C4	206,000	600
C5	190,000	85
C6	128,000	60
C7	120,000	55
C8	150,000	55
C9	71,000	60
Alternative pathway component		
Properdin	53,000	25
Factor B	90,000	225
Factor D	25,000	1
Inhibitors		
C1 Inhibitor	105,000	275
Factor I	88,000	34
Regulatory proteins		
C4-binding protein	560,000	8
Factor H	150,000	500
S protein (vitronectin)	80,000	500

generally given letter designations, as are other proteins that have major regulatory effects on the system.

The proteins of each pathway interact in a precise sequence. When a protein is missing, as occurs in some of the genetic deficiencies, the sequence is interrupted at that point. The early steps in the activation process are associated with the assembly of complement cleavage fragments to form enzymes that bind the next proteins in the sequence to continue the reaction cascade. These enzymes are designated with a bar placed over the symbol of the component to indicate active enzymatic activity.

THE CLASSIC COMPLEMENT PATHWAY

Initiation

The sequence of events that take place in the classic complement cascade is depicted in Fig 10–2. In most cases, the classic pathway is initiated by binding of antibody to an antigen. A single molecule of immunoglobulin M (IgM) on an antigenic surface or 2 molecules of IgG of appropriate subclasses bound side by side can bind and activate the first component of the pathway, **C1.** C1 is a macromolecular complex composed of 3 different proteins (C1q, C1r, and C1s) held together by calcium ions. Each C1 complex is composed of one C1q, 2 C1r, and 2 C1s chains. The

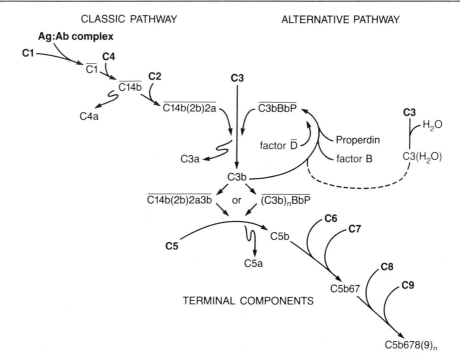

Figure 10–1. The complement cascade.

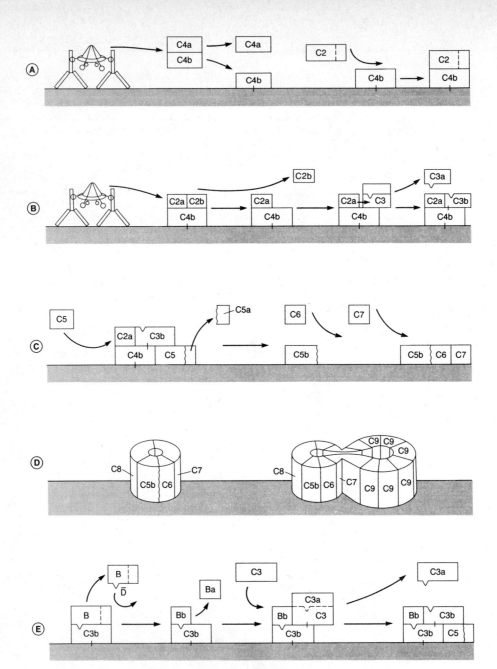

Figure 10–2. Diagram of the complement cascade. **A:** The classic complement pathway. A doublet of IgG antibody molecules on a surface can bind and activate C1, a 3-part molecule composed of C1q, C1r, and C1s. C1q has a core and 6 radiating arms, each of which ends in a pod. The pod recognizes and binds to the Fc fragment of the IgG. On activation the C1 binds and cleaves C4. The small fragment, C4a, is released. The large fragment, C4b, binds to the target to continue the cascade. In the presence of magnesium ion, C2 recognizes and binds to C4b. **B:** Once C2 is bound to C4b, it can be cleaved by C1. A small fragment, C2b, is released, and the large fragment, C2a, remains bound to the C4b. This newly formed complex of 2 protein fragments can now bind and cleave C3. This molecule is, in turn, cleaved into 2 fragments, C3a and C3b. The small fragment, C3a, is released, and the large fragment, C3b, can bind covalently to a suitable acceptor. C3b molecules that bind directly to the C4b continue the cascade. **C:** The complex formed of C2a, C4b, and C3b can bind and cleave C5. A small fragment of C5, C5a, is released. The large fragment, C5b, does not bind covalently. It is stabilized by binding to C6. When C7 binds, the complex of C5b, C6 and C7 becomes hydrophobic. It is partially lipid-soluble and can insert into the lipid of the cell membrane bilayer. **D:** When the C5b67 binds C8, a small channel is formed in the cell membrane. Multiple molecules of C9 can bind and markedly enlarge the channel. The channel has a hydrophobic outer surface and a hydrophilic central channel that allows passage of water and ions. **E:** The alternative complement pathway. In the presence of magnesium ion, C3b on a surface can bind factor B, just as C4b can bind C2. Factor D, a fluid-phase factor, can cleave bound factor B into 2 fragments, Ba and Bb. Ba is released. The C3bBb complex can now bind an additional molecule of C3 and cleave it, just as C4b2a can bind and cleave C3. C3a is released, and the new complex of C3bBbC3b, usually written (C3b)2Bb, can bind C5 to continue the cascade.

enzymatic potential of the complex resides in the C1r and C1s chains, each of which is an MW 85,000 pro-enzymatic form of a serine protease. Antibody binding is mediated by the much larger (MW 410,000) C1q portion of the complex, which binds the Fc portion of immunoglobulins. C1q can bind IgM, IgG1, IgG2, or IgG3. It does not bind IgG4, IgE, IgA, or IgD, so these antibody classes cannot activate the classic pathway.

C1q is itself composed of 6 identical subunits, each containing one copy each of 3 different polypeptide chains. Portions of these 3 chains closely resemble collagen and coil around one another to form a triple-helical collagenlike arm that is highly flexible. In the C1q complex, the 6 subunits are arranged to create a globular central core from which the 6 arms radiate outward (Fig 10–2). At the end of each arm is a podlike hand that is formed by the carboxyl termini of all three chains, and that mediates binding to the C_H2 domains in immunoglobulins of appropriate subclasses. The binding specificity of C1q has been exploited in creating clinical assays (called **C1q binding assays**) to detect immune complexes in serum.

If the antibody-binding sites (epitopes) on a target antigen are too low in density for proper arrangement of antibody molecules, C1 binding will not occur. This is seen with erythrocytes coated with anti-Rh$_o$ (D) antibody as a result of maternal-fetal **Rh incompatibility.** Although complement-activating subclasses of IgG are formed against such erythrocytes, complement is not usually activated and has no role in their destruction because the necessary IgG doublets do not form.

Binding of C1 to antibody results in activation of the proteolytic enzyme activities of C1r and, subsequently, C1s. Each of these polypeptides becomes activated because it is cleaved into 2 fragments, the shorter of which has protease activity. It is believed that the function of the activated C1r enzyme, $\overline{\text{C1r}}$, is to cleave C1s, which then develops enzymatic activity. $\overline{\text{C1s}}$ then cleaves the next component of the pathway, C4 (Fig 10–1 and 10–2A).

C4 & C2

C4 is a 3-chain molecule. The largest of the 3 chains, the α chain, is cleaved at a single site by $\overline{\text{C1s}}$, with the release of a small peptide, C4a. The larger peptide, consisting of most of the α chain together with the β and γ chains of C4, binds to the target cell to continue the complement cascade. Binding involves the formation of a covalent amide or ester bond between the target cell and the α chain of C4 (see the discussion of chemistry under C3 below). In the presence of magnesium ion, C4b on a target cell is capable of interacting with and binding the next component in the series, a single-chain molecule of MW 102,000, termed C2. C2 binds to C4b and, in the presence of $\overline{\text{C1s}}$, is cleaved. The larger cleavage fragment of C2 (C2a), which contains the enzymatic site,

remains in complex with C4b to continue the complement cascade (Fig. 10–2B). The complex of C4b and C2a develops a new capacity: the ability to bind and cleave the next component in the series, C3. For this reason it is termed the **classic pathway C3 convertase.** The peptide complex C4b2a is unstable and may release the C2a peptide as an enzymatically inactive fragment; however, target-bound C4b can accept another C2 and, in the presence of active C1, will regenerate a convertase capable of continuing the complement cascade. These early steps in the classic pathway are under tight regulation, as discussed below.

C3

The C3 convertase of the classic pathway binds and activates C3, a glycoprotein present at a concentration of about 1.2 mg/ml of plasma. C3 consists of 2 disulfide-linked chains, termed α and β (MW 110,000 and 75,000, respectively). Two amino acids in the C3 α chain are linked by a thiolester bond that lies buried in a hydrophobic pocket of the protein and twists the α chain into a strained configuration. When C3 is activated by the convertase, an inactive peptide C3a (MW 9,000) is cleaved from the α chain. As a result, the internal thiolester on the remaining C3b fragment becomes exposed to the surrounding medium. This highly reactive thiolester has a half-life of roughly 30–60 ms and, during this time, will react to form a covalent bond with any suitable acceptor in its vicinity.

If C3b bonds covalently to the adjacent C4b fragment on the target surface, the 2 (along with C2a) form a complex that can continue the complement cascade (Fig 10–2B). In addition, the presence of bound C3b strongly **opsonizes** the target particle, increasing its phagocytosis by cells that carry **C3b receptors** (CR1; see below). C3b also has a strong tendency to interact with nearby IgG molecules, and the dimer formed by C3b and IgG is a more potent opsonin than is C3b alone. If, on the other hand, the thiolester does not encounter a suitable acceptor, it reacts with water to form the conformationally altered inactive species **C3(H$_2$O)**; this rapid inactivation helps to ensure that the reactive form of C3b cannot diffuse a significant distance away from its target.

THE CLASSIC PATHWAY C5 CONVERTASE

The complex on a target surface consisting of C4b, C2a, and C3b ($\overline{\text{C4b2a3b}}$) has a newly expressed enzymatic activity: it can coordinate with and cleave C5, and so is called the **classic pathway C5 convertase.** Again, 2 fragments, C5a and C5b, are formed, with C5a being the smaller. The larger fragment (C5b) remains noncovalently associated with the $\overline{\text{C4b2a3b}}$

complex and is available to interact with later components. It is C5b that initiates the segment of the complement cascade that leads to membrane attack.

In summary, the early steps of the complement cascade lead to the generation of a series of enzymatically active peptides and peptide complexes. As each complex is formed, it has a different specificity from the preceding complex, and interacts with the next protein in the complement cascade. Each enzyme will interact with multiple molecules of the next substrate protein in the cascade of reactions either until it decays, as occurs with the C3 and C5 convertases, or until it is inhibited by regulatory proteins present on cells or in plasma. Thus, there is a potential for considerable biologic amplification: a limited number of antigen-antibody complexes will lead to the activation of large numbers of complement molecules.

Nonimmunologic Classic Pathway Activators

It is of interest that a number of nonimmunologic activators of the classic pathway exist. Certain bacteria (eg, certain *Escherichia coli* and *Salmonella* strains of low virulence) and viruses (eg, parainfluenza virus) interact with C1q directly, causing C1 activation and, in turn, classic pathway activation in the absence of antibody. Such an interaction obviously would aid the natural defense process of the host. Other structures, eg, the surface of urate crystals, myelin basic protein, denatured DNA, bacterial endotoxin, and polyanions such as heparin, also may activate the classic pathway directly. Such activation by urate crystals is thought to contribute to the inflammation and pain associated with gout.

THE ALTERNATIVE COMPLEMENT PATHWAY

C3 not only serves as a pivotal component of the classic pathway but also is the key component of the **alternative complement pathway.** This pathway provides yet another means of activating the complement cascade in the absence of bound antibodies. As described above, C3 can undergo hydrolysis of its thiolester bond to form a conformationally altered species called $C3(H_2O)$. Spontaneous decay of C3 to $C3(H_2O)$ is thought to occur continually but at a very low rate in the blood. In the presence of magnesium ions, $C3(H_2O)$ can bind another circulating protein called **factor B,** which is similar in many respects to C2; in fact, factor B and C2 are encoded by adjacent genes on chromosome 6 and may well have arisen through duplication of a single gene. The complex of $C3(H_2O)$ and factor B can be acted on by a third blood protein, **factor D,** which is a C1-like serine protease. As a result, factor B is cleaved, and the remaining complex acquires C3 convertase activity.

This initial complex can then cleave additional C3 proteins to produce highly reactive C3b.

This spontaneous sequence of reactions ensures that minute amounts of C3b are constantly being produced in the blood. Under normal circumstances, these fragments are rapidly inactivated by cleavage; stringent control mechanisms (see below) operate to limit the extent of the reaction and so prevent massive complement activation and damage to host cells. However, if these reactions happen to occur near a foreign particle, some C3b fragments may become covalently bound to its surface (Fig 10–2E). C3b is capable of binding factor B, which can then be acted on by factor D, forming a complex (C3bBb) called the **alternative pathway C3 convertase.** The C3 convertase, in turn, can bind and cleave an additional molecule of C3 to form a larger complex (denoted C3bBbC3b) that has **C5 convertase** activity. The latter complex then efficiently triggers subsequent steps in the complement cascade and so promotes an attack on the particle to which it is bound.

The alternative pathway C3 convertase (C3bBb) is extremely unstable and would ordinarily dissociate rapidly. In the blood, however, a protein called **properdin** binds to this convertase and stabilizes it, thus slowing its decay and allowing it to continue the complement cascade.

For many years, investigators have used a protein derived from cobra venom (**cobra venom factor**) to activate complement in the laboratory. Recent studies have shown that this protein is a fragment of cobra C3 and is a physiologic analog of C3b in this reptile. Cobra venom factor, when added to human plasma, functions just like human C3b to activate the alternative pathway. As described below, endogenous C3b is under tight regulatory control by other plasma proteins. By contrast, cobra venom factor is not inhibited by these regulators and therefore can induce massive complement activation.

THE LATE COMPONENTS C5–9 & THE MEMBRANE ATTACK COMPLEX

The late phase of the complement cascade (Fig 10–2C) begins when C5 is bound and then cleaved by either the alternative or classic pathway convertase into C5a and C5b. C5a is released and produces biologic effects, which are described in a later section. C5b continues the lytic sequence; however, it does not form a covalent bond with the surface of its target. C5b is rapidly inactivated unless it is stabilized by binding to the next component in the cascade, C6. The C5b6 complex can bind C7, the third protein involved in membrane attack. The C5b67 complex is strongly hydrophobic and will interact with nearby membrane lipids. It is capable of inserting into the lipid bilayer of cell membranes. In that location, one

C5b67 complex can accept one molecule of C8 and multiple molecules of C9, ultimately forming a cylindrical transmembrane channel, C5b678(9)n, which has been termed the **membrane attack complex (MAC)** (Fig 10–3). This structure has a hydrophobic outer surface, which associates with the membrane lipid of the bilayer, and a hydrophilic core through which small ions and water can pass. The ionic environment of the extracellular fluid then communicates with that inside the cell, so that once this complex is inserted into the membrane, the cell cannot maintain its osmotic and chemical equilibrium. Water enters the cell because of the high internal oncotic pressure, and the cell swells and bursts. The assembly of C5b–C8 appears to form a small membrane channel that is increasingly enlarged and stabilized by the binding of multiple molecules of C9. One such channel penetrating the erythrocyte membrane is sufficient to destroy the cell. Cells with more complex metabolic machinery can, to some extent, internalize and destroy complement complexes that form on the cell surface, thereby providing some protection against complement attack.

CONTROL MECHANISMS

The complement system has evolved to aid in the host defense process by directly damaging invading organisms and by producing tissue inflammation. Strict regulatory control of this system is of critical importance to prevent complement-mediated destruction of the individual's own tissues. When complement is involved in causing disease, it usually is functioning normally but is misdirected, ie, damaging to the host tissues. Many control proteins have evolved to defend against such attack.

The C1 Inhibitor

The first of these, **C1 inhibitor (C1INH),** recognizes activated $\overline{C1r}$ and $\overline{C1s}$ and destroys their activity. This glycoprotein (MW 105,000) not only inhibits $\overline{C1r}$ and $\overline{C1s}$, but also acts as an inhibitor of activated Hageman factor (see below) and of all the enzyme systems activated by Hageman factor fragments. Thus, C1INH regulates enzymes formed during activation of the kinin-generating system, the

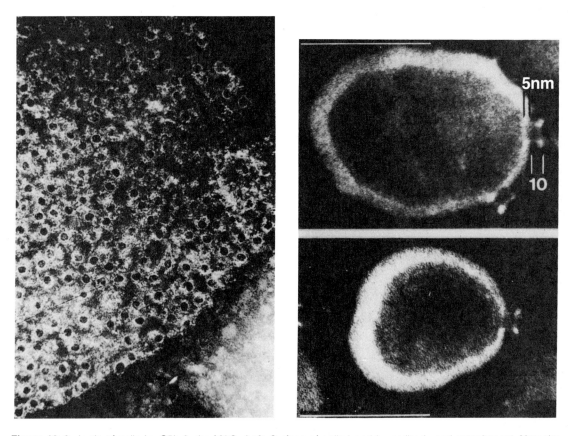

Figure 10–3. Lysis of cells by C5b-9, the MAC. **Left:** Surface of cells lysed by antibody and complement. Note the surface lesions. (Micrograph courtesy of R Dourmashkin.) **Right:** Two views of the purified lesions allowed to attach to lipid micelles. The hollow cylinder formed by the C5b–9 has allowed the electron-dense dye to enter the lipid droplet. (Photograph courtesy of S Bhakdi.)

clotting system, the fibrinolytic system, and the complement cascade. In each of these systems, C1INH binds physically to the active site of the enzyme to destroy its activity and in the process is consumed. Interestingly, during C1 inactivation the C1 is dissociated, with the C1INH binding to each of the C1r and C1s enzymatic sites and freeing C1q of its subunits. Since C1INH is consumed when acting as an inhibitor, 2 genes are necessary to provide the relatively high plasma concentration of the protein gene product required for effective inhibitor activity. A relative deficiency occurs in patients with **hereditary angioedema,** who have a defect in one of the 2 genes responsible for formation of C1INH. These patients have one-half to one-third the normal level of C1INH and have frequent attacks of angioedema—painless swelling of deep cutaneous tissues—whose cause is still uncertain. It may arise from activation of the kinin-generating system or from activation of the complement system, with generation of peptides that cause vascular leakage.

C4-binding Protein, Factor I & Factor H

C4-binding protein **(C4BP)** and a second protein, factor I, are responsible for regulation of C4b. C4BP binds to C4b and facilitates its cleavage by the proteolytic enzyme **factor I.** On target surfaces, C4BP is not required for C4b cleavage by factor I, but its presence may accelerate the cleavage process.

Factor I also acts proteolytically to inactivate C3b and C3(H$_2$O) (Fig 10–4). This activity requires a co-

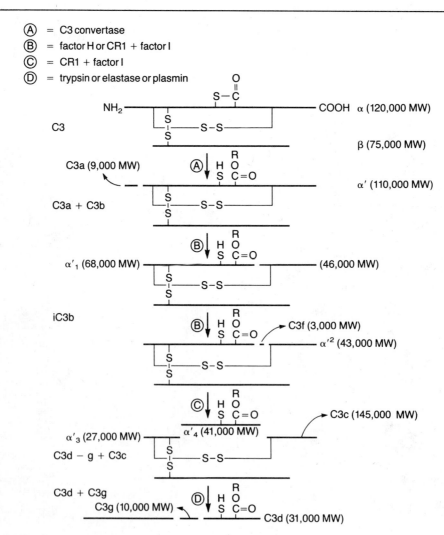

Figure 10–4. The C3 degradation pathway. The α and β chains of C3 are shown. Activation of C3 with the formation of C3a and C3b by the C3 convertases is shown (step A). C3b is degraded to iC3b by the action of factor H or CR1 plus factor I (step B). Two forms of iC3b have been described, differing in loss of a 3-kDa fragment. In the presence of CR1 and factor I, C3c is released and C3dg remains target bound (step C). C3dg can be further degraded to C3d by proteolytic enzymes (step D). Specific cellular receptors exist for each of these fragments.

factor termed **factor H.** Factor H acts as an obligate cofactor in the fluid phase and as an accelerator of C3 cleavage on cell surfaces (Fig 10–4). In the presence of factors H and I, the C3b or C3(H$_2$O) α chain is cleaved at 2 sites to form a partially degraded molecule, **iC3b.** This molecule, although inactive in continuing the complement cascade, is active as an opsonin and will be discussed further below. Under the appropriate conditions, as discussed below, factor I can cleave iC3b further to form a molecule termed C3dg, which also interacts with specific receptors that recognize this C3 degradation peptide.

Vitronectin (S Protein)

Yet another control protein, **S protein** (also called **vitronectin**), interacts with the C5b67 complex as it forms in the fluid phase and binds to its membrane-binding site to prevent the binding of C5b67 to biologic membranes. Following binding of S protein to fluid-phase C5b67, binding of C8 and C9 to the fluid-phase complex can proceed, but the complex does not insert into lipid membranes and does not lyse cells.

In the control of complement attack against host tissue, it would be beneficial if complement proteins such as C3b were rapidly degraded when bound to host cells but not degraded when bound to the surface of a microorganism. A process for accomplishing this goal has evolved. When deposited on a microorganism, C3b is often in a "protected site," which is protected from the action of the control proteins factors H and I. The C3b persists to activate the alternative pathway and destroy the organism. In contrast, on host cells C3b interacts with factors H and I and is degraded. The biochemical basis for this protection of C3b on an organism surface is not yet completely understood but appears to relate to the presence of charged carbohydrates such as sialic acid on mammalian cells, which may facilitate the binding of factor H.

GENETIC CONSIDERATIONS

Most of the genes encoding proteins of the classic and alternative pathways have been cloned, and their amino acid sequences have been determined. Moreover, the activation peptides have been studied in some detail. Allotypic variants of many of the proteins have been found that show genetic polymorphisms, as demonstrated by differences in surface charge. Almost all of the variants of complement proteins show autosomal codominant inheritance at a single locus. The genes for C4, C2, and factor B are located within the major histocompatibility locus on the short arm of chromosome 6 in humans and are termed class III histocompatibility genes. The significance of the intimate colocalization of histocompatibility genes and complement genes is unknown at present.

Interestingly, there are 2 C4 loci on each chromosome; thus, there are 4 C4 genes. The 2 loci code for proteins termed C4A and C4B, which differ in functional activity. Individuals with at least one null allele at one of the C4 loci are thought to be prone to the development of autoimmune disease. Genes for many of the regulatory proteins that interact with C4 and C3 are grouped as a supergene family on chromosome 1. This family is now known to encode factor H, C4-binding protein, decay-accelerating factor, CR1, and CR2. The gene products of this family each have a 60-amino-acid domain made up of shorter repeating segments that repeat multiple times in the molecule. They presumably originated from a common gene precursor. See Chapter 23 for a discussion of inherited complement component deficiencies with associated syndromes.

BIOLOGIC CONSEQUENCES OF COMPLEMENT ACTIVATION IN INFLAMMATION

In general, the larger fragments formed during complement component cleavage tend to continue the complement cascade whereas the smaller fragments mediate aspects of inflammation. For example, the cleavage of C3 and C5 generates C3a and C5a fragments, which consist of the first 77 and 74 amino acids of the C3 and C5 α chains, respectively. Cleavage of C4 generates C4a, a MW 77,000 amino acid fragment from the α chain of C4. All of these small activation peptides have **anaphylatoxic** activity: they cause smooth muscle contraction and degranulation of mast cells and basophils, with consequent release of histamine and other vasoactive substances that induce capillary leakage. **C5a** is the most potent of these anaphylatoxins.

C5a and C3a also have important immunoregulatory effects on T cell function, either stimulating (C5a) or inhibiting (C3a) aspects of cell-mediated immunity.

C5a has profound effects on phagocytic cells. It is strongly chemotactic for neutrophils and mononuclear phagocytes, inducing their migration along a concentration gradient toward the site of generation. It increases neutrophil adhesiveness and causes neutrophil aggregation. In addition, it dramatically stimulates neutrophil oxidative metabolism and the production of toxic oxygen species, and it triggers lysosomal enzyme release from a variety of phagocytic cells. Cellophane membranes used in **renal dialysis** machines and membrane oxygenators may activate the alternative pathway with C5a generation. This, in turn, may lead to neutrophil aggregation, embolization of the aggregates to the lungs, and pulmonary distress. It is suspected that C5a generation plays an important deleterious role in the development of **adult respiratory distress syndrome.**

The life span of these biologically potent peptides, C3a and C5a, is limited by a serum carboxy-peptidase that cleaves off the terminal arginine from the peptides, in most cases markedly reducing their activity.

COMPLEMENT RECEPTORS & RELATED MEMBRANE PROTEINS

C1q Receptors

The surfaces of most cells bear complement receptors. Receptors for the **C1q** component of C1 have been identified on neutrophils and monocytes, the majority of B lymphocytes, and a small population of lymphocytes lacking both B and T cell markers. Binding via this receptor has been shown to activate cells for a variety of cellular functions, including phagocytosis and oxidative metabolism. C1q can also augment the cytotoxicity of human peripheral blood lymphocytes to antibody-sensitized chicken erythrocytes and supports antibody-independent cytolytic activity by certain lymphoblastoid cell lines. The C1q receptor does not interact with C1q in intact C1 but interacts once the C1 has been dissociated by the C1 inhibitor.

C3 Receptors

The best-studied receptors are those that recognize C3 fragments (Table 10–2). Importantly, these receptors do not recognize native circulating C3 and are not blocked by the normal plasma protein. Receptors exist for C3b, iC3b, C3d, and C3dg. These receptors have a characteristic cellular distribution, with the C3b receptor (termed **CR1**) being prominent on erythrocytes, granulocytes, mononuclear phagocytes, and B lymphocytes in humans. In contrast, the C3bi receptor **(CR3)** is present only on phagocytic cells. The C3d receptor **(CR2)** is present on lymphoblastoid cells and B lymphocytes. These receptors bind the various C3 fragments as indicated. If the C3 is bound to an antigen or target particle, the antigen or target will bind via the C3 ligand to the surface of cells with the receptor. For phagocytic cells, binding of the target to the phagocyte surface can augment the ingestion process (see Chapter 1).

Thus, CR1 and CR3 are both important in the process of phagocytosis. However, they also serve several other functions. They both act as cofactors for the further degradation of C3 fragments by the serum enzyme factor I. In each case, C3 fragment bound to the receptor can be cleaved by factor I to the decay fragment C3dg. This fragment is not formed in the absence of complement receptors. CR3 is a member of the **integrin** protein family and plays a major role in cell adherence; phagocytes from CR3-deficient patients have marked abnormalities in adherence and ingestion. Another integrin, p150/95, binds C3b and

Table 10–2. Cellular receptors for C3 fragments.

Designation	Complement Component Recognized	Protein Structure	Cells	Function
CR1	C4b/C3b, iC3b	1 chain (MW 165,000–240,000)	Erythrocytes, phagocytes, B lymphocytes, some glomerular podocytes, eosinophils, Langerhans cells	Aids target cell ingestion by phagocytes; acts as cofactor in the metabolism of C3b, allowing factor I to cleave C3b to C3dg.
CR3	iC3b	2 chains, α (MW 170,000) and β (MW 95,000)	Phagocytes	Aids in ingestion; important in adherence of cells to surfaces; acts as cofactor for further degradation of C3bi.
CR2	C3d, C3dg	1 chain (MW 140,000)	B lymphocytes, some T cells, epithelial cells, follicular dendritic cells, NK and ADCC[1] effector lymphocytes	On B cells, has immunoregulatory properties; site of attachment of Epstein-Barr virus to lymphocytes and epithelial cells.
CR4	iC3b, C3dg	2 chains, α (MW 150,000) and β (MW 95,000)	Kupffer cells, other phagocytes	Not well studied; presumably aids in attachment and metabolism of C3 coated targets.
C3aR	C3a, C4a	?	Neutrophils, T cells, goblet cells, smooth muscle, mast cells, monocytes, eosinophils	Immunoregulation, anaphylatoxin (see text).
C3eR	C3e	?	Neutrophils	Causes release of PMNs from marrow stores.

[1]ADCC, antibody-dependent cell-mediated cytotoxicity (see Chapter 3).

C3dg and has recently been identified as **CR4.** Recently, a number of children with deficiency of all of the CR3-related proteins have been identified. They present with a history of delayed separation of the umbilical cord at birth and frequent soft-tissue and cutaneous infections by a variety of organisms, especially staphylococci and *Pseudomonas aeruginosa.*

CR2 (also designated **CD21**) is a receptor for the C3d and C3dg fragments of C3. It is present on B lymphocytes and nasal epithelial cells. It appears to function on B lymphocytes to facilitate differentiation. Interestingly, it serves as the site for attachment and cellular penetration of the **Epstein-Barr virus.**

Regulatory Molecules

Several other cellular membrane proteins act not as receptors but rather to control untoward complement activation. **Decay-accelerating factor (DAF)** is a single-chain membrane protein (MW 70,000) that is a potent accelerator of C3 convertase decay, but, unlike CR1 and CR3, it has no factor I cofactor activity. Functionally, the protein acts to limit membrane damage if, by chance, complement is activated at the cell surface. **C8-binding protein,** also known as **homologous restriction factor (HRF),** acts to prevent successful completion and membrane insertion of the MAC. This membrane protein therefore acts to prevent cell lysis at yet another step in the complement cascade. It is called homologous restriction protein because it recognizes C8 and C9 of the same species far better than it recognizes late components of other species. Human homologous restriction protein on cells will prevent the action of human C8 and C9 on those cells far better than it will prevent the action of C8 and C9 from other species. Any potential advantage of this function is completely obscure.

CD59 is yet another regulatory protein that prevents assembly of the complete C5b–9 complex on target cells and so prevents complement-mediated lysis. Interestingly, DAF, HRF, and CD59 are each bound to the cell surface by a **phosphoinositide glycosidic linkage** rather than by a transmembrane domain within the amino acid backbone of the protein. This phosphoinositide linkage is reported to give the protein far greater lateral mobility within the cell membrane, increasing its ability to intercept damage-causing complement complexes. In patients with **paroxysmal nocturnal hemoglobinuria,** phosphoinositide-linked proteins are incorrectly assembled or inserted into cellular membranes of hematologic cells, rendering these cells exquisitely sensitive to complement-mediated lysis.

Another protein, **membrane cofactor protein (MCP)** is present on most blood cells but not on erythrocytes. This protein, a product of the supergene C4b/C3b-binding family, acts as a cofactor to facilitate the cleavage of C3b and iC3b by factor I. It does not accelerate convertase decay or bind with sufficient affinity to act as a receptor.

THE KININ CASCADE

The kinin-generating system is a second important mediator-forming system in blood. Here there is one major final product, **bradykinin,** a nonapeptide with potent activity causing increased vascular permeability, vasodilatation, hypotension, pain, contraction of many types of smooth muscle, and activation of phospholipase A_2 with attendant activation of cellular arachidonic acid metabolism.

PROTEINS OF THE KININ CASCADE

Four plasma proteins make up the bradykinin-generating system: **Hageman factor, clotting factor XI, prekallikrein,** and **high-molecular-weight kininogen** (Fig 10–5). Factor XI circulates as a complex with high-molecular-weight kininogen in a molar ratio of 2:1. Prekallikrein also circulates in a complex with high-molecular weight kininogen in a molar ratio of 1:1. In contrast, Hageman factor circulates as an uncomplexed single-chain plasma protein.

STEPS IN KININ ACTIVATION

On interaction with a negatively charged surface such as is supplied experimentally by glass or naturally by many biologically active materials like the lipid A of gram-negative bacterial endotoxin, Hageman factor is cleaved and activated. The cleaved Hageman factor (αHFa) has proteolytic activity and can cleave additional molecules of Hageman factor to generate more αHFa. Cleavage of the single chain of Hageman factor (MW 80,000) yields heavy and light chains (MW 50,000 and 28,000, respectively) that remain linked by disulfide bonds. The active enzymatic site of Hageman factor resides in its light chain. Cleavage is also catalyzed by other proteolytic enzymes, particularly kallikrein. αHFa can interact with the complex of factor XI and high-molecular-weight kininogen to activate factor XI to factor XIa. This, in turn, can activate the intrinsic coagulation cascade. αHFa can also interact with the high-molecular-weight kininogen-prekallikrein complex to cleave the single-chain prekallikrein into a 2-chain molecule (kallikrein), with the chains associated via a disulfide linkage. The cleaved molecule now has proteolytic enzymatic activity associated with the lower-molecular-weight chain. To facilitate these cleavages of both factor XI and prekallikrein, high-molecular-weight kininogen complexes are bound to the surface, presumably near the Hageman factor.

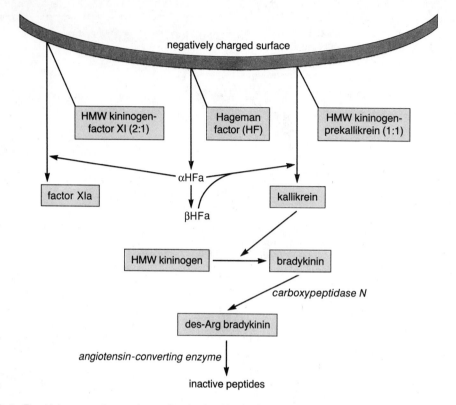

Figure 10–5. The kinin-generating pathway. Emphasized is the fact that complexes of high-molecular-weight (HMW) kininogen with both factor XI and prekallikrein associate on a surface with Hageman factor. The Hageman factor is activated and in turn is responsible for the activation of factor XI and prekallikrein. Active kallikrein cleaves high-molecular-weight kininogen to release bradykinin.

AMPLIFICATION & REGULATION OF KININ GENERATION

Active kallikrein is capable of further cleaving αHFa, with loss of the heavy chain but not the light chain. The resulting molecule, βHFa, remains capable of activating the high-molecular-weight kininogen-prekallikrein complex, but it does not remain surface-bound and does not interact efficiently with the high-molecular-weight kininogen–factor XI complex. Prekallikrein is also a single-chain glycoprotein that is converted to an active form by cleavage within a disulfide bridge, resulting in a 2-chain molecule with the chains linked by disulfide bonds. The enzymatic site resides in the light chain, and the surface-binding site is on the heavy chain. Active kallikrein can cleave high-molecular-weight kininogen at several sites to release bradykinin from the kininogen. Bradykinin has a short half-life, since it is rapidly attacked by carboxypeptidase N, which removes the C-terminal arginine to form the molecule termed des-Arg bradykinin. des-Arg bradykinin no longer has the smooth muscle-contracting activity of bradykinin and cannot induce capillary plasma leakage when in-

jected into skin, but it retains some of its vascular effects. des-Arg bradykinin is, in turn, cleaved by angiotensin-converting enzyme to form low-molecular-weight peptides that lack biologic activity.

PLASMA INHIBITORS OF KININ GENERATION

The inhibitors of this mediator-generating system include C1 inhibitor, α_2-macroglobulin, and α_1-proteinase inhibitor. C1 inhibitor and α_2-macroglobulin are the principal inhibitors of active kallikrein, with C1 inhibitor contributing most to inhibitory activity. C1 inhibitor and α_1-proteinase inhibitor are the 2 major inhibitors of factor XIa, and C1 inhibitor is the principal inhibitor of active Hageman factor.

LOW-MOLECULAR-WEIGHT KININOGEN & TISSUE KALLIKREINS

A low-molecular-weight kininogen also exists in plasma. This protein has an identical heavy chain to that of high-molecular-weight kininogen. Low-molecular-weight kininogen can act as a source of bradykinin, but it is not easily cleaved by kallikrein. However, there are tissue kallikreins—low-molecular-weight kallikreins found in multiple tissues—that can cleave low-molecular-weight kininogen to lysylbradykinin (bradykinin with an additional linked lysine). Presumably, lysylbradykinin undergoes the same degradation pathway as does bradykinin.

FUNCTIONS OF KININS IN DISEASE

The physiologic role of the kinin-generating system is uncertain, and in only a few cases do we understand its role in disease. Free bradykinin and lysylbradykinin have been found in nasal secretions during **rhinitis** and viral nasal inflammation, and it is reasonable to believe that both blood and tissue kalli-kreins contribute to its presence. It is believed that kinins, via their ability to cause smooth muscle contraction and capillary leakage, contribute to **asthma,** but this is by no means proven. Kinin generation has been found following antigen challenge of human lung fragments passively sensitized with specific IgE antibody, but the exact pathways involved in its generation are still uncertain. It has also been suggested that release of tissue kallikreins and activation of the kinin system is responsible for the severe pain of **pancreatitis.** The kinin-generating system has been reported to be involved in edema formation in **hereditary angioedema,** because kinins are present in fluid from suction-induced blisters over angioedema areas and because levels of circulating prekallikrein fall during attacks of this disease. Nevertheless, the kinin-forming system has not yet been conclusively proved to be responsible for the attacks of edema in hereditary angioedema.

REFERENCES

General
Borsos T: *The Molecular Basis of Complement Action,* Appleton-Century-Crofts, 1970.

Frank MM, Fries LF: Complement. Pages 679–702 in: *Fundamental Immunology,* 2nd ed. Paul WE (editor). Raven Press, 1989.

Harrison RA, Lachmann PJ: Complement technology. Chap 39 in: *Handbook of Experimental Immunology,* 4th ed. Vol. 1. Weir DM (editor). Blackwell, 1986.

Classic Pathway
Cooper NR: The classical complement pathway: Activation and regulation of the first complement component. Page 151 in: *Advances in Immunology.* Academic Press, 1985.

Kerr MA: The second component of human complement. *Methods Enzymol* 1981;**80:**54.

Tack BF: The β-Cys-τ-Glu thioester bond in human C3, C4, and α_2-macroglobulin. *Springer Semin Immunopathol* 1983;**6:**259.

Ziccardi RJ: The first component of human complement (C1): Activation and control. *Springer Semin Immunopathol* 1983;**6:**213.

Alternative Pathway
Pangburn MK, Muller-Eberhard HJ: The alternative pathway of complement. Springer *Semin Immunopathol* 1984;**7:**163.

Membrane Attack Complex
Mayer MM et al: Membrane damage by complement. *Crit Rev Immunol* 1981;**2:**133.

Muller-Eberhard HJ: The membrane attack complex of complement. *Annu Rev Immunol* 1986;**4:**503.

Control Mechanisms
Bock SC et al: Human C1 inhibitor: Primary structure, with DNA cloning, and chromosomal localization. *Biochemistry* 1986;**25:**4292.

Frank MM, Gelfand JA, Atkinson JP: Hereditary angioedema: The clinical syndrome and its management. *Ann Intern Med* 1976;**84:**580.

Genetic Considerations
Campbell RD et al: Structure, organization and regulation of the complement genes. *Annu Rev Immunol* 1988;**6:**161.

Perlmutter DH, Colton HR: Complement molecular genetics. Page 81 in: *Inflammation: Basic Principles and Clinical Correlates,* 2nd ed. Gallin JE, Goldstein IM, Snyderman R (editors). Raven Press, 1992.

Biologic Effects
Goldstein IM: Complement: Biologically active products. Page 63 in: *Inflammation: Basic Principles and Clinical Correlates,* 2nd ed. Gallin JE, Goldstein IM, Snyderman R (editors). Raven Press, 1992.

Hugli TE: Biochemistry and biology of anaphylatoxins. *Complement* 1986;**3:**111.

Hugli TE: Structure and function of the anaphylatoxins. *Springer Semin Immunopathol* 1984;**7:**193.

Reid KBM et al: Complement system proteins which interact with C3b or C4b. *Immunol Today* 1986;**7:**230.

Schapira M et al: Biochemistry and pathophysiology of human C1-inhibitor: Current issues. *Complement* 1986;**2:**111.

Cell Membrane Receptors & Regulatory Molecules
Berger M, Gaither TA, Frank MM: Complement receptors. *Clin Immunol Rev* 1983;**1:**471.

Pangburn MK, Schreiber RD, Muller-Eberhard HJ: Deficiency of an erythrocyte membrane protein with complement regulatory activity in paroxysmal nocturnal hemoglobinuria. *Proc Natl Acad Sci USA* 1983;**80:**5430.

Ross GD, Medof ME: Membrane complement receptors specific for bound fragments of C3. *Adv Immunol* 1985;**37:**217.

Schifferli JA, Ng YC, Peters DK: The role of complement and its receptor in the elimination of immune complexes. *N Engl J Med* 1986;**315:**488.

Zalman LS et al: Deficiency of the homologous restriction factor in paroxysmal nocturnal hemoglobinuria. *J Exp Med* 1987;**165:**689.

Kinins

Colman RW: Contact systems in infectious disease. *Rev Infect Dis* 1989;**4(suppl):**689.

Kozin F, Cochrane CH: The contact activation system of plasma: Biochemistry and pathophysiology. Pages 103–122 in: *Inflammation: Basic Principles and Clinical Correlates,* 2nd ed. Gallin JI, Goldstein IM, Snyderman R (editors). Raven Press, 1992.

Proud D, Kaplan AP: Kinin formation: Mechanisms and role in inflammatory disorders. *Annu Rev Immunol* 1988;**6:**49.

Inflammation

11

Abba I. Terr, MD

An immune response as it is usually described can be carried out entirely by lymphocytes and antigen-presenting cells. When such a response occurs in vivo, however, it often is accompanied by additional physiologic manifestations that may involve other cell types, extracellular proteins, or even other organ systems. For example, when an immunogen is injected into the skin, the resulting immune response is frequently accompanied by redness **(erythema)**, **warmth**, and **swelling** at the injection site. These signs reflect changes in blood vessels of the surrounding tissues: arterioles dilate so that local vascular perfusion is increased (producing erythema and warmth), and postcapillary venules become abnormally permeable, allowing vascular fluid to leak into the affected tissues to cause swelling **(edema).** In addition, various types of nucleated blood cells may migrate into the affected site to join in the response, becoming visible under the microscope as a **cellular infiltrate.** When a response occurs at or near a mucosal surface, glandular epithelial cells may dramatically increase their production of mucus or other secretions. If a response is intense and protracted, fibroblasts and endothelial cells at the site may proliferate and form a permanent scar. Additionally, some immune responses are accompanied by local or disseminated blood-clotting and coagulation, by activation of the serum complement or kinin cascades, or by systemic manifestations such as fever.

This multifaceted host reaction that results from and accompanies the "pure" immune response in vivo is termed **inflammation** or the **inflammatory response.** There are several distinct inflammatory pathways, each of which proceeds via a cascade of biologic events. Many of the individual steps in the inflammatory cascade are controlled by cytokines or other soluble regulatory molecules known as **inflammatory mediators.** A given mediator may not only produce effects directly but may also stimulate production of other mediators that control different aspects of the response. At the same time, other second-

ary events may be triggered by antigen-antibody complexes or by products of the activated complement cascade. Thus, each step in the process has the capability to induce subsequent steps, giving rise to an integrated response. The particular pathways and constellation of events that occur during an inflammatory response depend on many factors, including the nature of the inciting stimulus, its portal of entry, and the characteristics of the host. Not all inflammation is immunologically mediated. For example, some foreign substances can directly activate neutrophils and evoke neutrophil-mediated **acute inflammation** without the participation of lymphocytes (see Chapter 1). Even these reactions, however, may be controlled and modulated by the immune system in an immunized host through the opsonizing effect of antibodies.

An inflammatory response can be either beneficial or detrimental to the host. Increases in local vascular perfusion, for example, may have the beneficial effect of enhancing delivery of neutrophils, lymphocytes, and other circulating defensive cells to the site of an immune response. Similarly, leakage of protein-rich edema fluid into the site may help to dilute or inactivate a harmful immunogen, while increased glandular secretion helps flush foreign irritants off an epithelial surface. Localized clotting and coagulation may act to limit dissemination of an antigen through the circulation, and scarring is an integral component of the healing process. Inflammation is detrimental, on the other hand, when it temporarily or permanently injures host tissues and interferes with their normal functions. The terms **allergy** and **hypersensitivity** are used to describe the harmful effects of immunologically mediated inflammatory reactions that are directed against innocuous foreign substances such as dust, pollen, foods, or drugs. The pathogenic consequences of **autoimmune diseases** occur in part because of immunologically mediated inflammation directed against host tissues.

This chapter will describe immunologically medi-

Table 11–1. Inflammatory cells.

Circulating	Tissue-Resident
Lymphocytes	Mast cells
Neutrophils	Macrophages
Eosinophils	
Basophils	
Platelets	

ated inflammatory reactions, ie, those mediated either by antigen-specific lymphocytes or by preformed antibodies. The types of accessory cells and mediator substances that participate in these reactions will be considered first, and then the characteristics of the reactions themselves will be discussed. There are several distinct types of immunologic inflammatory reactions, each of which occurs through a specific mechanism and produces a characteristic pattern of associated phenomena. From a clinical standpoint, it is extremely important to recognize and understand these reaction patterns, since they offer insight into the pathologic processes at work in a given patient and provide clues that can guide the choice of appropriate therapy.

INFLAMMATORY CELLS

Any cell that participates in inflammatory reactions can be called an **inflammatory cell.** The term is thus applicable to many different cell types (Table 11–1). Some are long-term residents of normal tissues; others are circulating cells that enter tissues only in the course of an inflammatory response. Three types of inflammatory cells—neutrophils, macrophages, and lymphocytes—are the principal effector cells of most acute inflammatory or immune reactions and have been considered at length in earlier chapters. This section will focus on the properties of the other inflammatory cell types. Most of these cells express surface receptors for complement components, for the Fc portions of antibody molecules

(Table 11–2), and for various cytokines. As a result, their activities tend to be controlled directly or indirectly by ongoing immune responses or by activation of the complement cascade.

Eosinophils

Eosinophils are bone marrow-derived granulocytes whose clinical significance derives from their strong association with **allergic reactions** and with **helminthic parasite infections.** An eosinophil in blood or tissue can be recognized by its bilobed nucleus and by the characteristic eosinophilic granules in its cytoplasm. Human eosinophils are slightly larger than neutrophils, being 12–17 μm in diameter, but they contain substantially fewer specific granules (approximately 200 per cell). Eosinophil granules are spherical or round and 0.5 μm in diameter; they can be seen under the electron microscope to contain an electron-dense crystalloid core surrounded by a less dense amorphous matrix (Fig 11–1). The major contents of these granules include an **eosinophil peroxidase** (which is biochemically distinct from the myeloperoxidase of neutrophils but mediates the same reaction; see Chapter 1) and other enzymes that can generate toxic oxygen metabolites, a cytotoxic lysophosphatase called **Charcot-Leyden crystal protein,** and at least 3 other abundant basic proteins. One of the latter, called the **major basic protein,** has a strong affinity for acidic dyes such as eosin and is responsible for the intense red staining of the granules.

Circulating eosinophils normally make up about 1–3% of peripheral white blood cells. However, these circulating cells represent only a very small proportion of the total eosinophil population: it is estimated that, for every circulating eosinophil, there are approximately 200 mature eosinophils in the bone marrow and 500 in connective tissues throughout the body. Eosinophil production in the bone marrow is dependent not only on granulocyte-macrophage colony-stimulating factor (GM-CSF) and interleukin-3 (IL-3), which promote differentiation of all types of

Table 11–2. Inflammatory-cell immunoglobulin Fc receptors.

Receptor	Present on:					
	Neutrophils	Monocytes	Mast Cells	Basophils	Eosinophils	Platelets
IgM	−	−	−	−	−	−
IgG						
IgG1	+	+	−	?	+	+
IgG2	+	+	−	−	?	+
IgG3	+	+	−	−	?	+
IgG4	+	+	−	−	?	+
IgA	+	+	−	−	?	−
IgD	−	−	−	−	+	−
IgE	−	+	+	+	+	+
FcεRI	−	−	+	+	−	−
FcεRII	−	+	?	?	+	+

¹Symbols: +, receptor present; −, receptor absent; ?, presence unknown.

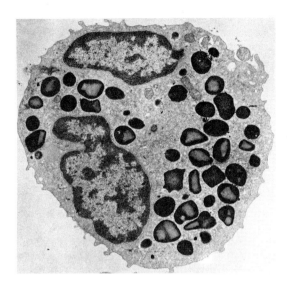

Figure 11–1. Electron micrograph of a mature human eosinophil. The numerous cytoplasmic granules stain darkly owing to the presence of peroxidase and contain characteristic central electron-dense crystalline cores with a surrounding amorphous matrix. The nucleus typically has 2 lobes. The cell is 15 μm in diameter. (Courtesy of Dorothy F. Bainton.)

granulocytes, but also on **IL-5,** which functions as a specific eosinophil growth factor (see Chapter 9). The life span of an eosinophil is relatively short: it has a marrow maturation time of 2–6 days, a circulating half-life of 6–12 hours, and a connective tissue residence time of only a few days. Increased concentrations of eosinophils **(eosinophilia)** in the blood can occur in several clinical settings but are most commonly encountered in allergic or parasitic diseases; the increase is thought to be mediated by IL-5. Eosinophilia of solid tissues also can occur in these disorders, as a result of chemokines and other mediators released locally by mast cells, macrophages, lymphocytes, and other cells. Intracellular and protozoan parasites do not evoke eosinophilic responses (see Chapter 50).

Eosinophils bear surface immunoglobulin E (IgE) receptors, but these are of the low-affinity **(FcεRII)** type and so are largely unoccupied when the serum IgE concentration is within the normal range (see Chapter 6). Approximately 10–30% of eosinophils from normal individuals also have low-affinity **(Fcγ-RIII)** or intermediate-affinity **(FcγRII)** IgG receptors (Table 11–2). In addition, 40–50% display receptors for complement components. These various receptor types enable an eosinophil to recognize and bind to particulate antigens that are coated with IgE, IgG, or complement derivatives, much as a neutrophil or macrophage recognizes an opsonized particle. Binding, in turn, leads to eosinophil activation, which

is characterized by (1) an increase in the number of surface Fc and complement receptors and certain other surface markers, (2) enhanced oxidative metabolism, (3) de novo synthesis and release of the arachidonate derivative leukotriene C_4 (LTC$_4$; see below) and certain other proinflammatory mediators, and (4) increased cytotoxic activity. Activation can also be induced or enhanced by contact with activated endothelial cells, by T cell-derived lymphokines (GM-CSF, IL-3, and IL-5), or by monokines such as IL-1 and tumor necrosis factor alpha (TNFα).

Activated eosinophils can phagocytose many types of particles in vitro (including bacteria, fungi, mycoplasmas, inert particles, and antigen-antibody complexes), but the evidence that they play a significant role as phagocytes in vivo remains inconclusive. Instead, they appear to act primarily by attaching themselves tightly onto an antibody-coated or complement-coated particle and discharging their granule contents onto its surface through **extracellular degranulation.** This occurs, for example, when eosinophils aggregate around a large tissue parasite such as *Trichinella, Schistosoma,* or *Fasciola.* The cationic granular proteins may attach themselves to the negatively charged surfaces of these parasites to exert their cytotoxic effects. For example, eosinophil peroxidase tends to attach itself in this manner and so concentrates production of toxic oxygen metabolites onto the target surface. Eosinophils also bind and attack large deposits of antigen-antibody complexes in the tissues (see below). Granular contents released during particularly intense responses can damage host tissues. For example, major basic protein is toxic to respiratory epithelium and is found in elevated concentrations in the sputum and airway secretions of people with asthma. Hexagonal, bipyramidal crystals of granule proteins, called **Charcot-Leyden crystals,** are also found in the sputum of asthmatics; they provide a useful clinical marker for eosinophil-mediated airway reactions.

Mast Cells

Mast cells are marrow-derived, tissue-resident cells that are essential for **IgE-mediated** inflammatory reactions (Table 11–3). Human mast cells are relatively large (10–15 μm in diameter) and heterogeneous in shape but generally are round, oval, or spindle-shaped, and they bear numerous surface projections (Fig 11–2). They possess a single round or oval eccentrically located nucleus. Their most distinctive feature under the light microscope is the presence in each cell of 50–200 densely packed granules that appear to fill the cytoplasm and that exhibit a distinctive purplish **(metachromatic)** coloration in hematoxylin-stained tissue preparations. Each granule is membrane-bounded and 0.1–0.4 μm in diameter; the granules contain relatively large amounts of **histamine, heparin, TNFα,** and other preformed inflammatory

Table 11–3. Properties of human mast cells and basophils.

	Mast Cells	Basophils
Cell diameter	5–7 μm	10–15 μm
Nucleus	Bilobed or multi-lobed	Round or oval; eccentric
Cell surface contour	Smooth with occasional short, broad projections	Numerous narrow projections
Predominant localization	Connective tissues	Blood
Lifespan	Weeks or months	Days
Terminally differentiated	No	Yes
Major granule contents	Histamine, chondroitin sulfate, neutral proteases, heparin, TNFα	Histamine, chondroitin sulfate, neutral proteases, major basic protein, Charcot-Leyden protein
Mediators that are synthesized and released after degranulation	TNFα, PAF, LTC$_4$, PGD$_2$	LTC$_4$

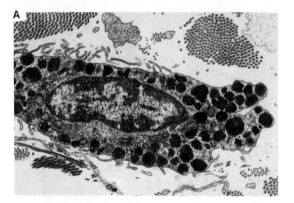

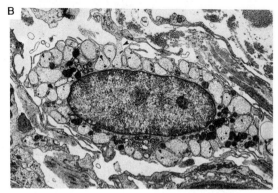

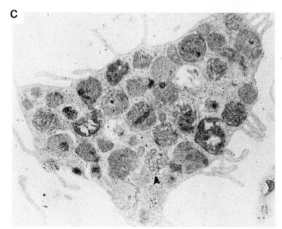

Figure 11–2. Electron micrographs of skin mast cells. **A:** An unstimulated mast cell. (Courtesy of Marc M. Friedman.) **B:** A mast cell activated 5 minutes earlier with ragweed antigen. Note the swollen, lucent appearance of the secretory granules. (Courtesy of Marc M. Friedman.) **C:** Cytoplasm of an unstimulated mast cell, showing the diverse appearances of the granules, which may contain crystalline, whorled, or granular material. (Courtesy of Karen Oetkon.) Each cell is 10–15 μm in diameter.

mediators that will be described later in this chapter. They also contain superoxide dismutase, peroxidase, and numerous acid hydrolases (such as β-hexosaminidase, β-glucuronidase, and arylsulfatase) that may act to degrade the extracellular matrix. Under the electron microscope, the granules may be seen to contain amorphous electron-dense granular zones as well as highly ordered crystalline arrays (Fig 11–2).

Mast cells express on their surfaces large numbers of high-affinity Fc receptors for IgE (**FcεRI**). As a result, the surface of each cell is decorated with lymphocyte-derived IgE molecules that have been adsorbed from the circulation and serve as receptors for specific antigens. Mast cells are scattered in connective tissues throughout the body but are found in especially large numbers beneath surface tissues such as the skin (which contains 10^4 mast cells/mm^3), lung alveoli (10^6 mast cells/g of tissue), gastrointestinal mucosa, and nasal mucous membranes. They are thus strategically positioned to detect inhaled or ingested antigens. When its surface IgE molecules bind antigens, a mast cell promptly undergoes activation, characterized by granule enlargement, solubilization of the crystalline structures within the granules, and then **degranulation** with release of granule contents into the surrounding tissues. Some of the substances within the granules induce local vascular permeability, smooth muscle contraction, and epithelial mucus secretion, whereas others act as chemotactic factors to attract other inflammatory cells. These regulatory factors are sometimes referred to as **mast cell mediators.** Some of the granular proteases and other enzymes may have nonspecific effects on an antigen, but otherwise mast cells do not appear to carry out any significant direct effector activities such as phagocytosis.

Histochemical and biochemical analyses indicate that mast cells at various body sites differ in the relative amounts of 2 neutral proteases in their cytoplasmic granules. The 2 proteases, called tryptase and chymase, together make up 25–70% of granule protein by weight; their physiologic substrates are undetermined. Most mast cells in the lungs and gastrointestinal mucosa contain only tryptase, whereas the majority in the skin and gastrointestinal submucosa contain both tryptase and chymase. This difference appears to be reversible and depends on factors in the local microenvironment; its functional significance is unknown.

Basophils

Basophils are circulating marrow-derived cells that have many of the same properties as tissue mast cells, although they represent an independent cell lineage. At 5–7 μm in diameter, they are the smallest cells of the granulocyte series and account for no more than 1% of nucleated cells in the marrow or peripheral blood. Like mast cells, basophils bear high-affinity Fc receptors for IgE (approximately 270,000 FcεRI receptors are present on each cell) and contain histamine-rich cytoplasmic granules. These 2 attributes distinguish mast cells and basophils from all other human cell types. However, basophils differ from mast cells morphologically and biochemically in several respects (Fig 11–3; Table 11–3).

Small to moderate numbers of basophils accumulate in tissues in a variety of inflammatory conditions involving the skin (such as late-phase cutaneous al-lergic responses, cutaneous basophil hypersensitivity reactions, and lesions of bullous pemphigoid), the small intestine (Crohn's disease), the kidneys (allergic interstitial nephritis, renal allograft rejection), nasal mucosa (allergic rhinitis), and eyes (allergic conjunctivitis). In view of these associations and the many similarities between basophils and mast cells, it is generally presumed that basophils participate in IgE-mediated reactions in a manner analogous to that of mast cells. Nevertheless, the importance of basophils in immunity and hypersensitivity has yet to be proven.

Platelets

Platelets are anucleate cytoplasmic fragments derived from bone marrow megakaryocytes and are the smallest circulating blood cells (2 μm in diameter). They have a 10-day life span in the circulation. Their primary function is in blood-clotting, but they also store and can release mediator substances that have important proinflammatory effects. During clot formation, platelets undergo an **activation** response that causes them to aggregate with one another and also to discharge the contents of the 3 types of storage granules in their cytoplasm (called dense bodies, α granules, and lysosomal granules, respectively) to the exterior. The released products may include various arachidonate metabolites (prostaglandin G_2 [PGG_2], PGH_2, and thromboxane A_2 [TXA_2]; see below), growth factors, and bioactive amines, as well as neutral and acid hydrolases. Occlusion of a blood vessel by platelet aggregates has the useful effects of entrapping leukocytes and preventing the spread of antigen through the circulation. Platelets express surface Fc receptors for IgG and also low-affinity **(FcεRII)** receptors for IgE. The latter receptor allows platelets to bind and secrete cytotoxic products (probably hydrogen peroxide or other oxygen metabolites) onto IgE-coated tissue parasites but without inducing platelet aggregation or degranulation. Antigen binding through the platelet FcεRII also induces production of **platelet-activating factor (PAF),** a potent inflammatory mediator (see below).

Endothelial Cells

Although not usually classified as inflammatory cells themselves, endothelial cells can participate actively in immune responses by promoting immigration and modulating the responses of circulating inflammatory cells. When endothelial cells are exposed to cytokines (such as IL-1, TNF, or gamma interferon [IFNγ]) or other products released at the site of an ongoing immune response, they may become activated and acquire increased adhesiveness for monocytes, neutrophils, and other circulating cells. Such increased adhesiveness is important in attracting leukocytes into the involved tissue (see Chapter 1). Activated endothelial cells sometimes express class II major histocompatibility complex (MHC) proteins

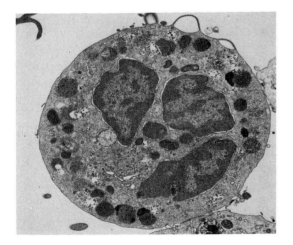

Figure 11–3. Electron micrograph of a peripheral blood basophil. The nucleus is multilobed, and the cytoplasmic surface is smooth with occasional short blunt folds or uropods. The cell is 5–7 μm in diameter. (Courtesy of Marc M. Friedman.)

Table 11–4. Some major inflammatory mediators.[1]

Vasoactive and smooth muscle-constricting mediators
  Histamine
  Arachidonate metabolites (PGD_2, LTC_4, LTD_4, TXE_4)
  PAF
  Adenosine
Chemotactic factors
  Chemokines
  PAF
  Complement components, especially C5a
  Arachidonate metabolites (LTB_4)
Enzymatic mediators
  Tryptase, others
Proteoglycan mediators
  Heparin

[1]The limited selection represented here omits many pro-inflammatory cytokines (see Chapter 9) and other mediators.

Table 11–5. Histamine receptors.

Receptor	Histamine Actions
H1	Increased post-capillary venular permeability Smooth muscle contraction Pulmonary vasoconstriction Increased cGMP levels in cells Enhanced mucus secretion Leukocyte chemokinesis Prostaglandin production in lungs
H2	Enhanced gastric acid secretion Enhanced mucus secretion Increased cAMP levels in cells Leukocyte chemokinesis Activation of suppressor T cells
H3	Histamine release inhibition Histamine synthesis inhibition

(and so may function as antigen-presenting cells) and can also secrete the cytokines IL-1 and GM-CSF, which modulate immune responses.

MEDIATORS OF INFLAMMATION

Inflammatory mediators are host-derived compounds that are secreted by activated cells and serve to trigger or enhance specific aspects of inflammation. Such compounds are said to be **proinflammatory;** ie, they promote inflammation. Many of the **cytokines** act as inflammatory mediators, as detailed in Chapter 9. This section will describe some of the other major mediators (Table 11–4), classifying them somewhat arbitrarily into 4 groups: (1) those with vasoactive and smooth muscle-constricting properties, (2) those that attract other cells and are termed chemotactic factors, (3) enzymes, and (4) proteoglycans. These categories are not mutually exclusive, and several mediators can be assigned to more than one group.

1. VASOACTIVE & SMOOTH MUSCLE-CONSTRICTING MEDIATORS

Histamine

Histamine (Fig 11–4) is an inflammatory mediator that is found preformed in the granules of mast cells and basophils. It is synthesized within these granules by the action of histidine decarboxylase on the amino acid histidine and may make up as much as 10% of granule contents by weight. Histamine is bound through ionic linkages to proteoglycans and proteins within the granules and is bound particularly tightly to mast cell heparin; however, it dissociates from these ligands when released to the extracellular space by degranulation. Histamine exerts its physiologic effects by interacting with any of 3 different target cell receptors, designated H1, H2, and H3. The receptors are expressed in a tissue-specific manner, and each produces characteristic effects (Table 11–5). Major effects mediated by the **H1 receptor** include contraction of bronchial, intestinal, and uterine smooth muscles and augmentation of vascular permeability in post-capillary venules. **Antihistamine** drugs used to treat allergies act by selectively blocking H1 receptor binding. In contrast, binding of **H2 receptors** augments gastric acid and airway mucus secretion and can be inhibited by such compounds as **cimetidine** and **ranitidine,** which are useful for treating peptic ulcer disease. **H3 receptor** binding principally affects histamine synthesis and release.

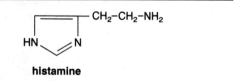

histamine

Figure 11–4. Chemical structure of histamine.

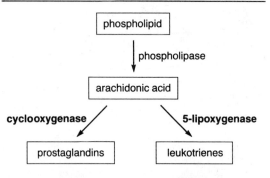

Figure 11–5. Major pathways of arachidonic acid formation and metabolism.

Arachidonic Acid Metabolites

The prostaglandins and leukotrienes are metabolites produced by enzymatic cyclooxygenation and lipoxygenation, respectively, of arachidonic acid (Fig 11–5). They constitute 2 major families of inflammatory mediators, whose members exhibit diverse vasoactive, smooth muscle-constricting, and chemotactic properties. Many **non-steroidal anti-inflammatory drugs,** such as **aspirin,** act primarily by blocking the synthesis of prostaglandins. At present, there are no inhibitors of leukotrienes that are sufficiently selective for clinical use.

Arachidonic acid is a 20-carbon fatty acid containing 4 double bonds (Fig 11–6). It can be liberated from membrane phospholipids either through the sequential action of phospholipase C and diacylglycerol lipase, or by the direct action of phospholipase A_2, on membrane phospholipids. Once liberated, arachidonic acid can be metabolized by either the cyclooxygenase or lipoxygenase pathway. Each of

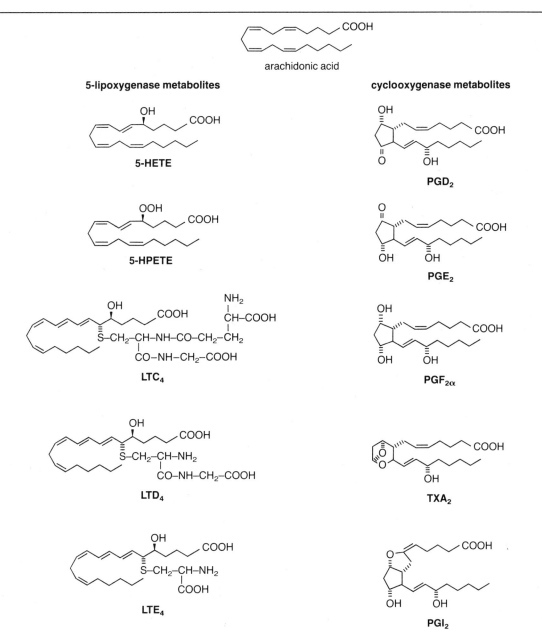

Figure 11–6. Chemical structures of arachidonic acid and of some principal 5-lipoxygenase and cyclooxygenase metabolites. Each of the compounds depicted is a physiologically active inflammatory mediator.

these pathways can give rise to many alternative products (Fig 11–6), each with its own spectrum of effects, and any of these metabolites may be produced by many different cell types in response to various stimuli. A complete discussion of the arachidonate metabolites is beyond the scope of this text, which will instead consider only a few representative mediators of this class that are involved in inflammation.

A. Cyclooxygenase Products: The main product of the cyclooxygenase pathway in connective-tissue mast cells is **prostaglandin D$_2$** (PGD$_2$). This mediator promotes local vascular dilatation and vascular permeability (although to a lesser extent than does histamine) and also is a chemoattractant for neutrophils. PGD$_2$ is thought to have a role, along with histamine, in mediating erythema and **wheal-and-flare** reactions in IgE-mediated allergic responses and may be responsible for the systemic flushing and hypotensive episodes that occur in patients with systemic mastocytosis. Basophils do not generate cyclooxygenase products.

B. Lipoxygenase Products: The 4 principal products of the lipoxygenase pathway are the **leukotrienes** LTB$_4$, LTC$_4$, LTD$_4$, and LTE$_4$ (Fig 11–6). These are the principal arachidonate metabolites released by mucosal mast cells. LTB$_4$ is a potent chemoattractant (see below). LTC$_4$, LTD$_4$, and LTE$_4$ collectively make up what was once termed "slow-reacting substance of anaphylaxis": they induce smooth muscle contraction, bronchoconstriction, and mucus secretion in the airways and the wheal-and-flare reaction in the skin. When injected intravenously, the last 2 compounds can cause hypotension and cardiac dysrhythmias. The leukotrienes are several hundred-fold more potent on a molar basis than is histamine and are therefore believed to have an important role in the genesis of allergic disorders.

Platelet-Activating Factor

PAF is a lipophilic organic mediator (Fig 11–7) that is released from activated mast cells and platelets and can also be produced by other activated cell types. It was originally named because of its ability to activate platelets, but it has since been found to have many other proinflammatory effects, including the ability to cause activation and degranulation of neutrophils and eosinophils. It is the most potent eosinophil chemoattractant known. Many of its effects appear to be indirect results of platelet activation. When injected into the skin, PAF causes a wheal-and-flare response and leukocyte infiltration. When inhaled, it causes acute bronchoconstriction, an eosinophilic infiltrate, and a state of nonspecific bronchial hyperreactivity that may persist for days or weeks following a single administration. Injected intravenously, it can cause widespread activation of neutrophils, platelets, and basophils, as well as profound hypotension.

The bioactive form of PAF, depicted in Fig 11–7, consists of a glycerol backbone linked to 3 substituents: (1) a long-chain alcohol, usually of 16–18 carbons; (2) an acetyl group; and (3) a phosphorylcholine moiety. Platelets and other cells normally store an inactive form of PAF that contains arachidonate at position 2; when a cell becomes activated, the arachidonate is excised and replaced by acetate to produce the active compound. Once outside the cell, PAF is rapidly degraded by plasma- and cell-associated hydrolases. Some inhibitors of PAF are currently being tested for therapeutic use, but none is yet available clinically.

Adenosine

The nucleoside adenosine (Fig 11–8) is liberated from degranulating mast cells and can then bind to surface adenosine receptors on many cell types. Its effects include bronchoconstriction and the induction of fluid secretion from intestinal epithelial cells. Blood adenosine concentrations may rise during acute asthmatic episodes.

2. CHEMOTACTIC MEDIATORS

Among the most important chemotactic mediators are the peptides that make up the **chemokine** family

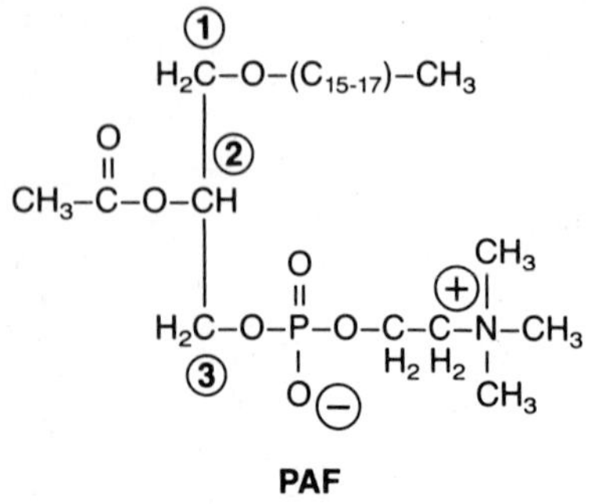

Figure 11–7. Chemical structure of the secreted, bioactive form of platelet-activating factor.

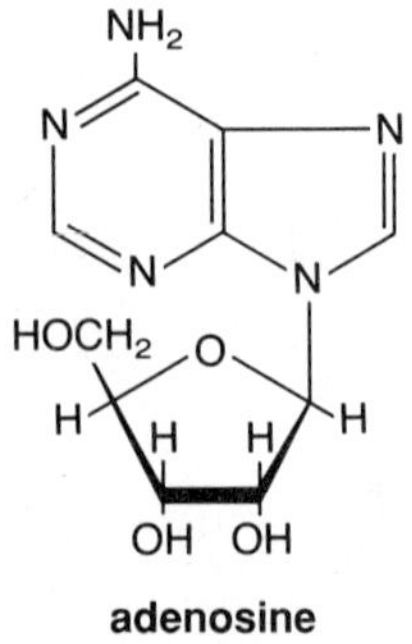

Figure 11–8. Chemical structure of adenosine.

of cytokines, which have been considered in detail in Chapter 9. Certain complement components, notably **C5a,** are also potent chemoattractants (see Chapter 10). In addition, several nonpeptide inflammatory mediators have been found to have significant chemoattractant activity. These include PAF and LTB_4 (see above), which, together with C5a, are potent neutrophil chemoattractants that are active at concentrations as low as 10^{-10} M. PAF also has strong chemoattractant effects on eosinophils.

3. ENZYMATIC MEDIATORS

A panoply of enzymes can be found in the storage granules of inflammatory cells and can be released to the exterior on degranulation. In addition to their effects on antigens and host tissues, a few of these can act to initiate the complement, clotting, or kinin cascade. For example, mast cell tryptase can cleave complement factor C3 to generate C3a, and it also acts on many clotting proteins. Other mast cell proteases can proteolytically activate kallikrein or kininogen (see Chapter 10).

4. PROTEOGLYCANS

Mast cell and basophil granules are rich in protein-polysaccharide complexes called proteoglycans, which form much of the structural matrix of these granules and also serve as binding sites for heparin and other mediators. These may be the primary functions of the chondroitin sulfate that is present in such granules. However, other proteoglycans also have intrinsic regulatory activity. For example, the major granular proteoglycan in human mast cells is heparin (MW 60,000), which has anticoagulant activity and also is capable of modulating tryptase activity (see above). Each human mast cell contains about 5 pg of heparin.

TYPES OF IMMUNOLOGICALLY MEDIATED INFLAMMATORY RESPONSES

Much of what is now known about inflammatory reactions in humans was derived from use of the **skin test**—a procedure in which a small amount of a purified antigen is injected beneath the skin and the response to the injection is then observed. Skin testing is widely used in clinical practice to assess whether patients are hypersensitive to particular antigens. It is also very useful experimentally for studying the mechanisms of immune reactions: for example, biopsies of test sites can be performed to examine the cellular infiltrates induced by an antigen, and fluids extracted from the sites can be assayed for inflammatory mediators.

More than a century of experience with skin testing in humans has revealed at least 4 distinct patterns of immunologically mediated inflammatory reactions (Table 11–6). Under the somewhat artificial conditions of the skin test, a single pure antigen may induce exclusively one type of reaction in a given patient. By contrast, responses against the more complex, multicomponent antigens encountered in nature often include 2 or more of these patterns simultaneously. Thus, these reaction patterns are not mutually exclusive but, rather, serve to highlight the major integrated pathways by which humans respond to foreign substances.

Table 11–6. Classes of immunologically mediated inflammation.

Type of Inflammation	Skin Test Terminology	Time to Maximal Reaction (hours)	Predominant Cellular Infiltrate	Principal Mediators	Principal; Mechanism Inducing the Inflammatory Response
Cell-mediated (CMI)	Delayed (DTH)	36	Lymphocytes, macrophages	Lymphokines	Lymphokines released from activated T_H cells induce primarily macrophage and T cell responses
Immune complex-mediated	Late	8	Neutrophils	Complement factor C5a	Immune complexes fix complement, inducing neutrophil reaction
IgE-mediated					
Immediate phase	Immediate	0.25	Eosinophils	Histamine, leukotrienes	Antigen binding to surface IgE leads to mast cell degranulation, with release of stored mediators
Late phase	Late	6	Eosinophils, neutrophils	PAF, TNFα, PGD_2, leukotrienes	Mediators synthesized and released by mast cells after degranulation.
Cutaneous basophil hypersensitivity	Delayed	36	Basophils	Unknown	Unknown

Cell-Mediated Immunity

Cell-mediated immunity (CMI) is the term applied to defensive reactions that are mediated primarily by activated T lymphocytes and macrophages. Reactions of this type are very common. They occur through the sequence of events outlined in Chapter 3, in which contact with antigen leads to activation, proliferation, and differentiation of T cells that have the appropriate specificities. Owing to the time required for these events to take place and for significant numbers of cells to be recruited into the response, CMI reactions develop rather slowly. Even in a highly immunized host, CMI responses exhibit a relatively long lag phase and do not achieve their maximal intensity until approximately 36 hours after exposure to the antigen. Consequently, CMI responses are also called **delayed-type hypersensitivity (DTH)** reactions.

The evolution of a DTH reaction is schematized in Fig 11–9. The reaction is initiated by activation of an antigen-specific TH cell, which then releases numerous immunoregulatory and proinflammatory lymphokines and other substances into the surrounding tissues. These compounds, together with bioactive substances released by the antigen-presenting cell, promote clonal expansion of the responsive TH cell and serve to attract additional inflammatory cells from the circulation. The chemoattracted cells may include antigen-specific and nonspecific T or B lymphocytes, as well as monocytes, neutrophils, eosinophils, and basophils. Some of the cytokines promote differentiation and activation of macrophages and so enhance the phagocytic, bactericidal, and antigen-presenting functions of these cells. Local blood vessels are induced to dilate, and this further enhances immigration of cells from the bloodstream. The coagulation-kinin systems also become activated, so that fibrin is formed and deposited at the site. Fibrin deposition is probably important in confining the inflammatory reaction to a discrete location and imparts a firm consistency **(induration)** that is characteristic of tissues undergoing DTH reactions.

Viewed under the light microscope, the site of an ongoing DTH reaction can be seen to contain a tissue infiltrate composed mainly of lymphocytes and macrophages, along with variable numbers of plasma cells and other inflammatory cells. This is sometimes referred to as a **chronic inflammatory infiltrate** to indicate the relatively long time (several days or more) needed for its development and to distinguish it from acute inflammatory infiltrates, which are composed primarily of neutrophils (see Chapter 1).

Certain types of antigens induce CMI with an especially pronounced macrophage response, leading to the formation of granulomas (see Chapter 1). Such **granulomatous inflammation** is therefore a subtype of CMI. It develops most commonly in response to particulate antigens that are large, insoluble, and resistant to elimination. These include foreign bodies (such as suture material, silica, talc, or mineral oil), fungi, metazoan parasites, or mycobacteria such as *Mycobacterium tuberculosis* or *M leprae*.

CMI reactions are encountered in many clinical settings, including numerous infectious diseases and certain types of vaccination sites, or following contact of many different types of chemicals with the skin or mucous membranes. CMI is also a major mechanism of allograft rejection and graft-versus-host disease and plays a role in some autoimmune disorders and in tumor immunity. Cytotoxic T cell reactions against virus-infected host cells are another example of this type of response. Indeed, immunity to infection by any type of intracellular pathogen is mediated by CMI; the types of organisms that provoke this type of immunity include viruses, fungi, protozoa, helminthic parasites, and some bacteria, such as *Chlamydia*.

Hypersensitivity diseases mediated by DTH are discussed in Chapter 28. The most common disease in this category is **allergic contact dermatitis.** In this disease, the sensitizing agents are usually haptens that form antigenic complexes when they bind to host proteins in the skin and are then processed and presented by Langerhans cells. Examples of common

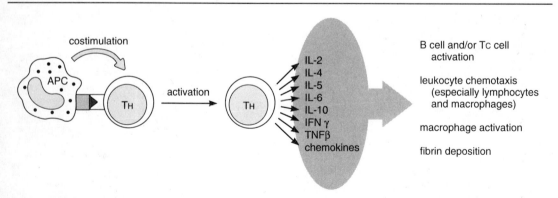

Figure 11–9. Schematic depiction of the immunologic events that give rise to a cell-mediated inflammatory response.

substances that act in this manner are pentadecyl cat-echol (the active immunogen in the oil of **poison ivy**) and **nickel** found in jewelry.

Despite their potential protective effects, pro-longed or intense CMI reactions can lead to perma-nent injury to host tissues. Perhaps for this reason, ac-tive feedback inhibition mechanisms exist that limit the intensity of CMI reactions. The mechanisms in-volved in this inhibition are unknown but appear to be antigenically nonspecific. Thus, persons with se-vere or widespread diseases that induce CMI are sometimes found to have reduced or absent cellular immunity to various unrelated antigens. This state of generalized, nonspecific depression of cellular im-munity is called **anergy.** It is usually defined clini-cally as the absence of DTH skin test reactivity to commonly encountered antigens or loss of a pre-viously positive DTH skin test. Anergy may occur in individuals with extensive granulomatous disorders such as miliary tuberculosis, severe coccidioidomy-cosis, lepromatous leprosy, or sarcoidosis. It also oc-curs in Hodgkin's disease. A temporary loss of CMI can occur during the acute phase of certain viral in-fections such as measles. Not surprisingly, CMI is also impaired in the various congenital forms of cel-lular immunodeficiency and in the acquired immune deficiency syndrome (AIDS).

Immune Complex-Mediated Inflammation

Immune complex-mediated inflammation refers to the inflammatory responses that occur when an anti-body binds to antigen and activates the complement cascade. Reactions of this type do not require the ac-tive participation of the lymphocytes that originally generated the antibody. Thus, they can occur rela-tively rapidly in an immunized host who has pre-formed circulating antibodies of the appropriate spec-ificity (Table 11–6). There are 2 classic types of immune complex-mediated reactions—the localized **Arthus reaction,** and systemic **serum sickness**—but their underlying mechanisms are similar. Each occurs through the sequence of complex formation, complex deposition, complement activation, and cellular infil-tration, as described below.

A. Immune-Complex Formation: The classic complement pathway is activated when antibody molecules of an appropriate class bind to an antigen in a spatial conformation that allows subsequent binding of complement component C1 (see Chapter 10). For this to occur, the chemical nature of the anti-gen is generally less important than the number and types of antibody molecules it binds. IgM antibodies, or IgG antibodies of any subclass except IgG4, can activate the classic pathway, whereas IgA, IgE, and IgD cannot. As few as one IgM or 2 IgG molecules can suffice to activate (or "fix") complement when bound to the surface of a particulate antigen, such as a bacterium or a virus-infected host cell.

By contrast, soluble molecular antigens will gener-ally fix complement only after they have been incor-porated into larger, multimeric **antigen-antibody complexes.** Such complexes (also called **immune complexes**) form because each immunoglobulin 4-chain unit contains 2 independent and identical anti-gen-binding sites and can therefore bind to 2 antigen molecules simultaneously. Thus, when soluble anti-gen and antibody molecules are present in an appro-priate molar ratio, they can cross-link one another to form a multimolecular lattice, as depicted in Fig 11–10. Because they contain numerous antibody molecules, immune complexes are often highly effi-cient at activating complement.

B. Complex Deposition: The physical proper-ties of immune complexes are strongly influenced by the molar ratios of the molecules they contain (see Chapter 12). Complexes formed with a substantial excess of either antigen or antibody are small and rel-atively soluble, whereas those formed at near-stoi-chiometric equivalence are larger and have a tendency to precipitate out of solution (the so-called **precipitin reaction**). Large, insoluble complexes of the latter type can form in the circulation when a large amount of antigen is introduced into the blood-stream of an immunized person. The complexes then tend to be deposited in tissues throughout the body, particularly in the internal elastic lamina of arteries and in perivascular regions. They also tend to become trapped as the serum is filtered through renal glomer-uli, and so they accumulate within the basement membranes of glomerular capillaries. Thus, massive systemic antigen exposure can lead to the widespread deposition of complement-fixing immune com-plexes. This is the pathogenic mechanism of **serum sickness.**

Alternatively, high concentrations of antigen-anti-body complexes can form at a discrete site where an-tigen is present in a solid tissue. This can occur, for example, when an antigen is injected into the dermis of an immunized person. The resulting complexes precipitate as focal deposits in the blood vessels and fix complement, producing a localized inflammatory response that is called the **Arthus reaction.**

C. Complement Activation and Cellular Infil-tration: The principal inflammatory factor derived from the complement cascade appears to be C5a, which is a powerful chemoattractant for neutrophils. When immune complexes in and around a blood ves-sel wall fix complement, C5a is released and stimu-lates neutrophilic infiltration (ie, acute inflammation) of the vessel. The resulting **vasculitis** has several components (Fig 11–10). Neutrophils release lyso-somal enzymes and toxic oxygen metabolites while phagocytosing the immune complexes, and these cause destruction of the vessel wall with associated microhemorrhages into the tissues. Endothelial cells swell and proliferate, platelets aggregate in the lumen, and fibrin is deposited in and around the ves-sel owing to activation of the coagulation cascade.

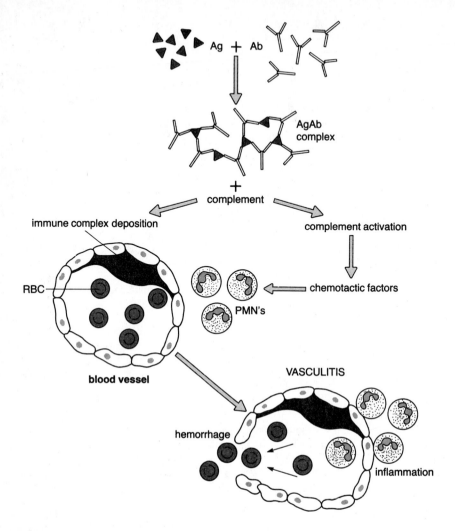

Figure 11–10. Schematic depiction of the immunologic events in immune complex-mediated inflammation. Ag, antigen; Ab, antibody; RBC, red blood cell; PMN, polymorphonuclear leukocyte.

Later in the progression of the injury, macrophages and lymphocytes also infiltrate the area, although the precise factors that attract them have not been determined.

Clinical Manifestations

As is true of all other types of inflammation, immune complex-mediated reactions can be beneficial, detrimental, or both. This type of inflammation often occurs in concert with other antibody-mediated phenomena (such as opsonization) during normal immune responses. In addition, it is the primary mechanism underlying several types of hypersensitivity. The Arthus reaction, for example, can frequently be observed at inoculation sites in persons who receive subcutaneous antigen injections as a treatment for allergy, and it also occurs occasionally as a response to insect bites or injected medications. These reactions

are generally limited to mild edema and cellular infiltration, with little or no vascular destruction. More severe Arthus reactions also occur in 2 autoimmune disorders—autoimmune thyroiditis and Goodpasture's syndrome—in which the action of anti-thyroglobulin antibodies and anti-glomerular basement membrane antibodies, respectively, can lead to destruction of the involved tissues.

Serum sickness is a systemic vasculitis of variable severity that is characterized clinically by fever, lymphadenopathy, arthralgias, and dermatitis. It once occurred commonly in persons receiving intravenous injections of large quantities of foreign immune serum—a widely used treatment for various infectious or toxic diseases prior to the antibiotic era. Today, it occurs occasionally among transplant patients who receive heterologous serum as a source of anti-lymphocyte or anti-thymocyte antibodies to suppress transplant rejection. Serum sickness also can occur as an allergic reaction to penicillin or other drugs or during the prodromal phase of some viral infections, most notably viral hepatitis.

A chronic form of serum sickness can be induced in animals by repeated intravenous infusions of antigen. Depending on the specific animal, antigen, and dosage regimen used, this can result in widespread vasculitis, glomerulonephritis, pulmonary alveolitis, or other lesions. This has been proposed as an experimental model for the immunopathogenesis of the human disorders systemic lupus erythematosus, rheumatoid arthritis, polyarteritis nodosa, and other diseases of unknown etiology that are characterized by the presence of circulating immune complexes and by vasculitis. However, the serum sickness model does not fully mimic the pathologic and clinical manifestations of these disorders, and the antigens responsible for vasculitis in the human diseases remain unknown.

The presence of circulating immune complexes does not always indicate disease. In fact, small quantities of immune complexes can be found in the serum of normal persons. The antigens responsible for these complexes are not all known, although at least some are antigens from ingested foods. The remainder may be other environmental antigens or autoantigens. Most such complexes are promptly eliminated through phagocytosis by splenic macrophages and other cells, whose surface Fc and complement receptors enable them to bind the IgG and C3 proteins present in these complexes. Immune-complex disease thus appears to require (1) large amounts of antigen; (2) generation of immune complexes large enough to activate complement; and (3) in some cases, impaired function of the phagocyte system, possibly because of abnormalities in the Fc or complement receptors.

IgE-Mediated Inflammation

IgE-mediated inflammation occurs when antigen binds to the IgE antibodies that occupy the FcεRI receptor on mast cells. Within minutes, this binding causes the mast cell to degranulate, releasing certain preformed mediators. Subsequently, the degranulated cell begins to synthesize and release additional mediators de novo. The result is a 2-phase response: an initial immediate effect on blood vessels, smooth muscle, and glandular secretion, followed a few hours later by cellular infiltration of the involved site. This type of inflammatory reaction is commonly referred to as **immediate hypersensitivity.**

As detailed above, IgE antibodies bind to mast cells via the numerous high-affinity Fcε receptors on the surface of each cell. The binding is noncovalent and reversible, so that the bound antibodies are in constant equilibrium with the pool of circulating IgE. As a result, each mast cell can bind many different antigens. The events that occur on binding are depicted in Fig 11–11. The response is initiated when a multivalent antigen binds and cross-links 2 or more IgE antibodies occupying FcεRI receptors. This cross-linking transmits a signal that activates the mast cell, resulting (as in other cell systems [see Chapter 2]) in activation of protein tyrosine kinases and increases in intracellular free calcium levels. These signaling events are complete within 2–3 minutes after antigen binding. Soon thereafter, cytoplasmic granules fuse with one another and with the surface membrane, discharging their contents to the exterior. Basophils are the only other cell type that express FcεRI receptors, but it is not known whether they contribute significantly to immediate hypersensitivity reactions.

The **immediate phase** of the inflammatory response is due mainly to preformed mediators (especially **histamine**) that are stored in the mast cell granules, and also to certain rapidly synthesized

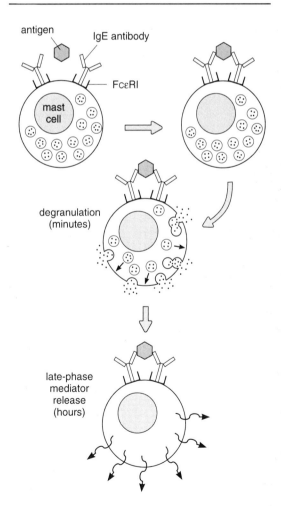

Figure 11–11. Schematic depiction of the immunologic events in an IgE-mediated inflammatory response.

arachidonate derivatives. It reaches maximal intensity within about 15 minutes after antigen contact. This phase is characterized grossly by erythema, localized edema in the form of a wheal, and **pruritus** (itching), all of which can be attributed to histamine. Microscopic examination at this stage reveals only vasodilation and edema. Manifestations of the **late phase** are due in part to presynthesized TNFα and in part to other mediators (principally PAF and various arachidonate metabolites) whose synthesis begins after the mast cell degranulates. The effects of these mediators become apparent about 6 hours after antigen contact and are marked by an infiltrate of eosinophils and neutrophils. Clinical features of the late phase include erythema, induration, warmth, pruritus, and a burning sensation at the affected site. Fibrin deposition probably occurs transiently, but there is no evidence of significant immunoglobulin or complement deposition. TNFα not only functions in the short term as a leukocyte chemoattractant but also can stimulate local angiogenesis, fibroblast proliferation, and scar formation during prolonged hypersensitivity reactions.

IgE-mediated inflammation is the mechanism underlying **atopic allergy** (such as hay fever, asthma, and atopic dermatitis), systemic **anaphylactic reactions,** and allergic **urticaria** (hives). It is also at least partially responsible for immunity to helminthic parasites. It may normally play a facilitative role as a first line of immunologic defense, since it causes rapid vasodilation and thus facilitates the entry of circulating soluble factors and cells to the site of antigen contact. Many serious sequelae of allergic disease can be ascribed to the actions of the chemoattracted leukocytes rather than to the mast cells themselves.

Cutaneous Basophil Hypersensitivity

The physiologic significance of cutaneous basophil hypersensitivity (previously called Jones-Mote hypersensitivity) is presently unknown. It is elicited by protein antigens that, when injected into the skin, produce a localized area of swelling which develops over the same time course as a DTH reaction but which is softer than a typical DTH lesion and is pruritic. Viewed under the microscope, the lesions reveal a prominent infiltrate of basophils but no granulomas or other features of DTH. Lesions of this type appear to be antibody-mediated, but their mechanism of formation is uncertain. Basophilic infiltrates are sometimes seen in renal allografts, suggesting that the process may be one component of transplant rejection.

REFERENCES

Barnett EV: Circulating immune complexes: Their biologic and clinical significance. *J Allergy Clin Immunol* 1986;**78:**1089.

Beer DJ, Rocklin RE: Histamine modulation of lymphocyte biology: Membrane receptors, signal transmission, and functions. *Crit Rev Immunol* 1987;**7:**55.

Braquet P, Rola-Pleszczynski M: Platelet-activating factor and cellular immune responses. *Immunol Today* 1987;**8:**345.

Erffmeyer JE: Serum sickness. *Ann Allergy* 1986;**56:**105.

Galli SJ: New concepts about the mast cell. *N Engl J Med* 1993;**328:**257.

Kinet JP: The high-affinity receptor for IgE. *Curr Opin Immunol* 1989;**2:**499.

Parker CW: Lipid mediators produced through the lipoxygenase pathway. *Annu Rev Immunol* 1987;**5:**65.

Samuelsson B et al: Leukotrienes and lipoxins: Structures, biosynthesis, and biological effects. *Science* 1987; **237:**1171.

Serafin WE, Austen KF: Current concepts: Mediation of immediate hypersensitivity reactions. *N Engl J Med* 1987;**317:**30.

Spencer DA: An update on PAF. *Clin Exp Allergy* 1992;**23:**521.

Stevens RL, Austen KF: Recent advances in the cellular and molecular biology of mast cells. *Immunol Today* 1989;**10:**381.

Valent P, Bettelheim P: The human basophil. *Crit Rev Oncol Hematol* 1990;**10:**327.

Weller PF: The immunobiology of eosinophils. *N Engl J Med* 1991;**324:**1110.

Section II.
Immunologic Laboratory Tests

Clinical Laboratory Methods for Detection of Antigens & Antibodies

12

R. P. Channing Rodgers, MD

One of the major challenges for modern medicine is the translation of basic advances in immunochemistry and immunobiology into diagnostic and therapeutic procedures that will be useful in the practice of clinical medicine. In the clinical immunology laboratory, tests that utilize a great many of the recently elucidated principles of basic immunology can be performed on a wide variety of samples taken from patients. The results of these laboratory procedures are then used by practicing physicians in the diagnosis, treatment, and prognosis of clinical disorders. Furthermore, qualitative and quantitative analysis of immune responses has led to better understanding of the pathogenesis of many clinical disorders. This understanding in turn has stimulated further basic scientific research in immunology. In fact, observations made by clinical investigators in immunology have frequently dramatically changed the course of basic research in immunology and related fields. An example is the impetus given to research on T cells and B cells by careful clinical descriptions of patients with thymic aplasia and hypogammaglobulinemia.

Over the past 3 decades, immunologic laboratory methods have gradually become increasingly more refined and simplified. Because of their inherent specificity and sensitivity, these methods have now achieved a central role in the modern clinical laboratory. The goals of laboratory medicine are to improve the availability, accuracy, and precision of a body of medically important laboratory tests, to ensure correct interpretation, to facilitate data transmission, and to assess the significance of new tests introduced into clinical medicine. A better understanding of the methods used in the immunology laboratory should provide the student and practitioner of medicine with a useful guide for correct application and interpretation of this body of knowledge.

In the present chapter, tests for the detection of antigens and antibodies in clinical practice are discussed. One should distinguish 2 separate uses of methods described. First, they can be used to detect immune responses and their pathology; second, they can use immunologic principles for quantitative and qualitative detection of antigens or antibodies. Most of the techniques described involve application in the clinical laboratory of the principles of immunochemistry. This chapter and the following one are not meant to be comprehensive laboratory manuals. Rather, the principles of the various immunologic methods and their application to selected clinical problems are reviewed. It is hoped that careful study of the chapters in this section in conjunction with the first section of this book will provide the reader with a solid background for an enhanced understanding of the detailed discussions of clinical immunology and descriptions of specific tests used in various disorders presented in clinical chapters that follow.

The topics covered in this chapter include the following:

(1) Immunodiffusion
(2) Electrophoresis and immunoelectrophoresis
(3) Immunochemical and physiochemical methods
(4) Binder-ligand assays
(5) Immunohistochemical techniques (immunofluorescence)
(6) Agglutination
(7) Complement assays
(8) Monoclonal antibodies
(9) Predictive value theory

IMMUNODIFFUSION

The purpose of all immunodiffusion techniques is to detect the reaction of antigen and antibody by the precipitation reaction. Although the formation of antigen-antibody complexes in a semisolid medium such as agar is dependent on buffer electrolytes, pH, and temperature, the most important determinants of the reaction are the relative concentrations of antigen and antibody. This relationship is depicted schematically in Fig 12–1. Maximal precipitation forms in the area of equivalence, with decreasing amounts in the zones of antigen excess or antibody excess. Thus, formation of precipitation lines in any immunodiffusion system is highly dependent on relative concentrations of antigen and antibody. The **prozone phenomenon** refers to suboptimal precipitation which occurs in the region of antibody excess. Thus, dilutions of antisera must be reacted with fixed amounts of antigen to obtain maximum precipitin lines. The prozone phenomenon is a cause of misinterpretation of immunoelectrophoresis patterns in the diagnosis of paraproteinemias when large amounts of antibodies are present.

Immunoprecipitation is a simple and direct means of demonstrating antigen-antibody reactions. The application of immunoprecipitation to the study of bacterial antigens launched the field of serology in the first part of the 20th century. In 1946, Oudin described a system of single diffusion of antigen and antibody in agar-filled tubes. This important advance was soon followed by Ouchterlony's classic description of double diffusion in agar layered on slides. This method is still in use today and has many applications in the detection and analysis of precipitating antigen-antibody systems.

Immunodiffusion reactions may be classified as single or double. In single immunodiffusion, either antigen or antibody remains fixed and the other reactant is allowed to move and complex with it. In double immunodiffusion, both reactants are free to move toward each other and precipitate. Movement in either form of immunodiffusion may be linear or radial. Specific examples are discussed in the remainder of this section.

Immunodiffusion has a clinical application in the quantitative and qualitative analysis of serum proteins, although this is now often done by more sensitive and automated methods such as nephelometry, ELISA, or RIA. Single radial diffusion in agar has largely been supplanted by these methods, which do not rely on immunoprecipitation or diffusion.

METHODS & INTERPRETATION

Double Diffusion in Agar

This simple and extremely useful technique (also called **Ouchterlony analysis**) is based on the principle that when antigen and antibody diffuse through a semisolid medium (eg, agar) they form stable immune complexes, which can be analyzed visually.

The test is performed by pouring molten agar onto glass slides or into Petri dishes and allowing it to harden. Small wells are punched out of the agar a few millimeters apart. Samples containing antigen and antibody are placed in opposing wells and allowed to diffuse toward one another in a moist chamber for 18–24 hours. The resultant precipitation lines that represent antigen-antibody complexes are analyzed visually in indirect light with the aid of a magnifying lens. When antigen and antibody are allowed to diffuse in a radial fashion, an arc that approximates a straight line is

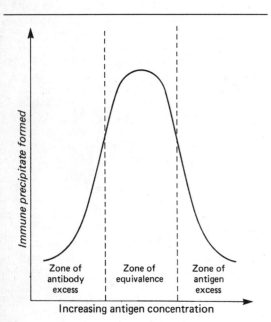

Figure 12–1. Antigen-antibody precipitin curve. Typical precipitin curve resulting from titration of increasing antigen concentration plotted against amount of immune precipitate formed. Amount of antibody is kept constant throughout.

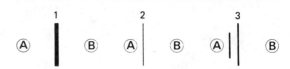

Figure 12–2. Reactions in simple double diffusion. In (1) antigen A and antibody B react equidistantly and intensely at equivalence. In (2) antigen A is present in reduced concentration or has not diffused as rapidly owing to size or charge, forming a precipitin line closer to the antigen well. In (3) a contaminant or impurity present in antigen A is reacting with antibody B.

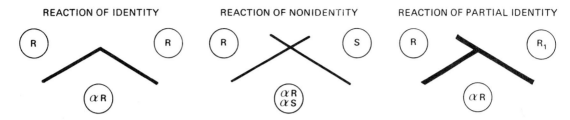

Figure 12–3. Reaction patterns in angular double immunodiffusion (Ouchterlony). R = antigen R, S = antigen S, R_1 = antigen R_1, αR = antibody to R, αS = antibody to S. Reaction of identity: Precisely similar precipitin lines have formed in the reaction of R with αR. Note that the lines intersect at a point. Reaction of nonidentity: Precipitin lines completely cross owing to separate interaction of αR with R and αS with S when R and S are non-cross-reacting antigens. Reaction of partial identity: αR reacts with both R and R_1 but forms lines that do not form a complete cross. Antigenic determinants are *partially* shared between R and R_1.

formed at the leading edges of the diffusing antigen and antibody. Examples of patterns produced in simple double diffusion are shown in Fig 12–2.

Double diffusion is commonly performed by placing antigen and antibody wells at various angles for comparative purposes. The 3 basic characteristic patterns of those reactions are shown in Fig 12–3. In addition to these 3 basic patterns, more complex interrelationships may be seen between antigen and antibody. The formation of a single precipitation line between an antigen and its corresponding antiserum can be used as a rough estimate of antigen or antibody purity. However, the relative insensitivity of the test and the limitation of immunodiffusion to *precipitating* antigen-antibody reactions partly restrict the applications of this technique. It is useful in demonstrating the identity of serologic reactions to antigens from various infectious agents with antibodies of known positive reactivity.

Double immunodiffusion in agar can also be used for semiquantitative analysis in human serologic systems where the specificity of the precipitation lines has already been determined. Such an analysis is performed by placing antibody in a central well surrounded circumferentially by antigen wells (Fig 12–4). Serial dilutions of antigen are placed in the

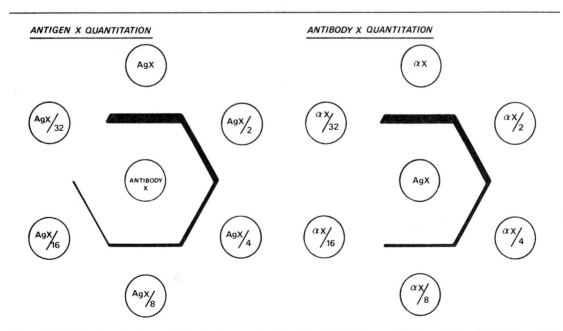

Figure 12–4. Semiquantitative analysis of antigen and antibody by double immunodiffusion. Antigen X (AgX) is serially diluted and placed circumferentially in wells surrounding the central well containing antibody against antigen X. Precipitin lines form with decreasing thickness until no longer visible at dilution of 1:32 of antigen X. On the right, a similar pattern is generated but with serial 2-fold dilutions of antibody X (αX). Formation of a single precipitin line indicates that a single antigen-antibody reaction has occurred.

surrounding wells, and the development of precipitation lines can be taken as a rough measure of antigen concentration. Alternatively, this form of analysis is very useful in determining the approximate precipitating titer of an antiserum by simply reversing the location of antigen and antibody in the pattern (Fig 12–4).

Single Radial Diffusion

Double immunodiffusion is only semiquantitative. In 1965, Mancini introduced a novel technique involving single diffusion for accurate quantitative determination of antigens. This technique grew out of the simple linear diffusion technique of Oudin by means of the incorporation of specific antibody into the agar plate. Radial diffusion is based on the principle that a quantitative relationship exists between the amount of antigen placed in a well cut in the agar-antibody plate and the resulting ring of precipitation. The technique is performed as diagrammed in Fig 12–5.

In the method described originally by Mancini, the *area* circumscribed by the precipitation ring was proportionate to the antigen concentration. This end point method requires that the precipitation rings reach the maximal possible size, which often requires 48–72 hours of diffusion. Alternatively, the single radial diffusion method of Fahey allows measurement of the rings prior to full development. In this modification, the logarithm of the antigen concentration is proportionate to the *diameter* of the ring.

A standard curve is experimentally determined with known antigen standards, and the equation that describes this curve can then be used for the determination of antigen concentration corresponding to any diameter size (Fig 12–6). The sensitivity of these methods is in the range of 1–3 μg/mL of antigen.

An important clinical application of single radial diffusion is in the measurement of serum proteins—for example, immunoglobulin concentrations. A monospecific antiserum directed only at Fc or H chain determinants of the immunoglobulin molecule must be incorporated into the agar to determine immunoglobulin concentrations, since L (light) chain determinants are shared among immunoglobulin classes. Owing to the relatively low concentrations of IgD and IgE in human serum, this technique is used primarily to determine the other 3 immunoglobulin classes, IgG, IgA, and IgM. However, by decreasing the amount of specific anti-immunoglobulin antiserum placed in the agar, so-called "low-level" plates can be produced that have increased sensitivity for detection of reduced levels of serum immunoglobulins (IgG, IgA, IgM, and IgD).

There are a number of common pitfalls in the interpretation of single radial diffusion tests for immunoglobulin quantitation: (1) Polymeric forms of immunoglobulin such as occur in multiple myeloma or Waldenström's macroglobulinemia diffuse more slowly than native monomers, resulting in underesti-

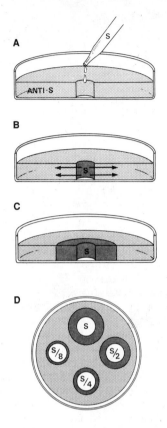

Figure 12–5. Single radial diffusion in agar (radial immunodiffusion). **A:** Petri dish is filled with semisolid agar solution containing antibody to antigen S. After agar hardens, the center well is filled with a precisely measured amount of material containing antigen S. **B:** Antigen S is allowed to diffuse radially from the center well for 24–48 hours. **C:** Where antigen S meets corresponding antibody to S in the agar, precipitation results. After reaction proceeds to completion or at a timed interval, a sharp border or a ring is formed. **D:** By serial dilution of a known standard quantity of antigen S—S/1, S/2, S/4, S/8—rings of progressively decreasing size are formed. The amount of antigen S in unknown specimens can be calculated and compared with standard in the timed interval (Fahey) method (Fig 12–5).

mation of immunoglobulin concentrations in these diseases. (2) High-molecular-weight immune complexes that may circulate in cryoglobulinemia or rheumatoid arthritis will result in falsely low values by a similar mechanism. (3) Low-molecular-weight forms such as 7S IgM in sera of patients with macroglobulinemia, systemic lupus erythematosus, rheumatoid arthritis, or ataxia-telangiectasia may give falsely high values. This phenomenon results from the fact that monomeric IgM diffuses more rapidly than the pentameric IgM parent molecule, which is used as the standard. (4) Reversed precipitation may

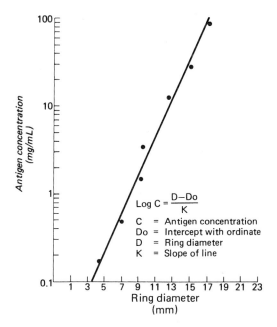

Figure 12–6. Standard curve for single radial diffusion. Relationship between ring diameter and antigen concentration is described by the line constructed from known amounts of antigen (Fig 12–5). Equation and curve for timed interval (Fahey) method.

occur in situations where the test human serum contains anti-immunoglobulin antibodies. In such a circumstance, diffusion and precipitation occur in 2 directions simultaneously and may result in falsely high values. This phenomenon has been well documented in the case of subjects with IgA deficiency who have antibodies to ruminant proteins. These proteins cross the IgA-deficient intestinal mucosa, thereby gaining access to lymphatic tissues and stimulating anti-IgA responses. The problem of IgA quantitation in this circumstance can be avoided by using anti-immunoglobulin from rabbits (ie, a nonruminant species).

APPLICATIONS: SERUM IMMUNOGLOBULIN LEVELS IN HEALTH & DISEASE

Serum immunoglobulin levels are dependent on a variety of developmental, genetic, and environmental factors. These include ethnic background, age, sex, history of allergies or recurrent infections, and geographic factors (eg, endemic infestation with parasites results in elevated IgE levels). The patient's age is especially important in the interpretation of immunoglobulin levels. Normal human infants are born with very low levels of serum immunoglobulins that they have synthesized; the entire IgG portion of cord serum has been transferred transplacentally from the mother (Fig 12–7). If an infection occurs in utero,

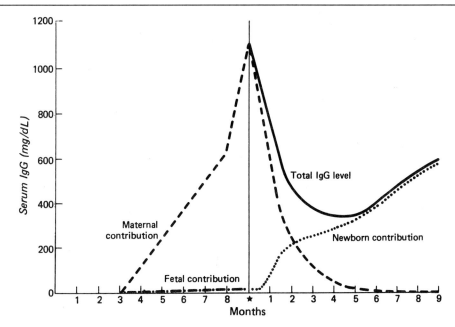

Figure 12–7. Development of IgG levels with age. Relationship of development of normal levels of IgG during fetal and newborn stages and maternal contribution. (Modified and reproduced, with permission, from Allansmith M et al: *J Pediatr* 1968;**72**:289.)

cord IgM and IgA are elevated. After birth, maternal IgG decays, resulting in a falling serum IgG level. This trend is reversed with the onset of significant autologous IgG synthesis. There is a gradual and progressive increase in IgG, IgA, and IgM levels until late adolescence, when nearly normal adult levels are achieved (Fig 12–8). Furthermore, it is clear that there is a great deal of variability in immunoglobulin levels in the healthy population (Fig 12–8).

In routine practice, only IgG, IgA, IgM, and IgE levels are ordinarily measured. Abnormalities of serum IgD concentrations have not clearly been associated with specific disease states. In fact, this immunoglobulin is the major B cell receptor for antigens and plays only a minor role as a circulating antibody. IgE levels, on the other hand, are useful in differential diagnosis of allergic, parasitic, and rare immunodeficiency states. Measurement of serum IgE levels requires sensitive methods such as RIA or enzyme-linked immunoassay. Measurement of serum IgG levels is particularly valuable in diagnosis and in monitoring immunoglobulin replacement in hypogammaglobulinemic patients.

Individual changes in serum immunoglobulin levels have been recorded in many diseases. A partial list of the instances of quantitative abnormalities in immunoglobulins is listed (Table 12–1). For a detailed discussion of immunoglobulin disorders, the reader is referred to Chapters 19 and 21, as well as other chapters in the Clinical section of this volume.

ELECTROPHORESIS & IMMUNOELECTROPHORESIS

The heterogeneity in human serum proteins can be readily analyzed by electrophoresis. The separation of proteins in an electrical field was perfected in 1937 by Tiselius, who used free or moving boundary electrophoresis. However, owing to the relative complexity of this method, zone electrophoresis in a stabilizing medium such as paper or cellulose acetate has replaced free electrophoresis for clinical use.

In 1952, a 2-stage method was reported that combined electrophoresis with immunodiffusion for the detection of tetanus toxoid by antiserum. Shortly thereafter, the now classic method of immunoelectrophoresis was introduced by Williams and Grabar and by Poulik. In this technique, both electrophoresis and double immunodiffusion are performed on the same agar-coated slide. Immunoelectrophoresis has become an important tool for clinical paraprotein analysis as well as a standard method for immunochemical analysis of a wide variety of proteins. More

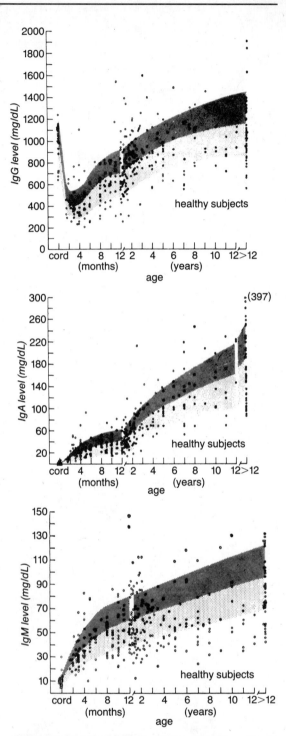

Figure 12–8. An example of variation of healthy subjects' serum levels of IgG, IgA, and IgM with age. Scattergrams of levels of IgG, IgA, and IgM in healthy subjects. Shaded areas are = 1 SD of the mean; each point represents one subject. (Reproduced, with permission, from Stiehm ER, Fudenberg HH: *Pediatrics* 1966;**37:**718.)

Table 12–1. Serum immunoglobulin levels in disease.[1]

Diseases	IgG	IgA	IgM
Immunodeficiency disorders			
Combined immunodeficiency	↓↓↔↓↓↓	↓↓↔↓↓↓	↓↓↔↓↓↓
X-linked hypogammaglobulinemia	↓↓↔↓↓↓	↓↓↔↓↓↓	↓↓↔↓↓↓
Common variable immunodeficiency	↓↔↓↓↓	↓↔↓↓↓	↓↔↓↓↓
Selective IgA deficiency	N	↓↓↓	N
Protein-losing gastroenteropathies	N↔↓↓↓	N↔↓↓↓	N↔↓↓↓
Acute thermal burns	N↔↓↓↓	N↔↓↓↓	N↔↓↓↓
Nephrotic syndrome	N↔↓↓↓	N↔↓↓↓	N↔↓↓↓
Monoclonal gammopathies (MG)			
IgG (eg, G-myeloma)	N↔↑↑↑	N↔↓↓↓	N↔↓↓↓
IgA (eg, A-myeloma)	N↔↓↓↓	N↔↑↑↑	N↔↓↓↓
IgM (eg, M-macroglobulinemia)	N↔↓↓↓	N↔↓↓↓	N↔↑↑↑
L chain disease (ie, Bence Jones myeloma)	N↔↓↓↓	N↔↓↓↓	N↔↓↓↓
Chronic lymphocytic leukemia	N↔↓↓↓	N↔↓↓↓	N↔↓↓↓
Infections			
Infectious mononucleosis	↑↔↑↑	N↔↑	↑↔↑↑
AIDS	↑↑	↑↑	↑↑
Subacute bacterial endocarditis	↑↔↑↑	↓↔N	↑↔↑↑
Tuberculosis	↑↔↑↑	N↔↑↑↑	↓↔N
Actinomycosis	↑↑↑	↑↑	↑↑↑
Deep fungus diseases	N	N↔↑	N
Bartonellosis	↑	↓↔N	↑↑↔↑↑↑
Liver diseases			
Infectious hepatitis	↑↔↑↑	N↔↑	N↔↑↑
Laennec's cirrhosis	↑↔↑↑↑	↑↔↑↑↑	N↔↑↑
Biliary cirrhosis	N	N	↑↔↑↑
Chronic active hepatitis	↑↑↑	↑	N↔↑↑
Collagen disorders			
Systemic lupus erythematosus	↑↔↑↑	N↔↑	N↔↑↑
Rheumatoid arthritis	N↔↑↑↑	↑↔↑↑↑	N↔↑↑
Sjögren's syndrome	N↔↑	N↔↑	N↔↑↑
Scleroderma	N↔↑	N	N↔↑
Miscellaneous			
Sarcoidosis	N↔↑↑	N↔↑↑	N↔↑
Hodgkin's disease	↓↔↑↑	↓↔↑	↓↔↑↑
Monocytic leukemia	N↔↑↑	N↔↑	N↔↑↑
Cystic fibrosis	↑↔↑↑	↑↔↑↑	N↔↑↑

N = normal, ↑ = slight increase, ↑↑ = moderate increase, ↑↑↑ = marked increase, ↓ = slight decrease, ↓↓ = moderate decrease, ↓↓↓ = marked decrease, ↔ = range.
[1]Modified and reproduced, with permission, from Ritzmann SE, Daniels JC (editors): *Serum Protein Abnormalities: Diagnostic and Clinical Aspects.* Little, Brown, 1975.

recently, immunofixation electrophoresis and electroimmunodiffusion methods have been introduced. Various electrophoretic methods and examples of their uses in clinical immunodiagnosis are described in the following paragraphs.

ZONE ELECTROPHORESIS

Proteins are separated in zone electrophoresis almost exclusively on the basis of their surface charge (Fig 12–9). The supporting medium is theoretically inert and does not impede or enhance the flow of molecules in the electrical field. Generally, paper, agarose, or cellulose acetate strips are used as supporting media. However, a major advantage of cellulose acetate is the speed of completion of electrophoretic migration (ie, 60–90 minutes compared with hours for paper). Additionally, cellulose acetate is optically clear; microquantities of proteins may be applied; and it is adaptable to histochemical staining procedures. For these reasons, cellulose acetate or agarose is preferred as the supporting medium for clinical zone electrophoresis.

In the technique itself, serum or other biologic fluid samples are placed at the origin and separated by electrophoresis for about 90 minutes, using alkaline buffer solutions. The strips are then stained for protein and scanned in a densitometer. In the densitometer, the stained strip is passed through a light beam. Variable absorption due to different serum protein concentrations is detected by a photoelectric cell and reproduced by an analog recorder as a tracing (Fig 12–9). Scanning converts the band pattern into peaks and allows for quantitation of the major peaks. Normal human serum is separated into 5 major elec-

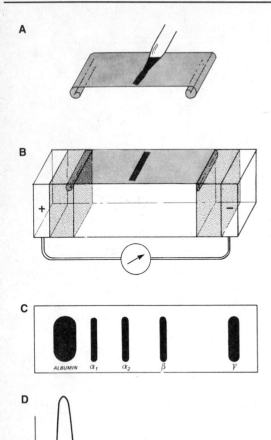

Figure 12–9. Technique of cellulose acetate zone electrophoresis. **A:** Small amount of serum or other fluid is applied to cellulose acetate strip. **B:** Electrophoresis of sample in electrolyte buffer is performed. **C:** Separated protein bands are visualized in characteristic position after being stained. **D:** Densitometer scanning from cellulose acetate strip converts bands to characteristic peaks of albumin, α_1-globulin, α_2-globulin, β-globulin, and γ-globulin.

trophoretic bands, ie, albumin, α_1-globulin, α_2-globulin, β-globulin, and γ-globulin, by this method.

Applications

Zone electrophoresis is useful in the diagnosis of human paraprotein disorders such as multiple myeloma and Waldenström's macroglobulinemia (Fig 12–10). In these disorders, an electrophoretically restricted protein spike usually occurs in the γ-globulin region of the electrophoretogram. Since in zone electrophoresis the trailing edge of immunoglobulins extends into the β region and occasionally the α re-

gion, spikes in these regions are also consistent with paraproteinemic disorders involving immunoglobulins.

A marked decrease in serum γ-globulin concentration such as occurs in hypogammaglobulinemia is sometimes detected by this technique (Fig 12–10). Reduction in IgA or IgM to very low levels cannot be detected by this method, since they represent such a relatively small fraction of total serum immunoglobulins. Free light chains are readily detectable in urine when present in increased amounts such as in Bence Jones proteinuria of myeloma (Fig 12–11). Zone electrophoresis in agarose gels has also been useful in the diagnosis of certain central nervous system diseases with alterations in cerebrospinal fluid proteins (Figs 12–12 and 38–3).

Oligoclonal bands in cerebrospinal fluid with restricted electrophoretic mobility have been detected in about 90% of clinically definite cases of multiple sclerosis. Agarose electrophoresis gel in conjunction with measurement of cerebrospinal fluid IgG/albumin ratios makes possible a fairly high degree of specificity for diagnosis of multiple sclerosis (see Chapter 38 and Fig 38–3).

Abnormalities in levels of serum proteins other than immunoglobulins may also be detected by serum protein electrophoresis. Hypoproteinemia involving all serum fractions occurs during excessive protein loss, usually in the gastrointestinal tract. Reduction in albumin alone commonly occurs in many diseases of the liver, kidneys, or gastrointestinal tract or with severe burns. α_1-globulin decrease may indicate α_1-antitrypsin deficiency, and an increase may reflect acute-phase reactions occurring in many inflammatory and neoplastic disorders. An increase in α_2-globulins usually reflects the nephrotic syndrome or hemolysis with increased hemoglobin-haptoglobin in the serum. Because of its relative insensitivity, zone electrophoresis is almost always a presumptive screening test for serum protein abnormalities. Specific quantitative biochemical or immunologic tests must be performed to definitively identify the particular protein.

IMMUNOELECTROPHORESIS

Immunoelectrophoresis combines electrophoretic separation, diffusion, and immune precipitation of proteins. Both identification and approximate quantitation can thereby be accomplished for individual proteins present in serum, urine, or other biologic fluid.

In this technique (Fig 12–13), a glass slide is covered with molten agar or agarose in an alkaline buffer solution. An antigen well and antibody trough are cut with a template-cutting device. The serum sample (antigen) is placed in the antigen well and is separated in an electrical field with a potential difference

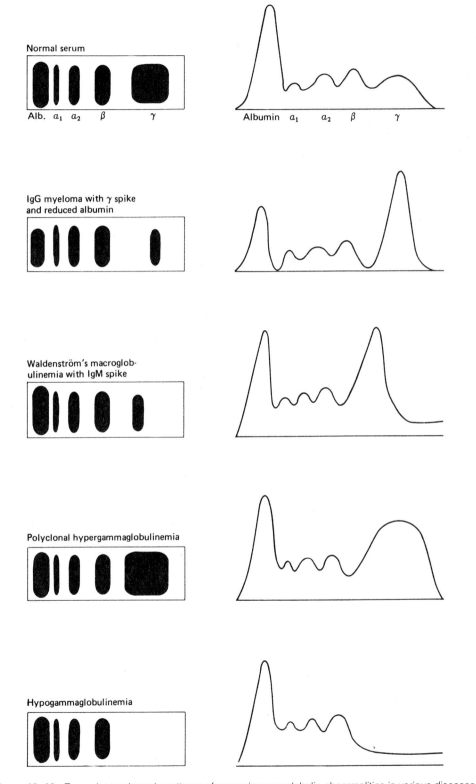

Figure 12–10. Zone electrophoresis patterns of serum immunoglobulin abnormalities in various diseases.

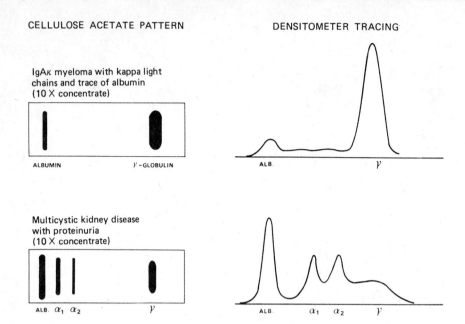

Figure 12–11. Zone electrophoresis patterns of urine abnormalities in various diseases.

of approximately 3.3 V/cm for 30–60 minutes. Antiserum is then placed in the trough, and both serum and antibodies are allowed to diffuse for 18–24 hours. The resulting precipitation lines may then be photographed or the slide washed, dried, and stained for a permanent record.

A comparison of the relationship of precipitation lines developed in normal serum by immunoelectro-

phoresis and zone electrophoresis is shown in Fig 12–14.

Applications

In the laboratory diagnosis of paraproteinemias, the results of zone electrophoresis and immunoelectrophoresis should be combined. The presence of a sharp increase or spike in the γ-globulin region on

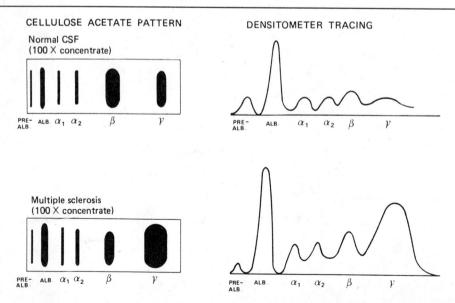

Figure 12–12. Zone electrophoresis patterns of cerebrospinal fluid from normal subject and multiple sclerosis patient.

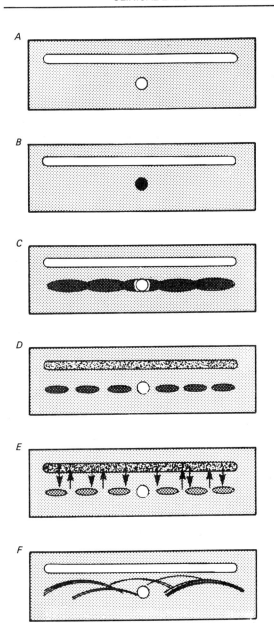

Figure 12–13. Technique of immunoelectrophoresis. *A:* Semisolid agar poured onto glass slide and antigen well and antiserum trough cut out of agar. *B:* Antigen well filled with human serum. *C:* Serum separated by electrophoresis. *D:* Antiserum trough filled with antiserum to whole human serum. *E:* Serum and antiserum diffuse into agar. *F:* Precipitin lines form for individual serum proteins.

zone electrophoresis strongly suggests the presence of a monoclonal paraprotein. However, it is necessary to perform immunoelectrophoresis to determine the exact H-chain class and L-chain type of the paraprotein. Several examples of the use of immunoelectrophoresis in demonstrating the identity of human serum paraproteins are shown in Fig 12–15.

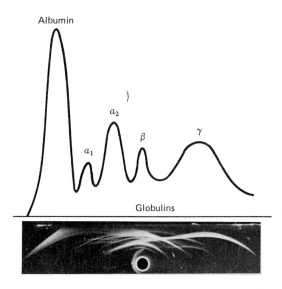

Figure 12–14. Comparison of patterns of zone electrophoresis and immunoelectrophoresis of normal human serum.

Immunoelectrophoresis distinguishes polyclonal from monoclonal increases in γ-globulin (Fig 12–15). Additionally, decreased or absent immunoglobulins observed in various immune deficiency disorders can be analyzed with this technique. However, a further quantitative analysis such as single radial diffusion, nephelometry, or RIA should be performed for measurement of immunoglobulin levels.

Immunoelectrophoresis can be used to identify L chains in the urine of patients with plasma cell dyscrasias or autoimmune disorders. Thus, with specific anti-κ and anti-λ antisera, the monoclonal nature of Bence Jones protein in myeloma can be confirmed.

Antisera to "free light chains" (κ or λ) obtained from the urine of myeloma patients occasionally reveal antigenic determinants not present on chains "bound" to heavy chains in the intact immunoglobulin molecule. In H-chain diseases, fragments of the immunoglobulin H chain are present in increased amounts in the serum (see Chapter 45). It was by careful analysis of immunoelectrophoretic patterns that Franklin initially discovered the existence of this rare but extremely interesting group of disorders. Immunoelectrophoresis is also helpful in identifying increased amounts of proteins present in the cerebrospinal fluid in patients with various neurologic diseases.

Immunofixation Electrophoresis

This technique involves separation of proteins electrophoretically in a gel, followed by immunoprecipitation in situ with monospecific antisera (Fig 12–16). Nonprecipitated proteins are removed by washing and the immunoprecipitation bands revealed with a

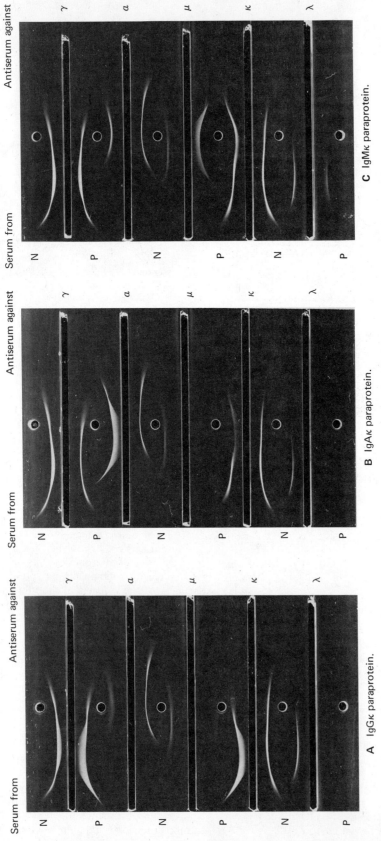

Figure 12–15. Immunoelectrophoresis patterns of serum in various diseases. **A:** IgGκ paraprotein. **B:** IgAκ paraprotein. **C:** IgMκ paraprotein.

A IgGκ paraprotein.

B IgAκ paraprotein.

C IgMκ paraprotein.

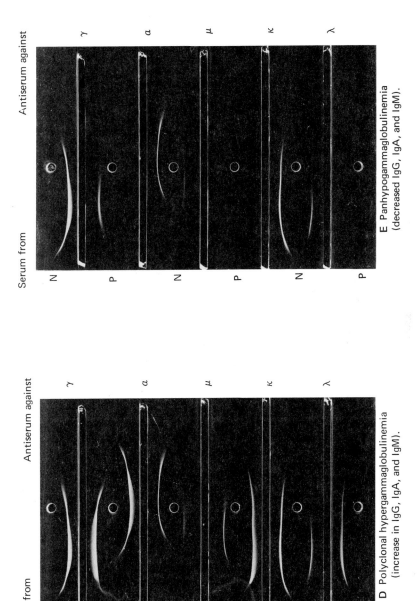

Figure 12–15. *Continued.* ***D:*** Polyclonal hypergammaglobulinemia. ***E:*** Panhypogammaglobulinemia. Individual patterns of serum from normal individuals (N) and patients with various serum protein abnormalities (P). In each case, N and P sera are reacted against antisera which are monospecific for γ, α, and μ heavy chains and κ and λ light chains.

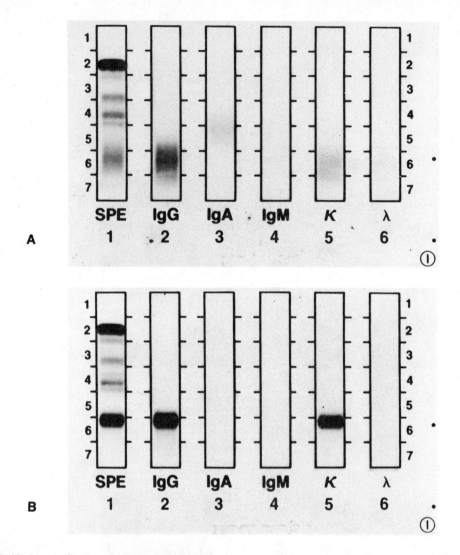

Figure 12–16. Immunofixation electrophoresis. **A:** Normal serum pattern. In lane 1 antibody to whole serum has detected normal serum proteins. In lanes 2–6 specific antibody to various light and heavy chains has detected the polyclonal immunoglobulins present in normal serum. The faint patterns for IgA, IgM, and κ reflect the relatively low concentrations of those molecules. **B:** IgG kappa paraprotein detected in serum from a patient with multiple myeloma. Note the very heavy IgG and kappa bands, which share the same position on the electropherogram. There is a reduction in other immunoglobulins, but other serum proteins are easily seen in lane 1.

protein stain. This method has been employed clinically to identify C3 conversion products and to identify paraproteins. This latter application is especially helpful for low-level IgM or IgA components, which may be buried in an excess of normal IgG. There are several modifications of this basic method, such as overlay with radioactive or enzyme-linked antibodies, that markedly increase its sensitivity. In clinical laboratories, its main use is for resolution of serum proteins in difficult diagnostic problems in which results of routine methods are equivocal. It is commonly used as a substitute for immunoelectrophoresis.

ELECTROIMMUNODIFFUSION

In immunodiffusion techniques described earlier in this chapter, antigen and antibody are allowed to come into contact and to precipitate in agar purely by diffusion. However, the chance of antigen and antibody meeting—and thus the speed of development of a precipitin line—can be greatly enhanced by electrically driving the 2 together. The technique of electroimmunodiffusion is useful in the serologic diagnosis of infectious diseases by serum **antigen** detection. Although numerous variations have been described coupling electrophoresis with diffusion, only 2 have as yet achieved any degree of clinical applicability. These are **one-dimensional double electroimmuno-diffusion** (counterimmunoelectrophoresis) and **one-dimensional single electroimmunodiffusion** (Laurell's rocket electrophoresis).

One-Dimensional Double Electroimmunodiffusion

This method is also known as countercurrent immunoelectrophoresis, counterimmunoelectrophoresis, and electroprecipitation. The basic principle of the method involves electrophoresis of antigen and antibody in opposite directions simultaneously from separate wells in a gel, with resultant precipitation at a point intermediate between their origins (Fig 12–17).

The principal disadvantages of double diffusion without electromotive force are the time required for precipitation (24 hours) and the relative lack of sensitivity. Double electroimmunodiffusion in one dimension can produce visible precipitin lines within 30 minutes and is approximately 10 times more sensitive than standard double diffusion techniques. However, this technique is only semiquantitative. Some of the antigens and antibodies detected by double electroimmunodiffusion are listed in Table 12–2.

One-Dimensional Single Electroimmunodiffusion

This method is also known as rocket electrophoresis or the Laurell technique. Its principal application has been to quantitate antigens other than immunoglobulins. In this technique, antiserum to the particular antigen or antigens one wishes to quantitate is incorporated into an agarose supporting medium on a glass slide in a fixed position so that antibody does not migrate. The specimen containing an unknown quantity of the antigen is placed in a small well. Electrophoresis of the antigen into the antibody-containing agarose is then performed. The resultant pattern of immunoprecipitation resembles a spike or roc-

Table 12–2. Examples of clinical applications of double electroimmunodiffusion.

Cryptococcus-specific antigen in cerebrospinal fluid
Meningococcus-specific antigen in cerebrospinal fluid
Haemophilus-specific antigen in cerebrospinal fluid
Fibrinogen
Cord IgM in intrauterine infection
Carcinoembryonic antigen (CEA)
α_1-Fetoprotein
Fungal precipitins

ket—hence the term rocket electrophoresis (Fig 12–18).

This pattern occurs because precipitation occurs along the lateral margins of the moving boundary of antigen as the antigen is driven into the agar containing the antibody. Gradually, as antigen is lost through precipitation, its concentration at the leading edge diminishes and the lateral margins converge to form a sharp point. The total distance of antigen migration for a given antiserum concentration is linearly proportionate to the antigen concentration. The sensitivity of this technique is approximately 0.5 µg/mL for proteins. Unfortunately, the weak negative charge of immunoglobulins prevents their electrophoretic mobility in this system unless special electrolytes and agar are employed. Several commercial systems are available for quantitating serum immunoglobulins and complement components by this technique.

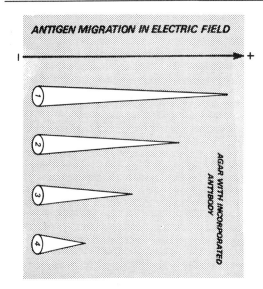

Figure 12–18. Single electroimmunodiffusion in one dimension (rocket electrophoresis, Laurell technique). Antigen is placed in progressively decreasing amounts in wells numbered 1–4. Electrophoresis is performed, and antigen is driven into antibody-containing agar. Precipitin pattern forms in the shape of a "rocket." The amount of antigen is directly proportionate to the length of the rocket.

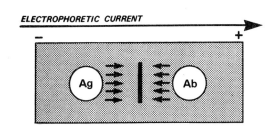

Figure 12–17. Double electroimmunodiffusion in one dimension. Antigen (Ag) and antibody (Ab) are placed in wells and driven together with an electric current. A precipitin line forms within a few hours after electrophoresis was begun.

IMMUNOCHEMICAL & PHYSICOCHEMICAL METHODS

Serum protein disorders can usually be effectively evaluated by immunodiffusion and electrophoretic methods. Occasionally, more detailed study of immunologically relevant serum constituents is necessary. In this section, we describe a number of the more complex immunochemical and physicochemical techniques that have proved to be important adjuncts in the characterization of serum protein and other disorders. These techniques may be available in the clinical laboratory; they include column chromatography, measurement of serum viscosity, and methods to detect cryoglobulins, pyroglobulins, and immune complexes.

CHROMATOGRAPHY

Chromatography is a technique of separating molecules, usually in a column, by partitioning them between a **liquid moving phase** and a **solid stationary phase,** which are in contact with each other. The sample containing materials to be separated is miscible with the moving phase. Chromatographic techniques are useful methods for protein fractionation and isolation of immunoglobulins. In these techniques, a sample is layered on the top of a glass cylinder or column filled with a synthetic gel and is allowed to flow through the gel. The physical characteristics of protein molecules result in retention in the gel matrix to differing degrees, and subsequent elution under appropriate conditions permits protein separation.

Ion Exchange Chromatography

Ion exchange chromatography separates proteins by taking advantage of differences in their electrical charges. The functional unit of the gel is a charged group absorbed on an insoluble backbone such as cellulose, cross-linked dextran, agarose, or acrylic copolymers. Diethylaminoethyl (DEAE), a positively charged group, is the functional unit of anion exchangers used for fractionation of negatively charged molecules (Fig 12–19). Carboxymethyl (CM), a negatively charged group, is the functional unit of cation exchangers used for fractionation of positively charged molecules. Changing the pH of the buffer passing through the column affects the charge of the protein molecule. Increasing the molarity of the buffer provides more ions to compete with the protein for binding to the gel. By gradually increasing the molarity or decreasing the pH of the elution buffer, the proteins are eluted in order of increasing number of charged groups bound to the gel. DEAE-cellulose chromatography is an excellent technique for isolation of IgG, which can be obtained nearly free of all other serum proteins.

Gel Filtration

Gel filtration separates molecules according to their size. The gel is made of porous dextran beads. Protein molecules larger than the largest pores of the beads cannot penetrate the gel pores. Thus, they pass through the gel in the liquid phase outside the beads and are eluted first. Smaller molecules penetrate the beads to different extents depending on their size and shape. Solute molecules within the gel beads maintain a concentration equilibrium with solute in the liquid phase outside the beads; thus, a particular molecular species moves as a band through the column. Molecules therefore appear in the column effluent in order of decreasing size (Fig 12–20).

IgM can be easily separated from other serum im-

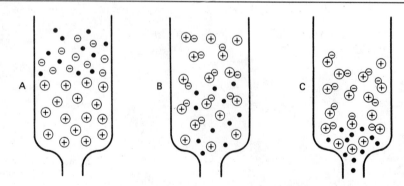

Figure 12–19. Principles of ion exchange chromatography. Three stages of protein separation by ion exchange chromatography are shown: **A:** The column bed is made up of a matrix of positively charged cellulose beads⊕. **B:** The negatively charged molecules ⊖ in the protein mixture bind to the column and are retained. **C:** The neutral molecules • pass between the charged particles and are eluted.

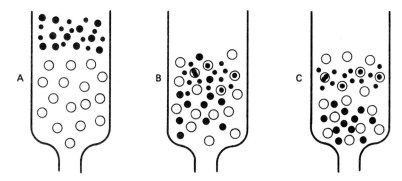

Figure 12–20. Principles of gel filtration chromatography. Three stages of protein separation by gel filtration are shown. **A:** Open circle ○ represents polymerized beads onto which a mixture of small ● and large ● protein molecules is layered. **B:** The molecules enter and pass through the column at different rates depending primarily on size and are separated by a simple sieving process. **C:** Larger molecules are eluted while smaller ones are retained.

munoglobulins by gel filtration. Fig 12–21 shows the separation of the IgM and the IgG components of a mixed IgM-IgG cryoglobulin. Gel filtration is widely used also to separate H and L chains of immunoglobulins or to isolate pure Bence Jones proteins from the urine of patients with multiple myeloma.

Affinity Chromatography

Affinity chromatography uses specific and reversible biologic interaction between the gel material and

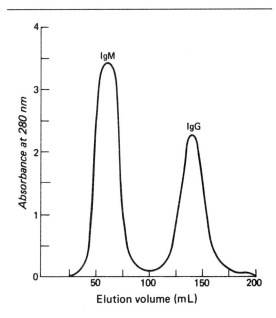

Figure 12–21. Separation of IgG-IgM mixed cryoglobulin by gel filtration. Two peaks are eluted from gel filtration column. The larger IgM molecules precede the smaller IgG molecules which were dissociated by dissolving the cryoprecipitate in an acidic buffer prior to application to the column. The absorbance at 280 nm measures the relative amount of protein in various eluted fractions.

the substance to be isolated. The specificity of the binding properties is obtained by covalent coupling of an appropriate ligand to an insoluble matrix, such as agarose or dextran beads. The gel so obtained is able to absorb from a mixed solution the substance to be isolated. After unbound substances have been washed out of the column, the purified compound can be recovered by changing the experimental conditions, such as pH or ionic strength.

Antigen-antibody binding is one of the reactions that can be applied to affinity chromatography. When the gel material is coupled to an antigen, a specific antibody can be purified. Alternatively, when a highly purified antibody can be coupled to the gel, the corresponding antigen can be isolated.

Protein A is a protein, isolated from the cell wall of some strains of *Staphylococcus aureus,* that specifically reacts with IgG molecules of subclasses 1, 2, and 4. It is used as a specific ligand for isolation of IgG or for isolation of IgG3 from a mixture of IgG molecules of all subclasses.

Cell separation can also be achieved by affinity chromatography. Subpopulations of T and B lymphocytes have been defined by characteristic surface markers (see Chapters 2 and 13) that can react with specific ligands. For example, B cells that bear surface immunoglobulins can be separated on an anti-immunoglobulin column. Immunoglobulin-positive cells are retained on the gel, and desorption is achieved by running through the column a solution of immunoglobulins that compete with the cells.

Currently, many of the chromatographic techniques described are done by high-performance (or pressure) liquid chromatography (HPLC). The principles are the same, but the moving phase is forced through a sealed column under pressure, resulting in a much more rapid, precise, and sensitive separation profile.

SERUM VISCOSITY

The measurement of serum viscosity is a simple and valuable tool in evaluation of patients with paraproteinemia. Normally, the formed elements of the blood contribute more significantly to whole blood viscosity than do plasma proteins. However, in diseases with elevated concentrations of serum proteins, particularly the immunoglobulins, the serum viscosity may reach very high levels and result in a characteristic symptom complex—the hyperviscosity syndrome. Serum viscosity is determined by a variety of factors including protein concentration; the size, shape, and deformability of serum molecules; and the hydrostatic state (solvation), molecular charge, and temperature sensitivity of proteins.

In clinical practice, serum viscosity is measured in an Ostwald viscosimeter. A few milliliters of serum are warmed to 37 °C and allowed to descend through a narrow-bore capillary tube immersed in a water bath at 37 °C. The rate of descent between calibrated marks on the capillary tube is recorded. The same procedure is repeated with distilled water instead of serum. The relative serum viscosity is then calculated according to the following formula:

$$\text{Relative serum viscosity} = \frac{\text{Rate of descent of serum sample (in seconds)}}{\text{Rate of descent of distilled water (in seconds)}}$$

Normal values for serum viscosity range from approximately 1.4 to 1.9. Similar measurements can be performed with plasma instead of serum. However, fibrinogen present in plasma is a major determinant of plasma viscosity, and variations in this protein, especially in the presence of nonspecific inflammatory states, can markedly affect the results. For this reason, measurement of serum viscosity is preferred.

Serum viscosity measurements are primarily of use in evaluating patients with Waldenström's macroglobulinemia, multiple myeloma, and cryoglobulinemia. In myeloma, aggregation or polymerization of the paraprotein in vivo often results in hyperviscosity. In general, there is a correlation between increased serum viscosity and increased plasma volume. However, the correlation between levels of relative serum viscosity and clinical symptoms is not nearly as direct. Increased serum viscosity may interfere with various laboratory tests that employ flow-through devices such as hematology counters and analyzers in clinical chemistry. Examples of disorders associated with increased serum viscosity are listed in Table 12–3.

Table 12–3. Disorders associated with increased serum viscosity.

Waldenström's macroglobulinemia
Essential macroglobulinemia
Multiple myeloma
Cryoglobulinemia
Hypergammaglobulinemic purpura
Rheumatoid diseases associated with immune complexes or paraproteinemias
Rheumatoid arthritis
Sjögen's syndrome
Systemic lupus erythematosus
HIV infection

CRYOGLOBULINS

Precipitation of serum immunoglobulins in the cold was first observed in a patient with multiple myeloma. The term "cryoglobulin" was introduced to designate a group of proteins that had the common property of forming a precipitate or a gel in the cold. This phenomenon was reversible by raising the temperature. Since those initial descriptions, cryoglobulins have been found in a wide variety of clinical situations. Purification and immunochemical analysis have led to classification of this group of proteins (Table 12–4). Type I cryoglobulins consist of a single monoclonal immunoglobulin. Type II cryoglobulins are mixed cryoglobulins; they consist of a monoclonal immunoglobulin with antibody activity against a polyclonal immunoglobulin. Type III cryoglobulins are mixed polyclonal cryoglobulins; ie, one or more immunoglobulins are found, none of which are monoclonal.

Technical Procedure for Isolation & Analysis

Blood must be collected in a warm syringe and kept at 37 °C until it clots. Serum is separated by centrifugation at 37 °C and then stored at 4 °C. When a cryoglobulin is present, a white precipitate or a gel appears in the serum after a variable period, usually 24–72 hours. However, the serum should be observed for 1 week to make certain that unusually late cryoprecipitation does not go undetected. The reversibility of the cryoprecipitation should be tested by rewarming an aliquot of precipitated serum.

The cryoprecipitate can be quantitated in several ways. Centrifugation of the whole serum in a hematocrit tube at 4 °C allows determination of the relative amount of cryoglobulin (cryocrit). Alternatively, the protein concentration in the serum before and after cryoprecipitation may be compared. The precipitate formed in an aliquot of serum may be isolated and dissolved in an acidic buffer and the cryoglobulin level estimated by the absorbance at 280 nm.

After isolation and washing of the precipitate, the components of the cryoglobulin are identified by immunoelectrophoresis or immunofixation electrophoresis. These analyses are performed at 37 °C, using

Table 12–4. Classification of types of cryoglobulins and associated diseases.

Type of Cryoglobulin	Immunochemical Composition	Associated Diseases
Type 1 monoclonal cryoglobulin	IgM IgG IgA Bence Jones protein	Myeloma, Waldenström's macroglobulinemia, chronic lymphocytic leukemia
Type II mixed cryoglobulin	IgM-IgG IgG-IgG IgA-IgG	Myeloma, Waldenström's macroglobulinemia, chronic lymphocytic leukemia, rheumatoid arthritis, Sjögren's syndrome, mixed essential cryoglobulinemia, hepatitis C
Type III mixed polyclonal cryoglobulin	IgM-IgG IgM-IgG-IgA	Systemic lupus erythematosus, rheumatoid arthritis, Sjögen's syndrome, infectious mononucleosis, cytomegalovirus infections, acute viral hepatitis, chronic active hepatitis, hepatitis C, primary biliary cirrhosis, poststreptococcal glomerulonephritis, infective endocarditis, leprosy, kala-azar, tropical splenomegaly syndrome

antiserum to whole human serum and antisera specific for γ, α, μ, κ, and λ chains. In this way, cryoglobulins can ordinarily be classified into the 3 types described above.

Clinical Significance

Type I and type II cryoglobulins are usually present in large amounts in serum (often more than 5 mg/mL). In general, they are present in patients with monoclonal paraproteinemias; eg, they are commonly found in patients with lymphoma or multiple myeloma. However, some are found in patients lacking any evidence of lymphoid malignancy, just as are "benign" paraproteins. Type III cryoglobulins indicate the presence of circulating immune complexes and are the result of immune responses to various antigens. They are present in relatively low concentrations (usually less than 1 mg/mL) in rheumatoid diseases and chronic infections (Table 12–4).

All types of cryoglobulins may be responsible for specific symptoms that occur as a result of changes in the cryoglobulin induced by exposure to cold. The symptoms include Raynaud's phenomenon, vascular purpura, bleeding tendencies, cold-induced urticaria, and even distal arterial thrombosis with gangrene.

Since type II and type III cryoglobulins are circulating soluble immune complexes, they may be associated with a serum sickness-like syndrome characterized by polyarthritis, vasculitis, glomerulonephritis, or neurologic symptoms. In patients with mixed essential IgM-IgG cryoglobulinemia, a rather distinctive syndrome may occur that is associated with arthralgias, purpura, weakness, and frequently lymphadenopathy or hepatosplenomegaly. This syndrome may be a sequela of hepatitis B infection. Glomerulonephritis is common. In some instances, it occurs in a rapidly progressive form and is of ominous prognostic significance.

Cryoglobulins may cause serious errors in a variety of laboratory tests by precipitating at ambient temperatures and thereby removing certain substances from serum. Complement fixation and inactivation and entrapment of immunoglobulins in the precipitate are common examples. Redissolving the cryoprecipitate usually does not fully restore activity to the serum, especially that of complement.

PYROGLOBULINS

Pyroglobulins are monoclonal immunoglobulins that precipitate irreversibly when heated to 56 °C. This phenomenon is different from the reversible thermoprecipitation of Bence Jones proteins and seems to be related to hydrophobic bonding between immunoglobulin molecules, possibly as a result of decreased polarity of the heavy chains. Pyroglobulins may be discovered incidentally when serum is heated to 56 °C to inactivate complement before routine serologic tests. Half of the cases involve patients with multiple myeloma. The remainder occur in macroglobulinemia and other lymphoproliferative disorders, systemic lupus erythematosus, and carcinoma and occasionally without known associated disease. They are not responsible for any particular symptom and have no known significance.

DETECTION OF IMMUNE COMPLEXES

The factors involved in deposition of immune complexes in tissues and production of tissue damage are discussed in Chapter 10. Subsequent chapters deal with the clinical manifestations of diseases associated with immune complexes, including rheumatic diseases (Chapter 31), hematologic diseases (Chapter 33), and renal diseases (Chapter 36). These clinical situations have in common the presence of detectable immune complexes in tissues or in the circulation.

Immune complexes are occasionally detected in

tissues by standard immunohistochemical staining techniques with specific antisera.

There are many methods for detecting circulating immune complexes in serum, most of which rely on the binding of such complexes to various complement components. None of these methods are used in routine clinical laboratory practice.

In a few disorders, eg, Lyme disease and HIV infection, antigen detection is hampered by its masking within immune complexes. Techniques to dissociate the antigen-antibody complexes have increased the apparent sensitivity of these antigen detection assays.

Clinical Usefulness

Initial enthusiasm regarding possible clinical benefits of measuring immune complexes has been tempered by their relative lack of diagnostic or prognostic specificity. Circulating complexes can occur in the absence of tissue deposition, and occasionally no serum complexes can be found despite tissue deposition. In addition, the considerable potential for uncovering causes of many idiopathic diseases by isolating and identifying the antigen in immune complexes has not yet been realized. Discrepancies among the results of various assays are common, and standards are generally lacking. Nevertheless, immune complexes have pathogenic roles depending on their size, immunoglobulin class, concentration, and affinity for cellular receptors.

NEPHELOMETRY

Nephelometry is measurement of light that is scattered from the main beam of a transmitted light source. This should not be confused with turbidimetry, which is the measurement of the decrease of light passing through a cloudy solution or suspension of material. In dilute solutions, the precipitation reaction between antigen and antibody produces increased reflection that can be measured by the scattering of an incident light. Devices to measure light scattering produced by reaction of diphtheria toxin and antitoxin were introduced by Libby in 1938, and this technique has received increasing application in the clinical laboratory.

Nephelometric determination of antigens is performed by addition of constant amounts of highly purified and optically clear specific antiserum to varying amounts of antigen. The resultant antigen-antibody reactants are placed in a cuvette in a light beam, and the degree of light scatter is measured in a photoelectric cell as the optical density (Fig 12–22). Accurate measurement of antigens can be made only in the ascending limb of the precipitin curve (Fig 12–1), where there is a direct linear relationship between antigen concentration and optical density. Thus, for accurate determination of solutions with high antigen

concentrations, the samples are diluted to various concentrations.

There are several different approaches to applying nephelometry in the clinical laboratory. Automated immunoprecipitation employs a fluorometric nephelometer in line with a series of flow-through channels that allow for the measurement of multiple samples simultaneously. Laser nephelometers use a helium-neon laser beam as the light source and sensitive detection devices to measure forward light scatter. Introduction of various electronic filters near the detection device ensures a high "signal-to-noise" ratio and a relatively high degree of sensitivity. A modified centrifugal fast analyzer equipped with a laser light source has also been used for scatter measurements. This method has the potential advantages of speed, small amounts of reagents required, and versatility for other assays.

Nephelometry is theoretically a rapid and simple method for quantitation of many antigens in biologic fluids. Disadvantages of the technique include the relatively high cost of optically clear, potent antisera of uniform specifications; high background resulting from sera containing lipids or hemoglobin; and the need for multiple dilutions, especially for high antigen concentrations. However, some of these potential sources of error are inherent in other immunoquantitative methods. Many of these inherent disadvantages can be overcome by the use of **rate nephelometry.** In this technique, a nephelometer electronically subtracts the background signal from that of an unreacted serum sample. More precise measurement of turbidity is achieved by taking several measurements rapidly during the ascending phase of the precipitation reaction. Nephelometers that combine many of these features are commercially available. The widespread use of such instruments—and nephelometric-grade reagents—has made this method cheaper and applicable to many immunochemical determinations.

BINDER-LIGAND ASSAYS

One of the most important analytic methods developed in the past quarter century is binder-ligand assay (also known as **ligand assay, competitive protein-binding assay,** and **saturation analysis**). The first ligand assay method was **radioimmunoassay (RIA),** developed by Berson and Yalow in 1959 to detect and quantitate human insulin, utilizing human anti-insulin antibodies. Their discovery that the body manufactures antibodies against endogenous substances went against a fundamental dictum of the time, which held that the body could not make anti-

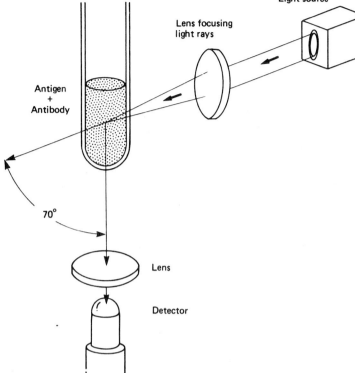

Figure 12–22. The principle of nephelometry for measurement of antigen-antibody reactions. Light rays from a laser or other high-intensity source are collected in the focusing lens and pass through the sample tube containing antigen and antibody. Light passing through the tube and emerging at a 70-degree angle is collected by another lens and focused into an electronic detector. This signal is converted to a digital recording of the amount of turbidity in the sample tube and can be mathematically related to either antigen or antibody concentration in the sample.

bodies against itself. This discovery was in certain respects as important as the application of these antibodies to a new assay method. Simultaneously, Ekins developed an assay for human thyroid hormone by using thyroid-binding globulin isolated from a patient with elevated levels of this binding protein. The basic principle of his assay was the same, although it used a serum carrier protein rather than an antibody.

Since their inception, ligand assays have revolutionized disciplines within biology and medicine. One can quantitate hormones, drugs, tumor markers, and allergens and antibodies associated with allergy. The rapid detection of bacterial and viral antigens and antibodies in infectious diseases such as hepatitis and AIDS is possible.

RADIOIMMUNOASSAY (RIA)

The chief goal of an assay is to determine the concentration of some molecule of interest, the **analyte.** Common to all of the ligand assays is the reaction of analyte with a binding protein, or **binder,** which most often is an **antibody.** In its role as a reactant with binder, the analyte is referred to as a **ligand.** Small analyte molecules are functionally **haptens,** which must be conjugated to carriers to be rendered immunogenic for the purpose of forming antibodies to be

used for their detection. The free haptenic analyte can be detected by these antibodies in the absence of the carriers. In certain assay designs, binder can react with multiple distinct ligands, including the analyte.

There is a bewildering array of ligand assay methods; only one member of the ligand assay family, RIA, will be described in full, followed by the broad chemical principles underlying some of the more important alternative ligand assay methods. Any ligand assay can be divided into 3 stages: calibration, interpolation, and quality control.

Calibration

A. Binder-Ligand Reaction: A number of reaction vessels are established, each containing a small fixed concentration of binder and a small fixed concentration of radioisotopically labeled analyte known as the **label** or **tracer** (Fig 12–23). Calibration requires a set of dilutions of analyte of known concentration; these are referred to as the **standards** or **calibrators.** Different known amounts of calibrator are then added to a series of antibody-label mixtures. The central event in RIA is the competition between the label and the unlabeled analyte for binding sites on an antibody. According to the degree of completion of the binder-ligand reaction, the assay is said to be either an **equilibrium assay** (the reaction is complete) or a **disequilibrium assay** (the reaction is in-

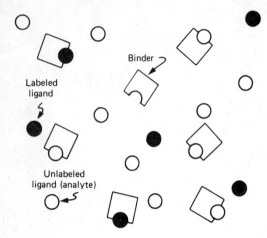

Figure 12–23. The binder-ligand reaction underlying RIA.

complete). The label is divided into 2 categories by the reaction: label that is bound to antibody (the **bound fraction**) and label that is free in solution (the **free fraction**). As the amount of analyte increases relative to the small fixed amount of label present, an increasing fraction of the label will be free.

B. Partitioning and Separation: The bound and free fractions are subjected to a **partitioning step,** after which they are physically separated. Partitioning methods that sequester the binder and binder-ligand complexes include **salting out** of protein (using ammonium or sodium sulfate), **protein denaturation/precipitation** by solvent (such as methanol, ethanol, or acetone), and **precipitation** by polyethylene glycol or by a **second antibody** directed against the primary antibody. Immobilization of the binder to a **solid phase** such as the assay reaction tube or a macroscopic particle allows for rapid separation of bound and unbound label or analyte. A common method of removing the free fraction is **adsorption of free ligand** (with talc, charcoal, silica, ion exchange resin, cellulose, Sephadex, or fuller's earth).

Following partitioning, the bound and free fractions are subjected to **physical separation** by centrifugation or filtration during which a small degree of mixing of bound and unbound fractions can occur.

C. Measurement of Response: In radioassays, the measurement is performed by **radioactive counting;** the method depends on the type of radiation emitted by the label. A **liquid scintillation counter** is used for alpha or beta emitters and a **solid crystal gamma counter** for gamma emitters. The final measurement, or some computed value derived from it, is known as the **response.** The choice of an appropriate response is dictated by the statistical requirements of data reduction. A commonly employed

value in RIA is the ratio of bound to total label, or B:T.

D. Creation of a Calibration Curve: The physical and chemical steps taken thus far are referred to as the **analytic method** of the assay. A relationship between calibrator concentration and assay response must now be established. Most currently encountered assay calibration curves are roughly symmetric sigmoid curves when plotted using a logarithmic concentration axis (Fig 12–24).

This sort of curve can usually be characterized by the 4-parameter logistic equation

$$y = \left[\frac{a - d}{a + (x/c^b)} \right] + d \qquad \dots(1)$$

where **a** = upper asymptote
d = lower asymptote
c = concentration corresponding to the response **(a + d)/2**
b = constant related to the slope at this point.

Earlier workers used a simplified form of this equation, the **logit transformation,** which lends itself well to manual plotting. If one defines a new response value as **y′ = (y − d)/(a − d)**, the logit transformation proceeds as follows:

$$Y = logit (y') = ln\left[\frac{y'}{1 - y'} \right] \qquad \dots(2)$$

Note the similarity of this approach to that of the von Krogh equation discussed later in this chapter. If the data really follow a symmetric sigmoid on the log-lin-

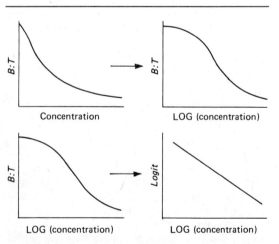

Figure 12–24. The logistic equation and the logit transformation. B:T = ratio of label bound to total label present.

ear plot, then a plot of Y versus log concentration will be a straight line. The term **b** in the 4-parameter logistic equation is simply the slope of the line in the logit-log coordinate system.

Interpolation of Test Concentrations

Once a calibration relationship is in hand, we are ready to estimate the concentration of analyte in **test specimen "unknowns."** These specimens are processed just as the calibrators were, and a response is obtained. This response is used in conjunction with the calibration curve to find a **concentration estimate** corresponding to the observed response; this process is known as **interpolation.**

Quality Control & Error Computations

The goal in obtaining an analyte concentration estimate is generally to answer a question such as "Is the analyte concentration higher (or lower) than a given dangerous or therapeutic level?" or "Is the concentration higher or lower than some previously measured concentration?" Because random errors are involved in any measurement, an assay result should be accompanied by statistically determined **confidence limits** to aid in such judgments. Such confidence limits define a zone within which the results would be expected to fall at some stated level of probability. Furthermore, it is desirable to control the level of both random and systematic error in assay results, and so certain quality control procedures should be followed with each assay batch to allow the rejection of results likely to contain extraordinarily large error. There are many varieties of quality control tests: one of them relies upon use of quality control specimens of known concentration in each assay batch.

TYPES OF ANALYTIC METHODS

Radioisotopic Labels

There has been an explosion of methods based on various modifications of this initial assay scheme, arbitrarily divided according to their labeling methods.

A. Immunoradiometric Assay (IRMA): In this method, the binder (generally an antibody) is labeled rather than the ligand.

B. Sandwich Assay: There are numerous variations of this technique. In its most basic form, the ligand reacts with an antibody that has been immobilized upon a solid surface. Then a radiolabeled second antibody is added, which reacts with the ligand at a different site. This method has the potential advantage of added chemical specificity because of the use of 2 distinct antigenic sites (Fig 12–25).

Enzymatic Labels

A. Enzyme-Multiplied Immunoassay (EMIT): The label consists of ligand conjugated to an enzyme, which remains active (Fig 12–26). Binding of anti-

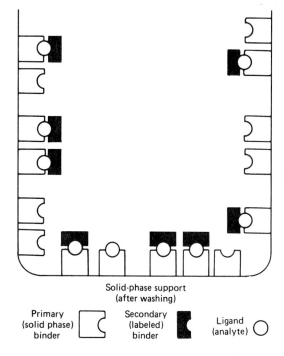

Figure 12–25. Sandwich assay.

body to the enzyme-ligand complex inactivates the enzyme; the presence of free ligand (analyte) competes with the enzyme-ligand complex for antibody, increasing the resulting enzymatic activity. Over a limited range, the enzyme activity will be approximately proportionate to the analyte concentration. This method has been widely used for therapeutic drug monitoring.

B. Enzyme-Linked Immunosorbent Assay (ELISA): This is an enzymatic variation on the sand-

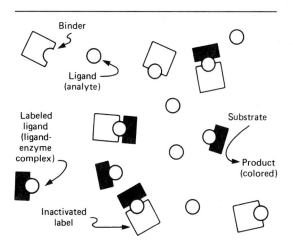

Figure 12–26. EMIT.

wich assay method. One is attempting to detect an antibody, so the roles of binder and ligand are reversed (Fig 12–27). The solid-phase component is an antigen. The antibody to be detected binds to this component, and then a second, enzyme-labeled antibody directed against the antibody to be detected is added. The substrate of the enzyme is added, and a colored reaction product is produced which can be easily measured spectophotometrically.

Fluorometric Labels

A. Fluorescence Polarization Immunoassay (FPIA): The label is coupled by means of the analyte to a fluorescein derivative to form tracer molecules (Fig 12–28). When free in solution, tracer molecules tumble randomly and so rapidly that when they are excited by polarized light, emitted light is unpolarized. When the tracer is bound to an antibody, the tumbling is slowed and the emitted light is more polarized. The degree of polarization will reflect the amount of label that is bound. Thus far, only small analytes have been measurable by this means.

Other Methods

Other methods employ liposomes or erythrocytes as solid supports, nephelometry for particle detection, metal atoms as labels (detected by atomic absorption), and electron-spin resonance ("spin labeling"). Enzymes from the blood-clotting cascade have been used to produce a colored product from a chromogenic substrate as a response. Solid-phase systems have been sped up by the use of ultrasound to en-

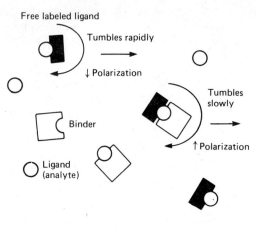

Figure 12–28. FPIA.

hance the reaction rate of the ligand with immobilized binder. Magnetic solid-phase support for antibody has been used to facilitate separation of bound and free fractions in an automated RIA method and in a manual sandwich assay. Bacteriophages have been used as labels, as have chemiluminescent substances (luminol and its derivatives). The latex agglutination assay is now commonly used for the rapid diagnosis of infectious agents. Microscopic latex spheres are coated with antibodies (or antigens), and agglutination (visible to the naked eye) is provoked by the presence of the corresponding antigen (or antibody).

A. Ultrasensitive Enzymatic Radioimmuno-assay (USERIA): A method of detecting cholera toxin and rotavirus that was 1000-fold more sensitive than ELISA or RIA was described in 1979. The method combines aspects of radiometric and enzymatic methods (Fig 12–29). A solid-phase antibody is reacted with the analyte or standard, and then a second antibody is added. A third antibody, conjugated to an enzyme (alkaline phosphatase), is then added to the system. Tritiated AMP is then added to the system, and after an incubation period, the tritiated adenosine produced by the enzyme is separated on a Sephadex column. The activity of the adenosine is counted and used as response.

B. Biotin-Avidin-Enhanced Immunoassays: In this method, 1000-fold greater sensitivity than RIA has been claimed (Fig 12–30). One of the more straightforward designs requires biotinylation of the binder. This process has a relatively low probability of interfering with binder performance owing to the chemically benign reaction (forming amide linkages) and to the low molecular weight (244) of biotin. There may be multiple biotin molecules per binder. The label, which may be enzymatic, radioisotopic, fluorometric, metallic, or of another type, is conjugated to avidin. Avidin is a small glycoprotein with an extremely high association constant for reaction with biotin. The label-avidin complex therefore asso-

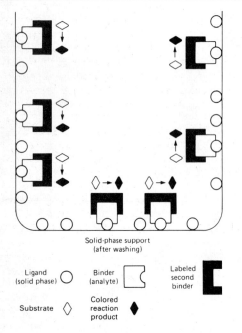

Solid-phase support
(after washing)

Ligand (solid phase) ○	Binder (analyte)	Labeled second binder
Substrate ◇	Colored reaction product ◆	

Figure 12–27. ELISA.

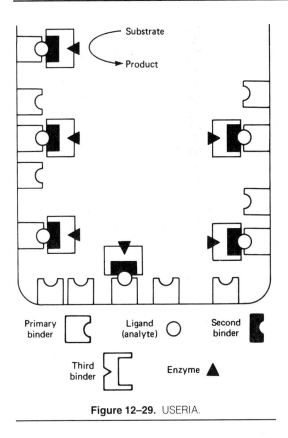

Figure 12–29. USERIA.

ciates with the binder. In another form, this assay employs avidin to bridge biotinylated binder-ligand complexes to a biotinylated label. Large complexes of avidin-biotin-label may also be attached to biotinylated binder. All of these methods are strategies for greatly increasing the amount of label per binder molecule.

COMPARING ANALYTIC PERFORMANCE OF DIFFERENT METHODS

The analytic performance of a given method is characterized by that assay's susceptibility to various forms of systematic error. For example, substances that mimic the presence of analyte or cross-react diminish assay specificity. Other substances can act as another binder or in some other way interfere with truthful measurement (**interference**). The amount of random error contained in the assay is expressed by the confidence limits around a particular assay determination. Random error determines the **sensitivity** of an assay, by which is meant the smallest amount of analyte that can be statistically distinguished from zero. It is best described in terms of the **lower detection limit,** which is the analyte concentration for which the confidence interval grazes zero. The precision of the assay, expressed as the width of the confidence interval, can be plotted against concentration to create an **imprecision profile,** which reveals assay error to be nonconstant; it is lowest at some point in mid-assay range and increases to either side.

It is difficult to compare the analytic performance of different ligand assay methods, since the workers involved often provide only scanty data, and many new methods are accompanied by exaggerated claims. A rigidly defined standard data reduction method would be of help, so that quantities such as analytic sensitivity and specificity would always be computed in the same manner.

Assay methods can be compared on the basis of the labeling method used. Two basic categories, **limited-reagent** (or **competitive**) **methods** and **excess-reagent** (or **noncompetitive**) **methods,** are examples. RIA is an example of the former category; here, labeled ligand and unlabeled ligand compete for a

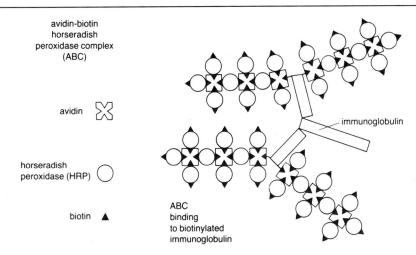

Figure 12–30. Biotin-avidin-enhanced assay.

limited amount of binder. The best achievable sensitivity of an RIA is of the order of 10^{-14} mol/L (this represents about 6×10^6 molecules in 1 mL of solution). A sandwich IRMA is an example of the latter category; a massive excess of labeled second antibody is added to the solid-phase binder-ligand complex. Excess-reagent methods are in principle capable of better sensitivity than are limited-reagent methods, but in practice IRMA has been less sensitive than RIA. ELISA and USERIA have achieved sensitivities 1 and 2 orders of magnitude lower than RIA. There is a general trend away from earlier methods such as RIA to methods that are more readily automated (there is particular interest in methods that do not require a physical separation step). It seems likely that a variety of different methods will remain in use to accommodate the properties of particular analytes: for example, until quite recently there remained analytes (such as vitamin B_{12}) for which RIA was the only analytic method available.

There are alternative chemical methods, such as HPLC, for many analytes. An important principle of ligand assay must be borne in mind—it measures the chemical (generally immunochemical) reactivity rather than the physiologic or functional activity of an analyte. This has sometimes been an advantage, where much new knowledge has been gained about the various forms of drugs and hormones capable of cross-reacting with the intended analyte.

GLOSSARY OF ASSAY TERMINOLOGY

Accuracy: The degree to which an analyte concentration estimate corresponds to the true value. This is rarely knowable absolutely. Inaccuracy is caused by a combination of random and bias errors.

Analyte: The substance to be measured.

Analyte concentration estimate: The concentration of analyte in a test specimen which is estimated by the assay procedure. Also sometimes known as **dose,** a term from the earlier biologic assay field.

Analytic method: The physical and chemical manipulations to which calibrators and test specimens are subjected to produce their corresponding assay response values.

Analytic sensitivity: A vague term generally associated with the ability to detect small concentrations but in fact used with multiple meanings, which has provoked immense needless debate. The use of some mathematically defined term such as the **lower detection limit** (see below) is recommended. Analogous to but not to be confused with **diagnostic sensitivity.**

Analytic specificity: A vague term associated with the ability to detect analyte as opposed to nonanalyte. The use of cross-reaction profiles is preferable. Analogous to but not to be confused with **diagnostic specificity.**

Batch: A single processing session in which a set of specimens is subjected to the assay analytic method.

Between-batch random error: The random error that accrues in an assay system, including within-assay random error and the additional sources of random error observed when comparing results obtained from repeated analysis of the same specimen in different batches of the same assay method.

Between-laboratory random error: The random error observed in measurements of the same specimen in different laboratories, including within-assay error, between-batch random error, and the additional sources of random error observed when comparing such results.

Bias: Systematic error. Causes include decay in the performance of the final detection device, specimen misidentification, decay of calibrators or test specimens, nonidentity of the chemical behavior of calibrators and test specimens (as with cross-reaction and interference), and others.

Calibration curve: The plotted or mathematically describable relationship between the response obtained from the analytic procedure and the analyte concentration.

Calibrators: Known concentrations of the analyte, used in creating the calibration curve. Also known as **standards.** There are multiple varieties.

Confidence interval: The analyte concentration range contained within a set of confidence limits.

Confidence limits: Statistically defined limits about an analyte concentration estimate, which reflect the random error inherent in the result. Example: 95% limits define a region within which, 95% of the time, the true estimate (in the absence of bias error) would be expected to fall (were the measurement with the accompanying computation of confidence limits to be repeated many times).

Continuous-response assay: An assay in which the response varies over a continuous range of values, or a discrete range so large as to be well approximated by a continuous range, as in radioimmunoassay.

Cross-reaction: The reaction with the specific assay binding substance by some chemical entity other than the analyte, in such a way as to falsify the measured amount of analyte.

Cross-reaction profile: A plot of the bias error in the estimated concentration of analyte as a function of the concentration of a specified cross-reacting species, at a given fixed concentration of analyte.

Cumulative sum chart: A type of quality control chart. The cumulative sum of deviations (from the expected value) of some quality control parameter is plotted. Various statistical tests are available to determine whether the plotted points may indicate a quality control problem.

Drift: A temporal shift in bias in assay results. This may sometimes be detected by placing quality control pool specimens at regular intervals in the assay batch.

Imprecision profile: A plot of imprecision (generally expressed as the width of a confidence limit of some specified level of certainty, and a given level of replication of calibrators and unknowns) versus analyte concentration. Also known as a **precision profile.**

Interference: Used in many different ways in clinical chemistry. For example, this term is used to refer to the bias error in a spectrophotometer reading produced by absorption of a given frequency of light by substances other than the one of primary interest. In ligand assays, the term usually refers to the presence of something that can mimic the chemical behavior of the binder, producing bias error. As an example, the presence of thyroid-binding globulin could interfere with a radioimmunoassay of thyroid hormone.

Interpolation: The process of reading the response for an unknown through the calibration curve to obtain an analyte concentration estimate.

Least squares (method of): A procedure for fitting a mathematical function to data in which the sum of the second powers of the vertical distances between the function and the data points is minimized.

Lower detection limit: The (statistically defined) lowest concentration distinguishable from the lowest calibrator concentration (the latter is generally zero). Should be reported along with its associated level of statistical confidence. Also referred to as the **minimum detection limit** or **minimum detectable dose.**

Outlier: Defined in 2 senses. First, a member of a replicate set that lies far from the other members of the set, presumably owing to some extraordinary error. Second, the mean of a replicate set for a calibrator that lies far from the calibration curve location suggested by the other calibrators, again presumably owing to some extraordinary error.

Parallelism testing: The process of determining whether the curve that can be drawn from the responses obtained from multiple dilutions of a test specimen can be superimposed upon the calibration curve by a simple multiplicative rescaling of the x axis of the test curve. Also referred to as **similarity testing,** which is perhaps more appropriate, since "parallelism testing" derives from the early days of biologic assay, when straight-line calibration relationships were used.

Pooled response-error relationship: A response-error relationship obtained by pooling information from a number of consecutive assay batches (generally 10–30) so as to achieve better estimates of the expected error than would be possible with the limited information available in a single batch. Often used to estimate the imprecision profile.

Power function: Plot of the probability of rejection of an assay result as a function of the amount of error present (either bias or random) for a specified quality control test.

Precision: A qualitative term concerned with the reproducibility of a result and hence with its random error. Avoidance of this term is recommended; the use of some precisely defined mathematic expression of random error, such as a set of confidence limits with its associated level of statistical significance, is preferred.

Quality control chart: A plot of some assay performance parameter, most often the measurement obtained for a quality control pool, plotted chronologically on a flow chart. Statistical tests may be performed to ascertain whether deviations from the average result would be so rare (if attributed to the usual amount of random error of the assay) as to represent a possible quality control problem. Also known as **Shewhart chart** and **Levey-Jennings chart.** See also **cumulative sum chart.**

Quality control pool: A large collection of material containing analyte stored so as to preserve it over a long period. Aliquots are taken and analyzed (with each assay batch in earlier assays, with decreasing frequency in some newer commercial assays) to assist in detecting exceptional error (particularly useful for bias).

Quantal-response assay: An assay in which the response is some value which varies over a discrete range of values (example: 1, 2, 3, ... n) rather than over a continuous range. An example is the type of biologic assay in which a small number of animals is employed and the response is the proportion of animals killed by a given dose of analyte. Requires statistical methods not discussed here.

Random error: Error arising from chance occurrences rather than systematic causes. Important sources in practice include pipetting, timing, and counting and detection errors. See also precision, imprecision, analytic sensitivity, lower detection limit, confidence limits.

Recovery: The amount of analyte detected when a known amount of calibrator is added to a previously assayed test preparation. Significant deviation from 100% suggests the presence of bias error.

Replicate: A repeated analysis of a calibrator, quality control specimen, or unknown, as when a specimen is said to be run in duplicate, triplicate, ... n-tuplicate. The only source of information about random errors.

Residual: The vertical distance between a data point (in assay, this is often the mean of replicates obtained for a given calibrator concentration) and the mathematic equation fitted to it. If the residual is properly weighted for the amount of data it represents and for its variance, it is referred to as a **studentized residual.**

Response: Some mathematical function of the final measurement taken from the assay analytic method.

Response-error relationship: A plot of the error in the selected response versus the response.

Run: Assay jargon for the process of analyzing a single assay batch.

Standard deviation: A measure of the random error inherent in a set of measurements of the same quantity (equal to the square root of the variance). Although the standard deviation may be computed for any given set of numbers, it is interpretable in strict probabilistic terms only if the data are drawn randomly from a gaussian population.

Test specimen: A sample, generally a biologic fluid, an aliquot of which is presented to the assay process in order to determine the concentration of analyte present.

Unknown: Test specimen.

Upper detection limit: The (statistically defined) highest concentration distinguishable from the highest calibrator concentration. Should be reported along with its associated level of statistical confidence.

Valid analytic range: The range between the upper and lower detection limits.

Variance: A measure of the random error inherent in a set of measurements of the same quantity, equal to the second power of the standard deviation.

Weighting: the use of some estimate of random error in the process of regression so as to take into account the relative error of the data being fitted; the final fit will pay more attention to data of higher precision than to data of lower precision. In assay work, the inverse of the variance (estimated from a pooled response-error relationship) should be employed.

Within-assay random error: The random error observed in assay results analyzed in a single batch.

IMMUNOHISTOCHEMICAL TECHNIQUES

IMMUNOFLUORESCENCE

Immunofluorescence can be applied as a histochemical or cytochemical technique for detection and localization of antigens in cells or tissues. Specific antibody is conjugated with fluorescent compounds without altering its immunologic reactivity, resulting in a sensitive tracer of tissue antigens. The conjugated antibody is added to cells or tissues and becomes fixed to antigens, thereby forming a stable immune complex. Unbound antibody is removed by washing, and the resultant preparation is observed in a fluorescence microscope. This adaptation of a regular microscope contains a high-intensity light source, excitation filters to produce a wavelength capable of causing fluorescence activation, and barrier filters to remove interfering wavelengths of light. When observed in the fluorescence microscope against a dark background, antigens bound specifically to fluorescent antibody can be detected by their bright color.

Fluorescence is the emission of light of one color, ie, wavelength, while a substance is irradiated with light of a different color. The emitted wavelength is at a lower energy level than the incident or absorbed light (Fig 12–31). Fluorochromes such as rhodamine or fluorescein used in clinical laboratories have characteristic absorption and emission spectra. Fluores-

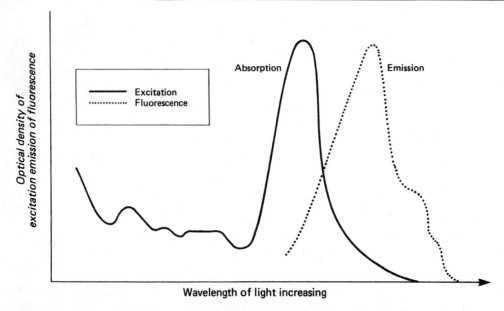

Figure 12–31. Absorption and emission spectra for a fluorescent compound.

cein isothiocyanate (FITC) is a chemical form of fluorescein that readily binds covalently to proteins at high pH primarily through ε-amino residues of lysine and terminal amino groups. Its absorption maximum is at 490–495 nm, and it emits its characteristic green color at 517 nm. Tetramethylrhodamine isothiocyanate, which emits red, has an absorption maximum at 550 nm and maximal emission at 580 nm (for rhodamine-protein conjugates). Consequently, different excitation and barrier filters must be used to visualize the characteristic green or red color of these fluorescent dyes. Generally, one wants to achieve an exciting wavelength nearly equal to that of the excitation maximum of the dye. Similarly, the barrier filter should remove all but the emitted wavelength spectrum. In practice, the actual brightness of fluorescence observed by the eye depends on 3 factors: (1) the efficiency with which the dye converts incident light into fluorescent light; (2) the concentration of the dye in the tissue specimen; and (3) the intensity of the exciting (absorbed) radiation.

Microscopes used for visualizing immunofluorescent specimens are modifications of standard transmitted light microscopes (Fig 12–32). In 1967, Ploem introduced an epi-illuminated system that employs a vertical illuminator and a dichroic mirror. In this system (Fig 12–33) the excitation beam is focused directly on the tissue specimen through the lens objective. Fluorescent light emitted from the epi-illuminated specimen is then transmitted to the eye through the dichroic mirror. A dichroic mirror allows passage of light of selected wavelengths in one direction through the mirror but not in the opposite direction.

There are several distinct advantages to the Ploem system. Fluorescence may be combined with transmitted light for phase contrast examination of the tissues, thereby allowing better definition of morphology and fluorescence. Also, interchangeable filter systems permit rapid examination of the specimen at different wavelengths for double fluorochrome staining, eg, red and green (rhodamine and fluorescein, respectively). This advantage in technique has resulted in superior sensitivity for examining cell membrane fluorescence in living lymphocytes.

Method & Interpretation

Virtually any antigen can be detected in fixed tissue sections or in live cell suspensions by immunofluorescence. It is the combination of high sensitivity and specificity, together with the use of histologic

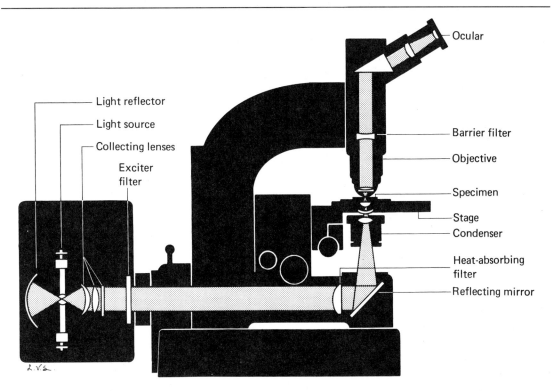

Figure 12–32. Fluorescence microscope with transmitted light. Light beam is generated by a mercury vapor lamp, reflected by a concave mirror, and projected through collecting lenses to the exciter filter, which emits a fluorescent light beam. A reflecting mirror directs the beam from underneath the stage, through the condenser into the specimen. A barrier filter removes wavelengths other than those emitted from the fluorescent compound in the specimen, and the fluorescence pattern is viewed through magnification provided by the objective and ocular lenses.

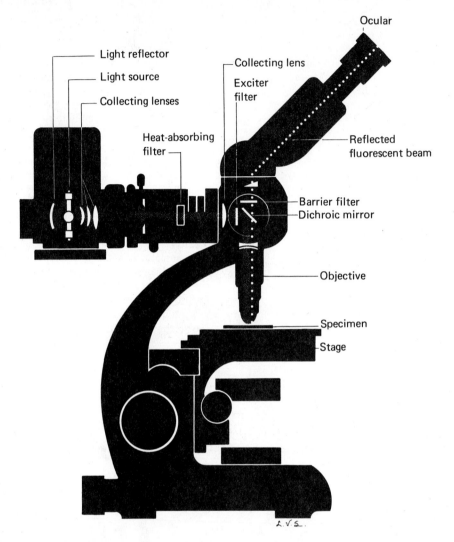

Figure 12–33. Fluorescence microscope with epi-illumination. The light beam is directed through the exciter filter and down onto the specimen. A dichroic mirror allows passage of selected wavelengths in one direction but not another. After reaching the specimen, the light is reflected through the dichroic mirror and emitted fluorescent light is visualized at the ocular.

techniques, that makes immunofluorescence so useful. The steps involved in immunofluorescence include preparation of immune antiserum or purified antibodies, conjugation with fluorescent dye, and, finally, the staining procedure.

For immunofluorescence, an antiserum to the antigen one wishes to detect is raised in heterologous species. Pure monoclonal antibodies can be used and are prepared as described below. Antisera should contain milligram amounts of antibody per milliliter. Specificity must exceed a level detectable in ordinary double diffusion or immunoelectrophoretic techniques. More sensitive methods available include hemagglutination inhibition, RIA, and ELISA. Unwanted antibodies present in either conjugates or an-

tiglobulin reagents for the test can usually be removed with insoluble immunoabsorbents or avoided entirely by use of monoclonal antibodies.

After obtaining antiserum of high potency and appropriate specificity, the γ-globulin fraction can be prepared by ammonium sulfate precipitation and DEAE-cellulose ion exchange chromatography. It is necessary to partially purify serum γ-globulin, since subsequent conjugation should be limited to antibody as much as possible. This will increase the efficiency of staining and avoid unwanted nonspecific staining by fluorochrome-conjugated nonantibody serum proteins that can adhere to tissue components.

Conjugation of γ-globulin depends largely on the particular dye to be combined with the antibody molecule. From a clinical laboratory standpoint, only fluorescein, rhodamine, and some phycobiliproteins have been used widely. Fluorescein, in the form of FITC, or rhodamine, as tetramethylrhodamine isothiocyanate, is either reacted directly with γ-globulin in alkaline solution overnight at 4 °C or dialyzed against γ-globulin. Unreacted dye is then removed from the protein-fluorochrome conjugate by gel filtration or exhaustive dialysis. If necessary, the resultant conjugate can be concentrated by lyophilization, pressure dialysis, or solvent extraction with water-soluble polymers. Thereafter, one must determine both the concentration of γ-globulin and the dye/protein or fluorescein/protein ratio of the compound. This is usually done spectrophotometrically with corrections for the alteration in absorbance of γ-globulin by the introduced fluorochrome.

Staining Techniques

A. Direct Immunofluorescence: (Fig 12–34) In this technique, conjugated antiserum is added directly to the tissue section or viable cell suspension.

B. Indirect Immunofluorescence: This technique allows for the detection of antibody in the serum. It eliminates the need to purify and individually conjugate each serum sample. The method is basically an adaptation of the antiglobulin reaction (Coombs test) or double antibody technique (Fig 12–34). Specificity should be checked as diagrammed and further established by blocking and neutralization methods (Fig 12–35).

Several additional variations in staining techniques have been used. These include (1) a conjugated anticomplement antiserum for the detection of immune complexes containing complement and (2) double staining with both rhodamine and fluorescein conjugates.

Immunofluorescence in which routine serologic procedures are used to detect antibody in human serum specimens has been widely applied (Table 12–5). Sensitivity is generally higher than with complement fixation and lower than with hemagglutination inhibition. Methods for detecting antibody by immunofluorescence include (1) the antiglobulin method, (2) inhibition of labled antibody-antigen reaction by antibody in test serum, and (3) the anticomplement method.

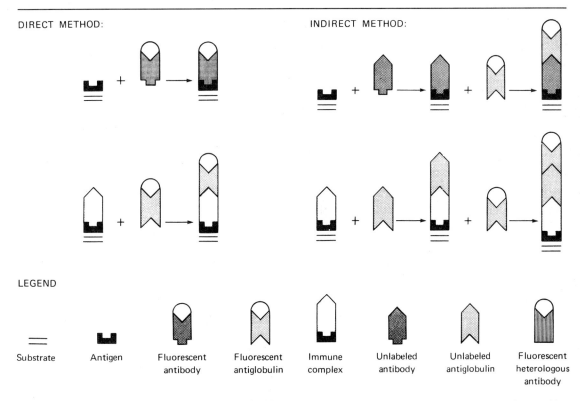

Figure 12–34. Mechanism of immunofluorescence techniques. *Direct Method* **(Top):** Antigen in substrate detected by direct labeling with fluorescent antibody. **(Bottom):** Antigen-antibody (immune) complex in substrate labeled with fluorescent antiglobulin reagent. *Indirect Method.* **(Top):** Incubation of antigen in substrate with unlabeled antibody forms immune complex. Labeling performed with fluorescent antiglobulin reagent. **(Bottom):** Immune complex in substrate reacted with unlabeled antiglobulin reagent and then stained with fluorescent antiglobulin reagent directed at unlabeled antiglobulin. (Modified and reproduced, with permission, from Nordic Immunology, Tilburg, The Netherlands.)

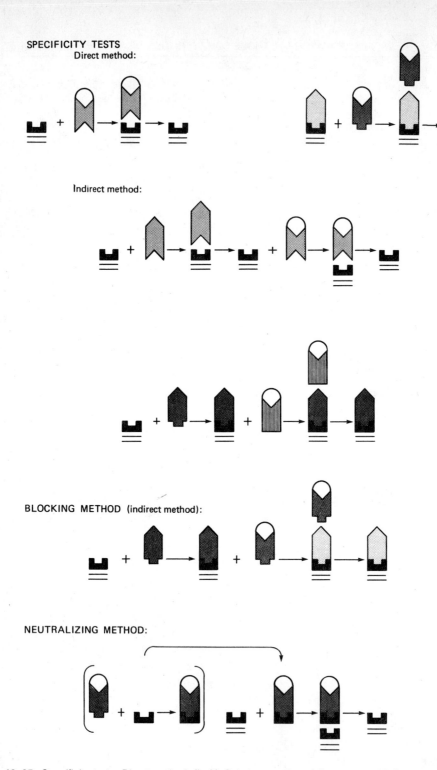

SPECIFICITY TESTS
Direct method:

Indirect method:

BLOCKING METHOD (indirect method):

NEUTRALIZING METHOD:

Figure 12–35. Specificity tests. *Direct method.* **(Left):** Substrate antigen fails to react with fluorescent antiglobulin reagent. No fluorescence results. **(Right):** Immune complex-substrate fails to react with fluorescent antibody directed against unrelated antigen. No fluorescence results. *Indirect method.* **(Top):** Unlabeled specific antiglobulin is replaced by unrelated antibody. In second step, fluorescent antiglobulin cannot react directly with antigen in substrate that has not bound specific antiglobulin. No fluorescence results. **(Bottom):** First step performed by reacting specific antibody with substrate antigen. In second stage, the specific conjugate is replaced by unrelated fluorescent heterologous antibody. No fluorescence results. *Blocking method.* Substrate antigen is incubated with unlabeled specific antibody prior to addition of specific fluorescent antibody. Decreased fluorescence results. *Neutralizing method.* Substrate antigen is incubated with specific fluorescent antibody after it is absorbed with specific antigen in substrate. No fluorescence results. Symbols are as in Fig 12–34. (Modified and reproduced, with permission, from Nordic Immunology, Tilburg, The Netherlands.)

Table 12–5. Clinical applications of immunofluorescence.

Identification of T and B cells in blood
Detection of autoantibodies in serum, eg, ANA
Detection of immunoglobulins in tissues
Detection of complement components in tissues
Detection of specific, tissue-fixed antibody
Rapid identification of microorganisms in tissue or culture
Identification of chromosomes of specific banding patterns
Identification of tumor-specific antigens on neoplastic tissues
Identification of transplantation antigens in various organs
Localization of hormones and enzymes
Quantitation of serum proteins and antibodies

C. Biotin-Avidin System: Avidin, a basic glycoprotein of MW 68,000, derived from egg albumin, has a remarkably high affinity (10^{15} kcal/mol) for the vitamin biotin. Biotin can easily be covalently coupled to an antibody and then reacted with fluorochrome-coupled avidin. After reaction of antigen with unlabeled antibody, the biotin-labeled second antibody is added. Since many molecules of biotin can be coupled to an antibody, the subsequent addition of fluorochrome-labeled avidin results in a firm bond with exceedingly bright fluorescence. Other advantages are lack of nonspecific binding of fluorochrome-coupled avidin to various substrates and general use of avidin conjugates in binding to biotin-labeled antibodies regardless of their species of origin or isotype.

Quantitative Immunofluorescence

Quantitative immunoassays using fluorochrome-labeled antigens and antibodies are available. The amount of light of a given wavelength emitted from a fluorescent specimen can be precisely measured by a microfluorometer. A number of assay methods have been introduced commercially in the field of quantitative immunofluorescence. Fluorescent immunoassay systems can be used to measure IgG, IgA, and IgM; C3 and C4; and antinuclear and anti-DNA antibodies. Immunoglobulins are measured by competitive binding of labeled specific antiserum for free and solid-phase antigen. The free antigen is present in patients' serum, whereas the bound immunoglobulin is fixed to a polymeric hydrophobic surface. The amount of fluorescent antibody bound to the solid-phase antigen is measured in a specially designed microfluorometer and converted to milligrams per deciliter by reference to a standard curve.

Serum antibodies to various cellular antigens such as DNA or nuclei can also be measured by an indirect fluorescence technique. Substrate (eg, DNA) is fixed to the polymer surface in solid phase and incubated with test sera. A second fluorescein anti-immunoglobulin reagent is then bound to the first antigen-antibody complex and the amount of bound fluorescence measured fluorometrically (Table 12–5).

OTHER IMMUNOHISTOCHEMICAL TECHNIQUES

Enzyme-Linked Antibody

In this method an enzyme is conjugated to antibody directed at a cellular or tissue antigen. The resulting conjugate is then both immunologically and enzymatically active. Use of these conjugates is entirely analogous to that for direct or indirect immunofluorescence techniques.

Horseradish peroxidase is usually the enzyme chosen for coupling to antibody. Tissues are first reacted directly with antibody-enzyme conjugate or directly with enzyme-linked antiglobulin reagent following incubation with unlabeled immune serum. Thereafter, the tissue is incubated with the substrate for the enzyme. The enzyme in this case is detected visually by formation of a black color after incubation with hydrogen peroxide and diaminobenzidine. One advantage of this method is that ordinary light microscopes may be used for anlaysis of tissue sections. Furthermore, enzyme-coupled antibody can be used for ultrastructural studies in the electron microscope.

Additional immunohistochemical techniques have been developed for localization of tissue or cellular antigens. One in particular, the peroxidase-antiperoxidase (PAP) method, has been used in surgical pathology for detecting enzymes and tumor-related antigens. This is a 3-step method. First, fixed slides are stained with rabbit antiserum to a tissue antigen to be measured. Next, an anti-rabbit immunoglobulin that reacts with the first antibody is applied. Finally, an immune complex, consisting of rabbit antibodies to peroxidase combined with peroxidase, is added. This immune complex reacts with the anti-rabbit bridging antibody. A peroxidase substrate is added, which forms the colored reaction product.

Other techniques being developed include hapten-coupled antibodies, the use of staphylococcal protein A as an intermediate reagent, and systems with more than one immunoenzymatic reagent, ie, double staining. Fixation difficulties and standardization of readily available reagents still limit the wider application of these potentially powerful techniques.

Ferritin-Coupled Antibody

Ferritin, an iron-containing protein, is highly electron-dense. When coupled to antibody, it can be used for either direct or indirect tissue staining. Ferritin-coupled antibody-antigen complexes in fixed tissue can then be localized with the electron microscope. Other electron-dense particles such as gold or uranium can also be introduced chemically into specific antitissue antibodies. These reagents have also been applied in immunoelectron microscopy.

Autoradiography

Radioactive isotopes such as ^{125}I that can be chemically linked to immunoglobulins provide highly sensitive probes for localization of tissue antigens. The antigens are detected visually after tissue staining by overlaying or coating slides with photographic emulsion. The appearance of silver grains as black dots has been used for subcellular localization of antigen both at light microscopic and ultrastructural levels. Autoradiography has also been applied to detection of proteins or immunoglobulins synthesized by cells in tissue culture.

Miscellaneous Methods

A variety of other methods have been described for localization of antigens in tissues. Many have not found widespread clinical application. In most cases, these techniques depend on secondary phenomena which occur as a result of the antigen-antibody interaction. These methods include the following:

(1) Complement fixation
(2) Conglutinating complement absorption test
(3) Antiglobulin consumption test
(4) Mixed hemadsorption
(5) Immune adherence
(6) Hemagglutination and coated particle reaction
(7) Immunoprecipitation

AGGLUTINATION

Agglutination and precipitation reactions form the basis of many techniques in laboratory immunology. Whereas precipitation reactions are quantifiable and simple to perform, agglutination techniques are only semiquantitative and somewhat more difficult. Important advantages of agglutination reactions are their high degree of sensitivity and the ability to assess end points visually. The agglutination of either insoluble native antigens or antigen-coated particles can be applied to measurement of a large variety of analytes.

According to Coombs, the 3 main requirements in agglutination tests are the availability of a stable cell or particle suspension, the presence of one or more antigens close to the surface, and the knowledge that "incomplete" or nonagglutinating antibodies are detectable with modifications, eg, antiglobulin reactions.

Agglutination reactions may be classified as either direct or indirect (passive). In the direct technique, a cell or insoluble particulate antigen is agglutinated directly by antibody. An example is the agglutination of group A erythrocytes by anti-A sera. Passive agglutination refers to agglutination of antigen-coated cells or inert particles which are passive carriers of otherwise soluble antigens. Examples are latex agglutination (fixation) for detection of rheumatoid fac-

tor and agglutination of DNA-coated erythrocytes for detection of anti-DNA antibody. Alternatively, **antigen** can be detected by coating latex particles or erythrocytes with purified **antibody** and performing so-called reversed agglutination. Another category of agglutination involves spontaneous agglutination of erythrocytes by certain viruses. This viral hemagglutination reaction can be specifically inhibited in the presence of antiviral antibody. Thus, viral hemagglutination can be used either to quantify virus itself or to determine by inhibition the titer of antisera directed against hemagglutinating viruses.

Inhibition of agglutination, if carefully standardized with highly purified antigens, can be used as a sensitive indicator of the amount of antigen in various tissue fluids. Hemagglutination inhibition using passive hemagglutination reactions can be semiautomated in microtiter plates and is sensitive for measuring antigens in concentrations of 0.1–10 µg/mL. With appropriate modification, passive hemagglutination with protein-sensitized cells can detect antibody at concentrations as low as 0.01 µg/mL.

AGGLUTINATION TECHNIQUES

Direct Agglutination Test

Erythrocytes, bacteria, fungi, and a variety of other microbial species can be directly agglutinated by antibody. Tests to detect specific antibody are carried out by serially titrating antisera in 2-fold dilutions in the presence of a constant amount of antigen. Direct agglutination is relatively temperature-independent except for cold-reacting antibody, eg, cold agglutinins. After a few hours of incubation, agglutination is complete and particles are examined either directly or microscopically for evidence of clumping. The results are usually expressed as a titer of antiserum, ie, the highest dilution at which agglutination occurs. Because of intrinsic variability in the test system, a titer usually must differ by at least 2 twofold dilutions ("2 tubes") to be considered significantly different from any given titer. Tests are carried out in small test tubes in volumes of 0.2–0.5 mL or in microtiter plates with smaller amounts of reagents.

Indirect (Passive) Agglutination Test

The range of soluble antigens that can be passively adsorbed or chemically coupled to erythrocytes or other inert particles has extended the application of agglutination reactions. Many antigens will spontaneously couple with erythrocytes and form stable reagents for antibody detection (Table 12–6). When erythrocytes are used as the inert particles, serum specimens often must be absorbed with washed, uncoated erythrocytes to remove heterophilic antibodies that would otherwise nonspecifically agglutinate them. The advantages of using erythrocytes for coating are their ready availability, sensitivity as indi-

Table 12–6. Substances that spontaneously adsorb to erythrocytes for hemagglutination.

Escherichia coli antigens
Yersinia antigens
Lipopolysaccharide from *Neisseria meningitidis*
Toxoplasma antigens
Purified protein derivative (PPD)
Endotoxin of *Mycoplasma* species
Viruses
Antibiotics, especially penicillin
Ovalbumin
Bovine serum albumin
DNA
Haptens, eg, DNCB

Table 12–7. Methods used to coat fresh and aldehyde-treated red blood cells with various antigens and antibodies for passive hemagglutination assay.[1]

Coupling Agent	Comments on Coupling	Antigens Commonly Coated
None	Simple adsorption	Penicillin, bacterial antigens including endo- and exotoxins, viruses, and ovalbumin.
Tannic acid	Adsorption possibly caused by changes analogous to enzymes. Most popular; usually satisfactory but often difficult and unreliable.	A wide spectrum of antigens: serum proteins, microbial and tissue extracts, homogenates, thyroglobulin, and tuberculin proteins.
Bisdiazotized benzidine (BDB)	Chemically stable covalent azo bonds.	Proteins and pollen antigens.
1,3-Difluoro-4, 6-dinitrobenzene (DFDNB)	Adsorption after modification of cell membrane.	Purified proteins and chorionic gonadotropin.
Chromic chloride (CrCl$_3$)	Proteins bound to erythrocytes by the charge effect of trivalent cations.	Proteins.
Glutaraldehyde, cyanuric chloride, tetrazotized O-dianisidine	Cross-linking and covalent coupling.	Various proteins and certain enzymes.
Tolulene-2,4-diisocyanate	Covalently bound.	Proteins.
Water-soluble carbodiimide	Covalently bound.	Proteins.

[1]Modified and reproduced, with permission, from Fudenberg HH: Hemagglutination inhibition: Passive hemagglutination assay for antigen-antibody reactions. In: *A Seminar on Basic Immunology*. American Association of Blood Banks, 1971.

cators, and storage capabilities. Erythrocytes can be treated with formalin, glutaraldehyde, or pyruvic aldehyde and stored for prolonged periods at 4 °C.

A list of general methods available for coating antigens to erythrocytes is presented in Table 12–7). Treatment of erythrocytes with tannic acid increases the amount of most protein antigens subsequently adsorbed. This higher density of coated antigen greatly increases the sensitivity of the agglutination reaction. Although highly purified antigens are required for immunologic specificity, slightly denatured or aggregated antigens coat tanned erythrocytes best.

Agglutination tests may be performed in tubes or microtiter plates. In antisera with very high agglutination titers, a prozone phenomenon may obscure the results. The prozone phenomenon produces falsely negative agglutination reactions at high concentrations of antibody as a result of poor lattice formation and steric hindrance by antibody excess. However, the use of standard serial dilutions eliminates this difficulty. Since IgM antibody is about 750 times as efficient as IgG in agglutination, the presence of high amounts of IgM can influence test results.

HEMAGGLUTINATION INHIBITION

The inhibition of agglutination of antigen-coated red blood cells by homologous antigen is a highly sensitive and specific method for detecting small quantities of soluble antigen in blood or other tissue fluids. The principle of this assay is that antibody preincubated with soluble homologous or cross-reacting antigens will be "inactivated" when incubated with antigen-coated erythrocytes. Thus, the test proceeds in 2 stages (Fig 12–36). Antibody in relatively low concentration is incubated with a sample of antigen of unknown quantity. After combination with soluble antigen, antigen-coated cells are added and agglutinated by uncombined or free antibody. (The degree of inhibition of agglutination reflects the amount of antigen present in the original sample.) Controls, including samples of known antigen concentration and uncoated erythrocytes, must be used. This hemagglu-

tination inhibition method has been used in the detection of HBsAg in hepatitis and in the detection of factor VIII antigen in hemophilia and related clotting disorders, but its use has been primarily in research, not clinical laboratories.

CLINICALLY APPLICABLE TESTS THAT INVOLVE AGGLUTINATION REACTIONS

Antiglobulin Test (Coombs Test)

The development of this simple and ingenious technique virtually revolutionized the field of immunohematology, and in various forms it has found widespread application in all fields of immunology. Antibodies frequently coat erythrocytes but fail to form the necessary lattice to produce agglutination. A typical example is antibody directed at the Rh determinants on human erythrocytes (see Chapter 15). However, the addition of an antiglobulin antiserum

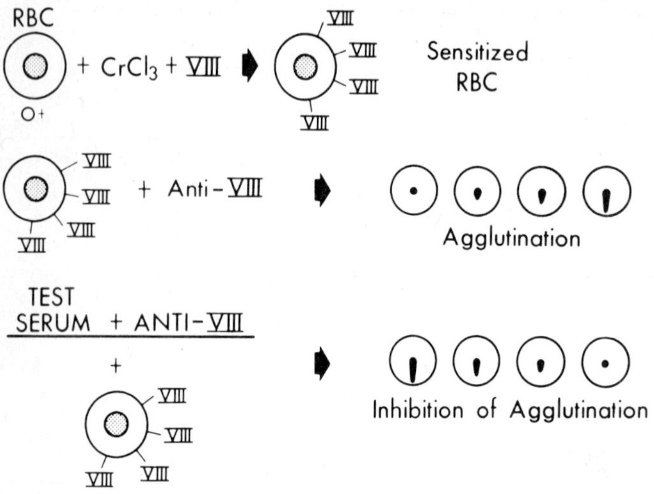

Figure 12–36. Hemagglutination inhibition. Human O-positive erythrocytes (RBC) are conjugated with coagulation factor VIII antigen by chromic chloride. The sensitized erythrocytes are reacted with specific antibody to factor VIII and are agglutinated. In the well of a V-shaped microtiter plate, agglutinated erythrocytes appear as discrete dots. Nonagglutinated cells form a streak when the plate is incubated at a 45-degree angle. Agglutination of sensitized red blood cells can be inhibited by the presence of homologous factor VIII antigen present in the test serum. With decreasing amounts of serum added to the test, the specific antibody agglutinates sensitized cells and forms a dot in the microtiter well. A semiquantitative estimation of the amount or titer of antigen in a test serum can be made in this way.

produced in a heterologous species (eg, rabbit anti-human γ-globulin) produces marked agglutination. Thus, the antiglobulin or Coombs test is used principally to detect subagglutinating or nonagglutinating amounts of antierythrocyte antibodies. However, more specific Coombs reagents directed at immunoglobulin classes, eg, anti-IgG, anti-IgA, or anti-L chains, may also be employed to detect cell-bound immunoglobulin. So-called non-gamma Coombs reagents, which are directed against various complement components, eg, C3 or C4, may also produce erythrocyte agglutination in the case of autoimmune hemolytic anemia. In some instances of this disorder, only complement components are bound to the erythrocyte and the regular antiglobulin reaction is negative. The **direct Coombs test** detects γ-globulin or other serum proteins that are adherent to erythrocytes taken directly from a sensitized individual. The **indirect Coombs test** is a 2-stage reaction for detection of incomplete antibodies in a patient's serum. The serum in question is first incubated with test erythrocytes, and the putative antibody-coated cells are then agglutinated by a Coombs antiglobulin serum. The major applications of Coombs tests include erythrocyte typing in blood banks, the evaluation of hemolytic disease of the newborn, and the diagnosis of autoimmune hemolytic anemia.

Bentonite Flocculation Test

Passive carriers of antigen other than erythrocytes have been widely used in serology for the demonstration of agglutinating antibody. Wyoming bentonite is a form of siliceous earth that can directly adsorb most types of protein, carbohydrate, and nucleic acid. After adsorption, many antigens are stable on bentonite for 3–6 months. Simple flocculation on slides with appropriate positive and negative control sera indicates the presence of serum antibody. Bentonite floc-

culation has been employed to detect antibodies to *Trichinella,* DNA, and rheumatoid factor.

Latex Fixation Test

Latex particles may also be used as passive carriers for adsorbed soluble protein and polysaccharide antigens. The most widespread application of latex agglutination (fixation) has been in the detection of rheumatoid factor. Rheumatoid factor is a pentameric IgM antibody directed against IgG (see Chapter 31). If IgG is passively adsorbed to latex particles, specific determinants on the IgG are revealed which then react with IgM rheumatoid factors. This method is more sensitive but less specific for rheumatoid factor than the Rose-Waaler test (see below).

Rose-Waaler Test

This passive hemagglutination test is also used for the detection of rheumatoid factor. Tanned erythrocytes (usually from sheep) are coated with subagglutinating amounts of rabbit IgG antibodies specific for sheep erythrocytes. Human rheumatoid factor will agglutinate these rabbit immunoglobulin-sensitized sheep erythrocytes by virtue of a cross-reaction between rabbit IgG and human IgG. The use of this test and latex fixation in the diagnosis of rheumatoid diseases (especially rheumatoid arthritis) is discussed in Chapter 31.

COMPLEMENT ASSAYS

Complement is one of the main humoral effector mechanisms of immune complex-induced tissue damage (see Chapter 11). Clinical disorders of complement function have been recognized for many decades, but their mechanism and eventual treatment have awaited elucidation of the complement sequence itself. The 9 major complement components of the classic pathway (C1–C9), several from the alternative pathway, and various inhibitors can now be measured in human serum. Clinically useful assays of complement consist primarily of CH_{50} or total hemolytic assays and specific functional or immunochemical assays for various components. Immunochemical means provide molecular concentrations in serum but do not provide data regarding the functional integrity of the various molecules.

It is worth emphasizing that the collection and storage of serum samples for functional or immunochemical complement assays present special problems as a result of the remarkable lability of some of the complement components. Rapid removal of serum from clotted specimens and storage at temperatures of −70 °C or lower are required for preservation of maximal activity.

Complement fixation or utilization, which occurs as a consequence of antigen-antibody reactions, provides a sensitive and useful means of detecting antigens or antibodies in serology.

HEMOLYTIC ASSAY

Specific antibody-mediated hemolysis of erythrocytes by complement is a relatively insensitive screening test for complement activity in human serum. However, it has limited usefulness, since a marked reduction in components is necessary to produce a reduction in the hemolytic assay. The hemolytic assay employs sheep erythrocytes (E), rabbit antibody (A) to sheep erythrocytes, and fresh guinea pig serum as a source of complement (C). Hemolysis is measured spectrophotometrically as the absorbance of released hemoglobin and can be directly related to the number of erythrocytes lysed. The amount of lysis in a standardized system employing E, A, and C describes an S-shaped curve when plotted against increasing amounts of added complement (Fig 12–37).

The curve is S-shaped, but in the mid-region, near 50% hemolysis, a nearly linear relationship exists between the degree of hemolysis and the amount of complement present. In this range, the degree of erythrocyte lysis is very sensitive to any alteration in complement concentration. For clinical purposes, measurement of total hemolytic activity of serum is taken at 50% hemolysis level. The CH_{50} is an arbitrary unit defined as the quantity of complement necessary for 50% lysis of erythrocytes under rigidly standardized conditions of sensitization with antibody (EA). CH_{50} test results are expressed as the reciprocal of the serum dilution giving 50% hemolysis. Variables that can influence the degree of hemolysis

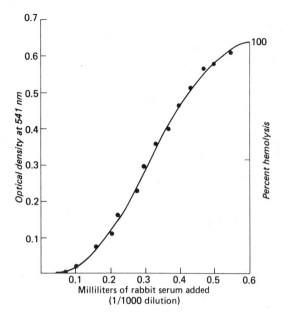

Figure 12–37. Relationship of complement concentration and erythrocytes lysed. Curve relating the percentage of hemolysis that results from increasing amounts of fresh rabbit serum (diluted 1:1000) as complement source is added to sensitized sheep erythrocytes (erythrocyte amboceptor [EA]). Hemolysis can be precisely determined by measuring the optical density of hemolysis supernates at 541 nm, the wavelength for maximal absorbance by hemoglobin.

include erythrocyte concentration, fragility (age) of erythrocytes, amount of antibody used for sensitization, nature of the antibody (eg, IgG or IgM), ionic strength of the buffer system, pH, reaction time, temperature, and divalent cation (Ca^{2+} or Mg^{2+}) concentrations.

The value for CH_{50} units in human serum may be determined in several ways. Usually, one employs the von Krogh equation, which converts the S-shaped complement titration curve into a nearly straight line.

The S-shaped curve in Fig 12–37 is described by the von Krogh equation:

$$X = K\left(\frac{Y}{1 - Y}\right)^{1/n}$$

where **X** = mL of diluted complement added,
    Y = degree of percentage lysis,
    K = constant,
    n = 0.2 ± 10% under standard E and A
      conditions.

It is convenient to convert the von Krogh equation to a log form that renders the curve linear for plotting of clinical results (Fig 12–38).

$$\log X = \log K + \frac{1}{n} \log \frac{Y}{1-Y}$$

The values of $Y/(1-Y)$ are plotted on a log-log scale against serum dilutions. The reciprocal of the dilution of serum that intersects the curve at the value $Y/(1-Y) = 1$ is the CH_{50} unit. Values for normal CH_{50} units vary greatly depending on particular conditions of the test employed. It should again be emphasized that the CH_{50} assay is relatively insensitive to reduction in specific complement components and may in fact be normal or only slightly depressed in the face of significant reduction in individual components.

MEASUREMENT OF INDIVIDUAL COMPLEMENT COMPONENTS

Functional Assays

Activation of the entire complement sequence of C1–C9 must occur to produce lysis of antibody-coated erythrocytes (EA). Thus, a general scheme can be proposed to determine the level of activity of individual complement components. Initially, one must obtain pure preparations of each of the individual components. These pure components are then added sequentially to EA until the step is reached just prior to the component to be measured. The test sample is added, and the degree of subsequent erythrocyte lysis

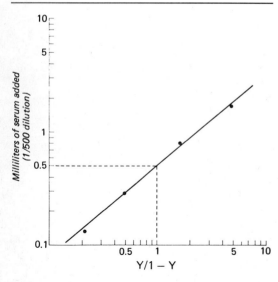

Figure 12–38. Determination of CH_{50} units from serum. Standard curve relating milliliters of serum 1:500 dilution to $Y/(1-Y)$ from von Krogh equation. When $Y/(1-Y) = 1.0$, the percentage of lysis equals 50%. In the example shown, 0.5 mL of 1:500 serum dilution has produced $Y/(1-Y) = 1.0$ or 50% lysis. The CH_{50} value for this serum equals 1000, since 1 mL of serum would have 1000 lytic units.

is then related to the presence of the later-acting components. Of course, all proximal components must be supplied in excess to measure more distally acting intermediates. Alternatively, the presence of genetically defined complement deficiencies has made available to the laboratory a further source of specifically deficient reagents for estimating individual component activity. A description of the technique of functional assays for complement components and their inhibitors is found in the monograph by Rapp and Borsos.

Immunoassays for Complement Components

Antibodies can be prepared against most of the major complement components and complement inhibitors, which allow immunochemical determination of complement components. Techniques that have been used for this purpose include electroimmunodiffusion (Laurell rocket electrophoresis), single radial diffusion, rate nephelometry, and ELISA. Although immunologic assay of complement components is independent of their biologic function, alterations in the chemical composition of complement components during storage may alter their behavior in these immunoassays. For example, in storage, C3 spontaneously converts to C3c, which has a smaller molecular size than native C3. Thus, when single radial diffusion of the timed interval variety is used, stored serum will give falsely high estimates because more rapid diffusion produces a larger ring diameter. Crucial to accuracy in clinical laboratory tests for complement is reliability of standards. In general, commercial sera prepared from large normal donor pools are adequate. However, since complement components are thermolabile when stored above $-70\ ^\circ C$, great care must be taken to ensure adequate refrigerated storage. In fact, the major source of error in complement determination is poor sample handling.

Measurement and significance of complement fragments or catabolic products are discussed in Chapter 11.

Significance of CH_{50} Units

A. Reduced Serum Complement Activity: Reduced amounts of serum complement activity have been reported in a variety of disease states (Table 12–8). The reduction in serum complement activity could be due to any one or a combination of (1) complement consumption by in vivo formation of antigen-antibody complexes, (2) decreased synthesis of complement, (3) increased catabolism of complement, or (4) formation of an inhibitor. Although complement has been demonstrated fixed to various tissues, eg, glomerular basement membrane, in association with antibody, tissue fixation of complement is apparently not an important mechanism in lowering serum complement activity. Isolated reduction in human serum levels of C1, C2, C3, C6, or C7 to 50%

Table 12–8. Diseases associated with reduced hemolytic complement activity.

Systemic lupus erythematosus with glomerulonephritis
Acute glomerulonephritis
Membranoproliferative glomerulonephritis
Acute serum sickness
Immune complex diseases
Advanced cirrhosis of the liver
Disseminated intravascular coagulation
Severe combined immunodeficiency
Infective endocarditis with glomerulonephritis
Infected ventriculoarterial shunts
Hereditary angioneurotic edema
Hereditary C2 deficiency
Paroxysmal cold hemoglobinuria
Myasthenia gravis
Infective hepatitis with arthritis
Allograft rejection
Mixed cryoglobulinemia (IgM-IgG)
Lymphoma

of normal only slightly reduces hemolytic activity. For this reason, many laboratories have switched from CH_{50} to a more simple immunochemical determination of the C3 level. In general, the reduction of the C3 level correlates positively with CH_{50} activity reduction.

B. Elevated Complement Levels: Although complement levels are elevated in a variety of diseases (Table 12–9), the significance of this observation is unclear. The most likely mechanism is overproduction.

The development of specific functional and immunologic methods for detecting complement components has led to the discovery of a variety of genetically determined disorders of the complement system. A discussion of the specific disease states which result from selective deficiency of the various complement components is found in Chapter 23.

COMPLEMENT FIXATION TESTS

The fixation of complement occurs during the interaction of antigen and antibodies. Thus, the con-

Table 12–9. Diseases associated with elevated serum complement concentrations.

Obstructive jaundice
Thyroiditis
Acute rheumatic fever
Rheumatoid arthritis
Periarteritis nodosa
Dermatomyositis
Acute myocardial infarction
Ulcerative colitis
Typhoid fever
Diabetes
Gout
Reiter's syndrome

sumption of complement in vitro can be used as a test to detect and measure antibodies, antigens, or both. The test depends on a 2-stage reaction system. In the initial stage, antigen and antibody react in the presence of a known amount of complement and complement is consumed (fixed). In the second stage, hemolytic complement activity is measured to determine the amount of complement fixed and thus the amount of antigen or antibody present in the initial mixture (Fig 12–39). The amount of activity remaining after the initial antigen-antibody reaction is back-titrated in the hemolytic assay (see above). Results are expressed as either the highest serum dilution showing fixation for antibody estimation or the concentration of antigen that is limiting for antigen determinations.

Extremely sensitive assays for antigen or antibody concentrations have been developed by using microcomplement fixation. However, these assays are too cumbersome and complex for routine clinical laboratory use.

Complement fixation tests (Fig 12–39) have received widespread application in both research and clinical laboratory practice. Table 12–10 lists some of the applications of complement fixation for either antigen or antibody determination. It should be recalled that all complement assay systems involving functional tests can be inhibited by anticomplementary action of serum. This may result from antigen-antibody complexes, heparin, chelating agents, and aggregated immunoglobulins, eg, as in multiple myeloma.

MONOCLONAL ANTIBODIES

The production of monoclonal antibodies by somatic cell hybridization of antibody-forming cells and continuously replicating cell lines created a revolution in immunology. The technique of hybridoma formation described by Köhler and Milstein in 1975 has allowed preparation of virtually unlimited quantities of antibodies that are chemically, physically, and immunologically completely homogeneous since each antibody is synthesized from cells derived from a single clone. These molecules are then generally

Table 12–10. Applications of complement fixation tests.

Hepatitis-associated antigen (HBsAg)
Antiplatelet antibodies
Anti-DNA
Immunoglobulins
L chains
Wassermann test for syphilis
Coccidioides immitis antigen

unencumbered by nonspecificity and cross-reactivity. In laboratory immunology, monoclonal antibodies are used to detect cellular and soluble antigens with RIA, ELISA, and immunofluorescence assay (IFA). Some well-established immunochemical methods such as immunodiffusion and immunoelectrophoresis probably do not require the degree of specificity afforded by monoclonal antibodies. The narrow specificity of monoclonal antibodies for single epitopes can theoretically limit their applicability.

TECHNIQUE OF MONOCLONAL ANTIBODY PRODUCTION

Hybridomas or somatic cell hybrids can readily be formed by fusing a single cell suspension of splenocytes or lymphocytes from immunized mice or rats to cells of continuously replicating tumor cells, eg, myelomas or lymphomas (Fig 12–40). The replicating cell line is selected for 2 distinct properties: (1) lack of immunoglobulin production or secretion, and (2) lack of hypoxanthine phosphoribosyl transferase (HPRT) activity. The cells are fused by rapid exposure to polyethylene glycol. Thereafter, 3 cell populations remain in culture: splenocytes, myeloma cells, and hybrids. The hybrids have the combined genome of the parent lines and eventually extrude chromosomes and acquire a diploid state. Selection for the hybrids is accomplished by awaiting natural death of the splenocytes. The myeloma cell line is killed, because in HAT medium, which contains hypoxanthine, aminopterin, and thymidine, HPRT cells cannot use exogenous hypoxanthine to produce purines. Aminopterin blocks endogenous synthesis of purines and pyrimidines, and the cells die. Hybrids begin to double every 24–48 hours, and colonies rapidly form.

The hybridoma cells are then cloned by limiting dilution methods and supernates assayed for antibody production, usually by ELISA or RIA. Recloning is performed to ensure monoclonality, and large numbers of cells are grown for antibody production. Extensive immunochemical and serologic studies are performed to ensure antibody specificity. Large quantities of antibody can be produced in serum-free tissue culture or in ascites fluid in syngeneic mice. Cells are stored in liquid nitrogen for further use.

Inter- as well as intraspecies hybridomas can be produced and propagated in long-term culture. For use in human therapeutic research, mouse hybridomas have usually been employed, but these regularly produce anti-murine antibody responses after infusions in humans. For this reason and for maximum specificity, human-to-human hybridomas have also been developed. Limitations in range of antibody specificities and technical difficulties in maintaining these hydridomas in culture need to be overcome.

Some examples of application of monoclonal antibodies in immunology are listed in Table 12–11.

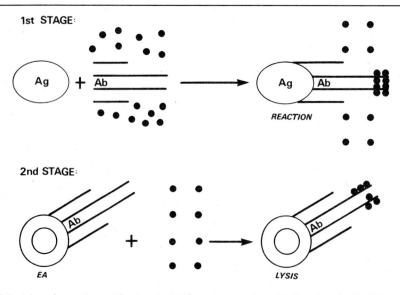

Figure 12–39. Principles of complement fixation. In the first stage, antigen (Ag) and antibody (Ab) are reacted in the presence of complement (●). The interaction of Ag and antibody fixes some but not all of the complement available. In the second stage, the residual or unfixed complement is measured by adding EA (erythrocyte amboceptor), which is lysed by residual complement. Thus, a reciprocal relationship exists between amounts of lysis in the second stage and antigen present in the first stage.

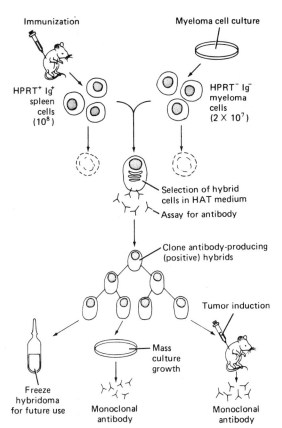

Figure 12–40. Formation of hybridomas between mouse cells and myeloma cells. Mouse myeloma cells that do not produce their own immunoglobulins and lack hypoxanthine and phosphoribosyl transferase (HPRT) are fused to splenocytes from an immunized mouse with polyethylene glycol. The hybrid cells are selected in hypoxanthine-aminopterin-thymidine (HAT) medium. Unfused myeloma cells are killed by HAT, and unfused splenocytes die out. The hybridomas are cloned, and antibody is produced in tissue culture or by ascites formation. (Reproduced, with permission, from Diamond BA, Yelton DE, Scharff MD: Monoclonal antibodies: A new technique for producing serologic reagents. *N Engl J Med* 1981;**304:**1344.)

COMPARATIVE SENSITIVITY OF QUANTITATIVE IMMUNOASSAYS

A major limitation of all quantitative immunoassays is their sensitivity. Exact lower limits of analyte detection vary with avidity, concentration, lots of antisera, temperature, length of reaction, and other factors. Nevertheless, it is useful to consider the approximate limits of sensitivity of various methods

Table 12–11. Applications of monoclonal antibodies.

Diagnostic (Many achieved; some experimental.)
 Leukocyte identification
 Lymphocyte subset determination
 HLA antigen detection
  Individual specificities of A, B, C, DR loci
  Framework specificities
 Viral detection and subtyping, eg, influenza variants
 Parasite identification
 Other microorganism detection
 Polypeptide hormone detection
 Relatedness of hormones, eg, hGH, hCS, hPRL
 Detection of carcinoembryonic protein, eg, CEA, AFP
 Detection of cardiac myosin for myocardial injury
 Typing of leukemias and lymphomas
 Detection of tumor-related antigens
 Immunohistochemical application in tissue sections
Therapeutic (Experimental; can be coupled to a toxin or radioisotope to enhance in vivo effects.)
 Antitumor therapy
  Individual tumor antigen-specific
  Anti-idiotype to surface immunoglobulin on B cell lymphomas
 Immunosuppression
  Organ transplantation
  Autoimmune and hypersensitivity diseases
  Treatment of GVH disease
 Fertility control
  Anti-hCG or antitrophoblast antibodies
  Drug toxicity reversal, eg, digitalis intoxication

available in the clinical immunology laboratory. The most commonly employed techniques are listed in Table 12–12 in order of increasing sensitivity.

PREDICTIVE VALUE THEORY

When *any* test is used to make a decision, there is some probability of drawing an erroneous conclusion. Predictive value theory can be used to deal with this problem. An example of its application in diagnosis of multiple sclerosis follows. This diagnosis is still made primarily by using the patient's history and physical findings. However, several laboratory tests are used as decision aids. One such test is the CSF IgG index, which is a ratio of ratios, [CSF IgG:albumin]:[serum IgG:albumin]. To simplify discussion, we have consolidated the patients into 2 groups, those with definite or probable multiple sclerosis, and all others. For every individual, 2 items of information are noted: (1) the diagnostic category (disease or no disease) and (2) the result of the laboratory test (normal or abnormal). This divides the results into 4 categories: **true positives** and **true negatives,** and **false positives** and **false negatives.** False-positive and false-negative results lead to erroneous conclusions.

Table 12–12. Relative sensitivity of assays for antigens and antibodies.[1]

Technique	Approximate Sensitivity (per dL)
Total serum proteins (by biuret or refractometry)	100 mg
Serum protein electrophoresis (zone electrophoresis)	100 mg
Analytic ultracentrifugation	100 mg
Immunoelectrophoresis	5–10 mg
Immunofixation	5–10 mg
Single radial diffusion	< 1–2 mg
Double diffusion in agar (Ouchterlony)	< 1 mg
Electroimmunodiffusion (rocket electrophoresis)	< 0.5 mg
One-dimensional double electroimmunodiffusion (counterimmunoelectrophoresis)	< 0.1 mg
Nephelometry	0.1 mg
Complement fixation	1 μg
Agglutination	1 μg
Enzyme immunoassay (ELISA)	< 1 μg
Quantitative immunofluorescence	< 1 pg
Radioimmunoassay (RIA)	< 1 pg

[1]Modified and reproduced, with permission, from Ritzmann SE: *Behring Diagnostics Manual on Proteinology and Immunoassays,* 2nd ed. Behring Diagnostics (New Jersey), 1977.

The results can be presented as a two-by-two contingency table as in Table 12–13.

Several basic terms are used in predictive value theory. **Diagnostic sensitivity** (not to be confused with analytic sensitivity, discussed in the context of ligand assay) is defined as the fraction of diseased subjects with abnormal test results. **Diagnostic specificity** is defined as the fraction of nondiseased subjects who have a normal laboratory test. The **positive predictive value** is the fraction of abnormal tests that represent disease, and **negative predictive value** is the fraction of normal tests that represent the absence of disease. Computing these values for the data in Table 12–13, we find

$$\text{Diagnostic sensitivity} = \frac{54}{64} = 0.84$$

$$\text{Diagnostic specificity} = \frac{110}{129} = 0.85$$

Table 12–13. A two-by-two contingency table.

Test Status	Disease Status		Totals
	Present	Absent	
Positive	54 (True positives)	19 (False positives)	73
Negative	10 (False negatives)	110 (True negatives)	120
Totals	64	129	193

Table 12–14. The effect of prevalence upon predictive value.

Test Status	Disease Status		Totals
	Present	Absent	
Positive	54 (True positives)	280 (False positives)	334
Negative	10 (False negatives)	1586 (True negatives)	1596
Totals	64	1866	1930

$$\text{Positive predictive value} = \frac{54}{73} = 0.74$$

$$\text{Negative predictive value} = \frac{110}{120} = 0.92$$

Note that diagnostic sensitivity and specificity reveal something about the test *given prior knowledge about the disease status,* whereas positive and negative predictive values estimate the *likelihood of disease given the test result.* Clearly, it is the latter case that is of interest when trying to make a diagnosis. In this context, it is vital to realize that although diagnostic sensitivity and specificity are qualities of a test, positive and negative predictive values are determined by both test performance and the prevalence of the disease in the patient population under study. Prevalence is defined as the proportion of the population afflicted by the disease in question. For the patient population in Table 12–13, the prevalence was (64/193 = 0.33), or 33%. Table 12–14 illustrates the effect of prevalence by presenting data for the CSF index in which the sensitivity and specificity have remained the same as in Table 12–13, but the prevalence of disease has decreased 10-fold, to 3.3%.

The positive and negative predictive values are now

$$\text{Positive predictive value} = \frac{54}{334} = 0.16$$

$$\text{Negative predictive value} = \frac{1586}{1596} = 0.99$$

Note that although the negative predictive value has increased slightly, there has been a substantial drop in the positive predictive value. The latter effect is due to the presence of a large number of false positives. For the population studied in Table 12–13 we could say that a positive test indicated disease in 74% of cases. For the population studied in Table 12–14, a positive test is associated with disease in only 16% of cases.

Predictive value theory applies only to dichotomous tests, ie, tests that are classified as normal or abnormal. In the case of the CSF index, this requires the selection of some diagnostic cutoff for the test results that separates normal from abnormal values.

The diagnostic sensitivity and specificity change as the cutoff is changed. More advanced decision theory provides more sophisticated tools for the analysis of tests reported as values from a continuous scale.

REFERENCES

General

Hudson L, Hay FC: *Practical Immunology,* 3rd ed. Blackwell, 1989.

IUIS/WHO Working Group: Use and abuse of laboratory tests in clinical immunology: Critical considerations of eight widely used diagnostic procedures. (Report of IUIS/WHO Working Group.) *Clin Exp Immunol* 1981;**46**:662.

Ritzmann SE (editor): *Protein Abnormalities.* Vol 1. *Physiology of Immunoglobulins.* Vol 2. *Pathology of Immunoglobulins.* Liss, 1982.

Rose NR et al: *Manual of Clinical Immunology,* 4th ed. American Society for Microbiology, 1992.

Voller A, Bartlett A, Bidwell D: *Immunoassays for the '80s.* University Park Press, 1981.

Weir DM (editor): *Handbook of Experimental Immunology,* 4th ed. 4 vols. Blackwell, 1986.

Immunodiffusion

Crowle AJ: *Immunodiffusion,* 2nd ed. Academic Press, 1973.

Deverill I, Reeves WG: Light scattering and absorption developments in immunology. *J Immunol Methods* 1980;**38**:191.

Ouchterlony O, Nilsson LA: Immunodiffusion and immunoelectrophoresis. Chapter 32 in: *Handbook of Experimental Immunology.* Vol 1. Weir DM (editor). Blackwell, 1986.

Stiehm ER, Fudenberg HH: Serum levels of immune globulins in health and disease: A survey. *Pediatrics* 1966;**37**:715.

Electrophoresis

Andrews AT: *Electrophoresis: Theory, Techniques and Biochemical and Clinical Populations,* 2nd ed. Oxford University Press, 1986.

Cawley LP et al: *Basic Electrophoresis, Immunoelectrophoresis and Immunochemistry.* American Society of Clinical Pathologists Commission on Continuing Education, 1972.

Gockman N, Burke MD: Electrophoretic techniques in today's clinical laboratory. *Clin Lab Med* 1986;**6**:403.

Jeppsson JO, Laurell CB, Franzen B: Agarose gel electrophoresis. *Clin Chem* 1979;**25**:629.

Ouchterlony O, Nilsson LA: Immunodiffusion and immunoelectrophoresis. Chapter 32 in: *Handbook of Experimental Immunology,* 4th ed. Vol 1. Weir DM (editor). Blackwell, 1986.

Roberts RT: Usefulness of immunofixation electrophoresis in the clinical laboratory. *Clin Lab Med* 1986;**6**:601.

Immunochemical & Physicochemical Methods

Brouet JC et al: Biological and clinical significance of cryoglobulins: A report of 86 cases. *Am J Med* 1974;**57**:775.

Somer T: Hyperviscosity syndrome in plasma cell dyscrasias. *Adv Microcirc* 1975;**6**:1.

Whicher JT, Warren C, Chambers RE: Immunochemical assays for immunoglobulins. *Ann Clin Biochem* 1984;**21**:78.

Williams RC: *Immune Complexes in Clinical and Experimental Medicine.* Harvard Univ Press, 1980.

Winfield JB: Cryoglobulinemia. *Hum Pathol* 1983; **14**:350.

Binder-Ligand Assay

Butt WR: *Practical Immunoassay: The State of the Art,* p 71–101. Dekker, 1984.

Dudley RA et al: Guidelines for immunoassay data processing. *Clin Chem* 1985;**31**:1264.

O'Sullivan MJ, Bridges JW, Marks V: Enzyme immunoassay: A review. *Ann Clin Biochem* 1979;**16**:221.

Rodgers RPC: Quality control and data analysis in binder-ligand assay. *Scientific Newsletters,* 1981.

Schall RF, Tenoso JH: Alternatives to radioimmunoassay: Labels and methods. *Clin Chem* 1981;**27**:157.

Immunohistochemical Techniques

Colvin RB, Bhan AK, McCluskey RT: *Diagnostic Immunopathology.* Raven Press, 1988.

Elias JM: *Immunohistopathology: A Practical Approach to Diagnosis.* ASCP Press, 1990.

Falini B, Taylor CR: New developments in immunoperoxidase techniques and their application. *Arch Pathol Lab Med* 1983;**107**:105.

Goldman M: *Fluorescent Antibody Methods.* Academic Press, 1968.

Kemeny DM: *A Practical Guide to ELISA.* Pergamon Press, 1991.

Nairn RC: *Fluorescent Protein Tracing.* 4th ed. Longman, 1976.

Robbins BA, Nakamura RM: Current status of fluorescent immunoassays. *J Clin Lab Anal* 1988;**2**:62.

Agglutination

Fudenberg HH: Hemagglutination inhibition. Pages 101–110 in: *A Seminar on Basic Immunology,* American Association of Blood Banks, 1971.

Herbert WJ: Passive hemagglutination with special reference to the tanned cell technique. Chapter 20 in: *Handbook of Experimental Immunology.* Weir DM (editor). Blackwell, 1978.

Complement Function

Cruse JM, Lewis RE Jr: *Complement Today.* Karger, 1993.

Harrison RA, Lachmann PJ: Complement technology. Chapter 39 in: *Handbook of Experimental Immunology,* 4th ed. Vol. 1. Weir DM (editor). Blackwell, 1986.

Morgan BP: *Complement: Clinical Aspects and Relevance to Disease.* Academic Press, 1990.

Ross GD: *Immunobiology of the Complement System: An Introduction for Research and Clinical Medicine.* Academic Press, 1986.

Whaley W (editor): *Methods in Complement for Clinical Immunologists.* Churchill Livingstone, 1985.

Monoclonal Antibodies

Beverley PCL: *Monoclonal Antibodies,* Churchill Livingstone, 1991.

Campbell AM: *Monoclonal Antibodies and Immunosensor Technology: The Production and Application of Rodent and Human Monoclonal Antibodies.* Elsevier, 1991.

Milstein C: Overview: Monoclonal Antibodies and 4 following chapters in section on Monoclonal Antibodies in: *Handbook of Experimental Immunology,* 4th ed. Vol 4. Weir DM (editor). Blackwell, 1986.

Peters JH, Baumgarten H: *Monoclonal Antibodies.* Springer Verlag, 1992.

Predictive Value Theory

Gottfried EL, Gerard S: Selection and interpretation of laboratory tests and diagnostic procedures. Chap 2, p 19–38, in: *Textbook of Clinical Diagnostics in Medicine.* Samly AH, Barondess JA, Douglas RG (editors). Lea and Febiger, 1987.

Griner PF et al: Selection and interpretation of diagnostic tests and procedures. *Ann Intern Med* 1981;**4:**553.

Hershey LA, Trotter JL: The use and abuse of the cerebrospinal fluid (CSF) profile in the adult: A practical evaluation. *Ann Neurol* 1980;**8:**426.

Sox HC Jr et al: *Medical Decision Making.* Butterworths, 1988.

Clinical Laboratory Methods for Detection of Cellular Immunity

13

Daniel P. Stites, MD

The immune system in humans has been divided into 2 major parts, one involving humoral immunity (antibody and complement) and the other cellular immunity. In many ways this separation is artificial, and many examples of the interdependence of cellular and humoral immunity exist. Nevertheless, dividing the immune system into parts in this way provides a conceptual and practical framework for the laboratory evaluation of immunity in clinical practice.

In the preceding chapter we reviewed methods of detecting antibodies and methods that primarily employ antibodies for antigen detection. The role of a variety of distinct cell types (see Chapter 2) in immune mechanisms in normal and diseased persons has become measurable in the clinical laboratory. Immunocompetent cells, including lymphocytes, monocyte-macrophages, and granulocytes, are all involved in the delayed hypersensitivity reactions that are so important in immunity to intracellular infection, tumor immunity, and transplant rejection. The clinical laboratory investigation of the number and function of these cells is still beset by difficulties in test standardization, biologic variability, the imprecise nature of many assays, and the complexity and expense of the procedures. Nevertheless, several tests that are of value in assessing cellular function have emerged for clinical use. Many of these assays employ sophisticated immunochemical methods for detecting cellular antigens or markers. Of great importance is the advent of monoclonal antibodies to detect various leukocyte subsets. Molecular biologic techniques such as Southern blots have recently been employed to detect either immunoglobulin gene or T cell receptor gene rearrangements as markers of specific B and T cell lineages are discussed in Chapter 14. Thus, we are witnessing an increasing fusion of biochemistry and molecular biology with cellular immunology.

The present chapter reviews the tests that have medical application in the detection of cell types and their corresponding functions. The intention is not to provide a comprehensive laboratory manual of all cellular immunologic procedures but to familiarize the reader with the principles, applications, and interpretation of assays with clinical applicability. Our understanding of cellular immunity continues to expand, and technologic advances in methods for its assessment have been developed. In chapter 17 special application of these and other tests for evaluating immune competence is described.

The topics discussed include (1) delayed hypersensitivity skin tests, (2) assays for T and B lymphocytes, (3) lymphocyte activation, (4) monocyte-macrophage assays, and (5) neutrophil function.

DELAYED HYPERSENSITIVITY SKIN TESTS

Despite the development of a multitude of complex in vitro procedures for the assessment of cellular immunity, the relatively simple intradermal test remains a useful tool, occasionally serving to establish a diagnosis. Delayed hypersensitivity skin testing detects cutaneous hypersensitivity to an antigen or group of antigens. However, when one is testing for an infectious disease, a positive test does not necessarily imply active infection with the agent being tested for. Delayed hypersensitivity skin tests are also of great value in the overall assessment of immunocompetence and in epidemiologic surveys. Inability to react to a battery of common skin antigens is termed **anergy,** and clinical conditions associated with this hyporeactive state are listed in Table 13–1.

Technique of Skin Testing
(1) Lyophilized antigens should be stored sterile at 4 °C, protected from light, and reconstituted shortly

Table 13–1. Clinical conditions associated with anergy.[1]

I. Immunologic deficiencies
  Congenital
    Combined deficiencies of cellular and humoral immunity
      Ataxia-telangiectasia
      Nezelof's syndrome
      Severe combined immunodeficiency
      Wiskott-Aldrich syndrome
    Cellular
      Thymic and parathyroid aplasia (DiGeorge's syndrome)
      Mucocutaneous candidiasis
  Acquired
    AIDS
    Sarcoidosis
    Chronic lymphocytic leukemia
    Carcinoma
    Immunosuppressive medication
    Rheumatoid diseases
    Uremia
    Alcoholic cirrhosis
    Biliary cirrhosis
    Surgery
    Hodgkin's disease and lymphomas
II. Infections
  Influenza
  Mumps
  Measles
  Viral vaccines
  Typhus
  Miliary and active tuberculosis
  Disseminated mycotic infection
  Lepromatous leprosy
  Scarlet fever
III. Technical errors in skin testing
  Improper antigen concentrations
  Bacterial contamination
  Exposure to heat or light
  Adsorption of antigen on container walls
  Faulty injection (too deep, leaking)
  Improper reading of reaction

[1]Modified from Heiss LI, Palmer DL: Anergy in patients with leukocytosis. *Am J Med* 1974;**56**:323.

before use. The manufacturer's expiration date should be observed.

(2) Test solutions should not be stored in syringes for prolonged periods before use.

(3) A 25- or 27-gauge needle usually ensures intradermal rather than subcutaneous administration of antigen. Multiple test devices that deliver up to 8 antigens simultaneously are also available, but these devices utilize a prick test, which has not been fully validated for delayed hypersensitivity skin testing. Subcutaneous injection leads to dilution of the antigen in tissues and thus can lead to a false-negative test.

(4) The largest dimensions of both erythema and induration should be measured with a ruler and recorded at both 24 and 48 hours.

(5) Hyporeactivity to any given antigen or group of antigens should be confirmed by testing with higher concentrations of antigen or, in ambiguous circumstances, by a repeat test with the intermediate dose.

Contact Sensitivity

Direct application to the skin of chemically reactive compounds results in systemic sensitization to various metabolites of the sensitizing compound. The precise chemical fate of the sensitizing compound is not known, but sensitizing agents such as dinitrochlorobenzene (DNCB) probably form dinitrophenylprotein complexes with various skin proteins. Sensitization with DNCB has been used experimentally in skin testing for delayed hypersensitivity in selected patients with suspected anergy. It is not a routine procedure and should be reserved for instances in which thorough delayed hypersensitivity testing with other antigens is negative. Concern regarding its possible toxicity and cross-sensitizing properties exists. Furthermore, its use as a diagnostic reagent is not currently approved by the FDA. Following application of DNCB to the skin, a period of about 7–10 days elapses before contact sensitivity can be elicited by a challenge dose applied to the skin surface. This sensitivity persists for years. The ability of a subject to develop contact sensitivity is a measure of cellular immunity to a new antigen to which the subject has not been previously exposed. Thus, the establishment of a state of cutaneous anergy in various disease states may be confirmed and extended by testing with DNCB.

Interpretation of contact sensitivity reactions depends on development of a flare, papular, or vesicular reaction at the site of challenge. Induration rarely occurs, since the test dose is not applied intradermally. In some clinical situations, a nonspecific depression in the inflammatory response can result in apparent anergy.

Patch testing is commonly employed by allergists and dermatologists to detect cutaneous hypersensitivity to various substances thought to be responsible for contact dermatitis. The test substance is applied in a low concentration and the area covered with an occlusive dressing. After 48 hours, the dressing is removed and the site examined for the presence of the inflammatory reaction described above. False-positive reactions can result from too high a concentration of the test substance, irritation rather than allergy, and allergy to the adhesive in the dressing. False-negative tests usually result from too low a concentration of the test substance or inadequate skin penetration. The results of patch testing must be carefully weighed with the clinical history and knowledge of the chemistry of the potential sensitizing agent. (See also Chapters 24 and 28).

Interpretation & Pitfalls

The inflammatory infiltrate that occurs 24–48 hours following intradermal injection of an antigen consists primarily of mononuclear cells. This cellular infiltrate and the accompanying edema result in induration of the skin, and the diameter of this reaction is an index of cutaneous hypersensitivity. A patient may also demonstrate immediate hypersensitivity to the same test antigen, ie, a coexistent area (wheal and flare) at 15–20 minutes and late-phase inflammation at 5–8 hours, but this usually fades by 12–18 hours (see Chapters 10 and 24). Induration of 5 mm or more in diameter is the generally accepted criterion of a positive delayed skin test. Smaller but definitely indurated reactions suggest sensitivity to a closely related or cross-reacting antigen. There is no definitive evidence that repeated skin testing can result in conversion of delayed hypersensitivity skin tests from negative to positive. However, with some antigens, intradermal testing can result in elevations of serum antibody titers and confuse a serologic diagnosis. For this reason, blood for serologic study should always be obtained before skin tests are performed.

False-negative results will be obtained in patients receiving systemic corticosteroids and possibly other immunosuppressive or anti-inflammatory drugs.

Delayed hypersensitivity skin testing is of relatively little value in establishing the diagnosis of defective cellular immunity during the first year of life. Infants may fail to react because of lack of antigen contact with the various test antigens. Consequently, in vitro assay for T cell numbers and function is much more useful in the diagnosis of congenital immunodeficiency disease (see Chapter 18). Genetic markers in the HLA-DR region are correlated with failure to respond to various tuberculin antigens.

Use of delayed and immediate hypersensitivity skin tests in diagnosis and management of allergies is discussed in Chapters 24–29).

Possible Adverse Reactions to Skin Tests

Occasional patients who are highly sensitive to various antigens will have marked local reactions to skin tests. If unusual sensitivity is suspected, a preliminary test should be performed with diluted antigen. Reactions include erythema, marked induration, and rarely, local necrosis. Patch testing may rarely result in sensitization. Systemic side effects such as fever or anaphylaxis are uncommon. Injection of corticosteroids locally into hyperreactive indurated areas may modify the severity of the reaction. Similarly, the painful blistering and inflammation that sometimes occur following surface application of contact sensitizers can be reduced by topical corticosteroids.

ASSAYS FOR HUMAN LYMPHOCYTES & MONOCYTES

The era of modern cellular immunology began with the discovery that lymphocytes are divided into 2 major functionally distinct populations. Evidence for the existence of T (thymus-derived) and B (bone marrow-derived) lymphocytes in humans originated from studies of other mammalian and avian species and analysis of lymphocyte populations in immunodeficiency diseases. Extensive studies of cell surface molecules with monoclonal antibodies and in vitro functional assays have provided direct evidence for the existence of these major lymphocyte types and a third type called natural killer (NK) cells.

The terms T lymphocyte and B lymphocyte usually denote the 2 major classes of immunocompetent cells in peripheral blood. During embryonic development, T lymphocytes arise in the thymus, migrate to peripheral lymphoid organs (lymph nodes and spleen), and circulate in the blood. B lymphocytes mature during embryogenesis from this origin in sites that are a functional equivalent of the avian bursa of Fabricius. T lymphocytes function as effector cells in cellular immune reactions, cooperate with B cells to form antibody (helper function), and suppress certain B cell functions (suppressor function). After appropriate antigenic stimulation, B lymphocytes differentiate into plasma cells that eventually secrete antibody. The notion that there is only one type of T cell or B cell has been found to be an oversimplification, since functionally distinct subclasses of T and B cells are now recognized. NK cells, a minor lymphocyte subpopulation, can also be assessed by cell surface markers and junctional assays.

Assays for T and B cells are currently in wide use in clinical immunology. Leukocytes are counted by microscopy or flow cytometry with specific antibodies to membrane antigens. The antibodies are conjugated either to fluorescent dyes or to enzymes that produce reactants. Such techniques can be applied either in tissue sections or in fresh suspensions of cells from blood, bone marrow, or other sites. Precise counting of T and B cells in human peripheral blood has made important contributions to our understanding of (1) immunodeficiency disorders, (2) autoimmune diseases, (3) tumor immunity, and (4) infectious disease immunity. It should be emphasized, however, that mere counting of T or B cells does not necessarily correlate with the functional capacity of these cells. At best, these assays provide a nosologic classification of immunocompetent cells; further evaluation of lymphocyte function usually should be performed to fully assess immunologic competence in clinical practice.

In 1983, the First International Workshop on Human Leukocyte Differentiation Antigens met and established a new nomenclature for immunologically defined cellular types and subtypes. They defined a series of **cluster of differentiation (CD)** types that define cellular antigens. In 1989, the fourth workshop refined and expanded this nomenclature. Definition of these CD types and relationship to other antigen or antibody designations are presented in Table 13–2. It should be emphasized that the CD nomenclature con-

Table 13–2. T cell differentiation antigens.

Cell Type Detected	CD Designation	Antibody Designation	Comments
Cortical thymocytes Langerhans cells	CD1	Leu 6 T6	Early T cell antigen also present on Langerhans cells, associated with β_2-microglobulin and not present on peripheral T cells.
E rosette-forming cells T cells NK cells	CD2	Leu 5 T11	Pan-T cell antigen SRBC receptor on T cells.
Mature T cells T cell antigen receptor	CD3	Leu 4	Also present on T cell in ALL and cutaneous T cell lymphoma.
Helper/inducer T cells Monocytes	CD4	Leu 3 T4	Can be further subdivided into helper and inducer subsets. Weakly expressed on monocytes.
Pan-T and -B cell subpopulation	CD5	Leu 1 T1 T101	B cells in CLL. B cells following marrow transplant. B cells secrete autoantibodies.
Mature T cells	CD6	T12	Malignant T cells.
Pan-T cells, thymocytes NK cells (some)	CD7	Leu 9 3A1	T cell leukemias.
Suppressor/cytotoxic T cells NK cells (some)	CD8	Leu 2 T8	Can be further subdivided into cytotoxic and suppressor subsets.

tinues to replace the more familiar, often proprietary, antibody designations, eg, CD4 for T4 or Leu 3.

Separation of Peripheral Blood Mononuclear Cells for Lymphocyte & Monocyte Assays

Tests for human mononuclear cells are ordinarily performed on purified suspensions of blood cells. An accepted procedure for obtaining mononuclear cell suspensions is density gradient centrifugation on Ficoll-Hypaque. This method results in a yield of 70–90% mononuclear cells with a high degree of purity but may selectively eliminate some lymphocyte subpopulations. Mononuclear preparations obtained by this method are relatively enriched in *monocytes*. These cells must be distinguished from lymphocytes by morphologic characteristics, phagocytic ability, endogenous enzymatic activity, or cell surface antigens (see below).

To avoid misinterpretation, results of tests for T, B, and NK cell markers on separated populations should generally be expressed as the number of cells per microliter of whole blood. Many published studies have indicated only the percentages of lymphocytes carrying a particular marker. Such a result could be due to an increase in the particular cell population or, alternatively, to a decrease in other populations. Thus, it is important that each laboratory establish standard absolute numbers of lymphocytes cells per microliter of whole blood from normal individuals.

Methods for assessing cellular phenotypes utilizing whole unseparated blood have been developed. Cells are stained with fluorochrome-conjugated monoclonal antibodies, and erythrocytes are lysed. The residual washed leukocytes are counted by flow cytometry or fluorescence microscopy. The whole-blood method has the advantage of simplicity and has largely replaced the counting of separated mononuclear cells. It is generally not useful for functional studies because of potential interference by erythrocytes or plasma proteins.

T LYMPHOCYTE ASSAYS

Human T Cell-Specific Markers

Production of heteroantisera to normal and malignant human T cells created the potential for direct immunochemical detection of cellular subpopulations by immunofluorescence and other sensitive techniques. However, with few exceptions, conventional antisera raised in animals to T cell subsets have lacked sufficient specificity owing to extensive cross-reactivity and broad response to species-specific rather than lineage-specific antigens on the immunizing cells. Some degree of improvement in the quality of these reagents was achieved by use of naturally occurring human antibody derived from sera of patients with various autoimmune diseases or by use of purified or continuously cultured T cell subpopulations. However, with the advent of monoclonal antibodies produced by murine hybridomas (see Chapter 12), a major breakthrough was achieved in identification of human T cells.

Monoclonal antibodies have been produced in many laboratories to class-specific and subclass-specific T cell antigens. These antibodies are highly specific and sensitive reagents for detecting cells in suspensions or fixed tissue sections. An enormous proliferation of abbreviations for these sera has occurred simultaneously with their commercial availability. The use of CD terminology for some of these markers is compared with more common proprietary designations in Table 13–2 and see appendix for more detailed listing of CD's. New antigens defining specialized subsets of T cells will continue to emerge for the current groupings.

A. Performance of Test:

1. Production of T cell antibodies–T cells from various sources—especially thymocytes, purified peripheral blood T cells, T leukemia cells, or T cells from continuous culture—can be used for immunization of rodents and subsequent production of monoclonal antibodies (see Chapter 12). Specificity must be shown by positive reaction with T cells and negative reaction with B cells and other cell types.

2. Detection of T cell antigens with specific antisera–Immunofluorescence or immunoenzyme staining of either live lymphocytes or frozen tissue sections is possible. Direct immunofluorescence is performed with fluorochrome-labeled immunoglobulin from hybridoma culture supernatants or purified antibodies from the hybridomas.

In vitro cytotoxicity of human T cells by specific antisera may also be used to estimate T cell populations. Methods for assessing T cell killing include trypan blue vital staining or ^{51}Cr release assay.

Methods to detect various CD molecules derived from either the surface or the interior of cells are being developed. Following lysis of mixed cell populations by detergents, the amounts of various CD molecules are quantified by ELISA, RIA, or other immunoassays.

B. Interpretation: The percentage or absolute number of T cells or T cell subsets is determined by their binding to various specific antibodies. Cells are counted by direct observation with a fluorescence or light microscope or by flow cytometry (see below). The latter analysis has essentially replaced microscopy in clinical laboratories as simpler and less expensive instruments are developed. The overwhelming advantages of objectivity, sensitivity, and speed make flow-cytometric analysis preferable to the tedious process of counting cells by microscopic observation.

T Cell subsets

Major subsets of T cells consist of helper and suppressor/cytotoxic types. However, helper cells (CD4) consist of at least 2 phenotypically and functionally distinct subtypes: naive cells, which are CD4+CD45RA+, and memory cells, which are CD4+CD45R0)+. These 2 subtypes of the CD4 class are recognized phenotypically by the simultaneous expression of CD4 molecules and either Leu 8 or TQ1 (which have not yet received CD designations). So far, no single reagent has been developed that can identify these populations.

Suppressor cells (CD8) can similarly be subdi-vided into so-called true suppressor cells (CD8+, CD11+), which influence B cell antibody function, and cytotoxic T cells (CD8+, CD11−). Combinations of monoclonal antibodies are thus also used to detect these 2 important T cell subsets.

Helper:Suppressor Cell Ratios (T$_H$/T$_S$ Ratio)

Largely because of the interest and concern generated by the AIDS (acquired immunodeficiency syndrome) epidemic, many laboratories express results of helper/inducer and suppressor/cytotoxic T cell counts as a ratio or quotient. Caution must be exercised in using this approach, since the ratio may vary depending on changes in either numerator or denominator or both. Also, standardization of normal values and the clinical significance of slight deviations from the reference range are not well understood. Diseases or conditions that have been reported to be associated with high or low helper:suppressor ratios are presented in Table 13–3. Obviously, this laboratory test is not diagnostic of any particular condition and has to be interpreted cautiously on the basis of the persistence or transience of the abnormality. In AIDS, for example, the reduction in the ratio seems to be permanent, whereas in some viral infections, eg, cytomegalovirus, it is reversible.

The use of absolute numbers or, in some instances, percentages of CD4 and CD8 cells is preferred. CD4 numbers are useful in AIDS prognosis and monitoring treatment. Levels of CD8 cells are transiently elevated in many viral infections.

E Rosette-Forming Cells

Human T cells were formerly identified by their ability to bind sheep erythrocytes (SRBC) to form rosettes (Fig 13–1). However, detection of this property has largely been replaced by more sensitive binding of monoclonal antibodies that identify the SRBC receptor, designated CD2.

Table 13–3. Helper:suppressor cell ratios in human peripheral blood.

Decreased in	Increased in
SLE with renal disease	Rheumatoid arthritis
Acute cytomegalovirus infection	Type I insulin-dependent diabetes mellitus
Burns	SLE without renal disease
GVH disease	Primary biliary cirrhosis
Sunburn or ultraviolet solarium exposure	Atopic dermatitis
Myelodysplasia syndromes	Sézary syndrome
Acute lymphocytic leukemia in remission	Psoriasis
Recovery from bone marrow transplant	Chronic autoimmune hepatitis
AIDS	
Herpes infections	
Infectious mononucleosis	
Measles	
Vigorous exercise	

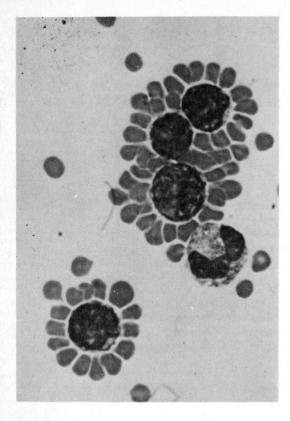

Figure 13–1. E rosette-forming cells. Lymphocytes from human peripheral blood that have formed rosettes with sheep erythrocytes. Such cells are T lymphocytes that bear the CD2 molecule. A granulocyte has failed to form a rosette. (Courtesy of M Kadin.)

B LYMPHOCYTE ASSAYS

B lymphocytes express a variety of cell surface molecules, which can be detected with either monoclonal antibodies or polyclonal antisera. Mature B cells express CD19, CD20, and HLA-DR. Immature B cells may express additional molecules such as CD10 (common acute lymphocytic leukemia antigen [CALLA]) (Table 13–4). Some B cell tumors, particularly chronic lymphocytic leukemia, express CD5, and CD5-bearing B cells may produce autoantibodies in systemic lupus erythematosus and rheumatoid arthritis. The use of B cell surface markers in tumor diagnosis is discussed in detail in Chapter 45.

Human B Cell-Specific Markers
A. Performance of Test: Monoclonal antibodies labeled with fluorochromes or enzymes are used to detect cells bearing the mature B cell markers CD19 and CD20. HLA-DR is also expressed on monocytes and activated on immature T cells. Fluorescence, or light microscopy in the case of enzyme-

linked monoclonal antibodies, may be used, but flow cytometry is currently the preferred method. Additional markers for subsets of B cells are available (see Table 13–4) but have limited clinical utility. Plasma cells generally fail to express B cell markers, but have a set of their own (eg, PC1 + PCA − 1), which can be detected with monoclonal antibodies.

B. Interpretation: No functional information directly emerges from enumeration of B cells. Special problems exist with the use of non-murine polyspecific antisera and Fc receptor binding (see below).

Surface Immunoglobulin
B lymphocytes have readily demonstrable surface immunoglobulin. This surface immunoglobulin is synthesized by the lymphocyte and under ordinary conditions does not originate from serum; ie, it is not cytophilic antibody. Lymphocytes generally bear monoclonal surface immunoglobulin, ie, immunoglobulin of a single H chain class and L chain type.

A. Performance of Test: Polyspecific antisera against all immunoglobulin classes permit detection of total numbers of B cells in a blood sample. Alternatively, a mixture of anti-κ and anti-λ antisera will detect total numbers of B cells. Monospecific antisera are developed by immunization with purified paraproteins and appropriate absorptions.

Tests for surface immunoglobulin-bearing B cells are performed by direct immunofluorescence with fluorochrome-labeled γ-globulin fractions derived from heterologous anti-immunoglobulin antisera or monoclonal antibodies. A major difficulty is to ensure the absence of all aggregated immunoglobulin in the test reagents (see below).

Generally, small amounts of anti-immunoglobulin antisera are mixed with purified lymphocyte suspensions for 20–30 minutes at 4 °C. After removal of unbound immunoglobulin, the presence of surface immunoglobulin is determined by counting in a fluorescence microscope or by flow cytometry.

Table 13–5 summarizes data on the numbers of surface immunoglobulin-bearing B cells in normal subjects. In certain disease states, eg, systemic lupus erythematosus, antilymphocyte antibody may be bound to B or T cells in vivo. To prove that surface immunoglobulin is a metabolic product of that cell, enzymatic removal and resynthesis of surface immunoglobulin may be performed in vitro.

B. Interpretation: The percentages of IgG-bearing lymphocytes are in fact considerably lower than previously reported. Falsely high levels are detected owing to formation of IgG–anti-IgG complexes at the cell surface with binding to B cells via the Fc receptor. When F(ab)'$_2$ anti-IgG reagents were prepared, the percentage of IgG-bearing cells was reduced from 5% to less than 1%.

The problem of binding of anti-immunoglobulin reagents to Fc receptors on B cells and monocytes is particularly severe with rabbit anti-human antisera. A

Table 13–4. B cell differentiation antigens.

Cell Type Detected	CD Designation	Antibody Designation	Comments
B cell subset T cells	CD5	Leu 1 T1 T101	B cell chronic lymphocytic leukemia B cell secretes autoantibodies
Immature B cells	CD10	CALLA J5	Pre-B cells Granulocytes Antigen is neural endopeptidase (encephalinase)
Immature and mature B cells	CD19	Leu 12 B4	
B cell tumors	CD20	Leu 16 B1	
B cells in mantle and germinal centers	CD22	Leu 14	

recent study suggests that nonspecific binding is almost eliminated by use of goat or sheep antisera to human immunoglobulins. The use of monoclonal murine antibodies to H and L chains also avoids this problem. Most investigators agree that IgM and IgD are the predominant surface immunoglobulins on human peripheral B lymphocytes.

Cytoplasmic Immunoglobulins

In some lymphoid cancers, particularly Waldenström's macroglobulinemia, chronic lymphocytic leukemia, or B cell lymphomas with leukemia, circulating lymphocytes with monoclonal intracytoplasmic immunoglobulins are detected. This immunoglobulin is usually identical to the molecule found on the surface of these cells and is occasionally present as a paraprotein in serum. Rarely, the intracellular immunoglobulin forms distinct crystals that appear as spindles or spicules within cytoplasm.

A group of patients with acute lymphocytic leukemias have been described with pre-B cells that express only intracytoplasmic IgM and no surface immunoglobulins at all. It is important to test for intracellular IgM, particularly in so-called null cell acute lymphocytic leukemia patients, since the group with pre-B cell leukemia is probably a distinct clinical subgroup with a different course and prognosis. Most of these cells react with CD19 antisera as well.

Intracellular immunoglobulins are detected by direct immunofluorescence with specific anti-heavy chain or -light chain sera or acetone- or ethanol-fixed cytocentrifuged preparations of purified lymphocytes.

Functional B Cell Assays

In the clinical laboratory, B cell function has been traditionally measured by the assessment of immunoglobulin levels or antibody titers, since these are the end products of B cell differentiation. However, 2 additional in vitro approaches to assessing functional abnormalities in B cells are now available. These are B cell activation by mitogens and immunoglobulin synthesis and secretion.

A. B Cell Activation by Mitogens: B cells can be stimulated to proliferate by several mitogens. Pokeweed mitogen (PWM) functions with T cell cooperation and is not a direct B cell test. However, staphylococcal protein A (Cowan 1 strain) (SAC) probably directly stimulates B cell activation. Measurement of this B cell attribute is analogous to phytohemagglutinin (PHA) or concanavalin A (Con A) stimulation described later for T cells.

B. Immunoglobulin Biosynthesis: B cell activation by antigens or mitogens results in small but detectable quantities of polyclonal immunoglobulins. Following 7–10 days of culture, these products are measured by radioimmunoassay (RIA) or enzyme-linked immunosorbent assay (ELISA) methods. Alternatively, B cells that produce immunoglobulins can be quantified by the reversed hemolytic plaque assay. In this assay, erythrocytes are coated with goat or rabbit anti-human immunoglobulins. They are mixed with putative immunoglobulin-producing lymphocytes and semisolid agar, and complement is

Table 13–5. Surface immunoglobulin-bearing B lymphocytes in normal adult blood.[1]

Surface Immunoglobulin	Mean % of Total Lymphocytes	Range
Total immunoglobulin	21	16–28
IgG	7.1	4–12.7
IgA	2.2	1–4.3
IgM	8.9	6.7–13
IgD[2]	6.2	5.2–8.2
IgE[3]	. . .	. . .
κ	13.9	10–18.6
λ	6.8	5–9.3

[1] From: WHO Workshop on Human T & B Cells. *Scand J Immunol* 1974;3:525.

[2] IgD and IgM are frequently expressed on the same cell.

[3] IgE B cells are extremely rare.

added. The presence of hemolytic plaques indicates the presence of immunoglobulin-producing cells.

B cells that have differentiated into plasma cells during an in vitro assay can be enumerated by staining for intracellular immunoglobulins by direct immunofluorescence in fixed smears of cultured cells.

The advantage of these in vitro B cell function tests is that they allow for delineation of immunoregulatory defects involving T or B cells by substitution of various cell populations among healthy and diseased cell donors. These assays are not routinely available in most clinical laboratories.

FLOW CYTOMETRY

Biochemical and biophysical measurements on single cells have been performed for years, primarily using visual analysis in various types of microscopes. Many of the immunohistochemical methods described in Chapter 12—and the cellular analysis methods discussed above—have become increasingly refined through the development of flow cytometers. A detailed description of the myriad applications of this general technique is beyond the scope of our discussion. In brief, flow cytometers are instruments capable of analyzing properties of single cells as they pass through an orifice at high velocity. Examples of measurements that can be made include physical characteristics such as size, volume, refractive index, and viscosity and chemical features such as content of DNA and RNA, proteins, and enzymes. Cell surface molecules are readily detected by immunofluorescence with monoclonal antibodies. These properties are detected by measuring light scatter, Coulter volume, and fluorescence. Instruments have been designed to analyze these properties and are combined with sophisticated electronics and computers. However, another class of even more sophisticated instruments—cell sorters—combine analytic capacity with the ability to sort cells on the basis of various preselected properties. One type of sorter, the fluorescence-activated cell sorter, has found many applications in immunologic research. Flow cytometers are now routinely found in clinical laboratories.

Cell Analysis by Flow Cytometry

Counting individual cells in complex mixtures is a tedious and imprecise technique even with monoclonal fluorescent antibodies and sophisticated microscopes. With the aid of a flow cytometer used as an analytic instrument, a single cell suspension may be analyzed for various measurements simultaneously at the rate of nearly 5000 cells per second. By combining light scatter or Coulter volume measurements with the powerful tool of fluorescently labeled monoclonal antibodies, subpopulations can be easily identified. A typical histogram produced by analysis of human T cells is shown in Fig 13–2. The number of

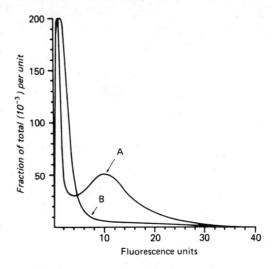

Figure 13–2. Single-color immunofluorescence histogram from flow-cytometric analysis of human T cells. Human lymphocytes were stained with fluorescently labeled anti-T cell antibody **(A)** and control nonreactive fluorescein isothiocyanate (FITC)-labeled antiserum **(B)**. In both patterns, a high, sharp peak of autofluorescence from unstained cells is observed near the y-axis. However, in the curve labeled **(A)** stained with anti-T cell antibody, a significant peak appears at about 11 fluorescence units. No such increase in the number or intensity of fluorescent cells is observed in the control **(B)** peak. (Modified and reproduced, with permission, from: Melamed MR, Mullaney PF, Mendelsohn ML: *Flow Cytometry and Sorting.* Wiley, 1979.)

cells under the curves can be determined and thereby the percentage of positive and negative cells in relation to an arbitrary threshold of fluorescent signal.

The use of 2 differently colored fluorochromes each coupled to a particular antibody allows simultaneous 2-color immunofluorescence of individual cells. Flow cytometers have been developed which can excite 2 different dyes that absorb light at similar wavelengths but emit light in orange and green. A "dot plot" graph of the results of simultaneous 2-color immunofluorescence in the analysis of activated DR antigen-positive suppressor/cytotoxic (CD8) cells in AIDS is shown in Fig 13–3.

Cells larger and smaller than lymphocytes can be "gated out" electronically so that the analysis concentrates solely on lymphocytes. With the addition of 90-degree light scatter, granulocytes can also be identified and gated out. This approach has allowed the development of whole-blood methods for lymphoid cell analysis.

Fluorescence-Activated Cell Sorters

A single cell suspension is isolated from blood or other tissues and labeled with either fluorescent anti-

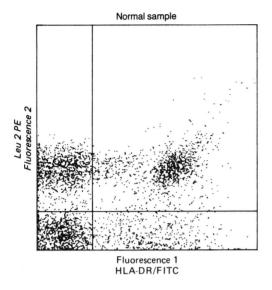

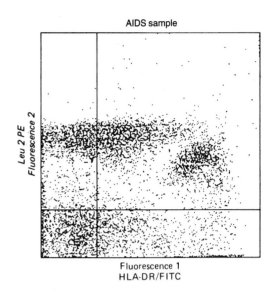

Figure 13–3. Presence of DR antigen on CD8+ (Leu 2+) cells. Simultaneous 2-color immunofluorescence analysis of human suppressor/cytotoxic T cells also bearing DR antigens. Human lymphocytes were stained with an FITC-labeled anti-DR antibody and a phycoerythrin-labeled anti-CD8 (Leu 2) antibody. The dot plot represents individual cells, with FITC-labeled cells on the x-axis and phycoerythrin-labeled cells on the y-axis. The coordinate of an individual dot thus indicates whether it is labeled with one or both antibodies. In addition, monocytes are labeled with antisera containing both fluorochromes and appear in both panels in the upper right quadrant. There is an increase in the number of doubly stained cells in AIDS versus the control panel.

body or another fluorochrome dye such as ethidium bromide, which specifically stains DNA (Fig 13–4). The cells are forced under pressure through a nozzle in a liquid jet surrounded by a sheath of saline or water. Vibration at the tip of the nozzle assembly causes the stream to break up into a series of droplets, and the size of the droplets can be regulated so that each will contain exactly one cell. The droplets are illuminated by the monochromatic laser beam and electronically monitored by fluorescence detectors. Droplets that emit appropriate fluorescent signals are electrically charged in a high-voltage field between deflection plates and are then sorted into collection tubes. Rapid, accurate, and highly reproducible separation of cells is thereby accomplished. Viability and sterility can be maintained, so that cells can be not only analyzed but also cultured or assayed functionally.

Clinical Applications of Flow Cytometry

The flow cytometer has had many applications in immunology. A partial list would include the following: (1) analysis and sorting of subpopulations of T and B cells by monoclonal fluorescent antibodies; (2) separation of various classes of lymphoid cells through sorting by size or antibody marker; (3) separation of live from dead cells; (4) cloning of individual cells by introducing microtiter plates in place of collection tubes; (5) analysis of cell cycle kinetics by various DNA stains: and (6) detection of rare cells such as monoclonal B cells in the blood of lymphoma

patients. Clinical applications are listed in Table 13–6. Computers are used to analyze multiple parameters measured simultaneously by the flow cytometer, including 2-color fluorescence, forward-angle light scatter, and 90-degree light scatter. Sophisticated data analysis and presentation software are available to produce clinically applicable information.

LYMPHOCYTE ACTIVATION

Lymphocyte activation or stimulation refers to an in vitro correlate of an in vivo process that regularly occurs when antigen interacts with specifically sensitized lymphocytes in the host. Lymphocyte transformation is a nearly synonymous term used first by Nowell in 1960 and later by Hirschhorn and others to describe the morphologic changes that resulted when small, resting lymphocytes were transformed into lymphoblasts on exposure to the mitogen PHA. Blastogenesis refers to the process of formation of large pyroninophilic blastlike cells in cultures of lymphocytes stimulated by either nonspecific mitogens or antigens.

Lymphocyte activation is an in vitro technique

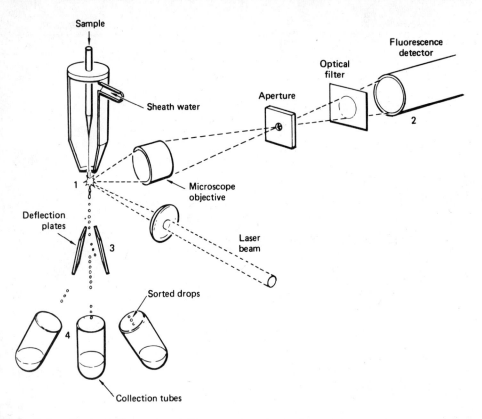

Figure 13–4. Cell purification by flow sorting. **1:** Flourescently stained cells are forced out of a small nozzle in a liquid jet. **2:** Cellular fluorescence, measured immediately below the nozzle, is used to select the cells to be sorted. **3:** The jet is broken into droplets. Droplets containing selected cells are electrically charged in a high- voltage field between deflection plates. **4:** The charged droplets are electrically deflected into collection tubes. (Courtesy of Joseph Grey, PhD.)

commonly used to assess cellular immunity in patients with immunodeficiency, autoimmunity, infectious diseases, and cancer. A myriad of complex biochemical events occur in lymphocytes following incubation with mitogens. These are substances that stimulate large numbers of lymphocytes and do not require a sensitized host, as is the case with antigens. These biochemical events include early membrane-related phenomena such as increased synthesis of phospholipids, increased permeability to divalent cations, activation of adenylate cyclase, and resultant elevation of intracellular cAMP. Synthesis of protein, RNA, and finally DNA occurs shortly thereafter. It is this last phenomenon, the increase in DNA synthesis, that eventually results in cell division and is the basis for most clinically relevant assays for lymphocyte activation. Convenience and custom have led clinical immunologists to use DNA synthesis rather than earlier events, eg, calcium influx or phospholipid metabolism, as a marker for lymphocyte activation.

Although the relationship between lymphocyte activation and delayed hypersensitivity is not always absolute, the method has found widespread use in clinical immunology. The in vivo delayed hypersen-

sitivity skin test is actually the result of a series of complex phenomena including antigen recognition, lymphocyte-macrophage interaction, release of lymphokines and monokines, and changes in vascular permeability. In vitro methods such as lymphocyte activation are useful for studying cellular hypersensitivity, since they permit analysis of specific stages in the immune response. In addition, they avoid challenge of the patient with potentially hazardous antigens such as drugs, transplantation antigens, or tumor antigens. Lymphocyte activation measures the *functional* capability of T or B lymphocytes to proliferate following antigenic challenge and is therefore a more direct test of immunocompetence than merely enumerating types of lymphocytes.

Lymphocyte responses can be suppressed or augmented by a variety of nonspecific factors present in human serum. This humoral modulation of responses to antigens or mitogens should be clearly differentiated from intrinsic suppression of cellular reactivity. Therefore, it is essential to avoid culture of lymphocytes in serum that may contain inhibitory substances. Their presence can usually be excluded by careful questioning of serum donors about their med-

Table 13–6. Clinical applications of flow cytometry.

Leukocyte phenotyping
  Diagnosis of congenital immunodeficiency diseases
  Assessment of prognosis of HIV-positive patients
  Monitoring of immunotherapy or chemotherapy in immun-
    odeficiency diseases
  Monitoring of immune reconstitution in bone marrow
    transplant recipients
Tumor cell phenotyping
  Diagnosis and classification of leukemias and lymphomas
  Determination of clonality of immunoglobulin-bearing cells
    from lymphomas and leukemias
  Differentiation of hematopoietic from nonhematopoietic
    tumors or cells
  Assessment of prognosis of cancers
DNA analysis
  Determination of aneuploidy
  Determination of cell cycle kinetics
Other applications
  Reticulocyte counting
  Platelet-associated immunoglobulin detection
  Leukocyte cross-matching in transplant recipients
  Cytogenetics

---

ications. If it is suspected that an individual's serum contains an inhibitor of lymphocyte activation, controls should be done with carefully washed cells obtained from that individual and cultured in normal serum. A partial list of serum suppressive factors and drugs that may influence in vitro lymphocyte responses is presented in Table 13–7. A note of caution

Table 13–7. Examples of lymphocyte suppressive factors in serum.

Serum proteins
  Albumin (high concentration)
  Specific antibodies to stimulating antigens
  Immunoregulatory globulin
  Alpha-1-acid glycoprotein
  Pregnancy-associated serum globulins
  C-reactive protein (CRP)
  Serum alpha globulin of amyloid (SAA)
  Alpha globulins in cancer, chronic infection, inflammatory
    diseases
  Alpha-fetoprotein (AFP)
  Low-density lipoprotein
  Antigen-antibody complexes
  HLA antibodies
  T cell antibodies
  Normal serum inhibitors (poorly characterized)
Hormones
  Glucocorticoids
  Progesterone
  Estrogens
  Androgens
  Prostaglandins
Drugs
  Aspirin
  Cannabis
  Chloroquine
  Ouabain
Others
  Interferon
  Cyclic nucleotides
  Cytokines

is warranted regarding the significance of this heterogeneous group of substances. Despite clear demonstration of substances with in vitro effects on lymphocyte responses, their in vivo action, particularly in view of the high concentrations often used in tissue culture, remains a matter of speculation.

METHODS & INTERPRETATIONS

Lymphocyte Activation by Mitogens

A number of plant lectins and other substances have been employed in assessing human lymphocyte function (Table 13–8). In contrast to studies in mice, there is no incontrovertible evidence that T or B lymphocytes are selectively activated by nonspecific mitogens. PHA and Con A are predominantly T cell mitogens, whereas pokewood mitogen stimulates B cells. Neither lipopolysaccharide nor anti-immunoglobulin antibody appears to be a potent B cell stimulant in humans. Staphylococcal protein A from *Staphylococcus aureus* cell walls is probably a specific stimulant of human B cells, possibly by triggering cells into DNA synthesis via the Fc receptor for IgG.

Anti-CD3 monoclonal antibody activates only those T cells that bear T cell receptor complex (see Chapter 8).

Lymphocyte Culture Technique for Mitogen Activation

Lymphocytes are purified from anticoagulated peripheral blood by density gradient centrifugation on Ficoll-Hypaque. Cultures are set up in triplicate or more in microtiter trays at a cell concentration of approximately 1×10^6 lymphocytes per milliliter. The culture medium is supplemented with 10–20% serum—either autologous, heterologous, or pooled human sera. Mitogens are added in varying concentrations on a weight basis, usually over a 2–3 log range. Cultures are incubated in a mixture of 5% CO_2 in air for 72 hours, at which time most mitogens have produced their maximal effect on DNA synthesis. DNA synthesis is measured by pulse-labeling the cultures with tritiated thymidine (^{3}H-Tdr), a nucleoside precursor that is incorporated into newly synthesized DNA. The amount of ^{3}H-Tdr incorporated relative to the rate of DNA synthesis is determined by scintillation counting in a liquid scintillation spectrophotometer. Scintillation counting yields data in counts per minute (cpm) or corrected for quenching to disintegrations per minute (dpm), which are then used as a standard measure of lymphocyte responsiveness. The cpm in control cultures are either subtracted from or divided into stimulated cpm, which yields a ratio commonly referred to as the stimulation index.

Obviously there are a multitude of technical as well as conceptual variables that can affect the results of this sensitive assay system. These include the con-

Table 13–8. "Nonspecific" mitogens that activate human lymphocytes.

Mitogen	Abbreviation	Biologic Source	Relative Specificity
Phytohemagglutinin	PHA	*Phaseolus vulgaris* (kidney bean)	T cells
Concanavalin A	Con A	*Canavalia ensiformis* (jack bean)	T cells (different subset from PHA)
Antilymphocyte globulin	ALG	Heterologous antisera	T cells + B cells
Anti-CD3 (MAb)	CD3	Hybridoma supernatant	T cell receptor-bearing cells
Staphylococcus protein A	SpA, SAC	*S aureus* (Cowan I strain)	B cells, T cell-independent
Pokeweed mitogen	PWM	*Phytolacca americana*	B cells, T cell-dependent
Streptolysin S	SLS	Group A streptococci	?(Probably T cells)

centration of cells, the geometry of the culture vessel, contamination of cultures with nonlymphoid cells or microorganisms, the dose of mitogen, the incubation time of cultures, and the techniques of harvesting cells.

The degree of lymphocyte activation is also a function of the cellular regulatory influences present in the culture. Suppressor or helper T, B, and mononuclear cells are all capable of modifying the final degree of proliferation in the specifically stimulated cell population. Some mitogens, particularly Con A, are known to activate suppressor T cells, which may reduce the proliferative response in such cultures.

Of additional importance in lymphocyte activation are culture time and dose-response kinetics. Since clinically important defects in cellular immunity are rarely absolute, quantitative relationships in lymphocyte activation are crucial. This is especially true when comparing the reduction of responsiveness of normal control subjects with that of a group of patients with altered lymphocyte function. With the use of microtiter culture systems and semiautomated harvesting devices, an attempt can be made to determine both dose- and time-response kinetics of either mitogen- or antigen-stimulated cultures (Figs 13–5 and 13–6).

Altered lymphocyte function can result in shifts in either time- or dose-response curves to the left or right. These shifts determine the optimal dose and optimal time of the lymphocyte response. Without such detailed analyses, it is usually impossible to accurately observe partial or subtle defects in lymphocyte responsiveness in various disease states. Cultures assayed at a single time with a single stimulant dose period are often grossly misleading.

Confusion may result from a nonstandardized format for presentation of data. Many laboratories present results of lymphocyte stimulation as a ratio of cpm in stimulated culture to those in control cultures—the so-called stimulation index. Others report "raw" cpm or dpm as illustrated in Figs 13–5 and 13–6. Neither method is entirely satisfactory. The stimulation index is a ratio, and marked changes can therefore result from changes in background or control cpm of the denominator. It is perhaps best to report data in both ways to permit better interpretations.

Antigen Stimulation

Whereas mitogens stimulate large numbers of lymphocytes, antigens stimulate far fewer cells that are specifically sensitized to the antigen in question. In

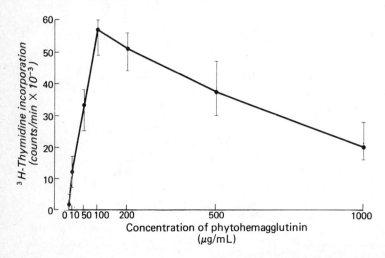

Figure 13–5. Dose-response curve for mitogen stimulation of 10^6 lymphocytes. Dose-response curve of a group of 10 normal adults whose peripheral blood lymphocytes were stimulated with varying concentrations of phytohemagglutinin for 72 hours. Lymphocytes were pulse-labeled with 2 μCi of tritiated thymidine 6 hours prior to harvesting. Counts per minute of tritiated thymidine incorporation were determined by liquid scintillation spectrometry and are plotted as the mean of 10 individual determinations ± 1 SD. A maximal response occurred at approximately 100–200 μg/mL of phytohemagglutinin.

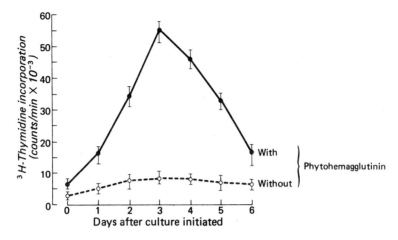

Figure 13–6. Time-response curve for mitogen stimulation of 10^6 lymphocytes. Time-response curve of peripheral blood lymphocytes from 10 normal adults stimulated in tissue culture for various lengths of time with an optimal concentration of phytohemagglutinin (100 μg/mL). Cultures were pulse-labeled with tritiated thymidine for 6 hours on the day of harvest. Maximal response occurred at 3 days after initiating the culture. Results are plotted as the mean ± 1 SD. of counts per minute.

most instances, only T cells respond to antigens in this test. A wide variety of antigens have been employed in lymphocyte activation, many of them also being used for delayed hypersensitivity skin testing (Table 13–9). In general, normal subjects show agreement between the results of skin tests and antigen-induced lymphocyte activation. However, in many conditions, the in vitro technique is apparently a more sensitive index of specific antigen-mediated cellular hypersensitivity. Furthermore, in vitro tests for T cell activation obviate the need for production of cytokines that produce dermal inflammation expressed as delayed hypersensitivity.

Lymphocyte Culture Technique for Antigen Stimulation

Culture methods are virtually identical to those described for mitogen stimulation. Additional factors to be considered include the possible presence in serum supplements of antibody directed against stimulating antigens. Antigen-antibody complexes may block or occasionally nonspecifically stimulate lymphocytes.

As in the case of mitogen-induced activation, time-

and dose-response kinetics are crucial in generating reliable data. Representative examples of such curves are shown in Figs 13–7 and 13–8. In contrast to mitogen-induced lymphocyte activation, antigen stimulation results in lower total DNA synthesis. Furthermore, the time of maximal response does not occur

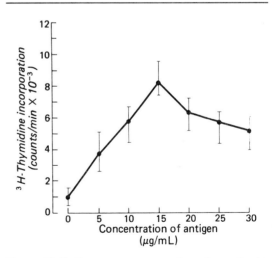

Figure 13–7. Dose-response curve for antigen stimulation of 10^6 lymphocytes. Dose-response curve of lymphocytes from 15 normal individuals with delayed hypersensitivity to the antigen. Cultures were harvested at 120 hours of culture after a 6-hour pulse with tritiated thymidine. Counts per minute were determined by scintillation spectrometry. Results are plotted as the mean ± 1 SD. from 15 skin test-positive subjects at various antigen concentrations. Maximum response is at 15 μg/mL of antigen.

Table 13–9. Antigens used to assess human cellular immunity in vitro.

PPD
Candida antigen
Streptokinase/streptodornase
Coccidioidin
Tetanus toxoid
Histoincompatible cells (MLC)
Trichophytin
Vaccinia virus
Herpes simplex virus

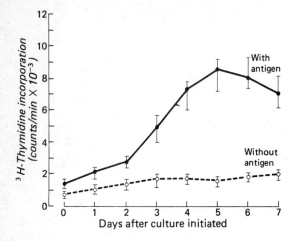

Figure 13–8. Time-response curve for antigen stimulation of 10^6 lymphocytes. Responses of peripheral blood lymphocytes from 15 normal adults with delayed hypersensitivity to the antigen. Cells were cultured as described in the legend to Fig 13–7. Antigen concentration for all cultures was 15 μg/mL. Maximal response occurred on days 5–7 of culture. Results are plotted as the mean ± 1 SD. for 15 individual determinations.

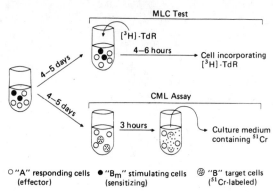

○ "A" responding cells (effector)   ● "Bₘ" stimulating cells (sensitizing)   ⊛ "B" target cells (^{51}Cr-labeled)

Figure 13–9. MLC and CML assays schematically represented. Cells (black and white balls) from separate individuals are cultured. In MLC, DNA synthesis in responding (noninactivated) cell is measured. In CML assay, the ability of "A" cells to kill ^{51}Cr-labeled "B" cells is measured. See the text for further explanation. [^{3}H]-TdR, tritiated thymidine. (Reproduced, with permission, from Bach FH, Van Rood JJ: The major histocompatibility complex: Genetics and biology. *N Engl J Med* 1976;**295**:806, 872).

until the culture has been allowed to continue for 5–7 days. Fig 13–8 clearly illustrates both the usefulness of and the necessity for performing careful time- and dose-response kinetics in assessing human lymphocyte function.

MIXED LYMPHOCYTE CULTURE & CELL-MEDIATED LYMPHOLYSIS

Mixed lymphocyte culture (MLC) is a special case of antigen stimulation in which T lymphocytes respond to foreign histocompatibility antigen on unrelated lymphocytes or monocytes. This test is performed as either a "one-way" or "2-way" assay (Fig 13–9). In the one-way MLC, the stimulating cells are treated with either irradiation (~ 2000 R) or mitomycin to prevent DNA synthesis without killing the cell. The magnitude of the response is then entirely the result of DNA synthesis in the nonirradiated or non-mitomycin-treated cells. In the 2-way MLC, cells from both individuals are mutually stimulating and responding, DNA synthesis represents the net response of both sets of cells, and the individual contributions cannot be discerned. The culture conditions, time of exposure, ^{3}H-Tdr pulse labeling, and harvesting procedures are usually identical to those for antigen stimulation. Controls include coculture of syngeneic irradiated and nonirradiated pairs and coculture of allogeneic irradiated pairs. The first control provides baseline DNA synthesis, and the second ensures adequate inactivation by irradiation (or mitomycin) of the stimulator cells.

In the use of MLC as a test for T cell function, difficulties in quantitation often arise owing to variations in stimulator cell antigens that determine the degree of genetic disparity between stimulator and responder cells. To overcome this difficulty and produce a more standardized test, frozen aliquots of viable pooled human allogeneic cells have been employed as stimulator cells.

The stimulating antigens on human cells are class I MHC molecules encoded by the HLA-D locus (see Chapter 5). Responding cells are primarily T lymphocytes with obligate macrophage cooperation. B cells can also respond in MLC, since a marked increase in immunoglobulin synthesis can be detected. MLC may be used as a histocompatibility assay (see Chapter 16) and as a test for immunocompetence of T cells, particularly in immunodeficiency disorders (see Chapters 20 and 21).

Cell-mediated lympholysis (CML) is an extension of the MLC technique in which cytotoxic effector cells generated during MLC are detected (Fig 13–9). This test involves an initial one-way MLC culture followed by exposure of stimulated cells to ^{51}Cr-labeled target cells specifically lysed by sensitized killer lymphocytes. These target cells are HLA-identical to the stimulator cells in MLC. Cytotoxicity is measured as the percentage of ^{51}Cr released in specific target cells compared with the percentage of ^{51}Cr released from control (nonspecific) target cells. Several lines of evidence indicate that cells which proliferate in MLC and killer cells which participate in CML assay are not identical. Killer cells are generated that have specificity for class I MHC antigens on target cells, whereas in class II MHC antigen differences determine the reaction. CML assays provide an additional measure of T cell function and can be used to estimate presensitization and histocompatibility in clinical transplantation (see also Chapter 16).

CLINICAL APPLICATION OF T & B CELL ASSAYS

Counting of T and B cells in peripheral blood and tissue specimens has limited application in both the diagnosis and investigation of pathophysiologic mechanisms of many disease states. Functional assays are even more limited in value primarily to studies of immune deficiency diseases. Current applications include the following.

(1) Diagnosis and classification of immunodeficiency diseases (see Chapters 18–22 and 52).

(2) Determination of origin of malignant lymphocytes in lymphocytic leukemia and lymphoma (see Chapter 45).

(3) Evaluation of immunocompetence and mechanisms of tissue damage in autoimmune disease, eg, systemic lupus erythematosus and rheumatoid arthritis (see Chapter 31).

(4) Detection of changes in cellular immune competence in HIV and other infections that may be of prognostic value (see Chapter 52).

(5) Monitoring of cellular changes following organ transplantation (see Chapter 57).

NATURAL KILLER (NK) CELLS

Natural killer (NK) cells can be enumerated by specific monoclonal antibodies using methods identical to those for T and B cells (see Chapter 17). Several monoclonal antibodies are available that detect either Fc receptors (CD16) or specific differentiation antigens (CD56, CD57) present on these cells. Some NK cells also express antigens from the CD2 T cell family. Functional testing is done by measuring the ability of these nonimmune cells to kill special target cells such as erythroleukemia cell line K562. Cytotoxicity is usually performed by using the ^{51}Cr release assay, similarly to cell-mediated lympholysis (Fig 13–9).

MONOCYTE-MACROPHAGE ASSAYS

The morphologic identification of normal peripheral blood monocytes in stained peripheral blood films ordinarily is quite simple. Monocytes are larger than granulocytes and most lymphocytes. They typically have round or kidney-shaped nuclei with fine, lightly stained granules. However, in suspension or even in tissue or blood specimens, additional markers may be required to differentiate monocytes from lymphocytes and primitive myeloid cells.

A reliable stain for monocytes is so-called nonspecific esterase, or α-naphthol esterase, which is present in monocytes but absent in most myeloid and lymphocytic cells. Monoclonal antibodies directed at specific differentiation antigens such as CD14 are available.

Functional attributes of monocytes are discussed in detail in Chapter 1. In the clinical laboratory, phagocytosis of particles or antibody-coated heat-killed microorganisms is useful for functional identification of monocytes.

NEUTROPHIL FUNCTION

Polymorphonuclear neutrophils (PMN) are bone marrow-derived leukocytes with a finite life span, which play a central role in defense of the host against infection. For many types of infections, the neutrophil plays the primary role as an effector or killer cell. However, in the bloodstream and extravascular spaces, neutrophils exert their antimicrobial effects through a complex interaction with antibody, complement, and chemotactic factors. Thus, in assessing neutrophil function, one cannot view the cell as an independent entity; its essential dependence on other immune processes, both cellular and humoral, must be taken into account.

Defects in neutrophil function can be classified as quantitative or qualitative. In quantitative disorders, the total number of normally functioning neutrophils is reduced below a critical level, allowing infection to ensue. Drug-induced and idiopathic neutropenia (see Chapter 33), with absolute circulating granulocyte counts of less than 1000/μL, are examples of this sort of defect. In these situations, granulocytes are functionally normal but are present in insufficient numbers to maintain an adequate defense against infection. In qualitative neutrophilic disorders, the total number of circulating PMN is either normal or sometimes actually elevated, but the cells fail to exert their normal microbicidal functions. Chronic granulomatous disease is an example of this type of disorder (see Chapter 22). In patients with chronic granulomatous disease the normal or increased numbers of circulating neutrophils are unable to kill certain types of intracellular organisms.

Phagocytosis by PMN can be divided into 5 distinct and temporally sequential stages: (1) motility, (2) recognition and adhesion, (3) ingestion, (4) degranulation, and (5) intracellular killing (Fig 13–10). The microbicidal activity of the neutrophil is the sum of the activity of these 5 phases. The clinical syndromes resulting from defects in many of the various stages in phagocytosis are discussed in Chapter 22. The laboratory tests used in clinical practice to evaluate phagocytic function in humans with various diseases will be discussed in terms of the 5 major steps in the process. It should be emphasized that for many neutrophil functions no standard assay exists; therefore, a variety of test choices depends on the local laboratory. The following sections will include examples of useful clinical tests of neutrophil function.

TESTS FOR MOTILITY

Neutrophils are constantly in motion. This movement can be either random or directed. Random or passive motion is the result of **brownian movement.** In **chemotactic movement** the cells are actively attracted to some chemotactic stimulus. Chemotaxins are produced by complement activation (C3a, C5a, C567; see Chapter 11), by fibrinolysis (fibrinopep-

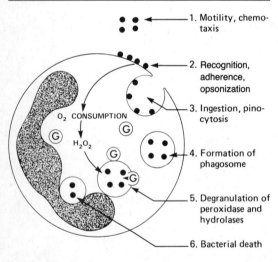

1. Motility, chemotaxis
2. Recognition, adherence, opsonization
3. Ingestion, pinocytosis
4. Formation of phagosome
5. Degranulation of peroxidase and hydrolases
6. Bacterial death

O_2 CONSUMPTION

H_2O_2

Figure 13–10. Steps in the progression of phagocytosis. Schematic representation of phagocytosis by a granulocyte. *1:* Bacteria attract phagocytic cells by chemotactic stimulus. *2:* Presence of opsonins (immunoglobulin and complement) facilitates recognition and surface attachment. *3:* Invagination of cell membrane with enclosed opsonized bacteria. *4:* Intracellular organelle, the phagosome, forms. *5:* Granules fuse with phagosomes and release enzymes into the phagolysosome. *6:* Bacterial death and digestion result. (Modified from Baehner: Chronic granulomatous disease. Page 175 in: *The Phagocytic Cell in Host Resistance.* Bellanti JA, Dayton DH [editors]. Raven Press, 1975.)

tide B), by microorganisms themselves (endotoxins), and by other leukocytes (lymphocyte chemotactic factor). Products of lipoxygenation of arachidonic acid, particularly LTB_4, are also chemoattractants. Relatively simple assays have been designed to assess leukocyte movement in vitro. An in vivo technique, the Rebuck skin window, preceded the development of in vitro assays and was one of the earliest methods developed for assessing leukocyte function.

Test for Random Motility

Random motility is tested for by the **capillary tube method.** Purified neutrophils in 0.1% human albumin solution at a concentration of 5 x 10^6/mL are placed in a siliconized microhematocrit tube. The tube is enclosed in a chamber specially constructed from microscope slides and embedded in adhesive clay. After being filled with immersion oil, the entire chamber is placed on the stage of a microscope. Motility is assessed by observing the leading edge of the leukocyte column in the microscope at hourly intervals. Measurements are expressed in millimeters of movement from the starting boundary of the packed leukocyte layer.

Test for Chemotaxis

Directional locomotion of neutrophils toward various chemotactic stimuli is quantitated by use of a Boyden chamber. Cells to be tested are placed in the upper chamber and are separated from the lower chamber containing a chemotactic substance by a filter membrane of small pore size. Neutrophils can enter the filter membrane but are trapped in transit through the membrane. After a suitable incubation period, the filter is removed and stained and the underside is microscopically examined for the presence of neutrophils.

Although this method is theoretically simple, there are numerous technical difficulties. These include nonavailability of filters of standard pore size, observer bias in quantitation of migrating neutrophils in the microscope, loss of cells that fall off or completely tranverse the filter, and failure of many workers to standardize cell numbers and serum supplements.

An additional method for measuring chemotaxis and random motility has been recently developed. This technique involves the radial migration of leukocytes from small wells cut into an agarose medium in a Petri dish. In many respects, the method is similar to single radial diffusion (see Chapter 12). Generally, 3 wells are cut into agarose. The cell population in question is placed in the center well. A chemoattractant is placed in an outer well, and a control nonattractant is placed in the remaining well. After several hours of migration, the distance from the center of the well originally containing cells to the leading edges of the migrating cells is measured.

In this way, the directed motility and the random motion can be quantitated. This method has achieved widespread application and in many laboratories has supplanted the somewhat more cumbersome Boyden chamber technique.

TESTS FOR RECOGNITION & ADHESION

As the neutrophil in an immune host approaches its target, by either random or directed motility, it recognizes microorganisms by the presence of antibody and complement fixed to the surface of the microorganisms. Enhancement of phagocytosis (opsonization) occurs under these circumstances. Adherence and aggregation of neutrophils are promoted by a series of membrane glycoproteins.

The family of membrane glycoproteins that function as adherence molecules includes LFA-1 (lymphocyte function associated antigen type 1), Mac-1 (macrophage 1) and p 150,95. These molecules all contain a common β subunit (CD18) and a unique α subunit. Mac-1 functions as a receptor for C3bi. Deficiencies of the β subunit have been described (see Chapter 23). Monoclonal antibodies to CD18 (the β subunit) are available, as well as those to specific α subunits: CD11a = LFA-1, CD11b = Mac-1, and CD11c = p 150,95. These molecules are present on granulocytes, monocytes, and some lymphocytes and can be readily measured by flow cytometry and immunofluorescence.

Tests to detect the presence of complement and antibody Fc receptors on neutrophils are rarely useful in clinical testing. The need for either antibody or complement (opsonins) coating of microorganisms for phagocytosis can be determined by employing sera devoid of either or both of these factors followed by an assay for ingestion and subsequent intracellular killing. Furthermore, IgG and complement receptors on neutrophils as well as mononuclear phagocytes can be readily detected by rosette formation with IgG-coated or complement-coated erythrocytes or by immunofluorescence with monoclonal antibodies.

TESTS FOR INGESTION

Ingestion of microorganisms by neutrophils is an active process that requires energy production by the phagocytic cell. Internalization of antibody-coated and complement-coated microorganisms occurs rapidly following their surface contact with neutrophils. Since subsequent intracellular events—ie, degranulation and killing—depend on the success of ingestion, tests for ingestion provide a rapid and relatively simple means of assessing the overall phagocytic process. Unfortunately, the term phagocytosis has often been used to denote *only* the ingestion phase of the

process. Thus, terms such as phagocytic index, which refer to the average number of particles ingested, really should be considered measurements of ingestion rather than of phagocytosis.

All tests to measure the ability of neutrophils to ingest either native or opsonized particles involve one of 2 general approaches. Either a direct estimate is made of the cellular uptake of particles by assaying the cells themselves, or the removal of particles from the fluid or medium is taken as an indirect estimate of cellular uptake.

Methods for quantitation of the ingestion of particles by cellular assays include (1) direct counting by light microscopy; (2) estimation of cell-bound radioactivity after ingestion of a radiolabeled particle; and (3) measurement of an easily stained lipid, eg, oil red O, after extraction from cells.

One disadvantage of many of these assays is that particles adherent to the neutrophil membranes are included as ingested particles. Other elements that influence results in performing ingestion assays include the presence of humoral factors (opsonins) which enhance uptake, the presence of serum containing acute-phase reactants which depress uptake, the need for constant agitation or tumbling of cells and particles to maximize contact and subsequent uptake, the type or size of the test particle used, and, finally, the ratio of particles to ingesting cells. No well-standardized assay is currently available for estimating particle ingestion.

TESTS FOR DEGRANULATION

Following ingestion of particles or microorganisms, the ingested element is bound by invaginated cell surface membrane in an organelle termed the **phagosome.** Shortly thereafter, lysosomes fuse with the phagosome to form a structure called the **phagolysosome.** Degranulation is the process of fusion of lysosomes and phagosomes with the subsequent discharge of intralysosomal contents into the phagolysosome.

Degranulation is an active process and requires energy expenditure by the cell. Thus, impairment of normal metabolic pathways of the neutrophil—especially oxygen consumption and the metabolism of glucose through the hexose monophosphate shunt—interferes with degranulation and subsequent intracellular killing.

A test for degranulation called frustrated phagocytosis has been developed and applied to the study of some neutrophil dysfunction syndromes. The frustrated-phagocytosis system (Fig 13–11) allows for examination of degranulation independently of ingestion. Heat-aggregated γ-globulin or immune complexes are fixed to the plastic surface of a Petri dish so that they cannot be ingested. Neutrophils are placed in suspension in Petri dishes with and without attached aggregated γ-globulin. The cell membranes

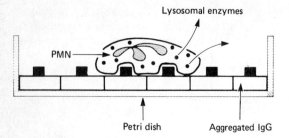

Figure 13–11. Assay of granulocyte degranulation by the "frustrated phagocytosis" method. The neutrophil is attached to aggregated IgG fixed to the bottom of a Petri dish. Lysosomal enzymes are discharged into supernatant as the cell attempts to phagocytose the IgG but is "frustrated." (Courtesy of S Barrett.)

Table 13–10. Antimicrobial systems of neutrophils.[1]

Acidic pH of phagolysosome
Lysozyme
Lactoferrin
Defensins
Cathepsin G
Myeloperoxidase-halogenation system
Hydrogen peroxide
Superoxide radical
Hydroxyl radical
Singlet oxygen

[1]For a further description of these systems, see Lehrer RI, et al: Neutrophils in host defense. *Ann Intern Med* 1988;**109:**127, and Boxer LA, Morganroth ML, Neutrophil function disorders. *Disease-a-Month* 1987;**33:**681.

of the neutrophils are stimulated by contact between γ-globulin and appropriate cell membrane receptors. This process results in fusion of intraleukocyte granules (lysosomes) with the cell membrane. As a result, intralysosomal contents are discharged into the suspending medium. The rate of release of lysosomal enzymes, particularly β-glucuronidase and acid phosphatase, is taken as an estimate of the rate of degranulation. Nonspecific cell death or cytolysis can be estimated by measuring the discharge of lactate dehydrogenase (a nongranule enzyme) into the medium. This assay system has been used to demonstrate retardation in the degranulation rate by neutrophils from patients with chronic granulomatous disease.

TESTS FOR INTRACELLULAR KILLING

The primary function of the neutrophil in host resistance is intracellular killing of microorganisms. This final stage of phagocytosis is dependent on the successful completion of the preceding steps: motility, recognition, ingestion, and degranulation. A variety of intraleukocytic systems make up the antimicrobial armamentarium of the neutrophil (Table 13–10). Obviously, a defect in intracellular killing could be the result of any one or a combination of these functions. However, in clinical practice 2 assays have received widespread use, ie, the Nitro Blue Tetrazolium dye reduction test and the intraleukocytic killing test. It is hoped that specific metabolic and antimicrobial assays for other intraleukocytic events will also become available in the future.

Nitro Blue Tetrazolium Dye Reduction Test

Nitro Blue Tetrazolium (NBT) is a clear, yellow, water-soluble compound that forms formazan, a deep blue dye, on reduction. Neutrophils can reduce the

dye following ingestion of latex or other particles subsequent to the metabolic burst generated through the hexose monophosphate shunt. The reduced dye can be easily measured photometrically after extraction from neutrophils with the organic solvent pyridine. The reduction of NBT to a blue substance thus forms the basis of the quantitative NBT test. The precise mechanism of NBT reduction is not known, but the phenomenon is closely allied to metabolic events in the respiratory burst following ingestion, including increased hexose monophosphate shunt activity, increased oxygen consumption, and increased hydrogen peroxide and superoxide radical formation. Since the generation of reducing activity in intact neutrophils parallels the metabolic activities following ingestion, NBT reduction is a useful means of assaying overall metabolic integrity of phagocytosing neutrophils. Failure of NBT dye reduction is a consistent and diagnostically important laboratory abnormality in chronic granulomatous disease. Neutrophils from these patients fail to kill certain intracellular microbes and fail to generate H_2O_2 or the superoxide radical.

Quantitative NBT Test

Isolated neutrophils are incubated in a balanced salt solution with latex particles and NBT. After 15 minutes of incubation at 37 °C, the reduced dye (blue formazan) is extracted with pyridine and measured spectrophotometrically at 515 nm. The change in absorbance between cultures of cells that actively phagocytose latex particles and those that do not is taken as an index of neutrophil function. The test is strikingly abnormal in chronic granulomatous disease (see Chapter 22). Various modifications of the quantitative NBT test have been developed as screening tests for chronic granulomatous disease. Prominent among these are so-called slide tests in which neutrophils, latex, and NBT are placed in a drop on a glass slide and the reduction to blue formazan assayed under the microscope. It can be performed on a single drop of blood, but abnormal results should be confirmed with the more precise quantitative method described above.

Chemiluminescence

Neutrophils emit small amounts of electromagnetic radiation following ingestion of microorganisms. This energy can be detected as light by sensitive photomultiplier tubes, such as those in liquid scintillation counters. During the respiratory burst, H_2O_2, superoxide radicals, and singlet oxygen are generated. Singlet oxygen, a highly unstable and reactive species, combines with bacteria or other intralysosomal elements to form electronically unstable carboxyl groups. As these groups relax to ground state, light energy is emitted. This entire process has been termed **chemiluminescence** and forms the basis of an important assay of neutrophil function. Similar to NBT, it requires all steps prior to actual bacterial killing to be intact. Recent studies show a precise correlation between light emissions and microbicidal activity. The oxidative steps in the biochemical pathways present in the neutrophil generate the chemiluminescence, which is easily detected in a liquid scintillation spectrometer with the coincidence circuit excluded.

In the test, neutrophils are incubated in clear, colorless balanced salt solution in the presence of an ingestible particle, eg, latex or zymosan, in a scintillation vial. Luminol, an intermediate fluorescent compound, can be added to intensify the light emissions. The emission of photons of light is measured as cpm in a scintillation counter over the next 10 minutes at 2-minute intervals. Studies with this technique have revealed markedly reduced chemiluminescence in chronic granulomatous disease (patients and carriers) and in myeloperoxidase-deficient patients. This method appears to be somewhat more sensitive than the quantitative NBT test and can probably be performed on very small numbers of cells. Newer methods employ a sample of whole blood, greatly simplifying the procedure by obviating the granulocyte separation steps. Many laboratories are substituting it for NBT reduction as a screening test for neutrophil dysfunction and in detection of carriers of chronic granulomatous disease.

Flow Cytometry

The neutrophil oxidative burst that follows ingestion produces hydrogen peroxide, which oxidizes various intracellular components. If 2′, 7′-dichlorofluorescein diacetate, a small nonpolar dye, is present during incubation of neutrophils, it is cleaved by esterases and trapped inside the cell. Hydrogen peroxide oxidizes the compound to fluorescent dichlorofluorescein, which can be easily detected by flow cytometry in a gated population of neutrophils.

This technique allows rapid, sensitive, and rela-

tively reproducible detection of patients with chronic granulomatous disease and generally allows discrimination between carriers and normal subjects. It has largely replaced the quantitative NBT tests in many laboratories.

Neutrophil Microbicidal Assay

Many strains of bacteria and fungi are effectively engulfed and killed by human neutrophils in vitro. Assuming that all of the stages of the phagocytic process that precede killing within the phagolysosome are intact, microbicidal assays are extremely useful tests for neutrophil function. As an example, the bactericidal capacity of neutrophils for the common test strain 502A of *S aureus* will be described in some detail.

Bacteria are cultured overnight in nutrient broth to make certain that they will be in a logarithmic growth phase. They are then diluted to give about 5 bacteria per neutrophil in the final test. Neutrophils are separated from whole heparinized blood by dextran sedimentation and lysis of erythrocytes with 0.84% NH_4Cl. Opsonin is provided as a 1:1 mixture of

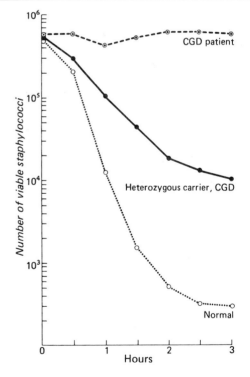

Figure 13–12. Bactericidal assay of granulocytes. Curves represent the number of viable intracellular organisms that survive after being ingested by granulocytes. Note the marked decline in bacterial survival in normal cells compared with reduced to absent killing by cells from patients and relatives with CGD (chronic granulomatous disease).

pooled frozen serum (−70 °C) and serum from freshly clotted blood. Bacteria, neutrophils, and opsonin are incubated in tightly capped test tubes and tumbled end over end at 37 °C. An aliquot of the entire mixture is sampled at zero time. After 30 minutes of incubation, antibiotics are added to kill extracellular bacteria. Aliquots of neutrophils with ingested organisms are sampled at 30, 60, and 120 minutes. Intracellular microorganisms are liberated by lysis of neutrophils by sterile water and the number of *viable* intracellular bacteria is estimated by serial dilutions and plating of lysed leukocytes. Results plotted as in Fig 13–12 show that normal neutrophils result in an almost 2-log reduction in viable intracellular *S aureus* cells 1 hour after incubation. Killing is virtually absent in cells from patients with chronic granulomatous disease and intermediate in heterozygous carriers.

By varying the test organism or the source of opsonin, this assay can be effectively used to measure a wide range of microbial activities and serum-related defects. Obviously, falsely "normal" killing will be

Table 13–11. Disorders of neutrophil function.

Leukocyte adherence deficiency
Chronic granulomatous disease (X-linked or autosomal recessive)
Job's syndrome
Chédiak-Higashi syndrome
Myeloperoxidase deficiency
Glucose-6-phosphate dehydrogenase deficiency
Acute leukemia
Down's syndrome
Premature infants
Transient neutrophil dysfunction
　Acute infections
　Ataxia-telangiectasia
　Cryoglobulinemia

the interpretation of the results if cells fail to ingest organisms normally. Thus, an independent assay for microbial ingestion must be performed prior to the neutrophil microbicidal test.

Some diseases with defective microbicidal activity demonstrable with this assay are listed in Table 13–11. For further details, see Chapter 22.

REFERENCES

General

Hudson L, Hay FC: *Practical Immunology,* 3rd ed. Blackwell, 1989.

Mishell BB, Shiigi SM: *Selected Methods in Cellular Immunology.* Freeman, 1980.

Rose NR, Conway de Macario E, Fahey JL (editors): *Manual of Clinical Laboratory Immunology,* 4th ed. American Society for Microbiology, 1992.

Virella G, Patrick CC, Goust JM: Diagnostic evaluation of lymphocyte functions of cell mediated immunity. *Immunol Series* 1993;**58**:291

Weir DM et al (editors): *Handbook of Experimental Immunology,* 4th ed. 4 vols. Blackwell, 1986.

Delayed Hypersensitivity Skin Tests

Ahmed RA, Blose DA: Delayed hypersensitivity skin testing: A review. *Arch Dermatol* 1983;**119**:934.

Frazer IH et al: Assessment of delayed-type hypersensitivity in man. A comparison of the "multitest" and conventional intradermal injection of six antigens. *Clin Exp Immunol* 1985;**35**:182.

Knapp W et al: *Leukocyte Typing IV.* Oxford, 1989.

Palmer DL, Reed WP: Delayed hypersensitivity skin testing: 1. Response rates in a hospitalized population. 2. Clinical correlates and anergy. *J Infect Dis* 1974; **130**:132, 138.

Assays for Human Lymphocytes & Monocytes

Adams DO, Edelson PJ, Koren HS (editors): *Methods for Studying Mononuclear Phagocytes.* Academic Press, 1981.

Bray RA, Landay AL: Identification and functional characterization of mononuclear cells by flow cytometry. *Arch Pathol Lab Med* 1989;**113**:579.

Fletcher MA, Klimas N, Morgan R: Lymphocyte proliferation. Chap 32, p 213, in: *Manual of Clinical Laboratory Immunology,* 4th ed. Rose NR, Conway de Macario E, Fahey JL (editors). American Society for Microbiology, 1992.

Smith D, DeShazo RD: Delayed hypersensitivity skin testing. Chap 30, p 202, in: *Manual of Clinical Laboratory Immunology,* 4th ed. Rose NR, Conway de Macario E, Fahey JL (editors). American Society for Microbiology, 1992.

Lymphocyte Activation

Stobo JD: Mitogens. Page 55 in: *Clinical Immunobiology.* Vol. 4, Bach FH, Good RA (editors). Academic Press, 1980.

Weiss A, Imboden J: Cell surface molecules and early events involved in T lymphocyte activation. *Adv Immunol* 1987;**4**:1.

Flow Cytometry & Cell Sorting

Braylan RC, Benson NA: Flow cytometric analysis of lymphomas. *Arch Pathol Lab Med* 1989;**113**:627.

Fleisher TA, Hagengruber C, Marti GE: Immunophenotyping of normal lymphocytes. *Pathol Immunopathol Res* 1988;**7**:305.

Keren DF: *Flow Cytometry in Clinical Diagnosis.* ASCP Press, 1989.

Kipps TJ, Meisenholder G, Robbins BA: New developments in flow cytometric analysis of lymphocyte markers. *Clin Lab Med* 1992;**2**:237.

McCarthy RC, Fetterhoff TJ: Issues of quality assurance in clinical flow cytometry. *Arch Pathol Lab Med* 1989;**113**:658.

Ryan DH, Fallon MA, Horan PK: Flow cytometry in the clinical laboratory. *Clin Chem Acta* 1988;**171:**125.

Neutrophil Function

Boxer LA, Morganroth ML: Neutrophil function disorders. *Disease-a-Month* 1987;**33:**681.

Horwitz MA: Phagocytosis of microorganisms. *Rev Infect Dis* 1982;**4:**104.

Lehrer RI et al: Neutrophils and host defense. *Ann Intern Med* 1988;**109:**127.

Synderman R, Gaetze EJ: Molecular and cellular mechanisms of leukocyte chemotaxis. *Science* 1981;**213:**830.

Wade BH, Mandell GL: Polymorphonuclear leukocytes: Dedicated professional phagocytes. *Am J Med* 1983;**74:**686.

Yang KD, Hill HR: Neutrophil function disorders: Pathophysiology prevention and therapy. *J Pediatr* 1991;**119:**343.

14

Molecular Genetic Techniques for Clinical Analysis of the Immune System

Tristram G. Parslow, MD, PhD

Genetic information in humans and most other organisms is encoded in the linear sequence of 4 nucleotide bases (abbreviated A, T, G, and C) along the strands of a DNA molecule. The sequence of the human genome is more than 3 billion DNA bases long, is divided among 23 chromosomes, and is present twice in each diploid nucleus. The human genome contains an estimated 100,000 genes, each comprising, on average, no more than a few thousand bases of coding sequence that specify a particular protein or structural RNA. The coding information of a typical human gene is rarely contained in a single, uninterrupted stretch of DNA but, instead, is divided into shorter coding segments called **exons**, which are separated by noncoding regions called **introns**. Individual genes are also widely separated from one another along the DNA, with noncoding sequences in between. Altogether, coding sequences are thought to make up only 5–10% of the human genome, and the function of the remaining sequences is, for the most part, unknown. The complete sequences of many human genes have been determined (by using techniques that lie outside the scope of this chapter), but the sequences that are known at present amount to only a tiny fraction of the entire genome.

During the past 2 decades, advances in nucleic acid chemistry and recombinant DNA technology have made it possible to analyze individual genes rapidly and precisely. The techniques involved are now commonplace in research and are gradually being adapted for use in clinical laboratories as well. DNA offers numerous advantages as a substrate for clinical analysis: it is a remarkably sturdy biomolecule that is fairly easy to handle; it can be obtained from either fresh or fixed tissue or blood specimens; and it can be manipulated and dissected in ways that are not possible with proteins. Most importantly, access to the information contained in DNA enables us to diagnose and investigate many disease processes at the most fundamental level. This chapter will summarize the basic concepts and practical techniques for analyzing

DNA from clinical specimens, along with some specialized applications to the immune system. At the end of the chapter, related techniques for studying cellular RNA are briefly discussed.

NUCLEIC ACID PROBES

Underlying the complexity of DNA is a simple but profound symmetry. Each DNA molecule is composed of two linear strands of bases, which are bound to one another side-by-side and coiled to form a double helix (Fig 14–1). The 2 strands are held together by hydrogen bonding between adjacent bases: A on one strand always binds to T on the other, and similar binding occurs between G and C. In normal DNA, the 2 strands are said to be **complementary** in that every base is appropriately paired to the corresponding position on the opposite strand. Bases within a strand are held together by strong covalent bonds, but the basepairing bonds between strands are relatively weak, so that the two strands can easily be separated ("**denatured**" or "melted apart") by heat or alkaline pH. When slowly returned to physiologic conditions, the strands reanneal spontaneously and in perfect alignment to re-form the original double-stranded helix.

This spontaneous pairing between complementary strands provides the basis for many of the techniques that are used to detect and characterize genes. These techniques employ short strands of known sequence as **probes** to detect strands with the complementary sequence. Probes of any desired sequence can readily be obtained in abundant quantities and at very high purity: single DNA strands up to about 100 bases long are easily prepared by using automated chemical synthesizers, whereas larger DNA sequences are generally introduced ("cloned") into bacteria to be replicated biologically. It is also possible to use probes made of RNA—a molecule that, for the purposes of this chapter, can be considered equivalent to single-

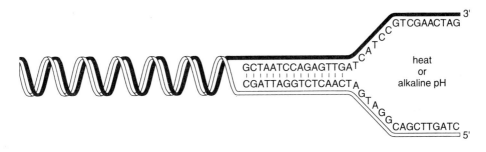

Figure 14–1. Structure of DNA. The molecule consists of 2 strands of covalently linked nucleotide bases, which are coiled around one another to form a double helix. The 2 strands are held together by relatively weak hydrogen bonds between bases. The strands will dissociate from one another when exposed to heat or alkaline pH but will spontaneously reassociate when returned to physiologic conditions.

stranded DNA—since these will also anneal specifically to a complementary DNA strand. RNA probes are most often prepared enzymatically by cloning the corresponding DNA sequence and using this as a template for in vitro transcription, ie, producing a complementary RNA strand from the template DNA.

Cellular DNA can be isolated by chemical extraction from a blood or tissue specimen followed by enzymatic treatment to remove traces of contaminating RNA or protein. Unless special precautions are taken, the extremely long strands of chromosomal DNA are usually sheared by mechanical forces into random fragments of roughly 50,000–100,000 bp during the purification process. To use a nucleic acid probe, this target DNA is first heated or exposed to alkali in order to separate the strands and then mixed with the labeled probe and returned to normal temperature and pH. As the molecules reassociate, some of the target strands will anneal (**"hybridize"**) to the probe rather than to the unlabeled complementary strand, forming labeled duplexes. To maximize the likelihood that a target strand will anneal to the probe rather than to its original partner, the hybridization reaction is usually carried out with a great molar excess of probe. The stability of the complex formed by a probe and its target is influenced by many factors, the most important of which are temperature, salt concentration, the length and base composition of the probe, and the presence of any mismatched bases. Under the conditions used in most assays, 2 strands must share at least 16–20 consecutive bases of perfect complementarity to form a stable hybrid. The probability of such a match occurring by chance is less than one in a billion (10^{-9}). Thus, nucleic acid probes possess an extraordinary degree of specificity: a typical probe is capable of recognizing and binding selectively to a single copy of its complementary sequence among the 3 billion bp in the human genome. DNA or RNA probes can easily by tagged with radioisotopes, fluorochromes, or enzymatic markers prior to use

(Fig 14–2) and can then act as "molecular stains" that recognize and bind only to the exact complementary sequence.

HYBRIDIZATION ASSAYS

Several different methods can be used to test whether a DNA specimen contains sequences complementary to a particular probe. One common approach takes advantage of the fact that, under certain conditions (eg, when exposed to ultraviolet light or when heated in the presence of high salt), DNA strands can be made to bind tightly onto nylon or nitrocellulose membranes. In a procedure called **dot blot hybridization** (Fig 14–3A), a solution of target DNA is denatured, spotted onto the surface of such a membrane, and then treated so that the separated DNA strands adhere irreversibly to the membrane. When immobilized in this manner, the target strands remain accessible on the membrane surface but are prevented from reannealing with one another. The membrane is then incubated with labeled probes under conditions where the probe does not adhere to the membrane but may hybridize with the target strands. Afterward, the filter is washed extensively to remove unhybridized probe. Any probe that has hybridized to the bound DNA can then be detected by autoradiography or enzymatic assay, depending on the particular label that it carries.

In an alternative approach, called a **nuclease protection** assay, target and probe DNAs are denatured, allowed to anneal together in solution, and then treated with an enzyme that specifically cleaves single-stranded but not double-stranded DNA. A probe will survive this enzymatic digestion only if it has become stably hybridized to the target DNA (Fig 14–3B).

The interaction between probe and target occurs with one-to-one stoichiometry, and this tends to limit the sensitivity of hybridization assays. One way of

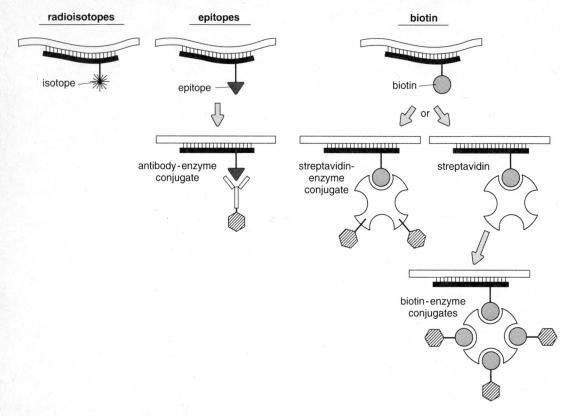

radioisotopes **epitopes** **biotin**

isotope

epitope

biotin

antibody-enzyme
conjugate

streptavidin-
enzyme
conjugate

streptavidin

or

biotin-enzyme
conjugates

Figure 14–2. Some methods for labeling and detecting DNA or RNA probes. Radioisotopes, small epitopes, or biotin can be incorporated covalently into one or more positions in a probe at the time of synthesis. The most commonly used radioisotopes for this purpose are ^{32}P and ^{35}S, which can be detected by autoradiography or scintillation counting. Probes labeled with epitopes or biotin can be detected by secondary labeling with an enzyme conjugated to a specific antibody or to the polyvalent biotin-binding protein streptavidin. One variation on the latter technique uses unconjugated streptavidin alone, which is then detected by binding of a biotin-enzyme conjugate. The enzyme used most commonly in these procedures is alkaline phosphatase, which can readily be assayed by its ability to generate chromogenic or chemiluminescent products.

maximizing the signal obtained is to incorporate multiple labels into a single probe, such as by radioactively labeling many bases in the probe (Fig 14–4). It may also be appropriate to use multiple probes that each recognize adjacent regions of a longer target sequence or to attach secondary probes onto a long, unhybridized "tail" on the primary probe (Fig 14–4). Still another approach is to use probes that form polyvalent complexes with an enzyme or fluorochrome marker, similar to those used in immunohistochemistry (see Chapter 12). For example, hybrids containing a probe that has been labeled with biotin can first be incubated with the polyvalent biotin-binding protein streptavidin and then secondarily tagged with many copies of a biotinylated marker enzyme (Fig 14–2). The use of enzymatic detection systems that produce colored or chemiluminescent products can itself greatly amplify the signal obtained. Even when such measures are taken, however, about 10^4–10^5 copies of

a target sequence must usually be present in a sample to be detectable by routine hybridization.

SOUTHERN BLOT

The simplest hybridization assays, such as the dot blot assay, indicate whether a particular sequence is present in the target DNA and may also give an estimate of its abundance. These assays are rarely used clinically, because easier and more sensitive tests can provide the same information (see Target Amplification Techniques, below). However, nucleic acid probes offer special advantages when they are used in conjunction with **restriction enzymes,** a class of bacterial enzymes that cut both strands of a linear DNA molecule at specific short recognition sequences, usually 4–6 bp long. For example, the enzyme *Eco*RI cuts only within the sequence GAATTC, whereas the

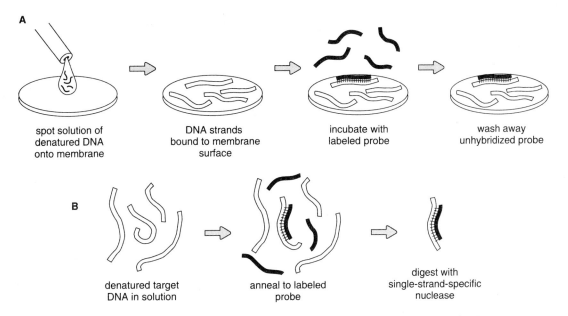

Figure 14–3. Two simple hybridization assays using nucleic acid probes. ***A:*** In the dot blot assay, denatured target DNA is attached to the surface of a nylon or nitrocellulose membrane and then incubated with a solution of labeled probe. ***B:*** In the nuclease protection assay, the reaction between probe and denatured target DNA takes place in solution; probes that have annealed to a target strand are detected by their ability to resist digestion by an enzyme (such as nuclease S1) that specifically digests single-stranded but not double-stranded nucleic acids.

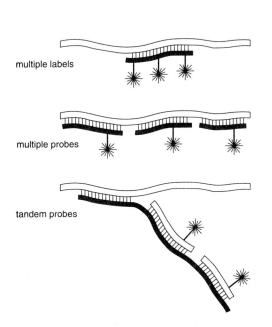

Figure 14–4. Some approaches for increasing the sensitivity of nucleic acid hybridization assays. These can be used singly or in combination.

enzyme *Bam*HI cleaves only GGATCC. Each restriction enzyme therefore cleaves long target DNA molecules into specific smaller segments called **restriction fragments,** whose number and length are determined by the sequence of the substrate DNA.

Because of the enormous size and complexity of the human genome, cleaving human DNA with a restriction enzyme yields millions of unique restriction fragments ranging up to tens of thousands of bases long. Nevertheless, the fragment that carries any particular gene can readily be identified, provided that a DNA probe complementary to the gene is available. The technique used for this purpose (Fig 14–5A) is called the **Southern blot,** after its inventor, E. M. Southern. DNA extracted from a tissue or blood specimen is first cleaved with one or more restriction enzymes, and the resulting DNA fragments are then subjected to electrophoresis through an agarose gel, which separates them according to length. Afterward, the gel is immersed in alkali solution to melt apart the complementary strands of each fragment. A sheet of nylon or nitrocellulose is then pressed firmly against the gel; the denatured DNA fragments bind tightly to this sheet and are drawn out of the gel. When the sheet is peeled away, it retains on its surface the immobilized DNA fragments, still arranged according to length as they had been in the gel but now exposed and accessible to further analysis. The sheet is then incubated with the labeled probe, which binds only to

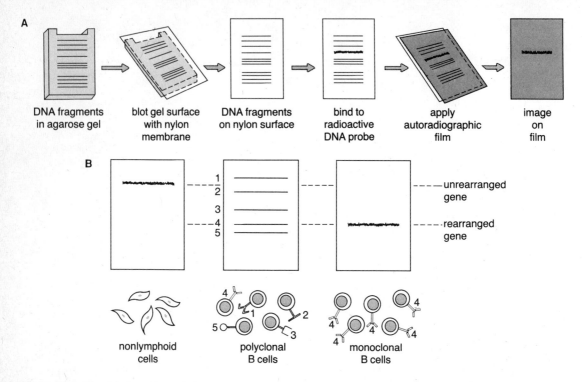

Figure 14–5. The Southern blot technique, and an application of this technique to determining clonality of lymphoid cell populations. **A:** The blotting technique is described in the text; it can be used to determine the size of DNA restriction fragments that encompass a specific gene. **B:** DNA rearrangement in lymphocytes alters the sizes of fragments bearing the immunoglobulin or T-cell receptor genes: the sizes of the rearranged fragments are characteristic of each B cell or T cell clone. This provides a means of detecting B or T cells and of assessing the clonal composition of lymphoid populations. The approach is illustrated for B cells by using an immunoglobulin gene. DNA isolated from nonlymphoid cells contains only unrearranged immunoglobulin genes, whereas DNA from normal lymphocyte populations reveals many different rearranged genes—one from each of the many independent B cell clones. Detection of only a single rearranged gene suggests that a lymphocyte population is monoclonal and therefore possibly malignant.

the fragment bearing its complementary sequence. Unbound probe is washed away, and the location of the remaining hybridized probe is determined by virtue of the label that it carries. The size of the bound target fragment can then be deduced from its location on the membrane, as this corresponds to the distance it migrated in the agarose gel.

The Southern blot reveals not only the presence of a particular sequence but also the size of the restriction fragment on which it lies. This size, in turn, is determined by the distribution of nearby restriction sites and so reflects the local DNA sequence.

GENE REARRANGEMENT ASSAY FOR LYMPHOCYTE CLONALITY

If all the cells in a population contain identical DNA, the restriction fragment carrying any given gene will have the same length in every cell, and all of these fragments will appear together as a single band on a Southern blot. This is the case for most cellular genes, including the immunoglobulin (Ig) and T cell receptor (TCR) genes of nonlymphoid cells. In lymphocytes, however, the Ig and TCR genes undergo specific rearrangements (see Chapter 7), which markedly alter the DNA sequences in and around these loci. Such rearrangements can be detected on the Southern blot by a shift in the size of the restriction fragment that carries an Ig or TCR gene. Moreover, because the size of the shifted fragment depends on the exact rearrangement that has occurred, it represents a unique and characteristic property of each lymphocyte clone—a molecular fingerprint that can be used to distinguish one lymphoid clone from another.

This provides a powerful means of estimating the clonal composition of lymphocyte populations (Fig 14–5B). In normal polyclonal lymphocyte populations, each of the innumerable clones contributes its own distinctively sized Ig or TCR fragment, but none of these is abundant enough to be detectable. Only when large numbers of clonally related cells are present do the rearranged genes appear in sufficient quantity to produce a detectable band. The presence of abnormally sized Ig or TCR bands on the Southern blot thus suggests the presence of a predominant clone of lymphoid cells, and this, in an appropriate setting, can be taken as evidence of lymphoid malignancy.

By using the Southern blot assay, clonal rearrangements of the Ig heavy-chain genes can be found in the neoplastic B cells in essentially all cases of B cell lymphoma regardless of histologic type. The clinical utility of this approach is somewhat limited, however, because B cell clonality can often be assessed more easily and cheaply by comparing the ratio of kappa (κ) and lambda (λ) light-chain proteins, using immunohistochemical stains (see Chapters 12 and 13). Nevertheless, the rearrangement assay is invaluable for demonstrating clonality in cases when malignant B cells either fail to express Ig protein or are heavily contaminated with polyclonal lymphocytes. Ig heavy-chain gene rearrangements are usually demonstrable in the lymphoid blast crisis of chronic myelogenous leukemia, in hairy cell leukemia, in "non-T, non-B" acute lymphoblastic leukemia, and in most null large cell lymphomas (see Chapter 45).

The analysis of TCR rearrangements has even greater potential usefulness, since no other practical method is available for assessing T cell clonality. For technical reasons, most clinical assays focus on the TCR β chain genes, which have been found to be clonally rearranged in nearly all cases of T cell leukemia and lymphoma, including plaque- or tumor-stage mycosis fungoides, Sézary syndrome, and adult T cell leukemia/lymphoma. The assay is especially useful for distinguishing reactive lymphadenopathy from T cell lymphoma (see Chapter 45).

Although Ig and TCR gene rearrangements are generally confined to the B and T cell lineages, respectively, the correlation is not absolute. Roughly 15% of poorly differentiated lymphoid malignancies harbor rearrangements of both TCR β and Ig heavy-chain genes—an example of lineage infidelity. Ig light-chain rearrangements, which occur later in normal ontogeny than heavy-chain rearrangements (see Chapter 7), are more specific for the B lineage but less sensitive for detecting clonality. Absence of any rearrangements argues strongly that a tumor is not of lymphoid origin. Specimens from separate lymphomatous lesions in a single patient usually show identical rearrangements. Because the rearrangements in recurrent cancers are identical to those seen prior to treatment, the Southern blot technique offers special advantages in monitoring remission and recurrence, since it may reveal persistence of a malignant clone that is not yet detectable morphologically.

The Southern assay for lymphocyte clonality has several limitations. Although it is potentially more sensitive than histologic examination (a clonal subpopulation can be detected even when diluted 100-fold with polyclonal cells), this degree of sensitivity requires prior knowledge of the position of an abnormal band on the gel. Faint bands seen in a case being analyzed de novo must be interpreted with great care, since they may represent technical artifacts. To minimize degradation of the DNA, fresh or frozen tissue must be used and processing must begin promptly. The method has been applied successfully to specimens obtained during fine-needle biopsies of lymph nodes, but obtaining sufficient DNA for a complete analysis generally requires a blood or tissue specimen that contains at least 25 million leukocytes.

It is also important to recognize that the TCR β locus includes far fewer V gene segments than are found in the Ig loci. This greatly increases the probability that unrelated T cell clones will coincidentally have the same rearrangement. Moreover, benign inflammatory responses to some antigens have been shown to use a particular TCR β V region preferentially and so might appear monoclonal by this assay. These facts may ultimately limit the validity of TCR rearrangements for diagnosing T cell neoplasia. More fundamentally, it is not clear that monoclonality signifies malignancy in every case. Therefore, as with any other single test, results from gene rearrangement analyses must always be interpreted in the context of all other available clinical and laboratory data.

IN SITU HYBRIDIZATION

Another specialized hybridization technique, called **in situ hybridization,** is based on the ability of labeled probes to bind target DNA in thin tissue sections or cytologic smears (Fig 14–6). This technique reveals not only the presence of a specific sequence but also its spatial distribution within tissues or individual cells. In brief, cells or tissues attached to the surface of a glass microscope slide are fixed, incubated with a labeled probe, and then washed to remove unbound probe. The specimen is then coated with a thin layer of photographic emulsion or chromogenic substrate that will reveal the location of any bound radiolabeled or enzymatically labeled probe. The assay is technically arduous and not very sensitive. It is sometimes used to detect abundant RNA species or viral DNA, which may be present in large amounts in a single infected cell. However, it is not well suited for examining most human genes, only 2 copies of which are present in each diploid cell.

TARGET AMPLIFICATION TECHNIQUES: POLYMERASE CHAIN REACTION

In the past, a major drawback of hybridization assays was their need for relatively large amounts of

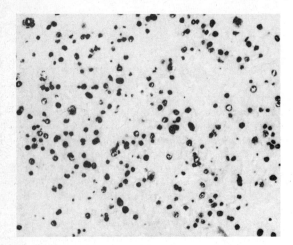

Figure 14–6. Detection of viral DNA in human cells by in situ hybridization. A lymph node biopsy specimen from a patient with Hodgkin's disease was fixed onto the surface of a glass slide and then hybridized with a biotinylated nucleic acid probe specific for sequences from Epstein-Barr virus. Hybridized probe was detected with streptavidin-conjugated alkaline phosphatase. The nuclei of cells that harbor the viral DNA stain darkly. (Courtesy of Lawrence M. Weiss.)

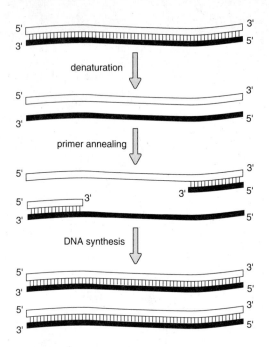

Figure 14–7. One cycle of DNA amplification by PCR. Each cycle consists of sequential heat denaturation, primer annealing, and DNA synthesis steps. Two different primers are used, and must be oriented as shown with respect to one another. DNA synthesis is performed with a thermostable DNA polymerase and proceeds unidirectionally from each primer. After one cycle, the region between the primers has been duplicated. If the process is repeated, the number of copies of this region increases exponentially, doubling with each cycle until the supply of primers is exhausted.

sample DNA to compensate for their low sensitivity. This problem has been surmounted in recent years by the development of powerful enzymatic techniques that can exponentially replicate specific DNA sequences in the test tube. With these techniques, it is now possible to analyze vanishingly small samples that initially contain fewer than 10 copies of the sequence of interest. The new methods take advantage of the chemical properties of nucleic acids and of highly specialized enzymes that can repair and replicate DNA in vitro.

Every single-stranded DNA molecule has 2 ends, called the 5′ and 3′ ends, whose chemical and biologic properties differ. In double-stranded DNA, the 2 strands are always antiparallel (ie, their 3′ and 5′ ends are in opposite orientation to one another). Cellular enzymes known as **DNA polymerases,** which elongate these strands during DNA replication, can do so only by adding new nucleotide bases sequentially onto the 3′ end of a preexisting strand, which serves as a **primer.** Moreover, most DNA polymerases will function only when the primer is annealed to a longer second strand, which serves as a **template** for DNA synthesis; the enzyme adds nucleotides in a sequence complementary to that of the template, producing a basepaired double helix.

These properties of DNA polymerases are exploited in a technique called the **polymerase chain reaction (PCR),** which can be used to replicate a particular region of target DNA selectively in vitro (Fig 14–7). Beginning with sample DNA from a very small number of cells, PCR can be used to synthesize multiple copies of a particular gene or gene segment that is present in those cells. PCR works best for copying regions less than about 2000 bp, and the DNA sequences flanking the region of interest must be known in advance. To use PCR, 2 short DNA primers (usually at least 16–20 bases long) are synthesized whose sequences are complementary to those of the flanking regions but on opposite strands; the 2 primers must be chosen so that their 3′ ends are directed toward one another (Fig 14–7). A vast molar excess of these primers is added to the sample DNA, which is then denatured by heating and allowed to anneal with the primers. A bacterial DNA polymerase is then added, which initiates synthesis at the 3′ end of each annealed primer and produces a new strand complementary to a portion of the adjacent template strand. Synthesis is continued for long enough that the newly synthesized strands extend through the entire region of interest. When the mixture is then denatured and reannealed again, each newly synthesized strand provides a new template for synthesis from the opposite primer. By repeated cycles of denaturation, annealing, and synthesis, the region between the 2 primers is amplified exponentially, with the number of double-stranded copies of this region doubling at each cycle. Under ideal conditions, 220,000 copies should theoretically be produced from a single original after only 20 cycles of PCR. This is enough copies to allow detection by routine hybridization techniques.

Automated, programmable instruments that can carry out the repeated thermal cycles necessary for PCR and that can accommodate multiple samples simultaneously are now widely available. The procedure is usually performed with **thermostable** DNA polymerases, isolated from thermophilic bacteria, since these can better withstand exposure to high temperature. PCR is widely used to facilitate detection of minute amounts of viral or bacterial DNA in clinical specimens, since it can often identify these microorganisms much more rapidly than conventional culture techniques. The technique can also be used to detect specific point mutations in human genes, provided that the approximate site of mutation is known. One limiting feature of this approach arises from the fact that the bacterial polymerases frequently make errors when synthesizing new strands and so can introduce mutations that are not present in the original sample.

Other strategies for exponentially amplifying DNA have been described. For example, the **ligase chain reaction (LCR)** uses DNA-repairing enzymes, called **DNA ligases,** whose function is to link preexisting DNA strands together by covalently joining the 5′ end of one to the 3′ end of another. Ligases will link 2 strands together only if they are already basepaired to a complementary strand that holds them in precise end-to-end alignment. LCR uses one pair of oligonucleotide strands whose sequences exactly match the 2 halves of the sequence of interest, along with a second pair of oligonucleotides whose sequences are complementary to the first (Fig 14–8). When denatured and allowed to reanneal to a target DNA, each pair of oligonucleotides binds to one of the target strands, and they are then permanently linked together by DNA ligase. At each subsequent cycle of denaturation and annealing, each linked pair of oligonucleotides can bring together the opposite pair, so that the number of linked pairs doubles with each cycle. LCR is usually performing with thermostable bacterial ligases and is somewhat more rapid than PCR, since no new DNA synthesis is required. The primers used are relatively short, and this severely limits the size of the target sequence that can be examined. However, since even a single base mismatch can prevent these short primers from annealing, the

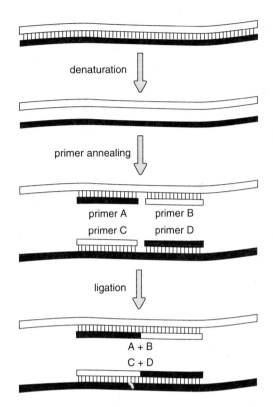

Figure 14–8. One cycle of DNA amplification by LCR. The process is similar to PCR, except that 4 different primers are required and a thermostable DNA ligase is used in place of DNA polymerase. With each cycle, pairs of primers bind to the target sequence and are then linked covalently by the ligase. In each subsequent cycle, a linked primer pair serves to bind the other 2 primers, so that the number of linked copies increases exponentially, doubling at each cycle.

LCR is very well suited for detecting point mutations in target DNA.

METHODS OF ANALYZING RNA

DNA and RNA probes can also be used to analyze the RNAs from a clinical specimen, and this can be highly advantageous for some purposes. Whereas DNA analysis can reveal the presence and structure of a particular gene sequence, RNA analysis indicates whether, and how strongly, it is being expressed. Another important advantage is sensitivity: a cell that expresses a particular gene often contains hundreds of copies of the RNA derived from it, and this RNA may be readily detectable even though the gene itself is not. Techniques such as in situ or dot blot hybridization can easily be adapted to search for specific sequences in cellular RNA. In a modified form of the Southern blot, called the **Northern blot,** a mixture of cellular RNAs can be separated according to length by agarose gel electrophoresis, transferred to the surface of a nylon or nitrocellulose membrane, and then hybridized to a labeled nucleic acid probe to determine the size and abundance of any particular RNA species.

However, RNA analysis also has some inherent limitations. Because expression of a given RNA varies widely depending on the lineage and physiologic state of a cell, it is critical to sample the right tissues at the right time. RNA is less durable than DNA (for example, it degrades rapidly and irreversibly at alkaline pH) and must be handled with correspondingly greater care. In addition, the number and types of enzymes that are available to manipulate RNA sequences are very limited. For some applications, it is necessary to begin by making a DNA copy of the target RNA, which then serves as the substrate for further analysis. For example, PCR amplification of RNA is carried out by a 2-stage procedure known as **reverse transcriptase PCR (RT-PCR).** The first stage employs an enzyme called reverse transcriptase, which synthesizes a DNA strand complementary to the RNA of interest by using one of the PCR primers as its primer. This complementary DNA is then used, in the second stage, as the starting material for PCR amplification by a conventional thermostable DNA polymerase.

OVERVIEW & PROSPECTS

Tests based on nucleic acid technology are a relatively new addition to the armamentarium of the clinical immunology laboratory, and it is not yet clear to what extent they will supplement or replace conventional assays. They are particularly well suited to the detection of viruses and other microorganisms in tissue specimens, since such organisms can often be recognized and positively identified by their unique RNA or DNA sequences much more quickly and inexpensively than by culture. Hence, PCR-based tests have already assumed an important role in microbiologic diagnosis, and it seems likely that this role will increase in the future. Immunologically important organisms that are currently assayed in this manner include Epstein-Barr virus, human immunodeficiency viruses, and human T-cell leukemia viruses (see Chapters 48 and 52).

DNA-based assays are also very useful for detecting large-scale chromosomal deletions or rearrangements that occur at fairly constant locations in the genome and that characterize several types of hematologic malignancies. Examples include the Philadelphia chromosome of chronic myelogenous leukemia, the t(14,18) of follicular lymphoma, and the t(8,14) and related anomalies of Burkitt's lymphoma (see Chapters 7 and 45). Detection of these rearrangements can be a useful adjunct in diagnosis and also provides a simple means to monitor disease progression or to search for minimal residual disease after therapy. The Southern blot assay for lymphocyte clonality has similar potential utility and may be especially useful for evaluating poorly differentiated malignancies; however, it is currently too labor-intensive and technically demanding to be adopted by many clinical laboratories. Clonality assays based on PCR technology are being developed. In addition, PCR, LCR, and related techniques can detect extremely subtle DNA anomalies, including single-base point mutations, and are likely to be used increasingly for the diagnosis of congenital immunodeficiencies and of hereditary predispositions to cancer or other disorders.

REFERENCES

Theory & Protocols

Barany F: Genetic disease detection and DNA amplification using cloned thermostable ligase. *Proc Natl Acad Sci USA* 1991;**88:**189.

Davey MP, Waldmann TA: Clonality and lymphoproliferative lesions. *N Engl J Med* 1986;**315:**509.

Eisenstein B: The polymerase chain reaction. A new method of using molecular genetics for medical diagnosis. *N Engl J Med* 1990;**322:**178.

Sambrook J, Fritsch EF, Maniatis T (editors): *Molecular Cloning: A Laboratory Manual,* 2nd ed. Cold Spring Harbor, 1989.

Southern EM: Detection of specific sequences among DNA fragments separated by gel electrophoresis. *J Mol Biol* 1975;**98:**503.

Specific Applications

Arnold A et al: Immunoglobulin-gene rearrangements as unique clonal markers in human lymphoid neoplasms. *N Engl J Med* 1983;**309:**1593.

Bakhshi A et al: Lymphoid blast crises of chronic myelogenous leukemia represent stages in the development of B-cell precursors. *N Engl J Med* 1983;**309:**826.

Cleary ML, Warnke R, Sklar J: Monoclonality of lymphoproliferative lesions in cardiac-transplant recipients. *N Engl J Med* 1984;**310:**477.

Cossman J et al: Gene rearrangements in the diagnosis of lymphoma/leukemia: Guidelines for use based on a multi-institutional study. *Am J Clin Pathol* 1991; **95:**347.

Flug F et al: T-cell receptor gene rearrangements as markers of lineage and clonality in T-cell neoplasms. *Proc Natl Acad Sci USA* 1985;**82:**3460.

Grody WW, Hilborne LH: Diagnostic applications of recombinant nucleic acid technology: Neoplastic disease. *Lab Med* 1992;**23:**19.

Reis MD et al: T-cell receptor and immunoglobulin gene rearrangements in lymphoproliferative disorders. *Adv Cancer Res* 1989;**52:**45.

Shibata D et al: Detection of specific t(14;18) chromosomal translocations in fixed tissues. *Hum Pathol* 1990;**21:**199.

Tawa A et al: Rearrangement of the T-cell receptor beta chain gene in non-T-cell non-B-cell acute lymphoblastic leukemia of childhood. *N Engl J Med* 1985;**313:**1033.

Waldmann TA: Rearrangements of genes for the antigen receptor on T cells as markers of lineage and clonality in human lymphoid neoplasms. *N Engl J Med* 1985;**313:**776.

Weiss LM et al: Clonal rearrangements of T-cell receptor genes in mycosis fungoides and dermatopathic lymphadenopathy. *N Engl J Med* 1985;**313:**539.

Weiss LM et al: Frequent immunoglobulin and T-cell receptor gene rearrangements in "histiocytic" neoplasms. *Am J Pathol* 1985;**121:**369.

Blood Banking & Immunohematology

Elizabeth Donegan, MD, & Edith L. Bossom, SBB

The ability to successfully transfuse whole blood, or more specific blood components, has saved countless lives and supported the advance of modern surgery and cancer chemotherapy. The first lifesaving transfusion was performed less than 200 years ago by James Blundell in 1818. Today, more than 22 million blood components, prepared from 14 million blood donations, are transfused in the USA annually. Transfusion is increasingly safe because blood group systems and their relationship to the immune response have been defined; techniques have been developed to separate, store, preserve, and test blood prior to infusion; and improved transfusion methods have been developed.

Nevertheless, transfusion continues to require the removal of blood from one human being for infusion into another. This "living transplant" carries with it the complexities of its human source and thereby brings with it the potential of untoward reaction in the recipient. Some risks of transfusion are now known, and others have yet to be described. Consequently, the need for transfusion must be judged carefully in light of these risks.

BLOOD GROUPS

The first blood group system was described at the turn of the twentieth century by Karl Landsteiner. He observed that erythrocytes from some individuals clumped when mixed with the serum of others but not with their own. Using this agglutination technique, he classified an individual's erythrocytes into 4 types: A, B, AB, and O. It is now recognized that A and B represent carbohydrate antigens on the erythrocyte. Group O individuals have neither of these antigens on their erythrocytes, whereas erythrocytes from AB individuals have both A and B antigens. The ABO system remains the most important blood group system for transfusion purposes.

Knowledge about blood groups has expanded to include a diverse and numerous array of antigenic determinants on erythrocytes. Today, more than 400 erythrocyte antigens belonging to 24 systems are known. Each blood group system has members; each member may be composed of one or more different antigens. Each antigen is controlled by one gene. The antigenic determinants of a group are produced either directly (for proteins) or indirectly (for carbohydrates) by alleles at a single gene locus or at a gene locus so closely linked to another that crossing over is extremely rare. For any antigen of a group, a single allele is present at that locus and others are therefore excluded. Antigens on erythrocyte surfaces are usually detected by reacting erythrocytes with known antisera. Since the genotype cannot be directly determined by measuring erythrocyte antigens, these tests define a phenotype. The number of antigenic determinants per erythrocyte and their ability to elicit an immune response vary from antigen to antigen.

ERYTHROCYTE ANTIGENS

H & ABO

Antigenic determinants of these systems are carbohydrate moieties whose specificity resides in the terminal sugars of an oligosaccharide. On erythrocyte and endothelial surfaces, most of the antigens are bound to glycoprotein, although some carbohydrate is also bound to membrane lipid. Genetic control is via the production of transferase enzymes that conjugate terminal sugars to a stem carbohydrate. The H and ABO systems have separate gene loci and are independent of one another (Fig 15–1).

The H gene codes for a fucosyl transferase enzyme that effects the addition of fucose to precursor chains and completes the stem chain. The last 3 sugars of the stem chain are called H substance. The *H* gene (hh) is rarely absent; this phenotype is called O_h or Bombay type. In the absence of a complete stem chain, addi-

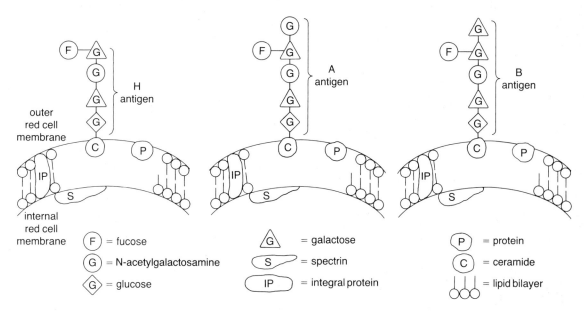

Figure 15–1. Chemical structure of A, B, and H blood groups.

tional sugars cannot be added despite the presence of A or B transferase, and high-titer anti-H is produced.

The ABO blood groups are determined by allelic genes A, B, and O (Table 15–1). The A group transferase conjugates N-acetylglucosamine to the completed stem chain. The B group transferase conjugates a terminal galactose. The O gene produces no transferase to modify the blood group substance (Fig 15–1).

Both groups A and B can be divided into subgroups. Eleven subgroups of A have been described, but most are rare. The most important are A_1 and A_2. Differences between subtypes of group A appear to be quantitative, ie, in the number of antigenic sites per erythrocyte surface. Of A blood, 78% is A_1 and 22% is A_2. A_1 cells carry about one million copies of A antigen on their surface, and A_2 cells carry 250,000 copies. AB blood can also be divided into A_1B and A_2B types. To detect weak variants of A, which may go undetected in routine testing, blood grouping often includes the use of O serum that contains an anti-A capable of detecting these weaker forms, eg, A_4. Although less frequently detected, subgroups of group B can also be distinguished. Subgroups of group B, like those of group A, demonstrate a continuum in the number of antigenic sites per erythrocyte surface.

The naturally occurring antibodies to groups A and B are thought to be stimulated by very common substances. Intestinal bacteria are known to have substances chemically similar to and therefore antigenically cross-reactive with A and B. These antibodies are first detected in children at 3–6 months of age, peaking at 5–10 years of age and falling with age and in some immunodeficiency states.

Two other systems directly interact with the ABO and H systems: Lewis and Secretor. Secretion of ABH substances in body fluids (saliva, sweat, milk, etc) is controlled by the allelic genes Se and se. These genes are independent of ABO and are inherited in a Mendelian dominant manner. Eighty percent of people are Se; they secrete Lewis and Sd antigens in addition to ABH substances. Typing of body fluids for these antigens has been useful in forensic investigations.

Rh

The Rhesus blood group system is second in importance only to the ABO system. Anti-Rh antibodies are the leading cause of hemolytic disease of the new-

Table 15–1. Routine ABO groupings.

			Frequency (%) in US Population			
Blood Group	Erythrocyte Antigens	Serum Antibody	White	Black	American Indian	Asian
O	H	Anti-A, Anti-B	45	49	79	40
A	A	Anti-B	40	27	16	28
B	B	Anti-A	11	20	4	27
AB	A and B	–	4	4	< 1	5

born and may also cause hemolytic transfusion reactions.

The mechanism of genetic control in this family of more than 40 antigens is still unclear. It is recognized that each person inherits one codominant Rh gene or gene complex from each parent, which produces a complex erythrocyte membrane material. The absence of antigens produced by the Rh gene is called the Rh_{null} phenotype and is associated with an erythrocyte membrane defect and hemolytic anemia. It is not clear whether Rh is a single gene that produces a single product having multiple antigenic specificities or whether it represents the simultaneous inheritance of 3 closely linked genes that produce 3 separate allelic erythrocyte antigens.

These divergent theories have given rise to differing systems of nomenclature. In the Wiener nomenclature, multiple Rh alleles are designated as either R or r with one of many superscripts. R alleles produce the antigen Rh_o in a particular phenotype in addition to 2 other antigens; r alleles denote the absence of Rh_o in another phenotype. In the Fisher and Race system (see Table 15–2), 3 allelic gene pairs are thought to commonly produce 5 antigens (the remaining antigens are rare variants). Each antigen (D, C, c, E, and e) has a corresponding designation in the Wiener system (ie, D = Rh_o, C = rh′, etc). C and c, as well as E and e, function as alleles. No d antigen is known; d describes the absence of D. The Rh antigens are inherited as 2 sets of 3, one from each parent (see below) (Table 15–3).

Clinically, Rh-positive (Rh^+) means the presence of D (Rh_o) and Rh-negative (Rh^-) indicates the absence of D (Rh_o). D is the most immunogenic of the Rh antigens. Slightly less than half of Rh^+ people are homozygous for D. Because there are no antisera to detect d, determination of zygosity depends on family studies. Roughly 15% of whites are Rh^-. Rh^- is less common in other races. Six weaker variants of D are described and are designated D^u. These weaker variants of D (D^u) can be missed in testing if blood is typed only with routine anti-D antisera but are detected if the indirect antiglobulin test is used. There is no harm in transfusing D^u individuals with Rh^- blood and Rh^- individuals are not sensitized with D^u-positive erythrocytes.

Other Erythrocyte Antigens

The majority of the remaining 20 blood group systems (representing more than 300 antigens) are rarely implicated in transfusion reactions. However, antibodies to the Kidd, Duffy, Kell, and MNS systems are known for their ability to cause hemolysis if antigen-positive blood is transfused into a sensitized recipient. The frequency of detecting shortened erythrocyte survival depends on the erythrocyte antigen and the antibody formed against it. The erythrocyte antigens more commonly involved in transfusion reactions are those that are both immunogenic and prevalent (high incidence). Low-incidence antigens, even if highly immunogenic, have a low likelihood of being transfused. In general, hemolytic antibodies are IgG and react at 37 °C (body temperature). IgM or cold-reacting antibodies rarely cause hemolysis.

Antibodies to Kidd antigens are a frequent cause of delayed hemolytic transfusion reaction. These anti-

Table 15–2. Frequencies of common Rh haplotypes.[1]

Fisher-Race Terminology for Phenotypes		Frequency in US Population (%)		
		White	Black	Asian
CDe	Rh-positive	0.42	0.17	0.70
CDE		0.14	0.11	0.21
CDE		0.00	0.00	0.01
CDe		0.04	0.44	0.03
Cde	Rh-negative	0.37	0.26	0.03
Cde		0.02	0.02	0.02
CdE		0.01	0.00	0.00
CdE		0.00	0.00	0.00

[1]Adapted and reproduced, with permission, from Mourant et al, *The Distribution of Human Blood Groups and Other Polymorphisms,* 2nd ed. Oxford University Press, 1976.

Table 15–3. Inheritance of ABO types.[1]

Parents		Offspring	Parents		Offspring
O × O (OO) (OO)	→	O (OO)	A × A (AA) (AA) (AO) (AO)	→	A or O (AA) (OO) (AO)
O × A (OO) (AA) (AO)	→	O or A (OO) (AO)	A × B (AA) (BB) (AO) (BO)	→	A, B, AB, or O (AO) (BO) (OO)
O × B (OO) (BB) (BO)	→	O or B (OO) (BO)	A × AB (AA) (AB) (AO)	→	A, B, or AB (AA) (BO) (AB) (AO)
O × AB (OO) (AB)	→	A or B (AO) (BO)	B × B (BB) (BB) (BO) (BO)	→	B or O (BB) (OO) (BO)
AB × AB (AB) (AB)	→	A, B, or AB (AA) (BB) (AB)	B × AB (BB) (AB) (BO)	→	A, B, or AB (AO) (BB) (AB) (BO)

[1]Phenotypes in bold; possible genotypes in italics below.

bodies are often difficult to identify in test systems because of poor reactivity. Four antigenic phenotypes have been described: $Jk^{(a+\ b-)}$, $Jk^{(a-\ b+)}$, $Jk^{(a+\ b+)}$, and $Jk^{(a-\ b-)}$. The $Jk^{(a-\ b-)}$ phenotype is rare except in some Pacific island populations.

The antigens of the Duffy system (Fy^a and Fy^b) are controlled by codominant alleles. Antibodies to Fy^a are more commonly associated with delayed hemolytic transfusion reactions than are those to Fy^b. Many blacks have a third allele, which produces the $Fy^{(a-\ b-)}$ phenotype. Duffy antigens on erythrocytes serve as receptors for the entry of *Plasmodium vivax* into the erythrocytes. $Fy^{(a-\ b-)}$ individuals who lack Duffy antigens are resistant to *P vivax* infection but not to *P falciparum* infection.

The Kell system, as first described, included the allelic pair K and k, k antigen being the more frequent. The system now includes 2 additional allelic pairs and several variants. The K antigen is highly immunogenic, with one of 20 individuals transfused with K^+ cells developing antibody. Antibodies to Kell antigen cause hemolytic disease of the newborn, hemolytic transfusion reactions, and, occasionally, autoimmune hemolytic anemia. Individuals of the McLeod phenotype lack Kx antigen, which is a precursor in the synthesis of Kell antigens. Absence of Kx results in the depressed expression of k. These individuals have erythrocyte and neuromuscular system abnormalities. The McLeod phenotype is also associated with some cases of chronic granulomatous disease (see Chapter 22).

METHODS FOR DETECTION OF ANTIGEN & ANTIBODIES TO ERYTHROCYTES

Antiglobulin Tests

Antibody or complement adsorbed onto erythrocytes is detected by using antibodies to human serum globulins (AHG). AHG reagents are produced either in animals or in tissue culture by using monoclonal antibody techniques (see Chapter 12). These reagents may be polyspecific (a mixture of antibodies to IgG, complement, and heavy and light chains) or monospecific (antibodies to specific immunoglobulin or components of complement). The direct antiglobulin test (DAT) detects antibody or complement coating the surface of erythrocytes, whereas the indirect antiglobulin test (IDAT) identifies antibody in serum.

To perform the DAT (Fig 15–2) erythrocytes are washed with saline to remove unbound antibody or complement and then incubated with AHG. If antibody is present on the erythrocytes, the Fab portion of AHG attaches to the Fc portion of the erythrocyte-bound antibody. Bridging of AHG Fab molecules between erythrocytes results in visually detectable agglutination. A positive test requires a minimum of 500 antibodies per erythrocyte surface unless more sensitive methods are used. The DAT is used in the investigation of autoimmune or drug-induced hemolytic anemia, hemolytic disease of the newborn, and suspected hemolytic transfusion reactions.

The IDAT detects **serum antibodies**, which can attach in vitro to erythrocytes (Fig 15–2). This test differs from the DAT in that before a DAT is performed, the serum to be tested is incubated with washed erythrocytes so that serum antibody, if present, binds to erythrocyte antigen. The erythrocytes are then washed to remove any unbound globulin, and AHG is added. If agglutination is observed, serum globulins to erythrocyte antigens are present. The IDAT is used by blood banks in 3 ways: (1) Recipient serum is tested by using panels of erythrocytes with known antigens on their surface to identify the presence and type of a recipient serum antibody. (2) Commercial serum reagents containing known erythrocyte antibodies are used to select blood donor cells that are free of specific erythrocyte antigens to transfuse recipients with identified erythrocyte antibodies. (3) Recipient serum is tested with blood donor cells to confirm the absence of an antigen-antibody reaction (cross-match).

Pretransfusion Testing

Blood is tested prior to transfusion to prevent clinically significant destruction of the recipient's erythrocytes. Clinically significant antibodies are those that are known to have caused unacceptably shortened erythrocyte survival in vivo or frank transfusion reaction. Generally, they are antibodies that react at 37 °C (body temperature) and that react in the antiglobulin test. Prior to transfusion, the recipient's erythrocytes and serum are tested for ABO and Rh_o (D) types and for antibodies to erythrocyte antigens, respectively (type and screen). Additionally, the recipient's serum is tested for compatibility with the erythrocytes from the intended donor (cross-match).

Type & Screen

ABO and Rh_o (D) **types** are determined by mixing the recipient's erythrocytes with anti-A, anti-B, and anti-D antisera. The ABO group is then confirmed by testing the recipient's serum against commercial A and B cells to detect isoagglutinins.

The recipient's serum is **screened** for alloantibodies that may not be demonstrated in the cross-match. In antibody screens, suspensions of O erythrocytes that contain known erythrocyte antigens on their surface are incubated with the recipient's serum. If antigen-antibody complexes are formed, hemolysis or agglutination of erythrocytes is observed. The screen is completed by the IDAT and again observed for agglutination.

In the **cross-match,** compatibility between donor and recipient is determined directly. Washed donor cells are combined with recipient serum, incubated,

Coombs tests

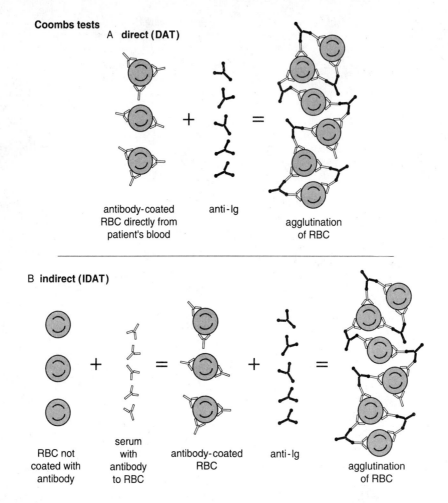

A **direct (DAT)**

antibody-coated
RBC directly from
patient's blood

anti-Ig

agglutination
of RBC

B **indirect (IDAT)**

RBC not
coated with
antibody

serum
with
antibody
to RBC

antibody-coated
RBC

anti-Ig

agglutination
of RBC

Figure 15–2. *A:* Schematic illustration of the technique for the direct Coombs test. ***B:*** Schematic illustration of the technique for the indirect Coombs test.

centrifuged, and observed for hemolysis or agglutination. If the recipient either has a history of previous erythrocyte antibody or has had antibody detected during the antibody screening procedure, the IDAT must be performed before a cross-match may be considered compatible.

These tests that detect antigen-antibody reactions with erythrocytes are performed most simply in saline solution. It is recognized that this causes some loss in test sensitivity for IgG antibodies owing to ionic repulsion forces between erythrocytes generated by clustering of Na^+ and Cl^- ions near erythrocyte surfaces. A variety of methods to increase the sensitivity of these tests have been developed. These procedures add different reagents, such as albumin, LISS (low-ionic-strength solution), or polybrene, to the test system or use enzyme-treated erythrocytes, all of which generally increase sensitivity.

TRANSFUSION REACTIONS

Blood transfusion has become increasingly safe and effective, but a variety of adverse reactions, only some of which are preventable, continue to occur (Table 15–4). Transfusions must be monitored during infusion for immediate reactions and over time to detect delayed reactions.

Hemolytic Reactions

The transfusion of erythrocyte-incompatible blood may cause immediate hemolysis. Hemolytic reactions are fatal in 10% of ABO-incompatible transfusions, which generally occur when large amounts of ABO-incompatible blood are transfused as a result of human error. Incompatible transfusions involving other blood groups are usually less severe. Clinically, reactions are often heralded by fever, chills, and burning

Table 15–4. Transfusion reactions.

Cause	Incidence	Manifestations	Treatment
Recipient erythrocyte antibodies			
Hemolytic (acute)	< 0.02%	Fever, chills, lowered blood pressure Pain in back or infusion site Hemoglobin in blood and urine	Stop transfusion; blood/urine to blood bank. Hydrate. Monitor hematocrit, liver, and renal function.
Hemolytic (delayed)		Lowered hematocrit, increased bilirubin; raised LDH days to weeks posttransfusion	Monitor hematocrit, also liver and renal function if severe.
Recipient leukocyte antibodies	< 2%		
Febrile		Temp raised ≥ 1°C, chills	Stop transfusion: rule out hemolytic reactions with patient's unit, blood/urine to blood bank; premedicate with antipyretics; give leukocyte-poor products if available.
Donor WBC antibodies		Noncardiac pulmonary edema, bronchospasm	Stop transfusion, treat symptoms; give leukocyte-poor products if available.
Plasma proteins Allergic	2–3%	Itching, urticaria, rarely asthma, bronchospasm, anaphylaxis	Stop transfusion; give antihistamines for urticaria; treat symptoms.

at the injection site. Reaction may progress to dyspnea and hypotension, with joint or back pain. Shock, generalized bleeding, and renal failure may follow.

Delayed hemolytic transfusion reactions occur 3–10 days posttransfusion. Many of these reactions are clinically undetected but are thought to occur in about one in 6000 transfusions. They result either from primary immunization to transfused erythrocyte antigens or from an anamnestic response in a previously sensitized individual whose antibody titers are undetectable at the time of transfusion. They are characterized by fever and anemia with elevated levels of bilirubin and a positive DAT.

Febrile Reactions

Febrile nonhemolytic reactions are caused by cytotoxic or agglutinating antibodies in the recipient, directed against donor leukocyte antigens. They are generally self-limiting and associated with fever of 38–39 °C and chills. They must be distinguished from fever associated with hemolytic transfusion reactions and from the high fever (> 40 °C) and rigors associated with bacterial contamination of blood components. Febrile transfusion reactions occur most frequently in multiply transfused recipients or in women sensitized to leukocytes from multiple pregnancies. Only one in 8 patients with a febrile reaction will have another reaction on subsequent transfusion. Recurrent febrile reactions are often controlled with antipyretics. Patients with uncontrolled febrile reactions may benefit from leukocyte-poor components prepared in a variety of ways to decrease the number of leukocytes transfused by as much as 90%.

High-titer leukocyte antibodies in either recipient or donor plasma can cause pulmonary edema (see Chapter 40). Recipient antibody to donor granulocytes or donor antibody to recipient granulocytes can cause granulocyte aggregates, which are filtered by the lungs. Antibodies adherent to granulocyte aggregates will activate complement.

Allergic Reactions

Allergic reactions to transfusion are generally characterized by itching, hives, and local erythema and only rarely are accompanied by cardiovascular instability. They are thought to be caused by infused plasma proteins and occur in 1–2% of transfusions. Patients with a history of allergy more frequently have allergic reactions to blood. Mild reactions can be treated with antihistamines, and the transfusion continued. Pretreatment with antihistamines often prevents these reactions if they are recurrent, but if they are severe, washed erythrocytes may be indicated. Anaphylactic reactions occur in some IgA-deficient recipients (see Chapter 19) after transfusion of as little as 10–15 mL of whole blood. Fortunately, these reactions are rare and are confined to individuals with high titers of anti-IgA. Reaction is due to the IgA present in transfused plasma and is prevented by transfusing washed erythrocytes.

Preventable transfusion reactions include those caused by bacterial contamination of blood components, congestive heart failure due to volume overload, and artificially produced donor erythrocyte destruction prior to infusion. Erythrocytes may be destroyed by inadvertent overheating or freezing of donor blood or mixing it with nonisotonic solutions.

Transfusion-Transmitted Infection

Transfusion may be complicated by a variety of infectious microorganisms, only some of which can be detected by current donor-screening methods (Table 15–5). The most frequently reported posttransfusion infections in developed countries are hepatitis and cytomegalovirus (CMV), HIV-1, and HTLV-I infections. In certain countries, posttransfusion malaria and Chagas' disease are significant problems. Elimination of potentially infected blood depends on successful donor screening by medical history, aseptic blood collection, and adequate laboratory testing of the donated blood. In the USA, all blood is tested for hepatitis by using HBsAg, anti-HBc, anti-hepatitis C virus (HCV), and alanine aminotransferase (ALT) and for syphilis, HIV-1/2, and HTLV-I/II by serologic means.

The incidence of posttransfusion hepatitis (PTH) is estimated to be < 1%. PTH is caused by hepatitis B virus in 5% of cases and by HCV in 95% of cases. Of transfusion recipients who develop posttransfusion hepatitis, 50% develop chronic hepatitis; 10% of these develop cirrhosis. All blood components can transmit hepatitis, except those that can be pasteurized, such as albumin and other plasma proteins.

CMV is transmitted to CMV-seronegative transfusion recipients by leukocytes contaminating some blood components, particularly erythrocytes and platelets. Whether transfusion of CMV-seropositive blood to CMV-seropositive recipients causes superinfection or other complications is unknown. Roughly 50% of blood donors are infected with CMV, which limits availability of CMV-negative blood. Posttransfusion CMV infection causes significant morbidity and mortality rates in severely immunocompromised patients. When possible, CMV-seronegative blood should be given to low-birth-weight infants (< 1250 g), CMV-seronegative pregnant women, and CMV-seronegative recipients of CMV-seronegative organ transplants.

HIV-1 infection due to transfusion has become increasingly infrequent with the initiation of donor HIV-1 antibody testing. HIV-1 can be transmitted by erythrocytes, platelets, cryoprecipitate, fresh-frozen plasma, and possibly other blood components. The risk of infection by transfusion is now estimated to be one in 225,000 per unit transfused. The virus can be transmitted by blood collected from donors who have been recently infected but have not yet formed antibody to HIV-1 and who have not voluntarily excluded themselves from donating blood. Even though HIV-2 infection is rare in the USA, isolated cases of HIV-2 infection are reported in parts of Europe and West Africa. Consequently, all US blood donations are screened for antibodies to both HIV-1 and HIV-2. Other retroviruses, HTLV-I and HTLV-II, are transmitted with 30% efficiency in cellular blood products. Prior to the availability of HTLV-I/II testing, one in 3500–5000 transfusion recipients were infected with HTLV-I/II. HTLV-I is a rare cause of posttransfusion spastic paraparesis. It is known to cause a form of T cell leukemia (see Chapter 45) and tropical spastic paraparesis in endemic populations. HTLV-II infection is not currently associated with a disease.

Other Diseases Transmitted by Transfusion

Epstein-Barr virus may be transmitted by transfusion. In most cases it results in asymptomatic seroconversion, but it can cause a mononucleosis syndrome. Transfusion-acquired delta hepatitis requires the presence of both the hepatitis delta virus and hepatitis B virus in the blood donor for transmission to a recipient (see Chapter 48). Because effective donor screening for HBsAg eliminates almost all of these donors, the risk of transmitting this agent is low.

Posttransfusion syphilis is now rare. There is a low incidence of syphilitic infection in blood donors, and all donors are screened for antibody. Since the organism does not survive cold storage for more than 48–72 hours, it can be transmitted only by fresh blood or platelets.

Malaria remains a disease of major worldwide importance. The parasite is present in erythrocytes of carriers sometimes for years after infection. There are no laboratory tests that are simple and sensitive enough available for screening the blood donor population. Because of this, blood banks in the USA rely on histories taken at the time of donation. Donors who have traveled to areas where malaria is endemic are deferred for 6 months (3 years if chemoprophylaxis is taken).

Other parasitic diseases reported to be transmitted by blood transfusion include the microfilariae *Wuchereria bancrofti, Acanthocheilonema persians, Mansonella ozzardi, Loa loa,* and *Brugia malayi.* Chagas' disease can be transmitted by *Trypanosoma cruzi. Toxoplasma gondii* can cause toxoplasmosis in transfusion recipients, and *Babesia microti* can cause babesiosis. Leishmaniasis is also reported as a posttransfusion infection.

Transfusion-transmitted bacterial infections are most frequently the result of inadequate decontami-

Table 15–5. Transfusion-transmitted infection.

Infection[1]	Risk/Unit Transfused
CMV infection	1:20–1:100
Hepatitis C	1:3300
Hepatitis B	1:200,000
HTLV-I/II	1:50,000–1:200,000
HIV-1 infection	1:225,000

[1]Rare infections include syphilis, malaria, Epstein-Barr virus infection, delta hepatitis, brucellosis, Chagas' disease, babesiosis, and leishmaniasis.

nation of skin at the time of blood collection but may also be caused by asymptomatic bacteremia in the donor or by contamination of the blood during storage and handling.

Immunologic Mechanisms of Transfusion Reactions

Hemolytic transfusion reactions are caused by antigen-antibody complexes on the erythrocyte membrane. These complexes activate Hageman factor (factor XIIa) and complement. Hageman factor, in turn, activates the kinin system (see Chapter 10). Bradykinins thus generated increase capillary permeability and dilate arterioles, causing hypotension. Complement is activated and leads to intravascular hemolysis as well as to histamine and serotonin release from mast cells. Hageman factor and free incompatible erythrocyte stroma activate the intrinsic clotting cascade, with consequent disseminated intravascular coagulation (DIC). Systemic hypotension with renal vasoconstriction and the formation of intravascular thrombi lead to renal failure. When complement activation is not complete, the reaction is less severe. Erythrocytes coated with C3b are cleared from the circulation by phagocytes, resulting in extravascular hemolysis, which takes place primarily in the liver.

Antileukocyte antibodies are either cytotoxic or agglutinating. These antibodies form complexes with antigens on leukocytes, activating complement. Activated complement generates vasoactive substances in the circulation. Endogenous pyrogens from destroyed granulocytes are also released into the circulation following cell lysis.

The mechanism of graft-versus-host disease depends on the engraftment of donor lymphocytes in the recipient. Donor lymphocytes recognize recipient tissue antigens as "foreign" and cause a clinical syndrome characterized by fever, skin rash, hepatitis, and diarrhea. Death may result. Engraftment can be prevented by irradiating lymphocyte-carrying components to preclude lymphocyte activation. Graft-versus-host disease occurs, rarely, in newborns undergoing exchange transfusion, patients with T cell immunodeficiencies, and patients severely immunosuppressed by intensive chemotherapy and irradiation (see Chapter 58). There are rare reports of graft-versus-host disease following transfusion of blood from a haplo-identical donor into an immunocompetent recipient. Consequently, designated blood donations collected from first-degree family members are now irradiated before transfusion.

Rh ISOIMMUNIZATION

The D antigen is a high-incidence, strongly immunogenic antigen, 50 times more immunogenic than the other Rh antigens. The prevalence of antibody formation to Rh+ blood depends on the dose of Rh+ cells: 1 mL of cells sensitizes 15% of individuals exposed; 250 mL sensitizes 60–70%. After the initial exposure to Rh+ cells, weak IgM antibody can be detected as early as 4 weeks. This is followed by a rapid conversion to IgG antibody. A second exposure to as little as 0.03 mL of Rh+ erythrocytes may result in the rapid formation of IgG antibodies.

The majority of potential transfusion reactions to Rh can be prevented by transfusing Rh− individuals with Rh− blood. Immunization and antibody formation to D antigen still occur owing to occasional Rh sensitization during pregnancy or to transfusion errors, particularly during emergencies. Immunization to other Rh antigens may occur because donor blood is typed routinely for D but not for other Rh antigens.

Hemolytic disease of the newborn occurs with the passage of Rh+ cells from the fetus to the circulation of the Rh− mother. Once anti-D antibody is formed in the mother, IgG but not IgM anti-D antibodies cross the placenta, causing hemolysis of fetal erythrocytes. Rh− mothers become sensitized during pregnancy or at the time of delivery as a result of transplacental fetal hemorrhage. The size and number of fetal hemorrhages increase as pregnancy progresses. Following delivery, 75% of women will have had transplacental fetal hemorrhage. The risk of transplacental fetal hemorrhage increases as the pregnancy progresses (3% in the first trimester, 45% in the second trimester, 64% in the third trimester). Some obstetric complications increase the risk of transplacental fetal hemorrhage: antepartum hemorrhage, toxemia of pregnancy, cesarian section, external version, and manual removal of the placenta. Total transplacental fetal hemorrhage can also occur following spontaneous or therapeutic abortion or amniocentesis. Overall Rh immunization occurs in 8–9% of Rh− women following the delivery of the first Rh+ ABO-compatible baby and in 1.5–2.0% of Rh− women who deliver Rh+ ABO-incompatible babies.

Rh Prophylaxis

Rh immunization can now be suppressed almost entirely if high-titer anti-Rh immunoglobulin (RhIg) is administered by 72 hours after the potentially sensitizing dose of Rh+ cells.

The protective mechanism of RhIG administration is not clear. RhIG does not effectively block Rh antigen from immunosuppressive cells by competitive inhibition, since effective doses of RhIG are known not to cover all Rh antigen sites. Intravascular hemolysis and rapid clearance of erythrocyte debris by the poorly immunoresponsive liver are also unlikely. Although this mechanism appears to explain the 90% protective effect of ABO incompatibility between mother and fetus, RhIG-induced erythrocyte hemolysis is extravascular. Rh+ fetal cells are removed primarily by highly phagocytic cells in the spleen and, to a lesser extent, the lymph nodes. The most likely mechanism is a negative modulation of the primary immune response. Antigen-antibody complexes are bound to cells bearing Fc receptors in the lymph nodes and spleen. These cells presumably stimulate suppressor T cell responses, which prevent antigen-induced B cell proliferation and antibody formation.

A prophylactic dose of 300 μg of RhIG intramuscularly prevents Rh immunization following exposure to up to 30 mL of Rh^+ erythrocytes. Initial recommendations were that 300 μg of RhIG be given to nonimmunized Rh^- mothers by 72 hours after delivery of an Rh^+ infant. The recommended dose is different in some other countries. Doses may have to be increased in cases of massive transplacental fetal hemorrhage. These recommendations have been extended to include prophylaxis for nonimmunized Rh^- mothers following abortion and amniocentesis and, in some other countries, routinely during pregnancy. The administration of RhIG to pregnant women has not been shown to have a detrimental effect on the fetus.

Large doses of RhIG can effectively suppress immunization following inadvertent transfusion of Rh^+ blood into Rh^- patients if given within 72 hours of transfusion. Once Rh immunization is demonstrated by the IDAT, administration of RhIG is ineffective.

BLOOD COMPONENT THERAPY

The transfusion of selective blood components has become increasingly important. More stringent screening and testing of blood donors has decreased the number of eligible donors at a time of increased need for blood. Increasing use of myelosuppressive chemotherapy for malignant diseases and organ transplantation requires more blood than ever before. The indications for transfusion are now assessed more critically. Blood transfusion is not entirely safe, and no transfusion should be given unless it is needed (Table 15–6).

Erythrocytes

The indications for erythrocyte transfusion and its effect depend on the clinical state of the recipient. One unit of erythrocytes is expected to increase the nonbleeding adult's hemoglobin by 1 g/dL and to increase the hematocrit by 3%. After senescent and damaged erythrocytes are cleared, 70–80% of transfused erythrocytes survive normally.

During acute blood loss, 1 hour or more is required for equilibration of intravascular and extravascular fluids and an accurate assessment of the fall in the hemoglobin level. Generally, a loss of 20% of blood volume can be corrected with crystalloid (electrolyte) solution alone, which can then be supplemented with colloid (protein) solution. Whole blood is indicated if blood loss exceeds one-third of blood volume. Operative blood loss of 1000–1200 mL rarely requires transfusion. If oxygen-carrying capacity is required in acute blood loss, packed erythrocytes are indicated.

A particular hemoglobin level is tolerated better in a patient with chronic anemia than in a patient with acute blood loss. Physiologic compensation by increased cardiac output and a shift of the oxyhemoglobin disassociation curve to the right for increased

Table 15–6. Guidelines for component therapy.[1]

Component	Indications for Use
Red blood cells	Use to increase O_2-carrying capacity; 1 unit will increase hemoglobin 1 g/dL in a 70-kg patient. Consider the degree of anemia, intravascular volume, and presence of coexisting cardiac, pulmonary, or vascular conditions. 1. If hemoglobin > 10 g/dL, transfusion is rarely indicated. 2. If hemoglobin < 7 g/dL, transfusion is usually indicated. 3. If hemoglobin is 7–10 g/dL, assess clinical status, mixed venous pO_2, and O_2 extraction ratio.
Platelets	Use to control or prevent bleeding due to low platelet count or abnormal platelet function; one concentrate will increase platelet count by ca 5000 platelets/mL. 1. Generally, patients with platelet counts > 10,000–20,000 should not receive platelets to prevent bleeding. 2. Actively bleeding patients with platelet counts > 50,000 generally will not benefit from platelets. 3. Generally, platelets are not indicated in massive transfusion or cardiac surgery.
FFP	Used to increase clotting factors in patients with documented deficiencies (PT/PTT > 1.5 × normal)[2], 1 unit will increase the level of any factor 2–3%. 1. FFP should not be used as a volume expander or nutritional source. 2. FFP is useful for treatment of factor II, V, VII, IX, X, and XI deficiencies when specific components are not available. 3. FFP is useful for patients with warfarin overdose who are actively bleeding or who require emergency surgery prior to vitamin K reversal. 4. FFP may be useful in massive blood transfusion (> 1 blood volume within a few hours). 5. FFP is useful as a source of antithrombin III in deficient patients undergoing surgery or heparin treatment, in infants with severe protein-losing enteropathy, and in patients with thrombotic thrombocytopenic purpura.

[1]Data from the following sources: Fresh frozen plasma—indication and risks, *JAMA* 1985;**253**:551; Platelet transfusion therapy, *JAMA* 1987;**257**:1777; and Perioperative red blood cell transfusion, *JAMA* 1988;**260**:2700.
[2]PT, prothrombin time; PTT, partial thromboplastin time.

oxygen delivery to tissues allow for adequate oxygenation in these cases.

Exchange transfusion of neonates is a special circumstance in which whole blood less than 7 days old is required to ensure tolerable levels of plasma electrolytes and adequate levels of 2,3-diphosphoglycerate. Preferably, the blood should be irradiated to prevent the rare occurrence of graft-versus-host-disease.

All erythrocyte components should be administered through blood filters. No medications of any kind, especially solutions containing calcium or glucose, should be infused with blood components.

Platelets

Platelets function to control bleeding by acting as hemostatic plugs on vascular endothelium. Platelet abnormalities that require transfusion may be either quantitative or qualitative. The vast majority of platelet transfusions are given to supplement small numbers of platelets due to increased production, to pooling, or to dilution.

Platelets are available as either random donor concentrates (recovered from a whole-blood donation) or as plateletpheresis (collected by using a cytopheresis machine). The transfusion of one concentrate is expected to increase the platelet count of a reasonably well 50-kg adult by 5000–10,000/µL. Plateletpheresis are equivalent to 6 concentrates. The survival of transfused platelets is decreased in patients who are actively bleeding; who have splenomegaly, fever, infection, or disseminated intravascular coagulation; or who are sensitized to platelet antigens. The transfusion of ABO-incompatible platelets is associated with slightly decreased platelet survival.

Transient thrombocytopenias, which are the result of treatment regimens for malignancy, are responsible for most platelet transfusions. Prophylactic platelets are often transfused when the platelet count falls below 20,000/µL. Since there is little significant bleeding when platelet counts are above 10,000/µL, prophylactic platelets may be given to patients with counts of less than 10,000/µL, or therapeutic platelets may be transfused during bleeding episodes. The potential benefit of single-donor plateletpheresis over pooled random-donor concentrates in delaying alloimmunization and increasing platelet counts has yet to be adequately studied.

Platelets have a limited role in preventing bleeding in surgical patients. Platelet counts between 50,000 and 60,000/µL result in adequate hemostasis. In the event of massive transfusion (15–20 units), the dilutional effect on the platelet count by stored blood must be considered and corrected if necessary. Stored blood does not contain platelets. Although a functional platelet abnormality during cardiac surgery has been described, controlled trials do not demonstrate the need for platelet transfusion if counts are above 60,000/µL, regardless of a history of recent aspirin consumption.

Plasma Products

Fresh-frozen plasma (FFP), stored plasma, and cryoprecipitate are valuable sources of coagulation factors. Stored plasma and FFP can often be used interchangeably. Levels of factors V and VIII in stored plasma are half those in FFP, but levels of other factors are equivalent. Cryoprecipitate is used as a source of factor VIII, von Willebrand factor, and fibrinogen.

FFP is used for treating isolated congenital factor deficiencies, with the exception of factor IX (for which it is relatively ineffective) and for correcting warfarin overdoses. It is also used to treat thrombotic thrombocytopenic purpura and for bleeding patients with C1 esterase inhibitor or bleeding patients with heparin-dependent antithrombin III deficiency who are heparin-resistant. Massively transfused patients with a prothrombin time or partial thromboplastin time greater than 1.5 times normal and platelet counts above 50,000/µL should also receive plasma. Plasma should not be used for volume expansion.

Cryoprecipitate is used in young hemophiliacs or patients with mild hemophilia to decrease the number of donor exposures compared with the use of factor concentrates. Cryoprecipitate and deamino-8-arginine vasopressin have proved to be useful in managing bleeding uremic patients.

REFERENCES

Anderson KC, Weinstein HJ: Transfusion-associated graft-versus-host disease. *N Engl J Med* 1990; **323**:315.

Barton JC: Nonhemolytic, noninfectious transfusion reactions. *Semin Hematol* 1981;**18**:95.

Bowman JM: The prevention of Rh immunization. *Transfusion Med Rev* 1988;**2**:129.

Bowman JM, Pollock JM: Failures of intravenous Rh immune globulin prophylaxis: An analysis of the reasons for such failures. *Transfusion Med Rev* 1987; **1**:101.

Chien S, Sung LA: Molecular basis of red cell membrane rheology. *Biorheology* 1990;**27**:327.

Dodd RY: The risk of transfusion-transmitted infection. *N Engl J Med* 1992;**327**:419.

Greenwalt TJ: Pathogenesis and management of hemolytic transfusion reactions. *Semin Hematol* 1981;**18**:84.

Huestis DW et al: *Practical Blood Transfusion.* Little, Brown, 1988.

Issitt PD: *Applied Blood Group Serology*, 3rd ed. Montgomery Scientific, 1985.

Mollison PL: *Blood Transfusion in Clinical Medicine*, 7th ed. Blackwell, 1983.

Mourant AE, Kopec AC, Domaniewska-Sobczak K: *The Distribution of Human Blood Groups and Other Polymorphisms*, 2nd ed. Oxford University Press, 1976.

Nance ST (editor): Blood safety: Current challenges. American Association of Blood Banks, 1992.

NIH Consensus Conference: Platelet transfusion therapy. *JAMA* 1987;**257:**1777.

NIH Consensus Conference: Perioperative red blood cell transfusion. *JAMA* 1988;**260:**2700.

NIH Consensus Conference: Fresh-frozen plasma. *JAMA* 1985;**253:**551.

Pineda AA, Brzica SM, Taswell HF: Hemolytic transfusion reaction: Recent experience in a large blood bank. *Mayo Clin Proc* 1978:**53:**378.

Sazama K: Reports of 355 transfusion-associated deaths: 1976 through 1985. *Transfusion* 1990;**30:**583.

Walker RH (editor): *Technical Manual for the American Association of Blood Banks*, 10th ed. American Association of Blood Banks, 1990.

Welbor JL, Hersch J: Blood transfusion reactions. *Postgrad Med* 1991;**90:**125.

Histocompatibility Testing

16

Beth W. Colombe, PhD

The human leukocyte antigen (HLA) system as we know it today has been defined largely by a single method, the complement-dependent lymphocytotoxicity test—a serologic assay. HLA antigens, encoded by the alleles of this genetic system, have been characterized through the reaction patterns of naturally occurring alloantibodies that bind to specific HLA antigens on target cells, fix complement, and then kill the cells. Through the discovery and testing of numerous alloantisera with lymphocytotoxic activity, the extensive polymorphism of the HLA system has been revealed. Table 16–1 lists the HLA antigens currently recognized by the World Health Organization.

Speculation on the amount of HLA polymorphism is now becoming resolved by applying the new techniques of molecular biology to HLA. Now the serologically defined polymorphisms of the HLA system have a molecular basis in the variations that exist in the exact sequences of nucleotides of genomic DNA and the amino acid sequences of the HLA antigens themselves. As more alleles are being sequenced, a new image of increasing complexity and allelic variation is emerging. For example, there are now 7 variants of HLA B27, 12 of A2, 6 of B35, 14 of DR4, etc. Whether such sequence differences have clinical significance remains to be determined. Despite these new advances, the majority of histocompatibility testing is currently focused upon the "classic" HLA specificities as defined serologically.

During the past 25 years, genetic and clinical studies have shown that HLA antigens are the major "transplantation antigens" that determine the compatibility of transplanted tissues and organs (Fig 16–1). Histocompatibility between individuals is based on the extent of matching of inherited HLA antigens and the degree of immunologic reactivity to these antigens in cellular and serologic cross-match testing. HLA matching and histocompatibility testing have an enormous practical influence on contemporary organ transplantation practices in clinical medicine.

HISTOCOMPATIBILITY TESTING & TRANSPLANTATION

The practice of testing for histocompatibility between an organ donor and the selected recipient is based on the presumption that tissue compatibility will promote graft acceptance and avoid immune rejection. The foundation for this assumption is the evidence that identical twins can accept and retain grafts from one another indefinitely, whereas grafts from all others are ultimately rejected in the absence of immunosuppressive therapy. Efforts to define the inherited basis for tissue compatibility have focused mainly on the HLA antigen system. It follows that the greater the identity of HLA antigens, the greater the histocompatibility of the graft with the recipient. Identification of HLA antigens is known as **tissue typing.** Cellular methods for tissue typing include the use of homozygous typing cells (HTC testing) and the mixed-lymphocyte culture (MLC) test for HLA compatibility. A state of histocompatibility between donor and recipient may also be inferred from absence of preformed antibodies and cytotoxic lymphocytes directed against the donor HLA antigens. Serologic testing for anti-donor antibodies is called cross-matching; cellular testing is done by the direct cell-mediated lympholysis (CML) assay.

Table 16–2 shows a flowchart that outlines a typical course of histocompatibility testing for a prospective kidney graft recipient. In the following sections, these various tests will be described, including the interpretation of results and rationale for use.

RATIONALE FOR TISSUE TYPING FOR TRANSPLANTATION

Comparison of the tissue types of a donor and the potential (unrelated) recipient usually reveals some degree of antigen mismatching because of the extensive polymorphism of the HLA antigen system.

Table 16–1. HLA antigen specificities.[1]

A	B	C	DR	DQ	DP
A1	B5	Cw1	DR1	DQ1	DPw1
A2	B7	Cw2	DR103	DQ2	DPw2
A203	B703	Cw3	DR2	DQ3	DPw3
A210	B8	Cw4	DR3	DQ4	DPw4
A3	B12	Cw5	DR4	DQ5(1)	DPw5
A9	B13	Cw6	DR5	DQ6(1)	DPw6
A10	B14	Cw7	DR6	DQ7(3)	
A11	B15	Cw8	DR7	DQ8(3)	
A19	B16	Cw9(w3)	DR8	DQ9(3)	
A23(9)	B17	Cw10(w3)	DR9		
A24(9)	B18		DR10		
A2403	B21		DR11(5)		
A25(10)	B22		DR12(5)		
A26(10)	B27		DR13(6)		
A28	B35		DR14(6)		
A29(19)	B37		DR1403		
A30(19)	B38(16)		DR1404		
A31(19)	B39(16)		DR15(2)		
A32(19)	B3901		DR16(2)		
A33(19)	B3902		DR17(3)		
A34(10)	B40		DR18(3)		
A36	B4005				
A43	B41		DR51		
A66(10)	B42				
A68(28)	B44(12)		DR52		
A69(28)	B45(12)				
A74(19)	B46		DR53		
	B47				
	B48				
	B49(21)				
	B50(21)				
	B51(5)				
	B5102				
	B5103				
	B52(5)				
	B53				
	B54(22)				
	B55(22)				
	B56(22)				
	B57(17)				
	B58(17)				
	B59				
	B60(40)				
	B61(40)				
	B62(15)				
	B63(15)				
	B64(14)				
	B65(14)				
	B67				
	B70				
	B71(70)				
	B72(70)				
	B73				
	B75(15)				
	B76(15)				
	B77(15)				
	B7801				
	Bw4				
	Bw6				

[1]Antigens as recognized by the World Health Organization. Antigens listed in parentheses are the broad antigens; antigens followed by broad antigens in parentheses are the antigen splits. Antigens of the Dw series are omitted.

When nuclear family members are tissue typed for a living-related transplant, only 25% of full siblings will be HLA identical to the transplant recipient, and parents and 50% of siblings will be matched at one haplotype. Cadaver donors will be genotypically complete mismatches to the random recipient, although there is a finite probability of complete or partial phenotypic identity. If the phenotypes of the patient and the cadaver are composed of the more common antigens, such as HLA-A1, -A2, and -B8, etc, the likelihood of HLA antigen matching increases.

A positive effect of HLA matching on kidney graft outcome has been clearly documented in reports from the two largest studies of renal transplant data: the UCLA Transplant Registry, Los Angeles, Calif, which has collected data on 106,000 transplants since 1970, and the Collaborative Transplant Study (CTS), Heidelberg, Germany, with data on 107,500 renal transplants since 1982. Both of these studies agree that the main factor that improves long-term (up to 10-year) renal allograft survival is donor-recipient matching for HLA antigens (Table 16–3). Table 16–3 indicates the decreasing graft survival obtained in primary renal transplants when the donor is HLA identical (sibling), one-half identical (parent), and completely mismatched and unrelated (cadaver).

Beneficial effects of HLA matching on short-term graft survival (1 year) are no longer apparent in the results from many individual transplant centers. Immunosuppression with cyclosporin has improved first-transplant graft survival of cadaver and one-haplotype-matched living-related transplants to near that of HLA-identical transplants: approximately 80–85% after 1 year.

Matching for the splits (subtypes) of HLA antigens may be even more significant for graft outcome than simple matching of the "generic" HLA antigens (for example, matching for B51 or B52 rather than for the broad B5 antigen). As shown in Table 16–4, from a recent CTS review of 33,000 transplants, matching for A and B locus antigen splits in conjunction with HLA-DR shows a striking correlation with graft survival. Table 16–4 shows percent graft survival for patients with 0, 3, and 6 mismatches for HLA-A, -B, and -DR antigens and the estimated half-life survival time for those grafts. Well-matched grafts (0 mismatches) survive approximately 60% longer than do completely mismatched (6 mismatches) grafts (half-life of 12.3 and 7.5 years, respectively).

Despite the dramatic improvement in 1-year survival, however, the ensuing rate of graft loss due to chronic rejection remains essentially unchanged; ie, half of cadaver grafts are still lost by 7.8 years, compared with 7.3 years in 1978. Thus, the use of cyclosporin has not established an operational state of long-term organ tolerance. It is estimated that if all kidneys were shared nationally, 25% of all waiting patients could be transplanted with kidneys with no

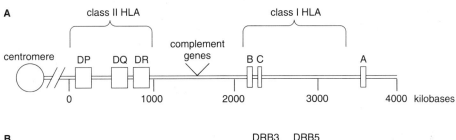

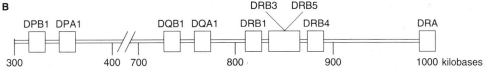

Figure 16–1. MHC genes on chromosome 6. **A:** Schematic representation of genes of the class I and II HLA regions. The region containing complement genes and genes for other factors, such as tumor necrosis factor (TNF), is indicated. **B:** Expanded view of class II HLA region showing genes for α and β chains of class II molecules. Pseudogenes have been omitted. The presence of genes for DRB3, DRB4, and DRB5 is dependent on the haplotype.

HLA-A, -B, or -DR mismatches. These statistics argue in favor of sharing organs on a regional and national scale to promote the most beneficial usage of scarce organ resources. To achieve this end, the National Organ Transplant Act of 1987 established the United Network for Organ Sharing (UNOS). UNOS links local and regional transplant procurement centers with a national registry of waiting recipients and establishes mandatory criteria for selection of recipients based on a point system for the following attributes: quality of HLA matching, degree of sensitization (panel-reactive antibody [PRA]), time on the waiting list, medical emergency status, and geographic factors.

In heart transplantation, distribution of hearts based on HLA matching is impractical because of the lack of availability of the organ. Retrospective analysis indicates an improvement in 3-year graft survival when there were less than 2 HLA-B and -DR mismatches compared with greater than 2 mismatches (83% and 70% survival, respectively). For liver transplantation, better HLA-matched livers are associated with fewer rejection episodes, but, paradoxically, liver graft survival results show no advantage from HLA matching and, possibly, a detrimental effect. The value of HLA matching for liver transplantation and for other organs, such as the pancreas, must await the collection of more data. Preliminary data for cornea transplantation do show that patients with pre-

Table 16–2. Flowchart of histocompatibility testing for the renal transplant patient.

A. Perform preliminary immunologic evaluation
   1. Patient
      HLA typing
      ABO/Rh typing
      Screening of serum for antibodies reactive with HLA antigens
      Testing of serum for autoantibodies
   2. Living related donors
      HLA typing
      ABO/Rh typing
      Cross-match with serum of patient to detect anti-donor antibodies
      MLC test with patient
B. Select living related donor
   This is based on:
      ABO compatibility
      Best match for HLA antigens
      Low stimulation of patient's cells in MLC test
      Negative preliminary cross-match
   If there is no appropriate living related donor, then
C. Place patient on waiting list for cadaver kidney
   Register patient with UNOS
   Screen serum sample monthly for antibodies reactive to HLA antigens
D. Select appropriate recipient for cadaver kidney
   HLA and ABO type cadaver donor
   Cross-match cadaver with ABO-compatible recipients
   Select candidates having no antibodies to donor's HLA antigens
E. Transplant: living-related and cadaver donors
   Cross-match with most recent patient sample drawn immediately pretransplant

Table 16–3. Effect of HLA matching on long-term renal allograft survival.[1]

Organ Donor	No. of Haplotypes Matched	% Graft Survival	
		4 year	10 year
HLA-identical sibling	2	85	70
Parent	1	70	50
Cadaver[2]	0	53	33

[1]Data from Terasaki PI (editor). *Clinical Transplantation* 1990, p 587. UCLA Tissue Typing Laboratory, 1990.
[2]Recipient treated with cyclosporin.

Table 16–4. Effect of HLA-A, -B, and -DR mismatches on primary renal graft survival.[1,2]

Number of Mismatches	Estimated 10-Year Graft Survival (%)	Half-Life of Graft (years)
0	53	12.3
3	42	9.4
6	32	7.5

[1]Data from G. Opelz, Collaborative Transplant Study, May 1992.
[2]Matching was done for split HLA-A and -B locus antigens.

viously rejected transplants will benefit from a well-matched transplant.

ANTIBODIES TO DETECT SENSITIZATION TO HLA ANTIGENS

Exposure to HLA antigens can occur as a consequence of blood transfusions, prior organ grafts, or pregnancy. The resultant formation of specific antibodies to those antigens is termed "sensitization." Reexposure to the previously immunizing antigens on a new allograft can produce rapid humoral and cellular immune responses, leading to hyperacute or accelerated rejection. Detection of such preformed specific antibodies is of paramount importance in evaluating the state of initial histocompatibility between recipient and donor, especially in the face of known HLA antigen mismatches. Two standard procedures have been developed, both of which involve the exposure of lymphocytes to the patient's serum. Antibody screening tests a serum sample against a panel of HLA-typed lymphocytes for anti-lymphocyte reactivity; cross-matching tests the patient's serum against the lymphocytes of a selected prospective organ donor to detect donor-specific antibodies.

SEROLOGIC METHODS IN HISTOCOMPATIBILITY TESTING

The simplest and fastest methods for histocompatibility testing are serologic; that is, they utilize blood serum that contains antibodies to HLA antigens. Anti-HLA antibodies are highly specific for the individual structural determinants that characterize the different antigens of the HLA system. Thus, when sera containing HLA antibodies are mixed with lymphocytes, the antibodies will bind only to their specific target antigens.

When the antigen-antibody complex is formed on the cell surface in the presence of complement, complement activation leads to cell lysis. Thus, cell death is an indicator of the shared specificity of antigen and antibody and is a "positive" test result. Detection of

this identity between antibody and antigen provides the answer to most basic questions in histocompatibility testing: (1) What are the HLA antigens of a particular cell? When the antibody specificity is known, as for the HLA typing reagents, and the cell is of unknown phenotype, the positive test results with specific antisera will identify the antigens of the cell. (2) Are there anti-HLA antibodies in a particular serum? When the serum is being tested for the presence of HLA antibodies, and when the HLA phenotype of the test cell is known, a positive test indicates anti-lymphocyte activity in the serum. From the pattern of reactions with a panel of HLA-typed cells, the specificity of the antibodies may be inferred. If the patient's serum reacts with the donor cell, the 2 individuals are incompatible.

Thus, through an iterative process of testing serum and typing cells, HLA antigens are defined, panels of typed lymphocytes are generated, and collections of HLA typing sera of known specificity are created.

TISSUE TYPING BY THE LYMPHOCYTOTOXICITY TEST

Tissue typing is accomplished by exposing the unknown cell to a battery of antisera of known HLA specificity. The typing sera are selected to give unequivocally strong positive scores to ensure reproducibility. When the cells are killed by the antiserum and complement, the cell is presumed to have the same HLA antigen as the specificity of the antibody.

Cell Isolation

Lymphocytes are the preferred cell type for HLA typing, antibody screening, and cross-matching. They are normally isolated from whole peripheral blood by buoyant density gradient separation (see Chapter 13), from buffy coat, or, in cadaveric testing, from lymph nodes and spleen. Care must be taken to prepare a cell suspension of excellent viability as well as one that is free of erythrocyte and platelet contamination. Although other cell types that bear HLA antigens, such as platelets, amniocytes, and fibroblasts, can be used for HLA typing in special circumstances, lymphocytes are the most responsive and reproducible target for the standard cytotoxicity assay.

The Complement-Dependent Lymphocytotoxicity Test: NIH Standard Method

Individual HLA antisera are predispensed in 1-μL quantities into the microtest wells of specifically designed plastic trays composed of 60 or 72 wells of 15 μL capacity. Replicates of the test tray are stored frozen for later use. Into a thawed test tray, 2000 isolated lymphocytes are dispensed per well, and the tray is incubated for 30 minutes at room temperature to allow anti-HLA antibodies to bind to their specific target HLA antigens. Complement (5 μL) is added, usually as rabbit serum, and the tray is incubated for another 60 minutes. To visualize the dead and live cells under phase contrast microscopy, a vital dye, eosin Y, is added, followed by formalin to fix the reaction. Live cells exclude the dye and appear bright and refractile, while dead cells take up the dye and are swollen and dark (Fig 16–2). In an alternative method known as fluorochromasia, the cells are prelabeled with a fluorochrome such as fluorescein diacetate (green) prior to plating. When the cells are killed in the positive test, the fluorescein leaks out and the cells "disappear." Positive results are compared with a negative well where all the cells are visible. A second fluorochrome of contrasting color such as ethidium bromide (red) may be added to visualize the dead cells.

Each test well is scored individually by inspection, with the percentage of dead cells per well being noted. The test is unequivocally positive when at least half of the cells are killed. (Table 16–5).

Table 16–5. Scoring the lymphocytotoxicity test for HLA typing.

% Dead Lymphocytes in Test Well	Score	Interpretation
0–10	1	Negative
11–20	2	Doubtful positive
21–50	4	Weak positive
51–80	6	Positive
81–100	8	Strong positive

Interpretation of the Tissue-Typing Test

An antigen is assigned by noting the patterns of reactivity of the individual sera and their specificities. The typing sera that reacted positively with the test cells should have antibody specificities in common. For an antigen to be assigned, the majority of sera of that specificity must be unequivocally positive. In phenotyping an individual for class I HLA, one expects to find patterns with 2 antigens each from the A, B, and C loci. When only a single antigen is identified at a locus, the individual may be homozygous for

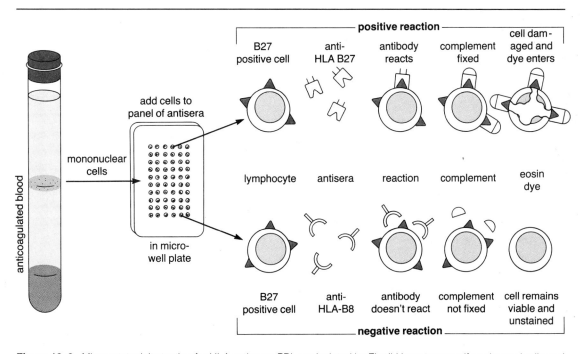

Figure 16–2. Microcytotoxicity testing for HLA antigens. PBL are isolated by Ficoll-Hypaque centrifugation and adjusted to 2×10^6 cells/mL. Then 1 μL of cells is added to each well of a tissue-typing plate that has been predispensed with a panel of HLA typing sera, each containing alloantibodies to specific HLA antigens. Illustrated are the reactions of HLA B27 cells with antisera specific for B27 (**upper**) and B8 (**lower**). B27 antibodies bind to B27 antigens on the cell surface, the antigen-antibody complex activates and fixes serum complement, the cell membrane is damaged, and the cell dies. Eosin dye penetrates the dead cells, staining them dark red under phase contrast microscopy, giving a positive test result. In contrast, the anti-B8 antibodies do not complex with the B27 antigen, the complement components are not activated, the cells remain undamaged, and eosin dye is excluded, resulting in a negative test. The cell is thus typed as B27-positive and B8-negative. Each test well is scored as percent dead cells (see Table 16–5) and the overall reaction pattern of the typing sera is interpreted to give the HLA antigen phenotype of the individual (see Table 16–6).

that allele or the laboratory has failed to identify the second antigen, usually owing to inadequacies in the array of typing sera. Table 16–6 shows a representation of HLA-typing test results.

TISSUE-TYPING REAGENTS: HLA ALLOANTISERA

Sources of HLA Typing Sera

The majority of HLA antisera are complex sera obtained from multiparous women. Maternal exposure to the mismatched paternal HLA antigens in the fetus gives rise to a polyclonal antibody response that frequently results in sera with multiple specificities. Consequently, several different antisera are used to type for a specific antigen. It is not unusual for a laboratory to use typing trays composed of more than 200 different sera to type a single individual for HLA-A, -B, -C, and -DR, -DQ antigens.

Placental fluid, a mixture of serum and tissue fluids, has proved to be a valuable second source of alloantisera for tissue typing. Antibodies of high titer can be recovered from the fluid shed from fresh placentae that have been refrigerated for 24 hours postdelivery. Attempts to immunize other animals, such as rabbits, for production of HLA antisera have largely failed. The xenoantisera reacted primarily with common human antigens such as the HLA-DR constant region. Thus, currently, the majority of HLA reagents are found among human sources by means of extensive serum-screening programs, a task undertaken by many tissue-typing laboratories. Through voluntary national and worldwide serum exchange programs, these reagents are distributed within the tissue-typing community for mutual benefit.

HLA antibodies are also found in the sera of patients exposed to HLA antigens through transfusions of blood and organ grafts. Generally, patients are not used as sources of HLA typing sera, since the quantities obtainable would be limited by their medical conditions.

MONOCLONAL ANTIBODIES TO HLA ANTIGENS

Recent efforts in numerous laboratories have resulted in a limited production of monoclonal antibodies to HLA specificities. It was hoped that hybridoma cell lines (see Chapter 12) would produce inexhaustible quantities of monospecific antibodies to HLA antigens. In reality, many murine monoclonal antibodies have been directed against human monomorphic framework determinants or to common epitopes rather than to the private polymorphic determinants of the individual HLA antigens. Unfortunately, most murine monoclonal antibodies do not fix complement. Non-complement-fixing antibodies can be used in assays that require only antigen binding, such as enzyme-linked immunosorbent assay (ELISA) and flow cytometry (see Chapters 12 and 13). Some monoclonal antibodies are reactive with more than one HLA specificity, indicating the existence of common antigenic determinants on HLA molecules.

SPECIFICITY OF HLA ANTIBODIES: PRIVATE & PUBLIC

An ideal HLA typing serum would be monospecific, that is, would have specificity for a single HLA antigen; however, in reality, the observed alloantibodies in a single serum are usually polyspecific. An alloantiserum can contain antibodies to multiple determinants on the immunizing antigen(s). Some determinants are the classic HLA **private** specificities that characterize each HLA allele (Table 16–1). Others are **public,** that is, are shared by several antigens that collectively constitute a cross-reacting antigen group (CREG group). Some complex sera can be rendered monospecific by dilution, whereas others lose all activity for all specificities simultaneously.

To determine the specificities of HLA antibodies, sera are tested against panels of cells of known HLA phenotype, a process termed "screening." The cell panel, usually from 40 to 60 cells, is preselected to provide a minimum of 2–3 representations of the most frequent HLA antigens. The antigens must be distributed among the cells so that the reaction pat-

Table 16–6. An example of HLA typing test results.[1]

Serum Name	Specificities	Score
A-001	A1	1
A-002	A1, A36	1
A-003	A1, A11	1
A-004	A2	1
A-005	A2, A28	6
A-006	A2, A28, B7	8
A-007	A3	8
A-008	A3	6
A-009	A3, A10, A11, A19	8
A-010	A11	1
A-011	A10, A11	1
A-012	A11, A1, A3 (weak)	4
B-001	B51, B52, B35	1
B-002	B51, B52	1
B-003	B51, B52, B53	1
B-004	B7, B42	8
B-005	B7, B27	8
B-006	B7, B55	8
B-007	B8	1
B-008	B8, B59	2
B-009	B44, B45, B21	6
B-010	B44, B45	8
B-011	B44	8
B-012	B45	1

[1]Interpretation: HLA phenotype is: A28, A3, B7, B44 (see Table 16–7).

tern for one antigen will not be entirely included within the pattern for a second antigen; for example, all of the HLA-A1 cells must not be the only HLA-B8 cells as well. If they were, the reaction patterns for both antibodies would be identical and the determination of A1 or B8, or both, could not be made with certainty. When the sera react with a subset of the panel, the specificity of the antibody is deduced by inspecting the HLA phenotypes of the positive cells. Table 16–7 illustrates the type of reaction patterns obtained on reagent or patient serum screens. The percent PRA is calculated as the ratio of the number of positive cells to the number of total panel cells multiplied by 100. PRA is indicative of the extent of sensitization of the patient to HLA. Note that the antibody specificities of sera with high PRA cannot be determined from these results. Special procedures must be used, such as dilution or treatment of the sera, or both, to determine antibody specificities.

TISSUE TYPING FOR CLASS II HLA ANTIGENS BY SEROLOGIC METHODS

Tissue typing for class II HLA antigens, HLA-DR and -DQ, is performed on lymphocyte preparations that are enriched for B lymphocytes. Special isolation procedures are required since approximately 80% of normal peripheral blood lymphocytes (PBL) are resting T cells that lack class II HLA antigens on their surface. The most widely used method for isolation of B cells for DR typing uses immunomagnetic beads coated with anti-DR antibodies. The beads are mixed with isolated PBL, and surface DR antigens on the B cells bind to beads coated with antibody. The plastic beads have a magnetic core so that application of a magnet to the side of the reaction tube will attract and hold the cells stationary in the tube while the unattached cells are discarded. The isolated B cells are

Table 16–7. An example of results of serum screening for class I HLA antibodies.[1]

Panel Cell HLA Antigens	Cytotoxicity Test Score for Patient Serum No:				
	1	2	3	4	5
A, A, B, B (locus)					
1, 2, 7, 60	1	1	8	1	8
2, 3, 8, 51	1	8	8	8	8
3, 29, 35, 44	1	8	1	6	8
30, 33, 55, 60	1	1	1	1	8
1, 30, 13, 51	1	1	1	8	8
24, 28, 35, 55	1	1	4	6	4
3, 28, 7, 44	1	8	4	1	6
2, 28, 35, 38	1	1	8	8	8

[1]PRA (panel-reactive antibody) was 0, 38, 50, 63, and 100%, for patient sera 1 through 5, respectively. PRA is calculated as (number of positive tests/number of cells tested) × 100. Analyzed antibodies were as follows (patient sera 1 through 5, respectively): None; A3; A2, weak A28; B51, B35; and Unknown (autoantibody?).

then washed, counted, and plated directly into DR typing trays for cytotoxicity testing.

Prior to the use of immunomagnetic beads, the most common method for B cell isolation was the adherence of B cells to nylon wool fibers. In this method, the PBL are passed through nylon-wool-packed columns made from plastic drinking straws or small syringes. The columns are filled with warm culture medium, and the cells are incubated in the wool for 30 minutes at 37 °C, allowing the B lymphocytes and macrophages to adhere to the fibers. The nonadherent T cells are then flushed out and saved for other tests. The B cells remaining are removed from the column by mechanical agitation of the wool and exposure to cooled medium. Nylon wool processing is normally used when large quantities of mixed lymphocytes must be processed for T and B cell lymphocyte testing, as in cadaver lymph node and spleen cell preparations. A minimum enrichment of 80% B cells is necessary for successful class II typing.

Antisera for Class II HLA Typing

Antisera for class II HLA tissue typing must be free of antibodies to class I HLA antigens. Unfortunately, the majority of HLA alloantisera contain mixtures of antibodies to class I and class II HLA antigens. Because their membranes have no class II antigens, pooled platelets are used as absorbents to clear HLA sera of any contaminating class I antibodies. Such manipulation of these sera can leave them diluted and operationally less reliable. Because B lymphocytes have more class I HLA antigens on their surface than do T cells, false-positive reactions from residual class I antibodies are possible. It is necessary that all absorbed class II antisera be thoroughly screened on T and B cells to ensure that absorption is complete. Overall, HLA typing sera for class II antigens are of poorer quality and in shorter supply than are reagents for class I typing. Currently, very few sera for HLA-DP typing are available. The antigens of the DP locus have been defined mainly by cellular assays (see below). Because of the paucity of good DR and DQ typing sera, serologic methods have had limited success in defining class II polymorphisms. Biochemical and molecular-biologic methods have provided significant new information. See the section on molecular HLA typing.

The complement-dependent cytotoxicity assay for class II HLA DR and DQ typing is performed with appropriate class II typing sera but is modified as follows: Initial incubation of cells and serum is performed at 37 °C for 60 minutes; after addition of complement, the mixture is incubated for 120 minutes at room temperature. The extended incubation times are used to promote binding of antibodies and complement. The temperature increase is used to avoid the false-positive reactions that can result from the binding of cold reactive nonspecific antibodies.

When immunoabsorbant beads are used for class II typing, the incubation times are generally decreased by approximately one-half, possibly because of the weakening of the cell membrane by attachment to the beads.

Variability in Tissue-Typing Results

HLA typing sera are not standardized by the usual practices of regulated quality control and licensure. The multiplicity of HLA antigens and the scarcity of the defining antisera make it impossible to license a standard reagent for each specificity. Each tissue-typing laboratory has the responsibility of obtaining the appropriate antisera and monitoring their performance. Typing sera are collected through serum exchange programs between laboratories, and new sera are discovered by means of extensive testing of sera from pregnant women, fluids recovered from placentae, and, occasionally, patient sera. Commercial typing trays are also available. Results with the laboratory's own serum trays may be compared with those of other collections of sera for confirmation of an HLA phenotype. All tissue-typing laboratories are required by the standards set by the American Society for Histocompatibility and Immunogenetics (ASHI) to control the quality of serologic and cellular reagents used for clinical testing. International and national quality control programs are available for typing, cross-matching, and serum analysis, and satisfactory performance is mandatory for ASHI accreditation of the laboratory.

A second variable in tissue typing is the serum complement, a reagent commercially available as the pooled serum from several hundred rabbits. Rabbit serum contains heterophile antibodies with anti-human lymphocyte activity that enhances its effectiveness in the cytotoxicity assay. Overabundance of these anti-human antibodies will render the complement innately cytotoxic and therefore produces false-positive results. As with typing sera, the individual laboratory must screen its source of complement to find one that promotes strong serum reactions without causing nonspecific toxicity. Because there is no standard complement source, it follows that the same serum tested in different laboratories has the potential of giving different results.

A third variable is the choice of method used to visualize the live and dead cells. Among these methods there are variations in incubation times and also in the definition of the end of the test period. Thus, in the exchange of typing sera between laboratories, it is important to note the method by which the serum was characterized.

CROSS-MATCHING

The purpose of the cross-match test is to detect the presence of antibodies in the patient's serum that are directed against the potential donor HLA antigens. If present, the antibodies signal that the immune system of the recipient has been sensitized to those donor antigens and is therefore primed to vigorously reject any graft bearing them. In the transplanted kidney, the main target of these antibodies is probably the HLA antigens on vascular endothelium of capillaries and arterioles. HLA antigen-antibody complexes on endothelium activate complement and lead to cell damage. Platelets then aggregate, eventually producing fibrin clots, which clog the vessels. This causes ischemic necrosis. Even weak, low-titer antibodies, particularly those directed against class I antigens, can contribute to graft rejection. Therefore, the ultimate goal of the cross-match is a test of both great sensitivity and specificity for HLA antigens.

Cross-Matching by Lymphocytotoxicity

A simple cross-match by the standard cytotoxicity method (see above) may be performed with donor PBL as targets. PBL cross-matches are usually included in the preliminary evaluation of potential living-related donors for renal graft recipients. PBL are normally about 80% T cells, which carry class I HLA antigens only, and 20% B cells and monocytes, which bear both class I and class II antigens. A strongly positive cross-match by cytotoxicity (50% or more cell death per well) clearly indicates the presence of antibodies to class I antigens. However, 10–20% cell killing could result from an antibody specific for class II or could be due to a weak anti-class I antibody. To resolve the specificity of the antibody, cross-matching is then performed on cell preparations enriched for either T or B lymphocytes.

Cross-Matching with Separated T & B Lymphocytes

A. T Cell Cross-Matches: T cell cross-matches are performed at room temperature and also at 37 °C in some laboratories to avoid the binding of cold-reactive antibodies, presumed to be autoreactive. A positive T cell cross-match by any method contraindicates transplantation, no matter how weak the reaction level; ie, a reaction of 4+ (20–50% dead cells per well above background) is considered just as positive a result as 6+ or 8+ (51% dead cells or greater).

Several methods to improve the sensitivity of T cell cross-matches by complement-dependent cytotoxicity have been developed. These include the following.

1.   Extended incubation–The simplest modification in the cytotoxicity assay to increase sensitivity is to extend the incubation time of cells, serum, and complement.

2.   The Amos wash step–This method interjects a wash step after the incubation of cells and serum and prior to the addition of complement to remove anti-complementary factors in the serum.

3.   Anti-human globulin (AHG)–The cytotoxicity of some antibodies may be enhanced by the addition of a second-step antibody, usually a polyclonal anti-human immunoglobulin reagent.

B. B Cell Cross-Matches: Cross-matching for antibodies to class II HLA antigens requires the use of B lymphocytes as targets and the same extended incubation times as HLA-DR and -DQ serologic typing. A positive B cell cross-match may result from antibodies binding to class I or class II HLA antigens. Moreover, B cells are a more sensitive indicator for weak class I antibodies, since they carry class I molecules in greater density than T cells do. Cross-matching by flow cytometry can readily distinguish between "true B" antibodies and weak class I antibodies of a positive B cell cross-match. The significance for transplant outcome of preformed antibodies to class II antigens is not yet clear. Successful transplantation into patients with low-titer anti-class II antibodies (titer of 1:1 or 1:2) has been reported, as has the acute rejection of grafts transplanted in the face of high-titer (1:8) antibodies. It is possible that the loss of grafts transplanted in the face of T-negative, B-positive cross-matches is due to the anti-class I component of these alloreactive sera.

C. Flow Cytometry Cross-Matching (See Chapter 13): Cross-matching by flow cytometry (FCC) has been shown to be up to 100 times more sensitive than visual serologic methods for the detection of HLA antibodies on lymphocytes. In this cross-matching application, T cells can be separated from B cells electronically through the use of a fluoresceinated antibody to a T cell surface antigen such as the CD3 T cell receptor complex. An electronic "gate" can be created so that only the fluorescently labeled T cells are selected. Donor lymphocytes are incubated with patient's serum to allow binding of any anti-donor antibodies. Antibody bound to the selected T cell population is detected by addition of an anti-human IgG directed to the F(ab)'$_2$ portion of the antibody and labeled with a fluorochrome of a different color from the T cell marking antibody (eg, green, if the anti-CD3 was red). The flow cytometer counts the number of labeled T cells and creates a histogram displaying the number of cells versus fluorescence intensity (Fig 16–3). Unlabeled cells lie near the origin, while labeled cells lie to the right of the origin on the x axis. A shift to the right of the T cell peak in the experimental test compared with the negative control indicates that anti-class I HLA antibody from the patient serum has bound to the donor T cells. FCCs can also be performed on B cells labeled with specific antibody to B cell antigen.

FCC is generally performed with the most recent and selected previously obtained sera for all cadaver waiting list patients who have rejected prior transplants or who have high PRAs, and for patients with living related donors in the event of a negative T cell and positive B cell serologic cross-match.

Occasionally, positive FCC cross-matches occur

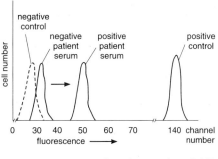

serum	mean channel no.	channel shift
negative control	27	—
negative patient	33	6
positive patient	50	23
positive control	140	113

Figure 16–3. Flow cytometry cross-match (FCC) with patient serum and donor T cells. A schematic composite tracing of a FCC fluorescence histogram illustrating representative peak positions for a negative and positive T cell FCC cross-match in relation to negative and positive control peaks. Peaks represent the number of cells (y axis) at a given fluorescence level (x axis) expressed as channel numbers. Donor lymphocytes are incubated with patient serum, and then a fluorescein isothiocyanate-labeled anti-human immunoglobulin is added, which fluorescently labels donor T cells that have bound patient antibody. When compared with the peak of T cells having no antibody bound, the fluorescent T cell peak is brighter and shifted to the right on the x axis. When the mean channel fluorescence of the T cell peak shifts to the right by more than 10 channels on a 256-channel scale, the cross-match is considered to be positive.

when both the serologic T and B cell cross-matches are negative. The nature of these antibodies is unknown and has been considered by some to be irrelevant to transplantation. For the unsensitized patient, such conclusions may be correct. However, for patients with high PRAs and those who have undergone previous transplants, caution (and further testing) is justified before the transplant is performed.

Cross-Matching for Autoantibodies

In cross-matching patient serum for donor compatibility, it is most important to distinguish nonspecific anti-lymphocyte antibodies, referred to as autoantibodies, from the specific anti-donor antibodies. The presence of autoantibodies is detected by the auto-cross-match, in which the patient's own serum and cells are combined in the standard cytotoxicity test. Autoantibodies can give a false-positive result in a donor cross-match, leading to the erroneous disqualification of that donor. Alternatively, preexisting autoantibodies can mask the presence of specific anti-donor antibodies. Autoantibody cross-matches are routinely performed in conjunction with all living-donor cross-matches for each serum that is tested.

CELLULAR ASSAYS FOR HISTOCOMPATIBILITY

In vivo, recognition of nonself antigens and destruction of cells bearing such markers is accomplished by cells of the immune system. Some of the clinically relevant class II HLA antigens that can trigger the immune response are not readily detected by the serologic methods discussed above. Instead, lymphocytes are used as discriminatory reagents for the HLA-Dw and -DP antigens and as indicators of histoincompatibility between donor and recipient. The functions of cellular recognition are utilized in the MLC, HTC, and primed lymphocyte typing (PLT) tests, and the dual functions of recognition and effector cell killing are used in the CML test.

MLC Test (See Chapter 13)

This is also known as the mixed-lymphocyte reaction (MLR). When the lymphocytes of 2 HLA-disparate individuals are combined in tissue culture, the cells enlarge, synthesize DNA, and proliferate, whereas HLA-identical cells remain quiescent. The proliferation is driven primarily by differences in the class II HLA antigens between the 2 test cells.

On the basis of MLC testing, class II antigens were originally described as a series of lymphocyte-activating determinants, products of the HLA-"D" locus (-Dw1, -Dw2, etc). No D locus products have ever been isolated, however, although several distinct "D region" loci (-DR, -DQ, and -DP) and their alleles have been identified. Dw "antigens" are now considered to be immunogenic epitopes formed by combinations of D region determinants that can be recognized by T cells. Distinct Dw types may represent unique haplotype combinations of various D region products.

Reactivity in MLC probably reflects the initial immune recognition step of graft rejection in vivo. The more immunogenic the D locus difference, the greater the cellular response in MLC and the more likely the rejection of the graft. Normally, both cells will proliferate, forming the 2-way MLC. To monitor the response of a single responder cell (the one-way MLC), the partner cell (stimulator) is inactivated by radiation or drugs (such as mitomycin C) that inhibit DNA synthesis (Fig 16–4). A maximum proliferative response usually occurs after incubation at 37 °C for 5–6 days. The culture is then pulsed with [³H]thymidine for 5–12 hours to label the newly synthesized DNA. Finally, the cells are harvested, washed free of unbound radioactivity, and counted in a beta counter.

A properly composed MLC test includes a checkerboard of one-way combinations of each cell serving as both stimulator and responder with all other cells. Each cell must be controlled for its ability to both stimulate and respond to HLA-mismatched cells. Normally, 2–4 unrelated control cells of known class II HLA type are tested individually with each family

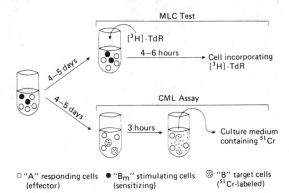

Figure 16–4. The MLC and CML tests. In the one-way MLC, responder PBLs are mixed 1:1 with irradiated stimulator cells and incubated at 37 °C in a humidified atmosphere with 5% CO_2. After 5 days, the culture is pulsed with [³H]thymidine ([³H]TdR) to label the nucleic acid in the responder cells. After 18 hours, cells are harvested and counted for internalized radioactivity. If the class II HLA antigens of the stimulator cells differ from those of the responder cells, the responder cells undergo blastogenesis, synthesize DNA, and proliferate. Increased sample radioactivity signals recognition of class II HLA differences. When responder and stimulator cells are class II identical, the proliferative responses are less than 20% of the maximum response to the mismatched controls and less than 2% over autologous (background) controls. (Reproduced, with permission, from Bach FH, Van Rood JJ: The major histocompatibility complex: Genetics and biology. *N Engl J Med* 1976;**295**:806, 872.)

member. The maximum response of each cell is obtained by exposure to a pool of irradiated stimulator cells of diverse HLA types.

Autologous controls combining self with irradiated self are also run to normalize the response of each cell to stimulators. Each test should be run in triplicate. It is absolutely necessary to perform the entire familial MLC at one time owing to the inherent variability of individual cellular responses from day to day.

Results are expressed as a stimulation index (SI) or relative response (RR). The SI is the ratio of counts per minute of the test over the autologous test for that cell:

$$SI = cpm \text{ of } \frac{\textbf{Responder vs Stimulator (irradiated)}}{\textbf{Responder vs Responder (irradiated)}}$$

A value of SI ≤ 2 is interpreted as HLA identity at HLA-D. The RR calculates the response in the experimental MLC relative to the maximum response of that cell elicited by the pool. Counts per minute of both are corrected by subtraction of the autologous control for the responder cell.

$$RR = \frac{\text{Responder vs Stimulator (irradiated)} - \text{Autologous control}}{\text{cpm of} \quad \text{Responder vs Pool (irradiated)} - \text{Autologous control}} \times 100$$

MLC testing can be useful in selecting the most compatible (least stimulatory) organ donor if several nonidentical family members (matched for zero or one haplotype) are available. The donor who is the least stimulatory to the patient is the preferred organ donor. The results of an intrafamilial MLC can address such questions as (1) Are 2 serologically identical DR antigens also functionally identical? (2) Is the individual with only one identifiable DR antigen a homozygote, or is the DR "blank" really a second DR antigen that was missed in the serologic testing? (3) Are the serologically assigned class II antigens consistent with the MLC results? If apparently HLA-identical individuals are reactive, there may have been a genetic recombination event.

The MLC test is frequently used to confirm apparent HLA identity in the living-related transplant situation and is especially useful if haplotyping could not be accomplished. When the HLA-identical recipient and donor are unrelated, as in voluntary bone marrow donation, MLC testing is extremely important in revealing hidden class II incompatibilities that could affect recipient tolerance to the graft and promote graft-versus-host disease.

HTC Test

MLC nonreactivity indicates HLA-Dw identity, and therefore the MLC test can be used to type for specific Dw alleles. Since most individuals to be tested are heterozygous at the D region, it follows that the stimulator cell must be homozygous for a given Dw antigen to result in MLC nonresponsiveness. Such HTCs have been identified in the random population, but the best source for HTCs is among the progeny of first-cousin marriages. True HTCs are rare and precious reagents, and few laboratories can afford to maintain the large cell panel necessary for complete and accurate testing.

The lymphocytes to be Dw typed are set up as responders in multiple MLC tests, each test with a different inactivated stimulator HTC. HTC testing can discriminate among the various subtypes of serologically identified DR antigens and thus can provide a finer definition of true class II HLA compatibility.

PLT Test

Lymphocytes already exposed (primed) to a specific antigen in a primary MLC will proliferate rapidly on reexposure to the same antigen. Thus, a primed cell can be used to test an unknown cell for the presence of the original stimulating antigen. With cells primed to class II HLA antigens, this assay can be used as an HLA typing test for D region antigens.

As in HTC typing, an extensive panel of specifically primed cells must be maintained for PLT testing. PLT was used to type for DP antigens, but this method has been supplanted by molecular typing methods and is now only rarely used.

CML Test

In primary MLC, exposure to nonself class I and class MHC II antigens can result in the generation of cytotoxic T lymphocytes (CTL). CTL kill their targets through direct contact, probably by the release of toxic mediators that lead to cell lysis. CD4 and CD8 CTL can be found infiltrating kidney allografts during rejection and are considered to be important effector cells in graft loss (see Chapter 57). To test for the capacity to generate CTL, a primary MLC is run with the patient as the responder and prospective donor cells as inactivated stimulators. After the MLC, the patient's cells are harvested and then reexposed in culture to fresh donor target cells that have been loaded with ^{51}Cr (Fig 16–4). Usually, the targets are preincubated with the mitogen phytohemagglutinin (PHA) for 6 days, since PHA-activated blast cells can incorporate more ^{51}Cr than resting lymphocytes can. CTL and targets are plated in effector:target-cell ratios of 100:1, 50:1, and 10:1. Control wells include targets alone to measure the spontaneous release of label and test wells containing target cells that are treated with detergent to release the maximum incorporated label. The test requires 4 hours of incubation in a humidified CO_2 atmosphere at 37 °C. At the conclusion, the supernatant of each test well is sampled and counted. In the experimental wells, the amount of ^{51}Cr released is corrected for the background level of spontaneously released label and compared with the maximum amount of label released:

$$\% \text{ Specific Release} = \frac{\text{cpm (Experimental)} - \text{cpm (Spontaneous)}}{\text{cpm (Maximum)} - \text{cpm (Spontaneous)}} \times 100$$

Elevated counts of 30–50% above spontaneous background are indicative of CTL activity.

Direct CML testing can be used to monitor posttransplant rejection by testing for the presence of activated circulating anti-donor CTL. The patient's PBL are placed directly in culture with ^{51}Cr-labeled donor cells as targets. An elevated donor cell lysis compared with pretransplant levels is considered evidence of circulating CTL, which are particularly prevalent during rejection.

CML testing has applications in living-related renal and bone marrow transplantation. The preferred kidney donor will be the one who fails to stimulate the recipient to form CTL. In bone marrow transplantation, the recipient is at risk for immune attack by the marrow donor (graft-versus-host disease). The capacity of the prospective donors to form CTL against the recipient may be assessed through MLC plus CML testing.

A summary of the serologic and cellular methods for histocompatibility testing is presented in Table 16–8. All of these methods are in current use and are accepted as appropriate (in some instances mandatory) procedures for clinical histocompatibility testing.

HISTOCOMPATIBILITY TESTING BY MOLECULAR-BIOLOGIC METHODS

Introduction

The classic polymorphisms of the HLA system have been inferred from the binding patterns of antibodies and reactions of lymphocytes activated by disparate MHC antigens. With the advent of gene cloning and DNA sequencing, these polymorphisms are known to derive from sequence differences localized to several variable regions in MHC molecules. In the class HLA II genes, the variable regions are found mainly in exon 2 of the coding regions but polymorphic regions also exist in the introns and flanking regions of the genes. Class II antigens can be characterized as a patchwork of combinations of these sequence polymorphisms. Thus many antigens share some of the same microsequences, a fact that accounts for the long-observed phenomenon of cross-reactivity of antisera and, more recently, the cross-hybridization of class II probes used in various HLA typing techniques. Clearly, the most definitive HLA typing method would be to completely sequence the DNA of the HLA genes of each individual. Undoubtedly, this will become the method of choice when automated sequencing technology becomes practical, affordable, and widely disseminated. Until then, there are alternative approaches that utilize knowledge of both the unique and the consensus sequences of HLA antigens.

HLA-typing methods can be characterized by the type of DNA on which the method operates and the type of polymorphism detected. Table 16–9 summarizes methods in current use. Mainly, the type of DNA is either genomic (ie, DNA isolated from the cell nucleus) or the amplified product of the polymerase chain reaction (PCR), a process that produces multiple copies of a specific subregion of HLA DNA (see below and Fig 16–6). The polymorphisms detected by the readout scheme are either allele-specific

Table 16–8. Serologic and cellular methods used in histocompatibility testing.

Test	Test Type and Components	Time	Application
Tissue typing			
Complement-dependent lymphocytotoxicity	Serologic (HLA antisera; complement; test cells)	3 h	Identification of class I and II HLA antigens.
MLC test	Cellular (donor and recipient cells combined in tissue culture)	6 d	Class II HLA antigen compatibility.
HTC test	Cellular (test cell and HTC combined in tissue culture)	6 d	Identification of HLA-D locus (Dw) antigens.
PLT	Cellular (lymphoctyes primed to specific DP antigen; test cells)	2 d	Identification of HLA-DP antigens.
Cross-matching			
PBL cross-match	Serologic (recipient serum; donor cells; complement; AHG optional)	3 h	Detection of preformed anti-donor antibodies in patient serum.
T/B cell cross-match	Serologic (purified donor T or B cells; recipient serum; AHG optional with T cells)	3–6 h	T cells: detection of anti-donor class I HLA antibodies; B cells: detection of antibodies to class I and II HLA.
CML test	Cellular (patient cells from primary MLC; fresh donor stimulators as targets)	4 h	Detection of anti-donor CTL.
FCC	Serologic (patient serum; donor cells; fluorescent anti-human immunoglobulin)	3–4 h	Detection of very weak and non-cytotoxic anti-donor antibodies.
Auto-cross-match	Serologic (patient PBL, T and B cells, and serum)	3–4 h	Detection of nonspecific anti-lymphocyte antibodies (autoantibodies).
Screening			
Screening for class I HLA antibodies	Serologic (patient serum; panel of HLA-typed T cells or PBL	3 h × 40 cells	Detection of class I HLA antibodies; identification of antibody specificity.
Screening for class II HLA antibodies	Serologic (patient serum absorbed; B cell panel typed for HLA-DR, DQ)	4 h × no. of cells plus absorption time	Detection of class II HLA antibodies; identification of antibody specificity.

Table 16–9. Molecular Histocompatibility Techniques.

Name	DNA Type Analyzed (Genomic or Amplified)	Primer Type (Group- or Allele-Specific)	Level of Antigen Identification (Generic[1] or Allele-Specific[2]
RFLP	Genomic		Generic
PCR-RFLP	Amplified	Group	Generic
PCR-SSOP	Amplified	Group	Allele
PCR, Nested	Amplified	Group/allele	Allele
PCR-SSP	Amplified	Group	Generic
Heteroduplex	Amplified	Group	

[1]Generic is equivalent to serologic typing.
[2]Allele-specific identifies an allele by its variable DNA sequences.

(specific for sequences unique to the generic HLA allele in question) or sequence-specific (specific for the microvariable regions of the HLA genes). Identification of HLA antigens can be either at the generic level, which is the same as serologic typing (DR1–DR18) or at the level of allelic subtypes as defined by direct sequencing of the genes. Table 16–10 shows the number of alleles of the class II loci, DRB1, DQB1, DQA1, DPA1, and DPB1, and indicates the nomenclature of the alleles by genetic locus. The complete DNA sequences have been determined for all of these alleles.

The first molecular method to be widely used to identify the generic (serologically defined) class II HLA antigens has been based on restriction fragment length polymorphisms (RFLP).

Table 16–10. Polymorphism of class II HLA alleles.

Locus	Antigen[1]	No. of Alleles	Nomenclature
DRB1	DR1	3	DRB1*0101 . . .
	DR15 (DR2)	3	DRB1*1501 . . .
	DR16 (DR2)	2	DRB1*1601 . . .
	DR3	3	DRB1*0301 . . .
	DR4	14	DRB1*1401 . . .
	DR11 (DR5)	6	DRB1*11011 . . .
	DR12	2	DRB1*1201 . . .
	DR13 (DR6)	6	DRB1*1301 . . .
	DR14 (DR6)	10	DRB1*1401 . . .
	DR7	2	DRB1*0701 . . .
	DR8	7	DRB1*0801 . . .
	DR9	1	DRB1*09011 . . .
	DR10	1	DRB1*1001
DRB3	DR52	4	DRB3*0101 . . .
DRB4	DR53	1	DRB4*0101
DRB5	DR51	4	DRB5*0101 . . .
DQA1	. . .[2]	13	DQA1*0101 . . .
DQB1	DQ5 (DQ1)	5	DQB1*0501 . . .
	DQ6 (DQ1)	6	DQB1*0601 . . .
	DQ2	1	DQB1*0201
	DQ3	5	DQB1*0301 . . .
	DQ4	2	DQB1*0401 . . .
DPA1		8	DPA1*0101 . . .
DPB1		32	DPB1*0101 . . .

[1]Equivalent antigens as defined serologically.
[2]No equivalent serologically defined antigens.

HLA Typing by RFLP

RFLP is currently used by many laboratories to identify the basic serologically defined class II HLA antigens. The technique of RFLP typing is based on the knowledge of the germline nucleotide sequences found in both coding (exons) and noncoding (introns and flanking) regions of class II HLA genes. These sequence differences serve as target sites for cleavage by bacterial restriction endonucleases. Such restriction sites are usually 4 or 6 bases in length, and more than 90 enzymes that can recognize a site of a unique nucleotide sequence are known. When isolated DNA is digested with a particular enzyme, the DNA of an HLA haplotype will be cut into fragments of different lengths depending on the locations of the restriction sites cut. Thus a new polymorphism consisting of a fragment length is created analogous to the classic HLA serological polymorphisms. It should be noted, however, that most of the sites cut lie in the introns of the HLA genes, so the resulting fragments are not equivalent to serologic polymorphisms. Subjecting the restriction digest fragments to gel electrophoresis separates them by size. The different-sized fragments are visualized by probing with cDNAs that hybridize with the consensus sequences within the fragments. This process of enzyme digestion, transfer of the fragments to a membrane by blotting of the gel, and hybridization by labeled probes is known as Southern blotting (Fig 16–5). Band patterns are produced that are diagnostic for most of the generic class II antigens. Locus-specific probes have been designed for the detection of the products of the different subloci of DR, DQ, and DP, eg, DRα, DPβ.

A. Uses and Limitations of RFLP Typing: RFLP typing cannot identify the many alleles now known to exist in class II HLA antigens (Table 16–10) such as the multiple subtypes of DR4, DR11, DR13, DR14, etc. Its main use has been to confirm and clarify serologically assigned DR and DQ types and to identify generic DP alleles. The method is time-consuming, usually requiring from 2 to 3 weeks and at least 5–10 µg of DNA.

RFLP analysis can reveal a new DR antigen by producing a novel banding pattern. Conversely, there

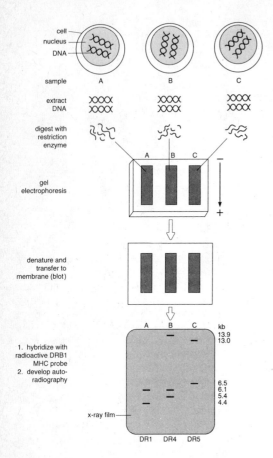

cell
nucleus
DNA

sample   A   B   C

extract
DNA

digest with
restriction
enzyme

gel
electrophoresis

denature and
transfer to
membrane (blot)

1. hybridize with
   radioactive DRB1
   MHC probe
2. develop auto-
   radiography

x-ray film

	A	B	C	kb
		—	—	13.9 13.0
			—	6.5 6.1
	—	—	—	5.4 4.4

DR1   DR4   DR5

Figure 16–5. Tissue typing by RFLP. A comparison of RFLP tissue typing of 3 samples, A, B, and C, is shown. Genomic DNA is extracted from the cells and digested with selected restriction endonucleases. Digests are dispersed by agarose gel electrophoresis, the DNA is denatured into single strands, and the gel pattern of fragments is transferred to a support membrane by blotting (Southern blot). The DNA fragments are hybridized with a radiolabeled HLA locus-specific probe (eg, DRB1) that will complex with DNA nucleotide sequences. After autoradiography, the restriction fragments that have hybridized with the probe appear as patterns of isolated bands of specific size (kilobases; kb). Control digests containing fragments of known size permit sizing of the bands. Many HLA alleles have characteristic band patterns (fragment length polymorphism) when digested with specific endonucleases. HLA antigens can be assigned from these patterns, as illustrated here for DR1, DR4, and DR5. (Reproduced, with permission, from Bidwell JL et al: A DNA RFLP typing system that positively identifies serologically well-defined and ill-defined HLA-DR and DQ alleles, including DRw10. *Transplantation* 1988;**45:**640.)

may be no enzymes capable of producing fragments that characterize some of the known HLA alleles.

Use of PCR in HLA Typing

PCR allows amplification of specific targeted regions of DNA. By providing multiple copies of selected DNA sequences, it forms the basis for newer HLA-typing methods such as oligonucleotide typing and sequence specific priming (discussed below). PCR provides several advantages for molecular HLA typing: it produces a useful amount of selected portions of the HLA gene and requires only a minute quantity of sample to initiate this process. The PCR product can then be used in various methods to detect internal polymorphisms of selected gene segments and thereby identify the HLA allele.

Currently, these methods are being applied only to VNTR (variable number tandem repeats) probing (see below) and class II HLA typing for clinical purposes. Because of the complexity of the class I alleles, a PCR-based typing system has not yet been finalized for HLA-A, -B, and -C locus products.

A. PCR Method: PCR is an automated method for amplification of a specific known DNA sequence. Two oligonucleotide primers are synthesized that are complementary to the 2 flanking regions of the DNA segment to be amplified. The upstream and downstream primers are different from one another and can range from 20 to 30 bp in length. The primers will hybridize to the flanking regions of the genes and "prime" the replication of the gene by thermostable polymerases. The PCR process involves the repetition of 3 steps: (1) denaturation of the sample DNA to single strands, (2) annealing of the sequence-specific oligonucleotide primers to the boundaries of the segment, and (3) extension of the primers by the polymerase to form new double-stranded DNA across the segment. It is a chain reaction since reaction products become the templates for the next cycle of the process (Fig 16–6). Repetition of the PCR will rapidly lead to the exponential accumulation of thousands of copies of the gene segment encompassed by the 5′ ends of the 2 primers. In a few hours, after approximately 25–30 cycles, more than one million copies of the chosen sequence are produced.

The reaction mixture includes template DNA, a mixture of nucleotides (deoxyribonucleoside triphosphates), the 2 PCR primers, *Taq* polymerase, and buffer.

B. Types of PCR Amplification:

1. Generic or group-specific amplification– Primers are directed at flanking sequences common to a group of alleles such as the DR4 group or to the alleles of the DRB3* (DR52) group. The product is a region of DNA known to contain sequence differences that characterize the alleles of the group. The product can be detected by oligonucleotide probes tailored to hybridize with, and thereby discriminate between, these specific allelic differences (successful hybridization indicates the presence of that allele) or

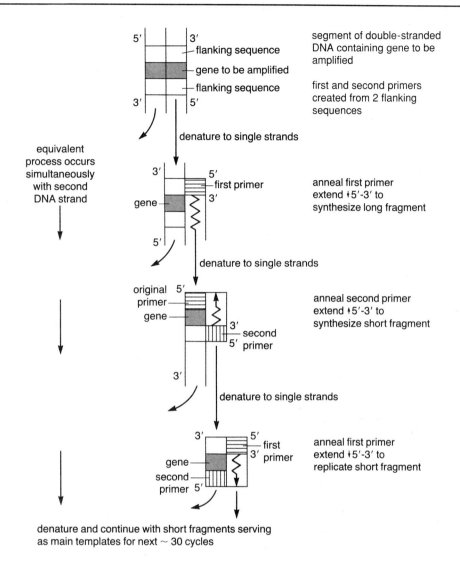

Figure 16–6. Amplification of DNA by the PCR. The segment of DNA that contains the gene of interest is sequenced, including upstream and downstream flanking regions. Primers are prepared with complementary sequences to the 2 flanking regions. The PCR amplification process has 3 steps: denaturation of the DNA to single strands; annealing of the primer to the flanking region of the gene; and extension of the primer across the gene segment, resulting in synthesis of a new copy of the gene. The new copies serve as templates for the subsequent cycles. As illustrated here, the original DNA sample is denatured into single strands and is mixed with the primers, nucleotides (deoxynucleoside triphosphates), and *Taq* polymerase. The first primer anneals to a flanking sequence. The polymerase extends 5′ to 3′ across the gene, creating a fragment of indeterminant length (the long fragment). The new DNA is denatured to 2 single strands. The second primer anneals to the long fragment (which contains the first primer) at the opposite flanking sequence. The polymerase extends the primer 5′ to 3′ across the gene, ending at the sequence of the first primer, creating the short fragment. From this point, subsequent cycles will amplify the short fragment geometrically, leading to a 10^6-fold replication at 30 cycles.

by application of allele-specific amplification to the group-specific product (nested PCR).

2. Allele-specific amplification (PCR-SSP)– A new method, which uses allele-specific PCR amplification, promises to simply and rapidly identify generic class II genes. This method utilizes the principle that PCR primers amplify a portion of DNA

most efficiently when they anneal perfectly to their complementary flanking sequences. Primers based on sequences specific for the DR alleles have been designed so that under proper conditions of annealing temperature and extension time, amplified product is produced only when an exact fit is made. If no product is produced, the DNA sample does not carry the sequence of the gene in question. After amplification, the sample is run on a minigel and examined with ethidium bromide for the presence or absence of product. This method, called PCR-SSP (sequence-specific primers) can identify the serologically defined DR antigens DR1–DR18, but is not yet capable of the high-resolution allele subtyping possible with oligonucleotide typing methods. All combinations of heterozygosity and homozygosity can be distinguished through use of an internal amplification control. The success of PCR-SSP clearly depends on the stringency of the experimental conditions.

A major advantage of PCR-SSP typing is that with the proper equipment, DR typing can be accomplished in under 3 hours with minimal sample manipulation and at reasonable cost. Molecular DR typing by this method will probably be included in the standard matching for cadaveric organ transplantation.

C. Typing for Class II Antigens with Sequence-Specific Oligonucleotide Probes: The amplified portions of HLA genes obtained from PCR can be further tested to reveal specific alleles within the amplified segment. The most sensitive method in current use is typing with synthesized oligonucleotide probes.

Oligonucleotide probes are short synthetic segments of single-stranded DNA, commonly 18–24 nucleotides long, complementary to known polymorphic sequences in HLA alleles. These probes hybridize only to their exactly complementary sequences under stringent hybridization conditions. Even a single base-pair difference causes the probes to break away from the pairing with the sample DNA. This property of perfect sequence specificity gives this method of class II HLA typing the greatest power for resolution of HLA alleles.

Multiple probes are required to identify an HLA allele because of the sharing of sequence polymorphisms. With the 11 International Histocompatibility Workshop collection of primers and probes to identify an allele in the DR52-related group consisting of alleles of the DR3, DR5, and DR6 groups, approximately 22 probes are required; DQB1 requires approximately 20, DQA1 requires 17, and DR1 and DR2 each require 7 probes. Alternative schemes have been proposed and are in current use. As more alleles are discovered, this number will certainly increase. The patterns produced by these probes can identify the complex collection of polymorphisms that is characteristic of a particular allele. Table 16–11 shows the hybridization patterns for DR4 alleles using the 11th International Histocompatibility Workshop probes.

Primer pairs are selected that amplify the DNA in the region which contains sequences present in the group of antigens of interest, for example, the DR4 group of alleles. Dots of amplified DNA product are allowed to adhere to a membrane in a "slot blot" (Fig 16–7A), applying as many dots as there are probes. The blots are then cut into strips, and each strip is exposed to a different labeled probe. Hybridization conditions must be optimized for each probe. After hybridization and development, the strips are reassembled and the pattern of hybridization signals is compared with the patterns for known alleles. Fig 16–7B shows a result comparing signals from 4 individual samples being typed for DR4 alleles.

Currently, there are several combinations of heterozygous alleles that share the same polymorphic sequences and therefore cannot be typed unambiguously with some sets of oligonucleotide probes. Other methods, such as sequencing of the amplified product (see HLA Typing by DNA Sequencing, below) are

Table 16–11. Oligonucleotide hybridization patterns for DR4 alleles.[1]

DR4 Allele	Pattern with Oligonucleotide Probe:										
	WS 1004	WS 3701	WS 3704	WS 5701	WS 5702	WS 7001	WS 7005	WS 7006	WS 7007	WS 8601	WS 8603
0401	+		+	+			+			+	
0402	+		+	+					+		+
0403	+		+	+		+		+			+
0404	+		+	+		+					+
0405	+		+		+	+				+	
0406	+	+		+		+		+			+
0407	+		+	+		+		+		+	
0408	+		+	+		+				+	
0409	+		+		+		+			+	
0410	+		+		+	+					+
0411	+		+		+	+		+			+

[1]Hybridization patterns for alleles of the DR4 group which illustrate that class II molecules are composites of polymorphic sequences. Oligonucleotide probes are from the 11th International Histocompatibility Workshop.

required for complete typing. HLA typing by the oligonucleotide method can reveal new antigens if an unexplained new pattern of hybridization occurs. More often, however, it will fail to detect a new sequence polymorphism since no probe has been synthesized for it.

A simpler method of oligonucleotide typing is to immobilize all the probes on a membrane and dot the amplified sample onto the probes, the so-called reverse dot blot technique. This method requires that all probes have the same hybridization conditions, a situation not yet achieved for most loci.

D. Other HLA Typing Methods Involving PCR-Amplified Products:

1. PCR-RFLP—Systems for DRB and DQB typing have been devised that treat the PCR-amplified product with bacterial restriction enzymes and use gel electrophoresis to visualize and identify the alleles. The region to be amplified is chosen to be specific to a group of antigens, such as the DQ1 subtypes, DQ5 and DQ6 (group-specific priming). Aliquots of the resultant product are each digested with a different enzyme chosen for the property of cleaving or not cleaving within the amplified sequence. The resulting fragments are separated on polyacrylamide gels and stained with ethidium bromide. Cleavage patterns characteristic for each allele, which can discriminate most but not all alleles, are visualized. If a second round of enzymes is used on the products of the first digestion, further discrimination is possible. This method is simpler than application of 10–30 (or more) oligonucleotide probes to immobilized PCR products but currently lacks fine resolution of alleles.

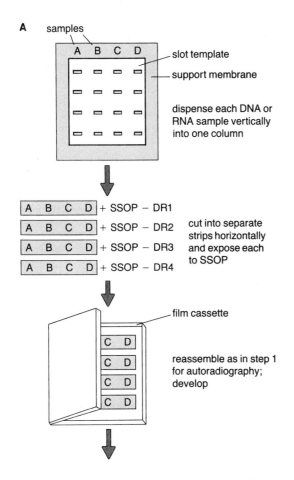

A samples

slot template

support membrane

dispense each DNA or RNA sample vertically into one column

A B C D + SSOP – DR1
A B C D + SSOP – DR2
A B C D + SSOP – DR3
A B C D + SSOP – DR4

cut into separate strips horizontally and expose each to SSOP

film cassette

reassemble as in step 1 for autoradiography; develop

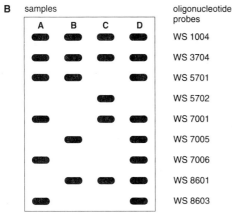

B samples

oligonucleotide probes

A	B	C	D	WS 1004
				WS 3704
				WS 5701
				WS 5702
				WS 7001
				WS 7005
				WS 7006
				WS 8601
				WS 8603

sample	results
A	DRB1* 0403
B	DRB1* 0401
C	DRB1* 0405
D	DRB1* 0401 + 0403

Figure 16–7. HLA typing by sequence-specific oligonucleotide probes. *(A)* Samples of DNA (or RNA) (A, B, C, or D) are dotted directly onto a support membrane by using a slotted template (the slot blot). Replicates of a single sample are placed into a single column of slots. After all samples have been dispersed, the membrane is cut horizontally into strips. Individual probes that are specific and diagnostic for individual HLA alleles, such as DR1 and DR2, are prepared. Each strip is hybridized with a different radiolabeled sequence-specific oligonucleotide probe (SSOP). The probes hybridize only to an exactly complementary nucleotide sequence in the sample. *(B)* The membrane is reassembled and developed by autoradiography. A band indicates the presence in the sample of the sequence of the corresponding HLA allele, and the antigen can be assigned, as illustrated here.

2. HLA typing by DNA sequencing (Sequence-based Typing)–

In this HLA typing method, PCR products derived from the second exon of HLA genes is directly sequenced to determine an HLA type. Total cellular RNA is prepared and then reverse transcribed to produce cDNA. RNA is used to avoid amplification of DNA present in pseudogenes, such as DRB2, since these genes are not transcribed. PCR primers composed of both conserved and nonconserved HLA sequences are used to produce the DNA to be sequenced. For the sequencing step, internal oligonucleotides are used for each locus to prime the sequencing reaction. After electrophoresis, the sequence ladders are produced for the DNA lying between the sequencing primer and the upstream or downstream amplification primer. Reading is initiated starting at a base located between 2 and 14 bases from the sequencing primer-binding site. Because of the complexity of the microsequence differences in HLA antigens, primers must be chosen that faithfully amplify DNA of all possible heterozygous combinations. Primers of conserved sequences will amplify all known alleles at DRB, DQA, and DQB. For DQ locus typing, any combination of DQA and DQB alleles will produce a unique sequence ladder. Typing for DRB1 alleles is more complex, since most haplotypes express alleles from more than one DRB locus (eg, DRB1*1501, DRB5*0101), necessitating the use of conserved-sequence primers that can generate up to 4 overlapping ladders (for DRB1, DRB3, DRB4, and DRB5) with complex sequences. A series of 5 different nonconserved primers were designed to permit unambiguous identification of sequences of all DRB alleles regardless of phenotypic combinations. With this protocol, the complete sequencing process can be performed in 16–24 hours. Complete sequencing of HLA alleles is a powerful tool that has revealed novel microheterogeneities within known alleles and will clearly identify novel alleles in the population.

Molecular Testing Methods for Histocompatibility & Genetic Identity Determination

A. Heteroduplex Analysis Applied to Histocompatibility Testing: Molecular HLA typing per se may not be required when only a preliminary assessment of genetic identity is desired, as between serologically identical siblings or when multiple donors are available for unrelated bone marrow transplantation.

1. Heteroduplex formation–A rapid method is available which utilizes the principle that denatured DNA strands reanneal into heteroduplexes, ie, to form a double helix in alternative combinations which are less than perfectly base pair matched. If the individuals are disparate genetically, mismatching at the polymorphic bases will modify the bending or increase the superhelical diameter of the DNA and cause a retardation in its migration in polyacrylamide gel electrophoresis. When denatured DNAs from 2 genetically disparate individuals are mixed, novel heteroduplexes will form, generating new band patterns in electrophoresis. Thus the genetic identity between 2 individuals can be quickly assessed by mixing PCR DNA from their HLA genes. Alternatively, a reference DNA for a single allele can be added to each sample, forming diagnostic bands, or the DNA can be enzymatically digested with a single endonuclease to differentiate the alleles in heterozygotes.

2. VNTR typing–The repetition of repeated DNA sequences in the genome, known as VNTR or DNA fingerprinting, is a genetic marker both in clinical and forensic applications. VNTRs are polymorphisms of fragment length and can be analyzed by Southern blotting of either genomic or PCR-amplified DNA. Primers to flanking regions of the repetitive sequence cluster will prepare adequate product for analysis when only minute or degraded forensic samples are available. Clinical applications include monitoring engraftment of bone marrow transplant recipients when the marrow donor is HLA-identical to the patient. Parentage testing can use either VNTR patterns or class II HLA alleleic typing to determine exclusion of an alleged father in cases of disputed paternity.

Molecular HLA typing methods provide the most accurate strategies for class II HLA typing and the determination of genetic identity. HLA typing for class I alleles is currently less well developed. The challenge for molecular methods is to produce an HLA typing result in a timely and cost-effective manner so that the benefits of precise molecular typing can be applied to the time-critical demands of organ donor testing for transplantation.

REFERENCES

General

Bodmer JG et al: Nomenclature for factors of the HLA system, 1991. *Tissue Antigens* 1992;**39:**161.

Marsh SGE, Bodmer JG: HLA class II nucleotide sequences, 1992. *Tissue Antigens* 1992;**40:**229.

Sasazuki T (editor): *HLA 1991.* Oxford Univ Press, 1992.

Zachary AA, Teresi GA (editors): *ASHI Laboratory Manual,* 2nd ed. American Society for Histocompatibility and Immunogenetics, 1990.

Zemmour J, Parham P: HLA class I nucleotide sequences, 1992. *Tissue Antigens* 1992;**40:**221.

Special Methods

Bodmer WF, Bodmer JG: Cytofluorochromasia for

HLA-A, -B, -C, and DR typing. Page 46 in: *Manual of Tissue Typing Techniques.* Ray JG (editor). NIH publication 80–545. US Department of Health, Education and Welfare, 1979.

Böyum A: Separation of leukocytes from blood and bone marrow. *Scand J Clin Lab Invest* 1968;**21(Suppl):**97.

Hirschberg H, Skare H, Thorsby E: Cell mediated lymphocytes: CML. A microplate technique requiring few target cells and employing a new method of supernatant collection. *J Immunol Methods* 1977; **16:**131.

Rudy T, Opelz G. Dithiothreitol treatment of crossmatch sera in highly immunized transplant recipients. *Transplant Proc* 1987;**19:**800.

Sheeky MJ, Bach FH: Primed LD typing (PLT)—technical considerations. *Tissue Antigens* 1976;**8:**157.

Terasaki PI et al: Microdroplet testing for HLA-A, -B, -C, and -D antigens. *Am J Clin Pathol* 1978;**69:**103.

Terashita GY: Flow cytometry crossmatching: An update. In *Clinical Transplants 1989.* Terasaki PI (editor). UCLA Tissue Typing Laboratory, 1989.

HLA & Transplantation

Mahoney RJ et al: The flow cytometry crossmatch and early renal transplant loss. *Transplantation* 1990;**49:**527.

Terasaki PI, Cecka M (editors): *Clinical Transplants 1991.* UCLA Tissue Typing Laboratory, 1991.

Tiercy J-M et al: Application of HLA-DR oligotyping to 110 kidney transplant patients with doubtful serological typing. *Transplantation* 1991;**51:**1110.

Molecular-Biologic Techniques

Bein G, Glaser R, Kirchner H: Rapid HLA-DRB1 genotyping by nested PCR amplification. *Tissue Antigens* 1992;**39:**68.

Bidwell JL et al: A DNA RFLP typing system that positively identifies serologically well-defined and ill-defined HLA-DR and DQ alleles, including DRw10. *Transplantation* 1988;**45:**640.

Carrington M et al: Typing of HLA-DQA1 and DQB1 using DNA single strand conformation polymorphism. *Hum Immunol* 1992;**33:**208.

Coen DM: The polymerase chain reaction. In *Current Protocols in Molecular Biology.* Supplement 16 15.0.3. Ausubel FM (editor). Greene Publishing, John Wiley & Sons, 1991.

Jeffreys AJ, Wilson V, Swee LT: Hypervariable 'minisatellite' regions in human DNA. *Nature* 1985; **314:**67.

Jeffreys AJ, Wilson V, Thein SL: Individual specific fingerprints of human DNA. *Nature* 1985;**316:**76.

Olerup O, Zetterquist H: HLA-DR typing by PCR amplification with sequence-specific primers (PCR-SSP) in 2 hours: An alternative to serological DR typing in clinical practice including donor-recipient matching in cadaveric transplantation. *Tissue Antigens* 1992;**39:**225.

Ota M et al: HLA-DRB1 genotyping by modified PCR-RFLP method combined with group-specific primers. *Tissue Antigens* 1992;**39:**187.

Santamaria P et al: HLA class II "typing": direct sequencing of DRB, DQB and DQA genes. *Hum Immunol* 1992;**33:**69.

Shaffer AL et al: HLA-DRw52-associated DRB1 alleles: Identification using polymerase chain reaction-amplified DNA, sequence-specific oligonucleotide probes, and a chemiluminescent detection system. *Tissue Antigens* 1992;**39:**84.

17 Laboratory Evaluation of Immune Competence

Daniel P. Stites, MD

The integrity of the human immune system depends on the presence of adequate numbers of functionally competent cells. These cells and their many secreted products interact in a complex manner to protect the host from invading microorganisms (for a summary, see Chapter 2). The several cardinal clinical manifestations of a failure in immune competence include (1) increased frequency of infections, (2) failure to clear infections rapidly despite adequate therapy, (3) dissemination of local infections to distant sites, and (4) occurrence of opportunistic infections. An increased risk of developing certain types of cancer may be a long-term consequence of immunodeficiency; however, the susceptibility to cancer in general and, particularly, the responsible mechanisms are still controversial (see Chapters 44 and 45). Similarly, development of autoimmunity could follow the loss of key suppressive regulatory influences within the immune system. Loss of such regulatory control can result in hypersensitivity or immune hyperfunction as a consequence of immunodeficiency (see Chapter 30).

UTILITY OF LABORATORY TESTS

A seemingly bewildering array of laboratory tests are available to finely dissect nearly every component of the immune response. Most assays have emerged from applications in basic or clinical immunology research. Relatively few such laboratory tests have developed established clinical reliability for diagnosis. To define a practical approach to clinical laboratory testing for immune competence, 2 key features of tests must be established: (1) sensitivity and specificity of the test for disease, and (2) technical accuracy of the testing procedure. Ideally, one needs to know predictive values that emerge from the sensitivities and specificities of the various tests in question (see Chapter 12). This usually requires extensive clinical investigation of large numbers of diseased patients and appropriate control subjects for each test. Unfortunately, this information is often lacking or difficult to obtain (see Chapter 12). Applications of quality control procedures, internationally accepted reagent standards, and uniformly accepted laboratory techniques are in many instances lacking. Nevertheless, a variety of relatively useful and technically reproducible laboratory tests are available in many clinical immunology laboratories. Appropriate use of these tests can lead to a very complete profile of a patient's immune competence. However, several important limitations regarding the application of laboratory tests, particularly in clinical contexts must be observed.

VARIABILITY OF TESTS

In contrast to its use for immunologic, epidemiologic, or other types of research, clinical laboratory testing for immunologic competence must always be interpreted in the context of a particular patient's history and physical examination. Ordinarily, the purpose of performing any laboratory test is to aid in a patient's diagnosis or management. Statistically speaking, abnormalities outside accepted reference ranges in laboratory tests in otherwise healthy individuals are to be expected. Many currently available tests have high inherent biologic and technical variability. The sources of biologic variability in test results include age, sex, race, diurnal variations, medications, nutritional status, intercurrent infections, and other less well-defined environmental factors. Technical variability is largely a function of instrumentation, reagents, and, especially, human error in sample labeling, preparation, and actual test performance. The presence of active disease, particularly of an infectious nature, can greatly influence immune-system test results. In general, then, immune-competence testing should be done during relatively disease-free intervals.

LIMITATIONS OF TESTING

Nearly all assays currently in clinical use are performed on blood cells or serum, even though blood is rarely, if ever, the site of functional immunologic activity. Obviously, the results must be interpreted somewhat narrowly with respect to the circulating blood compartment as the source of test materials. The populations of the cells of lymphoid tissues, such as bone marrow, lymph nodes, and spleen, may not be accurately reflected by their populations in blood. For freely diffusible humoral proteins, such as most antibodies that are in equilibrium with extracellular fluid, blood levels directly reflect tissue levels and do not present a problem. However, lymphocytes and monocytes may be sequestered extravascularly or not distributed in blood in the same proportions as in other organs. IgM antibodies are generally restricted to the intravascular and intralymphatic spaces as a result of their molecular size. The additional limitation of in vitro artifacts and the relatively crude nature of currently available in vivo tests must also be considered. Thus, new, relatively noninvasive techniques to measure immune-cell function and turnover in vivo are needed. Sampling cells or fluids from other sites such as bronchoalveolar lavage fluid, cerebrospinal fluid, lymph nodes, mucosal sites and secretions, and skin can give specialized insights into local immune competence in these organs. However, obtaining such specimens is often difficult. Special problems of technical standardization, inhomogeneity of samples (eg, bronchoalveolar lavage), lack of reference ranges, and continuous migration to and from these nonvascular sites make interpretation and measurement even more difficult. Stained tissue sections from biopsies allow for static cellular enumeration but are rarely if ever useful for making functional interpretations. Serum versus cerebrospinal fluid rations for albumin and IgG, for example, have been used to address the problem of compartmentalization and local antibody synthesis in the central nervous system (see Chapter 38).

In testing for immune competence, the clinical laboratory provides 2 types of quantitative information regarding various components of the immune system. These are (1) enumeration of various elements (eg, lymphocytes) and (2) functional competence of these elements, ie, the ability of T cells to proliferate in response to a particular recall antigen. A common pitfall in test interpretation is to confuse the mere *presence* of normal numbers or levels of a given immunologic element with *functional competence*. Thus, even though an individual's CD4 T cell counts are within the laboratory's reference range, their normality should not be assumed unless functional studies are performed. In addition, most currently used laboratory tests for immune competence are not antigen- or epitope-specific. Thus, finding a normal serum concentration of IgG, for example, provides no information about specific antibodies to particular bacterial antigens. In practice it is, of course, not possible to assess immune competence to a specific antigen if the antigen is not available in a form that can be used in the test or if the precise in vivo chemical nature of the antigen is unknown.

CLINICAL UTILITY OF TESTING

What are clinical situations in which performance of laboratory tests for evaluation of immune competence is indicated? Specific details of laboratory tests that are used for various diseases are included in the clinical chapters later in this volume. In general, these tests are useful in diagnosis, monitoring of treatment, and, occasionally, assessing prognosis in a limited group of clinical situations (Table 17–1). Most probably, additional applications will be defined in the future. Also, many additional tests and many other applications of the limited group of tests described below can be found in the research investigations of immune disorders in contrast to clinical laboratory testing.

SPECIFIC TESTING FOR IMMUNE COMPETENCE

A brief summary of one approach to testing basic elements of immune competence, including T cells, B cells, NK cells, complement, and phagocytes, is described. This is summarized in Table 17–2. There are obviously other tests available, and in some cases additional uses for the tests are described (see Table 17–4). The specific details of methods for detecting these elements and their functional states are presented in Chapters 12 and 13. "Normal" values or ref-

Table 17–1. Indications for laboratory testing for immune competence.

Clinical diagnosis, therapeutic monitoring, or prognosis of[1]:
1. Congenital and acquired immunodeficiency diseases (see Chapters 19–23, 45, and 52)
2. Immune reconstitution following bone marrow or other lymphoid tissue grafts (see Chapter 57)
3. Immunosuppression induced by drugs, radiation, or other means (see Chapter 58) for transplant rejection, cancer treatment, or autoimmune diseases
4. Autoimmune disorders (see Chapter 30), as a possible adjunct to diagnosis (rarely useful) or to monitor therapy
5. Immunization (see Chapter 55), to monitor efficacy or immune status
6. Clinical or basic research

[1]Tests must be interpreted in the clinical context, particularly in conjunction with a thorough history and physical examination.

Table 17–2. Summary of immune-competence testing.

Immune Cells	Detection or Enumeration	Function
T cells	FCM[1] with MAbs[2] for CD2, 3, or 5	Lymphocyte proliferation to mitogens or antigens, DHS[3] skin test
T cell subsets	FCM with MAbs for CD4 (helper inducer) and CD8 (suppressor cytotoxic)	Functional assays for help, suppression, cytotoxicity
B cells	FCM with MAbs for CD19, 20, anti-H and anti-L chains	Serum immunoglobulins or subclasses, antibodies especially postimmunization
NK cells	FCM with MAbs for CD16 or 56	K562 cellular cytotoxicity, ADCC
Complement	Immunochemical component detection	CH_{50} or specific hemolytic assay for components
Neutrophils	Morphologic or histochemical features by cell counter	Biochemical and microbicidal
Monocyte-macrophages	Morphologic histochemical features or MAb to CD14	Biochemical and microbicidal

[1]FCM, Flow cytometry.
[2]MAbs, monoclonal antibodies.
[3]DHS, Delayed hypersensitivity.

erence ranges for these tests are not given here because ordinarily they must be determined in individual laboratories.

T CELLS
(See Table 17–3)

Enumeration

The numbers and percentages of circulating T lymphocytes are maintained within fairly narrow limits by homeostatic mechanisms. Since T cells have no morphologically distinguishing features, they can be counted only by detection of lineage-specific molecules or antigenic markers. For all T cells, the most universal among these markers is CD3, a major structural component of the T cell receptor for antigens. Other cell surface markers are either incompletely expressed or specific for subsets of T cells. CD5 is also present on a subpopulation of B cells; CD2 can also be found on some natural killer (NK) cells; and CD7 is only weakly expressed on some mature T cells.

Technical Considerations

For accurate enumeration, flow cytometry is currently clearly the method of choice. Monoclonal anti-

bodies conjugated to fluorochromes directed at all known CD molecules on T cells are commercially available. Percentages of T cells in whole lysed blood are generally accurately determined by counting 10,000 cells per sample that are stained with fluorochrome-labeled monoclonal antibodies. Clearly, the accuracy of this technique is highly dependent on gating techniques to distinguish lymphocytes from other blood leukocytes. Manual counts of T cells by fluorescence microscopy are less desirable than flow cytometry, owing to the imprecision and laboriousness of cell-counting in a microscope. For calculation of absolute numbers of T cells, the percentage determined by immunofluorescence in a flow cytometer must be multiplied by the absolute lymphocyte count, usually determined by Coulter counting or manually in a hemacytometer. Lack of precision or accuracy in determining the absolute lymphocyte count from the leukocyte and differential count is a major source of technical variability in determining T cell counts.

Newly introduced flow cytometers can accurately determine absolute numbers of lymphocytes as well as immunofluorescently stained T cells. Techniques to measure total amounts of CD4, CD8, or other T cell-specific molecules by solubilization with detergents followed by ELISA have also been developed.

T Cell Subsets

The 2 major T cell subsets, CD4- and CD8-bearing cells, are enumerated by using fluorochrome-linked monoclonal antibodies and flow cytometry with lymphocyte gating (some monocytes also express low levels of CD4). It is now recommended that all such determinations be performed by simultaneous 2-color analysis with anti-CD3 monoclonal antibodies labeled with a second fluorochrome to ensure exclusion of non-T cells. Simultaneous 2-color analysis with additional monoclonal antibodies can resolve CD4 and CD8 into further subpopulations (see Chapter 13), but these finer distinctions are rarely of clinical value in assessing immune competence. One such example is the use of CD4 subsets in determining disease activity in multiple sclerosis by using the CD45R subset of CD4 cells, which decrease with disease activation, whereas CD45RO memory effector cells increase.

Functional Assays

A. All T Cells: Activation of T cells with nonspecific plant lectins or anti-CD3 monoclonal antibodies results in a complex series of biochemical events culminating in cellular DNA synthesis. Phytomitogens such as phytohemagglutinin, concanavalin A, and pokeweed mitogen are used for this purpose. Also, allogeneic cells can be used as relatively nonspecific stimulants in a mixed-lymphocyte culture (MLC). Anti-CD3, which directly interacts

Table 17–3. Summary of major tests for T cell immune competence.

Test	Technique	Parameters Measured	Limitations and Comments
Total T cells (numbers or percentages)	Flow cytometry with MAbs to CD2, CD3, or CD5	Percentage of cells bearing these epitopes in a particular gated mononuclear cell population	Need absolute lymphocyte count to convert to T cell numbers; no functional or clonal antigen specific information.
T cell subsets (numbers and percentages) Helper-inducer cells Suppressor-cytotoxic cells	Flow cytometry with MAbs to CD4, CD8, and CD3 simultaneously	Percentage of cells in mononuclear cell gate that bear these surface molecules	CD4 (but not CD3) also expressed on some monocytes; both subsets are functionally heterogeneous (eg, CD8 contains suppressor and cytotoxic T cells).
Lymphocyte proliferation to mitogens and allogenic cells	Lymphocyte culture with DNA synthesis detected by radioactive thymidine incorporation	Ability of polyclonal T cells to undergo activation to DNA synthesis	Does not define multiple possible defects in cellular physiology.
Antigens	Same	Clonal proliferation to epitopes	Avoids the need to perform skin test for DHS; relevant antigens may be unknown or unavailable for testing.

with membrane T cell receptors, can provide a particularly strong activation signal. Cellular responses are usually assessed by measuring radioactive thymidine uptake (see Chapter 15). Response to mitogen stimulation by these agents is macrophage-dependent but much less so than is the response to specific antigens.

B. T Cell Subsets: CD4 and CD8 cells do not proliferate in response to monoclonal antibodies to these epitopes. Complex functional tests to assess helper, suppressor, or cytotoxic functions of these cells are still predominantly in the realm of research laboratories but are occasionally useful in clinical situations (see below).

Antigen-specific T cells will proliferate in response to soluble or cell-bound antigens in vitro (see Chapter 13). This test is particularly useful when one wants to avoid direct in vivo contact with potentially toxic antigens by patch testing or delayed hypersensitivity intradermal tests.

C. Delayed Hypersensitivity Skin Tests: The ability to mount cutaneous delayed hypersensitivity to intradermally or epidermally applied antigens (patch testing) is dependent on both specific antigen-reactive and other relatively noncommitted T cells. Antigen-stimulated T cells release mediators that affect vascular permeability, monocyte function and movement, and proliferation of other noncommitted T cells. These cytokines and cells all contribute to local erythema and induration characteristic of this response. Thus, the delayed hypersensitivity skin test is not a measure solely of T cells. However, positive reactions to delayed hypersensitivity skin tests of one or more antigens mean that broadly reactive T cell immune competence is likely to be largely intact (see Chapter 13).

Additional tests for T cell function, which are not regularly available clinically, are listed in Table 17–4.

B CELLS

In contrast to assessing T cell competence, tests for B cell competence rely mainly on detecting the products of the B cell-plasma cell series, ie, immunoglobulins. Specific assays for antibody directed at selected epitopes of microorganisms are also available (Table 17–5).

Enumeration

A variety of specific B cell surface markers (CD antigens) that can be detected by monoclonal antibodies have been described. Initially, surface immu-

Table 17–4. Additional tests for T cell competence not regularly available clinically.

Lymphokine production
IL-2, IL-3, IL-5
Gamma interferon
IL-4
TNF
Receptors for lymphokines
IL-1
IL-2
Responsiveness to lymphokines
IL-1
IL-2
IL-4
Gamma interferon
Lymphocyte cytotoxicity
MHC restricted
MHC nonrestricted
Antigen-specific
Lectin (PHA)-dependent
Antibody-dependent cell-mediated cytotoxicity (ADCC)
Helper and suppressor T cell assays
Polyclonal immunoglobulin synthesis (pokeweed mitogen-induced)
Mitogen or antigen proliferation
T cell cytotoxicity
Lymphokine release or effect

Table 17–5. Summary of major tests for B cell immune competence.

Test	Technique	Parameters Measured	Limitations and Comments
Total B cells (numbers or percentages)	Flow cytometry with MAbs to CD19 or CD20 or antibodies to H or L chains	Percentage of cells that express these epitopes in a particular gated mononuclear cell population	Need absolute count to convert to B cell numbers; no functional or antigen-specific information.
Immunoglobulin concentrations (IgG, IgA, IgM)	Radial immunodiffusion or rate nephelometry with specific anti-H and anti-L chain antisera	Concentration of polyclonal immunoglobulin present in particular body fluid, eg, serum, cerebrospinal fluid, saliva	No clonal or antigen-specific information; results are highly age-dependent.
Antibody to specific epitopes or microorganisms	ELISA, radioimmunoassay, agglutination, precipitation, etc (see Chapter 12)	Titers of antibody to a specific epitope or group of epitopes on antigen from microorganisms	Deliberate immunization with pre- and postantibody titers useful; anti-A and anti-B are IgM isohemagglutinins.

noglobulins using either H- or L-chain-specific antisera were used. More recently, monoclonal antisera that detect CD19 or CD20 have also been used relatively interchangeably as pan-B cell markers. Additional antibodies that detect B cells from earlier stages of maturation or from other subsets are available (eg, CD22 and CD10) but are rarely useful in assessing B cell competence in peripheral blood of adults or even children. The coexpression of CD5 on T cells and CD1 on dendritic cells and thymocytes restricts the usefulness of these markers for B cell enumeration. Since plasma cells rarely circulate, antibodies directed at their special differentiation antigens, eg, PC-1 or PCA-1, are of use only in examining lymph nodes, spleen, bone marrow, or other lymphoid tissues. The typical morphologic features of plasma cells usually render them easily recognizable without immunohistochemical staining.

Technical Considerations

These are essentially the same as those discussed for T cells. Flow cytometry is the preferred method.

B Cell Subsets

B cells at early stages of maturation, eg, pre-B cells, do express unique surface markers and cytoplasmic μ chains. Detecting these cells is primarily of use in phenotyping B cell cancers or investigating the detailed pathogenic cellular mechanisms of B cell immunodeficiency diseases. Markers for other B cell subsets can be detected, but their clinical utility is unknown. Clonal or antigen-specific B cell detection has generally not been applied to assessment of clinical immunocompetence.

Functional Assays

The primary product of the B cell-plasma cell series is antibody, and, as such, measurement of immunoglobulins or specific antibodies provides the major route for assessing the function of B cell competence (see Chapter 12).

Immunoglobulin levels should be measured if a state of humoral immunodeficiency or B cell failure is suspected. The use of less specific tests such as protein electrophoresis or immunoelectrophoresis, which are only semiquantitative, is not recommended. These tests are used primarily in paraprotein diagnosis. Consideration of the patient's age is critical in interpreting immunoglobulin levels, since these levels are particularly susceptible to variation with age (see Chapter 12). Generally, IgG, IgA, and IgM levels are sufficient. Serum IgD levels are not useful in assessing immune competence, and, with the rare exception of the hyper-IgE syndrome with recurrent infections (see Chapter 22), IgE levels are also not helpful in diagnosis of immune deficiencies.

In some instances, particularly following deliberate immunization to test B cell competence, specific antibody is measured. Sera should be collected and frozen prior to administration of antigen and then subsequently some days or weeks later when serum antibody responses to the antigen in question are known to be elevated in the blood. Antibody should then be measured in both preimmunization and postimmunization specimens simultaneously. This approach can be used to detect primary antibody responses to antigens such as keyhole limpet hemocyanin or recall antigens such as polyvalent pneumococcal antigens of *Streptococcus pneumoniae,* tetanus toxoid, or influenza virus vaccine. One should never expose a suspected or known immunodeficient patient to live or attenuated viral vaccine, since this may result in virus dissemination followed by disease and possibly death.

Isohemagglutinins, anti-A and anti-B, are IgM antibodies directed at naturally occurring microbial polysaccharides that cross-react with antigens of the human ABH blood groups (see Chapter 15). In individuals older than 1 year, their titer is approximately 1:4. In incompatibly transfused or in utero-sensitized individuals, ABH antibodies may also be of IgG or other classes besides IgM. Rarely, the Schick test in diphtheria-immunized individuals can be used to measure specific IgG anti-diphtheria antibodies.

In vitro tests for immunoglobulin synthesis by mixed cultures of blood monocytes, T cells, and B cells have been extensively utilized in immunologic research. These tests depend on polyclonal immunoglobulin production induced by B cell mitogens such as pokeweed mitogen or staphylococcal protein A. By varying or eliminating selective T cell subsets or monocytes, suppression, helper, or antigen-presenting functions can be assessed. Currently, such intricate B cell functional assays have not achieved demonstrable routine clinical application.

IgG Subclasses

In some individuals with normal, reduced, or even elevated IgG levels, the level of one or more of the 4 IgG subclasses may be reduced (see Chapter 19). Since deficiency in some of these IgG subclasses, particularly IgG2, may be associated with recurrent infections, determination of their serum level is useful. Other possible indications and disease associations of IgG subclass deficiency are discussed in Chapter 19).

NK CELLS

NK cells represent a minor or third subpopulation (10–15%) of circulating peripheral-blood mononuclear cells. Some appear as large granular lymphocytes. Functionally, these cells kill a variety of autologous and allogeneic target cells without prior sensitization or known restriction by human leukocyte antigens (HLA antigens). They are thought to provide defense against viral infections and possibly some tumors. Recently, a few patients with selective absence of NK cells and recurrent infections (particularly herpesvirus infections) have been described. Chédiak-Higashi syndrome patients also have defective NK cells (see Chapter 22). Research is under way to elucidate possible antitumor effects of NK cells stimulated by interleukin-2 (IL-2) or other lymphokines, as well as their modulation within the neuroimmunologic axis.

Enumeration

Monoclonal antibodies to specific cell surface CD antigens of NK cells include CD56 (NKH1) and CD16 (FcIgG). These are used to count NK cells by microscopy or flow cytometry.

Functional Assays

NK cells kill "NK-sensitive" target cells in vitro. An example of such a target cell is the erythroleukemia cell line K562. Cytolysis by measurement of ^{51}Cr lysis is the most common test to detect NK cell function (see Chapter 13). NK cells also mediate antibody-dependent cellular cytotoxicity (ADCC). Assays for ADCC employ cytolysis of ^{51}Cr-labeled target cells (eg, erythrocytes) that are coated with either human or rabbit antibodies which contain γ-Fc regions, which bind FcIgG receptors present on NK cells.

NK cell enumeration and functional assays have not yet achieved widespread application in clinical laboratories.

COMPLEMENT

Genetic and some acquired deficiencies of complement are associated with a breakdown in host resistance to microorganisms (see Chapter 23). Complement is involved in host defense mechanisms in several ways, including (1) as an opsonin (C3a), (2) in lysing microorganisms (C1–C9), (3) in chemotaxis (C5a), and (4) in altering vascular permeability (C3a, C4a, C5a). Thus, any evaluation of host defense failure clearly should include measurement of complement.

Screening for Complement Deficiencies

Defects in C1–C9, properdin, and complement-regulatory factors have all been described. For components C3–C9 (inclusive), determination of hemolytic complement activity (CH_{50}) (see Chapter 12) will generally adequately screen for congenital lack of one of these components. In genetic defects of complement, eg, C6 deficiency, the entire activity of the protein is lost and hence the lytic function of the entire sequence is blocked. Thus, CH_{50} values approach zero. In acquired deficiency, variable reductions in CH_{50} occur depending on selective loss of the critical components of the lytic pathway. Defects in the alternative pathway proximal to C3 must be tested immunochemically or with specialized functional assays not ordinarily available in most clinical laboratories.

Identification of Specific Component Defects

Genetic or acquired reductions in specific components of either the classic or alternative pathway can be measured by either specific functional or immunochemical assays for these components (see Chapters 11 and 12). Generally, specific antisera are used in the clinical laboratory in either radial diffusion or nephelometric tests. Reduction in the CH_{50} or specific components can be the result of hypercatabolism or underproduction, or both, depending on the disease state. Functional assays such as chemotaxis or opsonization are usually performed in conjunction with the evaluation of phagocytic function.

PHAGOCYTIC CELLS

Polymorphonuclear leukocytes, particularly neutrophils (PMN) and monocyte-macrophages, play a crucial role in host defense against nearly all microorganisms. From an evolutionary standpoint, this is the oldest and most primitive form of immunity, predating antibody or T cell immunity by a considerable stretch of evolutionary development.

Enumeration

A. PMN: PMN are most readily counted by a routine leukocyte count and leukocyte differential. Although such counts can be made with a microscope, the use of automatic cell or Coulter counters provides much more accurate information. Morphologic assessments of neutrophils, particularly to assess maturity and granule content, also constitute an essential step in immune-competence evaluation. In cases of very low or high neutrophil counts, a bone marrow examination may be required to evaluate the integrity of granulocytopoesis.

B. Monocyte-Macrophages: Circulating monocytes can be counted by leukocyte counting and leukocyte differential similar to PMN. Histochemical stains, especially for nonspecific or α-naphthol es-

terase, are useful for identification. Monoclonal antibodies directed at CD14 or volume and light-scattering characteristics can be used to identify and count relative numbers of monocytes by flow cytometry.

Functional Assays

Granulocyte function includes a variety of stages outlined in Chapter 13. Screening for granulocytic function related to immune competence involves at least a biochemical assay for the hexose monophosphate shunt such as nitro blue tetrazolium dye reduction, chemiluminescence, or dichlorofluorescein fluorescence by flow cytometry.

More extensive microbicidal assays can be used to confirm defects in neutrophil function or to detect specific lesions related to particular microorganisms. The principles and examples of these assays are discussed in Chapter 13. Monocyte function can be assessed by similar biochemical or microbicidal tests with isolated enriched monocytes (see Chapter 13).

REFERENCES

General
Primary Immunodeficiency Diseases: Report of WHO Scientific Group. *Immunodef Rev* 1992;**3**:83.

Van der Valk P, Herman C: Biology of disease: Leukocyte functions. *Lab Invest* 1987;**57**:127.

Virella G, Patrick C, Goust JM: Diagnostic evaluation of lymphocyte functions and cell-mediated immunity. *Immunol Ser* 1993;**58**:291.

T and B Cell Assessment
Marti GE, Fleisher TA: Application of lymphocyte immunophenotyping in selected diseases. *Pathol Immunopathol Res* 1988;**7**:319.

Nicholson JKA: Using flow cytometry in the evaluation and diagnosis of primary and secondary immunodeficiency diseases. *Arch Pathol Lab Med* 1989;**113**:598.

Delayed Hypersensitivity Skin Tests
Ahmed AR, Blose DA: Delayed hypersensitivity skin testing: A review. *Arch Dermatol* 1983;**119**:934.

NK Cells
Biron CA, Byron KS, Sullivan JL: Severe herpes infections in an adolescent without natural killer cells. *N Engl J Med* 1989;**320**:1731.

Richards SJ, Scott CS: NK cells in health and disease: Clinical functional phenotypes and DNA genotypic characteristics. *Leukemia Lymphoma* 1992;**7**:377.

Ritz J: The role of natural killer cells in immune surveillance. *N Engl J Med* 1989;**320**:1748.

Immunoglobulins
French MAH: *Immunoglobulins in Health and Disease. Immunology and Medicine Series.* MTP Press, 1986.

Hamilton, RG: Human IgG subclass measurements in the clinical laboratory. *Clin Chem* 1987;**33**:1707.

Complement
Fries LF, Frank MM: Complement and relative proteins: Inherited deficiencies. In: *Inflammation: Basic Principles and Clinical Correlates,* 2nd ed. Gallin JI, Goldstein IM, Snyderman R (editors). Raven Press, 1992.

Ross SC, Denson P: Complement deficiency states and infections. *Medicine* 1984;**63**:243.

Phagocytic Cells
Borregaard N: The human neutrophil: Function and dysfunction. *Eur J Hematol* 1988;**41**:401.

Boxer LA, Morganroth ML: Neutrophil function disorders. *Disease-a-Month* 1987;**33**:681.

Mechanisms of Immunodeficiency 18

Arthur J. Ammann, MD

Four major components of the immune system assist the individual in defending against a constant assault by viral, bacterial, fungal, protozoal, and non-replicating agents that have the potential to produce infection and disease. These systems consist of antibody-mediated (B cell) immunity, cell-mediated (T cell) immunity, phagocytosis, and complement. Each system may act independently or in concert with one or more of the others.

Deficiency of one or more of these systems may be congenital (eg, X-linked infantile hypogammaglobulinemia) or acquired (eg, acquired hypogammaglobulinemia). Deficiencies of the immune system may be secondary to an embryologic abnormality (eg, DiGeorge's syndrome), may be due to an enzymatic defect (eg, chronic granulomatous disease), or may be of unknown cause (eg, chronic mucocutane-

Table 18–1. Causes of immunodeficiency.

Genetic patterns
  Autosomal recessive
  Autosomal dominant
  X-linked
  Gene deletions and rearrangements.

Biochemical and metabolic deficiency
  Adenosine deaminase deficiency
  Purine nucleoside phosphorylase deficiency
  Biotin-dependent multiple carboxylase deficiency
  Deficient membrane glycoproteins

Vitamin or mineral deficiency
  Biotin
  B_{12}
  Zinc

Arrest in embryogenesis

Autoimmune diseases
  Passive antibody (maternal to fetus)
  Active antibody (antibody to T cells)
  Active T cell (anti-B cell)

  Acquired immunodeficiency
    Post-viral infection
    Posttransfusion
    Multiple transfusions
    Chronic infection
    Nutritional deficiency
    Drug abuse
    Maternal alcoholism
    Radiation therapy
    Immunosuppressive therapy
    Cancer
    Chronic renal disease
    Splenectomy

Table 18–2. Clinical features associated with immunodeficiency.

Features frequently present and highly suspicious
  Chronic infection
  Recurrent infection (more than expected)
  Unusual infecting agents
  Incomplete clearing between episodes of infection or incomplete response to treatment

Features frequently present and moderately suspicious
  Skin rash (eczema, cutaneous candidiasis, etc)
  Diarrhea (chronic)
  Growth failure
  Hepatosplenomegaly
  Recurrent abscesses
  Recurrent osteomyelitis
  Evidence of autoimmunity

Features associated with specific immunodeficiency disorders
  Ataxia
  Telangiectasia
  Short-limbed dwarfism
  Cartilage-hair hypoplasia
  Idiopathic endocrinopathy
  Partial albinism
  Thrombocytopenia
  Eczema
  Tetany

Table 18–3. Classification of immunodeficiency disorders.

Antibody (B cell) immunodeficiency disorders
X-linked hypogammaglobulinemia (congenital hypogammaglobulinemia)
Transient hypogammagloublinemia of infancy
Common, variable, unclassifiable immunodeficiency (acquired hypogammaglobulinemia)
Immunodeficiency with hyper-IgM
Neutropenia with hypogammaglobulinemia
Polysaccharide antigen unresponsiveness
Selective IgA deficiency
Selective IgM deficiency
Selective deficiency of IgG subclasses
Secondary B cell immunodeficiency associated with drugs, protein-losing states
X-linked lymphoproliferative disease

Cellular (T cell) immunodeficiency disorders
Congenital thymic aplasia (DiGeorge's syndrome)
Chronic mucocutaneous candidiasis (with or without endocrinopathy)
T cell deficiency associated with purine nucleoside phosphorylase deficiency
T cell deficiency associated with absent membrane glycoprotein
T cell deficiency associated with absent class I or II MHC antigens or both (bare lymphocyte syndrome)
T cell receptor and signaling deficiencies
T cell deficiency associated with cytokine deficiencies

Combined antibody-mediated (B cell) and cell-mediated (T cell) immunodeficiency disorders
Severe combined immunodeficiency disease (autosomal recessive, X-linked, sporadic)
Cellular immunodeficiency with abnormal immunoglobulin synthesis (Nezelof's syndrome)
Immunodeficiency with ataxia-telangiectasia
Immunodeficiency with eczema and thrombocytopenia (Wiskott-Aldrich syndrome)
Immunodeficiency with thymoma
Immunodeficiency with short-limbed dwarfism
Immunodeficiency with adenosine deaminase deficiency
Immunodeficiency with nucleoside phosphorylase deficiency
Biotin-dependent multiple carboxylase deficiency
Graft-versus-host (GVH) disease
Acquired immunodeficiency syndrome (AIDS)

Phagocytic dysfunction
Chronic granulomatous disease
Glucose-6-phosphate dehydrogenase deficiency
Myeloperoxidase deficiency
Chédiak-Higashi syndrome
Job's syndrome
Tuftsin deficiency
Lazy leukocyte syndrome
Elevated IgE, defective chemotaxis, and recurrent infections
Immunodeficiency associated with natural killer cell defects

Table 18–4. Initial screening evaluation.

Antibody-mediated immunity
Quantitative immunoglobulin levels: IgG, IgM, IgA
Isohemagglutinin titer (anti-A and anti-B): measures IgM antibody function primarily
Specific antibody levels following immunization

Cell-mediated immunity
Leukocyte count differential: measures total lymphocytes
Total T cells and T cell subsets: measures total T cells, helper T cells, and suppressor T cells
Delayed hypersensitivity skin tests: measure specific T cell and inflammatory response to antigens

Phagocytosis
Leukocyte count with differential: measures total neutrophils
Nitroblue Tetrazolium (NBT), chemiluminescence, superoxide production: measures neutrophil metabolic function
Natural killer cell number and function

current bacterial otitis media and pneumonia are common in hypogammaglobulinemia. Patients with defective cell-mediated immunity are susceptible to fungal, protozoal, and viral infections that may present as pneumonia or chronic infection of the skin and mucous membranes or other organs. Systemic infection with uncommon bacterial organisms, normally of low virulence, is characteristic of chronic granulomatous disease. Other phagocytic disorders are associated with superficial skin infections or systemic infections with pyogenic organisms.

Numerous advances continue to be made in the identification and diagnosis of specific immunodeficiency disorders (Table 18–3). Screening tests are available for each component of the immune system (Table 18–4). These tests enable the physician to diagnose more than 75% of immunodeficiency disorders. The remainder can be diagnosed by means of more complicated studies (see Chapters 12 and 13), which may not be available in all hospital laboratories. There are still a number of individuals with an immunodeficiency disorder in whom the precise etiology or mechanism of immunodeficiency is unknown.

In addition to antimicrobial agents for the treatment of specific infections, new forms of immunotherapy are available to assist in the control of immunodeficiency or perhaps even to cure the underlying disease (Table 18–5). The usefulness of some of these treatment methods, such as bone marrow transplantation, is limited by the availability of suitable donors. The discovery of enzyme deficiencies (eg, adenosine deaminase deficiency) in association with immunodeficiency offers a potential new avenue of therapy by means of enzyme replacement. The most recent successful approach to treatment is that of gene therapy. Several patients with adenosine deaminase deficiency have been treated with their own cells transfected with the gene coding for adenosine deaminase.

Immunodeficiency disorders are discussed in the

ous candidiasis). The multiple causes of immunodeficiency are listed in Table 18–1.

In general, the symptoms and the physical findings of immunodeficiency are related to the degree of deficiency and the particular system that is deficient in function. General features are listed in Table 18–2. Features associated with specific immunodeficiency disorders are also listed in Table 18–2. The types of infections that occur often provide an important clue to the type of immunodeficiency disease present. Re-

Table 18–5. Treatment of immunodeficiency.

Treatment	B Cell Disorders	T Cell Disorders	Phagocytic Disorders
γ-Globulin.	X-linked hypogammaglobuline- mia; acquired hypogammaglobulinemia; sec- ondary hypogammaglobuline- mia when associated with infection. Do not use in selec- tive IgA deficiency.	Use only when absent antibody response is demonstrated. Not recommended for intramuscular use in Wiskott-Aldrich syn- drome. Gamma globulin does not transmit virus, eg, hepatitis, retrovirus.	Not recommended.
Hyperimmune γ-globulin.	Use in above disorders when specific exposure has occurred.	May be used when specific ex- posure has occurred.	May be used when spe- cific exposure has oc- curred.
Frozen plasma by intravenous in- fusion. Largely replaced by in- travenous γ-globulin. Risk of transmitting viral infections.	Replaced by gamma globulin.	Replaced by gamma globulin.	Not recommended.
Infusions of leukocytes.	Not recommended.	Not recommended.	Questionable value.
Infusion of erythrocytes.	Not recommended.	May be of benefit in certain en- zyme deficiencies associated with immunodeficiency (adeno- sine deaminase, purine nucleo- side phosphorylase). Irradiate to prevent GVH disease. Largely replaced by enzyme re- placement.	Not recommended.
Bone marrow transplant.	Not recommended.	Use only when T cell function is impaired. Histocompatible donor preferred.	Not recommended.
Fetal thymus transplantation.	Not recommended.	DiGeorge's syndrome. Rarely used at this time.	Not recommended.
Cultured thymus epithelium.	Not recommended.	Rarely used at this time.	Not recommended.
Fetal liver transplantation. (Pri- marily of historic interest.)	Not recommended.	Used in past in severe com- bined immunodeficiency in ab- sence of suitable bone marrow donor. Rarely used at this time.	Not recommended.
Thymosin, thymopentin, α_1 facteur thymique serique. (In- vestigational.)	Not recommended.	Limited evaluation to date. May enhance T cell function in a vari- ety of T cell disorders, including DiGeorge's syndrome. No effect in chronic candidiasis or severe combined immunodeficiency.	Not recommended.
Adenosine deaminase polyethyl- ene glycol.	Not recommended.	Specific for adenosine deami- nase deficiency.	Not recommended.
Gene therapy	Not used to date.	Used successfully in adenosine deaminase deficiency.	Not used to date.

next 4 chapters under the following categories: anti- body (B cell) deficiency, cellular (T cell) deficiency, combined T cell and B cell deficiency, and phago- cytic dysfunction. Complement factor deficiencies are discussed in Chapter 23. AIDS is discussed in

Chapter 52. In general, the terminology used for spe- cific deficiencies is based on the classification re- cently proposed by a committee of the World Health Organization (Table 18–3).

REFERENCES

Good RA, Pahwa RN (editors): The recognition of im- munodeficient disorders. (Symposium.) *Pediatr Infect Dis J* 1988;**7(Suppl):**S2.

Stiehm ER: *Immunologic Disorders in Infants and Chil- dren,* 3rd ed. Saunders, 1989.

Stiehm ER: New and old immunodeficiencies. *Pediatr Res* 1993; 33**(Suppl):**S2.

Symposium: Childhood immunodeficiency disorders: Diag- nosis, prevention, and management. *Clin Immunol Im- munopathol* 1986;**40:**1.

19

Antibody (B Cell) Immunodeficiency Disorders

Arthur J. Ammann, MD

Antibody immunodeficiency disorders comprise a spectrum of diseases characterized by decreased immunoglobulin levels ranging from complete absence of all classes to selective deficiency of a single class or subclass. There are also cases of specific antibody deficiency, particularly the inability to form antibody to polysaccharide antigens. The morbidity found in patients with antibody immunodeficiency disorders is dependent chiefly on the degree of antibody deficiency. Patients with hypogammaglobulinemia become symptomatic earlier and experience more severe disease than do patients with selective immunoglobulin deficiency. Screening tests for the specific diagnosis of antibody deficiency disorders are readily available in most hospital laboratories (see Table 18–4 and Chapter 12). They permit early diagnosis and prompt institution of appropriate treatment. Other procedures, such as quantitation of B cells in peripheral blood, determination of in vitro immunoglobulin production, and suppressor cell assays, may yield more precise diagnosis and insight into the cause or mechanism of the observed deficiency (Table 19–1). The exact role of these and other tests of B cell function has not been established for most clinical conditions.

X-LINKED INFANTILE HYPOGAMMAGLOBULINEMIA

Major Immunologic Features
- Symptoms of recurrent pyogenic infections usually begin by 5–6 months of age.
- IgG is less than 200 mg/dL, with absence of IgM, IgA, IgD, and IgE.
- B cells are absent in peripheral blood.
- Patients respond well to treatment with gamma globulin.

General Considerations
In 1952 Bruton described a male child with hypogammaglobulinemia, and this is now recognized

as the first clinical description and precise diagnosis of an immunodeficiency disorder. The disorder is easily diagnosed by using standard laboratory tests that demonstrate marked deficiency or complete absence of all 5 immunoglobulin classes. Male infants with this disorder usually become symptomatic following the natural decay of transplacentally acquired maternal immunoglobulin at about 5–6 months of age. They suffer from severe chronic bacterial infections, which can be controlled readily with gamma globulin and antibiotic treatment. The prevalence of this disorder in the USA is not precisely known, but estimates in the United Kingdom suggest that it is one case per 100,000 population. Two female siblings with congenital hypogammaglobulinemia have been reported.

Immunologic Pathogenesis
Extirpation of the bursa of Fabricius in birds results in complete hypogammaglobulinemia. Several investigators think that the human equivalent of the bursa, the source of B cell precursors, is the gastrointestinal tract-associated lymphoid tissue (tonsils, adenoids, Peyer's patches, and appendix), whereas others assign this role to stem cells in fetal liver and bone marrow. In X-linked infantile hypogammaglobulinemia, a stem cell population is presumed to be absent, resulting in the complete absence of B lymphocytes and plasma cells. However, investigations have provided some evidence of pre-B cells in the marrow and peripheral blood of patients, suggesting that the defect may be at a later stage of B cell differentiation. These pre-B cells do not secrete immunoglobulin. The genetic defect has recently been defined and consists of a defect in the enzyme tyrosine kinase. This should result in more precise diagnosis, the ability to diagnose the disorder in utero, and eventual gene therapy.

The individual immunoglobulin isotypes are a result of immunoglobulin heavy (H)-chain diversity. The formation of individual H chains is a result of somatic rearrangement of variable (V), diversity (D),

Table 19–1. Evaluation of antibody-mediated immunity.

Test	Comment
Protein electrophoresis	For presumptive diagnosis of hypogammaglobulinemia or to evaluate for paraproteins.
Quantitation of immunoglobulins	Best procedure for quantitation of IgG, IgM, IgA, and IgD.
Enzyme-linked immunosorbent assay (ELISA)	IgE quantitation.
Isohemagglutinins	For evaluation of IgM function. Expected titer of > 1:4 after 1 year of age.
Specific antibody response	For evaluation of immunoglobulin function. Immunize with tetanus or diphtheria toxoid or typhoid. Do not immunize with live virus if immunodeficiency is suspected.
B cell quantitation with monoclonal antibody	Normally 10–25% (total IgG-, IgM-, IgD-, and IgA-bearing cells) of total circulation lymphocytes.
In vitro immunoglobulin synthesis with T cell subsets	Determines helper/suppressor T cell function in hypogammaglobulinemia.

and joining (J) segment genes, as described in Chapter 6. In some forms of X-linked infantile hypogammaglobulinemia, a truncated μ chain is produced as a consequence of premature transcription prior to D-J segment rearrangement. A second form has been shown to be a result of failure of V_H gene rearrangement, resulting in the production of truncated μ and α H chains.

Clinical Features

A. Symptoms and Signs: Patients with X-linked infantile hypogammaglobulinemia usually remain asymptomatic until 5–6 months of age, at which time the passively transferred maternal IgG reaches its lowest level. The loss of protection from maternal antibodies usually coincides with the age at which these children are increasingly exposed to pathogens. Initial symptoms consist of recurrent bacterial otitis media, bronchitis, pneumonia, meningitis, dermatitis, and, occasionally, arthritis or malabsorption. Many infections respond promptly to antibiotic therapy, and this response occasionally will delay the diagnosis of hypogammaglobulinemia. The most common organisms responsible for infection are *Streptococcus pneumoniae* and *Haemophilus influenzae;* other streptococci and certain gram-negative bacteria are occasionally responsible. Although patients normally have intact T cell immunity and respond normally to viral infections such as varicella and measles, there have been reports of paralytic poliomyelitis and progressive encephalitis following immunization with

live vaccines or exposure to wild virus. Fatal echovirus infection has been reported in patients with congenital hypogammaglobulinemia. The encephalitis in a few patients has responded to treatment with intravenous gamma globulin or plasma. A relationship of echovirus infection, dermatomyositis, and hypogammaglobulinemia has been proposed. These observations suggest that some patients with hypogammaglobulinemia may also be unusually susceptible to some viral illnesses.

An important clue to the diagnosis of hypogammaglobulinemia is the failure of infections to respond completely or promptly to appropriate antibiotic therapy. In addition, many patients with hypogammaglobulinemia have a history of continuous illness; ie, they do not have periods of well-being between bouts of illness.

Occasionally, patients with hypogammaglobulinemia may not become symptomatic until early childhood. Some of these patients may present with other complaints, such as chronic conjunctivitis, abnormal dental decay, or malabsorption. The malabsorption may be severe and may cause retardation of both height and weight. Frequently, the malabsorption is associated with *Giardia lamblia* infestation. A disease resembling rheumatoid arthritis has been reported in association with hypogammaglobulinemia. This occurs principally in untreated infants or is an indication for more intensive therapy with gamma globulin.

Physical findings usually relate to recurrent pyogenic infections. Chronic otitis media and externa serous otitis, conjunctivitis, an abnormal degree of dental decay (Fig 19–1), and eczematoid skin infections are frequently present. Despite the repeated infec-

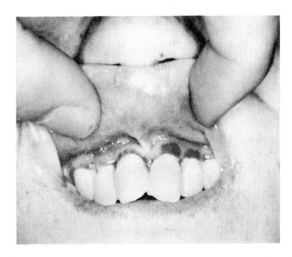

Figure 19–1. Early periodontal disease in a child with hypogammaglobulinemia. Recurrent ear infections and dental disease were the first manifestations of susceptibility to infection.

tions, lymphadenopathy and splenomegaly are absent.

B. Laboratory Findings: The diagnosis of X-linked infantile hypogammaglobulinemia is based on the demonstration of absence or marked deficiency of all 5 immunoglobulin classes. Although the diagnosis is suspected from serum protein electrophoresis and established by immunoelectrophoresis (see Chapter 12), specific quantitation of immunoglobulins is necessary, especially during early infancy. Total immunoglobulin levels are usually below 250 mg/dL. The IgG level is usually below 200 mg/dL, while IgM, IgA, IgD, and IgE levels are extremely low or undetectable. Rarely, patients have complete absence of IgG, IgA, IgM, and IgD but normal amounts of IgE. It is unusual for patients with hypogammaglobulinemia to have depressed levels of IgG and normal levels of IgM or IgA. Before a diagnosis of immunodeficiency is established in a patient with hypogammaglobulinemia, failure to make antibody following antigenic stimulation should be demonstrated. The diagnosis is difficult in infants under 6 months of age because of maternal IgG in the serum.

Isohemagglutinins that result from natural immunization are normally present in infants of the appropriate blood group by 1 year of age. Titers of anti-A and anti-B should be greater than 1:4 in normal individuals. Antibody to a specific antigen may be measured following immunization, but a patient suspected of having an immunodeficiency disorder should never be immunized with live attenuated viral vaccine. Although lymph node biopsies have been recommended in the past, this is probably unnecessary with currently available diagnostic studies. Rarely, an intestinal biopsy to determine the presence or absence of plasma cells may be necessary to assist in the diagnosis in difficult cases. In X- linked infantile hypogammaglobulinemia, there are no plasma cells in the lamina propria of the gut. There is a complete absence of circulating B cells, with normal to increased numbers of T cells. T cell immunity is intact. Delayed hypersensitivity skin tests are usually positive; isolated peripheral blood lymphocytes respond normally to phytohemagglutinin (PHA) and to allogeneic cells in mixed lymphocyte culture (MLC).

C. Other Tests: X-ray of the lateral nasopharynx has been suggested as a method of demonstrating the lack of lymphoid tissue, but this rarely adds significant information to the findings on physical examination. X- rays of the sinuses and chest should be obtained at regular intervals to monitor the course of the patient and to determine the adequacy of treatment. Pulmonary function studies should also be performed on a regular basis, when the patient is old enough to cooperate. Patients with hypogammaglobulinemia who have gastrointestinal tract symptoms should be investigated for the presence of *G lamblia* and other causes of malabsorption.

Immunologic Diagnosis

Total immunoglobulin levels are below 250 mg/dL; the IgG level is below 200 mg/dL, and IgM, IgA, IgD, and IgE levels are markedly reduced or absent. B cells are absent in peripheral blood, and there are no plasma cells containing immunoglobulins in tissue and lymph nodes. Lymph nodes are markedly depleted in B-cell-dependent areas. No antibodies are formed following specific immunization. T cell numbers and functions are intact. Natural killer (NK) cell activity is normal.

Molecular Diagnosis

It is now possible to establish a genetic diagnosis of the tyrosine kinase defect.

Differential Diagnosis

A diagnosis of X-linked infantile hypogammaglobulinemia may be difficult to establish in the age range of 5–9 months unless new molecular techniques are available. By this time most infants have lost their maternal immunoglobulins and are susceptible to recurrent infections. The majority of normal infants during this time have IgG levels below 350 mg/dL but usually show some evidence of IgM and IgA production (usually >20 mg/dL). If the diagnosis appears uncertain, several approaches may be taken. Immunoglobulin levels may be determined again 3 months after the initial values. If there is an increase in IgG, IgM, or IgA, it is highly unlikely that the patient has hypogammaglobulinemia. Alternatively, the patient may be immunized with killed vaccines, and specific antibody levels determined. The most difficult diagnostic problem is the differentiation of prolonged physiologic hypogammaglobulinemia from X-linked infantile hypogammaglobulinemia. In the former, the hypogammaglobulinemia may sometimes be severe enough to require treatment, and immunoglobulin levels may be as low as those of patients with congenital hypogammaglobulinemia. Normal production of immunoglobulins may not occur until as late as 18 months of age in patients with physiologic hypogammaglobulinemia. In most instances these patients will begin to produce their own immunoglobulin despite concurrent gamma globulin administration. This is manifested by increasing levels of IgG as well as IgM and IgA. Since IgM and IgA make up less than 10% of commercial gamma globulin, a gradual increase in these levels argues strongly against a diagnosis of congenital hypogammaglobulinemia. The best way to avoid mistaking congenital hypogammaglobulinemia for prolonged physiologic hypogammaglobulinemia in infants is to compare immunoglobulin levels with those in age-matched controls and to obtain sequential measurements of immunoglobulins at 3-month intervals during the first year of diagnostic uncertainty. Rarely, patients with human immunodeficiency virus (HIV) infection have hypogammaglobulinemia.

A number of familial syndromes of hypogamma-globulinemia and neutropenia have been described. The number is significant, and it is not certain whether this is an association or a secondary manifestation as a consequence of recurrent infection.

Patients with severe malabsorption—particularly protein-losing enteropathy—may have severely depressed levels of immunoglobulins because of enteric loss. In most instances, a diagnosis of protein-losing enteropathy can be established by the demonstration of a concomitant deficiency of serum albumin. Occasionally, however, patients with severe malabsorption and primary hypogammaglobulinemia also lose albumin through the intestinal tract. Under these circumstances, a diagnosis can best be made by obtaining an intestinal biopsy. Patients with protein-losing enteropathy have normal numbers of plasma cells containing intracellular immunoglobulins in the gut and in other lymphoid tissues. These patients also have normal numbers of circulating B cells.

Polyarthritis may be a presenting feature in patients with hypogammaglobulinemia. Most patients with juvenile rheumatoid arthritis have elevated levels of immunoglobulins. Patients with arthritis and hypogammaglobulinemia usually respond promptly to gamma globulin therapy. Patients with chronic lung disease should also be suspected of having cystic fibrosis, asthma, α-antitrypsin deficiency, or immotile cilia syndrome.

Treatment

Replacement gamma globulin therapy consists primarily of the use of intravenous gamma globulin. Although manufacturing techniques may vary for the different preparations that have been approved for clinical use, their compositions are similar. All contain almost exclusively IgG, with only trace amounts of IgM and IgA. Some preparations contain a more physiologic representation of the IgG subclasses and therefore may be useful in the treatment of IgG subclass deficiencies. All of the preparations may contain small amounts of other nonantibody proteins. Intramuscular gamma globulin is prepared in a manner similar to that of intravenous gamma globulin, but with the omission of chemical treatment steps that prevent it from aggregating or stimulating the complement pathway in vivo. Although intramuscular gamma globulin is safe to use by local injection, it will cause severe anaphylactoid reactions if given intravenously. Even though it is inexpensive to use and easy to administer, it has been largely replaced by intravenous gamma globulin because larger amounts of the latter can be safely given to patients. The use of intramuscular gamma globulin has been largely relegated to preventing hepatitis and other infectious diseases in normal individuals.

Starting doses of intravenous gamma globulin range from 100 to 200 mg/kg given intravenously once each month. The total amount given is dependent on the control of symptoms. Patients whose symptoms are not controlled on lower doses may have the total dose increased to as much as 400 mg/kg given on a monthly basis or even as frequently as every week. During an acute illness, such as meningitis or pneumonia, gamma globulin may be given as frequently as every day if the patient fails to respond appropriately to antibiotics plus standard doses of gamma globulin. If a patient with an acute illness has not received gamma globulin for 2 weeks, it is advisable to provide a repeat maintenance dose. The maximum dose of intravenous gamma globulin has not been defined, but certain factors should be considered when doses larger than 400 mg/kg are used or the frequency of administration is greater than once a week. Pulmonary function may be acutely impaired when large amounts of intravenous gamma globulin have been administered to children with pulmonary disease. Also, there are no data to suggest that giving excess amounts of passive antibody is therapeutically advantageous.

The half-life of intravenous gamma globulin is between 15 and 25 days. Serum levels of IgG approaching normal can be achieved for the first 2–4 days following intravenous administration, but they return to abnormal values after 2–3 weeks. Weekly administration results in stabilization of levels, but this has not been shown to be of clinical benefit. Because there are limitations in the amount of gamma globulin that can be given intramuscularly, this method of administration does not result in an increase in serum IgG levels.

Reactions to intravenous gamma globulin are rare. Patients occasionally experience dyspnea, sweating, increased heart rate, or abdominal pain. In most instances these symptoms subside when the infusion rate is temporarily reduced.

Anaphylactoid reactions to gamma globulin administration have been observed. These are not mediated through the IgE allergic pathway, since most patients with hypogammaglobulinemia do not form IgE antibodies. The chief causes of these reactions are aggregate formation in the gamma globulin preparation and inadvertent intravenous administration of intramuscular preparations. Patients who have repeated reactions to gamma globulin should first be treated with an alternative preparation obtained from a different commercial source. If reactions continue, it may be necessary to centrifuge the preparation to remove aggregates prior to administration.

Therapeutic gamma globulin is prepared from pools of serum obtained from donors screened for absence of viruses causing hepatitis or acquired immunodeficiency syndrome (AIDS).

Additional therapy may be necessary in patients who fail to respond to maximum doses of gamma globulin. Continuous use of antibiotics may be necessary. Prophylactic broad-spectrum antibiotics such as ampicillin in low to moderate doses may be effective in controlling recurrent infection. Physical therapy with postural drainage should be used for patients with chronic lung disease or bronchiectasis.

Occasionally, a patient with hypogammaglobulinemia may be discovered who has minimal or no symptoms. These patients should receive gamma globulin therapy, even though they have not experienced repeated infection, to avoid future infections that may subsequently cause permanent complications.

Malabsorption, occasionally found in patients with hypogammaglobulinemia, usually responds to treatment with gamma globulin, intravenous fresh-frozen plasma, or both. If *G lamblia* is found, the patient should be treated with metronidazole in doses of 35–50 mg/kg/d in 3 divided doses for 10 days (for children) or 750 mg orally 3 times a day for 10 days (for adults).

Complications & Prognosis

Although patients with congenital hypogammaglobulinemia have survived to the second and third decades, the prognosis must be guarded. Despite what may appear to be adequate gamma globulin replacement therapy, many patients develop chronic lung disease. The presence of severe infection early in infancy may result in irreversible lung damage. Patients who recover from meningitis may have severe neurologic handicaps. Patients with severe pulmonary infection frequently develop bronchiectasis and chronic lung disease. Regular examinations and prompt institution of therapy are necessary to control infections and to prevent complications. Fatal echovirus infections of the central nervous system have been reported even in patients receiving gamma globulin therapy. Some of these infections have been associated with dermatomyositis. Some patients may develop leukemia or lymphoma.

TRANSIENT HYPOGAMMAGLOBULINEMIA OF INFANCY

Under normal circumstances, maternal IgG is passively transferred to the infant beginning at week 16 of gestational life. At the time of birth, the serum IgG level in the infant is usually higher than that in the mother. IgA, IgM, IgD, and IgE are not placentally transferred under normal circumstances. In fact, the presence of elevated levels of IgM or IgA in cord blood suggests premature antibody synthesis, usually a sign of intrauterine infection. Over the first 4–5 months of life, there is a gradual decrease in the serum IgG level and a gradual increase in the serum IgM and IgA levels (Fig 19–2). The IgM level usually rises more rapidly than the IgA level. Almost all infants go through a period of hypogammaglobulinemia at approximately 5–6 months of age. At this time, the serum IgG level reaches its lowest point (approximately 350 mg/dL), and many normal infants begin

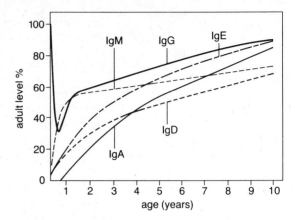

Figure 19–2. Development of serum immunoglobulins with increasing age. Levels are expressed as percentages of adult levels. Maternally acquired IgG levels decrease rapidly over the first 6 months of age. IgM levels increase more rapidly than IgA, IgD, and IgE levels.

to experience recurrent respiratory tract infections. Occasionally, an infant may fail to produce normal amounts of IgG at this time, resulting in transient hypogammaglobulinemia, or so-called physiologic hypogammaglobulinemia. The presence of normal serum levels of IgM and IgA argues strongly against a diagnosis of X-linked hypogammaglobulinemia. However, some infants with transient hypogammaglobulinemia may also fail to produce normal amounts of IgM or IgA.

Additional studies may be of no diagnostic usefulness, since many infants fail to respond to immunization at this age and isohemagglutinin titers may be low. Under these circumstances, a lymph node or intestinal biopsy may assist in establishing the diagnosis. Patients with congenital hypogammaglobulinemia lack plasma cells containing immunoglobulins in the intestinal tract and in peripheral lymph nodes. In addition, patients with congenital hypogammaglobulinemia lack circulating B cells, whereas children with physiologic hypogammaglobulinemia do not. If the patient is not experiencing severe recurrent infection, it is best to wait 3–5 months and repeat immunoglobulin measurements rather than to perform invasive procedures. In the presence of an increasing IgG, IgM, or IgA level, congenital hypogammaglobulinemia is unlikely. If the patient has been treated with gamma globulin to prevent severe or recurrent infection, measurement of IgM and IgA levels assumes greater importance. Because commercial gamma globulin contains primarily IgG, the administration of gamma globulin will not affect serum levels of IgM and IgA. Increasing levels of these immunoglobulin classes indicate that the patient had transient hypogammaglobulinemia. Hypogammaglobulinemia may persist for as long as 2 years.

The cause of transient hypogammaglobulinemia is not known. In some cases, IgG anti-Gm antibodies have been demonstrated during the last trimester of pregnancy in women who have previously had infants with transient hypogammaglobulinemia. It is postulated that these antibodies cause suppression of the infant's endogenous immunoglobulin production in a manner similar to the suppression of normal erythrocyte production from placental transfer of antibody against Rh factors. Recent studies indicate that patients with transient hypogammaglobulinemia have normal numbers of B cells but a transient deficiency in the number and function of helper T cells.

Occasionally, these infants become sufficiently symptomatic that they must be treated just like those with X-linked infantile hypogammaglobulinemia. Gamma globulin therapy may be required for as long as 18 months. Routine immunization should not be given during the period of transient hypogammaglobulinemia. The continued administration of gamma globulin will not delay the development of normal IgG. Once a normal immune system has been established, the complete series of pediatric immunizations should be administered.

COMMON, VARIABLE UNCLASSIFIABLE IMMUNODEFICIENCY (Acquired Hypogammaglobulinemia)

Major Immunologic Features
- Recurrent pyogenic infections occur, with onset at any age.
- There is increased incidence of autoimmune disease.
- The total immunoglobulin level is less than 300 mg/dL, with the IgG level below 250 mg/dL.
- B cell numbers are usually normal.

General Considerations
Patients with acquired hypogammaglobulinemia present clinically like patients with X-linked infantile hypogammaglobulinemia, except that they usually do not become symptomatic until 15–35 years of age. In addition to increased susceptibility to pyogenic infections, they have a high prevalence of autoimmune disease. These patients also differ from those with congenital hypogammaglobulinemia in that they have a higher than normal prevalence of abnormalities in T cell immunity, which in most instances progressively deteriorates with time. Acquired hypogammaglobulinemia affects both males and females and may occur at any age.

Immunologic Pathogenesis
The cause of acquired hypogammaglobulinemia is unknown. Most patients have an intrinsic defect in B cells. Peripheral blood lymphocytes from some pa-

tients with acquired hypogammaglobulinemia have an inhibiting effect on the immunoglobulin synthesis in cells from normal patients, suggesting that the course of this disorder may reside at the level of suppressor T cells. Other patients have diminished numbers of helper T cells. Some studies have shown a heterogeneity of arrested B cell development ranging from normal proliferative B cell responses and IgM-secreting cells to absent proliferative responses. Two enzymatic abnormalities have been described. In some patients there is a failure of glycosylation of the heavy-chain IgG. In others, a deficiency of 5′-nucleotidase has been found. The latter abnormality is most probably secondary to alterations in T cell:B cell ratios rather than being a primary defect. An X-linked lymphoproliferative disorder associated with acquired hypogammaglobulinemia has been described following Epstein-Barr virus (EBV) infection. Genetic studies of acquired hypogammaglobulinemia have demonstrated an autosomal recessive mode of inheritance in certain families in which abnormal lymphocyte metabolism has been shown to be inherited. In most instances, however, there is no clear-cut evidence of genetic transmission. An increased prevalence of other immunologic disorders, including autoimmune disease, has been observed in families of patients with acquired hypogammaglobulinemia. The presence of normal numbers of circulating peripheral blood B cells in most of these patients suggests that the disorder is a result of diminished synthesis or release of immunoglobulin rather than production of fewer cells synthesizing immunoglobulin.

Clinical Features
A. Symptoms and Signs: Recurrent sinopulmonary infection is the initial presentation of acquired hypogammaglobulinemia in most cases. These may be chronic rather than acute and overwhelming, as in X-linked infantile hypogammaglobulinemia. Infections may be caused by pneumococci, *H influenzae*, or other pyogenic organisms. Chronic bacterial conjunctivitis may be an additional presenting complaint. Some patients develop severe malabsorption prior to the diagnosis of hypogammaglobulinemia. The malabsorption may be severe enough to cause protein loss sufficient to produce edema. Giardiasis, cholelithiasis, and achlorhydria are additional findings.

Autoimmune disease has been a presenting complaint in some patients with acquired hypogammaglobulinemia. A rheumatoid arthritis-like disorder, systemic lupus erythematosus (SLE), idiopathic thrombocytopenic purpura, dermatomyositis, hemolytic anemia, hypothyroidism, Graves' disease, and pernicious anemia have been reported in association with acquired hypogammaglobulinemia.

In contrast to patients with X-linked infantile hypogammaglobulinemia, those with acquired hypogammaglobulinemia may have marked lymphadenopathy and splenomegaly. Intestinal lymphoid nodular hyperplasia has been described in association with malabsorption. Other abnormal physical findings relate to the presence of chronic lung disease or intestinal malabsorption. Leukemia, lymphoma, and gastric carcinoma occur with increased frequency.

B. Laboratory Findings: Immunoglobulin measurements may show slightly higher IgG levels than are reported in X-linked infantile hypogammaglobulinemia. Total immunoglobulin levels are usually below 300 mg/dL, and the IgG level is usually below 250 mg/dL. IgM and IgA may be absent or present in significant amounts. The Schick test is useful to demonstrate a lack of normal antibody response, but it should be performed following booster immunization with diphtheria antigen. Blood group isohemagglutinins are absent or present in low titers (<1:10). The failure to produce antibody following specific immunization establishes the diagnosis in patients who have borderline immunoglobulin values. Live attenuated vaccines should not be used for immunization. Peripheral blood B lymphocytes are usually present in normal numbers in patients with acquired hypogammaglobulinemia, in contrast to their absence in patients with X-linked infantile hypogammaglobulinemia.

Although most patients with acquired hypogammaglobulinemia have intact cell-mediated immunity, a significant number demonstrate abnormalities as evidenced by absent delayed hypersensitivity skin test responses, depressed responses of isolated peripheral blood lymphocytes to PHA and allogeneic cells, and decreased numbers of T cells. Many patients also demonstrate reduced in vitro production of interleukins (IL) including IL-2, IL-4, and IL-5. Other patients have reduced CD4/CD8 ratios with increased numbers of CD8 cells bearing the CD57 receptor. NK cell activity is normal. A few patients have been found to have abnormal macrophage-T cell interaction. Repetition of these tests is important, because the immunodeficiency appears to progressively involve cell-mediated immunity, resulting in additional immunologic deficiencies.

Biopsy of lymphoid tissue demonstrates a lack of plasma cells. Although some lymph node biopsies may reveal lymphoid hyperplasia, there is a striking absence of cells in the B cell-dependent areas similar to that seen in congenital hypogammaglobulinemia.

C. Other Tests: Other tests that may be abnormal in these patients relate to associated disorders. The chest x-ray usually shows evidence of chronic lung disease, and sinus films show chronic sinusitis. Pulmonary function studies are abnormal. Patients with malabsorption may have abnormal gastrointestinal tract biopsies, with blunting of the villi similar to that seen in celiac disease. Studies for malabsorption may indicate a lack of normal intestinal enzymes and an abnormal D-xylose absorption test. Occasionally, autoantibodies are found in patients who have an as-

sociated autoimmune hemolytic anemia or SLE. Autoantibodies are not found in those with an associated pernicious anemia, but biopsies of the stomach demonstrate marked lymphoid cell infiltration. Lymphoreticular cancers and thymomas have occurred in some patients.

Immunologic Diagnosis

The total immunoglobulin level is below 300 mg/dL, with the IgG level below 250 mg/dL. IgM and IgA may be absent or present in normal amounts. The antibody response following specific immunization is absent. Isohemagglutinins are depressed, and the Schick test is reactive. The number of circulating peripheral blood B cells is usually normal but may be decreased.

Cell-mediated immunity may be intact or may be depressed, with negative hypersensitivity skin tests, depressed responses of peripheral blood lymphocytes to PHA and allogeneic cells, and decreased numbers of circulating peripheral blood T cells. The CD4/CD8 ratio may be reduced. The number of B cells in the peripheral blood may be normal or diminished. There is occasionally an increased number of null cells, ie, lymphocytes lacking surface markers for either T or B cells.

Differential Diagnosis

The clinical presentation of patients with X-linked infantile hypogammaglobulinemia and those with acquired hypogammaglobulinemia may be similar. This does not present a major clinical problem. Severe malabsorption in protein-losing enteropathy may cause hypogammaglobulinemia, but these patients always have a concomitant deficiency of serum albumin. Differentiating between protein-losing enteropathy and acquired hypogammaglobulinemia may be difficult under circumstances where protein-losing enteropathy is accompanied by gastrointestinal loss of lymphoid cells. In both groups of patients, antibody responses and cell-mediated immunity may be impaired. When the presenting feature of acquired hypogammaglobulinemia is an autoimmune disease, there may be a delay in recognizing and treating the immune deficiency. In most instances, however, patients with autoimmune disease have normal or elevated immunoglobulin levels. Patients with chronic lung disease should also be investigated for cystic fibrosis, chronic allergy, α_1-antitrypsin deficiency, or immotile cilia syndrome. Patients with HIV infection may occasionally develop hypogammaglobulinemia. If HIV infection is suspected in a patient with hypogammaglobulinemia, HIV should be sought by means of viral culture or polymerase chain reaction (PCR) techniques rather than antibody testing.

Treatment

The treatment of acquired hypogammaglobulinemia is identical to that of X-linked infantile hypogammaglobulinemia (see Table 18–5). Gamma globulin and continuous administration of antibiotics are usually required. Intravenous gamma globulin at 100–200 mg/kg is given once each month. If symptoms are not controlled, the dose may be increased to 400 mg/kg per week or the original dose may be given more frequently. Gamma globulin should always be given during an acute illness. During acute illnesses, it can be given weekly or daily. Patients should be monitored at regular intervals with chest x-rays and pulmonary function tests to determine the adequacy of therapy. Pulmonary physical therapy is an essential part of treatment in patients with chronic lung disease.

Specific treatment of malabsorption problems may be required. Some patients respond to treatment with gamma globulin. In others, the malabsorption may be associated with secondary enzymatic deficiencies that resemble celiac disease. These patients may respond to dietary restrictions. If the malabsorption is associated with *G lamblia* infection, metronidazole therapy should be used.

Caution should be exercised in the treatment of associated autoimmune disorders. The use of corticosteroids and immunosuppressive agents in a patient with immunodeficiency may result in markedly increased susceptibility to infection. Splenectomy has been used in the treatment of hypogammaglobulinemia and hemolytic anemia, but the mortality rate from overwhelming infection is high.

Complications & Prognosis

Patients with acquired hypogammaglobulinemia may survive to the seventh or eighth decade. Women with this disorder have had normal pregnancies and delivered normal infants (albeit hypogammaglobulinemic until 6 months of age). The major complication is chronic lung disease, which may develop despite adequate gamma globulin replacement therapy. An increased prevalence of malignant disease, including leukemia, lymphoma, and gastric carcinoma, has been observed. Patients who develop acquired T cell deficiencies have increasing difficulty with infection characteristic of both T and B cell deficiencies.

IMMUNODEFICIENCY WITH HYPER-IgM

This syndrome, characterized by an increased level of IgM (ranging from 150 to 1000 mg/dL) associated with a deficiency of IgG and IgA, is relatively rare and in most instances appears to be inherited in a X-linked manner. However, several cases have been reported of an acquired form that affects both sexes. It has been postulated that in the normal individual there is a sequential development of immunoglobulins, initiated by IgM production and subsequently re-

sulting in the production of IgG and IgA. Arrest in the development of immunoglobulin-producing cells after the formation of IgM-producing cells would be a possible cause. This hypothesis has been confirmed by several investigative groups who have shown that the X-linked form is associated with a genetic defect in the CD40 ligand on T cells. The normal sequence of IgM to IgG antibody production is dependent on the binding of the protein CD40 to the CD40 ligand on T cells. A defective ligand interferes with binding and antibody production. The hyper-IgM syndrome may be present congenitally or make a late appearance. It has also been reported in association with EBV. Inheritance may be X-linked or autosomal dominant or recessive.

Patients present with recurrent pyogenic infections, including otitis media, pneumonia, and septicemia. Some have recurrent neutropenia, hemolytic anemia, or aplastic anemia.

Laboratory evaluation reveals a marked increase in the serum IgM level, with absence of IgG and IgA. Isohemagglutinin titers may be elevated, and the patient may form antibodies following specific immunization. Detailed studies of cell-mediated immunity have not been performed, but some reports indicate that it is intact. Patients with this disorder may develop an infiltrating neoplasm of IgM-producing plasma cells.

Treatment is similar to that of X-linked infantile hypogammaglobulinemia (see Table 18–5). Because so few cases have been reported, it is difficult to determine the prognosis.

Since the genetic defect has been recognized, it should be easier to establish a diagnosis in utero and early in infancy. It should also be possible to detect the carrier state.

SELECTIVE IgA DEFICIENCY

Major Immunologic Features

- IgA level is below 5 mg/dL, with other immunoglobulin levels normal or increased.
- Cell-mediated immunity is usually normal.
- There is increased association with allergies, recurrent sinopulmonary infection, gastrointestinal tract disease, and autoimmune disease.

General Considerations

Selective IgA deficiency is the most common immunodeficiency disorder. The prevalence in the normal population has been estimated to vary between 1:800 and 1:600. Considerable debate exists about whether individuals with selective IgA deficiency are "normal" or have significant associated diseases. Studies of individual patients and extensive studies of large numbers of patients suggest that absence of IgA predisposes to a variety of diseases. The diagnosis of selective IgA deficiency is established by finding a serum IgA level of less than 5 mg/dL.

Immunologic Pathogenesis

The cause of selective IgA deficiency is not known. An arrest in the development of B cells has been suggested on the basis of the observation that these patients have increased numbers of B cells with both surface IgA and IgM or surface IgA and IgD. An associated IgG_2 subclass deficiency has been found in some patients, and this has been used to explain the varied clinical manifestations related to antibody deficiency. The presence of normal numbers of circulating IgA-bearing B cells suggests that this disorder is associated with decreased synthesis or release of IgA or impaired differentiation to IgA plasma cells rather than with the absence of IgA B lymphocytes. Utilizing the concept of sequential immunoglobulin production (IgM to IgG to IgA), selective IgA deficiency could result from an arrest in the development of immunoglobulin-producing cells following the normal sequential development of IgM to IgG. The variety of diseases associated with selective IgA deficiency may be the result of enhanced or prolonged exposure to a spectrum of microbial agents and nonreplicating antigens as a consequence of deficient secretory IgA. The continuous assault by these agents on a compromised mucosal immune system could result in an increased incidence of infection, autoantibodies, autoimmune disease, and cancer. Recently, an increased prevalence of HLA-A1, -B8, and -Dw3 has been found in patients with IgA deficiency and autoimmune disease.

Lymphocyte culture studies in IgA-deficient patients have demonstrated that IgA cells synthesize but fail to secrete IgA. Some individuals have suppressor T cells that selectively inhibit IgA production by normal lymphocytes.

Acquired IgA deficiency and susceptibility to sinopulmonary tract infections occur frequently in patients treated with phenytoin or penicillamine. In at least some instances, the IgA level returns to normal when the drug therapy is stopped.

Clinical Features

A. Symptoms and Signs:

1. Recurrent sinopulmonary infection–The most frequent presenting symptoms are recurrent sinopulmonary viral or bacterial infections. Patients occasionally present with recurrent or chronic right middle lobe pneumonia. Pulmonary hemosiderosis occurs with increased frequency and may be erroneously diagnosed as chronic lung infection.

2. Allergy–In surveys of selected atopic populations the prevalence of selective IgA deficiency is 1:400–1:200, compared with a prevalence of 1:800–1:600 in the normal population. Although the reasons for this association are not known, the absence of

serum IgA may result in a significant reduction in the amount of antibody competing for antigens capable of combining with IgE. Alternatively, patients who lack IgA in their secretions may more readily absorb allergenic proteins, thereby enhancing the formation of IgE antibodies. Allergic diseases in patients with selective IgA deficiency are often more difficult to control than the same allergies in other patients. Allergic symptoms in these patients may be "triggered" by infection as well as by other environmental agents.

An increase in circulating antibody to bovine proteins, sometimes associated with circulating immune complexes, including complexes with human antibody to bovine immunoglobulin, has been found in patients with selective IgA deficiency. This has been interpreted as providing additional evidence for abnormal gastrointestinal tract absorption. However, removal of cow's milk from the diet is usually not effective in ameliorating symptoms.

A unique form of allergy exists in these patients. Certain patients with selective IgA deficiency develop high titers of antibody directed against IgA. Anaphylactic reactions from infusion of blood products containing IgA occur in some of these patients. The prevalence of antibodies directed against IgA in patients, however, is much higher (30–40%) than the prevalence of such anaphylactic transfusion reactions. Most patients who have anti-IgA antibodies have not had a history of gamma globulin or blood administration, suggesting that these antibodies are "autoantibodies" or that they arise from sensitization to breast milk, passive transfer of maternal IgA, or cross-reaction with bovine immunoglobulin from ingestion of cow's milk.

3. Gastrointestinal tract disease–An increased prevalence of celiac disease has been noted in patients with selective IgA deficiency. The disease may present at any time and is similar to celiac disease unassociated with IgA deficiency. Intestinal biopsies show an increase in the number of IgM-producing cells. An anti-basement membrane antibody has also been found with increased incidence. Ulcerative colitis and regional enteritis have also been reported in association with selective IgA deficiency. Pernicious anemia has been found in a significant number of patients who also have antibodies to both intrinsic factor and gastric parietal cells.

4. Autoimmune disease–A number of autoimmune disorders are associated with selective IgA deficiency. They include SLE, rheumatoid arthritis, dermatomyositis, pernicious anemia, thyroiditis, Coombs-positive hemolytic anemia, Sjögren's syndrome, and chronic active hepatitis. Although the association of IgA deficiency and certain autoimmune disorders may be fortuitous, the increased prevalence of IgA deficiency in patients with SLE and rheumatoid arthritis (1:200–1:100) is statistically significant.

The clinical presentation of patients with autoimmune disease associated with selective IgA deficiency does not appear to differ significantly from that of individuals with the identical disorder and normal or elevated levels of IgA. Because patients with selective IgA deficiency are capable of making normal amounts of antibody in the other immunoglobulin classes, they usually have the autoantibodies that characterize the specific autoimmune disease (antinuclear antibody, anti-DNA antibody, antiparietal cell antibody, etc).

5. Selective IgA deficiency in apparently healthy adults–Patients with selective IgA deficiency are capable of making normal amounts of antibody of the IgG and IgM classes. Many are entirely asymptomatic, although long-term follow-up of some of these patients indicates that they may develop significant disease with time. There are several reasons why some patients remain asymptomatic. A small percentage of patients with selective IgA deficiency have normal amounts of secretory IgA and normal numbers of plasma cells containing IgA along the gastrointestinal tract. IgA-deficient patients have increased amounts of low-molecular-weight (7S) IgM in their secretions, which may subserve the secretory antibody function in place of IgA antibodies. Finally, patients with selective IgA deficiency may have different exposures to pathogens and noxious agents in the environment.

6. Selective IgA deficiency and genetic factors–Both an autosomal recessive and an autosomal dominant mode of inheritance of IgA deficiency have been postulated. IgA deficiency appears with greater than normal frequency in families with other immunodeficiency disorders such as hypogammaglobulinemia. Partial deletion of the long or short arm of chromosome 18 (18q syndrome) or ring chromosome 18 has been described in selective IgA deficiency. However, many patients with abnormalities of chromosome 18 have normal levels of IgA in their serum. Selective IgA deficiency has been reported in one identical twin but not the other. In a study of familial IgA deficiency, an association with HLA-A2, -B8, and -Dw3 was described. Other studies have shown an increase in association with HLA-A1 and -B8.

7. Selective IgA deficiency and cancer–Selective IgA deficiency has been reported in association with thymoma, reticulum cell sarcoma, and squamous cell carcinoma of the esophagus and lungs. Several patients with IgA deficiency and cancer also had concomitant autoimmune disease and recurrent infection.

8. Selective IgA deficiency and drugs–Phenytoin and other anticonvulsants have been implicated as a possible cause of some cases of selective IgA deficiency or hypogammaglobulinemia, and these patients are frequently symptomatic with recurrent sinopulmonary infections. Withdrawal of the drug does not always result in a return to normal IgA

levels. In vitro production of IgA by peripheral blood lymphocytes in these patients may be normal or deficient. Deficient T-cell/B-cell interaction is found in some patients.

B. Laboratory Findings: Selective IgA deficiency is defined as a serum level of IgA below 5 mg/dL, with normal or increased levels of IgG, IgM, IgD, and IgE. Some patients with IgA deficiency may also have IgG2 subclass deficiency. Because there are a number of methods for measuring immunoglobulin levels, each laboratory should establish standards for detection of low IgA levels. B cells from these patients are capable of forming normal amounts of antibody following immunization. In most instances, absence of IgA in the serum is associated with absence of IgA in the secretions and with the presence of normal secretory component. Increased amounts of 7S IgM may be found in the serum and secretions. As discussed above, some patients have autoantibodies including antibodies directed against IgG, IgM, and IgA. The number of circulating peripheral blood B cells (including IgA-bearing B cells) is normal. Increased numbers of suppressor T cells have been found in some patients.

Cell-mediated immunity is normal in most patients. Delayed hypersensitivity skin tests, the response of isolated peripheral blood lymphocytes to PHA and allogeneic cells, and the number of circulating T cells are normal. A few patients have low levels of T cells, diminished production of T cell interferon, and decreased lymphocyte mitogenic responses.

Other laboratory abnormalities are those typical of the associated diseases. Individuals who have chronic sinopulmonary infection may have abnormal x-rays and abnormal pulmonary functions. Patients with IgA deficiency and celiac disease show appropriate pathology on gastrointestinal tract biopsies, impaired D-xylose absorption, and antibody directed against basement membrane in some cases. Patients with IgA deficiency and autoimmune disease have characteristic autoantibodies, eg, anti-DNA, antinuclear, antiparietal cell, and a positive Coombs test. An increase in circulating immune complexes has been described.

Differential Diagnosis

Selective IgA deficiency must be distinguished from other more severe immunodeficiency disorders with a concomitant deficiency of IgA. Forty percent of patients with ataxia-telangiectasia have IgA deficiency. These patients usually have cellular immunodeficiency as well. If IgA deficiency is found during the first years of life, a definitive diagnosis may not be possible because the complete ataxia-telangiectasia syndrome may not be present until the patient is 4–5 years old. Other immunodeficiency disorders that have been associated with selective IgA deficiency are chronic mucocutaneous candidiasis and cellular immunodeficiency with abnormal immunoglobulin synthesis (Nezelof's syndrome) and selective deficiency of IgG2. A careful history should be obtained to rule out IgA deficiency secondary to drugs, especially anticonvulsants or penicillamine.

Treatment

Patients with selective IgA deficiency should not be treated with gamma globulin. Therapeutic gamma globulin contains only a small quantity of IgA, and this is not likely to reach mucosal secretions through parenteral administration. Furthermore, IgA-deficient patients are capable of forming normal amounts of antibody of other immunoglobulin classes. Finally, they recognize injected IgA as foreign, so that gamma globulin infusions in these patients enhance the risk of development of anti-IgA antibodies and subsequent anaphylactic transfusion reactions. There is as yet no means by which the deficient IgA can be safely replaced. Patients with combined IgA and IgG subclass deficiency with documented impaired antibody formation have been treated with gamma globulin, but its efficacy has yet to be documented. Patients with recurrent sinopulmonary infection should be treated aggressively with broad-spectrum antibiotics to avoid permanent pulmonary complications. Patients with SLE, rheumatoid arthritis, celiac disease, etc, are treated in the same fashion as patients with the same diseases without IgA deficiency.

Transfusion reactions in patients with selective IgA deficiency may be minimized by several means. Packed washed (3 times) erythrocytes should be used to treat anemia. Although this does not completely eliminate the possibility of a transfusion reaction, it will decrease the risk. Alternatively, patients may be given blood from an IgA-deficient donor whose blood type matches the recipient's. Preserving the patient's own plasma and erythrocytes for future use is recommended if possible.

Complications & Prognosis

IgA-deficient patients have survived to the sixth or seventh decade without severe disease. Most individuals, however, become symptomatic during the first decade of life. Recognition of the potential complications and prompt therapy for associated diseases will increase longevity and reduce the morbidity rate. Regular follow-up examinations are necessary for early detection of associated disorders and complications. A very few patients have developed normal IgA levels after years of IgA deficiency.

SELECTED IgM DEFICIENCY

Selective IgM deficiency is a rare disorder associated with the absence of IgM and normal levels of other immunoglobulin classes. IgM-bearing B cells are present in normal numbers. Some patients have decreased helper T cell activity. Some patients are capable of normal antibody responses in the other immunoglobulin classes following specific immunization, whereas others respond poorly. Cell-mediated immunity appears to be intact, but there has been an insufficient number of detailed studies to confirm this.

The cause of selective IgM deficiency is unknown. Increased suppressor T cell activity specific for IgM has been described. The absence of IgM in the presence of IgG and IgA has yet to be explained, since it appears to contradict the theory of sequential immunoglobulin development. The disorder has been found in both males and females.

Patients with selective IgM deficiency are susceptible to autoimmune disease and to overwhelming infection with polysaccharide-containing organisms (eg, pneumococci, H influenzae). They may also have chronic dermatitis, diarrhea, and recurrent respiratory infections. Insufficient data are available to determine appropriate therapy. It would appear logical to manage these patients in a manner similar to the way an infant is managed following splenectomy, ie, either immediate antibiotic (penicillin or ampicillin) treatment of all infections or continuous antibiotic treatment. If patients are unable to form antibody to specific antigens, gamma globulin therapy should be given.

SELECTIVE DEFICIENCY OF IgG SUBCLASSES

Major Immunologic Features

- One or more IgG subclasses are deficient.
- T cell immunity is normal.
- Patients have recurrent bacterial infections.
- The condition is sometimes associated with other immunodeficiencies such as selective IgA deficiency or ataxia-telangiectasia.

General Considerations

IgG antibodies exist in 4 isotypic variants identified by antigenic differences of the Fc portion of the immunoglobulin molecule. These are termed IgG1, IgG2, IgG3, and IgG4 and make up approximately 65, 20, 10, and 5% of the total serum immunoglobulin levels, respectively (Fig 19–3). IgG subclasses develop independently, with IgG1 and IgG3 maturing more rapidly than IgG2 or IgG4. Deletion of constant heavy-chain genes or abnormalities of isotype switching may result in deficiencies of one or more of the IgG subclasses.

Clinically, patients have recurrent respiratory tract infections and repeated pyogenic sinopulmonary infections with S pneumoniae, H influenzae, and Staphylococcus aureus. Some patients develop or present with evidence of autoimmune diseases such as SLE

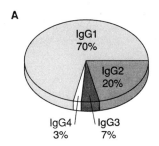 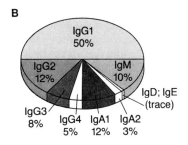

Figure 19–3. Normal distribution of serum immunoglobulins. **A:** Percentages of IgG subclasses relative to total IgG. **B:** Percentages of immunoglobulin classes and subclasses relative to total immunoglobulin.

or pulmonary hemosiderosis. As selective deficiency of IgG subclasses may be found in other immunodeficiency disorders such as ataxia-telangiectasia or selective IgA deficiency, other features of immunodeficiency may predominate.

IgG2-IgG4 deficiency is usually found in individuals with recurrent infections or autoimmune disease who are either normoglobulinemic or hypergammaglobulinemic. A few healthy individuals with this deficiency have been described. It is also found in some patients with ataxia-telangiectasia.

IgG2 deficiency is associated with recurrent sinopulmonary infections and an inability to respond to polysaccharide antigens (such as pneumococcal or *H influenzae* polysaccharide). However, the patient does respond normally to protein antigens such as tetanus or diphtheria toxoid.

IgG3 deficiency is found in a small percentage of individuals with recurrent infections who are screened by specific IgG subclass determinations for antibody deficiency. Familial occurrence of IgG3 deficiency has been reported.

IgG4 deficiency is also associated with recurrent respiratory infections and/or manifestations of autoimmune disease. It occurs with approximately the same frequency in individuals with recurrent respiratory tract infections as does IgG3 deficiency.

A diagnosis of one or more IgG subclass deficiencies is made by the finding of significantly low levels of one or more IgG subclasses compared with those in age-matched normal controls. The total IgG concentration may be normal, low, or elevated. The response to immunization may be variable, ranging from normal to a selective inability to respond to polysaccharide antigens. T cell immunity is usually intact.

Most patients with selective IgG subclass deficiency respond to treatment with gamma globulin administered in a manner similar to that used in the treatment of hypogammaglobulinemia. However, the decision to commit a patient to lifelong treatment is a difficult one and should not be based on immunoglobulin levels alone. Rather the antibody response

following immunization and the clinical course should also be taken into account.

X-LINKED LYMPHOPROLIFERATIVE SYNDROME (Duncan's Syndrome)

Major Immunologic Features
- Patients are susceptible to fatal EBV infection.
- Hypogammaglobulinemia develops.
- Lymphoma develops.

General Considerations

The X-linked lymphoproliferative syndrome is a disease that renders individuals unusually susceptible to several serious outcomes of EBV infection: (1) fatal infectious mononucleosis, with severe liver disease and hepatitis accounting for most of the deaths; (2) fatal infectious mononucleosis with lymphoma; (3) infectious mononucleosis with immunodeficiency; and (4) lymphoma. Approximately 63% of patients develop fatal infectious mononucleosis, 29% develop immunodeficiency, and 24% develop lymphoma. The mortality rate associated with this syndrome is 85% by 10 years of age and 100% by 40 years of age.

Immunologic abnormalities include inverted helper/suppressor T cell ratios, deficient proliferative responses of mononuclear cells to mitogenic stimulation, defective gamma interferon production, and decreased NK cell activity. Abnormalities of B cell immunity include hypogammaglobulinemia, failure to switch from IgM- to IgG-specific antibody following immunization with bacteriophage, and lack of antibody to EBV, especially to EBV nuclear antigen (EBNA). These abnormalities are found primarily in long-term survivors. In contrast, patients who die early as a result of EBV infection may have normal T cell and B cell immunity prior to infection, suggesting that the immune defect in X-linked lymphoproliferative syndrome is probably a progressive one.

There is no effective treatment to prevent the progression of the immunodeficiency in this syndrome. If hypogammaglobulinemia develops, gamma globulin therapy should be given. Recently, the genetic defect has been located by restriction fragment length polymorphism mapping. In the future it should be possible to identify carriers of the genetic defect, provide appropriate genetic counseling, and diagnose the disease in utero.

REFERENCES

X-Linked Infantile Hypogammaglobulinemia

Marx J: Tyrosine kinase defect also causes immunodeficiency. *Science* 1993;**259**:897.

Rosen FS, Janeway CA: The gamma globulins. 3. The antibody deficiency syndromes. *N Engl J Med* 1966;**275**:709.

Siegel RL et al: Deficiency of T helper cells in transient hypogammaglobulinemia of infancy. *N Engl J Med* 1981;**305**:1307.

Van Maldergem L et al: Echovirus meningoencephalitis in X-linked hypogammaglobulinemia. *Acta Paediatr Scand* 1989;**78**:325.

Common Variable Hypogammaglobulinemia

Cunningham-Rundles C: Clinical and immunologic analyses of 103 patients with common variable immunodeficiency. *J Clin Immunol* 1989;**9**:22.

Hermans PE, Diaz-Buxo JA, Stobo JD: Idiopathic late-onset immunoglobulin deficiency: Clinical observations in 50 patients. *Am J Med* 1976;**61**:221.

Jaffe JS et al: T cell abnormalities in common variable immunodeficiency. *Pediatr Res* 1993;**33(suppl)**:S24.

Ochs H: Intravenous immunoglobulin therapy of patients with primary immunodeficiency syndromes. Pages 9–14 in: *Immunoglobulins: Characteristics and Uses of Intravenous Preparations.* US Department of Health and Human Services, 1981.

Saiki O et al: Three distinct stages of B cell defects in common varied immunodeficiency. *Proc Natl Acad Sci USA* 1982;**79**:6008.

White WB et al: Immunoregulatory effects of intravenous immune serum globulin therapy in common variable hypogammaglobulinemia. *Am J Med* 1987;**83**:431.

X-Linked Immunodeficiency with Hyper-IgM

Arrufo A et al: The CD40 ligand, gp39, is defective in activated T cells from patients with X-linked hyper IgM syndrome. *Cell* 1993;**72**:291.

Eskola J et al: Regulatory T-cell function in primary humoral immunodeficiency states. *J Clin Lab Immunol* 1989;**28**:55.

Ohno T et al: Selective deficiency in IL-2 production and refractoriness to extrinsic IL-2 in immunodeficiency with hyper-IgM. *Clin Immunol Immunopathol* 1987;**45**:471.

Stiehm ER, Fudenberg HH: Clinical and immunologic features of dysgammaglobulinemia type 1. *Am J Med* 1966;**40**:895.

Selective IgA Deficiency

Ammann AJ, Hong R: Selective IgA deficiency: Presentation of 30 cases and a review of the literature. *Medicine* 1971;**50**:223.

Ferreira A et al: Anti-IgA antibodies in selective IgA deficiency and in primary immunodeficient patients treated with gamma-globulin. *Clin Immunol Immunopathol* 1988;**47**:199.

Oxelius VA et al: IgG subclass deficiency in selective IgA deficiency. *N Engl J Med* 1981;**305**:1476.

Selective IgM Deficiency

Guill MF et al: IgM deficiency: Clinical spectrum and immunologic assessment. *Ann Allergy* 1989;**62**:547.

IgG Subclass Deficiency

Heiner DC: Recognition and management of IgG subclass deficiencies. *Pediatr Infect Dis J* 1987;**6**:235.

Ochs HD, Wedgwood RJ: Disorders of the B-cell system. Pages 226–256 in: *Immunologic Disorders in Infants and Children.* Stiehm ER (editor). Saunders, 1989.

Ochs HD, Wedgwood RJ: IgG subclass deficiencies. *Annu Rev Med* 1987;**38**:325.

Schur PH et al: Selective gamma-G globulin deficiencies in patients with recurrent pyogenic infections. *N Engl J Med* 1970;**283**:631.

X-Linked Lymphoproliferative Syndrome

Grierson H, Putillo DT: Epstein-barr virus infections in males with X-linked lymphoproliferative syndrome. *Ann Intern Med* 1987;**106**:538.

Webster AD et al: Viruses and antibody deficiency syndromes. *Immunol Invest* 1988;**17**:93.

T Cell Immunodeficiency Disorders 20

Arthur J. Ammann, MD

Immunodeficiency disorders associated with isolated defective T cell immunity are rare. These diseases were formerly called cellular immunodeficiencies. In most patients, defective T cell immunity is accompanied by abnormalities of B cell immunity. This reflects the collaboration between T cells and B cells in the process of antibody formation. Thus, almost all patients with complete T cell deficiency have some impairment of antibody formation. Some patients with T cell deficiency have normal levels of immunoglobulin but fail to produce specific antibody following immunization. These patients are considered to have a qualitative defective in antibody production.

Patients with cellular immunodeficiency disorders are susceptible to a variety of viral, fungal, and protozoal infections. These infections may be acute or chronic.

Screening tests utilized to evaluate T cell immunity are listed in Table 18–4. The availability of additional tests for the evaluation of T cell immunity (Table 20–1) permits more precise diagnosis in many instances.

CONGENITAL THYMIC APLASIA (DiGeorge's Syndrome, Immunodeficiency With Hypoparathyroidism)

Major Immunologic Features

- There is congenital aplasia or hypoplasia of the thymus.
- Lymphopenia reflects a decreased number of T cells.
- T cell function in peripheral blood is absent.
- Antibody levels and function are variable.
- Treatment with thymus graft is successful.

General Considerations

DiGeorge's syndrome is one of the few immunodeficiency disorders associated with symptoms immediately following birth. The complete syndrome consists of the following features: (1) abnormal facies consisting of low-set ears, "fish-shaped" mouth, hypertelorism, notched ear pinnae, micrognathia, and an antimongoloid slant of eyes (Fig 20–1); (2) hypoparathyroidism; (3) congenital heart disease; and (4) cellular immunodeficiency. Initial symptoms are related to associated abnormalities of the parathyroids and heart and may result in hypocalcemia and congestive heart failure, respectively. If the diagnosis of DiGeorge's syndrome is suspected because of these early clinical findings, confirmation may be obtained by demonstrating defective T cell immunity. The importance of early diagnosis is related to the complete reconstitution of T cell immunity that can be achieved following a fetal thymus transplant or thymic factor therapy (Table 18–5).

Immunologic Pathogenesis

During weeks 6–8 of intrauterine life, the thymus and parathyroid glands develop from epithelial evaginations of the third and fourth pharyngeal pouches (Fig 20–2). The thymus begins to migrate caudally during week 12 of gestation. At the same time, the philtrum of the lip and the ear tubercle become differentiated along with other aortic arch structures. It is likely that DiGeorge's syndrome is the result of interference with normal embryologic development at approximately 12 weeks of gestation. In some patients, the thymus is not absent but is in an abnormal location or is extremely small, though the histologic appearance is normal. It is possible that such patients have "partial" DiGeorge's syndrome, in which hypertrophy of the thymus may take place with subsequent development of normal immunity. Following thymic transplantation, there is rapid T cell reconstitution, lack of graft-versus-host (GVH) reaction, and lack of cellular chimerism, suggesting that patients lack a thymic humoral factor capable of expanding their own T cell immunity.

Table 20–1. Evaluation of cell-mediated immunity.

Test	Comment
Total lymphocyte count	Normal at any age: >1200/μL.
Delayed hypersensitivity skin test	Used to evaluate specific immunity to antigens. Suggested antigens are *Candida,* mumps, purified protein derivative, and streptokinase-streptodornase (4 units/0.1 mL).
Lymphocyte response to mitogens (PHA), antigens, and allogeneic cells (mixed-lymphocyte culture)	Used to evaluate T cell function. Results are expressed as stimulated counts divided by resting counts (stimulated index).
Total T cells using monoclonal antibodies to CD3, CD2, or CD4 plus CD8	Used to quantitate the number of circulating T cells. Normal: >60% of total lymphocytes.
Monoclonal antibody to T cells and T cell subsets (CD4 and CD8)	Determines total number of T cells as well as T cell subsets, eg, helper/suppressor.
Cytokine production (IL-1, IL-2, lymphotoxin, tumor necrosis factor, etc)	Used to detect specific cytokine production from subsets of mononuclear cells as an index of function.
Helper/suppressor T cell function	Provides information on T cell regulation of immunity.

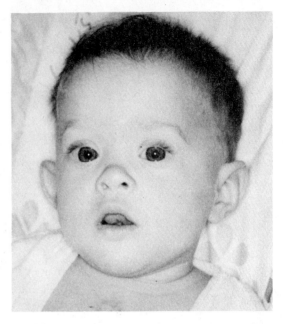

Figure 20–1. Infant with DiGeorge's syndrome. Prominent are low-set and malformed ears, hypertelorism, and fish-shaped mouth. Also note the surgical scar from cardiac surgery.

Clinical Features

A. Symptoms & Signs: The most frequent presenting sign in patients with DiGeorge's syndrome occurs in the first 24 hours of life with hypocalcemia that is resistant to standard therapy. Various types of congenital heart disease have been described, including interrupted aortic arch, septal defects, patent ductus arteriosus, and truncus arteriosus. Renal abnormalities may also be present. Some patients have the characteristic facial appearance described above. Patients who survive the immediate neonatal period may then develop recurrent or chronic infection with various viral, bacterial, fungal, or protozoal organisms. Pneumonia, chronic infection of the mucous membranes with *Candida,* diarrhea, and failure to thrive may be present.

Spontaneous improvement of T cell immunity occasionally occurs. These patients are considered to have "partial" DiGeorge's syndrome, but the reason for the spontaneous improvement in T cell immunity is not known. Patients have also been suspected of having DiGeorge's syndrome on the basis of hypocalcemia and congenital heart disease with or without the abnormal facies but have been found to have normal T cell immunity. Subsequently, these patients may develop severe T cell deficiency.

B. Laboratory Findings: Evaluation of T cell immunity can be performed immediately after birth

in a patient suspected of having DiGeorge's syndrome. The lymphocyte count is usually low (<1200/μL) but may be normal or elevated. In the absence of stress during the newborn period, a lateral-view x-ray of the anterior mediastinum may reveal absence of the thymic shadow, indicating failure of normal development. Delayed hypersensitivity skin tests to recall antigens are of little value during early infancy, because sufficient time has not elapsed for sensitization to occur. T cells are markedly diminished in number, and the peripheral blood lymphocytes fail to respond to phytohemagglutinin (PHA) and allogeneic cells.

Studies of antibody-mediated immunity in early infancy are not helpful, because immunoglobulins consist primarily of passively transferred maternal IgG. Although it is believed that some of these patients have a normal ability to produce specific antibody, the majority have some impairment of antibody formation. Sequential studies of both T cell and B cell immunity are necessary, since spontaneous remissions and spontaneous deterioration of immunity with time have been described.

A diagnosis of hypoparathyroidism is established by the demonstration of low serum calcium levels, elevated serum phosphorus levels, and an absence of parathyroid hormone. Congenital heart disease may be diagnosed immediately following birth and may be mild or severe. Other congenital abnormalities in-

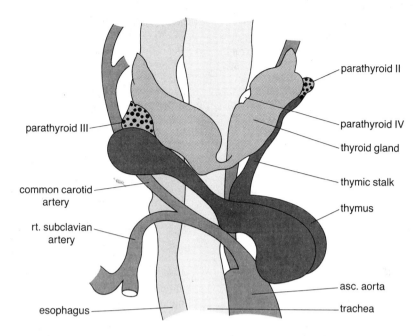

parathyroid II

parathyroid IV

thyroid gland

thymic stalk

thymus

parathyroid III

common carotid artery

rt. subclavian artery

asc. aorta

esophagus

trachea

Figure 20–2. Embryologic development of the thymus and parathyroid glands from the third and fourth pharyngeal pouches.

clude esophageal atresia, bifid uvula, and urinary tract abnormalities.

Immunologic Diagnosis

T cell immunity is usually absent at birth, as indicated by lymphocytopenia, depressed numbers of circulating T cells, and no response of peripheral blood lymphocytes to PHA and allogeneic cells. Rarely, normal T cell immunity may develop with time or previously normal T cell immunity may become deficient. In some patients, studies of T cell functions are variable and range from diminished T cell numbers with normal function to a complete absence of T cell immunity.

Some patients with DiGeorge's syndrome have normal B cell immunity as indicated by normal levels of immunoglobulins and a normal antibody response following immunization. However, some patients have low immunoglobulin levels and fail to make specific antibody following immunization. Live attenuated viral vaccines should not be used for immunization. Natural killer (NK) cell activity is normal.

Rarely, a patient presents with the immunologic features of severe combined immunodeficiency, ie, absent T cell and B cell immunity. The presence of hypocalcemia or congenital abnormalities of the third and fourth aortic arch establishes the diagnosis.

Differential Diagnosis

Many infants with severe congenital heart disease and subsequent congestive heart failure develop transient hypocalcemia. These infants should be suspected of having DiGeorge's syndrome. When the characteristic facial features are found in addition to the hypocalcemia and congenital heart disease, an even stronger suspicion is present. Studies of T cell immunity will usually establish a diagnosis, except in infants with DiGeorge's syndrome who have developed effective T cell immunity with time. It is essential that all infants with congenital heart disease and hypocalcemia be monitored until they are at least 1 year old. The hypocalcemia associated with DiGeorge's syndrome is usually permanent, in contrast to that seen in congenital heart disease with congestive heart failure. Congenital hypoparathyroidism is usually not associated with congenital heart disease. However, both in this disorder and in DiGeorge's syndrome, levels of parathyroid hormone are low to absent and the patients are resistant to the standard treatment for hypocalcemia. Low parathyroid hormone levels may also be found in transient hypocalcemia in infancy. Two patients with DiGeorge's syndrome are known to have had spontaneous remissions of their hypoparathyroidism.

Immunologic studies in DiGeorge's syndrome and in severe combined immunodeficiency disease may be identical in the newborn period. The presence of hypocalcemia, congenital heart disease, and an abnormal facies differentiate DiGeorge's syndrome from severe combined immunodeficiency disease.

Patients with the fetal alcohol syndrome may have similar facial and cardiac abnormalities to those in patients with DiGeorge's syndrome, as well as recurrent infections associated with decreased T cell immunity.

Treatment

Fetal thymus transplantation was previously the treatment of choice. This resulted in permanent reconstitution of T cell immunity. The technique of thymus transplantation varied from local implantation in the rectus abdominis muscle to implantation of a thymus in a Millipore chamber. The thymus was also minced and injected intraperitoneally. Because patients with DiGeorge's syndrome have been observed to develop a GVH reaction following administration of viable immunocompetent lymphocytes, fetal thymus glands older than 14 weeks of gestation were not used. Thymocytes from glands younger than 14 weeks of gestation lack cells capable of GVH reaction but can provide needed stem cells or thymic epithelial cells for further T cell development. Patients have been reported to be successfully treated with thymosin and thymus epithelial transplants. Some patients undergo spontaneous resolution of the T cell immunodeficiency. Intravenous immunoglobulin therapy should be used if antibody deficiency exists and to control recurrent infection.

The hypocalcemia is rarely controlled by calcium supplementation alone. Calcium should be administered orally in conjunction with vitamin D or parathyroid hormone.

Congenital heart disease frequently results in congestive heart failure and may require immediate surgical correction. If surgery is performed prior to the availability of a fetal thymus transplant, any blood given should be irradiated with 3000 R to prevent a GVH reaction.

Complications & Prognosis

Prolonged survivals have been reported following successful thymus transplantation or spontaneous remission of immunodeficiency. Sudden death may occur in untreated patients or in patients initially found to have normal T cell immunity. Congenital heart disease may be severe, and the infant may not survive surgical correction. Death from GVH disease following blood transfusions has been observed in patients in whom a diagnosis of DiGeorge's syndrome was not suspected.

CHRONIC MUCOCUTANEOUS CANDIDIASIS
(With & Without Endocrinopathy)

Major Immunologic Features

■ Onset may be either with chronic candidial infec-

tion of the skin and mucous membranes or with endocrinopathy.
■ Delayed hypersensitivity skin tests to *Candida* antigen are negative despite chronic candidal infection.

General Considerations

Chronic mucocutaneous candidiasis affects both males and females. A familial occurrence has been reported, suggesting an autosomal recessive inheritance. The disorder is associated with a selective defect in T cell immunity, resulting in susceptibility to chronic candidal infection. B cell immunity is intact, resulting in a normal antibody response to *Candida* and, in some patients, the development of autoantibodies associated with idiopathic endocrinopathies. The disorder may appear as early as 1 year of age or may be delayed until the second decade.

Various theories have been proposed to explain the association of chronic candidal infection and the development of endocrinopathy. Initially it was believed that hypoparathyroidism predisposed to candidal infection. Subsequently it was found that many patients developed severe candidal infection without evidence of hypoparathyroidism. A basic autoimmune disorder has been postulated, with the suggestion that the thymus also functions as an endocrine organ and that the thymus and other endocrine glands are involved in an autoimmune destructive process.

Clinical Features

A. Symptoms & Signs: The initial presentation of chronic mucocutaneous candidiasis may be either chronic candidal infection or the appearance of an idiopathic endocrinopathy. If candidal infection appears first, several years to several decades may elapse before endocrinopathy occurs. Other patients may present with the endocrinopathy first and subsequently develop the infection. Candidal infection may involve the mucous membranes, skin, nails, and, in older patients, the vagina. In severe forms, infection of the skin occurs in a "stocking-glove" distribution and is associated with the formation of granulomatous lesions (Fig 20–3). Patients are usually not susceptible to systemic candidiasis. Rarely, they may develop infection with other fungal agents.

Other symptoms are related to the specific endocrinopathy. Hypoparathyroidism is the most common and is associated with hypocalcemia and tetany. Addison's disease is the next most common. A variety of other endocrinopathies have been reported, including hypothyroidism, diabetes mellitus, and pernicious anemia. Occasionally, there is a history of acute or chronic hepatitis preceding the onset of endocrinopathy. Additional disorders include pulmonary fibrosis, ovarian failure, adrenocorticotropic hormone (ACTH) deficiency, and keratoconjunctivitis.

B. Laboratory Findings: Studies of T cell im-

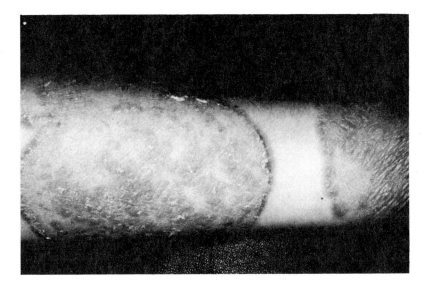

Figure 20–3. Chronic *Candida* infection in a patient with mucocutaneous candidiasis. Note the well-demarcated areas of involvement.

munity reveal a specific although variable defect. Patients usually have a normal total lymphocyte count. Peripheral blood lymphocytes respond normally to PHA, allogeneic cells, and antigens other than *Candida* antigens. The least severe T cell defect is an absent delayed hypersensitivity skin test response to *Candida* antigen in the presence of documented chronic candidiasis. Other patients may have additional defects, including the inability to form migration inhibitory factor (MIF) in response to *Candida* antigens or inability of lymphocytes to be activated by *Candida* antigens and decreased suppressor T cell activity. B cell immunity is intact, as demonstrated by the presence of normal or elevated levels of immunoglobulins, increased amounts of antibody directed against *Candida,* and autoantibody formation. Occasionally, selective absence of IgA or elevated levels of immunoglobulins may be observed. Plasma inhibitors of T cell function and increased numbers of suppressor T cells have been reported in some cases. Isolated cases have been described with neutrophil chemotaxis or macrophage abnormalities.

Other laboratory abnormalities are related to the presence of endocrinopathies. Hypoparathyroidism is associated with decreased serum calcium levels, elevated serum phosphorus levels, and low or absent parathyroid hormone levels. Increased skin pigmentation may herald the onset of Addison's disease prior to disturbances in serum electrolytes. An ACTH stimulation test is useful to document the presence of Addison's disease. Other abnormalities of endocrine function include hypothyroidism, abnormal vitamin B_{12} absorption, and diabetes mellitus. Abnormal liver function studies may indicate chronic hepatitis. Occasionally, iron deficiency is present, which, when treated, results in improvement in the candidal infection. Autoantibodies associated with specific endocrinopathy are usually present before and during the development of endocrine dysfunction. They may be absent when complete endocrine deficiency is present. Patients should be evaluated on a yearly basis for endocrine function because the endocrinopathies are progressive.

Immunologic Diagnosis

Major aspects of T cell immunity are normal, as indicated by a normal response of peripheral blood lymphocytes to PHA and allogeneic cells. Activation of lymphocytes and MIF production in response to antigens other than *Candida* antigens is normal. T cell numbers are normal. In some patients, only the delayed hypersensitivity skin test response to *Candida* antigens is absent. Other patients have absent MIF production or an absence of lymphocyte activation by *Candida* antigens. Plasma inhibitors of cellular immunity may also occur. B cell immunity is intact with normal production of antibody to *Candida.*

Differential Diagnosis

Children with chronic candidal infection of the mucous membranes may have a variety of immunodeficiency disorders. Detailed studies of B cell and T cell immunity differentiate between chronic mucocutaneous candidiasis, in which there is a selective deficiency of T cell immunity to *Candida* antigens, and other disorders in which T cell immunity may be completely deficient. Patients with DiGeorge's syndrome (thymic aplasia and hypoparathyroidism) present early in infancy, whereas chronic mucocutaneous candidiasis with hypoparathyroidism is a disorder of later onset and progressive nature. Patients with late-onset idiopathic endocrinopathies should be considered to have chronic mucocutaneous candidiasis, even though candidal infection is not present at the time of diagnosis. These patients may develop chronic candidal infection as late as 10–15 years after the onset of endocrinopathy.

Treatment

There is no treatment to prevent the development of idiopathic endocrinopathy. The physician must be alert to the gradual development of endocrine dysfunction—particularly Addison's disease, which is the major cause of death. Chronic skin and mucous membrane candidal infection is difficult to treat. Topical treatment with a variety of antifungal agents has been attempted but has usually been unsuccessful. Local miconazole therapy has provided control in some patients in recent trials. Courses of intravenous amphotericin B have resulted in improvement in a significant number of patients, but this form of treatment is limited by the renal toxicity of the drug. Oral clotrimazole is occasionally beneficial. Oral ketoconazole, an antifungal agent, has been successfully used. The efficacy of transfer factor therapy with or without amphotericin B is unproven. Two patients refractory to all other forms of therapy were successfully treated with fetal thymus transplants.

Complications & Prognosis

Patients may survive to the second or third decade but usually experience extensive morbidity. Individuals with severe candidal infection of the mucous membranes and skin develop serious psychologic difficulties. Systemic infection with *Candida* usually does not occur. Rarely, patients may develop systemic infection with other fungal agents. Hypoparathyroidism is difficult to manage, and complications are frequent. Addison's disease is the major cause of death and may develop suddenly without previous symptoms.

IMMUNODEFICIENCY ASSOCIATED WITH NATURAL KILLER (NK) CELL DEFICIENCY

NK cells are negative for the T cell receptor-CD3 complex but have receptors for the Fc portion of the immunoglobulin molecule (CD16) and a member of the complement/lymphocyte adhesion molecule (CD11b). In addition, they have the NKH-1 (CD56) determinant, which identifies the large granular lymphocyte population that NK cells resemble morphologically. NK cells spontaneously lyse a number of target cells, including tumor cells, but when activated by interleukin-2 (IL-2) or gamma interferon, they will lyse a broad range of virus-infected cells. It is therefore believed that these cells play a role in host defense against cancer and microbial infection.

Deficiency of NK cells is not confined to a single defined immunodeficiency disorder, although there are isolated case reports of what appear to be selective NK deficiencies. NK cell deficiency has been documented in the Chédiak-Higashi syndrome, the X-linked lymphoproliferative syndrome, the chronic fatigue syndrome, and leukocyte adhesion molecule (CD11/CD18) deficiency. NK cell deficiency has also been detected in primary immunodeficiency diseases, primarily in severe combined immunodeficiency disease and other T cell disorders, suggesting an association between NK and T cell defects.

Although NK cell deficiency has been detected most consistently in the X-linked lymphoproliferative syndrome, which is associated with fatal Epstein-Barr virus infection, cancer, and hypogammaglobulinemia, there has been a report of a female child who had recurrent severe infections with herpes viruses, including varicella, cytomegalovirus infection, and herpes simplex. Immunologic evaluation was normal, except for deficient NK cell numbers and function. The peripheral blood mononuclear cells were unable to mediate spontaneous or IL-2-induced NK cell functions. This case suggests that isolated defects in NK cell function exist. No specific treatment to correct the NK cell defect was attempted. Acyclovir was used to treat the acute infections, and the patient was maintained on intravenous gamma globulin.

REFERENCES

Thymic Aplasia With Hypoparathyroidism

Barrett DJ et al: Clinical and immunologic spectrum of the Di-George syndrome. *J Clin Lab Immunol* 1981;**6**:1.

DiGeorge AM: Congenital absence of the thymus and its immunologic consequences: Concurrence with congenital hypoparathyroidism. In: *Immunologic Deficiency Diseases in Man.* Bergsma D, McKusick FA (editors). National Foundation—March of Dimes Original Article Series. Williams & Wilkins, 1968.

Radford DJ et al: Spectrum of DiGeorge syndrome in patients with truncus arteriosis: Expanded DiGeorge syndrome. *Pediatr Cardiol* 1988;**9**:95.

Chronic Mucocutaneous Candidiasis

Arulanantham K, Dwyer JM, Genel M: Evidence for defective immunoregulation in the syndrome of familial candidiasis endocrinopathy. *N Engl J Med* 1979; **300:**164.

Kirkpatrick CH: Chronic mucocutaneous candidiasis. Antibiotic and immunologic therapy. *Ann NY Acad Sci* 1988;**544:**471.

Kirkpatrick CH, Rich RR, Bennett JE: Chronic mucocutaneous candidiasis: Model building in cellular immunity. *Ann Intern Med* 1971;**74:**955.

Mobacken H, Moberg S: Ketoconazole treatment of 13 patients with chronic mucocutaneous candidiasis: A prospective three year trial. *Dermatologica* 1986; **173:**229.

Natural Killer Cell Deficiency

Biron CA, Byron KS, Sullivan JL: Severe herpes virus infections in an adolescent without natural killer cells. *N Engl J Med* 1989;**320:**1731.

Ritz J: The role of natural killer cells in immune surveillance. *N Engl J Med* 1989;**320:**1789.

Stiehm ER: New and old immunodeficiencies. *Pediatr Res* 1993;**33(Suppl):**S2.

Combined Antibody (B Cell) & Cellular (T Cell) Immunodeficiency Disorders

Arthur J. Ammann, MD

Combined immunodeficiency diseases are variable in cause and severity. Defective T cell and B cell immunity may be complete, as in severe combined immunodeficiency disease, or partial, as in ataxia-telangiectasia. The distinct clinical features of ataxia-telangiectasia serve to further differentiate the disorder from severe combined immunodeficiency disease and also suggest that these disorders do not have the same cause. Enzymatic deficiencies in the purine pathway have been described in association with combined immunodeficiency, and specific genetic mutations of single amino acids are responsible in many instances. These discoveries have provided additional evidence for a diverse origin of combined immunodeficiency disease.

Studies of both T cell and B cell immunity are necessary to completely evaluate patients with combined immunodeficiency disorders (see Tables 18–4, 19–1, and 20–1). In addition, analysis of erythrocyte and leukocyte enzymes (adenosine deaminase and nucleoside phosphorylase, respectively) can assist appropriate classification.

The onset of symptoms in patients with combined immunodeficiency diseases is usually early in infancy. These patients are susceptible to a very wide spectrum of microorganisms. Immunotherapy is frequently difficult and often not available.

SEVERE COMBINED IMMUNODEFICIENCY DISEASE

Major Immunologic Features

- The onset of symptoms occurs by 6 months of age, with recurrent viral, bacterial, fungal, and protozoal infections.
- X-linked, autosomal, and sporadic forms occur.
- Both T cell and B cell immunity are absent.

General Considerations

The immunologic deficiency includes the absence of T cell and B cell immunity, resulting early in susceptibility to infection by virtually all types of microorganisms. Without treatment, patients rarely survive beyond 1 year of age before succumbing to one or more opportunistic infections. The disease is inherited in 2 forms: an X-linked recessive form (X-linked lymphopenic agammaglobulinemia) and an autosomal recessive form (Swiss-type lymphopenic agammaglobulinemia). The exact prevalence of this disorder is not known, and many patients die before the diagnosis is made. Because the immune system of patients with this disorder may be made completely normal by bone marrow transplantation, early diagnosis is crucial to prevent irreversible complications.

Immunologic Pathogenesis

The basic defect of the various genetic forms is not known. The successful use of histocompatible bone marrow transplantation has provided support for the concept of a basic stem cell defect. However, the defect may reside in the failure of the thymus and bursa equivalent to develop normally secondary to the absence of a cytokine or differentiation factor.

Clinical Features

A. Symptons and Signs: Without treatment, patients with severe combined immunodeficiency disease usually succumb to overwhelming infection within the first year of life. Early findings include failure to thrive, chronic diarrhea, persistent thrush (oral candidiasis), pneumonia, chronic otitis media, and sepsis. The microorganisms that result in acute and chronic infection include viruses, bacteria, fungi, and protozoa. Infants with this disease are particularly susceptible to *Candida,* cytomegalovirus, and *Pneumocystis carinii* infection. When smallpox immunization was routinely administered, many of these infants developed progressive vaccinia. Death from progressive poliomyelitis following attenuated-virus immunization has been documented. During the first several months of life, patients may be partially protected from bacterial infections by the transplacental passive transfer of maternal IgG antibodies. They subsequently develop susceptibility to a wide variety of gram-positive and gram-negative organisms.

As these patients lack T cell immunity entirely, they are susceptible to graft-versus-host (GVH) reactions that may develop following maternal infusion of cells during gestation or delivery, infusion of viable cells in the form of blood transfusions, or attempts at immunotherapy (see the discussion of GVH disease below). The presence of an acute or chronic GVH reaction, as a consequence of blood transfusion or engraftment of maternal cells, may complicate the diagnosis of severe combined immunodeficiency disease. Some of these patients have been misdiagnosed as having an acute viral illness, histiocytosis X, or other chronic disorders.

Physical findings relate to the degree and type of infections present. Pneumonia, otitis media, thrush, dehydration, skin infections, and developmental retardation may be present. Lymphoid tissue and hepatosplenomegaly are absent unless the disease is complicated by GVH reaction.

B. Laboratory Findings: All tests of T cell immunity are abnormal. The thymus is absent roentgenographically, lymphopenia is usually present, T cell numbers are markedly depressed, and the response of isolated peripheral blood lymphocytes to phytohemagglutinin (PHA) and allogeneic cells is absent. Rarely, there is a proliferative response to allogeneic cells. T cell subset analysis varies considerably. Specific antigens on T cells are absent in some patients, whereas in others they show developmental arrest at the prothymocyte level. Delayed hypersensitivity skin tests are not useful for diagnosis, because in most cases the patient is too young for sufficient time to have elapsed for antigen exposure and sensitization to occur. During the first 5–6 months of life, a diagnosis of severe combined immunodeficiency disease may be difficult to establish because of the presence of maternal IgG. However, most normal infants who have had repeated infection will develop significant amounts of serum IgM, IgA, or both. If the diagnosis is doubtful, it may be necessary to immunize the patient to determine specific antibody responses. Patients suspected of having immunodeficiency diseases should never be immunized with attenuated live virus vaccines. In the majority of patients with severe combined immunodeficiency, B cells are absent or markedly reduced from birth. A subgroup of patients exists in whom B cell numbers may be elevated. Natural killer (NK) cell activity may be normal or deficient. Adenosine deaminase activity is normal.

Biopsy of lymphoid tissue is rarely necessary to establish a diagnosis. If biopsies are needed, they should be performed with strict antiseptic measures because secondary infection is frequent. Biopsy of lymph nodes (if they can be found) demonstrates severe depletion of lymphocytes, without corticomedullary differentiation and without follicle formation. Biopsy of the intestinal tract shows a complete absence of plasma cells.

Patients who have pulmonary infiltrates that do not respond to antibiotic therapy or who have rapid respiration and low arterial blood Po_2 should be suspected of having *P carinii* infection regardless of whether the x-ray is abnormal. Because this disorder can be treated, it is important to establish an early diagnosis. Some debate exists about whether the diagnosis is best made by means of concentrated-sputum examination, bronchoscopy, needle biopsy, or open-lung biopsy. In some instances, open-lung biopsy provides the most complete information. Cytomegalovirus infection should be considered in all patients. Cultures of blood, mucous membranes, and stools for predominant bacteria may be important in determining subsequent treatment. Individuals who have been inadvertently immunized with live polio-virus vaccine should have stools cultured for polio-virus.

Patients frequently have anemia and lymphopenia. Complications such as chronic systemic infection and GVH reaction may result in multiple abnormalities, including elevation of liver enzyme levels, jaundice, chronic diarrhea with subsequent electrolyte abnormalities and dehydration, pulmonary infiltrates, cardiac irregularities, and abnormal cerebrospinal fluid analysis.

Immunologic Diagnosis

Severe combined immunodeficiency disease is associated with complete absence of T cell and B cell immunity. Evaluation of T cell immunity reveals lymphopenia; absence of thymus shadow; depressed T cell numbers; absence of peripheral blood lymphocyte responses to PHA, allogeneic cells, and antigens; and absence of response to delayed hypersensitivity skin tests. Evaluation of B cell immunity reveals hypogammaglobulinemia, absence of antibody response following immunization, and few or no circulating B cells (rarely, elevated B cell numbers are found).

Differential Diagnosis

Severe combined immunodeficiency disease must be differentiated from other immunodeficiency disorders with defects in T cell and B cell immunity. The early onset of symptoms and the complete absence of both T cell and B cell immunity found in severe combined immunodeficiency disease usually result in a specific diagnosis. Combined immunodeficiency associated with the absence of an enzyme (adenosine deaminase) in the purine pathway may be differentiated from severe combined immunodeficiency disease by specific determination of adenosine deaminase activity. This disorder initially is usually less severe clinically and immunologically. The presence of a GVH reaction in a patient with severe combined immunodeficiency disease may complicate the diagnosis. If chronic dermatitis is present in association with hepatosplenomegaly and histiocytic infiltration, the condition may be mistaken for Letterer-Siwe syndrome. Some patients may present with chronic diarrhea and pigmentary skin changes, resulting in an erroneous diagnosis of acrodermatitis enteropathica (see the discussion of GVH disease below). Omenn's syndrome closely resembles severe combined immunodeficiency with GVH disease and is believed by some not to be a distinct syndrome.

Treatment

Aggressive diagnostic measures are necessary to establish the cause of chronic infection before treatment can be instituted. Open-lung biopsy should be performed if *P carinii* infection is suspected. The treatment of choice for *P carinii* infection consists of pentamidine and trimethoprim-sulfamethoxazole given simultaneously. Specific antibiotic treatment is necessary for suspected bacterial infection. Superficial candidal infection is treated with topical antifungal drugs, but systemic infection requires intravenous amphotericin B or ketoconazole therapy.

Complications must be avoided. Immunization with live attenuated virus should not be performed. Blood products containing potentially viable lymphocytes should be irradiated with 3000–6000 R prior to administration (see the discussion of GVH disease below). Prophylactic trimethoprim-sulfa-methoxazole should be used to prevent *P carinii* infection.

During the initial period of evaluation, gamma globulin may be administered in doses of 0.2–0.4 mL/kg intramuscularly once a month or as frequently as once a week. Severely ill patients appear to improve with the use of intravenous gamma globulin in doses of 100–400 mg/kg every 1–4 weeks. Definitive treatment consists of transplantation of histocompatible bone marrow. Because of the inheritance of the histocompatibility antigens, the usual donor for a bone marrow transplant is a histocompatible sibling. The bone marrow must be matched for human leukocyte antigens (HLA) A, B, C, and DR by the mixed leukocyte reaction (MLR). Despite careful matching, a GVH reaction may develop. Several techniques have been used in performing bone marrow transplantation, including intraperitoneal injection and intravenous infusion of filtered bone marrow. The dose of bone marrow cells administered has varied, but injection of as few as 1000 nucleated cells per kilogram has resulted in successful immunologic reconstitution. Transplantation of unmatched marrow has previously resulted in a fatal GVH reaction. However, the use of unmatched marrow from nonsibling donors, prepared by lectin separation of cells or marrow treated with monoclonal antibody to deplete cells responsible for GVH disease, has resulted in successful immune reconstitution with minimal GVH disease.

In the absence of a histocompatible bone marrow donor, other forms of therapy have been used. Long-term survivors of fetal-liver (<9 weeks' gestation) transplants and of fetal-thymus (<14 weeks' gestation) transplantation have been observed. In both of these techniques, the use of older fetal liver or thymus will result in a fatal GVH reaction, probably because of the presence of mature immunocompetent cells. Thymus epithelial transplants and combined fetal-liver and fetal-thymus transplants have also been used. In most instances these approaches have been replaced by bone marrow transplantation.

Complications & Prognosis

Patients with severe combined immunodeficiency disease are unusually susceptible to infection with many microorganisms and will die before 1 year of age if untreated. If the diagnosis is not made immediately, the patient may receive live attenuated poliovirus immunization and succumb to progressive poliomyelitis. In other instances, patients may receive unirradiated blood products and die of complications of GVH disease. Following successful bone marrow transplantation, 10-year survivals with maintenance of normal T cell and B cell function have been recorded. Patients have survived as long as 1 year following fetal-liver transplantation and as long as 6 years following fetal-thymus transplantation. Complete reconstitution of immunity in patients receiving fetal organ transplantation has not yet been achieved.

T CELL MEMBRANE SIGNALING & CYTOKINE DEFECTS

Major Immunologic Features

- Phenotypic characteristics of other T cell immunodeficiency disorders are present.
- Symptoms vary from mild to severe infections.
- Multiple, newly defined abnormalities are present in the T cell signaling pathway.

General Considerations

T cells are inactivated following interaction with an antigen-presenting cell (APC), a step that is dependent on cell-to-cell contact. The T cell receptor (TCR) binds to the MHC of the APC, resulting in the expression of cytokine receptors and cytokine secretion. In addition, there are multiple intracellular events including the accumulation of phosphorylated substrates (especially tyrosine phosphorylation) and increases in concentrations of Ca^{2+}. Many immune functions are dependent on appropriate secretion of cytokines such as IL-2, tumor necrosis factor, gamma interferon, and transforming growth factor beta. T cells play an important role in the secretion and regulation of cytokines. As basic research defines the T cell signaling pathways, activation events, and specific cytokines, defects in these functions will be described in increasing numbers of patients.

1. T CELL MEMBRANE DEFECTS

At least 4 cases have been described, all of whom had significant recurrent infections with varying degrees of immunodeficiency. T cell proliferative responses to antigens and mitogens are abnormal. All patients had abnormalities of the TCR, but the portion of the TCR affected and the levels of expression varied. The precise molecular defect leading to the abnormal TCR phenotypic expression has not been delineated.

2. T CELL IMMUNODEFICIENCY WITH ABNORMAL CYTOKINE PRODUCTION

Over 16 patients have been described, all of whom have T cell immunodeficiency of various degrees and recurrent infection. These patients are distinguished from those with other forms of immunodeficiency by their inability to produce specific cytokines following in vitro stimulation of peripheral blood mononuclear cells. The most common deficiency, although still rare, is deficient production of IL-2. One patient responded to treatment with recombinant IL-2. A single patient was described with deficient production of multiple cytokines including abnormalities of IL-2, IL-3, IL-4, and IL-5. Since many cytokines are now available for clinical use, it will be important to identify these patients and determine whether their immunodeficiency can be corrected.

CELLULAR IMMUNODEFICIENCY WITH ABNORMAL IMMUNOGLOBULIN SYNTHESIS (Nezelof's Syndrome)

Major Immunologic Features
- Patients are susceptible to viral, bacterial, fungal, and protozoal infection.
- T cell immunity is depressed or absent.
- There are various degrees of B cell immunodeficiency associated with various combinations of increased, normal, or decreased immunoglobulin levels.

General Considerations
The disorders included in this classification are diverse and probably do not all have the same cause. Many of the patients, if they could be restudied or evaluated in detail with newer diagnostic techniques, might be found to have a specific defect such as a cytokine deficiency or TCR abnormality. Features include marked deficiency of T cell immunity and various degrees of deficiency of B cell immunity. Disorders with specific clinical symptoms or laboratory abnormalities, such as ataxia-telangiectasia and Wiskott-Aldrich syndrome, and those associated with enzyme deficiency, such as adenosine deaminase deficiency, are excluded here. Most of the cases included in this category are sporadic and do not have a defined inheritance pattern.

Immunologic Pathogenesis
There does not appear to be a specific genetic pattern. The syndrome is sporadic in distribution and occurs in both males and females. The presence of moderate to severe deficiencies of T cell immunity with various degrees of B cell immunodeficiency suggests that the primary defect is within the thymus, but, as has been recently discovered, thymus developmental abnormalities may simply be secondary to more fundamental defects such as abnormal IL-2 receptors.

Clinical Features
A. Symptoms & Signs: Patients are susceptible to recurrent fungal, protozoal, viral, and bacterial infections. The spectrum of infection is similar to that found in patients with congenital hypogammaglobulinemia and other forms of combined immunodeficiency. Patients frequently have marked lymphadenopathy and hepatosplenomegaly, in contrast to patients with congenital hypogammaglobulinemia and severe combined immunodeficiency disease.

B. Laboratory Findings: T cell immunity is abnormal, but the degree of deficiency may vary. Lymphopenia may be present, but occasionally a normal lymphocyte count is obtained. T cell numbers are moderately to markedly decreased. The lymphocyte response to PHA and specific antigens may be absent or slightly depressed, and the lymphocyte response to allogeneic cells may vary from zero to normal. B cell immunity is abnormal. The 5 immunoglobulin classes may be present in various combinations of increased, normal, or decreased amounts. Total circulating B cells are usually present in normal numbers, although the distribution among various types of surface immunoglobulin- bearing B cells may vary. Despite the presence of normal or elevated levels of immunoglobulin, there is no antibody response following specific immunization. Antibodies to specific antigens may be present, however, indicating that at one time some of these patients may have been able to form antibody. Isohemagglutinins may be absent or normal, and the Schick test may be either reactive or nonreactive.

Biopsy of lymphoid tissue in these patients may reveal the presence of plasma cells. The lymph nodes may be large and may contain numerous histiocytes and macrophages with granuloma formation.

Immunologic Diagnosis

The principal immunologic features in this group of disorders are moderate to marked reductions in the number of total lymphocytes and T cells and a diminished response of peripheral blood lymphocytes to PHA, allogeneic cells, and specific antigens. There is usually no response to delayed hypersensitivity skin tests. Variable degrees of B cell deficiency are present, consisting of various combinations of elevated, normal, or low levels of specific immunoglobulin classes. The antibody response to specific antigens is usually absent. Some evidence of prior antibody formation may be found, eg, the presence of isohemagglutinins. The number of total circulating B cells is usually normal. Detailed studies of cytokine production and TCR expression should be performed.

Differential Diagnosis

Because there is a lack of uniformity in the clinical and laboratory presentation of these patients, it is necessary to rule out other disorders with definite clinical or laboratory associations. The clinical features of ataxia-telangiectasia are usually present by 3–4 years of age, and an elevated level of alpha-fetoprotein is usually present by 1 year of age. Patients with Wiskott-Aldrich syndrome have thrombocytopenia from birth and can be excluded on this basis. Patients with severe combined immunodeficiency disease have complete absence of T cell and B cell immunity. Immunodeficiency disorders with associated enzyme deficiencies may have a similar presentation and are excluded on the basis of enzyme analysis of erythrocytes or leukocytes. Patients with short-limbed dwarfism are excluded on the basis of characteristic clinical and radiologic features. Patients with cellular immunodeficiency and abnormal immunoglobulin synthesis do not develop endocrine abnormalities and can therefore be distinguished from patients with DiGeorge's syndrome and chronic mucocutaneous candidiasis, who are capable of normal antibody synthesis. Culture of human immunodeficiency virus (HIV) or antibody to HIV is necessary to distinguish a child with acquired immunodeficiency syndrome (AIDS) from one with this disorder.

Treatment

Aggressive treatment of infection is necessary. Patients failing to show an antibody response after immunization (even if immunoglobulin levels are normal) should receive gamma globulin once a month (see the discussion of the treatment of hypogammaglobulinemia above). Continuous broad-spectrum antibiotic coverage may be useful. Aggressive pulmonary therapy is important to prevent chronic lung disease.

Although histocompatible bone marrow transplantation would appear to be curative in these patients, few successes have been reported. This appears to be due to a lack of histocompatible donors rather than the complications of transplantation. Thymus transplantation and the use of several thymus factors have been reported to provide reconstitution of T cell immunity and partial reconstitution of B cell immunity. Since cytokine therapy may be possible in the future, it would be important to clearly define potential specific immune abnormalities.

Patients should not be immunized with attenuated live viral vaccines. All blood products should be irradiated with 3000 R.

Complications & Prognosis

Patients do not develop the severe complications observed in severe combined immunodeficiency disease. A GVH reaction is possible, but none has been reported. Some of these patients, however, may develop progressive encephalitis following immunization with live attenuated virus. Chronic lung disease, chronic fungal infection, and later development of cancer are long-term complications. Survival beyond 21 years has been recorded.

IMMUNODEFICIENCY WITH ATAXIA-TELANGIECTASIA

Major Immunologic Features

- Clinical onset occurs by 2 years of age.
- Complete syndrome consists of ataxia, telangiectasia, and recurrent sinopulmonary infection.
- Selective IgA deficiency is present in 40% of patients.
- There is a predisposition to malignancies including lymphoma, lymphoid leukemia, T cell leukemia, and epithelial cell malignancies.

General Considerations

Ataxia-telangiectasia is inherited in an autosomal recessive manner. It is associated with characteristic features, including ataxia, telangiectasia, recurrent sinopulmonary infection, and abnormalities in both T cell and B cell immunity. The disorder was first considered to be primarily a neurologic disease; it is now known to involve the neurologic, vascular, endocrine, and immune systems.

Immunologic Pathogenesis

There is no unifying theory that explains the multisystem abnormalities present in ataxia-telangiectasia. It is unlikely that there is a fundamental immunologic defect. Rather, the multisystem abnormalities may be a result of a specific genetic defect that affects DNA repair and alters the function of many organ systems. Abnormalities that may result are abnormal collagen (deficient in hydroxylysine); elevated alpha-fetoprotein level, indicative of a defect in organ maturation; enhanced susceptibility of cells to radiation damage; and defective DNA repair. Clones of lymphocytes with structural rearrangements of band q11 of chromosome 14 and bands q32–35 and p13–15 of chromosome 7 have been consistently found. These chromosome markers may be found in malignant cell lines isolated from ataxia-telangiectasia patients. It is of interest that the structural rearrangements are at the locations that bear the TCR genes. There appears to be a consensus that the ataxia-telangiectasia gene is localized to chromosome 11q22–23, although the exact gene has not yet been identified. Spontaneously occurring chromosomal translocations involving break points in T cell receptor genes have been described and suggest a possible defect in recombination. The disorder is progressive, with both the neurologic abnormalities and the immunologic deficiency becoming more severe over time.

Clinical Features

A. Symptoms & Signs: The onset of ataxia may occur at 9 months to 1 year of age or may be delayed as long as age 4–6 years. Telangiectasia is usually present by 2 years of age but has been delayed until 8–9 years of age (Fig 21–1). As patients grow older, additional neurologic symptoms develop, consisting of choreoathetoid movements, dysconjugate gaze, and extrapyramidal and posterior column signs. Telangiectasia may develop first in the bulbar conjunctiva and subsequently appear on the bridge of the nose, on the ears, or in the antecubital fossae. Recurrent sinopulmonary infections may begin early in life, or patients may remain relatively symptom-free for 10 years or more. There is increased susceptibility to both viral and bacterial infections. Secondary sexual characteristics rarely develop in patients at puberty, and most patients appear to develop mental retardation with time.

B. Laboratory Findings: Various degrees of abnormalities in T and B cell immunity have been described. Lymphopenia may be present, T cell numbers may be normal or decreased, and the response of lymphocytes to PHA and allogeneic cells may be normal or decreased. There may be no response to de-layed hypersensitivity skin tests. IgG2, IgG4, or IgA2 subclass deficiency is present in some patients. In still other patients, IgE may be absent. Antibody responses to specific antigens may be depressed. The number of circulating B cells is usually normal. NK cell activity is normal.

Other laboratory abnormalities relate to associated findings. Abnormalities have been shown on pneumoencephalography. Endocrine studies have shown decreased 17-ketosteroids and increased follicle-stimulating hormone (FSH) excretion. An insulin-resistant form of diabetes has been found. Cytotoxic antibodies to brain and thymus have been found. Cytotoxic antibodies to brain and thymus have been found. Increased levels of alpha-fetoprotein have been found in all patients tested, but may not be specific for the disease, as increased levels have also been found in other immunodeficiency disorders. Alpha-feto-protein levels are also high in normal infants until 1 year of age. Many patients have elevated titers to Epstein-Barr virus (EBV) antigens.

Immunologic Diagnosis

Selective IgA deficiency is found in 40% of patients. IgA2, IgG2, or IgG4 subclass deficiency has also been described. IgE deficiency and variable deficiencies of other immunoglobulins may also be found. The antibody response to specific antigens may be depressed. Variable degrees of T cell deficiency are observed; these usually become more severe with advancing age.

Differential Diagnosis

If the onset of recurrent infection occurs before the development of ataxia or telangiectasia, it may be difficult to differentiate this disorder from cellular immunodeficiency with abnormal immunoglobulin synthesis. If a patient has a gradual onset of cerebellar ataxia unassociated with telangiectasia and immunologic abnormalities, it may take years before a diagnosis can be established with certainty. Usually, by the age of 4 years, the characteristic recurrent sinopulmonary infections, immunologic abnormalities, ataxia, and telangiectasia are present simultaneously. Because selective IgA deficiency is the most common immunodeficiency disorder detected and many patients with selective IgA deficiency have no associated symptoms, it may take several years before a diagnosis of ataxia-telangiectasia can be excluded. Alpha-fetoprotein levels are normal in patients with IgA deficiency.

Treatment

Early treatment of recurrent sinopulmonary infections is essential to avoid permanent complications. Some patients may benefit from continuous broad-spectrum antibiotic therapy. In patients who develop chronic lung disease, aggressive physical therapy is beneficial. Successful bone marrow transplantation

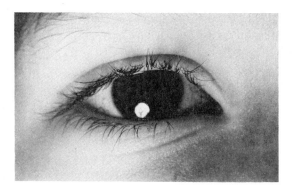

Figure 21–1. Telangiectasis of the conjunctivae and over the bridge of the nose in a child with ataxia-telangiectasia.

has not been performed, but this is probably related to the lack of histocompatible bone marrow donors. Fetal thymus transplantation has provided some benefit in a limited number of patients. Thymic factor therapy has been used on an experimental basis to treat a limited number of patients. The use of intravenous gamma globulin in a patient unable to form antibody may result in a reduced number of infections (see Chapter 19).

Attenuated viral vaccines should not be given. All blood products should be irradiated with 3000 R prior to administration.

Complications & Prognosis

Long-term survivors develop progressive deterioration of neurologic and immunologic functions. The oldest patients have reached the fifth decade of life. The chief causes of death are overwhelming infection and lymphoreticular or epithelial cell cancer (carinoma of the stomach, liver, and ovaries). Leukemias, some with associated abnormalities of chromosome 14, have been reported in 24% of patients (Fig 21–2), and non-Hodgkin lymphomas have been reported in 45% of patients. As these patients reach the second decade, morbidity becomes severe, with chronic lung disease, mental retardation, and physical debility being the principal problems. Heterozygote carriers as well as family members have an increased incidence of cancer.

IMMUNODEFICIENCY WITH THROMBOCYTOPENIA, ECZEMA, & RECURRENT INFECTION (Wiskott-Aldrich Syndrome)

Major Immunologic Features
- Complete syndrome consists of eczema, recurrent pyogenic infection, and thrombocytopenia.
- It can be diagnosed at birth by demonstration of thrombocytopenia in a male infant with a positive family history.
- The serum IgM level is usually low, with elevated serum IgA and IgE levels.

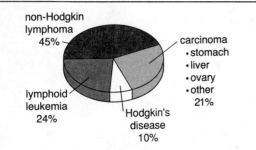

Figure 21–2. Relative percentages of cancers reported in patients with ataxia-telangiectasia.

- Thrombocytopenia is characterized by small platelets.
- The incidence of lymphoid malignancies is increased.

General Considerations

Patients may become symptomatic early in life, with bleeding secondary to thrombocytopenia. Subsequently they develop recurrent bacterial infection in the form of otitis media, pneumonia, and meningitis. Eczema usually appears by 1 year of age. The disease is progressive, with increasing susceptibility to infection and cancer. It is inherited in an X-linked manner. At autopsy, the thymus and lymph nodes have an abnormal architecture, with depletion of T cells, poor follicle formation, and poor corticomedullary differentiation.

Immunologic Pathogenesis

Two of the earliest abnormalities are thrombocytopenia and hypercatabolism of immunoglobulin. There are several hypotheses linking thrombocytopenia, eczema, and recurrent infection. It has been suggested that there are abnormal α granules of platelets and macrophages in patients and carriers. Another suggestion is that the inability of patients to respond to polysaccharide antigens results in immunologic attrition. This, however, does not explain the thrombocytopenia or eczema. An MW 115,000 surface glycoprotein termed sialophorin is absent, present at reduced levels, or abnormal in lymphocytes from patients. Normally this glycoprotein is present in lymphocytes, monocytes, and platelets, and its absence is believed to result in early senescence of cells. More recently, a reduced surface cell expression of CD23 and aberrant CD23 proteolysis has been described. CD23 is involved in the differentiation of immune cells, inhibition of monocyte migration, B cell proliferation, and IgE production. Thus, an abnormality of CD23 might result in many of the hematologic and immunologic defects described.

Clinical Features

A. Symptoms & Signs: Recurrent infection usually does not start until after 6 months of age. Patients are susceptible to infection with capsular polysaccharide-type organisms (eg, *Pneumococcus, Meningococcus,* and *Haemophilus influenzae*), which cause meningitis, otitis media, pneumonia, and sepsis. As the patients become older, they become susceptible to infection with other types of organisms and may have recurrent viral infection. Eczema is usually present by 1 year of age and is typical in distribution (Fig 21–3). It may be associated with other allergic manifestations. Frequently, it is secondarily infected. Thrombocytopenia is present at birth and may result in early manifestations of bleeding. Bleeding is usually increased during episodes of infection

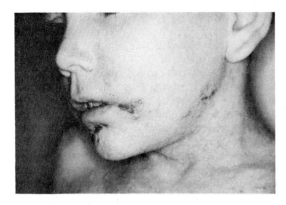

Figure 21–3. Chronic facial eczema in a child with Wiskott-Aldrich syndrome.

and is associated with a decrease in the platelet count. The bleeding tendency becomes less severe as the child becomes older.

B. Laboratory Findings: Thrombocytopenia is present at birth, and this fact is helpful in diagnosis. The platelet count may range from 5000 to 100,000/μL. Platelets are small in Wiskott-Aldrich syndrome, in contrast to those in other disorders associated with thrombocytopenia, eg, idiopathic thrombocytopenia, in which they are larger than normal. Anemia is frequently present and may be Coombs-positive. An increased incidence of chronic renal disease has been reported.

Immunologic Diagnosis

The earliest detected immunologic abnormality consists of hypercatabolism of immunoglobulins. Studies of B cell immunity demonstrate normal IgG levels, decreased IgM levels, increased IgA and IgE levels, few or absent isohemagglutinins, normal numbers of B cells, and an inability to respond to immunization with polysaccharide antigen. paraproteins are frequently observed. T cell immunity is usually intact early in the disease but may decline with advancing years.

Differential Diagnosis

When the complete syndrome is present, there is little doubt about the diagnosis. Idiopathic thrombocytopenia in a male child may be difficult to differentiate from Wiskott-Aldrich syndrome. In idiopathic thrombocytopenia, the immunoglobulins, isohemagglutinins, and response to polysaccharide antigens are normal. Small platelets favor the diagnosis of Wiskott-Aldrich syndrome. Male patients with eczema and recurrent infection have normal immunologic studies and normal platelet counts, although they may have elevated levels of serum IgA and IgE.

Treatment

Infections should be treated promptly and aggressively with antibiotics effective against the most common organisms. Corticosteroids should not be used to treat the thrombocytopenia, since they will enhance the susceptibility to infection. Splenectomy has been fatal in this disease, but there have been recent attempts to use splenectomy and continuous antibiotic prophylaxis to prevent both bleeding and infectious complications. Treatment of immunodeficiency is difficult. Intramuscular gamma globulin is not used, because of the thrombocytopenia and potential bleeding at injection sites, but intravenous gamma globulin can be given (see Chapter 19). Successful bone marrow transplantation has been achieved.

Complications & Prognosis

With aggressive therapy, the long-term prognosis has improved. Immediate complications are related to bleeding episodes and acute infection. As patients become older, they become susceptible to a wider spectrum of microorganisms. Chronic keratitis secondary to viral infection is frequent. Lymphoreticular cancers, especially of the central nervous system, occur in older patients. Myelogenous leukemia occurs more frequently in this disorder than in other immunodeficiency disorders.

IMMUNODEFICIENCY WITH THYMOMA

Major Immunologic Features

- Recurrent infections occur.
- Acquired hypogammaglobulinemia may precede or follow thymoma.

General Considerations

Recurrent infection may be the presenting sign if the thymoma is associated with immunodeficiency. This takes the form of sinopulmonary infection, chronic diarrhea, dermatitis, septicemia, stomatitis, and urinary tract infection. Thymoma has also been associated with muscle weakness (when found in conjunction with myasthenia gravis), aplastic anemia, thrombocytopenia, diabetes, amyloidosis, chronic hepatitis, and the development of nonthymic cancer.

Patients with acquired hypogammaglobulinemia should be observed at regular intervals for the development of thymoma, which is usually detected on routine chest x-rays. Occasionally, the thymoma is detected prior to the development of immunodeficiency. Marked hypogammaglobulinemia is usually present. The antibody response following immunization may be abnormal. Some patients have deficient T cell immunity as assayed by delayed hypersensitivity skin tests and response of peripheral blood lymphocytes to PHA. Increased activity of suppressor cells has been found in some patients. In patients who have aregenerative anemia, pure erythrocyte aplasia is seen on marrow aspiration. Thrombocytopenia, granulocytopenia, and autoantibody formation are occasionally observed. In 75% of cases, the thymoma is of the spindle cell type. Some tumors may be malignant.

In no instance has the removal of the thymoma resulted in improvement of immunodeficiency. This is in contrast to pure erythrocyte aplasia and myasthenia gravis, which may improve following removal of the thymoma. Gamma globulin is beneficial in controlling recurrent infections and chronic diarrhea (see Chapter 19).

The overall prognosis is poor, and death secondary to infection is common. Death may also be related to associated abnormalities such as thrombocytopenia and aplastic anemia.

IMMUNODEFICIENCY WITH SHORT-LIMBED DWARFISM

Major Immunologic Features
- Both T and B cell immunodeficiency may be found.
- Recurrent systemic infections occur.
- Prognosis is variable.

General Considerations
Three forms of immunodeficiency with short-limbed dwarfism exist. Type I is associated with combined immunodeficiency, type II with T cell immunodeficiency, and type III with B cell immunodeficiency.

The clinical features of each type vary with the degree of immunodeficiency. In short-limbed dwarfism associated with combined immunodeficiency, symptoms of infection are identical to those seen in severe combined immunodeficiency disease. Susceptibility to viral, bacterial, fungal, and protozoal infection is observed. Patients usually die in the first year of life. Patients with short-limbed dwarfism and T cell immunodeficiency are susceptible to recurrent sinopulmonary infection, fatal varicella, and progressive vaccinia, and they may develop a malabsorptionlike syndrome. Patients with short-limbed dwarfism and B cell immunodeficiency experience recurrent pyogenic infections in the form of pneumonia, sepsis, otitis media, and meningitis. In all patients, short-limbed dwarfism is characterized by short extremities and pudgy hands (Fig 21–4). The head is normal in size, which distinguishes this disorder from achondroplasia. During infancy, redundant skin folds are often seen around the neck and large joints of the extremities. Patients with short-limbed dwarfism and T cell immunodeficiency may also have cartilage-hair hypoplasia, manifested by light, thin, and sparse hair.

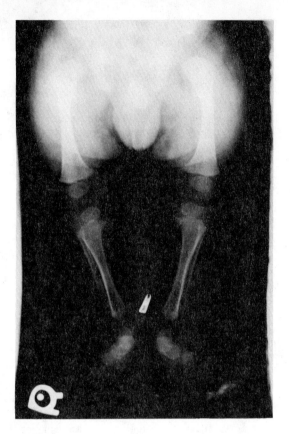

Figure 21–4. X-ray of extremities in a child with cartilage-hair hypoplasia and immunodeficiency. Note the redundant skin folds.

Immunologic abnormalities vary with the degree of immunodeficiency. In short-limbed dwarfism associated with combined immunodeficiency, T cell and B cell immunity are absent. In short-limbed dwarfism associated with T cell immunodeficiency, T cell immunity is deficient as measured by delayed hypersensitivity skin tests and responsiveness of peripheral blood lymphocytes to PHA, allogeneic cells, and varicella antigens, whereas B cell immunity is intact. In short-limbed dwarfism associated with B cell immunodeficiency, B cell immunity is absent and T cell immunity is intact.

Radiologic abnormalities consist of scalloping, irregular sclerosis, and cystic changes in the metaphyseal portions of long bones (Fig 21–4). Aganglionic megacolon has been reported. Patients with cartilage-hair hypoplasia have reduced hair diameters and lack the pigmented central core.

Treatment of these disorders is individualized to the associated immunodeficiency (eg, severe combined immunodeficiency, cellular immunodeficiency, and antibody immunodeficiency).

The prognosis varies with the degree of immunodeficiency. There have been no survivors with severe combined immunodeficiency disease. Patients with T cell immunodeficiency may survive to the fourth or fifth decade only to succumb to overwhelming varicella infection. The prognosis in patients with antibody immunodeficiency is similar to that of patients with X-linked hypogammaglobulinemia, but loss of T cell function may occur over time.

IMMUNODEFICIENCY WITH ENZYME DEFICIENCY

1. ADENOSINE DEAMINASE & NUCLEOSIDE PHOSPHORYLASE DEFICIENCY

Major Immunologic Features
- Recurrent and severe viral, bacterial, fungal, and protozoal infections occur.
- There are varied degrees of T and B cell immunodeficiency.
- Purine enzyme activity is absent or reduced.

General Considerations
Patients with enzyme deficiency and immunodeficiency may have clinical and laboratory abnormalities identical to those of patients with immunodeficiency and normal enzyme activity. Enzyme deficiency as a cause of immunodeficiency probably accounts for fewer than 15% of immunodeficiency disorders at present. It is almost certain that additional enzyme deficiencies will be discovered.

Adenosine deaminase and purine nucleoside phosphorylase are necessary for the normal catabolism of purines (Fig 21–5). Adenosine deaminase catalyzes the conversion of adenosine and deoxyadenosine to inosine and deoxyinosine. Nucleoside phosphorylase catalyzes the conversion of inosine, deoxyinosine, guanosine, and deoxyguanosine, to hypoxanthine and guanine. Several mechanisms have been postulated to explain the means whereby these enzyme deficiencies result in immunodeficiency. Experimental evidence indicates that adenosine, in increased amounts, may result in increased cyclic AMP (cAMP) activity, which is known to be associated with inhibition of lymphocyte function. Adenosine has also been shown to be toxic to cells in culture as a result of pyrimidine starvation. There is also evidence that exogenous adenosine can lead to the intracellular accumulation of S-adenosylhomocysteine, which acts as a potent inhibitor of DNA methylation. However, the most likely mechanism of inhibition of lymphocyte function is a result of the accumulation of deoxyadenosine and subsequently deoxy-ATP, which results in inhibition of ribonucleotide reductase and subsequent depletion of deoxyribonucleoside triphosphates. In purine nucleoside phosphorylase deficiency,

deoxygunaosine has been shown to result in the accumulation of deoxy-GTP. Again, this most probably results in inhibition of ribonucleotide reductase. These mechanisms have great importance in devising potential biochemical treatment for these disorders.

The degree of combined immunodeficiency is variable. The spectrum of immunologic aberrations varies from complete absence of T cell and B cell immunity, as observed in patients with severe combined immunodeficiency disease (85–90% of patients), to mild abnormalities of T cell and B cell function. Clinically, the phenotypic expression correlates with the degree of enzyme deficiency. Patients with the most complete form of enzyme deficiency have SCID. About 10–15% of patients have a delayed onset, some until 5–8 years of age. Routine neonatal screening has resulted in the detection of "partial" adenosine deaminase deficiency in immunologically normal individuals. Patients with enzyme deficiencies should be evaluated completely to determine the extent of the immunologic deficiency. As a result of the marked variability in immunodeficiency, there is considerable variation in the age at onset, severity of symptoms, and eventual outcome. Patients with adenosine deaminase deficiency and severe combined immunodeficiency may have radiologic abnormalities that include concavity and flaring of the anterior ribs, abnormal contour and articulation of posterior ribs and transverse processes, platyspondylisis, thick growth arrest lines, and an abnormal bony pelvis. Patients with nucleoside phosphorylase deficiency and T cell immunodeficiency have normal bone x-rays, absent T cell immunity, normal B cell immunity, a history of recurrent infection, and autoantibody formation. They are susceptible to fatal varicella and vaccinia infections.

The mode of inheritance of these enzyme defects appears to be autosomal recessive. The carrier state can be demonstrated in both sexes by diminished adenosine deaminase or nucleoside phosphorylase activity. With the identification of the precise genetic defects in these disorders, intrauterine and carrier diagnosis will be more precise. The enzymes are absent in erythrocytes, leukocytes, tissue, and cultured fibroblasts in these patients. An intrauterine diagnosis of adenosine deaminase deficiency can be made. Patients may not be immunodeficient at birth.

The specific genetic defect(s) for both adenosine deaminase and nucleoside phosphorylase have been described. In most instances a mutation in a single nucleotide, which results in a single amino acid change, is responsible.

Treatment of this disorder is similar to that of severe combined immunodeficiency or combined immunodeficiency. Several successful bone marrow transplants have been performed, with subsequent return of immunologic function. The patients' cells continue to have absent enzyme activity following transplantation.

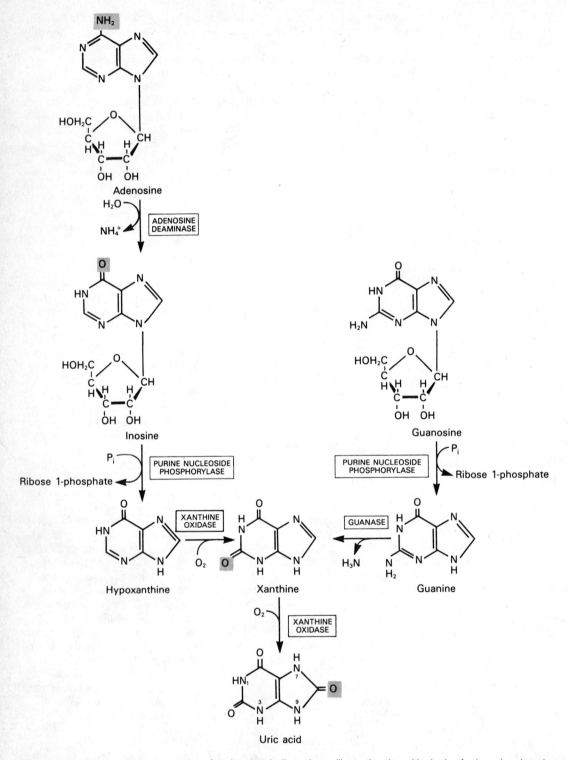

Figure 21–5. Schematic representation of purine metabolic pathway illustrating the critical role of adenosine deaminase and purine nucleoside phosphorylase. (Reproduced, with permission, from Murray RK et al: *Harper's Review of Biochemistry.* 22nd ed. Appleton & Lange, 1990.)

Some patients with adenosine deaminase deficiency have been successfully treated by monthly infusions of irradiated erythrocytes as a source of enzyme. Other patients have responded partially or not at all. Biochemical treatment of a single nucleoside phosphorylase-deficient patient with oral uridine was unsuccessful. Deoxycytidine therapy was evaluated in a single patient without any evidence of success. Others have responded partially to thymosin, thymus transplantation, or both. Additional patients have been successfully treated with bovine adenosine deaminase plus polyethylene glycol to prolong the enzyme half-life and reduce immunogenicity of the enzyme. This method proved to be associated with fewer complications than repeated red blood cell transfusions. Several patients have been successfully treated with autologous, genetically corrected T cells.

2. 5′-NUCLEOTIDASE DEFICIENCY

There have been several reports of decreased activity of 5′-nucleotidase and immunodeficiency. This enzyme deficiency has been described in association with acquired hypogammaglobulinemia, X-linked hypogammaglobulinemia, Wiskott-Aldrich syndrome, AIDS, and selective IgA deficiency. However, 5′-nucleotidase may be a differentiation marker of lymphocytes—in particular B lymphocytes—and the deficiency may therefore reflect a diminished number of B cells or an abnormality of maturation in the peripheral circulation of these patients.

3. TRANSCOBALAMIN II DEFICIENCY

Several patients have been described with a deficiency of transcobalamin II, a vitamin B_{12}-binding protein necessary for the transport of vitamin B_{12} into cells. These patients were found to have hypogammaglobulinemia, macrocytic anemia, lymphopenia, granulocytopenia, thrombocytopenia, and severe intestinal malabsorption. Vitamin B_{12} treatment resulted in the reversal of all of the manifestations of the disorder. Specific antibody synthesis occurred following administration of vitamin B_{12}.

4. BIOTIN-DEPENDENT CARBOXYLASE DEFICIENCIES

Patients with infantile chronic mucocutaneous candidiasis, ataxia, alopecia, intermittent lactic acidosis, and increased excretion of β-hydroxypropionate, methylcitrate, β-methylcrotonylglycine, and 3-β-hydroxyisovalerate in the urine have been described. Immunologic abnormalities in both B cell and T cell function were found. A second (neonatal) form has been described that is associated with severe acidosis and multiple episodes of sepsis. An intrauterine diagnosis has been made, and intrauterine therapy with biotin has been given. Treatment with biotin, 10 mg/d, reduced the abnormal metabolites in the urine and reversed the alopecia, ataxia, and chronic candidiasis. Multiple biotin-dependent carboxylase deficiencies may be one of several causes of the chronic mucocutaneous candidiasis syndrome with abnormal T cell function or severe recurrent sepsis. Biotin deficiency and immunodeficiency may also be a result of nutritional deficiencies and has been found in patients receiving hyperalimentation without biotin supplementation and in individuals on diets high in avidin (raw eggs), which binds biotin and prevents absorption.

GRAFT-VERSUS-HOST (GVH) DISEASE

GVH disease occurs when there is an unopposed attack of histoincompatible cells on an individual who is unable to reject foreign cells. The requirements for the GVH reaction are (1) histocompatibility differences between the graft (donor) and host (recipient), (2) immunocompetent graft cells, and (3) immunodeficient host cells. A GVH reaction may result from the infusion of any blood product containing viable lymphocytes, as may occur in maternal-fetal blood transfusion, intrauterine transfusion, therapeutic whole-blood transfusions or transfusions of packed erythrocytes, frozen cells, platelets, fresh plasma, or leukocyte-poor erythrocytes, or from transplantation of fetal thymus, fetal liver, or bone marrow. The onset of the GVH reaction occurs 7–30 days following infusion of viable lymphocytes. Once the reaction is established, little can be done to modify its course. In the majority of immunodeficient patients a GVH reaction is fatal. The exact mechanism by which a GVH reaction is produced is not known. Biopsy of active GVH lesions usually demonstrates infiltration by mononuclear cells and eosinophils as well as phagocytic and histiocytic cells. The GVH reaction may appear in 3 distinct forms: acute, hyperacute, and chronic.

In the acute form of GVH reaction, the initial manifestation is a maculopapular rash, which is frequently mistaken for a viral or allergic rash (Fig 21–6). Initially, it blanches with pressure and then becomes diffuse. If the rash is persistent, it will begin to scale. Diarrhea, hepatosplenomegaly, jaundice, cardiac irregularity, central nervous system irritability, and pulmonary infiltrates may occur during the height of the reaction. Enhanced susceptibility to infection is also present and may result in death from sepsis.

In the hyperacute form of GVH reaction, the rash may also begin as a maculopapular lesion, but then it rapidly progresses to a form resembling toxic epider-

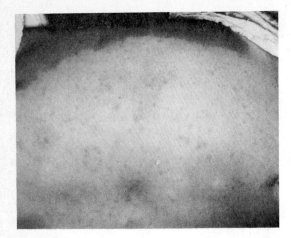

Figure 21–6. Maculopapular rash in early GVH disease in an infant with severe combined immunodeficiency disease.

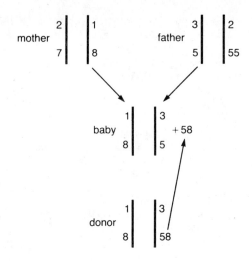

Figure 21–7. Inheritance of HLA antigens from the parents of a child with GVH disease and detection of additional antigen from the blood donor.

mal necrolysis, usually associated with severe diarrhea. This has not been associated with staphylococcal infection. Clinical and laboratory abnormalities similar to those found in the acute form may be observed. Death occurs shortly after the onset of the reaction.

The chronic form of GVH reaction may be a result of maternal-fetal transfusion or attempts at immunotherapy with histocompatible bone marrow transplantation. The clinical and laboratory features may be markedly abnormal or only slightly so. Interference with normal nail growth results in a dysplastic appearance. Chronic desquamation of the skin is usually present. Hepatosplenomegaly may be prominent, along with lymphadenopathy. Chronic diarrhea and failure to thrive are common. Secondary infection is a frequent complication. On biopsy of skin or lymph nodes, histiocytic infiltration may be found, leading to an erroneous diagnosis of Letterer-Siwe disease. Patients with Letterer-Siwe disease have normal immunoglobulin levels and normal T cell immunity, but patients with chronic GVH disease have severe immunodeficiency. Chronic GVH disease has also been confused with acrodermatitis enteropathica.

The diagnosis is suggested by the diffuse clinical abnormalities present in a patient who is known to have cellular immunodeficiency and who has received a transfusion of potentially immunocompetent cells in the preceding 5–30 days. The diagnosis is established by the demonstration of sex chromosome or HLA chimerism (Fig 21–7). On occasion, patients with known GVH disease fail to have detectable chimerism. Incubation of peripheral blood mononuclear cells with interleukin-2 may result in detectable chimerism.

There is no adequate treatment of GVH disease once it is established. Corticosteroids merely serve to enhance the susceptibility to infection. Antilymphocyte globulin also results in further suppression of immunity. Cyclosporin, a more specific immunosuppressive agent, may be useful. Experimentally, treatment with monoclonal antibody to tumor necrosis factor or gamma interferon reduces the severity of GVH disease. Since treatment is inadequate, prevention is essential. Any patient who is suspected of having cellular immunodeficiency and who requires the administration of a blood product should receive cells that have been subjected to 3000–6000 R of radiation to destroy viable lymphocytes and thus prevent GVH disease. Blood products to be irradiated include whole blood, packed erythrocytes, lymphocyte-poor erythrocytes, platelets, and fresh plasma. Interestingly, GVH disease has not yet been described in patients with AIDS despite the severe T cell immunodeficiency. This may be a result of HIV-1 infection of graft T cells, preventing the establishment of a graft.

IMMUNODEFICIENCY WITH CELL MEMBRANE ABNORMALITIES

A number of immunodeficiency disorders have now been linked to deficiencies of an essential cell membrane component. Undoubtedly, more of these abnormalities will be discovered. The 3 primary syndromes that have been described include the bare lymphocyte syndrome, LFA-1/Mac-1 glycoprotein deficiency, and gpL-115 glycoprotein deficiency.

1. BARE LYMPHOCYTE SYNDROME

Major Immunologic Features
- Susceptibility to viral infections occurs.
- Class I or class II HLA antigens, or both, are absent.
- Immunologic features are similar to those of combined immunodeficiency disease.

General Considerations

Patients with the bare lymphocyte syndrome have deficient expression of HLA molecules associated with immunodeficiency. A description of the HLA genes of the major histocompatibility complex (MHC) on the short arm of chromosome 6, the families of cell surface proteins encoded by these genes, their expression on cells of the immune system, and their role in the immune response is found in Chapter 5. Absence or low-level expression of class I or class II antigens, or both, occurs in the bare lymphocyte syndrome and is thought to be the primary reason for the impaired immunity observed in these patients.

Immunologic Pathogenesis

The bare lymphocyte syndrome is a rare disorder, occurring primarily in families from the Mediterranean area, and is often the product of a consanguineous union. It is inherited in an autosomal recessive manner. The first case was discovered by an inability to HLA type the patient's cells. From detailed investigations of subsequent patients, it is unlikely that the bare lymphocyte syndrome represents a single disorder; rather, it is a collection of genotypic abnormalities with various phenotypic expressions. The defect in patients is a result of abnormally low or absent expression of class I or class II HLA antigens, or both. In patients with deficient cell surface class II antigen expression, both the presence and absence of the class II gene has been found. In some instances, when the gene is present, class II antigens can be induced following stimulation of cells in vitro with antigens or gamma interferon. In other studies, it has been shown that there is an abnormality of the *trans*-activating class II regulatory gene that lies outside the major histocompatibility locus. Other investigators have shown that the class II-deficient variant is a deficiency in a DNA-binding protein referred to as the X-box-binding protein (RF-X), which may play an important role in the regulation of class II gene transcription.

Clinical Features

A. Symptoms & Signs: Individuals may be entirely healthy or symptomatic with features similar to those observed in patients with combined immunodeficiency. The symptoms include opportunistic infections, chronic diarrhea, recurrent viral infections, oral candidiasis, central nervous system viral infection, aplastic anemia, and growth failure.

B. Laboratory Findings: Lymphopenia with diminished T cell numbers and function is found in severe cases. The response of peripheral blood lymphocytes to antigens is usually reduced, while the response to mitogens may be normal. B cell numbers are normal or elevated.

Immunological Diagnosis

Routine typing for histocompatibility antigens will reveal the absence or decreased expression of HLA class I or class II antigens, or both. An intrauterine diagnosis can be established in the presence of a family history of the syndrome by analyzing fetal blood cells or chorionic villus biopsy material. To assist in bone marrow transplantation and matching, HLA genotyping was performed in several patients by using restriction enzyme fragments and specific HLA probes.

Differential Diagnosis

The bare lymphocyte syndrome should not be confused with other combined immunodeficiency diseases. In rare instances, severe leukopenia associated with another form of immunodeficiency may make HLA typing difficult.

Treatment

Severe forms of the bare lymphocyte syndrome require bone marrow transplantation. Determining an appropriate match for transplantation may be difficult and may require special techniques such as DNA hybridization. Supportive therapy is similar to that for severe combined immunodeficiency, with the use of intravenous gamma globulin and prophylactic trimethoprim-sulfamethoxazole. Immunotherapy with delta interferon may be of use in selected patients, as delta interferon results in the expression of HLA antigens following incubation of cells in vitro in certain forms of the syndrome.

Complications & Prognosis

Without appropriate treatment, patients may succumb to overwhelming infection, opportunistic infection, or progressive viral infection. Some individuals remain asymptomatic throughout their lives and have normal immunologic function.

2. LEUKOCYTE ADHESION DEFICIENCY (LFA-1/Mac-1, p150, and p95 GLYCOPROTEIN DEFICIENCY)

Major Immunologic Features
- Recurrent bacterial infections occur.
- There is an abnormal inflammatory response with an inability to form pus.

■ Cell surface integrins (glycoproteins) LFA-1/Mac-1, p150, and p95 are deficient.

General Considerations

Patients with leukocyte adhesion deficiency have recurrent pyogenic infections, with onset in the first weeks of life. Common microbial agents of these infections include *Staphylococcus aureus, Pseudomonas aeruginosa, Klebsiella, Proteus,* and enterococci. Delayed separation of the umbilical cord is common. As patients become older, they develop recurrent skin infections, sinusitis, vaginitis, perianal abscesses, periodontal disease, tracheobronchitis, pneumonia, recurrent progressive necrotic soft tissue infections, and septicemia. The disease may be fatal in the first years of life, or it may follow a more protracted course. The inheritance pattern is autosomal recessive.

The cause of the immunologic and clinical abnormalities is a deficiency of the LFA-1/Mac-1, p150, and p95 family of integrins. LFA-1 (lymphocyte function-associated antigen 1) and Mac-1 (macrophage 1) glycoproteins are found on the surface of cells, along with a third glycoprotein referred to as p150,95 (molecular weight designations). They function as adhesion molecules and are present on lymphocytes, monocytes, granulocytes, and large granular lymphocytes. Mac-1 functions as a complement receptor (CR3) for a cleaved form of complement (C3bi). It has been identified with monoclonal antibodies termed OKM-1 OKM-10, and Leu 15.

LFA-1, Mac-1, and P150,95 have a common β chain but have distinct α chains termed L1 (LFA-1 molecule), M1 (Mac-1 molecule), and X1 (p150,95 molecules) (Fig 21–8). It is believed that a deficiency in the β subunit is responsible for the decreased expression of LFA-1/Mac-1 glycoproteins. The genetic defect is on chromosome 21. Single amino acid mutations have been demonstrated in the common β chain region in some patients. An additional abnormality in phenotypically similar patients has been described, consisting of an absence of the Siayl-Lewis X ligand of E-selectin.

Deficiency of the adherence integrins results in several immunologic abnormalities. In vivo and in vitro chemotaxis of granulocytes and in vitro cell spreading are abnormal. Zymosan-induced chemiluminescence, but no phorbol myristate acetate-induced chemiluminescence, is abnormal. Antibody-

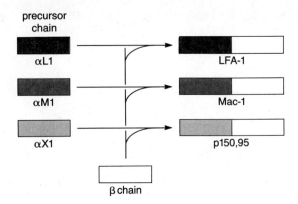

Figure 21–8. Comparative structures of leukocyte adhesion glycoproteins.

dependent cellular cytotoxicity and NK cell functions are also abnormal in some patients. Lymphocytes do not respond well to the mitogens PHA and concanavalin A. Following immunization, impaired antibody responses are observed.

Treatment of leukocyte adhesion deficiency is directed toward the specific infectious agents involved. As patients are infected with common pathogenic organisms but not with the opportunistic ones, they should respond to appropriate antibiotic therapy. Early aggressive treatment should be used, and prophylactic therapy should be given under certain circumstances, such as dental procedures.

3. DEFICIENT gpL-115 MEMBRANE GLYCOPROTEIN

Patients have been described who had a clinical syndrome of recurrent viral, protozoal, and bacterial infections. These patients had normal levels of serum immunoglobulins. A decreased response of lymphocytes to mitogens and specific antigens was described. Lymphocytes were also characterized as having a reduced cell volume. The disorders are X-linked immunodeficiencies. There is considerable molecular heterogeneity in gpL-115. Similar abnormalities, affecting both lymphocytes and platelets, are found in patients with Wiskott-Aldrich syndrome.

REFERENCES

Severe Combined Immunodeficiency Disease

Hitzig WH: Congenital thymic and lymphocytic deficiency disorders. In: *Immunologic Disorders in Infants and Children.* Stiehm ER, Fulginiti V (editors). Saunders, 1973.

Pahwa R et al: Recombinant interleukin 2 therapy in severe combined immunodeficiency disease. *Proc Natl Acad Sci USA* 1989;**86**:50969.

Pahwa SG, Pahwa RN, Good RA: Heterogeneity of B lymphocyte differentiation in severe combined immunodeficiency disease. *J Clin Invest* 1980;**66**:543.

Cellular Immunodeficiency With Abnormal Immunoglobulin Synthesis

Lawlor EJ et al: The syndrome of cellular immunodeficiency with immunoglobulins. *J Pediatr* 1974; **84**:183.

Ataxia-Telangiectasia

Baxter GD, Kumar S, Lavin MF: T cell receptor gene rearrangement and expression in ataxia-telangiectasia B lymphoblastoid cells. *Immunol Cell Biol* 1989; **67**:57.

Boder E, Sedgwick RP: Ataxia-telangiectasia: A familial syndrome and progressive cerebellar ataxia, oculocutaneous telangiectasia and frequent pulmonary infection. *Univ South Cal Med Bull* 1957;**9**:15.

Bridges BA, Harnden DG: Untangling ataxia-telangiectasia. *Nature* 1981;**289**:222.

Swift M et al: Breast and other cancers in families with ataxia-telangiectasia. *N Engl J Med* 1987;**316**:1289.

Taylor, AMR et al: Fifth International Workshop on Ataxia-Telangiectasia. *Cancer Res* 1993;**53**:438.

Wiskott-Aldrich Syndrome

Cooper MD et al: Wiskott-Aldrich syndrome: Immunologic deficiency disease involving the afferent limb of immunity. *Am J Med* 1968;**44**:489.

Parkman R et al: Complete correction of the Wiskott-Aldrich syndrome by allogeneic bone marrow transplantation. *N Engl J Med* 1978;**298**:921.

Parkman R et al: Surface protein abnormalities in lymphocytes and platelets from patients with Wiskott-Aldrich syndrome. *Lancet* 1981;**2**:1387.

Reisinger D, Parkman R: Molecular heterogeneity of a lymphocyte glycoprotein in immunodeficient patients. *J Clin Invest* 1986;**79**:595.

Shelley CS et al: Molecular characterization of sialophorin (CD43), the lymphocyte surface sialoglycoprotein defective in Wiskott-Aldrich syndrome. *Proc Natl Acad Sci USA* 1989;**86**:2819.

Simon HU et al: Defective expression of CD23 and autocrine growth-stimulation in Epstein-Barr virus (EBV) transformed B cells from patients with Wiskott-Aldrich syndrome (WAS). *Clin Exp Immunol* 1993;**91**:43.

Immunodeficiency with Thymoma

Soppi E et al: Thymoma with immunodeficiency (Good's syndrome) associated with myasthenia gravis and benign IgG gammapathy. *Arch Intern Med* 1985;**145**:1704.

Waldmann TA et al: Thymoma, hypogammaglobulinemia and absence of eosinophils. *J Clin Invest* 1967; **46**:1127.

Immunodeficiency with Short-Limbed Dwarfism

Ammann AJ, Sutliff W, Millinchick E: Antibody mediated immunodeficiency in short-limbed dwarfism. *J Pediatr* 1974;**84**:200.

Lux SE et al: Chronic neutropenia and abnormal cellular immunity in cartilage-hair hypoplasia. *N Engl J Med* 1970;**282**:234.

Polmar SH, Pierce GF: Cartilage hair hypoplasia: Immunological aspects and their clinical implications. *Clin Immunol Immunopathol* 1986;**40**:87.

Combined Immunodeficiency with Enzyme Deficiency

Blaise RM: Development of gene therapy for immunodeficiency: Adenosine deaminase deficiency. *Pediatr Res* 1993;**33**:S49.

Cowan MJ, Ammann AJ: Immunodeficiency associated with inherited metabolic disorders. *Clin Haematol* 1981;**10**:139.

Cowan MJ et al: Multiple biotin-dependent carboxylase deficiencies associated with defects in T cell and B cell immunity. *Lancet* 1979;**1**:115.

Giblet ER et al: Nucleoside phosphorylase deficiency in a child with severely defective T cell immunity and normal B cell immunity. *Lancet* 1975;**1**:1010.

Hershfield MS et al: Enzyme replacement therapy with polyethylene glycol adenosine deaminase in adenosine deaminase deficiency: Overview and case reports of three patients, including two now receiving gene therapy. *Pediatr Res* 1993;**33**:S42.

Hirschhorn R: Overview of biochemical abnormalities and molecular genetics of adenosine deaminase deficiency. *Pediatr Res* 1993;**33**:S35.

Hirschhorn R, Martin DW: Enzyme defects in immunodeficiency diseases. *Semin Immunopathol* 1978; **1**:299.

Levy Y et al: Adenosine deaminase deficiency with late onset of recurrent infections: Response to treatment with polyethylene glycol-modified adenosine deaminase. *J Pediatr* 1988;**113**:312.

Meuwissen HJ, Pollara B, Pickering RJ: Combined immunodeficiency disease associated with adenosine deaminase deficiency. *J Pediatr* 1975;**86**:169.

Morgan G et al: Heterogeneity of biochemical, clinical and immunologic parameters in severe combined immunodeficiency due to adenosine deaminase deficiency. *Clin Exp Immunol* 1987;**70**:491.

Shanon A et al: Combined familial adenosine deaminase and purine nucleoside phosphorylase deficiencies. *Arch Dis Child* 1988;**63**:931.

Bare Lymphocyte Syndrome

Marcadet A et al: Genotyping with DNA probes in combined immunodeficiency syndrome with defective expression of HLA. *N Engl J Med* 1985;**312**:1287.

Reigh W et al: Congenital immunodeficiency with a regulatory defect in MHC class II gene expression lacks a specific HLA-DR promoter binding protein, RF-X. *Cell* 1988;**53**:897.

T Cell Membrane, Signal, and Cytokine Defects

Alarion B et al: Familial defect in the surface expression of the T-cell receptor–CD3 complex. *N Engl J Med* 1988;**319**:1203.

Castigli E et al: Severe combined immunodeficiency with selective T-cell cytokine genes. *Pediatr Res* 1993; **33**:52.

Chatila T et al: An immunodeficiency characterized by

defective signal transduction in T lymphocytes. *N Engl J Med* 1989;**320:**696.

Stiehm ER: New and old immunodeficiencies. *Pediatr Res* 1993;**33:**52.

Leukocyte Adhesion Deficiency

Etzioni A et al: Brief report: Recurrent severe infections caused by a novel leukocyte adhesion deficiency. *N Engl J Med* 1992;**327:**1789.

Kishimoto TK et al: Heterogeneous mutations in the beta subunit common to the LFA-1, Mac-1, and p150,95 glycoproteins cause leukocyte adhesion deficiency. *Cell* 1987;**50:**193.

Marlin SD et al: LFA-1 immunodeficiency disease. *J Exp Med* 1986;**164:**855.

Springer TA: The LFA-1, Mac-1 glycoprotein family

and its deficiency in an inherited disease. *Fed Proc* 1985;**44:**2660.

Sullivan KE, Stobo JD, Peterlin P: Molecular analysis of the bare lymphocyte syndrome. *J Clin Invest* 1985;**76:**75.

Wacholtz MC, Patel SS, Lipsky PE: Leukocyte function-associated antigen 1 is an activation molecule for human T cells. *J Exp Med* 1989;**170:**431.

Wardlaw AJ et al: Distinct mutations in two patients with leukocyte adhesion deficiency and their functional correlates. *J Exp Med* 1990;**172:**335.

Deficient gpL-115 Membrane Glycoprotein

Parkman R et al: Immune abnormalities in patients lacking a lymphocyte surface glycoprotein. *Clin Immunol Immunopathol* 1984;**33:**363.

Phagocytic Dysfunction Diseases

22

Arthur J. Ammann, MD

Phagocytic disorders may be divided into extrinsic and intrinsic defects. The extrinsic category includes deficiencies of opsonins secondary to deficiencies of antibody and complement factors, suppression of the total number of phagocytic cells by immunosuppressive agents, interference of phagocytic function by corticosteroids, and suppression of the number of circulating neutrophils by autoantibody directed specifically against neutrophil antigens. Other extrinsic disorders may be related to abnormal neutrophil chemotaxis secondary to complement deficiency or abnormal complement components. The intrinsic phagocytic disorders are the result of enzymatic deficiencies within the metabolic pathway necessary for killing of bacteria. These include chronic granulomatous disease with abnormalities in the respiratory burst pathway, myeloperoxidase deficiency, and glucose-6-phosphate dehydrogenase deficiency.

Phagocytic disorders may also result from abnormalities of adhesion molecules, resulting in recurrent severe bacterial infections. However, leukocyte adhesion abnormalities also result in T cell dysfunction, and so these abnormalities are discussed in Chapter 21.

Susceptibility to infection in phagocytic dysfunction syndromes may range from mild recurrent skin infections to severe, overwhelming, fatal systemic infection. Characteristically, all of these patients are susceptible to bacterial infection and do not have difficulty with viral or protozoal infections. Some of the more severe disorders may be associated with overwhelming fungal infections.

Numerous tests can now be performed to evaluate phagocytic dysfunction (see Chapter 13). Screening tests are listed in Table 18–4, and definitive studies are listed in Table 22–1.

CHRONIC GRANULOMATOUS DISEASE

Major Immunologic Features

- There is susceptibility to infection with organisms normally of low virulence, eg, *Staphylococcus epidermidis, Serratia marcescens, Aspergillus.*
- Inheritance is X-linked (autosomal variant occurs).
- Onset of symptoms occurs by 2 years of age: draining lymphadenitis, hepatosplenomegaly, pneumonia, osteomyelitis, and abscesses.
- Diagnosis is established by quantitative nitroblue tetrazolium test, quantitative killing curve, superoxide generation, or chemiluminescence.

General Considerations

Chronic granulomatous disease (CGD) is inherited as an X-linked disorder, with clinical manifestations appearing during the first 2 years of life. An autosomal variant of the disease has been described. Patients are susceptible to infection with a variety of normally nonpathogenic and unusual organisms. Characteristic abnormal laboratory studies will detect both patients and female carriers of the disease. Female carriers are usually asymptomatic. Early diagnosis and aggressive therapy have improved the prognosis for these patients.

Immunologic Pathogenesis

There are several different genetic forms of CGD based on different biochemical abnormalities and patterns of inheritance. However, the functional defect, which occurs in the respiratory burst, is similarly abnormal in the various forms and results in characteristic clinical abnormalities. The respiratory burst in neutrophils and monocytes is triggered by opsonized microorganisms or other appropriate stimuli, resulting in an increase in intracellular oxygen consumption with conversion of oxygen to hydrogen peroxide, oxidized halogens, and superoxide and hydroxyl radicals (Fig 22–1). Patients with the various forms of chronic granulomatous disease are unable to

Table 22–1. Evaluation of phagocytosis.

Test	Comment
Quantitative Nitroblue tetrazolium (NBT)	Used for diagnosis and screening of chronic granulomatous disease and for detection of carrier state.
Quantitative intracellular killing curve	Used for diagnosis of chronic granulomatous disease. Can be performed with organisms isolated from the individual patient.
Chemotaxis	Abnormal in a variety of disorders associated with frequent bacterial infection. Does not provide a specific diagnosis. Performed by using a Boyden chamber and a microscopic or radioactive technique to determine cell migration. Rebuck skin window provides a qualitative result in vivo.
Chemiluminescence	Abnormal in chronic granulomatous disease and myeloperoxidase deficiency.
Enzyme tests	Deficiencies of specific enzymes: glucose-6-phosphate dehydrogenase, alkaline phosphatase, myeloperoxidase.
Membrane glycoproteins	Deficient in leukocyte adhesion (intergrin) disorders and associated with abnormal leukocyte adherence.

generate a respiratory burst after stimulation of neutrophils and monocytes and are therefore unable to kill certain microorganisms.

The central enzyme in the respiratory burst is NADPH oxidase. This enzyme is composed of 4 subunits with both cytosol and membrane components. Defects in any component lead to CGD. Certain classes of redox groups participate in electron transport by the respiratory burst oxidase. Cytochrome b is deficient in the X-linked form of the disease (about 60% of the cases) but is present in what appears to be the autosomal form of the disease (about 30% of the

① NADPH oxidase
$$NADPH + 2O_2 \xrightarrow{\text{NADPH oxidase}} NADP^+ + 2O_2^- + H^+$$

② superoxide dismutase
$$O_2^- + O_2^- + 2H^+ \xrightarrow{\text{superoxide dismutase}} H_2O_2 + O_2$$

③ myeloperoxidase
$$H_2O_2 + Cl^- \xrightarrow{\text{myeloperoxidase}} H_2O + OCl^-$$

Figure 22–1. Respiratory burst resulting in the generation of superoxide (O_2^-), hydrogen peroxide (H_2O_2), and hypochlorite (OCl^-).

cases). However, a number of other biochemical variants have been described, including a low-affinity NADPH oxidase. Additional defects include deficiency of the flavoprotein component of the NADPH-dependent superoxide-generating oxidase and lack of neutrophil cytosolic factors required for activation of oxidative metabolism. Because the various abnormalities overlap, it is difficult to determine the inheritance of CGD in the absence of detailed genetic studies and a strong family history. Genetic and biochemical studies suggest that there are 4 major forms of CGD: (1) X-linked with deficiency of cytochrome b_{588} (designated by international investigators as CGD X91), (2) autosomal recessive with deficiencies in the cytosolic NADPH oxidase (designated CGD A47), (3) autosomal recessive with deficient alpha cytochrome b_{588} (designated CGD A22), and (4) deficiencies in the cytosolic component p67-phox (designated CGD A67). The basic genetic defects are a consequence of multiple mutations on different chromosomes (16q24, Xp21.1), all resulting in similar biochemical and clinical features.

Clinical Features

A. Symptoms & Signs: In the majority of patients, the diagnosis can be established before 2 years of age. The most frequent abnormalities consist of marked lymphadenopathy, chronic infected ulcerations, hepatosplenomegaly, chronic draining lymph nodes, and at least one episode of pneumonia. Other manifestations include rhinitis, conjunctivitis, dermatitis, ulcerative stomatitis, perianal abscess, osteomyelitis, chronic diarrhea with intermittent abdominal pains, esophageal stenosis, and intestinal obstruction. Chronic and acute infection occurs in lymph nodes, skin, lungs, intestinal tract, liver, and bone. A major clue to early diagnosis is the finding of normally nonpathogenic or unusual organisms. Organisms responsible for infection include *S aureus, S epidermidis, Serratia marcescens, Pseudomonas, Escherichia coli, Candida* and *Aspergillus.*

B. Laboratory Findings: The most widely available tests for diagnosis are the quantitative nitroblue tetrazolium (NBT) test and chemiluminescence assays. Patient leukocytes have absent NBT dye reduction and reduced chemiluminescence, whereas carriers may have normal or reduced values. Patients with CGD are unable to kill certain intracellular bacteria at a normal rate. The leukocyte-killing curves for organisms to which these individuals are susceptible usually indicate little or no killing over a period of 2 hours (Fig 22–2). Other abnormal findings include decreased oxygen uptake during phagocytosis and abnormal bacterial iodination. Natural killer (NK) cell activity is normal.

The blood leukocyte count is usually elevated even if the patient does not have active infection. Hypergammaglobulinemia is present, and antibody function is normal. T cell immunity is normal. Com-

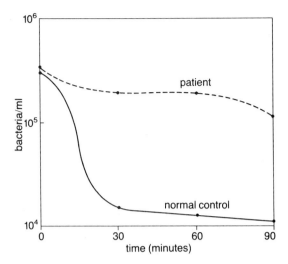

Figure 22–2. Bacterial killing curves in normal control and in patient with chronic granulomatous disease. The patient's phagocyte cells are unable to kill significant numbers of bacteria following an in vitro incubation period of 90 minutes.

plement factors may be elevated. During episodes of pneumonia, the chest x-ray is frequently severely abnormal. Liver function tests may be abnormal as a result of chronic infection. Pulmonary function tests are usually abnormal following episodes of pneumonia and may not return to normal for several months. Several patients have been reported to have a rare Kell blood group, the "McLeod" phenotype. Histologic examination of the infected area often reveals an accumulation of pigmented histiocytes.

Immunologic Diagnosis

A diagnosis can be established by using the quantitative NBT dye reduction assay or quantitative chemiluminescence and confirmed by using specific bactericidal assays (see Chapter 13). These assays may also be used to identify the carrier state and to establish an intrauterine diagnosis. Both male and autosomal variants of chronic granulomatous disease have abnormal test results. B cell immunity, T cell immunity, and complement are normal. Chemiluminescence is the best method for detecting the carrier state. Several instances of an intrauterine diagnosis have been reported by using fetal blood and NBT or chemiluminescence test.

Differential Diagnosis

Few clinical disorders are confused with CGD. Two other disorders with abnormal enzymatic function are associated with clinical symptoms and laboratory features similar to those of CGD. One of these is the autosomal variant of CGD associated with deficient glucose-6-phosphate dehydrogenase. Myelo-

peroxidase deficiency may have some similar clinical features. Any child presenting with osteomyelitis, pneumonia, liver abscess, or chronic draining lymphadenopathy associated with a normally nonpathogenic or unusual organism should be suspected of having CGD.

Treatment

Aggressive diagnostic measures and therapy are necessary for long-term survival and diminished morbidity. Blood cultures, aspiration of draining lymph nodes, liver biopsy, and open-lung biopsy should be used to obtain a specific bacterial diagnosis. Therapy should be instituted immediately, while results of cultures are pending. The choice of antibiotics should be appropriate for the spectrum of bacterial infections, such as a combination of penicillin and gentamicin or penicillin and chloramphenicol. These would cover the majority of organisms, but not *Candida* or *Aspergillus,* for which amphotericin B is the treatment of choice. Amphotericin B therapy should be given intravenously, starting with high doses in the range of 1 mg/kg/d. Newer antifungal agents with reduced toxicity should be considered. The ultimate survival of the patient is dependent on early and intensive therapy. Treatment with antibiotics may be prolonged, requiring 5–6 weeks of total therapy. Additional therapy has included the use of leukocyte infusions, but experience has been extremely limited. Several investigators have used continuous anti-infective therapy with sulfisoxazole. A single successful bone marrow transplant has been performed. Recently, patients have been treated prophylactically with gamma interferon, which increases the respiratory burst activity of neutrophils and monocytes.

Complications & Prognosis

Chronic organ dysfunction may result from severe or chronic infection. Examples are abnormal pulmonary function, chronic liver disease, chronic osteomyelitis, and malabsorption secondary to gastrointestinal tract involvement. The mortality rate in CGD has been considerably reduced by early diagnosis and aggressive therapy. Survival into the second decade and beyond has been recorded. Female carriers have an increased incidence of systemic and discoid lupus erythematosus.

GLUCOSE-6-PHOSPHATE DEHYDROGENASE DEFICIENCY

Glucose-6-phosphate dehydrogenase deficiency is inherited in an X-linked manner. Complete absence of leukocyte glucose-6-phosphate dehydrogenase activity has been associated with a clinical picture similar to that of CGD. The defect in leukocytes is believed to be a result of deficient generation of

NADPH needed as a reducing equivalent for the oxidase. Some investigators have demonstrated decreased hexose monophosphate shunt activity and decreased hydrogen peroxide production in the leukocytes. Leukocytes are unable to kill certain organisms at a normal rate, similar to the situation in chronic granulomatous disease. The susceptibility of these patients to microorganisms is similar to that of patients with CGD. Glucose-6-phosphate dehydrogenase deficiency differs in that the onset is later, both males and females are affected, and hemolytic anemia is present. The laboratory diagnosis is based on the demonstration of deficient leukocyte glucose-6-phosphate dehydrogenase. The NBT test, the leukocyte intracellular killing curve, the production of hydrogen peroxide, and the consumption of oxygen are all abnormal. Treatment and prognosis are similar to those of chronic granulomatous disease. This disorder should be distinguished from the more common erythrocyte deficiency of this enzyme, which is associated with hemolytic anemia but without recurrent infections.

MYELOPEROXIDASE DEFICIENCY

Several patients with complete deficiency of leukocyte myeloperoxidase have been described. Myeloperoxidase is one of the enzymes necessary for normal intracellular killing of certain organisms. It catalyzes the oxidation of microorganisms by intracellular H_2O_2 in the presence of halides (Fig 22–1). The leukocytes of these patients have normal oxygen consumption, hexose monophosphate shunt activity, and superoxide and hydrogen peroxide production. The intracellular killing of organisms is delayed, but may reach normal levels with increased in vitro incubation times. Chemiluminescence of leukocytes is decreased. Susceptibility to candidal and staphylococcal infections has been the chief problem. The diagnosis can be established by using a peroxidase stain of peripheral blood. No specific treatment is available other than appropriate antibiotic therapy.

ALKALINE PHOSPHATASE DEFICIENCY

Several patients have been reported who have recurrent bacterial infection associated with absent leukocyte alkaline phosphatase activity. There is a modest reduction in bactericidal activity.

CHÉDIAK-HIGASHI SYNDROME

Chédiak-Higashi syndrome is a multisystem autosomal recessive disorder. Symptoms include recurrent bacterial infections with a variety of organisms,

hepatosplenomegaly, partial albinism, central nervous system abnormalities, and a high incidence of lymphoreticular cancers.

The characteristic abnormality of giant cytoplasmic granular inclusions in leukocytes and platelets is observed on routine peripheral blood smears under ordinary light microscopy. Additional abnormalities include elevated Epstein-Barr virus (EBV) antibody titers, abnormal neutrophil chemotaxis, decreased NK cell activity, and abnormal intracellular killing of organisms (including streptococci and pneumococci as well as the organisms found in CGD). The killing defect is manifested in vitro by delayed intracellular killing. Oxygen consumption, hydrogen peroxide formation, and hexose monophosphate shunt activity are normal. Abnormal microtubule function, abnormal lysosomal enzyme levels in granulocytes, and protease deficiency in granulocytes, have been described and are associated with increased levels of leukocyte cyclic AMP (cAMP). Abnormal leukocyte function in vitro has been corrected by ascorbate, but the results of treatment in vivo are contradictory. Improved granulocyte function in vitro has also been observed after treatment with anticholinergic drugs.

There is no definitive treatment other than specific antibiotic therapy against infecting organisms. The prognosis is poor because of progressive increased susceptibility to infection and neurologic deterioration. Most patients die during childhood, but survivors to the second and third decades have been reported.

JOB'S SYNDROME

Job's syndrome was originally described as a disorder of recurrent cold staphylococcal abscesses of the skin, lymph nodes, or subcutaneous tissue (Fig 22–3). The first patients were fair-skinned, red-haired girls of Italian descent. Initial descriptions also included eczematoid skin lesions, otitis media, and chronic nasal discharge. Few signs of systemic infection or inflammatory response occurred in association with the infection. Additional reports of Job's syndrome indicated that the disorder might be a variant of CGD. However, most of the patients do not have abnormal immunologic tests. Patients with hyper-IgE, syndrome have clinical and laboratory features similar to those of Job's syndrome; in fact, these may be the same disorder (see below). Treatment consists of appropriate antibiotic therapy. The prognosis is uncertain.

TUFTSIN DEFICIENCY

Tuftsin disease has been reported as a familial deficiency of a phagocytosis-stimulating tetrapeptide

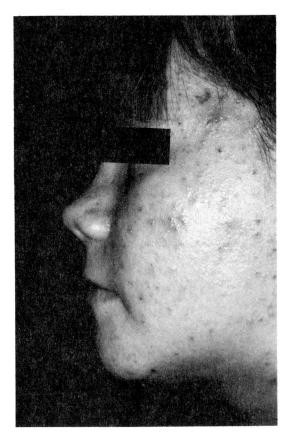

Figure 22–3. Coarse facial features, multiple small abscesses, and "saddle" nose in a female with Job's syndrome.

that is cleaved from a parent immunoglobulinlike molecule (termed leukokinin) in the spleen. Tuftsin also appears to be absent in patients who have been splenectomized. Local and severe systemic infections occur with *Candida, S aureus,* and *Streptococcus pneumoniae.* Tuftsin levels are determined only in a few specialized laboratories. There is no treatment, and the prognosis is uncertain. Gamma globulin therapy appeared to be beneficial in the 2 families in which it was tried.

ELEVATED IgE, DEFECTIVE CHEMOTAXIS, ECZEMA, & RECURRENT INFECTION (Hyper-IgE Syndrome)

These patients—both males and females—have an early onset of eczema and recurrent bacterial infections in the form of abscesses involving the skin, lungs, ears, sinuses, and eyes. Systemic infection

may involve other areas. Organisms causing infection include *S aureus, Candida, H influenzae, Streptococcus pneumoniae,* and group A streptococci. Laboratory findings consist of eosinophilia, IgE concentrations in excess of 5000 IU/mL, diminished antibody response following immunization, and normal lymphocyte response to phytohemagglutinin (PHA) and concanavalin but reduced response to antigens and allogeneic cells by mixed lymphocyte culture (MLC). Abnormalities of chemotaxis are present in some but not all patients. Patients have been shown to have decreased numbers of suppressor T cells with increased spontaneous IgE production in vitro. Increased amounts of IgE antibody and decreased amounts of IgA antibody to *Staphylococcus* antigens are found. Antibiotic therapy is indicated for specific infections. The prognosis is unknown, although patients have survived to adulthood.

LEUKOCYTE MOVEMENT DISORDERS

A number of patients have been described who have decreased leukocyte chemotaxis and recurrent infections (usually bacterial). In some cases, there is a deficiency of IgG and an IgG inhibitor of chemotaxis. Defective actin polymerization was found in association with defective neutrophil phagocytosis and locomotion. Abnormal chemotaxis has been found in congenital ichthyosis. Mannosidosis, a storage disease manifested by mental retardation and recurrent infections, in associated with abnormal chemotaxis and delayed phagocytosis. Mannose, which accumulates within leukocytes, may interfere with cell function. Similar abnormalities have been described in type IB glycogen storage disease.

MISCELLANEOUS PHAGOCYTIC DISORDERS

A variety of rare phagocytic disorders have also been described. They are usually associated with recurrent skin infections and systemic bacterial infections. Diagnosis of these rare disorders is usually made by sophisticated tests, which are not available in most medical centers. Abnormalities that have been described include decreased lactoferrin granules, abnormal polymerization of actin, and deficiency of specific granules. Because of the rarity of these disorders, there is insufficient information on which to base recommendations regarding treatment and prognosis. Phagocytic disorders that result from abnormalities of leukocyte adhesion molecules (integrins) also have T cell defects and are discussed in Chapter 21.

REFERENCES

Chronic Granulomatous Disease

Cheson BD, Curnutte JT, Babior BM: The oxidative killing mechanism of the neutrophil. *Prog Clin Immunol* 1977;**3:**1.

Curnutte JT, Babior BM: Chronic granulomatous disease. *Adv Hum Genet* 1987;**16:**229.

de Boerm et al: Cytochrome b558 negative, autosomal recessive chronic granulomatous disease: Two new mutations in the cytochrome b558 light chain of the NADPH oxidase (p22-phox). *Am J Hum Genet* 1992; **51:**1127.

Johnston RB, Baehner RL: Chronic granulomatous disease: Correlation between pathogenesis and clinical findings. *Pediatrics* 1971;**48:**730.

Lomax KJ et al: Recombinant 47-kilodalton cytosol factor restores NADPH oxidase in chronic granulomatous disease. *Science* 1989;**245:**409.

Orkin SH: Molecular genetics of chronic granulomatous disease. *Annu Rev Immunol* 1989;**7:**277.

Glucose-6-Phosphate Dehydrogenase Deficiency

Cooper MR et al: Complete deficiency of leukocyte glucose-6-phosphate dehydrogenase with defective bactericidal activity. *J Clin Invest* 1972;**51:**769.

Quie PG, Abramson JS: Disorders of the polymorphonuclear phagocytic system. Pages 343–383 in: *Immunologic Disorders in Infants and Children.* Stiehm ER (editor). Saunders, 1989.

Myeloperoxidase Deficiency

Czarnetzki BM: Disorders of phagocyte killing and digestion (CGD, G-6-PD and myeloperoxidase deficiencies). *Curr Probl Dermatol* 1989;**18:**101.

Lehrer RI, Cline MJ: Leukocyte myeloperoxidase deficiency and disseminated candidiasis: The role of myeloperoxidase in resistance to *Candida* infection. *J Clin Invest* 1969;**48:**1478.

Nauseef WM: Myeloperoxidase deficiency. *Hematol Oncol Clin North Am* 1988;**2:**577.

Chédiak-Higashi Syndrome

Ganz T et al: Microbicidal/cytotoxic proteins of neutrophils are deficient in two disorders: Chédiak-Higashi syndrome and specific granule deficiency. *J Clin Invest* 1988;**82:**552.

Haliotis T et al: Chédiak-Higashi gene in humans. 1. Impairment of natural-killer function. *J Exp Med* 1980;**151:**1039.

Stolz W et al: Chédiak-Higashi syndrome: Approaches in diagnosis and treatment. *Curr Probl Dermatol* 1989;**18:**93.

Stossel TP, Root RK, Vaughn M: Phagocytosis in chronic granulomatous disease and the Chédiak-Higashi syndrome. *N Engl J Med* 1972;**286:**120.

Tuftsin Deficiency

Constantopoulos A: Congenital tuftsin deficiency. *Ann NY Acad Sci* 1983;**419:**214.

Phillips JH, Babcock GF, Nishioka K: Tuftsin, A naturally occurring immunopotentiating factor. 1. In vitro enhancement of murine natural cell-mediated cytotoxicity. *J Immunol* 1981;**126:**915.

Spirer Z et al: Tuftsin stimulates IL-1 production by human mononuclear cells, human spleen cells and mouse spleen cells in vitro. *J Lab Clin Immunol* 1989; **28:**27.

Increased IgE, Defective Chemotaxis, & Recurrent Infections

Durkin HG et al: Control of IgE responses. *Clin Immunol Immunopathol* 1989;**50:**S52.

Hill HR, Quie PG: Raised serum IgE levels and defective neutrophil chemotaxis in three children with eczema and recurrent bacterial infections. *Lancet* 1974;**1:**183.

Kraemer MJ et al: In vitro studies of the hyper-IgE disorders: Suppression of spontaneous IgE synthesis by allogeneic suppressor T lymphocytes. *Clin Immunol Immunopathol* 1982;**25:**157.

Leung DY, Geha RS: Regulation of the human IgE antibody response. *Int Rev Immunol* 1987;**2:**75.

Matter L et al: Abnormal immune response to *Staphylococcus aureus* in patients with *Staphylococcus aureus* hyper IgE syndrome. *Clin Exp Immunol* 1986;**66:**450.

Leukocyte Movement Disorders

Boxer LA, Henley-Whyte ET, Stossel TP: Neutrophil action dysfunction and abnormal neutrophil behavior. *N Engl J Med* 1974;**291:**1093.

Quie PG, Abramson JS: Disorders of the polymorphonuclear phagocytic system. Pages 343–383 in: *Immunologic Disorders in Infants and Children.* Stiehm ER (editor). Saunders, 1989.

Complement Deficiencies

23

Michael M. Frank, MD

As discussed in detail in Chapter 10, there are 2 major pathways of complement activation. In each pathway, peptides derived from several complement components assemble to form a complex enzyme capable of binding and cleaving C3, the principal component formed by complement activation. Once these pathways have joined at the level of the component C3, they proceed together to interact with C5, C6, C7, C8, and C9 to produce a lytic lesion when activated at a cell surface. These later-acting components have together been termed the membrane attack complex, since they form a C5b–9 complex that inserts into biologic membranes to cause lysis. There are a limited number of patients with a genetically controlled deficiency of one of the components of the classic, alternative, or terminal attack pathways. In addition, there are patients who are known to have defects in control proteins that regulate a number of steps in the cascade. The major clinical features of each are shown in Table 23–1. For the most part, the consequences of these defects can be predicted from a knowledge of the mechanisms of activation and the biologic activities of the various complement components.

In general, defects of components of the 2 pathways behave as autosomal recessive traits. Individuals with one normal gene have about half-normal levels of the deficient proteins. Affected individuals are those with little or no gene product; they are the product of 2 heterozygous deficient parents. A few complement components composed of subunits are encoded by multiple genes. Individual independently inherited genes code for C1q, C1r, and possibly C1s as well as C8 α-γ chain and C8 β chain. Inheritance of these also follows an autosomal recessive pattern. Since there is a broad range of plasma concentrations for many of the components in normal individuals, it is not always possible to distinguish heterozygous individuals from normal individuals on the basis of their plasma complement component levels. In most cases, heterozygous individuals are phenotypically normal, except as noted below. When an individual

with the homozygous phenotype is totally deficient in one of the proteins of the classic pathway or one of the terminal components, the lytic pathway is interrupted at the point at which that component must function and the complement titer (CH50) is zero; ie, the quantity of serum required to lyse an antibody-sensitized sheep erythrocyte is infinite. Similarly, with a defect in the alternative-pathway components or terminal components, the alternative-pathway titer is zero.

ALTERNATIVE-PATHWAY COMPONENT DEFICIENCIES

The alternative complement pathway is believed to be the older pathway phyogenetically and to provide the first line of host defense to bacterial attack, before the host has had sufficient time to respond to the infection by developing antibody. For that reason it might be expected that defects in the early steps of the alternative pathway might predispose individuals toward serious infection. The individual's ability to bind and activate C3 to provide adequate opsonic and other complement functions is compromised, and such patients have frequent infections with high-grade pathogens (eg, pneumococci, *Haemophilus influenzae,* and staphylococci). Relatively few such individuals have been reported. An increased incidence of neisserial infection, in addition to infections with high-grade pathogens, has been reported in properdin deficiency.

CLASSIC-PATHWAY COMPONENT DEFICIENCIES

Since the alternative pathway provides a first line of defense against bacterial infection, one might expect that the deficiencies in the early steps of the classic pathway would not be associated with frequent se-

Table 23–1. Inherited complement and complement-related protein deficiency states.

Deficient Protein	Observed Pattern of Inheritance at Clinical Level	Reported Major Clinical Correlates[1]
C1q	Autosomal recessive	ACUD
C1r	Probably autosomal recessive	ACUD
C1s	Found in combination with C1r deficiency	ACUD
C4	Probably autosomal recessive (2 separate loci C4A and C4B)[2]	ACUD
C2	Autosomal recessive, HLA-linked	ACUD
C3	Autosomal recessive	ACUD
C5	Autosomal recessive	Recurrent disseminated neisserial infections, SLE
C6	Autosomal recessive	Recurrent disseminated neisserial infections
C7	Autosomal recessive	Recurrent disseminated neisserial infections, Raynaud's phenomenon
C8 (β chain or α-γ chains)	?Autosomal recessive	Recurrent disseminated neisserial infections
C9	Autosomal recessive	Recurrent disseminated neisserial infections
Properdin	X-linked recessive	Recurrent pyogenic infections, fulminant meningococcemia
Factor D	?	Recurrent pyogenic infections
C1 inhibitor	Autosomal recessive	Hereditary angioedema, increased incidence of several autoimmune diseases[3]
Factor H	Autosomal recessive	Glomerulonephritis
Factor I	Autosomal recessive	Recurrent pyogenic infections, ACUD
CR1	Autosomal recessive[4]	Association between low erythrocyte CR1 and SLE, ACUD
CR3	Autosomal recessive[5]	Leukocytosis, recurrent pyogenic infections, delayed umbilical cord separation

[1]A significant number of individuals with complement deficiencies, especially C2 and the terminal components, are clinically well. A significant number of patients with defects in C5–9 have had autoimmune disease. ACUD, autoimmune collagen vascular disease (SLE, glomerulonephritis).

[2]Individuals lacking C4A or C4B are designated "q0" (quantity 0). Thus, individuals can be C4Aq0 or C4Bq0. Such individuals are reported to have a higher than normal incidence of autoimmune diseases. Similarly, heterozygous C2 deficient individuals are reported to have an increased incidence of autoimmune disease.

[3]Includes approximately 85% of cases with silent alleles and 15% with alleles encoding for dysfunctional variant C1 inhibitor protein.

[4]Homozygosity for low (not absent) numerical expression of CR1 on erythrocytes is detectable in vitro and appears to be associated with SLE. An acquired defect in CR1 numbers may also be operative.

[5]Low but not absent leukocyte CR3 is detectable in both parents of most CR3-deficient children.

vere infections, and this is the case. Nevertheless, it has become increasingly clear, as the relatively few patients with defects in this portion of the cascade have been observed for more prolonged periods, that these individuals do not have normal host resistance. Patients with deficiency of early classic-pathway components generally recover from infections well, but they are at a clear disadvantage when other defense mechanisms are inadequate. They are more likely to die of overwhelming infection than are persons with normal levels of all complement components.

C3 & TERMINAL-COMPONENT DEFICIENCIES

C3 is critical to both the classic and alternative pathways, and, as might be expected, patients with C3 deficiency are prone to develop overwhelming sepsis with high-grade pathogens. Patients with defects in the later-acting terminal components respond quite well to most infectious agents. Their opsonic function, mediated by both the classic and alternative pathways, is intact. However, they have a much higher than normal frequency of disseminated meningococcal and gonococcal (neisserial) infections. Presumably, the lytic function of the late-acting components is required to defend adequately against these highly encapsulated organisms. It is interesting that neisserial infections in individuals with deficiencies in late-acting components follow a quite different course from those in noncomplement-deficient individuals. These infections tend to occur in relatively older individuals, involve different groups of neisserial organisms (untypable and Y type organisms), and are less likely to be lethal than infections that occur in normal individuals. Presumably, such complement-deficient patients synthesize antibody to the organisms, and this antibody provides partial but not complete protection. Individuals with no antibody to the organisms are far more likely to die of overwhelming sepsis than are individuals with antibody.

A large group of C9-deficient individuals has been discovered by mass screening in Japan. The consequences of this defect in the Japanese population are still being evaluated, but it is striking that no major medical illnesses have been reported. It should be recalled that lytic lesions usually can be formed in target cells by the action of the C5–C8 component. The function of C9 is to enlarge and stabilize the C5678 lytic lesion, but the action of C5–C8 on the infecting organism may be sufficient to protect against disease.

COMPLEMENT DEFICIENCIES & AUTOIMMUNITY

Patients missing proteins of the classic or alternative pathway, as well as some individuals with late-component defects, have an unexpectedly high incidence of autoimmune disease, particularly systemic lupus erythematosus (SLE) and glomerulonephritis. It is currently believed that one of the biologic consequences of complement activation is to cause antigen-antibody complexes, once they have bound complement, to adhere to circulating erythrocytes via the erythrocyte complement receptor CR1. Presumably, such complexes, adherent to the erythrocyte surface, are less likely to escape from the circulation into the tissues, where they can cause tissue damage.

The genes for at least 3 complement proteins, C4, C2, and factor B, are located within the major histocompatibility locus on chromosome 6 in humans (class 3 histocompatibility genes). One of these genes, C4, normally exists in 2 copies on each chromosome, coding for 2 different gene products, C4A and C4B. These 2 proteins have biochemical differences, and they differ in their efficiency in mediating complement attack. It is quite common to find individuals missing one or more of the C4 alleles and others deficient in one of the C2 genes. Many investigators have found that such individuals who are heterozygous for the deficiency are more prone to develop the signs and symptoms of autoimmune disease than are normal controls. In particular, individuals missing the C4A alleles and designated C4AqO (for C4A quantity 0) are far more likely to develop SLE. Because the C4B allele is much more active hemolytically and because the range of normal values is wide, these individuals can be identified only by specific characterization of the circulating protein by methods not available in most hospital laboratories.

COMPLEMENT REGULATORY FACTOR DEFICIENCIES

Regulatory proteins that control complement activation may also be deficient. The best-studied and most common of these deficiencies is the partial deficiency of the control protein C1 inhibitor (C1INH). This protein functions to inactivate the subcomponents of C1, C1r, and C1s following their activation by stoichiometrically binding to the enzymatic sites on these proteins. The C1 inhibitor also acts to inactivate activated Hageman factor and its enzymatically active fragments, as well as those pathways activated by Hageman factor, the intrinsic clotting pathway (factor XI), the kinin-generating pathway (kallikrein), and the fibrolytic pathways (plasmin).

HEREDITARY ANGIOEDEMA

The disease of C1INH deficiency, hereditary angioedema, is characterized by recurrent attacks of edema of subcutaneous and submucosal tissues. It particularly affects the extremities and the mucosa of the gastrointestinal tract. Typically, attacks last for 1–4 days and are harmless, although when they involve the bowel wall they usually induce severe abdominal pain. Occasionally, attacks affect subcutaneous and submucosal tissue in the region of the upper airway. In this case they may be associated with respiratory obstruction and asphyxiation. Attacks are sporadic, but in some patients they may be induced by emotional stress or physical trauma. Although attacks usually begin in childhood, they seldom become severe until puberty.

Diagnosis is important, because patients respond poorly to the drugs usually used to treat episodic angioedema: epinephrine, antihistamines, and glucocorticoids. Diagnosis is established by the demonstration of low antigenic or functional levels of C1 esterase inhibitor. Such patients usually have normal levels of C1, low levels of C4 and C2, and normal levels of C3. The actual mechanism of angioedema formation is unknown; investigators have implicated both the complement- and kinin-generating systems in the production of attacks.

Two classes of drugs provide effective therapy. Plasmin inhibitors are fairly effective, although they do not correct the biochemical abnormality (low C4 and C2 levels), suggesting that their principal action is not the inhibition of enzymatic C1. Their mode of action is unknown. The second class of drugs that has proved useful is the group of anabolic steroids or impeded androgens. These agents, particularly the drug danazol, cause an increase in C1 inhibitor, presumably owing to increased synthesis. This leads to a rise in C4 and C2 levels toward normal, and in most patients the drug completely alleviates symptoms. All the useful oral androgens appear to have similar clinical activity, although the effect on levels of C1 inhibitor, C4 and C2 is much less striking with some.

Hereditary angioedema is different from most hereditary complement deficiency diseases in that it results from autosomal dominant rather than recessive inheritance. Individuals with this disease have defective production of C1INH by one of the 2 genes present on chromosome 11. Approximately 85% of patients have one nonproductive gene and have one-third to one-half the normal levels of C1INH. The other 15% of patients have a gene mutation that leads to production of an abnormal C1INH product with no functional activity of the abnormal gene product. The product of one normal gene does not appear to be sufficient to control activation of the various mediator pathways. Hereditary angioedema is treated effectively in most patients by administration of androgens or anabolic steroids. Although the mechanism of action of these drugs is not formally proven, they appear to act by inducing synthesis of the C1INH protein by hepatocytes, thereby correcting the defect. These drugs markedly diminish the frequency and severity of angioedema attacks. For unknown reasons, drugs that inhibit active plasmin are also therapeutically useful. They improve the clinical manifestations but do not correct the C1INH deficiency.

There are rare patients with an acquired form of C1 esterase inhibitor deficiency who present with clinical findings of recurrent angioedema similar to the patients with the inherited form of the disease. In most cases, this is due either to the formation of a monoclonal autoantibody to the C1INH protein that blocks normal C1 inhibitor function or to excessive activation of C1 with utilization of C1INH at a higher rate than the rate of resynthesis. The latter may occur during the course of an autoimmune disease such as SLE or may occur in the setting of a cancer, where it appears that the malignant cell synthesizes molecules that activate C1 and deplete C1 inhibitor. Interestingly, diseases associated with depletion of C1 inhibitor also often respond to treatment with anabolic steroids. Whereas patients with the inherited form of C1 esterase inhibitor deficiency have normal plasma levels of C1 and C3 and markedly depressed levels of C4 and C2, patients with the acquired form have profoundly depressed C1 titers, reflecting the marked activation and utilization of C1 that, in turn, depletes C1 inhibitor.

Patients have also been described who are deficient in the C3 regulatory factors H and I. These individuals also have a higher than expected incidence of infections, reflecting the fact that normal degradation of C3b does not occur, alternative-pathway activation is poorly regulated, and C3 is abnormally consumed. Thus, these individuals act as if they were partially deficient in C3 and other alternative-pathway regulatory factors. They also would be expected to have an abnormally high incidence of autoimmune disease.

COMPLEMENT RECEPTOR DEFICIENCIES

There are many cell membrane-bound complement-regulatory factors. In general, inherited deficiencies of these proteins are rare. A group of children have been identified who fail to express the iC3b receptor (CR3) on their cell surface or who have low expression of the protein. These children fail to express the 3 CD11 membrane proteins. These 3 proteins have different α chains (CD11a, b, and c) and the same β chain (CD18), which is coded for by a gene on chromosome 21, and are members of an adhesion-promoting group of molecules termed **integrens.** The β chain is important in protein transport and this inherited defect causes a failure to transport synthesized CD11/18 proteins to the cell surface. All of these children have phagocytes with defective cell-cell adhesion properties and defective adhesion to glass and other surfaces. The children show abnormal separation of the umbilical cord after birth and have frequent infections, often of the skin.

Acquired deficiencies of cell membrane–bound complement regulatory factors exist. The best studied is the group of defects associated with the acquired disease paroxysmal nocturnal hemoglobinuria (PNH). The regulatory proteins delay-accelerating factor (DAF), homologous restriction factor (HRF), and CD59 are bound to the cell by a glycosidic linkage rather than by a hydrophobic, membrane–spanning domain. The formation of this linkage is abnormal in patients with PNH, and all proteins bound to the cell by similar linkages are absent from progeny of a proportion of the marrow stem cells. Thus affected erythrocytes from PNH patients are missing some or all of the regulatory proteins that prevent formation of the membrane attack complex on autologous cells and are highly susceptible to complement-mediated lysis.

It has been reported that individuals with SLE have decreased numbers of CR1 on their cell surfaces as an inherited defect, but this point remains controversial. Clearly, the expression of CR1 on erythrocytes is an inherited trait, with some individuals showing larger numbers of receptors than others.

COMPLEMENT ALLOTYPE VARIANTS

Many of the complement proteins exist in allotypic forms, with many inherited variants that can be detected by difference in their electrophoretic mobility. Some of these electrophoretic variants show a predilection for certain disease states, especially autoimmune disease. Whether this reflects a change in function of the complement protein caused by a mutation that leads to the electrophoretic variant or a linkage of the gene for one complement variant to other nearby disease-causing genes on the same chromosome that segregate together is not clear. Nevertheless, these cases of linkage disequilibrium have been well documented in population studies.

REFERENCES

General Reviews

Agnello V: Complement deficiency states. *Medicine* 1978;**57**:1.

Ross SC, Densen P: Complement deficiency states and infection: Epidemiology, pathogenesis and consequences of neisserial and other infections in an immune deficiency. *Medicine* 1984;**63**:243.

Complement Deficiency & Infection

Alper CA et al: Increased susceptibility to infection associated with abnormalities of complement-mediated functions and of the third component of complement (C3). *N Engl J Med* 1970;**282**:349.

Densen P et al: Familial properdin deficiency and fatal meningococcemia correction of the bactericidal defect by vaccination. *N Engl J Med* 1987;**316**:922.

Ellison RT et al: Prevalence of congenital or acquired complement deficiency in patients with sporadic meningococcal disease. *N Engl J Med* 1983;**308**:913.

Ellison RT et al: Underlying complement deficiency in patients with disseminated gonococcal infection. *Sex Transm Dis* 1987;**14**:201.

Figuera JE, Densen P: Infectious diseases associated with complement deficiencies. *Clin Microbiol Rev* 1991;**4**:359.

Fine DP et al: Meningococcal meningitis in a woman with inherited deficiency of the ninth component of complement. *Clin Immunol Immunopathol* 1983;**28**:413.

C9 Deficiency in Population Studies

Inai S et al: Deficiency of the ninth C1 component of complement in man. *J Clin Lab Immunol* 1979;**2**:85.

Complement Deficiency & Autoimmunity

Berger M et al: Circulating immune complexes and glomerulonephritis in a patient with congenital absence of the third component of complement. *N Engl J Med* 1983;**308**:1009.

Berliner S et al: Familial systemic lupus erythematosus and C4 deficiency. *Scand J Rheumatol* 1981;**10:280.**

Glass D et al: Inherited deficiency of the second component-complement rheumatic disease association. *J Clin Invest* 1976;**58**:853.

Genetics & HLA Linkage

Colten HR: Genetics and synthesis of components of the complement system. Page 163 in: *Immunobiology of the Complement System.* Ross GD (editor). Academic Press, 1986.

Dawkins RL et al: Disease associations with complotypes, supratypes and haplotypes. *Immunol Rev* 1983;**70**:1.

Howard PF et al: Relationship between C4 null genes, HLA-D region antigens, and genetic susceptibility to systemic lupus erythematosus in Caucasian and black Americans. *Am J Med* 1986;**81**:187.

Rich S et al: Complement and HLA: Further definition of high-risk haplotypes in insulin dependent diabetes. *Diabetes* 1985;**34**:504.

Hereditary Angioedema & Acquired C1 Inhibitor

Alsenz J, Bork K, Loos M: Autoantibody-mediated acquired deficiency of C1 inhibitor. *N Engl J Med* 1987;**316**:1360.

Frank MM, Gelfand JA, Atkinson JP: Hereditary angioedema: The clinical syndrome and its management. *Ann Intern Med* 1976;**84**:580.

Frank MM et al: Epsilon aminocaproic acid therapy of hereditary angioneurotic edema: A double-blind study. *N Engl J Med* 1972;**286**:808.

Gelfand JA et al: Acquired C1 esterase inhibitor deficiency and angioedema: A review. *Medicine* 1979; **58**:321.

Gelfand JA et al: Treatment of hereditary angioedema with danazol: Reversal of clinical and biochemical abnormalities. *N Engl J Med* 1976;**295**:1444.

Rosen FS et al: Genetically determined heterogeneity of the C1 esterase inhibitor in patients with hereditary angioneurotic edema. *J Clin Invest* 1971;**50**:2143.

Schapira M et al: Biochemistry and pathophysiology of human C1 inhibitor: Current issues. *Complement* 1985;**2**:111.

CD11/CD18 Deficiency

Anderson DC et al: The severe and moderate phenotypes of heritable Mac-1, LFA-1 deficiency: Their quantitative definition and relation to leukocyte dysfunction and clinical features. *J Infect Dis* 1985;**152**:668.

Mechanisms of Hypersensitivity

Abba I. Terr, MD

Allergy refers to certain diseases in which immune responses to environmental antigens cause tissue inflammation and organ dysfunction. The clinical features of each allergic disease reflect the immunologically induced inflammatory response in the organ or tissue involved. These features are generally independent of the chemical or physical properties of the antigen. The diversity of allergic responses arises from the involvement of different immunologic effector pathways, each of which generates a unique pattern of inflammation. The classification of allergic diseases is based on the type of immunologic mechanism involved. This chapter will cover mechanisms, classification, and clinical evaluation of the allergic diseases.

DEFINITIONS

An **allergen** is any antigen that causes allergy. The term is used to denote either the antigenic molecule itself or its source, such as pollen grain, animal dander, insect venom, or food product. **Hypersensitivity** and **sensitivity** are often used as synonyms for allergy. **Immediate hypersensitivity** and **delayed hypersensitivity** are the terms formerly used to define antibody-mediated allergy and T lymphocyte-mediated allergy, respectively.

PREVALENCE

Allergy is common throughout the world. The predilection for specific allergic diseases, however, varies among different age groups, sexes, and races. The prevalence of sensitivity to specific allergens is determined both by genetic predilection and by geographic and cultural factors responsible for exposure to the allergen.

ALLERGENS

Any foreign substance capable of inducing an immune response is a potential allergen. Many different chemicals of both natural and synthetic origin are known to be allergenic. Complex natural organic chemicals, especially proteins, are likely to cause antibody-mediated allergy, whereas simple organic compounds, inorganic chemicals, and metals more frequently cause T cell-mediated allergy. In some cases the same allergen may be responsible for more than one type of allergy. Exposure to the allergen may be through inhalation, ingestion, injection, or skin contact.

Allergies caused by certain allergens are encountered frequently in clinical practice, whereas others are rare. Examples of common allergens are the protein Amb a I in ragweed pollen and pentadecylcatechol in poison ivy. Sensitization of a specific individual to a particular environmental allergen is the result of a complex interplay of the chemical and physical properties of the allergen, the mode and quantity of exposure, and the unique genetic makeup of the individual.

SUSCEPTIBILITY TO ALLERGY

A clinical state of allergy affects only some of the individuals who encounter each allergen. The occurrence of allergic disease on exposure to an allergen requires not only prior sensitization but also other factors that determine the localization of the reaction to a particular organ (Table 24–1). This is particularly evident in atopic allergy, where sensitization may cause disease localized to the nasal mucosa, the bronchial mucosa, the skin, the gastrointestinal tract, or a combination of 2 or more of these sites (see Fig 25–1). The nonimmunologic factors involved in the expression of clinical atopic disease are not yet known, although a disturbance in autonomic control,

Table 24–1. Factors that determine expression of disease in allergy.

Allergen Exposure	Allergic Sensitization	Target Organ Susceptibility	Clinical Disease	Type of Disease
− or +	−	−	−	No disease
+	+	−	−	Asymptomatic sensitivity
+	+	+	+	Allergic disease
− or +	−	+	+	Nonallergic disease

such as β-adrenergic blockade or cholinergic hyper-reactivity in the target tissue, has been postulated.

Most of the diseases in which allergy is expressed, eg, asthma, rhinitis, atopic dermatitis, contact dermatitis, anaphylaxis, and urticaria-angioedema, can occur in the absence of allergy. Recognition of these nonimmunologic diseases is important in differential diagnosis. In some cases, environmental triggers are nonspecific or cannot be identified. In other cases a specific environmental agent activates inflammatory mediators nonimmunologically. Examples of the latter phenomenon include direct mast cell release of histamine by opiate drugs, aspirin-induced asthma (possibly an aberrant metabolism of arachidonic acid), anaphylactoid reactions from radioiodinated contrast media, urticaria from eating shellfish and berries, and occupational isocyanate asthma. In these examples, no allergen-specific immunologic sensitivity has been shown to be responsible for the reaction, even though the disease occurs in only a limited percentage of the exposed population.

MECHANISMS & CLASSIFICATION OF ALLERGIC DISEASE

Allergy is an immunologic phenomenon. The disease results when an exposure to the allergen induces an immune response, referred to as "sensitization" rather than immunization (Fig 24–1A). Once sensitization occurs, an individual will not be symptomatic until there is an exposure to the allergen. Then the reaction of allergen with specific antibody or sensitized effector T lymphocyte induces an inflammatory response, producing the symptoms and signs of the allergic reaction (Fig 24–1B).

Among the currently recognized pathways of immunologically induced inflammation (see Chapter 11), 3 different ones are responsible for the known allergic diseases: (1) the IgE/mast cell/mediator pathway, (2) the IgG or IgM immune complex/complement/neutrophil pathway, and (3) the effector T lymphocyte/lymphokine pathway. Specific diseases associated with each of these processes are shown in

Table 24–2 and are discussed in the following 3 chapters. A brief description of the immunologic mechanisms is given here. More detailed information can be found in the first section of this book.

THE IgE/MAST CELL/MEDIATOR PATHWAY

IgE antibodies have a unique configuration on the Fc portion of the molecule for fixation to mast cells (Fig 24–2). Fixation occurs at a high-affinity mast cell surface receptor, FcεRI. The allergic reaction is initiated when the polyvalent allergen molecule reacts with antibodies occupying these receptors. The result is a bridging of FcεRI, thereby altering the cell surface membrane. This, in turn, signals intracellular events causing release and activation of mediators of inflammation: histamine, leukotrienes, chemotactic factors, platelet-activating factor, and proteases. Mast cell activation is modulated by intracellular cyclic nucleotides and is accompanied by cell degranulation. The released activated mediators act locally and cause increased vascular permeability, vasodilation, smooth muscle contraction, and mucous gland secretion. These biologic events account for the salient clinical features of the **immediate phase,** occurring in the first 15–30 minutes following allergen exposure. Over the succeeding 12 hours there is a progressive tissue infiltration of inflammatory cells, proceeding

Table 24–2. Classification of allergic diseases based on immunologic mechanisms.

1. **Allergic disease caused by IgE antibodies and mast cell mediators**
   a. Atopic diseases
      1. Allergic rhinitis
      2. Allergic asthma
      3. Atopic dermatitis
      4. Allergic gastroenteropathy
   b. Anaphylactic diseases
      1. Systemic anaphylaxis
      2. Urticaria-angioedema
2. **Allergic disease caused by IgG or IgM antibodies and complement activation**
   a. Serum sickness
   b. Acute hypersensitivity pneumonitis
3. **Allergic disease caused by sensitized T lymphocytes**
   a. Allergic contact dermatitis
   b. Chronic hypersensitivity pneumonitis

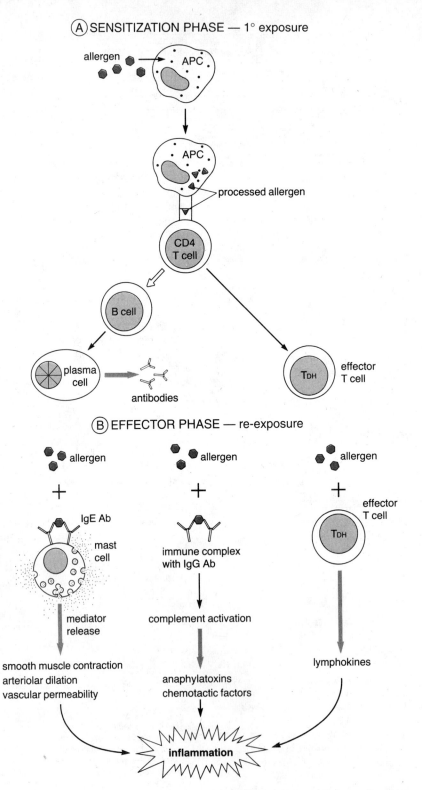

Figure 24–1. Role of the immune system in allergy. **A:** Sensitization phase, showing immunologic response to allergen from unsensitized (nonallergic) state to sensitized (allergic) state. **B:** Effector phase, showing reaction on reexposure of allergen to specific antibody or to specifically sensitized effector T cell.

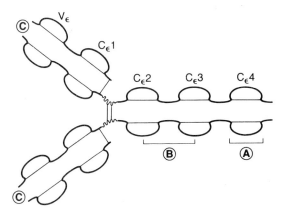

Figure 24–2. Schematic diagram of the IgE antibody molecule. The structure is similar to that of IgG, but there is an additional H chain domain (**A**), accounting for its higher molecular weight. The regions of the molecule containing the site for fixation to mast cell FcεRI (**B**) and the allergen-binding sites (**C**) are indicated.

from neutrophils to eosinophils to mononuclear cells in response to other chemical mediators and biochemical events not yet fully delineated. The period of 6–12 hours after allergen exposure is designated the **late phase** of the IgE response and is characterized by clinical manifestations of cellular inflammation.

This mechanism is responsible for the atopic diseases, anaphylaxis, and urticaria. The reaction can be triggered by extremely small amounts of allergen.

THE IgG OR IgM/COMPLEMENT/ NEUTROPHIL PATHWAY

IgG or IgM antibodies form complexes with antigen, and such complexes cause tissue inflammation. This pathway contributes to the pathogenesis of many human diseases, including certain allergic diseases. Allergen-antibody complexes activate the complement system through the classic pathway via receptors on C1q for the Fc portion of the IgG or IgM antibody molecule. Complement activation generates anaphylatoxins and chemotactic peptides, which cause increased vascular permeability and infiltration of neutrophils. Activated neutrophils generate additional inflammatory and toxic products. Macrophages are also recruited and become activated, contributing further to tissue inflammation and injury.

This mechanism is responsible for the cutaneous Arthus reaction, serum sickness, and the acute phase of hypersensitivity pneumonitis (extrinsic allergic alveolitis). Because immune complexes in moderate antigen excess are the most efficient for activating C1q, relatively large quantities of allergen are required to initiate the reaction.

THE EFFECTOR T LYMPHOCYTE/ LYMPHOKINE PATHWAY

Some allergic diseases are not mediated by antibody but, rather, by reaction of allergen with the effector T lymphocyte sensitized to the specific allergen from a prior exposure. The effector T cell has the CD4 phenotype, and when it encounters the allergen it is activated to generate lymphokines; this results in the accumulation over several days of a mononuclear cell infiltrate.

Other immunologic pathways leading to inflammation have been studied so far only at an in vitro level but have not yet been clearly identified as the primary pathogenetic mechanism of human disease. These potential mechanisms for allergy are listed in Table 24–3. They may play a secondary role in diseases caused by the 3 primary pathways described above.

CLINICAL EVALUATION

GENERAL CONSIDERATIONS

When allergy is suspected, the diagnostic process is aimed at determining whether the disease is caused by allergy and, if so, to identify the type of allergy and each of the responsible allergens. Many straightforward cases of seasonal hay fever caused by pollen or contact dermatitis caused by poison ivy can be diagnosed easily and quickly, but more complex or obscure allergic diseases require considerable detective work. History, physical examination, and appropriate laboratory tests are required, as in the diagnosis of any medical condition.

HISTORY

The history is essential. It is critically important to correlate results of specific allergy testing to the patient's history. Whenever allergy is suspected, the physician should be prepared first to obtain a detailed

Table 24–3. Immunologic pathways potentially capable of allergen-antibody activation.

1. Alternative complement pathway activation via IgA antibodies
2. Anaphylatoxins (C3a, C5a, C4a) generated by classic or alternative pathway complement activation
3. IgG4 antibody activation of mast cells for mediator release
4. Complement activation of the kininogen-kallikrein-kinin system

description of the symptoms and the timing and environmental locations associated with appearance and disappearance of those symptoms. Allergen exposure may occur through inhalation, ingestion, injection, or skin or mucous membrane contact. Variations in symptoms during the course of a day, week, month, and year and the association with home, work, school, or vacation trips are useful clues in diagnosis of the common inhalant and occupational allergies. When inhalant allergy is suspected, an environmental history should include details of work, hobbies, pets, and the influence of weather and climate on respiratory symptoms. A history of medication usage and dietary habits is relevant for possible ingested allergens. Drugs and insect bites and stings may cause allergy by injection. When allergic contact dermatitis is suspected, the physician should inquire especially about exposure to plants, perfumes, cosmetics, clothing, topical medications, work, and hobbies.

Other important historical data are the age of onset, the course of the illness, and the effect of hormonal factors such as puberty, menstrual-cycle variations, and pregnancy. The influence of prior treatments such as antihistamine drugs, antibiotics, and corticosteroids may help to distinguish allergic from nonallergic conditions. The presence of other known allergies and results of prior allergy evaluations in the patient, as well as family history of allergy, may also be helpful.

Many allergists use standard questionnaires for part or all of the history. If the questionnaire is self-administered, the patient's answers should be reviewed by the physician.

PHYSICAL EXAMINATION

Allergic diseases are often episodic, because signs and symptoms are dependent upon exposure to the allergen. Objective signs of allergy are therefore present when the physical examination is performed during the period of allergen exposure. A negative physical examination performed during a period of allergen avoidance does not mean that the patient does not have allergy. The examination should be thorough enough to rule out other causes for the patient's symptoms. In allergic dermatoses the appearance, distribution, and extent of the skin lesions will direct the questioning to likely environmental sources of the allergen.

LABORATORY TESTING

A variety of laboratory tests are available to supplement the history and physical examination. There are procedures for quantitating the extent of functional and anatomic effects on a particular organ, for sampling fluids or tissues for evidence of disease, and

for establishing the presence of specific immune responses.

1. TESTS OF AIRWAY FUNCTION

The standard pulmonary-function tests quantitate the amount of obstructive airway and restrictive lung disease in patients with respiratory allergy. Reversible airway obstruction can be shown by bronchodilator response in a patient with current airway obstruction or by bronchoconstrictor response in a patient without baseline airway obstruction. Tests of nasal airway resistance are available but are not suitable for routine use. Tympanometry may aid in diagnosis of otitis media complicating allergic rhinosinusitis.

Airway hyperirritability in patients with asthma can be quantitated by bronchoprovocation tests with inhalation of certain chemicals (histamine, methacholine) or with physical stimuli (exercise). The former are more sensitive but may be positive in non-asthmatics under certain conditions, whereas the latter are more specific to asthma but less sensitive.

The usual measurement used for the various bronchoprovocation tests is a fall in 1-second forced expiratory volume (FEV_1), which can be rapidly and reproducibly measured by spirometry. Increasing doses of aerosolized methacholine or histamine are delivered by nebulizer, and the provocative dose causing a 20% fall in FEV_1 is designated PD_{20}.

Physical challenges with exercise, cold dry isocapnic hyperventilation, or ultrasonically nebulized distilled water have also been standardized for detecting nonspecific bronchial hyperirritability. The mechanisms involved are not understood precisely, although these physical stimuli possibly stimulate bronchial mast cells to release mediators non-immunologically, whereas histamine and methacholine act directly on bronchial smooth muscle. In all cases of nonspecific testing, maximal bronchoconstriction is achieved in about 5 minutes, with reversion to baseline in 15–20 minutes without a late-phase response (Fig 24–3). Rarely, methacholine may produce a prolonged, severe episode of asthma that requires treatment. The procedures can be performed in an outpatient setting, but emergency equipment should be available in the event of a severe induced asthma attack.

Any one of these tests can be used to assist in diagnosis of asthma in patients with a history of symptoms but negative tests for reversible airway obstruction. Under these conditions a negative methacholine challenge test rules out asthma. However, a positive test indicating airway hyperirritability may be obtained in other conditions such as (1) allergic rhinitis, especially during the pollen season; (2) following a viral respiratory infection or recent immunization with influenza or live measles vaccine; (3) in some relatives of asthmatics; and (4) in a small portion of

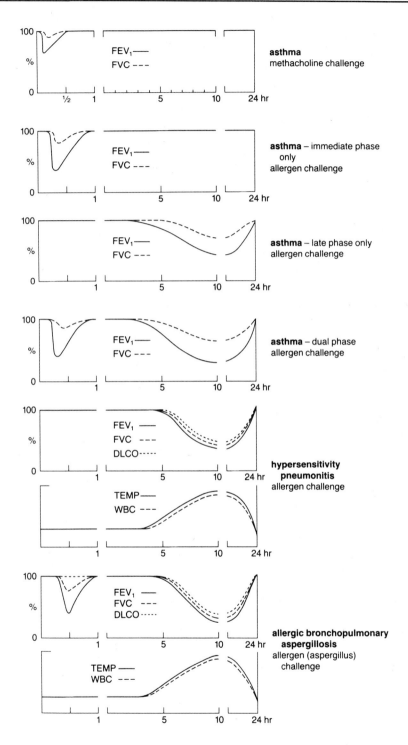

Figure 24–3. Bronchial provocation tests for detection of nonspecific bronchial hyperirritability (methacholine challenge) or immunologic reactivity (allergen challenge). Shown are the responses in patients with asthma (IgE antibody sensitivity), hypersensitivity pneumonitis (principally T cell-mediated sensitivity), and allergic bronchopulmonary aspergillosis (combined IgE and IgG antibody sensitivities). FEV$_1$, forced expiratory volume in 1 second; FVC, forced vital capacity; DLCO, diffusing capacity for carbon monoxide; TEMP, temperature; WBC, leukocyte count.

the normal population. The test has been especially helpful in diagnosis and screening for potential occupational asthma. Recent clinical studies suggest that it might be used in monitoring allergen immunotherapy for asthma.

2. ANATOMIC TESTS

Visualization of paranasal sinuses, lungs, and the gastrointestinal tract may require x-ray, computed tomography, or endoscopy.

3. TISSUE DIAGNOSIS

When appropriate, samples of nasal or sinus secretions, sputum, bronchoalveolar fluid, gastrointestinal secretions, stool, or blood can be examined for inflammatory cell content. These studies, as well as histopathology of biopsy specimens from tissues of patients with suspected allergic disease, may confirm the type of inflammation associated with a particular type of allergic response, but they do not identify the causative allergen.

4. ALLERGY SKIN TESTING

A variety of skin test methods are used in the clinical diagnosis of each type of allergic disease. The skin test is a bioassay for the presence or absence of an immune response to a specific allergen that sets off a particular effector mechanism of inflammation and a visible transient skin lesion. The skin is a convenient organ to test, since it is equipped with all of the elements necessary for eliciting a localized controlled allergic reaction, even though the disease is targeted to another organ.

For diagnosis, skin testing occupies an intermediate position between in vitro tests, which demonstrate specific immune response only, and in vivo provocation tests, which demonstrate the ability of the diseased target organ to respond immunologically to the allergen. Skin tests require some skill in performance and interpretation, but they have many advantages. The tests are convenient, inexpensive, and safe if done properly. Results are available with no delay beyond the time required for the allergic response. There is no possibility of sample (ie, patient) error. Many suspected allergens can be tested simultaneously. Discomfort is usually minimal.

The principal disadvantage of skin testing is the need to discontinue certain inhibitory drugs. Occasionally, skin testing is prohibited for lack of available skin because of generalized dermatitis. The procedure may be unacceptable to some small children and adults. The potential for a systemic reaction or flare of the disease exists, but these are exceedingly unlikely with proper precautions.

Patch Tests

The patch test stimulates allergic contact dermatitis on a small patch of skin to which a known concentration of allergen is applied. It is therefore a true provocative test of the disease. In most cases of allergic contact dermatitis, the allergen is a chemical that couples to skin protein, yielding a hapten-protein conjugate. This conjugate then reacts with sensitized cutaneous T lymphocytes to liberate lymphokines, which produce localized cell-mediated inflammation at the site of contact with the test allergen.

A. Method: The concentration of allergen, usually a chemical, is determined by prior testing of several allergic and nonallergic subjects. It must be high enough to elicit a positive reaction in the former but not high enough to cause skin irritation in the latter. Two test methods are available. In the open patch method a drop of acetone extract is applied to the skin. The acetone quickly dries, depositing the test chemical on the skin site, which is left uncovered and inspected after 48 hours. In the closed patch method the allergen in petrolatum is applied to a pad taped to the skin. After 48 hours the pad is removed and the site is inspected. A positive test consists of erythema, papules, or vesicles. If the test is negative, the site should be examined again at 72 and 96 hours, because weak reactions may appear later. Multiple tests can be performed simultaneously. Preferred areas for testing are the back, forearms, or upper arms.

About 20 chemicals cause most cases of allergic contact dermatitis (see Chapter 28). Textbooks on contact dermatitis should be consulted for proper concentrations of many other known contact sensitizers.

Systemic corticosteroid drugs inhibit cell-mediated hypersensitivity and should be discontinued prior to testing. Antihistamines and other antiallergy drugs need not be discontinued.

B. Indications: The patch test is indicated for diagnosis of allergic contact dermatitis if the cause is not apparent by history and distribution of the lesions. When the disease is caused by a topical medication, cosmetic, or other product containing a number of chemical components, each component should be tested separately so that allergen elimination can be specific.

C. Adverse Effects: A strongly positive test in a patient with severe allergy may cause considerable itching and discomfort, in which case the patch should be removed in less than 48 hours. Patch testing during the active phase of contact dermatitis may exacerbate the disease. Whenever possible, the dermatitis should be cleared by treatment before the test is begun. Occasionally the test itself can induce sensitivity, so the selection of test allergens should be limited to those suspected clinically.

D. Photopatch Test: This is a test for photoallergic contact dermatitis. The procedure is identical to the patch test, except that the test site is exposed to ultraviolet light or sunlight after the patch is removed, and the reaction is read after 24 hours and again after 48 hours. A control site is a patch test to the allergen without light exposure.

Cutaneous Tests

The cutaneous test (prick test, puncture test, epicutaneous test) introduces into the dermis, at a single point, a minute quantity of allergen sufficient to react with IgE antibodies fixed to cutaneous mast cells for release of mediators to produce a visible wheal and erythema (Fig 24–4A). It is the procedure least likely to produce systemic anaphylaxis, because of the small amount of allergen introduced into the skin. For the same reason it is also unlikely to elicit an Arthus or cell-mediated skin reaction.

For routine diagnosis in atopic and anaphylactic diseases, a single drop of concentrated aqueous allergen extract in buffered saline diluent at pH 6.0 is placed on the skin, which is then pricked lightly with a needle point at the center of the drop. After 20 minutes the reaction is graded and recorded as indicated in Table 24–4. A negative diluent control must be included. Positive controls of histamine or a nonspecific mast cell mediator-releasing agent such as codeine, or both, may be included. The skin of the back, volar aspect of the forearms, or upper arms can be used. Fifty or more allergens can be tested at one time on the back, but test sites should be at least 3.5 cm apart. A result of 2+ or greater is positive. A result of 0 or 1+ should be repeated by using the intracutaneous method. A late phase reaction is not usually elicited by prick testing.

Another cutaneous testing method is the scratch test, in which a short linear scratch is made in the skin, to which the allergen is then applied. It is not recommended because it frequently causes nonspecific irritation, it is painful, and occasionally it causes scarring.

Any drug with antihistaminic (H_1-receptor blocking) activity must be discontinued for an appropriate period (24 hours or longer, depending upon the drug) prior to testing. The new nonsedating antihistamines have long half-lives and inhibit skin testing for weeks. Some drugs prescribed for other diseases, notably the tricyclic antidepressants, are potent antihistaminics. Corticosteroids, theophylline, sympathomi-

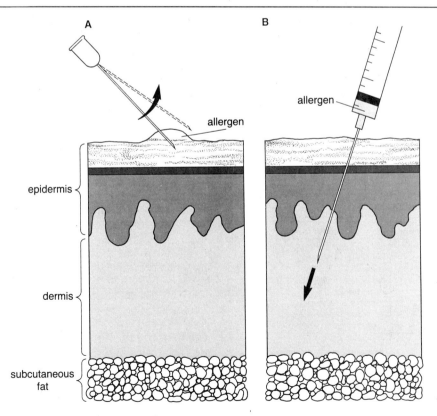

Figure 24–4. The technique of allergy skin testing. **A:** Cutaneous test. **B:** Intradermal test.

metic drugs, and cromolyn do not inhibit immediate skin test reactions and need not be withdrawn prior to testing.

Intradermal Tests

In the intradermal skin test (intracutaneous test), a measured quantity of allergen is introduced into the skin for detection of IgE-mediated (atopic or anaphylactic), IgG-mediated (immune complex), or effector T lymphocyte-mediated (cellular or delayed hypersensitivity) responses (Fig 24–4B). It is therefore used in diagnosis of several different types of allergic diseases.

Intradermal tests should be applied to the arm only, so that a tourniquet can be used in the event of an unexpected systemic reaction. The allergen extract must be nontoxic and free of microbial contaminants. A tuberculin syringe with 27-gauge needle is used, and the volume to be injected depends on the immunologic effector mechanism under study.

For IgE-mediated sensitivities, the recommended volume ranges from 0.005 to 0.02 mL, but is usually 0.01 mL. Larger volumes are unnecessary and cause confusing results. In most cases, intradermal testing in suspected IgE-mediated diseases is performed only for allergens giving negative or at most 1+ responses to prior prick testing (see above), since the intradermal test is approximately 1000 times more sensitive. The reaction is read in 20 minutes (Table 24–4). A 1:500 (wt/vol) dilution of most common inhalant allergens is satisfactory for diagnosis of atopic allergy. A negative diluent control is necessary. A positive histamine or histamine-release control, or both, is optional but recommended if the patient has recently taken antihistamines.

After the immediate wheal-and-erythema subside, a late-phase 6–12 hour reaction appears in some cases. The diagnostic significance of the late-phase skin reaction is currently uncertain.

Serial dilution (skin endpoint) titration is a semi-quantitative form of intradermal testing in which 5- or 10-fold increasing concentrations of allergen extract are tested for each allergen until a positive result occurs. Skin test sensitivity correlates roughly with clinical target organ sensitivity, but the main purpose of serial titration is to determine a starting dose for immunotherapy that will avoid the risk of systemic reaction. It is routinely used in testing for Hymenoptera insect venom anaphylaxis. Some physicians titrate atopic allergens in testing, but this is not recommended because it requires many more injections than the standard 2-stage prick and single-dose intradermal test, which can be quantitated by the size of the reaction.

Antihistamine drugs inhibit the intradermal wheal-and-erythema skin test reactions, as discussed above.

Intradermal testing can be used to detect circulating IgG antibodies in a suspected Arthus reaction. The cutaneous Arthus reaction is grossly similar to the late-phase IgE antibody reaction in appearance and timing, except that there is no preceding immediate-phase wheal-and-erythema and a high concentration of injection allergen is required to elicit a positive test. Immune-complex allergic reactions are infrequent in clinical practice (see Chapter 27), and IgG antibodies can usually be detected in vitro, so the Arthus skin test has not been standardized and is rarely used. A preliminary prick test should be done so that the procedure can be withheld if the patient has a significant (coincidental) IgE sensitivity to the allergen.

The tuberculin test is an intradermal test for cell-mediated hypersensitivity or immunity. It is performed by injecting 0.10 mL of the test allergen intradermally. There is a delayed (onset after 12 hours or more) response of erythema, induration, and tenderness. A positive test consists of induration 10 mm or greater in diameter of 48 hours. The test is not used in clinical diagnosis of cell-mediated allergies (see Chapter 13), but it is used extensively for detecting immunity in certain infections and in assessing cellular immunodeficiency (see Chapter 17).

Passive Transfer of the Skin Test

The immediate wheal-and-erythema skin test reaction in atopy or anaphylaxis can be transferred from the allergic patient to a nonallergic subject by injecting serum containing the IgE antibody from the former into the skin of the latter, proving an antibody causation for the disease. This is known as the Prausnitz-Küstner reaction. Cell-mediated skin test reactions, on the other hand, can be transferred by specifically sensitized effector T lymphocytes and not by serum antibodies. These serum or cell passive transfer procedures have been invaluable in research and have been used to a limited extent in the past for diagnosis. Their use in clinical practice is no longer justified, because of the risk of transmitting blood-borne microorganisms and the availability of the other testing methods discussed below.

Table 24–4. Wheal-and-erythema skin tests.

Test	Reaction	Appearances
Prick	Neg	No wheal or erythema.
	1+	No wheal; erythema < 20 mm in diameter.
	2+	No wheal; erythema > 20 mm in diameter.
	3+	Wheal and erythema.
	4+	Wheal with pseudopods; erythema.
Intracutan-eous	Neg	Same as control.
	1+	Wheal twice as large as control; erythema < 20 mm in diameter.
	2+	Wheal twice as large as control; erythema > 20 mm in diameter.
	3+	Wheal 3 times as large as control; erythema.
	4+	Wheal with pseudopods; erythema.

5. IN VITRO TESTS

The need for in vitro diagnostic tests for allergies that use blood (or occasionally other body fluids) stems from the potential danger, the perceived discomfort, and the subjectivity of in vivo tests. In vitro tests can provide precision, reproducibility, and efficiency. Blood samples can be stored so that serial testing of samples drawn at different times can be performed simultaneously under identical conditions. In vitro tests are especially well suited for large-scale population screening and for testing allergens that are potentially toxic or irritating. They are useful in situations in which in vivo testing is thwarted by other factors, eg, the inability to do skin tests in a patient with extensive dermatitis or in an uncooperative child.

In vitro tests, however, frequently measure only isolated components of the complex events in an allergic reaction (Fig 24–5). The clinical expression of allergy requires not only an immune response (the sensitized state), but also a properly reactive target tissue or organ, and exposure to a sufficient amount of allergen. The reaction can be further modified by extraneous factors such as age, endogenous endocrine hormone output, psychologic factors, and medications. All in vitro tests have limitations in sensitivity and are dependent on the quality of the allergen and reagents and on other technical factors. Results of any test must always be interpreted in the context of the history, physical examination, and other diagnostic procedures.

Tests for IgE Antibodies

Quantitative measurement of allergen-specific IgE antibodies in serum requires special methods to detect the extremely minute quantities (picograms per milliliter) found in allergic patients. The standard technique is the **radioallergosorbent test (RAST).** This is a 2-phase (solid/liquid) system using an insolubilized allergen that is incubated first in the test serum to react with allergen-specific antibodies and then in radiolabeled heterologous anti-human IgE to detect the allergen-specific antibodies of the IgE isotype. The method is diagrammed and described in Fig 24–6. The test requires purified preparations of allergens and anti-human IgE. The RAST uses a cellulose disk as the insoluble immunosorbent to which protein allergens are coupled covalently with cyanogen bromide. There are a number of modifications of this method in which other immunosorbents and other detection labeling systems (various chemicals detected by fluorescence or colorimetry) are used.

Disadvantages of these in vitro methods are both biologic and technical. The quantity of serum IgE antibody is not necessarily a direct reflection of the biologically relevant mast cell-fixed antibody. The test result may be falsely positive in patients with a high total IgE level because of nonspecific binding of allergen to some immunosorbents, and it may be falsely low in desensitized patients with high levels of IgG antibody. Like all other allergy tests, results must be interpreted in the context of the clinical history and examination.

Tests for IgG Antibodies

These are discussed in Chapter 12.

Tests of Immune Complexes

These are discussed in Chapter 12.

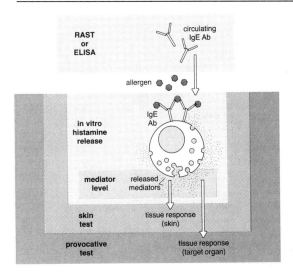
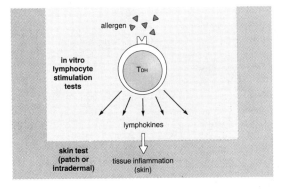

A **B**

Figure 24–5. Schematic diagram showing the components of IgE-mediated (**A**) and T cell-mediated (**B**) allergic reactions that are detected by various diagnostic procedures.

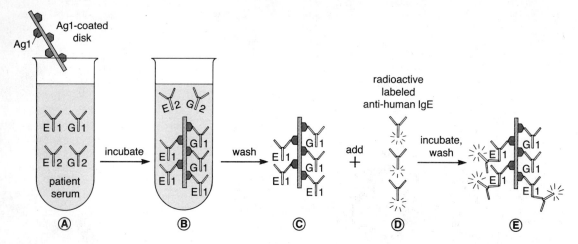

Figure 24–6. Diagram of radioallergosorbent test (RAST). **A:** A disk coated with the test allergen (Ag1) is incubated with serum of a patient with allergy to Ag1, as well as to other allergens (Ag2). **B:** IgE antibodies to Ag1 (E1) and IgG antibodies to the same allergen (G1) react with the Ag1-coated disk, whereas IgE and IgG antibodies (E2, G2) do not, and they remain in the serum. **C,D:** After being washed, the disk is incubated with a radiolabeled heterologous antibody to human IgE. **E:** After the disk is washed to remove unreacted labeled anti-IgE, the amount of radioactivity measured in a gamma counter is proportionate to the quantity of specific IgE antibody (E1) in the patient's serum. IgG antibodies to the same allergen (G1) on the disk do not react with the anti-human IgE antibody.

Lymphocyte Stimulation

This is discussed in Chapter 13.

6. PROVOCATIVE TESTS

Occasionally it is desirable to test the target (respiratory, gastrointestinal, or cutaneous) tissue responsiveness to the allergen under controlled conditions. The patch test for immediate contact urticaria or delayed contact dermatitis is such a procedure. In the nasal provocation test, changes in nasal airway resistance and visible signs of congestion and rhinorrhea are observed after exposure to quantitative allergen challenge. Timed changes in bronchial airway flow rate or resistance are measured by bronchial provocation. Oral challenge with food or drug may be done to observe subjective gastrointestinal symptoms, appearance of skin eruptions, or objective changes in airway resistance.

A positive provocation test does not prove an immunologic basis for the disease, and except for patch testing, they are not used for routine diagnosis. Provocation testing is, however, an invaluable research tool for studying pathogenetic mechanisms and drug efficacy in allergic disease.

Allergen Bronchoprovocation Testing

Inhalational challenge with aerosolized allergen extracts to provoke a bronchial or pulmonary reaction under controlled conditions in the laboratory is of limited use in clinical practice. It is applicable in testing for allergic asthma and hypersensitivity pneumonitis (Fig 24–3).

The method of nebulizing and delivering known quantities of allergen extract is the same as for the methacholine challenge test (see above). Aqueous allergen extracts in several dilutions are prepared in buffered saline. An initial titration skin testing is necessary to determine a safe starting dose for bronchial challenge.

For testing in patients with allergic asthma, a measurement sensitive to acute airway obstruction is used, as in the methacholine challenge, and the dose-response result is presented in the same fashion. Usually the change in FEV_1 is expressed by determination of PD_{20} (the provocative dose of allergen that causes a 20% fall in FEV_1). Provocation tests have been done with the common inhalant atopic allergens, occupational allergens, and various chemicals. A fall in FEV_1 begins in 10 minutes or less, peaks at 20–30 minutes, and then returns to baseline. This immediate-phase asthmatic response occurs slightly later after allergen challenge than is the case for methacholine, histamine, or physical challenge. It is likely to be more severe and unpredictable, and it may require treatment with an inhaled bronchodilator drug. There may be a late-phase asthmatic response beginning at 4–6 hours, peaking at 8–12 hours, and clearing by 24 hours. Allergen challenges may cause isolated early or late responses, or both. Therefore, pulmonary function monitoring should be continued at hourly intervals after the immediate phase has subsided. Because of the possibility of late-phase responses, allergen bronchoprovocation should be performed in a hospital with appropriate facilities for detecting and treating these reactions. A positive late-phase response may increase the patient's nonspecific bronchial hyperirritability for several days, so if a second allergen is to be tested, this should be done at least 1 week later.

The indications for provocation testing in clinical practice are limited. For routine diagnosis of atopic asthma, bronchoprovocation with allergen gives results that correlate well with skin tests, but patients with only allergic rhinitis may also have specific bronchial response to inhaled allergen extract. A positive test to a suspected causative agent of occupational asthma does not necessarily mean that the asthma is immunologic. For example, bronchoprovocation with isocyanates produces specific immediate and late asthmatic responses in workers with clinical isocyanate asthma, even though the illness does not correlate well with an IgE (or other) immune response to this chemical. Allergen bronchoprovocation may be useful to monitor desensitization therapy.

Allergen bronchoprovocation is especially helpful in cases of suspected hypersensitivity pneumonitis. The method of delivery of allergen is the same as in tests for asthma, but pulmonary function measurements should be sensitive to measures of restrictive lung disease. The fall in forced vital capacity (FVC) and diffusing capacity for CO, as well as fever and leukocytosis, begin 4–6 hours after challenge, reach maximum effect at 8 hours, and return to normal values by 24 hours in patients with acute hypersensitivity pneumonitis.

To quantitate and standardize allergen challenges, it is necessary to use aerosolized aqueous extracts. The procedure therefore does not stimulate natural allergic asthma or hypersensitivity pneumonitis caused by particulate allergens, as in the case of pollen and mold asthma, in which the inhaled material is in the form of particles up to 60 μm in diameter. Particles of this size, when inhaled naturally, do not reach the tracheobronchial tree, in contrast to liquid aerosols 1–5 μm in diameter, which do so readily.

Nasal Provocation Testing

An objective quantitative test of nasal mucosal reactivity to allergen or nonimmunologic stimulus is not available for routine diagnosis because of technical difficulties in assessing nasal reactivity. Present methods of rhinomanometry for measuring nasal airway resistance are limited by artifacts and poor patient acceptance. Nasal airflow is subject to anatomic factors, atmospheric conditions, psychologic stimuli, and physiologic fluctuations. Quantitation of rhinorrhea, sneezing, or itching is crude and subjective.

Nasal provocation testing has been useful in research but not in clinical practice.

Elimination Diet Testing

Dietary elimination and challenge with foods suspected of causing urticaria or exacerbating atopic dermatitis, asthma, and gastrointestinal or other symptoms are commonly used by allergists. The procedure is not standardized but, rather, is tailored to each individual diagnostic situation. Elimination diets aim to alleviate ongoing symptoms. One or more foods, depending on the history, are eliminated until symptoms disappear. If symptoms are intermittent, a preliminary diet-symptom record may reveal the food(s) to be eliminated. If necessary, all natural foods are eliminated and nutrition is maintained by artificial diet, but restrictive diets should not be continued for more than 2 weeks. If symptoms clear, the eliminated foods are reintroduced one at a time to determine which food or foods provoke the allergic reaction or symptoms. A positive food challenge is repeated several more times for verification, but a single negative result generally rules out allergy to that food. There are no standard time limits for elimination or challenge, but, traditionally, most allergists accept a positive challenge within 2 hours to the same food on 3 successive trials as valid proof of a cause-and-effect relationship, although other information would be necessary to determine the mechanism. The clinical features of the induced reaction and evidence by skin or in vitro test of the relevant immune response will distinguish allergic reactions from toxic, digestive, metabolic, or psychologic responses to the food.

These elimination challenge maneuvers are subjective and greatly prone to erroneous diagnosis of food allergy because of physician and patient bias. A history of an acute allergic reaction to a single food allergen, supplemented if necessary by elimination and challenge testing and accompanied by IgE antibody detected by skin or in vitro test, is sufficient for diagnosis and therapeutic elimination of that food. In other situations in which delayed reactions, atypical or elusive symptoms and signs, and multiple suspect foods might lead to a nutritionally inadequate therapeutic elimination diet, the method of double-blind oral provocation testing should be employed.

Oral Provocation Testing

Double-blind food challenges are critical in defining the role of foods in allergic diseases. The procedure is simple and inexpensive enough to be used in clinical practice, although it is time-consuming. Patients with a history of anaphylaxis to a food should not be deliberately challenged.

Freeze-dried foods are packed into large opaque gelatin capsules. Each capsule can contain up to 600 mg of dry food. Lactose or a food to which the patient is not allergic can be used as a placebo control. The patient swallows a specified dose determined by the number of capsules and is observed for symptoms, signs, and an appropriate objective measure such as a pulmonary function test. The observation time and measurements are based on the history. The order and frequency of active and placebo challenges are determined by a double-blind protocol. If a severe reaction is anticipated, increasing doses are given, starting as low as 10 mg of dried food and increasing to an amount corresponding to the amount suspected to cause a reaction by history. As much as 8 g can be consumed in capsule form by most patients. Some foods can be disguised in flavored milk shakes. A negative double-blind food challenge should be confirmed by an open dietary trial of the same food, since freeze-drying and encapsulating the food could conceivably change its allergenicity. When properly performed, this procedure is a powerful tool for avoiding an unsubstantiated diagnosis of food allergy when the test is negative. It is important to remember that a positive response shows only an intolerance to the food and does not prove an allergic pathogenesis.

REFERENCES

General

deShazo RD, Smith DL (editors): Primer on allergic and immunologic diseases, second edition. *JAMA* 1992;**268**:2785. (Entire issue.)

Middleton E et al. (editors): *Allergy: Principles and Practice,* 4th ed. Mosby, 1993.

Patterson R (editors): *Allergic Diseases: Diagnosis and Management,* 4th ed. Lippincott, 1993.

Ricci M, Rossi O: Dysregulation of IgE responses and airway allergic inflammation in atopic individuals. *Clin Exp Allergy* 1990;**20**:601.

Samter M (editor): *Immunologic Diseases,* 4th ed. Little, Brown, 1988.

Diagnosis

Adkinson NF: The radioallergosorbent test in 1981: Limitations and refinement. *J Allergy Clin Immunol* 1981;**67**:87.

AMA Council on Scientific Affairs: In vivo diagnostic testing and immunotherapy for allergy. Part I. *JAMA* 1987;**258**:1363.

AMA Council on Scientific Affairs: In vivo diagnostic testing and immunotherapy for allergy. Part II. *JAMA* 1987;**258**:1505.

AMA Council on Scientific Affairs: In vivo testing for allergy. Report II. *JAMA* 1987;**258**:1639.

Berstein M et al: Double-blind food challenge in the diagnosis of food sensitivity in the adult. *J Allergy Clin Immunol* 1982;**70**:205.

Bock SA et al: Appraisal of skin tests with food extracts for diagnosis of food hypersensitivity. *Clin Allergy* 1978;**8**:559.

Bruce CA et al: Diagnostic tests in ragweed-allergic asthma: A comparison of direct skin tests, leukocyte histamine release and quantitative bronchial challenge. *J Allergy Clin Immunol* 1974;**53**:230.

Cockcroft DW: Bronchial inhalation tests. I. Measurement of nonallergic bronchial responsiveness. *Ann Allergy* 1985;**55**:527.

Cockcroft DW: Bronchial inhalation tests. II. Measurement of allergic and occupational bronchial responsiveness. *Ann Allergy* 1987;**59**:89.

Terr AI: In vivo tests for immediate hypersensitivity. *Annu Rev Med* 1988;**39**:135.

Townley RJ, Hopp RJ: Inhalation methods for the study of airway responsiveness. *J Allergy Clin Immunol* 1987;**80**:111.

The Atopic Diseases

25

Abba I. Terr, MD

GENERAL CONSIDERATIONS

Definition

Atopy refers to an inherited propensity to respond immunologically to many common naturally occurring inhaled and ingested allergens with the continual production of IgE antibodies. Allergic rhinitis and allergic asthma are the most common manifestations of clinical disease following exposure to these environmental allergens. Atopic dermatitis is less common. Allergic gastroenteropathy is still rarer and may be transient. Two or more of these clinical diseases can coexist in the same patient at the same time or at different times during the course of the illness. Atopy can also be asymptomatic (Fig 25–1).

Nonallergic rhinitis, asthma, and eczematous dermatitis occur in a significant number of patients without atopy, ie, in the absence of IgE-mediated allergy. There is a statistical association of elevated total serum IgE and blood and tissue eosinophilia with atopy, but these features are not always present in atopy, and they frequently occur in a variety of nonatopic conditions.

IgE antibodies also cause **nonatopic allergic diseases**—anaphylaxis and urticaria-angioedema (see Chapter 26)—and they are important in acquired immunity to parasites. A low level of IgE production is present in the normal population.

Thus, the definition of atopy is restricted to a condition with certain specific immunologic and clinical features. Nevertheless, it is a condition that affects a significant portion of the general population, usually estimated at 10–30% in developed countries. The etiology of atopy involves complex genetic factors. Clinical disease requires both genetic predisposition and environmental allergen exposure.

Immunology

A detailed description of the immunopathogenesis of IgE-mediated diseases is given in Chapter 11. Both **mast cells** and **basophils** have high-affinity IgE cell membrane receptors for IgE (**FcεRI**). Mast cells are abundant in the mucosa of the respiratory and gastrointestinal tracts and in the skin, where atopic reactions localize. The physiologic effects of the mediators released or activated immunologically by these cells are responsible for the functional and pathologic features of the immediate and late phases of atopic diseases. The important mediators of IgE allergy are histamine, chemotactic factors, prostaglandins, leukotrienes, and platelet-activating factor.

In allergic rhinoconjunctivitis the reaction occurs entirely at the local tissue level. Contact with allergenic particles such as pollen grains, fungus spores, dust, or skin scales from a pet is followed promptly by absorption of soluble allergenic protein at the mucosal surface. There, the relevant IgE antibody on the mucosal mast cell reacts with allergen, causing prompt mediator release and clinical symptoms. It is not clear whether the bronchial reaction in asthma requires inhalation of smaller particles, such as pollen fragments, capable of reaching the lower respiratory airways or whether allergic asthma is initiated by soluble allergen reaching the bronchial mucosa through the circulation. In atopic dermatitis, ingestion of allergenic food can flare the skin lesions, in which case exposure to the allergen must be via the circulation. The dermatitis can also be activated by direct topical exposure in instances of house dust mite allergy.

Atopic patients typically have multiple allergies; ie, they have IgE antibodies to and symptoms from many environmental allergens. As expected, the total serum IgE level is higher on average in the atopic population than in a comparable nonatopic population, although there is sufficient overlap that a normal serum IgE concentration does not rule out atopy. In general, total IgE in serum is higher in patients with allergic asthma than in those with allergic rhinitis and higher still in those with atopic dermatitis. Some nonatopic diseases are associated with a high serum total IgE (Table 25–1). Although measurement of total serum IgE is not a useful diagnostic indicator of

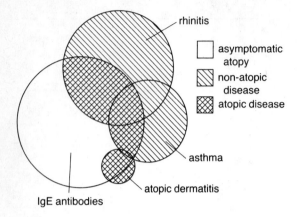

Figure 25–1. Interrelationships of atopy, atopic diseases, and IgE antibodies to environmental allergens.

atopy and does not measure specific IgE antibody, several studies show that the presence of IgE in cord serum is a predictor of subsequent atopy.

Since mast cell-bound and not circulating IgE antibodies are functionally important in initiating atopic reactions upon exposure to allergen, measurement of the total quantity of IgE fixed to high-affinity mast cell and basophil receptors (FcεRI) might be more relevant to atopy. There is no technique for making such a measurement currently, but estimates of skin mast cell-bound IgE by threshold-dilution skin testing with heterologous anti-IgE show that the tissue IgE level is much higher in atopic individuals than in the normal population.

It has been suggested that antibodies of the IgG4

Table 25–1. Diseases associated with elevated total serum IgE.

Disease	Possible Explanation of Elevated IgE
Allergic rhinitis	Multiple atopic allergies.
Allergic asthma	Multiple atopic allergies.
Atopic dermatitis	Multiple allergies and linkage to a non-MHC gene.
Allergic bronchopulmonary aspergillosus	Unknown; varies with disease activity.
Parasitic diseases	IgE antibodies associated with protective immunity.
Hyper-IgE syndrome	Unknown.
Ataxia-telangiectasia	T-suppressor cell defect?
Wiskott-Aldrich syndrome	Unknown.
Thymic alymphoplasia	Unknown.
IgE myeloma	Neoplasm of IgE-producing plasma cells; IgE is monoclonal.
Graft-versus-host reaction	Transient T suppressor cell defect?

subclass may also fix to mast cells and basophils. The mast cell affinity for IgG4 appears to be low, and evidence that IgG4 antibodies can trigger mediator release in the presence of allergens is controversial. There is no indication that human atopic disease pathogenesis involves IgG4 antibodies.

Etiology

The etiology of atopy is unknown. Epidemiologic, family, and twin studies, as well as animal experiments, provide substantial evidence that genetic factors are involved in the propensity for atopy, in the regulation of total IgE production, and in the production of IgE antibodies to specific epitopes. However, a genetic basis for the various disease manifestations is not established. Several family studies have shown associations of human leukocyte antigen (HLA) types with enhanced production of antibody of IgE (and other) isotypes to a particular allergen. Genetic control of the total level of serum IgE is independent of genes in the major histocompatibility complex (MHC).

One theory based on the study of in vitro IgE antibody production by blood lymphocytes suggests that atopic allergy may arise through abnormal regulation by helper and suppressor T lymphocytes of the differentiation of B cells committed to IgE production into IgE antibody-secreting plasma cells. These regulatory T cells exert their effect through the secretion of protein IgE-binding factors that either enhance or suppress the differentiation of B cells.

A second theory suggests that the defect in atopy resides at the level of absorption of environmental allergens at respiratory and gastrointestinal surfaces prior to processing of the allergen for the immune response. The theory proposes that there is a normal protective mucosal barrier to exogenous antigens which is defective in atopy. Some support for this theory comes from the observation that levels of IgG antibodies to inhalant and food allergens are higher in atopic than nonatopic individuals, although these IgG antibodies are not believed to cause disease.

A third theory of atopy proposes a single defect for both the enhanced production of allergen-specific IgE antibodies and the hyperreactivity of target tissues to the mediators released from mast cells by IgE antibody. Immune cells and bronchial smooth muscle cells are both under autonomic control. Thus, an inherited (or perhaps acquired) **autonomic imbalance** such as β-adrenergic blockade or cholinergic overactivity could account for both enhanced IgE antibody production and target organ hyperreactivity. There is no direct evidence for defective autonomic control of IgE antibody production in atopy, although there is some indirect evidence for functional β-adrenergic blockade in the asthmatic airway and in atopic eczematous skin.

Substantial evidence points to the critical role of **cytokines** in the ability of CD4 T lymphocytes to induce IgE antibody production by B cells. Interleukin-4 (IL-4) enhances while gamma interferon (IFN γ) suppresses IgE responses. Thus, a fourth theory would involve up- or down-regulation of these and other cytokines by as yet unidentified etiologic factors in atopy.

Environmental factors play a role in etiology. An accumulation of clinical experience suggests that the initial age of exposure to a particular food or pollen may determine the intensity of the subsequent IgE antibody response. A concurrent viral respiratory infection during environmental allergen exposure may have an adjuvant effect on both specific and total IgE production. Tobacco smoking may exert a similar effect. However, if the total level of serum IgE at the time of birth predicts future development of atopy, acquired factors would probably have only a secondary or permissive role.

Finally, the relationship between IgE-mediated atopic allergy and IgE-mediated immunity in **helminthiasis** offers an interesting opportunity to speculate about etiology. Atopic allergy is a prominent clinical problem in developed countries which are largely free of helminthic infestation. In populations in which these infections are endemic, serum IgE levels are typically high because of ongoing IgE stimulation, and it can be assumed that tissue mast cells are chronically saturated with parasite-specific IgE antibodies. The IgE mast cell-mediated immune mechanism has a selective advantage for the host under these circumstances. In a population free of parasitic infections, however, the IgE immune system may be vestigial for immunity but still available to react adversely to innocuous environmental allergens.

ATOPIC ALLERGENS

The allergens responsible for atopic disease are derived principally from natural airborne organic particles, especially plant pollens, fungal spores, and animal and insect debris, and from ingested foods. The ability of different pollens, molds, or foods to sensitize for IgE allergy varies, so that some of these environmental allergens are intrinsically more sensitizing than others, irrespective of the amount of exposure.

Pollen Allergens

The allergenic pollens are from wind-pollinated (anemophilous) flowering plants. There are far fewer of these plants than insect-pollinated (entomophilous) plants, but they discharge large numbers of lightweight, buoyant pollens that are dispersed over a wide area by wind currents. Within each local geographic area the common allergenic trees, grasses, and weeds pollinate during specific and predictable seasons, producing the corresponding seasonal respiratory symptoms in allergic patients.

The number of pollen-producing plants potentially capable of causing allergy is enormous, but those of proven allergenicity are limited. The major taxa and representative examples are listed in Table 25–2. Within each botanic subclass there are many species that cause allergy. Natural, cultivated, and ornamental plants all may produce allergenic pollen. Plants with attractive flowers are generally insect-pollinated, producing small amounts of heavy pollen that does not become airborne, and thus they are usually not the cause of inhalant allergy.

Allergenic pollen grains are mostly spherical, 15–50 μm in diameter, and they can usually be identified morphologically by light microscopy (Fig 25–2). Air sampling for identifying and quantitating pollens is done by volumetric impaction devices such as the rotorod or rotoslide sampler (Fig 25–3). Several representative examples of pollen seasons are shown in Fig 25–4.

Mold Allergens

Fungi are multicellular eukaryotic organisms that are abundant and ubiquitous. They are saprophytic, growing on a variety of dead or decaying organic material, where they flourish in direct relation to temperature and humidity. They reproduce sexually or asexually, producing airborne spores, some of which are allergenic.

Allergy to fungal spores is an important cause of disease in many atopic patients. However, specific diagnosis is hampered by the confusing taxonomic classification and nomenclature because of the enormous biologic complexity of fungi in their morphologic, reproductive, and ecologic behavior. It is difficult to obtain pure spores of many species for immunologic testing. Seasonal patterns of spores in air samples are poorly defined, making clinical correlation especially problematic. Mold spores range in

Table 25–2. Botanic classifications of pollinating plants frequently associated with atopic respiratory allergy.[1]

Botanic Classification[2]	Common Names of Typical Plants
Division Microphyllophyta	Club mosses
Division Pteridophyta	Ferns
Division Pinophyta	
Subdivision Pinicae	Conifers
Division Magnoliophyta	Flowering plants
Class Liliopsida	
Subclass Commelinidae	Grasses, sedges
Subclass Arecidae	Palms, cattails
Class Magnoliopsida	
Subclass Hamamelididae	Nettles, beeches
Subclass Caryophyllidae	Chenopods, sorrels
Subclass Dilleniidae	Willows, poplars
Subclass Rosidae	Maples, ashes
Subclass Asteridae	Ragweeds, sages

[1]Adapted and reproduced, with permission, from Weber RW, Nelson HS: Pollen allergens and their interrelationships. *Clin Rev Allergy* 1985;3:291.
[2]Classification system of Takhtajan.

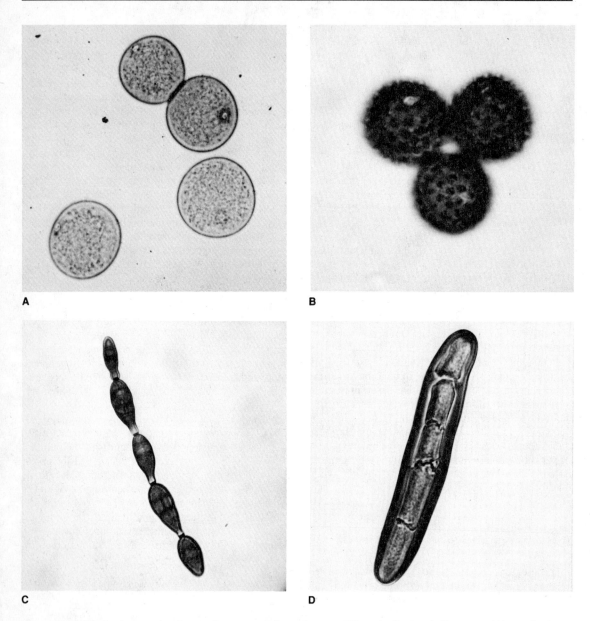

Figure 25–2. Photomicrographs of several common pollens. **A:** grass (30 μm in diameter); **B:** ragweed (20 μm in diameter); **C:** *Alternaria* mold spores (70 μm in length); **D:** *Helminthosporium* mold spores (80 μm in length). (Courtesy of William R. Solomon, MD.)

size from 1 to 100 μm in diameter (Fig 25–2). Volumetric impaction samplers that are used for pollen counting are inefficient in trapping spores, so sampling by these devices does not yield quantitative data for spores. Table 25–3 lists some of the fungi most frequently associated with atopic allergy.

Arthropod Allergens

There are more than 50,000 species of mites. The house dust mites, *Dermatophagoides pteronyssinus*

and *D farinae,* are the most common of all of the known atopic allergens. These tiny arachnids, barely visible to the naked eye, are found in house dust samples throughout the world but are most prevalent in warm, humid climates. They are especially abundant in bedding, upholstery, and blankets, where their natural substrate, desquamated human skin scales, are likely to be found. The two species cross-react extensively but not completely. House dust contains other uncharacterized allergens, but they are of minor im-

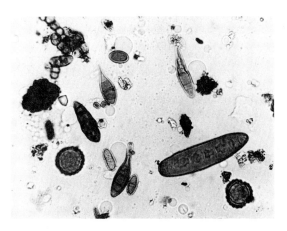

Figure 25–3. Typical "catch" of a volumetric air sampler showing pollen grains, mold spores, insect debris, plant particles, dust, and unidentified particles. (Courtesy of William R. Solomon, MD.)

portance compared with *Dermatophagoides* spp. IgE antibodies and environmental exposure to these mite allergens correlate especially well with atopic asthma and atopic dermatitis, because exposure is by inhalation and dermal contact, respectively.

Other allergenic mites such as *Euroglyphus maynei, Lepidoglyphus destructor,* and *Acarus siro*—storage mites that infest grains—may cause occupational allergy in grain handlers.

Various species of cockroaches are insect pests in homes and restaurants, especially in large cities where there is overcrowding and poor hygiene. Several studies have now documented high rates of sensitivity to cockroach allergen among allergic patients in inner-city populations; this often occurs as an isolated allergy. Other "endemic" causes of respiratory allergy are the emanations and debris of certain insects that swarm in huge numbers seasonally in specific locales. Examples of such insects include caddis fly and mayfly at the eastern and western ends, respectively, of Lake Erie; the green nimitti midge, *Cladotanytarsus lewisi,* in the Sudan; and Lepidoptera in Japan.

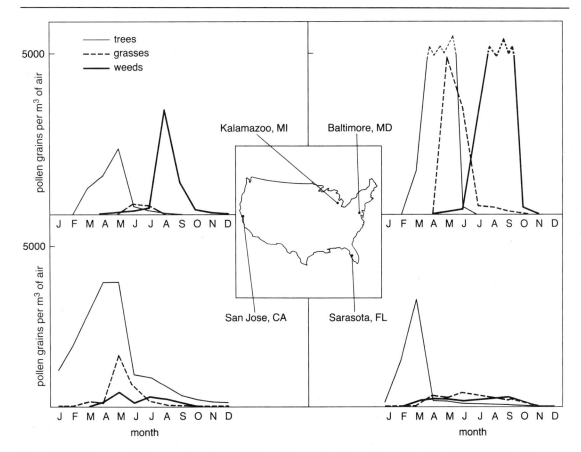

Figure 25–4. Representative examples of quantitative pollen counts at four different locations in the US during the same year (1984). Data from the American Academy of Allergy and Immunology Pollen and Mold Committee.

Table 25–3. Common fungal aeroallergens.

Basidiomycetes	Botrytis
Ustilago	Helminthosporium
Ganoderma	Stemphylium
Alternaria	Cephalosporium
Cladosporium	**Phycomycetes**
Aspergillus	Mucor
Sporobolomyces	Rhizopus
Penicillium	**Ascomycetes**
Epicoccum	Eurotium
Fusarium	Chaetomium
Phoma	

Animal Allergens

Atopic allergy to household pets, especially cats and dogs, has always been easily recognized because patients sensitive to these animals experience immediate intense attacks of asthma when in the same house with an animal to which they are allergic. Other animals encountered in domestic, occupational, and recreational settings also cause allergy. The source of the allergen may be in the dander (horse, dog), saliva (cat), or urine (rodents).

Food Allergens

Allergenic components of foods can induce IgE antibodies that may be responsible for either atopic or nonatopic (anaphylactic) reactions. IgE antibodies to foods frequently exist in atopic patients without causing any reaction when the food is eaten. The factors that operate to convert asymptomatic sensitivity to symptomatic disease are currently unknown. IgG antibodies to many food antigens occur in most people, but they have no known pathogenic significance.

Virtually any food is capable of causing allergy on ingestion, and many have been shown to do so in isolated cases, but certain foods are more likely to be allergenic than others. Seafoods are a particularly prominent cause of allergy in areas where fish is a staple in the diet. Crustaceans and mollusks are an important cause of anaphylaxis and anaphylactoid reactions. Legume, cow's milk, and egg white allergies are also common. Wheat, corn, chocolate, and citrus fruits, on the other hand, are often implicated in causing a variety of symptoms that are not characteristic of allergy in patients lacking IgE antibodies to these foods.

The allergenicity of a particular food protein can be changed by heating or cooking. A reaction can occur to the raw food only or to the cooked form only, or to both.

Occupational allergy, especially asthma from the inhalation of airborne food allergens, is a significant problem for many food handlers.

Allergen Extracts

Pollens, molds, foods, and animal and insect emanations are biologically complex materials made up of a mixture of numerous chemicals, many of which have allergenic potential. Aqueous extracts used in testing for IgE antibodies in allergic patients may contain a number of different allergens in addition to nonallergenic soluble compounds. There is an ongoing effort to isolate, purify, analyze, characterize, name, and standardize every important atopic allergen. To date more than 75 allergen proteins causing human IgE-mediated disease have been isolated and purified, and many have been cloned. Availability of these purified materials will help to resolve clinical problems such as cross-reactivity among plants or foods. Purified allergens are essential reagents for research studies on structure-function relationships and for genetic studies.

Crude aqueous extracts are useful for clinical testing and immunotherapy. For many years, standardization of extracts has been based on weight/volume or total protein content, neither of which reflects the allergen content accurately. Recently, standardization of allergen content either by endpoint skin test titration or by radioallergosorbent test (RAST) inhibition has been introduced, and the term Allergen Unit (AU) is now used to denote bioequivalence. A comparison of these methods is shown in Table 25–4.

ALLERGIC RHINITIS

Major Immunologic Features

■ Allergic rhinitis is the most common clinical expression of atopic hypersensitivity.

■ IgE-mediated allergy is localized in the nasal mucosa and conjunctiva.

■ Pollens, fungal spores, dust, and animal danders are the usual atmospheric allergens.

General Considerations

Allergic rhinitis (also known as allergic rhinoconjunctivitis or hay fever) is the most common manifestation of an atopic reaction to inhaled allergens. More than 20 million persons in the US suffer from this disease. It is a chronic disease, which may first appear at any age, but the onset is usually during childhood or adolescence.

Epidemiology

Allergic rhinitis occurs in 10–12% of the US population. The prevalence and morbidity rate are influ-

Table 25–4. Approximate equivalence of different methods for expressing allergen content in extracts used for testing and immunotherapy.

Method	Units
Weight/volume (W/V)	1:20
Protein nitrogen units/mL (PNU/mL)	10,000
Allergy units/mL (AU/mL)	100,000
Noon units/mL	100
Micrograms of protein/mL	100

enced by the geographic distribution of the common allergenic plants and dust mite. The disease affects both sexes equally. It persists for many years if untreated. It is never fatal, but it does cause considerable morbidity and time lost from school or work.

Clinical Features

A. Symptoms: A typical attack consists of profuse watery rhinorrhea, paroxysmal sneezing, nasal obstruction, and itching of the nose and palate. Postnasal mucus drainage causes sore throat, clearing of the throat, and cough. There is usually an accompanying allergic blepharoconjunctivitis, with intense itching of the conjunctiva and eyelids, redness, tearing, and photophobia. In some patients, conjunctivitis may occur in the absence of nasal symptoms. The disease occurs seasonally in patients with pollen allergy. It may be present year-round if the sensitivity is to a perennial allergen such as house dust, or there may be perennial symptoms with seasonal exacerbations in patients with multiple allergies. Diurnal variation may suggest a household allergen, and symptoms that disappear on weekends suggest an occupational allergy. Severe attacks are often accompanied by systemic malaise, weakness, fatigue, and, sometimes, muscle soreness after intense periods of sneezing. Fever is absent. Swelling of the nasal mucosa may lead to headache because of obstruction of the ostia of the paranasal sinuses.

B. Signs: Rhinoscopy shows a pale, swollen nasal mucosa with watery secretions. The conjunctivae are hyperemic and edematous. There may be eyelid swelling from edema. Lower-eyelid ecchymoses—probably from eye-rubbing—are called "allergic shiners." These changes revert to normal when there is no allergen exposure and the patient is asymptomatic.

C. Laboratory Findings: Eosinophils are numerous in the nasal secretions, but this is not diagnostic, since nasal eosinophilia is found in some patients with nonallergic rhinitis and in those with asthma. Blood eosinophilia is present during symptomatic periods. The presence of any eosinophils in conjunctival scrapings, however, is probably diagnostic. Sinus x-rays, tympanometry, and audiometry may be indicated if an associated sinusitis or otitis media is suspected.

Immunologic Diagnosis

The diagnosis of allergic rhinitis is established by the history and physical findings during the symptomatic phase. Diagnosis of the specific allergic sensitivities in each case is then determined by skin testing for a wheal-and-flare response or by in vitro testing. Selection of allergens for detection of specific IgE antibodies by skin or in vitro test is based on the patient's history and on the known local environmental allergens.

Differential Diagnosis

Chronic nonallergic (vasomotor) rhinitis is a common disorder of unknown cause in which the primary complaint is nasal congestion, usually associated with postnasal drainage. It differs from allergic rhinitis by the absence of sneezing paroxysms or eye symptoms, and rhinorrhea is minimal. Congestion may be unilateral or bilateral, and it often shifts with position. Symptoms occur year-round and are generally worse in cold weather or in dry climates. The nasal mucosa is unusually sensitive to irritants such as tobacco smoke, fumes, and smog. Symptoms usually begin in adult life. The disease is more common among women, and it may begin during pregnancy. Examination shows swollen, erythematous nasal mucosa and strands of thick, mucoid postnasal discharge in the pharynx. Allergy skin tests are negative or unrelated to the symptoms. In nonallergic vasomotor rhinitis, the nasal secretions may or may not contain eosinophils, so nasal eosinophilia is not a reliable sign of allergy but may indicate a preasthmatic state. There is a good therapeutic response to decongestants and humidification, but antihistamines are usually not effective.

Rhinitis medicamentosa denotes the severe congestion that occurs from the rebound effect of excessive use of sympathomimetic nasal sprays or nose drops. In this disease, the mucosa is often bright red and swollen, but these changes are reversible with complete avoidance of nose drops or sprays, even if they have been used excessively for many years.

Infectious rhinitis is almost always due to a virus, and most patients with allergic rhinitis can distinguish their allergic symptoms from those of the common cold, which usually produces fever, an erythematous nasal mucosa, and an exudate in the nasal secretions that is polymorphonuclear rather than eosinophilic. Primary bacterial or fungal infections of the nasal passages are rare.

Some hormones may produce nasal congestion. This is common in pregnancy or with the use of oral contraceptive drugs. Nasal congestion occurs frequently in myxedema. Certain drugs produce nasal congestion (Table 25–5.)

Anatomic obstructions may occur from foreign

Table 25–5. Drugs that may cause nasal congestion.

Drug	Presumed Mechanism
Oral contraceptives	Unknown
Reserpine	Norepinephrine depletion
Guanethidine	Norepinephrine release blockade
Propranolol	Adrenergic blockade
Thioridazine	α-Adrenergic blockade
Tricyclic antidepressants	Norepinephrine uptake blockade
Aspirin (rarely)	Idiosyncratic generation of vasodilating arachidonate metabolite?

bodies in the nose, tumors, nasal septal deviation or spurs, and nasal polyps. Nasal polyposis is a constitutional condition independent of atopy and allergic rhinitis, but it is associated with asthma, aspirin sensitivity, sinusitis, and eosinophilia. Nasal polyps also occur in children with cystic fibrosis. Anatomic lesions are best detected by fiberoptic rhinoscopy after the application of a topical decongestant.

Vernal keratoconjunctivitis is a disease of unknown cause that usually affects children, producing giant papillary excrescences of the palpebral conjunctivae with symptoms of intense itching and a stringy exudate. The exudate contains eosinophils, mast cells, basophils, and plasma cells, suggesting an immunologic basis, but search for an allergic cause is usually unrewarding. Reversible giant papillary conjunctivitis is caused in some patients by the use of soft contact lenses.

Immunologic Pathogenesis

Soluble allergens from inhaled pollens, spores, and other aeroallergenic particles are rapidly eluted on contact with the moist mucous membranes of nasal mucosa and conjunctivae. Contact with the corresponding IgE antibody on local mast cells and basophils releases the various mast cell-associated mediators described in Chapter 11. Symptoms of sneezing, rhinorrhea, congestion, and pruritus appearing within minutes are caused by the effects of endogenously liberated histamine, leukotrienes, and prostaglandin D_2 in the early-phase allergic response. Chemotactic factors produce an inflammatory exudate that produces the more persistent congestion and nonspecific tissue hyperirritability of the late-phase response. The hyperirritability lowers the nasal threshold to both allergic and irritant stimuli such as temperature changes, irritant particles and gases, sunlight, and ingested alcohol, thereby accentuating the effect of other allergens and prolonging symptoms after cessation of the allergen exposure.

A significant number of patients with allergic rhinitis have a coexisting bronchial hyperreactivity in the absence of clinical signs of asthma. It is not known whether this is an intrinsic abnormality related to atopy or an acquired defect from allergen exposure, possibly a component of the late allergic response. The absence of symptomatic asthma may be explained by effective compensating homeostatic mechanisms that are defective or inoperative in asthmatic patients.

Treatment

Treatment consists of environmental measures to avoid allergen exposure, drugs, and desensitization. For any atopic disease, prophylactic treatment by avoidance of allergens is usually the most effective means of treatment. However, avoidance is not always possible or practical, and so medications are needed to control symptoms. In some cases, the immune response itself can be altered by desensitization therapy.

A. Environmental Measures: Avoidance of an allergen is recommended on the basis of a clinical history of symptomatic allergy and not because of a positive skin test alone. Appropriate measures in individual cases may be the removal of household pets, control of house dust exposure by frequent cleaning, and avoidance of dust-collecting toys or other objects in the patient's bedroom. Air-cleaning devices with high-efficiency particle filters may be helpful. Dehumidification and repair of leaking pipes or roofs may be necessary to prevent mold growth. Avoidance of pollen and outdoor molds is not possible unless the patient is able to stay in an air-conditioned home or office. In some cases, the patient might arrange a vacation trip to a pollen-free area during the peak pollen season.

In cases of occupational allergy, every effort should be made to modify the patient's work routine and to employ industrial hygiene measures to avoid allergen exposure; however, if these measures fail, a change in the patient's job may be necessary.

B. Drug Treatment: Antihistamines are the most commonly used drugs in allergic rhinitis, although their use is restricted by side effects. New nonsedating antihistamines avoid the most troublesome side effects. Orally administered nasal decongestants may be helpful, either alone or in combination with antihistamines. Sympathomimetic and antihistaminic eye drops are useful for allergic conjunctivitis. Administration of cromolyn by nasal sprays or conjunctival drops 4 times daily is beneficial and is virtually free of any immediate or long-term toxicity.

Systemic corticosteroids can be extremely effective in relieving symptoms of allergic rhinitis, but since the disease is a chronic, recurrent, benign condition, these drugs should be used with extreme care. The patient with very severe symptoms lasting for only a few days or several weeks each year who does not respond to antihistamines can be given oral prednisone for 1 or 2 weeks in a dosage just high enough to suppress symptoms. Flunisolide or beclomethasone by nasal spray may be equally effective without causing significant systemic corticosteroid effects. Side effects of nasal burning and epistaxis from nasal corticosteroid sprays are more annoying than dangerous, but the potential for mucosal atrophy and septal perforation with prolonged use requires periodic monitoring. Corticosteroid eye drops should be used very sparingly for brief periods only to control acute severe allergic conjunctivitis, with careful monitoring by an ophthalmologist.

C. Desensitization: Allergen injection therapy has been shown in many prospective double-blind controlled trials to be effective in treating allergic rhinitis. Because of the length of treatment required and the potential danger of serious systemic reactions, injection treatment is used in patients whose symptoms are uncontrolled despite appropriate environmental measures and symptomatic medications. The procedure, which is discussed more fully in Chapter 56, must be individualized and coordinated with environmental and drug treatment to be most effective; therefore, it should be initiated and monitored by a trained allergist.

Complications

Sinusitis as a concomitant or complication of allergic rhinitis is a controversial issue. The diagnosis of sinusitis is difficult because of frequent discrepancies between paranasal sinus symptoms and radiographic evidence of pathology. Mild sinus membrane thickening (less than 6 mm) is frequent in allergic rhinitis and could represent noninfectious allergic inflammation. Significant thickening, opacification, and airfluid levels usually indicate an infectious sinusitis. Obstruction of the sinus ostia by swollen nasal membranes, whether caused by allergy, a common cold, or nonallergic vasomotor rhinitis, can cause secondary sinus infection, but to date there is no direct evidence that the sinus mucosa per se is a target organ in atopy.

Otitis media with or without effusion is common in children, and its causes are multifactorial, usually involving eustachian tube dysfunction and anatomic factors. The disease does not appear more frequently in atopic than in nonatopic children or adults. It is unlikely that inhaled allergen reaches the middle ear or eustachian tube, although tubal obstruction by swollen nasopharyngeal allergic mucosa or dysfunction caused by the allergic mediators could prolong or exacerbate the disease.

Nasal polyps are likewise observed with similar frequency in atopic and normal individuals. Although polyposis is not a complication of allergic rhinitis, management can be hampered by untreated nasal allergy, and vice versa.

Prognosis

Although no definitive studies have been done on the course of untreated allergic rhinitis, symptoms can be expected to recur or persist for many years if not for life. The severity of the symptoms is dependent upon the degree of exposure to the allergen. A patient with a pollen allergy who moves to an area where that pollen-producing plant does not grow will no longer by symptomatic.

ASTHMA

Major Immunologic Features

- Allergic asthma is a manifestation of IgE-mediated allergy localized in the bronchus.
- Important immunologically released or activated mediators are histamine, leukotrienes, and eosinophil chemotactic factor.
- Hyperirritability of bronchial mucosa amplifies the bronchoconstricting effects of mediators.

Definition

Asthma (also known as reversible obstructive airway disease) is a disease characterized by hyperresponsiveness of the tracheobronchial tree to respiratory irritants and bronchoconstrictor chemicals, producing attacks of wheezing, dyspnea, chest tightness, and cough that are reversible spontaneously or with treatment. The disease is chronic and involves the entire airway, but it varies in severity from occasional mild transient episodes to severe, chronic, life-threatening bronchial obstruction. There is an associated eosinophilia in the blood and in respiratory secretions. Episodes of asthma are triggered immunologically by allergen inhalation in patients with atopic allergy.

General Considerations

It is important to understand the role of allergy in asthma. Asthma and atopy may coexist, but only about half of the asthmatic population has atopy and a smaller percentage of atopic patients have asthma. All asthmatic patients—regardless of the presence or absence of atopy—have the cardinal features that define asthma: airway hyperreactivity, reversible airway obstruction, and eosinophilia. In those with allergic asthma, attacks are triggered by allergen exposure as well as by other nonallergic factors.

Asthma and atopy are not wholly independent, however, because asthma occurs more frequently among atopic than nonatopic individuals, especially during childhood. It is not known whether predisposition to the 2 conditions is genetically linked or whether atopy enhances the clinical expression of an undefined asthmatic predisposition. A recent large-scale epidemiologic study showed that, contrary to abundant previous evidence, there is a positive statistical correlation of asthma and IgE antibodies in all age groups. Nonetheless, by tradition and clinical usefulness, asthma is often classified into extrinsic and intrinsic subgroups.

A. Extrinsic Asthma: This is also known as allergic, atopic, or immunologic asthma. As a group, patients with extrinsic asthma generally develop the disease early in life, usually in infancy or childhood. Other manifestations of atopy—eczema or allergic rhinitis—often coexist. A family history of atopic disease is common. Attacks of asthma occur during pollen seasons, in the presence of animals, or on exposure to house dust, feather pillows, or other allergens, depending on the patient's particular allergic sensitivities. Skin tests show positive wheal-and-flare reactions to the causative allergens. Total serum IgE concentration is frequently elevated but is sometimes normal.

B. Intrinsic Asthma: This is also known as nonallergic or idiopathic asthma. It characteristically appears first during adult life, usually after an apparent respiratory infection, so that the term "adult-onset asthma" is sometimes applied. This term is misleading, because some nonallergic asthmatics first develop the disease during childhood and some allergic asthmatics become symptomatic for the first time as adults when they are exposed to the relevant allergen. Intrinsic asthma pursues a course of chronic or recurrent bronchial obstruction unrelated to pollen seasons or exposure to other allergens. Skin tests are negative to the usual atopic allergens. The serum IgE concentration is normal. Blood and sputum eosinophilia is present. Personal and family histories are usually negative for other atopic diseases. Other schemes for classifying asthma into subgroups, eg, aspirin-sensitive, exercise-induced, infectious, and psychologic, merely define external triggering factors that affect certain patients more so than others.

Epidemiology

Asthma is a worldwide disease that has been recognized for centuries, but prevalence figures vary, in part because of differences in definition and methods of case-finding. It is a common disease, which affects approximately 5% of the population of Western countries. There is no reason to suspect that the rate in Asia and Africa is substantially different. Onset during childhood is predominantly before the age of 5 years, and it affects boys more than girls (by about 3:2). The childhood-onset form is usually of the allergic variety. Adult onset may be at any age, but typically it occurs in the fifth decade. Ordinarily it is of the intrinsic type, and it affects women more than men (by about 3:2).

Some recent studies suggest that the prevalence is increasing, but this may reflect better diagnosis and not a true change in incidence. Death caused by asthma—about 2000–3000 cases per year in the US—is relatively infrequent, but there are reports recently from several countries, including the US, of increasing asthma mortality rates and some evidence of increasing morbidity rates, despite substantial advances in symptomatic therapy.

Although not a major cause of mortality, asthma remains a leading cause for time lost from work and school.

Clinical Features

A. Symptoms: Asthma may begin at any age. It is characterized by attacks of wheezing and dyspnea that can range in severity from mild discomfort to life-threatening respiratory failure. Some patients are symptom-free between attacks, whereas others are never entirely free of airway obstruction. The asthmatic attack causes shortness of breath, wheezing, and tightness in the chest, with difficulty in moving air during inspiration but more so during expiration. Coughing is usually present, and with prolonged asthma the cough may produce thick, tenacious spu-

tum that can be either clear or yellow. In children, coughing, especially at night, may be the only symptom to suggest the diagnosis. Fever is absent, but fatigue, malaise, irritability, palpitations, and sweating are occasional systemic complaints.

B. Signs: Physical examination during the attack shows tachypnea, audible wheezing, and use of the accessory muscles of respiration. The pulse is usually rapid, and blood pressure may be elevated. Pulsus paradoxus indicates severe asthma. The lung fields are hyperresonant, and auscultation reveals diminished breath sounds, wheezes, and rhonchi but no rales. The expiratory phase is prolonged. In a severe attack with high-grade obstruction, breath sounds and wheezing may both be absent. These are ominous signs, especially if accompanied by pallor and peripheral cyanosis, excitement or anxiety, and inability to speak. Chronic severe asthma in young children may lead to a structural barrel chest deformity.

C. Laboratory Findings: An increased total eosinophil count in the peripheral blood is almost invariably present unless suppressed by corticosteroids or sympathomimetic drugs. There is eosinophilia in nasal secretions. Sputum examination reveals eosinophils, Charcot-Leyden crystals, and Curschmann's spirals.

The chest x-ray may be normal during the attack or may show signs of hyperinflation, and there may be transient scattered parenchymal densities indicating focal atelectasis caused by mucus plugs in scattered portions of the airway. Total serum IgE is usually elevated in childhood allergic asthma and normal in adult intrinsic asthma, but this test lacks specificity in individual cases as a diagnostic screen for either asthma or atopy (Fig 25–5).

Pulmonary function tests show the abnormalities of airway obstructive disease. Flow rates and 1-sec-

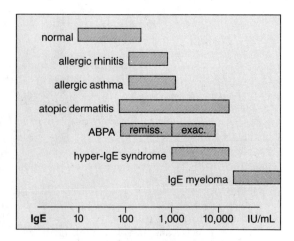

Figure 25–5. Total serum IgE levels in normal individuals and patients with various allergies and IgE disorders. Abbreviations: ABPA, Allergic bronchopulmonary aspergillosis; remiss., remission; exac., exacerbation.

ond forced expiratory volume (FEV_1) are decreased, vital capacity is normal or decreased, and total lung capacity and functional residual capacity are usually normal or slightly increased but may be decreased with extreme bronchospasm. Following administration of an aerosolized sympathomimetic bronchodilator, ventilation improves with significant increase in flow rates and FEV_1, indicating the reversible nature of the bronchial obstruction. The lack of response in a patient already receiving large doses of sympathomimetic drugs does not rule out reversibility, and the test should be repeated at a later date after improvement from additional treatment such as hydration, corticosteroids, and chest physical therapy.

Repeated tests of ventilatory function are helpful in the long-term management of the asthmatic patient. Serial determinations of FEV_1, maximal expiratory flow rate, or peak flow rate are easily done in the office or clinic, and they will often detect airway obstruction that may not be apparent to the patient or to the physician on auscultation of the chest.

Inexpensive peak flow rate measurement devices are valuable for daily monitoring at home and work. Information can be used to uncover possible allergens and irritants in the patient's environment and as early warning of a worsening condition requiring more intensive treatment.

Bronchial provocation testing has made a significant contribution to pathophysiologic and pharmacologic research in recent years. These procedures are not necessary for routine diagnosis but are helpful in special circumstances (see Chapter 24). Nonspecific bronchial hyperirritability can be demonstrated by using quantitative challenges with methacholine, histamine, cold air, or exercise. These tests of bronchial hypersensitivity are almost always positive in asthma, but they are not by themselves diagnostic of the disease, since bronchial hyperirritability occurs in a significant number of patients with allergic rhinitis, in normal subjects following viral respiratory infections, and in a small percentage of normal individuals. Since the procedure provokes an asthma attack, it should not be used in the presence of significant bronchial obstruction or if asthma can be diagnosed by other criteria.

Bronchial provocation by inhaling allergens to diagnose specific atopic sensitivities is sometimes useful in suspected occupational asthma, for which measurement of a dose-response effect under controlled conditions is desirable. This may be the case when the patient encounters several potential allergens at work. The patient should be monitored in a hospital for this procedure because of possible severe late-phase reactions.

Pathology

Autopsy on fatal asthma shows hyperinflation of the lungs, hypertrophy and hyperplasia of bronchial smooth muscle, and excessive mucus secretion. Death is usually caused by asphyxiation from mucus plugging of the airways. Microscopic examination shows hypertrophy and hyperplasia of submucosal glands and bronchial smooth muscle, mucosal infiltration with an edematous and mixed cellular inflammatory response especially rich in eosinophils, and epithelial desquamation within mucus plugs. Similar but less intense pathology exists during asymptomatic periods. The pathology therefore reflects both the early phase (smooth muscle contraction, edema, hypersecretion) and late phase (cellular inflammation) of the IgE-mediated allergic response. The gross and microscopic pathology of allergic asthma is indistinguishable from that of nonallergic asthma.

Immunologic Pathogenesis

The cause of asthma is not known. Pathogenesis of the asthmatic attack involves both allergic and nonallergic mechanisms. There is evidence that bronchoconstriction is mediated by an autonomic (vagal) reflex mechanism involving afferent receptors in the bronchial mucosa or submucosa which respond to irritants or chemical mediators and efferent cholinergic impulses, causing bronchial muscle contraction and hypersecretion of mucus. The mast cell-associated mediators (histamine, leukotrienes, prostaglandins, kinins, platelet-activating factor, and chemotactic factors) have properties that can explain the pathologic and functional abnormalities of the asthmatic attack. In the asthmatic patient, the afferent receptors appear to be sensitized to respond to a low threshold of stimulation. It has been proposed that the hyperirritable state of the bronchial mucosa results from defective functioning or blockade of its β-adrenergic receptor, preventing a homeostatic bronchodilating response from endogenous catecholamines. Bronchial hyperirritability is enhanced further during the late phase of the asthmatic reaction.

The linkage between allergen-IgE antibody interaction and release, activation, and secretion of mediators from the mast cell is now firmly established. The means by which nonallergic stimuli such as irritants and viral infections stimulate mast cells is unknown at present, and it is possible that other cells and mediators are involved in nonallergic asthma.

The variety of nonspecific agents that initiate an asthma attack is extensive. Some of these factors are listed in Table 25–6. Some of these items have been shown to increase the underlying bronchial hyperirritability as well, making the patient more sensitive to the effects of other triggers.

Approximately 10% of asthmatic patients have **aspirin sensitivity.** In these patients, ingestion of aspirin is followed in 20 minutes to 3 hours by an asthmatic attack, which is caused by an idiosyncratic pharmacologic response to the drug. Other nonsteroidal anti-inflammatory drugs cause a similar reaction. These anti-inflammatory drugs inhibit cyclooxygenase, the initial enzyme in the synthesis of prosta-

Table 25–6. Nonspecific triggers of asthma.

Infections
Viral respiratory infections
Physiologic factors
Exercise
Hyperventilation
Deep breathing
Psychologic factors
Atmospheric factors
SO_2
NH_3
Cold air
O_3
Distilled water vapor
Ingestants
Propranolol
Aspirin
Nonsteroidal anti-inflammatory drugs
Sulfites
Experimental inhalants
Hypertonic solutions
Citric acid
Histamine
Methacholine
Prostaglandin $F_{2\alpha}$
Occupational inhalant
Isocyanates

glandins from cell membrane arachidonic acid, and the quantitative ability of these drugs to provoke asthma is directly related to the ability to inhibit cyclooxygenase, indomethacin being the most potent and acetaminophen the least. Nasal polyposis is common in aspirin-sensitive patients.

The mechanism of aspirin-sensitive asthma is idiosyncratic and not immunologic. Since aspirin and related compounds normally inhibit the cyclooxygenase pathway of biosynthesis of prostaglandin E_2 (a bronchodilator) from arachidonic acid, it is suspected that in this disease an idiosyncratic response to these drugs favors the local synthesis of either prostaglandin F_{2a} (a bronchoconstrictor) or leukotrienes via the lipoxygenase pathway.

The clinical significance of immediate and late phases of the IgE response is especially clear in asthma. Bronchospastic episodes that occur within minutes upon allergen exposure and are promptly relieved by bronchodilators correspond to the immediate-phase response. Chronic asthma that is poorly responsive to β-adrenergic agonists and theophylline, associated with enhanced nonspecific airway hyperirritability, and dependent on corticosteroids for reversal, is characteristic of the late-phase allergic response. Bronchial provocation challenge with many of the usual inhaled aeroallergens, ie, pollens, fungi, and dust mite, produce dual early and late asthmatic reaction in untreated allergic asthma.

Exercise-induced and hyperventilation-induced bronchoconstriction in asthmatic patients is a consequence of water loss from the airway, which increases the osmolarity of fluid overlying the mucosal epithelial cells. This stimulates mast cells to release mediators, which, in turn, contract bronchial smooth muscle either directly or indirectly through vagal afferent receptor stimulation. Airway cooling, which occurs from inhaling cold air, exaggerates the effect of water loss.

The conceptual model of allergen-IgE antibody-induced allergic disease as discussed in Chapters 11 and 24 is well established. It requires direct contact of allergen with antibodies fixed to tissue mast cells, which then release mediators locally in the target tissues, where the inflammatory pathology and clinical symptoms and signs localize. In atopy the allergen molecule is often encountered as a component of an airborne particle such as a pollen grain or mold spore. In allergic rhonconjunctivitis these particles easily impact on the target conjunctiva and nasal mucosa, completing the direct contact model. In allergic asthma, however, particles at the upper end of this size range would not ordinarily be expected to penetrate as far as the tracheobronchial tree. However, recent immunochemical air-sampling methods have shown that pollen and spore fragments and even droplets containing allergen are inhaled as a significant portion of the ambient allergen load inhaled by the allergic patient.

The allergens commonly associated with allergic asthma and allergic rhinitis are generally similar. However, individual patients may tend to react with rhinitis to pollens and with asthma to molds and animal dander. Very young asthmatic children frequently have food-induced asthma without rhinitis.

Allergic asthma is the usual manifestation of IgE-mediated occupational disease. New occupational inhalant allergens are continually being discovered. A partial list is shown in Table 25–7. Occupational asthma may also arise from nonimmunologic sensitivity or irritation to many other substances that fail to induce IgE antibody or other immune responses. In these cases, the cause and pathogenesis are unknown, but possible mechanisms that have been suggested include toxic chemical injury to the bronchial mucosa, irritant stimulation of mast cells or vagal irritant receptors, and β-adrenergic blockade. Patients with atopic allergy to specific allergens, eg, animals, are obviously precluded from working in a job in which they are exposed to these allergens. However, most cases of occupational asthma—both IgE-mediated and nonimmunologic—occur in nonatopic workers, showing that an unusual high-dose exposure to a potential allergen in an occupational setting can override the requirement for genetic predisposition of atopy.

Immunologic Diagnosis

The diagnosis of asthma is made by history, physical examination, and pulmonary function tests to show reversible bronchial obstruction. Blood and sputum examination for eosinophilia is confirmatory. Chest x-rays are useful primarily to exclude other

Table 25–7. Occupational allergens causing IgE-mediated allergic asthma.[1]

Allergen	Occupational Exposure
Animal products	
Cows, pigs, poultry, mice, hamsters, rabbits, rats, guinea pigs, bats, dogs, cats, horses	Animal/insect breeders, laboratory workers, veterinarians, breeders
Insect dusts	
Mealworms, storage mites, silk filatures, locusts, bees, cockroaches, flies	Grain handlers, sewerage workers, beekeepers
Sea creatures	
Crabs, shrimp, seasquirt body fluid, fish feed, *Echinodorus plamosus* larvae	Processors, breeders
Plant products	
Dusts, flours, cotton dust, grain dusts, grain flours	Cotton mill and textile workers, grain elevator and bakery workers
Fruits, seeds, leaves, pollens	
Castor beans, green coffee beans	Coffee processors, seamen, laboratory workers
Weeping fig, sunflower pollen, tobacco	Producers, agricultural workers
Organic dyes and inks	
Vegetable, dusts, gums, extracts	
Western red and eastern white cedar (plicatic acid), California redwood, exotic woods	Carpenters, sawmill workers
Colophony (abietic acid)	Electronics workers
Microbial agents	
Alginates, fungal allergens, humidifier contaminants, protozoa, fungi, bacteria	Biotechnology industry, laboratory, office workers
Enzymes	
Subtilisin, papain, pineapple bromelain, pepsin, hog trypsin, pancreatic extracts	Detergent manufacturers, pharmaceutical workers, food processors
Therapeutic agents	
Antibiotics and related compounds, penicillins, cephalosporins, tetracycline, phenylglycine acid chloride, sulfonamides, spiramycin	Pharmaceutical workers, poultry chick breeders
Pharmaceuticals and related compounds	
α-Methyldopa, amprolium hydrochloride, cimetidine, furanbased binder, glycyl compound (salbutamol intermediate), psyllium (bulk laxative)	Pharmaceutical workers, nurses
Piperazine	Medical and veterinary workers
Sterilizing agents	
Chloramine, sulfone chloramides, hexachlorophene	Abattoir, kitchen, hospital workers
Inorganic chemicals	
Metal fumes and salts	Metalworkers
Aluminum, chromium, cobalt, fluoride, nickel, platinum, stainless steel, welding fumes, vanadium, zinc	Chemical industry workers, metal refiners, platers, grinders, welders
Ammonium persulfate	Beauticians
Organic chemicals	
Amines (diamines, ethanolamines, tetramines)	Chemical, electronic, plastic, rubber industry workers, photographers, beauticians, fur handlers
Anhydrides (phthalic, tetrachlorophthalic, trimellitic), azobisformamide, azodicarbonamide	Plastics industry workers, food wrappers

[1]Modified and reproduced, with permission, from Butcher BT, Salvaggio JE: *J Allergy Clin Immunol* 1986;**78**:547.

cardiopulmonary diseases. The methacholine challenge test is reserved for instances in which the history is equivocal and pulmonary function is normal.

The history is the primary diagnostic tool for evaluating the presence of allergy and identifying the relevant allergens. In general, inhalant allergens that are important in allergic rhinitis are also implicated in allergic asthma. These include pollens, fungi, animal danders, house dust, and other household and occupational airborne allergens. In young children and infants, allergy to foods may also cause asthma. History and physical findings of other atopic diseases—atopic dermatitis or allergic rhinitis—as well as a family history of atopy increase suspicion that asthma may involve atopic allergy. Skin testing for wheal-and-flare reactions will verify the specific sensitivities. RAST or other in vitro tests may be used in unusual situations when skin testing is contraindicated. Bronchoprovocation allergen testing is used primarily in difficult diagnostic cases of suspected occupational lung disease.

Differential Diagnosis

Chronic bronchitis and emphysema (chronic obstructive lung disease) produce airway obstruction that does not respond to sympathomimetic bronchodilators or corticosteroids, and there is no associated eosinophilia in the blood or sputum. In children acute bronchiolitis, cystic fibrosis, aspiration of a foreign body, and airway obstruction caused by a congenital vascular anomaly must be considered. Benign or malignant bronchial tumors or external compression from an enlarged substernal thyroid, thymus enlargement, aneurysm, or mediastinal tumor may cause wheezing. Acute viral bronchitis may produce enough bronchial inflammation with symptoms of obstruction and wheezing that it may be termed asthmatic bronchitis. Cardiac asthma is a term used for intermittent dyspnea (resembling allergic asthma) caused by left ventricular failure. Carcinoid tumors may occasionally cause attacks of wheezing because of release of serotonin or activation of kinins produced by the neoplasm.

Treatment

Since the cause of asthma is unknown, cure of the basic defect, the hyperirritable bronchial mucosa, is not possible. The aim of treatment is symptomatic control. Environmental measures, drugs, and allergen desensitization may be required.

A. Environmental Control: Irritants such as smoke, fumes, dust, and aerosols should be avoided. If the diagnostic evaluation indicates allergy to animal danders, feathers, molds, or house dust, these should be eliminated from the house.

B. Drug Treatment:

1. Sympathomimetics–β-Adrenergic bronchodilator drugs are effective and are used in the acute attack or for long-term management. Epinephrine has both α- and β-adrenergic effects, but it has a long history of efficacy in acute asthma attacks. It acts rapidly and is given subcutaneously in a dose of 0.2–0.5 mL of 1:1000 aqueous solution. Its duration of action is short, so that if repeated injections are required, long-acting epinephrine (1:200 in suspension) or terbutaline can be used. Albuterol, pirbuterol, metaproterenol, and isoetharine are selective β-adrenergic bronchodilators that are given by inhalation in aerosol. They are available as solutions to be administered by a hand-held nebulizer, in an intermittent positive-pressure breathing device, or in metered-dose pressurized inhalers, but patients must be cautioned that overuse can lead to paradoxic bronchial constriction and worsening of asthma. The β-adrenergic drugs terbutaline, metaproterenol, and albuterol are available as oral sympathomimetic drugs for achieving sustained bronchodilation in chronic asthma. Side effects of nervousness, muscle-twitching, palpitations, tachycardia, and insomnia can occur with all of them.

2. Xanthines–Theophylline and related compounds are especially effective as bronchodilators when used in combination with sympathomimetic drugs. Intravenous aminophylline, 250–500 mg, can be administered fairly rapidly in an acute asthmatic attack, and various oral forms of theophylline are available for long-term use. Absorption of theophylline varies with the drug preparation, the age of the patient, and other factors such as smoking and heart failure. Serum theophylline determination should be utilized to obtain a therapeutic level of 10–20 μg/mL.

3. Corticosteroids–Glucocorticoids are remarkably effective in the treatment of asthma. Even when all other forms of treatment have failed, the response to adequate steroid treatment is so dependable that failure of response might be considered grounds for questioning the diagnosis of asthma. The therapeutic effect in asthma is anti-inflammatory, but the precise mechanism of action is unknown, and these drugs are just as effective in reversing asthma in nonallergic patients as in patients suffering allergen-induced attacks. Despite their effectiveness, however, systemic corticosteroids should not be considered primary drugs in the treatment of asthma, and in practice they should be given only when other forms of treatment prove inadequate. The dangers of long-term steroid therapy must be kept in mind by any physician prescribing the drugs.

Treatment is started at high dosage and continued until the obstruction is alleviated, with return of physical findings and flow rates to normal. The dose necessary to achieve this varies with the individual patient, but 30–60 mg of prednisone daily is usually sufficient. An occasional steroid-resistant patient may require a much higher dose because of an abnormally accelerated rate of drug catabolism. After complete clearing of the attack, the daily dose is reduced by slow tapering over many days or weeks to avoid a recurrence of asthma. Long-term alternate-day maintenance therapy minimizes adrenocortical suppression, but not all steroid-dependent asthmatic patients can be controlled in this fashion.

Beclomethasone dipropionate, triamcinolone acetonide, and flunisolide, highly potent corticosteroid drugs, are available in aerosolized form for inhalation. They are effective as long-term maintenance therapy for many steroid-dependent asthmatic patients. Many experts today recommend regular long-term inhaled corticosteroids as primary anti-inflammatory prophylaxis in virtually all asthmatic patients. Adrenocortical suppression and systemic side effects are usually slight. When they are used to replace a systemic steroid drug, the dosage of systemic drug must be tapered very slowly to avoid adrenal insufficiency. Inhaled corticosteroids are not useful for treatment of an acute asthma attack.

4. Cromolyn sodium–This drug is available as a powder administered in 20-mg doses by inhalation in a specially designed inhaler or micronized in a metered-dose inhaler. It is not a bronchodilator but is believed to inhibit the release of mediators of immediate hypersensitivity in the lung. It is administered as a long-term prophylactic treatment. It is more effective in younger patients with allergic asthma than in adults, and it frequently prevents exercise-induced bronchospasm. Cromolyn will not reverse an acute attack.

5. Other drugs–Antibiotics are used if secondary bacterial bronchitis or pneumonia occurs. Expectorants and hydration are helpful for thick, tenacious sputum. Inhaled ipratropium bromide, an anticholinergic drug with minimal side effects because of poor absorption, may help to eliminate the asthmatic cough.

C. Desensitization: The effectiveness of injection treatment in pollen hay fever has been shown in several controlled studies, and most allergists believe that allergic asthma responds just as well (see Chapter 56).

D. Treatment of Status Asthmaticus and Respiratory Failure: A severe attack of asthma unresponsive to repeated injections of epinephrine or other sympathomimetic drugs, termed status asthmaticus, is a medical emergency requiring immediate hospitalization and prompt treatment. Factors leading to this condition include respiratory infection, excessive use of respiratory-depressant drugs such as sedatives or opiates, overuse of aerosolized bronchodilators, rapid withdrawal of corticosteroids, and ingestion of aspirin in aspirin-sensitive asthmatic patients.

Immediate determination of arterial blood gases and pH with repeated measurements until the patient responds satisfactorily is necessary for optimal treatment. Injections of terbutaline or epinephrine are continued. If the patient has not been receiving oral theophylline, 250–500 mg of aminophylline may be given intravenously for 10–30 minutes initially, followed by slow intravenous drip with careful attention to toxic symptoms. Serum theophylline determinations are used to maintain the optimal therapeutic level of 10–20 μg/mL of serum. Intravenous corticosteroids are indicated if the patient has previously received steroids, if the attack was caused by aspirin, if excessive aerosolized bronchodilator was a factor in the attack, or if significant CO_2 retention exists. Intravenous hydrocortisone at 4 mg/kg or methylprednisolone at 1 mg/kg, repeated every 2–4 hours, should be given until the patient can be maintained on oral prednisone at 60–80 mg daily in divided doses.

Dehydration usually accompanies status asthmaticus and may give rise to inspissated mucus plugs that further impair ventilation. During the first 24 hours, up to 3–4 L of intravenous fluid may be necessary for rehydration. Oxygen should be supplied by tent, face mask, or nasal catheter to maintain arterial Po_2 at about 80–100 mm Hg. Expectorants and chest physical therapy are helpful adjuncts to eliminate mucus plugs. Sedatives should be avoided even in the anxious patient because of the danger of respiratory depression. Antibiotics are used only for concomitant bacterial infection.

Respiratory failure, indicated by an arterial Po_2 level above 65 mm Hg and arterial blood pH below 7.25, may require mechanical assistance of ventilation in addition to all the measures listed above. This should be performed by a team of physicians, nurses, and technicians experienced in this form of respiratory therapy.

Complications & Prognosis

The disease is chronic, and its severity may change in an unpredictable fashion. Some children apparently "outgrow" asthma in the sense of becoming asymptomatic, but they may continue to show evidence of bronchial lability, and symptoms can reappear later in life. The acute attack can be complicated by pneumothorax, subcutaneous emphysema, rib fractures, atelectasis, or pneumonitis. There is no evidence that emphysema, bronchiectasis, pulmonary hypertension, and cor pulmonale result from longstanding uncomplicated asthma.

Allergic Bronchopulmonary Aspergillosis

This disease occurs almost exclusively in patients with a history of asthma who harbor *Aspergillus* endobronchially and who develop a heterogeneous form of hypersensitivity with both IgE and IgG antibodies to *Aspergillus* antigens (see Chapter 27).

ATOPIC DERMATITIS

Major Immunologic Features
- It often accompanies atopic respiratory allergy.
- The clinical course is usually independent of allergen exposure.
- Very high serum levels of IgE may occur.

Definition

Atopic dermatitis (also known as eczema, neurodermatitis, atopic eczema, or Besnier's prurigo) is a common chronic skin disorder specific to a subset of patients with the familial and immunologic features of atopy. The essential feature is a pruritic dermal inflammatory response, which induces a characteristic symmetrically distributed skin eruption with predilection for certain sites. There is frequent overproduction of IgE by B lymphocytes, possibly caused by abnormal T lymphocyte regulation. Patients often have multiple IgE antibodies to environmental inhalant and food allergens, but the role of these allergens in the dermatitis is uncertain.

General Considerations

Atopic dermatitis is classified as a cutaneous form of atopy because it is associated with allergic rhinitis and asthma in families (and frequently in the same patient) and the serum IgE concentration is often high. However, the severity of the dermatitis does not always correlate with exposure to allergens to which the patient reacts positively on skin testing, and allergy desensitization is not effective in this disease. There is evidence for an underlying target organ (ie, skin) abnormality that might be a metabolic or biochemical defect, possibly linked genetically to the high level of serum IgE. Some studies also suggest a partial deficiency in T cell immunity. Atopic dermatitis may begin at any age. Onset at 3–6 months of age is typical, but it may first appear during childhood or adolescence and occasionally during adult life.

Clinical Features

A. Symptoms: The disease almost always begins in infancy or early childhood. Many cases clear by 2 years of age. Persistence into later childhood and adult life is marked by frequent cycles of remission and exacerbation. Itching is the cardinal symptom. It often worsens at night and is provoked by temperature changes, sweating, exertion, emotional stress, and embarrassment. There is a strong family history of atopy. Scratching and rubbing cause the typical eczematous skin eruption to flare. Itching is also exacerbated by irritants such as wool and by drying agents such as soap and defatting solvents. Ingestion of allergenic foods may cause acute exacerbations. The disease may improve spontaneously during the summer.

B. Signs: The skin is typically dry and scaly. Active skin lesions are characterized by intensely pruritic inflamed papules (prurigo), erythema, and scaling. Scratching produces weeping and excoriations. Chronic lesions are thickened and lichenified. Distribution of the lesions is dependent on age. In infancy, the forehead, cheeks, and extensor surfaces of the extremities are usually involved. Later, the lesions show a flexural pattern of distribution, with predilection for the antecubital and popliteal areas and the neck. The face, especially around the eyes and ears, is often affected when distribution is more widespread. Staphylococcal pustules are common. Stroking of the skin produces white dermographism, in contrast to the normal erythema-and-whealing of the triple response of Lewis.

C. Laboratory Findings: Elevated total serum IgE, sometimes extremely high, occurs in 60–80% of cases. A normal level does not rule out the diagnosis.

Epidemiology

Approximately 0.7% of the US population currently have active disease, but the prevalence in children is 4–5%, equally distributed between the sexes. Racial predilection and geographic distribution have not been studied.

Pathology

Grossly, the lesion begins acutely with an erythematous edematous papule or plaque with scaling. Itching leads to weeping and crusting, then to chronic lichenification. Microscopically, the acute lesion is characterized by intercellular edema, and the dermis is infiltrated with mononuclear cells and CD4 lymphocytes. Neutrophils, eosinophils, plasma cells, and basophils are rare, and vasculitis is absent, but degranulated mast cells can be seen. The chronic lesion features epidermal hyperplasia, hyperkeratosis, and parakeratosis. The dermis is infiltrated with mononuclear cells, Langerhans cells, and mast cells. There may be focal areas of fibrosis, including involvement of perineurium of small nerves.

Immunologic Diagnosis

The history and physical examination are almost always sufficient to make the diagnosis. Marked elevation of serum IgE is confirmatory, but a normal IgE level does not rule out atopic dermatitis. Biopsy is usually not required.

Because of the uncertainty about specific allergic sensitivities in pathogenesis, skin or in vitro allergy tests will usually produce positive results that may reflect concomitant respiratory allergies or asymptomatic sensitivities rather than causes of the skin disease. In some children with atopic dermatitis there may be positive skin tests to foods that cause acute exacerbation of eczema when those foods are given in a double-blind placebo-controlled oral challenge test. Blood T lymphocyte subset counts are not useful in diagnosis.

Differential Diagnosis

Localized neurodermatitis (lichen simplex chronicus) and allergic or irritant contact dermatitis produce similar eczematous changes of the skin. Seborrhea and dermatophytoses are occasionally confused with atopic dermatitis. Pompholyx (dyshidrosis) with secondary eczema may simulate atopic dermatitis of the hands.

Immunologic Pathogenesis

There is an intrinsic skin abnormality in atopic dermatitis, perhaps analogous to the hyperirritable airway in asthma. Some evidence suggests hyperreactivity to cholinergic stimuli, which might relate to the reduced threshold of the itch response. Increased numbers of mast cells and increased histamine content in the skin have been reported, but the other mast cell-associated chemical mediators have not been thoroughly examined for a role in this disease. Blood basophil counts are normal. Injection of methacholine intradermally initially produces a normal wheal and erythema; this is followed in 2–5 minutes by blanching because of edema. The delayed-blanch response is typical but not diagnostic of atopic dermatitis.

A. Defective Lymphocyte Regulation: Much indirect information suggests a defect in cell-mediated immunity. Delayed hypersensitivity skin test responses to recall antigens, in vitro lymphocyte responses to mitogen and allergen, and the autologous mixed lymphocyte reaction have all been reported to be deficient. Decreased prevalence of naturally acquired and experimentally induced allergic contact dermatitis and increased susceptibility to herpes simplex virus, vaccinia virus, warts, molluscum contagiosum, and dermatophyte skin infections are consistent with a defect in the T cell effector mechanism. Furthermore many investigations have shown that excessive production of IgE by peripheral blood B lymphocytes in this disease can be accounted for by deficiency in CD8 T lymphocytes. It has been suggested that a defective CD4 helper T lymphocyte population could explain the failure of CD8 T lymphocytes to function as suppressors of IgE production and to achieve sufficient cytotoxicity for effective immunity against secondary skin infections.

B. The Role of Allergy: Atopic respiratory diseases with hypersensitivity to environmental allergens, eosinophilia, elevated serum IgE levels, and a family history of allergy are frequently associated with atopic dermatitis. Nevertheless, it is often difficult to attribute the dermatitis to allergy. The skin lesions rarely flare during pollen seasons, although in some patients there is an association with exposure to house dust, animals, or other environmental allergens. More commonly, food allergy is implicated in dermatitis in children. Milk, corn, soybeans, fish, nuts, and cereal grains are frequently implicated, but other foods may occasionally be important allergens also. Recent controlled food challenges have shown clear-cut exacerbations of the early inflammatory pruritic lesions in selected cases, although the responsible food cannot always be detected by skin testing.

C. Association with Systemic Disorders: Eczema indistinguishable from atopic dermatitis is found in children with phenylketonuria. The skin lesions of Letterer-Siwe disease are also very similar. Atopic dermatitis without allergy is a feature of several immunologic deficiency disorders, especially Wiskott-Aldrich syndrome, ataxia-telangiectasia, and X-linked hypogammaglobulinemia (see Chapters 18–20).

Treatment

Atopic dermatitis is a chronic disease requiring constant attention to proper skin care, environmental control, drugs, and avoidance of allergens when indicated. Because dry skin enhances the tendency to itch, frequent application of nonirritating topical lubricants is the most important preventive measure. Small areas of active eczema respond well to topical corticosteroids, but acute involvement of large areas of skin may warrant a brief course of systemic corticosteroids beginning with a high dose and tapering slowly after the acute eruption clears. Oral antihistamines help to control itching. If their sedative effect precludes use during the daytime, a bedtime dose will help to control involuntary scratching during sleep. Frequent bathing or washing, irritating fabrics such as wool, and harsh detergents should be avoided. The hands and fingernails must be kept clean to prevent secondary infection, and if infection does occur, an appropriate antibiotic should be prescribed.

Complications & Prognosis

Atopic dermatitis that persists beyond childhood has an unpredictable tendency to remit spontaneously, even after years of involvement. This is not related to the severity of involvement, the presence or absence of allergy, or treatment. Allergic rhinitis and asthma are not complications but, rather, additional manifestations of the underlying atopic disease.

The most frequent complication is secondary infection, almost always by *Staphylococcus,* as a result of scratching. In the past, the most serious complication was eczema vaccinatum from exposure to vaccinia virus by inadvertent vaccination or contact with a recently vaccinated person in the family or classroom. Eczema herpeticum is a similar condition caused by herpes simplex virus. Topical antibiotics or antihistamines may cause secondary contact dermatitis. Hand dermatitis occurs from excessive contact with water, soap, and solvents in the home and the workplace.

Ophthalmic complications include atopic keratoconjunctivitis, keratoconus, and atopic cataracts.

ALLERGIC GASTROENTEROPATHY

Major Immunologic Features

- Some atopic patients have localized IgE reactions in the gut to an ingested food.
- Gastrointestinal loss of serum proteins and blood may lead to edema and anemia.
- The condition is rare in adults; it is more common but transient in infants.

Definition

Allergic gastroenteropathy (also known as eosinophilic gastroenteropathy) is an unusual atopic manifestation in which multiple IgE food sensitivities are associated with a local gastrointestinal tract mucosal reaction. This produces acute gastrointestinal symptoms, eosinophilia, and gastroenteric loss of fluid, protein, and blood. Extraintestinal allergic symptoms, such as asthma and urticaria, may also be provoked by foods. Other atopic manifestations in the patient and family usually are present.

General Considerations

Allergic gastroenteropathy is the least common expression of atopy. Ingested food allergen reacting with local IgE antibodies in the jejunal mucosa liberates mast cell mediators, causing gastrointestinal symptoms shortly after the meal. Continued exposure to the food produces chronic inflammation, resulting in gastrointestinal protein loss and hypoproteinemic edema. Blood loss through the inflamed intestinal mucosa may be significant enough to cause iron deficiency anemia. In some patients, extraenteric manifestations of atopy may be produced by the same food allergen.

Epidemiology

Very few cases have been reported, but the disease has been described in infants, children, and adults. It is a very rare cause of gastrointestinal symptoms.

Immunologic Pathogenesis

The pathogenesis is that of atopy, as discussed above. The condition may occur more commonly in infants than in adults because of the much greater permeability of the infantile gastrointestinal mucosa to intact proteins. This may account for the transient nature of allergic gastroenteropathy in infants and young children.

The allergic reaction occurs locally in the upper gastrointestinal mucosa. Ingested food allergens react with IgE antibodies fixed to mucosal mast cells, thereby liberating mediators responsible for hyperemia, increased vascular permeability, and smooth muscle contraction. This results in acute symptoms, chronic loss of blood and plasma protein, and intestinal malabsorption.

Clinical Features

A. Symptoms and Signs: Nausea, vomiting, diarrhea, and abdominal pain occur within 2 hours after ingestion of the allergenic food, and these symptoms resolve on avoidance of the food. Rhinitis, asthma, or urticaria may accompany the intestinal symptoms. Chronic or repeated exposures to allergenic foods in undiagnosed disease may lead to blood loss anemia, abdominal distension, and voluminous foul stools from steatorrhea, edema from hypoalbuminemia, and systemic symptoms of anorexia, weight loss, and weakness. Children may experience growth retardation. Most patients have other manifestations of atopy, including atopic dermatitis, asthma, and allergic rhinitis, and there is usually a family history of atopy.

B. Laboratory Findings: Blood counts show hypochromic microcytic iron deficiency anemia and eosinophilia. Stool examination will reveal gross or occult blood and Charcot-Leyden crystals. Serum albumin is low, and total serum IgE may be elevated. Gastrointestinal x-rays may show mucosal thickening and edema of the small bowel.

Immunologic Diagnosis

A history of chronic or recurrent gastrointestinal symptoms associated with specific foods in an atopic patient should raise a suspicion of this diagnosis, especially if there is accompanying evidence of gastrointestinal blood loss, iron deficiency anemia, intestinal malabsorption, protein-losing enteropathy, other manifestations of atopy, or high serum total IgE.

In reported cases the causative food allergens have been single or multiple. Milk is the usual cause in children. Nursing infants may react to food allergens in breast milk from the maternal diet. The suspected food allergens identified by history can be tested for IgE antibodies by a skin test or RAST. Tests for antibodies to other foods may uncover other allergies, but these should be confirmed by elimination and challenge, preferably performed double-blind. Peroral jejunal biopsy may be necessary in difficult cases.

Pathology

An eosinophilic inflammatory infiltrate in the lamina propria of the upper gastrointestinal tract mucosa is present following allergen exposure and resolves with allergen avoidance.

Differential Diagnosis

Gastrointestinal allergy is overdiagnosed. Patients with food-related gastrointestinal symptoms—even atopic patients—are much more likely to have nonallergic food intolerance. Primary gastrointestinal diseases, reactions to food contaminants, and psychologic food aversion must be considered. Inflammatory bowel diseases, intestinal lymphangiectasia, and primary immunoglobulin deficiencies may produce similar symptoms. In children, lactase and other carbohydrate enzyme deficiencies, phenylketonuria, pancreatic deficiency from cystic fibrosis, and maple syrup urine disease should be ruled out by appropriate tests.

Treatment

Elimination of the allergenic food from the diet is curative. In some cases of milk allergy, boiled milk may be tolerated if the protein allergen is heat-labile. Corticosteroid treatment usually inhibits the reaction, but long-term steroid therapy should be necessary only for patients who do not respond to the elimination diet. There are reports that oral cromolyn in a dose of 200–400 mg given before the allergenic food is eaten inhibits the gastrointestinal allergic reaction, but there are no long-term studies on this form of treatment.

Complications

The major complications of this disease are edema and anemia. Unlike intestinal lymphangiectasia, significant gastroenteric loss of plasma immunoglobulins and lymphocytes does not occur, so susceptibility to infection is usually not a problem. Persistent disease activity may lead to secondary reversible lactose intolerance. Malnutrition can result from undiagnosed disease.

Prognosis

The infantile form of allergic gastroenteropathy is usually transient, but the duration of the disease is unpredictable and is not related to severity of the reaction. No long-term follow-up studies on adults are available.

REFERENCES

General

Hopkin JM: Genetics of atopy. *Clin Exp Allergy* 1989;**19**:263.

Ishizaka K: IgE-binding factors and regulation of the IgE antibody response. *Annu Rev Immunol* 1988;**6**:513.

Leskowitz S, Salvaggio J, Schwartz H: A hypothesis for the development of atopic allergy in man. *Clin Allergy* 1972;**2**:237.

Marsh DG, Meyers DA, Bias WB: The epidemiology and genetics of atopic allergy. *N Engl J Med* 1981;**305**:1551.

Terr AI: The atopic worker. *Clin Rev Allergy* 1986;**4**:267.

Allergens

Anderson JA, Sogn DD (editors): *Adverse Reactions to Foods*. NIH Publication no. 84–2442. US Department of Health and Human Services, 1984.

Anderson MC, Baer H, Ohman JL: A comparative study of the allergens of cat urine, serum, saliva, and pelt. *J Allergy Clin Immunol* 1985;**76**:563.

Burge HA: Fungus allergens. *Clin Rev Allergy* 1985;**3**:319.

Platts-Mills TAE, Rawk F, Chapman MD: Problems in allergen standardization. *Clin Rev Allergy* 1985;**3**:271.

Solomon WR: Aerobiology of pollinosis. *J Allergy Clin Immunol* 1984;**74**:449.

Weber RW, Nelson HS: Pollen allergens and their interrelationships. *Clin Rev Allergy* 1985;**3**:291.

Yunginger JW: Allergenic extracts: Characterization, standardization, and prospects for the future. *Pediatr Clin N Am* 1983;**30**:795.

Allergic Rhinitis

Allansmith MR, Ross RN: Ocular allergy. *Clin Allergy* 1988;**18**:1.

Busse W (editor): New directions and dimensions in the treatment of allergic rhinitis. *J Allergy Clin Immunol* 1988;**82**:889.

Druce HM, Kaliner MA: Allergic rhinitis. *JAMA* 1988;**259**:260.

Fireman P: Newer concepts in otitis media. *Hosp Pract* 1987;**22**:85.

Friedlaender MH: Ocular allergy. *J Allergy Clin Immunol* 1985;**76**:645.

Mullarkey MF, Gill JS, Webb DR: Allergic and nonallergic rhinitis: Their characterization with attention to the meaning of nasal eosinophilia. *J Allergy Clin Immunol* 1980;**65**:122.

Mygind N, Anggard A: Anatomy and physiology of the nose—pathophysiologic alterations in allergic rhinitis. *Clin Rev Allergy* 1984;**2**:173.

Norman PS: Allergic rhinitis. *J Allergy Clin Immunol* 1985;**75**:531.

Todd NW: Allergy as a cause of otitis media. *Immunol Allergy Clin N Am* 1987;**7**:371.

Asthma

Barnes PJ: New concepts in the pathogenesis of bronchial hyperresponsiveness and asthma. *J Allergy Clin Immunol* 1989;**83**:1013.

Busse WW: The relationship between viral infections and the onset of allergic diseases and asthma. *Clin Exp Allergy* 1989;**19**:1.

Chan-Yeung M, Lam S: Occupational asthma. *Am Rev Respir Dis* 1986;**133**:686.

Chapman ID, Foster A, Morley J: The relationship between inflammation and hyperreactivity of the airways in asthma. *Clin Exp Allergy* 1993;**23**:168.

Cherniak RM: Continuity of care in asthma management. *Hosp Pract* 1987;**22**:119.

Cohen SH: Advances in the diagnosis and treatment of asthma. Clinical evaluation—allergy and immunology. *Chest* 1985;**87(Suppl)**:S26.

Hargreave FE et al: The origin of airway hyperresponsiveness. *J Allergy Clin Immunol* 1986;**78**:825.

König P: Inhaled corticosteroids—their present and future role in the management of asthma. *J Allergy Clin Immunol* 1988;**82**:297.

Lenfant C, Sheffer AL: Guidelines for the diagnosis and management of asthma. *J Allergy Clin Immunol* 1991;**88(Suppl)**:425. [Entire issue.]

Li JTI, O'Connell EJ: Viral infections and asthma. *Ann Allergy* 1987;**59**:321.

Mathison DA, Stevenson DD, Simon RA: Precipitating factors in asthma: Aspirin, sulfites, and other drugs and chemicals. *Chest* 1985;**87(Suppl)**:S50.

McFadden ER Jr: Clinical physiologic correlates in asthma. *J Allergy Clin Immunol* 1986;**77**:1.

McFadden ER: Therapy of acute asthma. *J Allergy Clin Immunol* 1989;**84**:151.

Ohman JL: Allergen immunotherapy in asthma: Evidence for efficacy. *J Allergy Clin Immunol* 1989;**84**:133.

Pattemore PK, Johnston SL, Bardin PG: Viruses as precipitants of asthma symptoms. J. Epidemiology. *Clin Exp Allergy* 1992;**22**:325.

Rachelefsky GS, Siegel SC: Asthma in infants and children—treatment of childhood asthma. Part II. *J Allergy Clin Immunol* 1985;**76**:409.

Scoggin C: Exercise-induced asthma. *Chest* 1985;**87(Suppl)**:S48.

Siegel SC, Rachelefsky GS: Asthma in infants and children. Part I. *J Allergy Clin Immunol* 1985;**76**:1.

Summer WR: Status asthmaticus. **Chest** 1985;**87(Suppl)**:S87.

Atopic Dermatitis

Businco L, Sampson HA (editors): International symposium on atopic dermatitis: An update. *Allergy* 1989;**44(Suppl 9)**:1.

Hanifin JM: Atopic dermatitis. *J Allergy Clin Immunol* 1984;**73**:211.

Oakes RC, Cox AD, Burgdorf WH: Atopic dermatitis: A review of diagnosis, pathogenesis, and management. *Clin Pediatr* 1983;**7**:467.

Sampson HA: The role of food allergy and mediator release in atopic dermatitis. *J Allergy Clin Immunol* 1988;**81**:635.

Sampson HA: Pathogenesis of eczema. *Clin Exp Allergy* 1990;**20**:459.

Stone SP, Muller SA, Gleich GJ: IgE levels in atopic dermatitis. *Arch Dermatol* 1973;**108**:806.

Allergic Gastroenteropathy

Gryboski JD: Gastrointestinal aspects of cow's milk protein intolerance and allergy. *Immunol Allergy Clin N Am* 1991;**11**:773.

Hutchins P, Waler-Smith JA: The gastrointestinal system. *Clin Immunol Allergy* 1982;**2**:43.

Min K-U, Metcalfe DD: Eosinophilic gastroenteritis. *Immunol Allergy Clin N Am* 1991;**11**:799.

Scudamore HH et al: Food allergy manifested by eosinophilia, elevated immunoglobulin E level, and protein-losing enteropathy: The syndrome of allergic gastroenteropathy. *J Allergy Clin Immunol* 1982;**70**:129.

Walker WA, Hong R: Immunology of the gastrointestinal tract. (2 parts.) *J Pediatr* 1973;**83**:517, 711.

Anaphylaxis & Urticaria

26

Abba I. Terr, MD

The atopic diseases (see Chapter 25) are characterized by a genetic predisposition to the production of IgE antibodies to common environmental antigens. Anaphylaxis and urticaria also are caused by IgE antibodies, but they lack the genetically determined propensity and the target organ hyperresponsiveness of atopy, and they have no special predilection for the atopic individual. The immunologic pathogenesis for all IgE-mediated diseases is the same, but separate consideration of atopic and nonatopic diseases is important clinically. There are differences in the allergens, mode of exposure to the allergen, genetic factors that influence etiology, diagnostic methods, prognosis, and treatment.

Allergic gastroenteropathy, described in Chapter 25, has features of anaphylaxis, but it is included in the chapter on atopic diseases because it occurs almost exclusively in patients with other atopic manifestations.

ANAPHYLAXIS

Major Immunologic Features

- Systemic anaphylaxis is the occurrence of an IgE-mediated reaction simultaneously in multiple organs.
- The usual causative allergen is a drug, insect venom, or food.
- The reaction can be evoked by a minute quantity of allergen and is potentially fatal.

General Considerations

A. Definitions: **Anaphylaxis** is an acute, generalized allergic reaction with simultaneous involvement of several organ systems, usually cardiovascular, respiratory, cutaneous, and gastrointestinal. The reaction is immunologically mediated, and it occurs upon exposure to an allergen to which the subject had previously been sensitized. **Anaphylactic shock** refers to anaphylaxis in which hypotension,

with or without loss of consciousness, occurs. **Anaphylactoid reaction** is one in which the symptoms and signs of anaphylaxis occur in the absence of an allergen-antibody mechanism. In this case, the endogenous mediators of anaphylaxis are released in vivo through a nonimmunologic mechanism.

B. Epidemiology: Anaphylaxis has no known geographic, racial, or sex predilection. It occurs at the rate of 0.4 cases per million per year in the general population, although in hospitals the prevalence is reported to be 0.6 per 1000 patients. The latter figure shows that medications and biologic products are a major cause.

C. Pathology: Grossly there is urticaria and angioedema. The lungs are diffusely hyperinflated, with mucus plugging of airways and focal atelectasis. The microscopic appearance of the lungs is similar to that in acute asthma, with hypersecretion of bronchial submucosal glands, mucosal and submucosal edema, peribronchial vascular congestion, and eosinophilia in the bronchial walls. Pulmonary edema and hemorrhage may be present. Bronchial muscle spasm, hyperinflation, and even rupture of alveoli may be seen microscopically. An important feature of human anaphylaxis is edema, vascular congestion, and eosinophilia in the lamina propria of the larynx, trachea, epiglottis, and hypopharynx. Myocardial ischemia has been found in a high proportion of cases, probably secondary to shock. Occasionally, myocardial infarction occurs. A direct effect of anaphylaxis on the myocardium or coronary arteries has not been shown. The liver, spleen, and other visceral organs are often grossly congested and microscopically hyperemic and edematous. Eosinophils are found in the splenic sinusoids, liver, lamina propria of the upper respiratory tract, and pulmonary blood vessels. Pulmonary edema and intra-alveolar hemorrhage may occur.

Death is usually attributable to asphyxiation from upper airway edema and congestion, irreversible shock, or a combination of these factors. Death occurring after many hours of shock may be from the effects of the late phase of the IgE allergic reaction or secondary to the failure of other organs.

D. Immunologic Pathogenesis: Anaphylaxis requires the presence of IgE antibodies and exposure to the allergen, but it is clear that it occurs in only a very small proportion of patients satisfying these requirements. In some cases the mode and quantity of allergen exposure are important. One example is the inadvertent injection of atopic allergens to atopic persons—a well-recognized risk of diagnostic skin testing and allergen immunotherapy. However, in most instances in which drugs, foods, or insect venoms are the cause, nonimmunologic potentiating factors such as an increased reactivity of mast cells, basophils, or target organs can only be surmised.

Anaphylaxis is the sudden systemic result of the allergen-IgE antibody mast cell-mediator release sequence detailed in Chapters 11 and 24. The result is a sudden profound and life-threatening alteration in functioning of the various vital organs. Vascular collapse, acute airway obstruction, cutaneous vasodilation and edema, and gastrointestinal and genitourinary muscle spasm occur almost simultaneously, although not always to the same degree.

E. Anaphylactic Shock: Hypotension and shock in anaphylaxis reflect generalized vasodilatation of arterioles and increased vascular permeability with rapid transudation of plasma through postcapillary venules. This shift of fluid from intravascular to extravascular spaces produces hypovolemic shock with edema (angioedema) in skin and various visceral organs, pooling of venous blood (especially in the splanchnic bed), hemoconcentration, and increased blood viscosity. Low cardiac output diminishes cardiac return and produces inadequate coronary artery perfusion. Low peripheral vascular resistance can lead to myocardial hypoxia, dysrhythmias, and secondary cardiogenic shock. Stimulation of histamine H_1 receptors in coronary arteries may cause coronary artery spasm. Some patients experience anginal chest pains and, occasionally, myocardial infarction during anaphylaxis. After a prolonged period of shock, organ failure elsewhere may ensue, particularly the kidneys and central nervous system. In some cases shock occurs rapidly before extensive fluid shifts would be expected to occur, suggesting that neurogenic reflex mechanisms might be involved.

F. Urticaria & Angioedema: Histamine and other mediators stimulate receptors in superficial cutaneous blood vessels, causing the swelling, erythema, and itching that characterize urticaria, a hallmark cutaneous feature of systemic anaphylaxis. Increased permeability of subcutaneous blood vessels causes the more diffuse swelling of angioedema, which may account for a substantial volume of fluid loss from the intravascular compartment.

G. Lower Respiratory Obstruction: Bronchial muscle spasm, edema and eosinophilic inflammation of the bronchial mucosa, and hypersecretion of mucus into the airway lumen occur in some patients with anaphylaxis and are indistinguishable from an acute asthmatic attack. Both histamine and leukotrienes have bronchoconstrictor activity, but the former affects the larger proximal airways preferentially, and the latter affects peripheral airways. Airway obstruction leads to impairment of gas exchange with hypoxia, further compounding the vascular effects of anaphylaxis. If this is left untreated, acute cor pulmonale and respiratory failure may occur.

H. Other Effects: Histamine acts on gastrointestinal and uterine smooth muscle, causing painful spasm. Hageman factor-dependent pathways may be activated by basophil and mast cell enzymes during anaphylaxis. One such enzyme has kallikrein activity and has been called basophil kallikrein of anaphylaxis, cleaving bradykinin from high-molecular-weight kininogen. Bradykinin has potent vascular permeability as well as vasodilating, smooth muscle-contracting, and pain-inducing properties, and it is occasionally found in anaphylactic states. Hageman factor activation of the intrinsic clotting mechanism may also explain some of the coagulation abnormalities found in systemic anaphylaxis.

Clinical Features

A. Symptoms & Signs: The reaction begins within seconds or minutes after exposure to the allergen. There may be an initial fright or sense of impending doom, followed rapidly by symptoms in one or more target organ systems: cardiovascular, respiratory, cutaneous, and gastrointestinal.

The cardiovascular response may be peripheral or central. Hypotension and shock are symptoms of generalized arteriolar vasodilatation and increased vascular permeability producing decreased peripheral resistance and leakage of plasma from the circulation to extravascular tissues, thereby lowering blood volume. In some patients without previous heart disease, cardiac arrhythmias may occur. Without prompt treatment by intravascular fluid replacement, prolonged shock may lead to the secondary effects of hypoxia in all vital organs. Death can result from blood volume depletion and irreversible shock or from a cardiac arrhythmia.

The respiratory tract from the nasal mucosa to the bronchioles may be involved. Nasal congestion from swelling and hyperemia of the nasal mucosa and profuse watery rhinorrhea with itching of the nose and palate simulate an acute hay fever reaction. The hypopharynx and larynx are especially susceptible, and obstruction of this critical portion of the airway by edema is responsible for some of the respiratory deaths. Bronchial obstruction from bronchospasm, mucosal edema, and hypersecretion of mucus results in an asthmalike paroxysm of wheezing dyspnea. Obstruction of the smaller airways by mucus may lead to respiratory failure.

The skin is a frequent target organ, with generalized pruritus, erythema, urticaria, and angioedema. Angioedema often involves the eyelids, lips, tongue, pharynx, and larynx. The conjunctival and oropharyngeal mucosa are erythematous and edematous. Occasionally, urticaria persists for many weeks or months after all other symptoms have subsided.

Gastrointestinal involvement occurs because of contraction of intestinal smooth muscle and mucosal edema, resulting in crampy abdominal pain and sometimes nausea or diarrhea. Similarly, uterine muscle contraction may cause pelvic pain. Abortion can result if the patient is pregnant.

Hemostatic changes can occur but are not often investigated. The intrinsic coagulation pathway is activated, resulting in the possibility of disseminated intravascular coagulation and depletion of clotting factors. Thrombocytopenia may occur, possibly because platelets aggregated by platelet-activating factor (PAF) are sequestered from the circulation. In some cases, circulating heparin or other anticoagulants have been demonstrated.

Convulsions, with or without shock, have been reported rarely. In cases of fatal anaphylaxis, death usually occurs within 1 hour of onset.

B. Laboratory Findings: Laboratory tests are seldom necessary or helpful initially, although certain tests may be used later to assess and monitor treatment and to detect complications. Immediate emergency treatment should never be delayed pending results of laboratory studies. The blood cell counts may be elevated because of hemoconcentration. Eosinophil counts may be elevated but are usually normal or low because of the compensatory effect of endogenous or exogenous catecholamines and glucocorticoids. Chest x-ray will show hyperinflation, with or without areas of atelectasis caused by airway mucus plugging. The electrocardiogram may show a variety of abnormalities, including conduction abnormalities, atrial or ventricular dysrhythmias, ST-T wave changes of myocardial ischemia or injury, and acute cor pulmonale. Myocardial infarction may be evidenced by electrocardiographic and serum enzyme changes. Plasma histamine and serum tryptase levels may be elevated.

Clinical Diagnosis

The diagnosis of systemic anaphylaxis in a patient observed during an acute attack should be established or suspected as rapidly as possible by the symptoms and physical findings of hypotension, urticaria, angioedema, and laryngeal or bronchial obstruction, or any combination of these. Appropriate treatment should be instituted as soon as the condition is suspected. After the reaction is successfully treated, diagnostic efforts are directed to the cause.

Immunologic Diagnosis

The history is essential in determining the allergen responsible for an anaphylactic reaction. Skin testing

or in vitro tests establish the presence of an IgE immune response to an allergen. This information is not in itself diagnostic but must be consistent with the history to establish the cause of the reaction. Ingestion of a food or drug; parenteral administration of a drug, vaccine, blood product, or other biologic material; or an insect sting occurring shortly (usually 1 hour or less) before the onset of symptoms raises suspicion that this is the cause. If the patient has experienced more than one episode, evidence of exposure to a common allergen should be sought.

Identification of the specific allergen may require persistent detective work. A reaction to drinking milk may be caused by penicillin contamination. A reaction to a viral vaccine may be caused by egg white from the egg embryo in which the virus was cultured. Occasionally, a reaction occurs after injection of 2 agents with anaphylactic potential (eg, penicillin and horse serum) or after a meal including several different "allergenic" foods such as fish, legumes, nuts, or berries.

The diagnosis is confirmed by detecting the presence of IgE antibody to the suspected allergen. In most cases, the immediate wheal-and-flare skin test is the most reliable procedure, especially if the allergen is a protein. Systemic reactions to skin tests have occurred in highly sensitive individuals, so testing should be done initially by the cutaneous-prick method. If the test is negative, intradermal testing to diluted sterile extracts of known potency can then be done.

To minimize the risk of anaphylaxis from the skin test itself, serial-titration testing with 10-fold-increasing concentrations of allergen is recommended when testing with protein allergens. Table 26–1 lists several recommended starting concentrations.

Skin testing in cases of suspected Hymenoptera venom anaphylaxis has been shown to be reliable if freshly reconstituted lyophilized venom extracts are used for testing. Testing with standard food extracts may yield false-negative reactions if the allergen is labile. Prick testing with direct application of the food itself to the skin may yield a positive test, but some foods contain vasoactive chemicals produce false-positive reactions.

Skin testing with haptenic drugs is generally not reliable. Certain drugs cause nonspecific histamine release, producing a wheal-and-flare reaction in normal individuals (Table 26–2). Immunologic activation of mast cells requires a polyvalent allergen, so a negative skin test to a univalent haptenic drug does not rule out anaphylactic sensitivity to that drug.

Table 26–1. Starting intracutaneous skin test concentrations.

Allergen	Starting Concentration
Hymenoptera venoms	0.001 μg/mL
Insulin	0.001 U/mL
Horse serum	1:1000 dilution

Table 26–2. Drugs that cause nonspecific wheal-and-flare skin reactions.

Aspirin
Codeine
Curare
Histamine
Hydralazine
Meperidine
Morphine
Polymyxin B
Stilbamidine

Table 26–3. Some foods that cause anaphylaxis.

Crustaceans	**Seeds**
Lobster	Sesame
Shrimp	Cottonseed
Crab	Caraway
Mollusks	Mustard
Clams	Flaxseed
Fish	Sunflower
Legumes	**Nuts**
Peanut	**Berries**
Pea	**Egg white**
Beans	**Buckwheat**
Licorice	**Milk**

IgE antibodies to major and minor penicillin allergy determinants are detected by wheal-and-flare skin tests. Penicilloyl-polylysine (6×10^{-5} M solution) elicits a positive skin test in most patients with "major determinant sensitivity," ie, a history of late urticaria or drug rash but not anaphylaxis. "Minor determinant sensitivity" indicates anaphylaxis to penicillin. The test mixture of minor penicillin allergy determinants is not presently marketed, although a skin test using penicillin G (1000 units/mL) is usually positive in persons with documented anaphylaxis. The test is not recommended if there is an unequivocal history of penicillin anaphylaxis, because of risk of anaphylaxis to the test.

In vitro tests to detect the presence of circulating IgE antibody may be helpful if the test is positive, but a negative result does not rule out anaphylactic sensitivity, because the high affinity of IgE antibodies for mast cell receptors may result in a level of circulating IgE antibodies too low for detection by in vitro methods. The radioallergosorbent test (RAST) is the most frequently used in vitro test for IgE antibody, but it can be used only for protein allergens. Technical factors account for a significant number of false-positive and false-negative results.

The presence of IgE antibodies, whether detected by a skin test or an in vitro test, does not diagnose the cause of anaphylaxis without correlation with the patient's history.

Allergens

The allergens responsible for anaphylaxis are different from those commonly associated with atopy. They are usually encountered in a food, a drug, or an insect sting. Foods and insect venoms are complex mixtures of many potential allergens. In only a few cases have the allergens been identified chemically. The same allergen or allergenic epitope may exist naturally in more than one food, drug, or venom, resulting in cross-reactivity.

A. Foods: Any food can contain an allergen that could cause anaphylaxis. Table 26–3 lists some of the more common ones. Peanuts, nuts, fish, and egg white lead the list in frequency.

B. Drugs: Any drug is capable of causing anaphylaxis, although the risk is minimal for most people. Table 26–4 lists drugs and diagnostic agents

reported to cause anaphylaxis in patients with drug-specific IgE antibody. Heterologous proteins and polypeptides are the most likely to induce this type of sensitivity. However, most drugs used today are organic chemicals, which function immunologically as haptens. Anaphylaxis can occur from parenteral, oral, or topical drug administration. In some cases the amount needed to cause a systemic reaction can be extremely small; eg, a reaction in penicillin-allergic patients has been produced by minute amounts of penicillin in the milk obtained from penicillin-treated cows.

Anaphylaxis to blood and blood components may be caused by food allergens in donor blood or, rarely, by passive transfer of IgE antibodies to a food or drug when the transfusion recipient ingests that allergen shortly before or after the transfusion.

C. Insect Venoms: Anaphylaxis occurs from stings of Hymenoptera insects (Table 26–5), occasionally from biting insects such as deer flies, kissing bugs, and bedbugs, and rarely from snake venom. The venom of Hymenoptera insects is a complex bio-

Table 26–4. Some drugs and diagnostic agents that cause anaphylaxis.

Heterologous proteins and polypeptides	Haptenic drugs
Hormones	Antibiotics
Insulin	Penicillin
Parathormone	Streptomycin
Adrenocorticotropic	Cephalosporin
hormone	Tetracycline
Vasopressin	Amphotericin B
Relaxin	Nitrofurantoin
Enzymes	Diagnostic agents
Trypsin	Sulfobromophthalein
Chymotrypsin	Sodium dehydrocholate
Chymopapain	Vitamins
Penicillinase	Thiamine
Asparaginase	Folic acid
Vaccines	Others
Toxoids	Barbiturates
Allergy extracts	Diazepam
Polysaccharides	Phenytoin
Dextran	Protamine
Iron-dextran	Aminopyrine
Acacia	Acetylcysteine

Table 26–5. Hymenoptera insects.

Honeybee (*Apis mellifera*)
Yellow jacket (*Vespula* spp)
Hornet (*Dolichovespula* spp)
Wasp (*Polistes* spp)
Fire ant (*Solenopsis* spp)

logic fluid containing several enzymes and other active constituents. There are multiple allergens for human anaphylaxis, some specific to a particular species and others cross-reactive among species and genera. Allergens in honeybee venom include phospholipase A, hyaluronidase, phosphatase, and melittin.

The sting of a single insect is sufficient to produce a severe, even fatal anaphylactic reaction in sensitive patients. Sensitization occurs from prior stings, and if patients are allergic to a common or cross-reacting antigen they may have an anaphylactic reaction after being stung by any species of Hymenoptera insect. There is no evidence that other allergic diseases, including atopy and drug anaphylaxis, predispose to Hymenoptera anaphylaxis.

D. Other Allergens: There have been several cases of anaphylaxis occurring in women during intercourse because of allergy to a glycoprotein allergen in seminal fluid. There is one report of a woman sensitized to exogenous progesterone administered as a drug. She subsequently had anaphylaxis to endogenous progesterone and was cured by oophorectomy.

Latex allergy has recently become a significant cause of anaphylaxis and contact urticaria among medical personnel and children with spina bifida or urogenital birth defects. The allergen is derived from the rubber tree *Hevea brasiliensis*. IgE antibodies in affected patients are detected best by skin test, and these patients must carefully avoid all sources of latex products.

Anaphylactoid Reactions

A reaction clinically and pathologically identical to anaphylaxis can occur without the participation of an IgE antibody and corresponding allergen. This phenomenon is called an anaphylactoid reaction. (The term "anaphylactoid" is sometimes used inappropriately to refer to mild IgE-mediated anaphylactic reaction.)

A. Exercise-Induced "Anaphylaxis": A number of cases have been described. In some the reaction occurs only in association with eating, sometimes related to a specific food. During exercise the plasma histamine level rises, suggesting that nonimmunologic mast cell stimulation might be triggered by an endogenous factor, possibly endorphin. The reason for individual susceptibility is unknown, although a familial tendency has been reported, possibly because of a genetic defect. Many cases, however, are transient, suggesting a role for acquired factors.

B. Cholinergic Anaphylactoid Reaction. Exercise, emotions, and overheating provoke reactions in patients with this rare condition. The plasma histamine level rises when there is an increase in core body temperature. Patients may have a positive methacholine urticarial skin test. A proposed mechanism is an abnormal reactivity of mast cells to the compensatory cholinergic response in thermoregulation when the core body temperature is elevated. This disease is an exaggerated form of cholinergic urticaria, described later in this chapter.

C. "Aggregate Anaphylaxis": Administration of gamma globulin for prophylaxis in patients with common variable immunodeficiency or other immunodeficiency diseases can cause anaphylactoid reactions. High-molecular-weight aggregated gamma globulin is probably responsible, since immunoglobulin aggregates can activate complement through the classic pathway. Ultracentrifugation of the preparation to eliminate aggregates prevents such reactions. Aggregated immunoglobulins generate anaphylatoxins C3a, C4a, and C5a from the parent complement components C3, C4, and C5, respectively, in a manner similar to the effect of antigen and corresponding specific IgG or IgM complement-activating antibodies. Anaphylatoxins are capable of activating mast cells for mediator release, thereby producing the anaphylactoid reaction.

D. Non-IgE Anaphylaxis: Some patients with selective absence of IgA produce IgG anti-IgA antibodies following transfusion of IgA-containing plasma in whole blood or blood products. In such patients, subsequent administration of transfused IgA may cause anaphylaxis, presumably from complement activation and anaphylatoxin generation by circulating complexes of IgA and anti-IgA. An alternative explanation would involve antibodies of the IgG4 subclass. Several laboratories have reported that IgG4 antibodies can activate mast cells for mediator release in the presence of antigen. There is no direct proof yet that IgG4 "short-term sensitizing" antibodies are involved in systemic anaphylaxis.

E. Anaphylactoid Reactions From Ionic Compounds: Radiographic iodinated contrast media, especially when used for intravenous pyelography or cholangiography, produce anaphylactoid reactions that are frequently mild, causing only hives or itching. However, they may be severe, causing shock. In one case in 100,000, these reactions are fatal. The reaction can occur on first exposure and does not necessarily recur on subsequent exposure. Attempts to demonstrate specific antibodies to the compounds have been unrewarding. The reaction may be related to the ionic nature of these compounds, since newer nonionic contrast media appear less likely to cause such reactions.

The antibiotic polymyxin B is also a highly charged ionic compound that causes anaphylactoid reactions in some patients.

F. Other Causes: Polysaccharides such as dextran, gums, and resins produce anaphylactoid reactions by unknown mechanisms, probably direct mast cell activation. Certain drugs, especially the opiates, curare, and *d*-tubocurarine, behave similarly (Table 26–6).

G. Idiopathic Anaphylaxis. A few patients experience recurrent attacks of anaphylaxis without evidence of exposure to an antecedent allergen. Exhaustive exploration of the history and careful observation of subsequent attacks will sometimes reveal an unsuspected allergen, but most of these cases appear to be truly idiopathic. Recurrent idiopathic anaphylaxis, like idiopathic chronic urticaria-angioedema, occurs predominantly in women between 20 and 60 years of age.

Differential Diagnosis

Anaphylactic and anaphylactoid reactions are identical in presentation. The former is produced by an antigen-antibody reaction, whereas the latter is caused by nonimmunologic release of mediators, so that the distinction must be determined by demonstrating whether the causative substance is an allergen.

Anaphylactic shock must be differentiated from other causes of circulatory failure, including primary cardiac failure, endotoxin shock, and reflex mechanisms. The most common form of shock that simulates anaphylactic shock is vasovagal collapse, which may occur from the injection of local anaesthetics, particularly during dental procedures. In this case, there is pallor without cyanosis, nausea, bradycardia, and an absence of respiratory obstruction and cutaneous symptoms.

The Jarisch-Herxheimer reaction occurs several hours after antimicrobial treatment of syphilis or onchocerciasis. It is characterized by fever, shaking chills, myalgias, headaches, and hypotension. Unlike anaphylaxis, it can be prevented by pretreatment with corticosteroids.

Aspirin and nonsteroidal anti-inflammatory drugs affect a certain subset of asthmatic patients, producing an acute asthmatic reaction that may include nasal congestion, erythema, facial swelling, and shock. Sulfite additives in certain foods and drugs may affect some asthmatics with a similar anaphylactic-like reaction. These nonimmunologic phenomena are discussed in Chapter 25.

Treatment

Treatment of anaphylaxis and anaphylactoid reactions is the same. It must be started promptly, so a high index of suspicion is necessary, and the diagnosis must be made rapidly. Once anaphylaxis is suspected, aqueous epinephrine, 1:1000 solution, is injected intramuscularly or subcutaneously in a dose of 0.2–0.5 mL for adults or 0.01 mL/kg of body weight for children. The dose is repeated in 15–30 minutes, if necessary. If the reaction was caused by an insect sting or injected drug, 0.1–0.2 mL of epinephrine, 1:1000 solution, can be infiltrated locally to retard absorption of the residual allergen. When anaphylaxis occurs in a patient receiving a β-adrenergic blocking drug, the reaction may be especially resistant to epinephrine, so that higher doses may be required. A tourniquet should be applied proximally if the injection or sting is on an extremity. The patient should then be examined quickly but thoroughly to assess the involved target organs, so that subsequent treatment is appropriate to the physiopathologic abnormalities.

A. Shock: The patient should be recumbent with the legs elevated in Trendelenberg's position. An intravenous line, preferably by catheter, facilitates drug administration. Intravenous epinephrine can be given in a dose of 1–5 mL, 1:10,000 solution, for adults and 0.01–0.05 mL/kg for children if systolic blood pressure is below 60. Other vasopressor drugs, such as dopamine, can be administered while blood pressure and pulse rate are being monitored. The specific treatment for shock, however, is fluid infused rapidly. Normal saline may be satisfactory, although as much as 6 L or more in 12 hours may be necessary. Initially, 1 L should be given every 15–30 minutes while vital signs and urine output are monitored. Plasma or other colloid solutions might be required. It may be necessary to monitor fluid replacement by measuring central venous pressure.

B. Laryngeal Edema: Examination of the airway for the presence of laryngeal obstruction should be done early. Establishing an effective airway is lifesaving. Passage of an endotracheal tube may be difficult because of the swelling. Puncture of the cricothyroid membrane with a 14- or 16-gauge short needle will provide an airway, but it is too dangerous to attempt in a child. Cricothyrotomy is the preferred

Table 26–6. Drugs and additives that cause anaphylactoid reactions.

Nonsteroidal anti-inflammatory drugs
  Aspirin
  Aminopyrine
  Fenoprofen
  Flufenamic acid
  Ibuprofen
  Indomethacin
  Mefenamic acid
  Naproxen
  Tolmetin
  Zomepirac

Opiate narcotics
  Morphine
  Codeine
  Meperidine

Mannitol
Radiographic iodinated contrast media
Curare and *d*-tubocurarine
Dextran

method if treatment must be done outside a hospital. In the hospital, surgical tracheostomy is preferred.

C. Bronchial Obstruction: The treatment is the same as for acute asthma. Intravenously, aminophyllin at 6 mg/kg in 20 mL of dextrose in water given over 10–15 minutes serves as a loading dose, to be followed by 0.9 mg/kg/h. If the patient is an asthmatic and is receiving theophylline currently, a lower dose is necessary, and theophyllin blood levels should be monitored. If bronchospasm persists, nebulized β-adrenergic bronchodilators can be given by intermittent positive-pressure breathing. Hydrocortisone or methylprednisolone injections intramuscularly are used if the patient has recently received steroid therapy for asthma or for another condition. Oxygen by nasal catheter at 4–6 L/min is necessary in Pa_{CO_2} is less than 55 mm Hg. In the event of respiratory failure with Pa_{CO_2} above 65 mm Hg, intubation and mechanical assistance of ventilation are necessary.

D. Urticaria, Angioedema, & Gastrointestinal Reactions. These manifestations are not life-threatening and respond well to antihistamines. If they are mild, an oral antihistamine tablet is adequate. If they are severe, diphenhydramine, 50 mg (1–2 mg/kg for children), can be given intramuscularly or intravenously.

Monitoring treatment is vital in severe cases of anaphylaxis. Measurement of vital signs, examination of upper and lower airway potency, measurement of arterial blood gases, and electrocardiography are best accomplished in the emergency room or intensive care unit. All patients should be observed for 24 hours after satisfactory treatment, except in very mild cases.

Histamine H_2 receptor-blocking drugs, such as cimetidine or ranitidine, have been advocated as an adjunct to H_1 receptor antagonists, but their effectiveness has yet to be evaluated. Corticosteroid drugs have no antianaphylactic actions and should not be expected to alleviate the immediate acute life-threatening manifestations, although there may be special indications, as noted above. Complications such as cardiac arrythmias, hypoxic seizures, and metabolic acidosis are treated in the usual way.

The management of anaphylaxis from a Hymenoptera insect sting is the same as for any anaphylactic reaction. In honeybee stings, the venom sac and stinger usually remain in the skin and should be removed promptly by scraping with a knife or fingernail. Local reactions usually require only cold compresses to ease pain and reduce swelling, but extensive local inflammation may require brief corticosteroid therapy.

Prevention

A. Avoidance: Once the diagnosis of anaphylaxis has been established and the cause has been determined, prevention of future episodes is essential.

In the case of food or drug allergy, the allergen and potential cross-reacting allergens must be thoroughly avoided. Insect-sensitive patients should avoid outdoor food and garbage, flowers, perfumes, mowing the lawn, and walking barefoot outdoors. Pretreatment with antihistamines and corticosteroids prior to radiography requiring administration of a contrast medium reduces the risk of a reaction in patients who have experienced a prior radiographic anaphylactoid reaction. Patients with IgA deficiency who require blood products should be transfused from donors with absent IgA (see Chapter 19).

Any physician or nurse who administers drugs by injection should be prepared to treat a possible anaphylactic reaction by having appropriate drugs available, and patients should remain under observation for 15–20 minutes after any injection.

B. Anaphylaxis Kit: Patients with anaphylactic sensitivity to Hymenoptera insects or food should carry at all times a small kit containing a preloaded syringe of epinephrine and an antihistamine tablet. Epinephrine or a β-adrenergic drug in a metered-dose inhaler is not a reliable means of protection for anaphylactic shock.

C. Desensitization: Hymenoptera venom desensitization has been shown to be highly effective, as judged by responses to subsequent natural stings. Treatment is recommended for patients who have experienced systemic anaphylaxis after a sting and who have a significant positive skin test to one or more venoms. The maintenance dose for venom desensitization, 100 μg of each venom, is usually achieved in 12 weeks or less on weekly increasing doses. It should be continued at intervals of 4–6 weeks indefinitely. Some patients maintain long-lasting protection after discontinuing a 5-year course of desensitization. However, reliable criteria for determining the optimal treatment duration in every case are not currently known.

Insulin-allergic diabetic patients and the occasional penicillin-sensitive patient may require desensitization.

Complications

Death from laryngeal edema, respiratory failure, shock, or cardiac arrhythmia usually occurs within minutes after onset of the reaction, but in occasional cases irreversible shock persists for hours. Permanent brain damage may result from the hypoxia of respiratory or cardiovascular failure. Urticaria or angioedema may recur for months after penicillin anaphylaxis. Myocardial infarction, abortion, and renal failure are other potential complications.

Prognosis

It is usually assumed that in anaphylaxis each succeeding exposure results in a more severe reaction. However, experience with cases of anaphylaxis to penicillin, Hymenoptera venom, and food indicates that this not necessarily the case. If sufficient time elapses without allergen exposure, there may be a decrease or loss or sensitivity in some patients. There is no method to predict changes in sensitivity, but it can sometimes be documented by periodic testing. Immunotherapy for stinging-insect sensitivity is strikingly effective in favorably altering the prognosis, and desensitization can occasionally abrogate penicillin anaphylaxis for a short time to permit the drug to be used safely. The prognosis must always be guarded by the knowledge that IgE immunologic memory may be lifelong. Anaphylactoid drug reactions follow various courses. Patients who react adversely to radiographic iodinated contrast media will usually tolerate subsequent exposure to the same contrast medium without reaction, but statistically a reaction is more likely to occur in a patient who had experienced a prior reaction.

URTICARIA & ANGIOEDEMA

Major Immunologic Features
- Acute urticaria-angioedema is a cutaneous form of anaphylaxis.
- IgE-mediated allergies to foods or drugs are common causes.
- Chronic or recurrent disease is usually non-immunologic and of unknown cause.

General Considerations

Urticaria (also known as hives) and angioedema (also known as angioneurotic edema) can be considered a single illness characterized by vasodilatation and increased vascular permeability of the skin (urticaria) or subcutaneous tissues (angioedema). It is a localized cutaneous form of anaphylaxis and is one of the manifestations of systemic anaphylaxis. The same IgE antibody mechanism is responsible for the pathogenesis of allergic urticaria-angioedema and for that of systemic anaphylaxis, and the lists of the usual allergens are very similar. Idiopathic (nonallergic) urticaria-angioedema is analogous to the anaphylactoid reaction. In contrast to anaphylaxis, urticaria is a benign condition and is much more common.

A. Epidemiology. Urticaria affects about 20% of the population, usually as a single or occasional acute attack.

B. Pathology. A variety of histopathologic lesions have been described, but these correlate poorly with the clinical presentation. They include edema, nonnecrotizing vasculitis, necrotizing vasculitis, perivasculitis, and a variety of different inflammatory reactions in the skin.

C. Pathogenesis: Urticaria and angioedema are the visible manifestations of localized cutaneous or subcutaneous edema from the increased permeability of blood bessels, probably postcapillary ven-

ules. Since injection of histamine into the skin produces the spontaneous wheal, erythema, and pruritus of a typical urticarial lesion, it is generally accepted that endogenous histamine liberation is the mechanism responsible for the disease. The fact that subcutaneous tissue is looser and contains fewer nerve endings explains the more diffuse swelling and less severe itching in angioedema. Elevated levels of histamine in venous blood draining areas of induced urticaria have been repeatedly demonstrated. Other mediators from mast cells, particularly leukotrienes, are also believed to contribute to the pathophysiology.

D. Immunologic Pathogenesis: Many cases of acute urticaria and angioedema have been shown to have an allergic cause. In these cases, allergen-specific IgE antibody fixed to cutaneous or subcutaneous mast cells triggers mediator release or activation when allergen is encountered, as in anaphylaxis or atopy. Other potential immunologic pathways for mast cell mediator liberation, eg, the complement-derived anaphylatoxin pathway, have not been shown to operate in this disease. Idiopathic urticaria-angioedema and the various physical urticarias described below lack an allergen-antibody etiology. The precise means by which cutaneous mast cells are stimulated under these circumstances is unknown.

Clinical Features

A. Symptoms & Signs: Urticaria appears as multiple areas of well-demarcated edematous plaques that are intensely pruritic. They are either white with surrounding erythema or red with blanching when stretched. Individual lesions vary in diameter from a few millimeters to many centimeters. They are circular or serpiginous. Regardless of the duration of the illness, individual lesions are evanescent, lasting from 1 to 48 hours. They may appear anywhere on the skin surface but often have a predilection for areas of pressure. Angioedema appears as diffuse areas of nondependent, nonpitting swelling without pruritus, with predilection for the face, especially the periorbital and perioral areas. Swelling can occur in the mouth and pharynx as well.

Acute urticaria lasts for a few hours or at most a few days and is most likely to be associated with an identifiable cause, including allergy, nonspecific drug effect, infection, or physical factors. Chronic or recurrent urticaria persists with a variable course over a period of many weeks to years. Urticaria and angioedema may appear together in the same patient.

B. Laboratory Findings: There are no abnormal laboratory tests, except for the specific procedures described below.

Clinical Diagnosis

The diagnosis is immediately apparent on inspection of the skin.

Immunologic Diagnosis

A complete medical and environmental history and physical examination are usually necessary to determine the cause. Allergic urticaria may arise from exposure to allergens by ingestion or injection (most commonly), direct skin contact (less frequently), and inhalation (rarely). The discussion on common allergies in anaphylaxis earlier in this chapter applies to acute allergic urticaria.

Food allergy is diagnosed by careful dietary history, use of elimination diets, and appropriate food challenges. Drug allergy requires close scrutiny of the patient's recent drug history, elimination of suspected drugs, and occasionally deliberate challenge, although skin testing is helpful for certain drugs such as penicillin. The diagnosis of cold urticaria is made by applying an ice cube to the forearm for 5 minutes and observing localized urticaria after the skin has been rewarmed. Similar tests with application of heat, ultraviolet light, vibration, pressure, or water to a test area of the skin are appropriate if the history suggests these causes.

Cholinergic urticaria is suggested by the typical appearance of the lesions and exercise provocation. The methacholine skin test is positive in only one-third of patients.

Diagnostic tests for parasitic or other infections, lymphomas or other neoplasms, or connective tissue diseases are generally indicated only if the history and physical examination would have suggested such diseases in the absence of urticaria. It should be emphasized that in most cases of chronic recurrent urticaria, no cause is found even with the most diligent search.

Causes

A. Allergy: Ingestant allergens are much more frequent causes of urticaria than are inhalants. Any food or drug can cause hives. Occult sources of drugs such as penicillin in milk and the use of proprietary medications such as laxatives, headache remedies, and vitamin preparations must be considered. Food and drug additives are occasionally responsible. Insect sting allergy may cause urticaria without any other signs of systemic anaphylaxis.

B. Physical Causes: Dermographism, the whealing reaction that is an exaggerated form of the triple response of Lewis, occurs following scratching or stroking of the skin in 5% of the population. Another common phenomenon, unrelated to dermographism, is the appearance of hives after showering.

Cold urticaria may be induced locally by cooling of the skin on contact with cold. The hives often appear only upon rewarming. Occasionally generalized hives are provoked by cooling a portion of the body. Patients are in danger of shock when swimming in cold water. The diagnostic ice cube test is described above. Occasionally the reaction can be passively transferred by serum to the skin of an unaffected individual.

Familial cold urticaria is a rare autosomal dominant disorder in which cold produces fever, chills, joint pains, and hives.

Urticaria and angioedema induced by heat, sunlight, water, or vibration are different syndromes and are rare. Pressure urticaria is a common feature of all forms of urticaria. However, delayed-pressure urticaria resulting from prolonged sustained pressure producing painful swelling is a distinct entity.

Cholinergic urticaria is a disease of unknown cause in which small (1–3-mm) wheals with prominent surrounding flare appear after exercise, heat, or emotional stress. Elevated body temperature is necessary for the reaction, which is believed to be initiated by a cholinergic response that triggers mast cell release. Other symptoms including hypotension and gastrointestinal cramping may accompany the urticaria and angioedema.

C. Vasculitis: Urticaria is reported as a symptom in some patients with systemic lupus erythematosus (SLE), systemic sclerosis, polymyositis, leukocytoclastic vasculitis, palpable purpura, hypocomplementemia, or cryoglobulinemia, but there is as yet no convincing explanation for the association.

D. Neoplasms: Urticaria or angioedema is occasionally reported in a patient with neoplasm, especially Hodgkin's disease and lymphomas, but a cause-and-effect relationship is difficult to document. Rarely, angioedema from C1 esterase deficiency is caused by a lymphoma. This is discussed in Chapter 23.

E. Cyclooxygenase Inhibitors: Aspirin and nonsteroidal anti-inflammatory drugs frequently precipitate acute or chronic urticaria. They also potentiate idiopathic urticaria or urticaria from other causes. The mechanism is unknown. There are many reports that food and drug additives, most notably tartrazine yellow dye and the preservative sodium benzoate, also cause or exacerbate hives, but the evidence is unimpressive.

F. Emotions: Precipitation of hives by emotional stress or other psychologic factors is a frequent clinical observation, but explanation of this phenomenon requires further study.

G. Idiopathic Urticaria-Angioedema: This category encompasses most cases of chronic urticaria-angioedema, because exhaustive diagnostic studies are unrevealing in the large majority of patients with recurrent urticaria lasting for more than 6 weeks.

Differential Diagnosis

The characteristic appearance of urticaria and angioedema, coupled with a history of rapid disappearance of the individual lesions, leaves little chance of incorrect diagnosis.

Multiple insect bites may evoke wheals, but careful inspection will show the bite punctum at the center of the lesion. Angioedema can be distinguished from ordinary edema or myxedema by its absence from dependent areas of localization and by its evanescent appearance.

Hereditary angioedema is a rare condition that produces periodic swelling and may be accompanied by abdominal pain and laryngeal edema. Urticaria does not occur in this disease. The disease is suspected when there is a similar family history of recurrent episodes unrelated to exposure to allergens. The diagnosis is made by finding decreased serum C4 and is confirmed by the absence of C1 esterase inhibitor activity in the serum. It is described in greater detail in Chapter 23.

Urticaria pigmentosa is an infiltration of the skin with multiple mast cell tumors that appear as tan macules which urticate when rubbed or stroked. It may be accompanied by visceral mast cell tumors (systemic mastocytosis).

Treatment

Urticaria caused by foods or drugs is treated by avoidance of the offending agents, although hyposensitization to a drug might be attempted in the rare instances in which no alternative drug is available. Urticaria associated with infection is self-limited if the infection is adequately treated. In cases of physical allergy, protective measures to avoid heat, sunlight, or cold must be advised.

Drug treatment is a useful adjunct in the management of all patients, whether or not the cause has been found, but a good response to symptomatic treatment should not deter the physician from efforts to find an underlying cause. Antihistamine drugs are the principal method of treatment, but they must be given in adequate dosage. H_1 receptor antagonists have a proven but inconsistent effectiveness in treating urticaria. The combined use of H_1 and H_2 receptor blockers is frequently recommended but of unproven value for this disease. Epinephrine injections may relieve hives transiently and should be used in treating angioedema involving the pharynx or larynx. Corticosteroids are usually ineffective and should not be used to treat urticaria of unknown cause.

Complications & Prognosis

Urticaria is a benign disease. Since it is a cutaneous form of anaphylaxis, an excessive dose of allergens or physical triggering agent could result in life-threatening systemic anaphylaxis. Angioedema can obstruct the airway if localized in the larynx or adjacent structures.

REFERENCES

Anaphylaxis

Casale TB, Keahery TM, Kaliner M: Exercise-induced anaphylactic syndromes: Insights into diagnostic and pathophysiologic features. *JAMA* 1986;**255**:2049.

Reisman RE, Lieberman P: Anaphylaxis and anaphylactoid reactions. *Immunol Allergy Clin N Am* 1992;**12**:501 (Entire issue).

Sheffer AL: Anaphylaxis. *J Allergy Clin Immunol* 1985;**75**:227.

Slater J: Latex allergy—what do we know? *J Allergy Clin Immunol* 1992;**90**:3.

Smith PL et al: Physiologic manifestations of human anaphylaxis. *J Clin Invest* 1980;**66**:1072.

Valentine MD: Insect venom allergy: Diagnosis and treatment. *J Allergy Clin Immunol* 1984;**73**:299.

Wiggins CA, Dykewicz MS, Patterson R: Idiopathic anaphylaxis: Classification, evaluation and treatment of 123 patients. *J Allergy Clin Immunol* 1988;**82**:849.

Urticaria & Angioedema

Hirschmann JV et al: Cholinergic urticaria. *Arch Dermatol* 1987;**123**:462.

Kauppinen I, Juntunen K, Lanki H: Year book: Urticaria in children: Retrospective evaluation and follow-up. *Allergy* 1984;**39**:469.

Matthews KP: Urticaria and angioedema. *J Allergy Clin Immunol* 1983;**72**:1.

Soter NA, Wasserman SI: Physical urticaria/angioedema: An experimental model of mast cells activation in humans. *J Allergy Clin Immunol* 1980;**66**:358.

Wanderer AA et al: Clinical characteristics of cold-induced systemic reactions acquired in cold urticaria syndromes: Recommendations for prevention of this complication and a proposal for a diagnostic classification of cold urticaria. *J Allergy Clin Immunol* 1986;**78**:417.

Immune-Complex Allergic Diseases   27

Abba I. Terr, MD

This chapter will discuss allergic diseases mediated by immune complexes of allergen with IgG or IgM antibodies. Activation of complement by immune complexes generates chemotactic and vasoactive mediators that cause tissue damage by a combination of immune-complex deposition, alterations in vascular permeability and blood flow, and the action of toxic products from inflammatory cells. The pathology of immune complexes has been extensively studied in animals, and the process is detailed in Chapter 11. Tissue injury caused by immune complexes is believed to occur also in certain nonallergic diseases discussed elsewhere in this book. These include systemic lupus erythematosus (see Chapter 31), vasculitis (see Chapter 34), glomerulonephritis (see Chapter 36), rheumatoid arthritis (see Chapter 31), and acute allograft rejection (see Chapter 57).

The classic immune-complex allergic diseases are the cutaneous Arthus reaction and systemic serum sickness. In allergic bronchopulmonary aspergillosis a 2-phase immunologic mechanism is involved, in which immune complexes of *Aspergillus* antigens and IgG antibodies produce bronchial inflammation and bronchopulmonary tissue destruction in the presence of a concomitant IgE response to the allergen.

THE ARTHUS REACTION

In 1903 Arthus showed that the intradermal injection of a protein antigen into a hyperimmunized rabbit produced local inflammation which progressed to a hemorrhagic necrotic lesion that ulcerated. Later investigations established that the Arthus phenomenon is a localized cutaneous inflammatory response to the deposition of immune complexes in dermal blood vessels. It therefore serves as a model system for all immune complex-mediated diseases.

Arthus reactions are rare in humans. Hemorrhagic necrosis at the site of injection of a drug or an insect bite or sting could suggest an Arthus reaction, but the distinction from a toxic reaction or secondary infection requires laboratory or immunohistochemical evidence of the relevant immune complexes. A limited form of the Arthus reaction occurs commonly at the site of allergy desensitization injections after sufficient doses of injected allergens have been given to generate IgG "blocking" antibodies (see Chapter 25). Because the level of IgG antibodies achieved in allergy therapy is relatively low, the cutaneous and subcutaneous tissue inflammation produces only mild erythema and induration. This begins several hours after the injection and usually subsides in less than 24 hours.

The immunologic pathogenesis is dependent on antigen and antibody concentrations necessary to form immune complexes capable of initiating complement activation. Intermediate-size complexes activate complement most readily and therefore are the most damaging to tissues. Large insoluble complexes are rapidly cleared by the mononuclear phagocyte system, and small complexes fail to activate complement receptors. Immune complexes activate complement through fixation of the Fc portion of antibody with the Fc receptor on C1q. C3a and C5a anaphylatoxins are liberated. These molecules activate mast cells to release permeability factors, permitting localization of the immune complexes along the endothelial cell basement membrane. A coincidental IgE antibody response could theoretically achieve the same effect as complement-generated anaphylatoxins. Chemotactic factors from various complement components attract neutrophils. Neutrophils, macrophages, lymphocytes, and other cells with membrane Fc receptors are activated. Activated neutrophils are especially important in the Arthus reaction. They release toxic chemicals such as oxygen-containing free radicals, generate proteolytic enzymes from cytoplasmic granules, and phagocytose the immune complexes.

SERUM SICKNESS

Major Immunologic Features

■ Serum sickness is a systemic immune-complex complement-dependent reaction to an extrinsic antigen.

■ The severity of the disease is antigen dose-dependent.

■ The typical reaction produced by heterologous serum can occur in milder forms from other drugs.

General Considerations

Serum sickness (also known as serum disease) was a common disease when heterologous antiserum was used as passive immunization in the treatment of a number of infectious and toxic illnesses in the pre-antibiotic era. Today, "serum therapy" with heterologous (usually equine) serum or gamma globulin is restricted to passive immunization for a very few toxic diseases and the use of antilymphocyte or antithymocyte globulin for immunosuppressive therapy. Vaccines, other protein drugs, and bee stings may cause serum sickness. A mild serum sickness reaction is occasionally caused by nonprotein drugs, especially sulfonamides, penicillin, and cephalosporins.

A. Definition. Serum sickness is an acute, self-limited allergic disease caused by immune complex-activated complement-generated inflammation after injection of a protein or haptenic drug. The cardinal features are fever, dermatitis, lymphadenopathy, and joint pains.

B. Epidemiology. Serum sickness is caused by therapeutic injection of foreign material that is potentially antigenic as well as therapeutic. Therefore, its prevalence depends on the prevalence of certain forms of medical treatment. Therapeutic injections or large quantities of heterologous serum produce serum sickness in proportion to the dose. The attack rate was approximately 90% when a 200-mL dose of horse serum was given. Fractionated gamma globulin is less likely than is whole serum to cause the disease. There are no prevalence statistics available today, but reports of serum sickness are now uncommon.

C. Immunologic Pathogenesis: The pathogenesis of human serum sickness is believed to be similar to the mechanism of "one-shot" serum sickness produced experimentally in immunized rabbits (Fig 27–1). Following a single large dose of injected antigen there is a brief period of equilibration between blood and tissues followed by slow degradation of antigen over several days as the primary antibody response is initiated. Antibody synthesis leads to antibody release into the circulation, where antigen-antibody complexes gradually form under conditions of moderate antigen excess. Intermediate-sized complexes deposit in small blood vessels in various organs, triggering the events that are described above

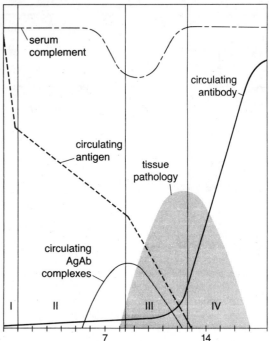

Figure 27–1. Immunologic events in experimental "one-shot" serum sickness in rabbits. The pathogenesis of human serum sickness is similar. A single high dose of antigen is given intravenously on day 0. **Phase I:** Equilibration of antigen between blood and tissues. **Phase II:** Primary antibody response. Near the end of this phase, antibody combines with antigen to form circulating immune complexes. **Phase III:** Tissue pathology and progression of clinical disease. Circulating complexes activate complement and deposit in tissues. The serum complement level falls transiently, and residual antigen is rapidly cleared from the blood. **Phase IV:** Remission. Antigen is no longer available, and the level of circulating antibody rises. No further immune complexes form, complement levels return to normal, pathologic lesions repair, and symptoms subside.

in the Arthus reaction. This gives rise to the clinical and pathological manifestations of disease. Free antigen is removed more rapidly from the circulation as antibody production and immune-complex formation increases. The circulating complexes then shift to antibody excess, thereby decreasing in size and clearing more rapidly. Finally, free antibody circulates, no further lesions appear, and healing takes place.

The optimal conditions for serum sickness occur during the primary antibody response of the previously immunized host. With subsequent exposures to the same antigen, the anamnestic antibody response facilitates rapid antigen clearance and greatly reduces the amount and persistence of immune complexes in the circulation.

Clinical Features

A. Symptoms & Signs: Primary serum sickness begins 4–21 days (usually 7–10 days) after initial exposure to the causative antigen. The first sign is often a pruritic rash, which may be urticarial, maculopapular, or erythematous. There may be angioedema, and the injection site usually becomes inflamed. Fever, lymphadenopathy, arthralgias, and myalgias complete the clinical presentation. Joint swelling and redness may occur, and occasionally there are headache, nausea, and vomiting. Recovery takes 7–30 days. Clinically significant cardiac or renal involvement is unusual. There may be neurologic involvement, usually in the form of mononeuritis involving especially the brachial plexus. Rarely there may be polyneuritis, Guillain-Barré syndrome, or even meningoencephalitis.

Secondary serum sickness occurs in patients previously sensitized to the antigen. There is a short latent period of only 2–4 days, and the clinical course of the disease may be brief but the manifestations could be severe.

Serum sickness reactions to most drugs used today are much milder than the disease that was caused by horse serum injections.

B. Laboratory Findings: There is slight leukocytosis. Plasma cells in the bone marrow are increased in number and may appear in the blood. There may be eosinophilia, but this is not characteristic. The erythrocyte sedimentation rate is increased. Circulating immune complexes and reduced levels of serum complement components are often detected in disease caused by heterologous serum, but they are not usually detected in drug-induced serum sickness (for detection methods, see Chapter 12). Mild proteinuria, hematuria, and casts; transient electrocardiographic abnormalities; and pleocytosis are not unusual.

Immunologic Diagnosis

There is no specific diagnostic test. The diagnosis is made on the basis of a compatible history of typical symptoms at an appropriate interval after drug administration, along with the physical and laboratory evidence. The disease is almost always benign and self-limited, with good prospects for complete recovery, so invasive tests such as tissue biopsy are not indicated.

Serum IgG and IgE antibodies specific to the relevant antigen may be detected in the time course illustrated in Fig 27–1 if confirmation of the diagnosis is required.

Treatment

Treatment should be conservative and symptomatic. Aspirin and antihistamines are effective. A short high-dose course of oral corticosteroids is warranted if symptoms are severe.

Complications & Prognosis

Complications are rare. Occasionally laryngeal edema may cause respiratory obstruction. The neuritis rarely is permanent.

ALLERGIC BRONCHOPULMONARY ASPERGILLOSIS

Major Immunologic Features

- Both IgE and IgG antibodies to *Aspergillus* are involved in the pathogenesis of pulmonary disease.
- IgE antibodies are directed to spore allergens.
- IgG antibodies are directed to mycelial allergens.
- There is nonspecific elevation of serum IgE level during acute exacerbations of disease.

General Considerations

Allergic bronchopulmonary aspergillosis (ABPA) is an unusual but not rare illness of young atopic adults with allergic asthma and is caused by a concomitant IgE and IgG antibody response to the ubiquitous fungus *Aspergillus fumigatus*. Airborne spores of this organism prevail both indoors and outdoors year-round in many geographic areas. The disease may occur in infants and children. It causes bronchiectasis and other destructive lung changes, but tissue damage can be prevented if the condition is diagnosed and treated properly.

A. Epidemiology: It is estimated that ABPA occurs in 1–2% of patients with asthma. Most cases have been reported in the USA and United Kingdom, but the disease probably occurs throughout the world. Prevalence rates are not available. With rare exceptions, it is a disease of persons with atopic asthma, but it is also associated with cystic fibrosis (see below). It has not been reported as an occupational disease. There is no known genetic predilection other than that related to atopy, and no human leukocyte antigen (HLA) association has been found.

B. Immunologic Pathogenesis: *A fumigatus* is ubiquitous in the air and soil, and it may be found indoors where moisture and organic matter favor mold growth. Occasional cases are caused by *A ochraceous* or *A terreus*. Exposure to *Aspergillus* is universal, but there is no evidence that excessive environmental exposure causes the disease. However, high-dose exposure may trigger acute attacks in the sensitized subject.

The pathogenesis of the disease is not entirely clear. There is general consensus that ABPA is an allergic disease that requires both IgE and IgG antibodies to *Aspergillus* and that their corresponding immunologic effector mechanisms cause the tissue damage (see Chapter 11). Inhalation of *Aspergillus* spores causes an immediate IgE-mediated bronchospastic reaction to an allergen in the spore, thereby trapping the organisms in the intraluminal mucus of the larger proximal bronchi. When the spores germinate and produce mycelia, the reaction of IgG antibodies to a different mycelial antigen produces tissue damage and inflammation, probably from immune complex-activated complement-derived products. Repeated episodes weaken the bronchial wall, leading to focal bronchiectasis. The significance of pathologic evidence of T cell-mediated inflammation in disease pathogenesis is unknown. The inflammatory process extends to peribronchial lung parenchyma, causing acute inflammatory infiltrates and ultimately chronic parenchymal destruction and fibrosis.

C. Pathology: The disease is confined to the lungs, where pathologic effects are 2-fold: those of the underlying asthma, and those associated with the acute inflammatory episodes and its sequelae. *Aspergillus* hyphae and inflammatory cells can be found in mucus plugs. The adjacent bronchial wall is infiltrated with mononuclear cells and eosinophils. A similar infiltrate affects peribronchial tissues, producing areas of interstitial pneumonia. There is a notable absence of granulocytic inflammation and vasculitis. Immunofluorescence studies have generally not shown immune-complex deposits, although these have been demonstrated in the late-onset skin test site in this disease (see below). The reason for this discrepancy, which weakens the argument for immune-complex pathogenesis, is not clear, but it may reflect the timing of the biopsy studies. Areas of chronic inflammation show noncaseating granulomas. Bronchiectasis and pulmonary fibrosis are late effects in the disease. The pathology, like the clinical manifestations, is variable.

Clinical Features

A. Symptoms & Signs: The clinical picture of ABPA is that of asthma with superimposed acute episodes of fever, cough productive of mucus plugs, chest pains, and malaise. There may be hemoptysis. Other nonspecific symptoms include headache, arthralgias, and myalgias. Some patients present with chronic lung damage, which suggests that the acute inflammatory episodes may be asymptomatic. Physical findings are those of asthma, as well as rales over areas of pulmonary infiltration.

B. Laboratory Findings: The diagnosis of ABPA is readily confirmed by objective evidence for the appropriate immune responses. Intradermal skin testing elicits a dual IgE antibody-mediated wheal-and-flare reaction to *A fumigatus* extract, followed by an Arthus reaction. Immunofluorescence at the height of the late response 6–12 hours after the intradermal injection shows deposition of immunoglobulins and C3, distinguishing this response from a late-phase IgE reaction. Prick testing may not be sensitive enough to elicit the IgG antibody Arthus re-

sponse, but it is usually sufficient for detecting the immediate IgE wheal-and-flare.

Serum precipitins to *Aspergillus* are found in about 70% of cases, and most of the remainder will be positive if the serum is concentrated 5-fold. IgG and IgE antibodies in serum can also be detected by radioallergosorbent test (RAST) or enzyme-linked immunosorbent assay (ELISA).

The total serum IgE level is characteristically high in this disease, and the level varies directly with disease activity. The mechanism for this is not known, but IgE levels have important diagnostic and prognostic significance. The majority of the excess IgE cannot be accounted for by *Aspergillus*-specific antibody, suggesting that some aspect of the active phase of ABPA inhibits T lymphocytes with suppressor activity for IgE-bearing B lymphocytes. Eosinophilia is present in blood and sputum, as in any case of asthma. Smear and culture of mucus plugs or sputum may yield the *Aspergillus* organism.

Pulmonary-function testing reveals reversible airway obstruction, but the acute inflammatory episodes can be distinguished from simple asthma by reduction in diffusing capacity. In chronic disease, obstruction may be only partially reversible and a restrictive component may be prominent. Bronchial provocation testing with *Aspergillus* extract produces a dual immediate bronchospastic component followed by a late-phase obstructive-restrictive component accompanied by fever and leukocytosis (see Fig 24–3).

The chest x-ray may reveal a variety of abnormalities but it may also be normal. There is no pathognomonic radiologic finding in this disease. Abnormalities that do occur may be found in many other lung diseases. During the acute phase, mucus plugs may produce focal areas of atelectasis or even segmental or lobar collapse. The peribronchial inflammation appears as migratory infiltrates especially in the upper lobes and hilar areas. Chronic disease from repeated acute insults can cause volume loss, particularly in the upper lobes. Bronchiectasis revealed by bronchography or tomography is saccular and proximal, less commonly cylindric.

Clinical Diagnosis

The diagnosis of ABPA is made on the basis of certain clinical and laboratory findings. There is no single diagnostic test. Table 27–1 lists diagnostic criteria. The diagnosis is definite when all 7 major criteria are met and probable when 6 are met. All major and minor criteria can be found in other illnesses, but the critical important of a definitive diagnosis is the necessity of corticosteroid therapy in this disease to prevent irreversible pulmonary damage. Any patient with a history of asthma and recurrent pulmonary infiltrates not otherwise explained should be given a diagnostic skin test with *Aspergillus*. Absence of the immediate reaction virtually rules out ABPA, but if the test is positive, a search for serum precipitins and radiographic evidence of bronchiectasis is indicated.

Differential Diagnosis

A fumigatus can cause other respiratory diseases. Invasive aspergillosis is an opportunistic infection that may complicate immunosuppression caused by drugs or disease (as discussed in Chapter 53). Aspergilloma is a localized growth of the organism invading a lung cavity or cyst. It typically induces a very marked precipitating antibody response, with a negative Arthus skin test, probably because of antibody excess at the skin site. *Aspergillus* hypersensitivity pneumonitis is a rare cause of farmer's lung. Finally, the organism is an atopic allergen in some cases of allergic asthma.

The variable clinical and radiologic features of the disease mimic other pulmonary diseases, including asthma with periodic mucus plugging or intercurrent viral infections, tuberculosis, hypersensitivity pneumonitis, pulmonary infiltration with eosinophilia (PIE syndrome), mucoid impaction, and bronchocentric granulomatosis.

ABPA in Cystic Fibrosis

By using the criteria of Table 27–1, the diagnosis of ABPA is made more frequently in children with cystic fibrosis than in the atopic asthmatic population. It is difficult to be sure whether this reflects a fundamental predisposition or a secondary opportunistic effect. Both atopy and *Aspergillus* infections are prevalent in children with cystic fibrosis, setting the stage for the necessary immune response involved in the pathogenesis of ABPA. Markedly elevated and fluctuating serum IgE levels, eosinophilia, and dramatic x-ray resolution of infiltrates with corticosteroid treatment are important diagnostic clues that ABPA is present in this disease.

Treatment

The diagnosis is important, because prompt high-dose systemic corticosteroid therapy causes prompt resolution of the acute allergic inflammatory episode and prevents the occurrence of long-term irreversible bronchial and parenchymal lung tissue damage. The mechanism of the therapeutic effect can only be surmised, but it is probably anti-inflammatory rather than immunosuppressive. An initial dose of 60 mg of prednisone daily in divided doses should be maintained until there is clinical and radiologic cure of the episode, after which a slowly tapering dose with maintenance at 20–30 mg once on alternate days should prevent relapses. It is useful to monitor total serum IgE levels, which fall during remissions and rise again with recurrences. There is some evidence that the serum IgE rise might precede the clinical exacerbation. Serial chest x-rays should also be part of the monitoring process.

The concurrent asthma is treated in the standard fashion, including desensitization if indicated. Injections of *Aspergillus* extract, however, should probably be avoided because this might theoretically enhance the IgG antibody response and hence worsen the disease. Inhaled corticosteroids are not indicated for acute attacks, but they can be used to control the asthma between attacks. Chest physiotherapy and inhaled bronchodilators are helpful adjuncts to improve expectoration of mucus plugs, but antifungal drugs are of unproven benefit.

Complications & Prognosis

Table 27–2 is a scheme for staging untreated disease. The course is variable and unpredictable and may depend upon factors of environmental exposure, so that not all patients proceed through all stages. Nevertheless, early recognition and adequate treatment prevent deterioration in pulmonary function and subsequent development of chronic airway obstruction and restrictive disease with pulmonary fibrosis. Occasionally, aspergilloma develops in a bronchiectatic or emphysematous cyst in ABPA. Cor pulmonale is likely to occur in stage V disease.

Table 27–1. Diagnostic criteria for ABPA.[1]

Major criteria
1. Episodic bronchial obstruction
2. Peripheral blood eosinophilia
3. Positive immediate skin reactivity
4. Serum precipitating antibodies
5. Elevated serum IgE
6. History of pulmonary infiltrates
7. Central bronchiectasis

Minor criteria
1. *A fumigatus*-positive sputum culture
2. History of expectorating brown plugs or flecks
3. Arthus (late) skin reactivity

[1]Reproduced, with permission, from Slavin RG: Allergic bronchopulmonary aspergillosis. *Clin Rev Allergy* 1985;**3**:167.

Table 27–2. Proposed stages of increasing severity and chronicity in ABPA.[1]

Stage	Description
I	Acute episode responsive to systemic corticosteroids
II	Remission
III	Recurrent exacerbations
IV	Recurrent exacerbations with steroid-dependent severe asthma
V	Pulmonary fibrosis, irreversible obstruction, advanced x-ray changes, cavitation and upper lobe contraction, severe bronchiectasis, emphysema

[1]Reproduced, with permission, from Patterson, R et al: Allergic bronchopulmonary aspergillosis: Staging as an aid to management. *Ann Intern Med* 1982;**96**:286.

REFERENCES

Serum Sickness

Bielory L et al: Human serum sickness: A prospective analysis of 35 patients treated with equine antithymocyte globulin for bone marrow failure. *Medicine* 1988;**67**:40.

Erffmeyer JE: Serum sickness. *Ann Allergy* 1986; **56**:105.

Naguwa SM, Nelson BL: Human serum sickness. *Clin Rev Allergy* 1985;**3**:117.

Allergic Bronchopulmonary Aspergillosis

Greenberger PA, Patterson R: Allergic bronchopulmonary aspergillosis and the evaluation of the patient with asthma. *J Allergy Clin Immunol* 1988;**81**:646.

Laufer P et al: Allergic bronchopulmonary aspergillosis in cystic fibrosis. *J Allergy Clin Immunol* 1984;**73**:44.

Patterson R et al: Allergic bronchopulmonary aspergillosis: Staging as an aid to management. *Ann Intern Med* 1982;**96**:286.

Cell-Mediated Hypersensitivity Diseases

28

Abba I. Terr, MD

Acquired immunity to many infectious diseases is mediated by specifically sensitized effector T lymphocytes (TDH cells). This is dramatically evident in the marked susceptibility to recurrent infections by many bacterial, fungal, viral, and other pathogens that characterizes patients with congenital (see Chapters 21 and 22) and acquired (see Chapter 52) T cell deficiency. The effector T lymphocyte also is responsible for certain forms of allergy, frequently referred to as delayed hypersensitivity.

This chapter will discuss a very common form of T cell-mediated allergy, allergic contact dermatitis, and a much less common disease, hypersensitivity pneumonitis. Allergic contact dermatitis is a pure form of T cell hypersensitivity, whereas hypersensitivity pneumonitis is a complex disease that may assume several forms clinically with a corresponding immunologic complexity involving antibodies, T cells, and a combination of both, depending upon factors of allergen dose and the form and the duration of allergen exposure. Hypersensitivity pneumonitis is included in this chapter because T cell mechanisms rather than antibody-mediated mechanisms are predominant in most clinically recognized cases.

ALLERGIC CONTACT DERMATITIS

Major Immunologic Features
- It is mediated by specifically sensitized T cells.
- It is caused most often by contact with haptenic chemicals.
- Patch testing is efficient and accurate in diagnosis.

General Considerations
A. Definition: Allergic contact dermatitis (also known as eczematous contact allergy) is an eczematous skin disease caused by cell-mediated hypersensitivity to an environmental allergen. Both sensitization and elicitation of the reaction involve contact of the allergen with the skin. Allergens caus-

ing the disease are numerous, are common, and include both natural and synthetic chemicals.

B. Epidemiology: The disease occurs worldwide and affects both sexes and all age groups. The most common allergen, pentadecylcatechol, found in poison ivy and poison oak, affects 50% of the US population clinically and another 35% subclinically.

C. Immunologic Pathogenesis: Allergic contact dermatitis is mediated by cutaneous T cell hypersensitivity. In this process, the Langerhans cell, a skin macrophage, functions as the antigen-processing cell at the local site of allergen penetration. It is uncertain whether the site of origin of the sensitized T lymphocyte is the skin, the regional lymph nodes, or elsewhere. Sensitization on primary contact takes several days. Once sensitization occurs, it lasts for years, if not for life, and is generalized. Reactions can be elicited anywhere on the skin. In some instances systemic reactions have been provoked when the allergen enters the body by ingestion or injection.

Many important sensitizing allergens are organic chemicals, and some are metals. It is assumed that they function as haptens, but the source and nature of the host carrier protein in the skin are unknown.

D. Pathology: The inflammatory response is allergic contact dermatitis is characterized by perivenular cuffing with lymphocytes, epidermal-cell vesiculation and necrosis, appearance of basophils and eosinophils, interstitial fibrin deposition, and dermal and epidermal edema.

Clinical Features
A. Symptoms & Signs: The skin eruption appears acutely as erythema, swelling, and vesiculation. In severe cases there may be extensive blistering, scaling, and weeping. In chronic milder disease, papules and scaling are more prominent. The lesion is pruritic or frankly painful if severe. The rapidity of onset after contact is directly proportionate to the degree of sensitivity and may range from 6 hours to several days.

The location of the eruption on the skin is helpful in diagnosing the cause. Certain areas of skin, such as the eyelids, react more easily than others, such as the palms. Metal dermatitis, usually caused by sensitivity to nickel, appears in discrete patches corresponding to the area of contact with jewelry, watches, or metal objects on clothing. A variety of allergens, such as dyes and fabric finishes, are found in clothing, causing a skin eruption on areas of skin covered by the apparel. Volatile allergens affect exposed areas, usually the face and arms. *Rhus* dermatitis from poison oak or poison ivy produces an especially severe disease with prominent vesicles and bullae, and there are characteristic streaks of vesicles corresponding to brushing of the skin by the plant leaves.

B. Laboratory Findings: There are none.

Allergens

The list of known allergens is enormous and theoretically unlimited. All types of chemicals can produce this disease, but metallic inorganic compounds and organic chemicals are the most likely, in contrast to the protein allergens that dominate in the other types of allergic conditions. The reason for this is unknown but is probably associated with the unique handling of foreign materials by the skin. The most common contact allergens are listed in Table 28–1.

Clinical Diagnosis

Diagnosis is suggested by the physical appearance of the eruption and distribution of lesions. By history, reactions may appear suddenly or present as a chronic, low-grade, smoldering dermatitis. The history must then be directed to monitoring exposures in the home, work, and recreational environment for possible allergens.

Table 28–1. Common contact allergens and concentrations used in patch testing.

Benzocaine 5%
Mercaptobenzothiazole 1%
Colophony 20%
p-Phenylenediamine 1%
Imidazolidinyl urea 2%
Cinnamic aldehyde 1%
Lanolin alcohol 30%
Carba mix 3%
Neomycin sulfate 20%
Thiuram mix 1%
Formaldehyde 1%
Ehtylenediamine dihydrochloride 1%
Epoxy resin 1%
Quaternium 15 2%
p-tert-Butylphenol formaldehyde resin 1%
Mercapto mix 1%
Black rubber mix 0.6%
Potassium dichromate 0.25%
Balsam of Peru 25%
Nickel sulfate 2.5%

Immunologic Diagnosis

The diagnosis is confirmed by patch testing, a time-honored, well-standardized procedure which is both an immunologic skin test and a provocation test that reproduces the disease "in miniature." Standard patch test allergens in concentrations that elicit allergic but not irritant reactions are available commercially for a number of the common contact sensitizers (Table 28–1). Reactions are read in 48 hours for localized eczema at the patch test site (Table 28–2).

Differential Diagnosis

Eczema refers to a general pattern of response of the skin to a variety of injurious stimuli. Scratching of the skin from any pruritic dermatosis can cause eczematization. The most common causes are atopic dermatitis; localized or generalized neurodermatitis; skin infection by bacteria or fungi; primary contact irritation by chemicals, foods, saliva, sweat, or urine; and dyshidrosis.

Treatment

The disease responds to systemic corticosteroids, which should be given as early as possible. Small localized areas of involvement can be treated with a topical steroid cream. Applications of cool, wet dressings containing Burow's solution (aluminum acetate) are helpful for acute lesions. Chronic lichenified dermatitis requires a potent fluorinated steroid ointment with an occlusive dressing. Extensive areas of involvement or severe bullous lesions should be treated with a brief oral burst of high-dose prednisone or with intramuscular triamcinolone or methylprednisolone. An antibiotic may be indicated for secondary infection. Antihistamines are generally not effective for controlling the pruritus.

Prognosis

A cure is to be expected if the correct allergen is identified and avoided. However, exposure to a cross-reacting allergenic chemical may cause a recurrence. Chromate allergy tends to be chronic, despite avoidance.

Prevention

The only means of prevention of the dermatitis in a sensitized patient is avoidance. The Landsteiner-Chase phenomenon of tolerance to contact sensitivity in guinea pigs by prior oral ingestion of allergen has

Table 28–2. Patch test interpretation.

Result	Interpretation
−	No reaction
±	Mild erythema
+	Definite erythema
+ +	Erythema and papules
+ + +	Erythema, papules, and vesicles

no practical application in humans. Some patients with mild nickel sensitivity can tolerate jewelry that is treated with a protective coating. *Rhus* dermatitis can probably be lessened, if not prevented, if the skin is thoroughly washed with water immediately after contact.

Desensitization with oral or injected *Rhus* extract or pentadecylcatechol has advocates in clinical practice, but there is, as yet, no sound evidence of effectiveness. Some patients appear to lose sensitivity after repeated natural exposure, a phenomenon known as "hardening," but this also remains to be documented.

PHOTOALLERGIC CONTACT DERMATITIS

Major Immunologic Features
- Allergen requires activation by ultraviolet light.
- Immunologic mechanism is identical to that of allergic contact dermatitis.

General Considerations
A. Definition: Photoallergic contact dermatitis is an uncommon eczematous skin disease caused by cell-mediated hypersensitivity to certain environmental chemicals that require sunlight activation to render them allergenic. The skin eruption appears on sun-exposed areas of the skin only.

B. Epidemiology: The disease has been associated primarily with drugs or chemical constituents of topical products such as soaps, cosmetics, and topical drugs. It therefore appears from time to time in epidemic form when a new product is introduced. The epidemic subsides when the product is withdrawn from the market once the photosensitivity potential is discovered.

C. Immunologic Pathogenesis: The mechanism is identical to ordinary allergic contact dermatitis, except that the causative chemical agent must be activated by the ultraviolet component of sunlight to become allergenic. The mechanism of allergen activation is unknown. Two theories have been proposed. Ultraviolet radiation may cause an alteration in tertiary structure to generate the necessary allergen epitope, or, alternatively, free radicals generated by ultraviolet light may be necessary for binding of the hapten chemical to skin carrier protein.

D. Pathology: The pathology is indistinguishable from that of allergic contact dermatitis.

Clinical Features
The dermatitis varies in its clinical appearance from an exaggerated sunburn to typical eczema to a severe vesiculobullous dermatosis. The distribution corresponds to sunlight exposure, but severe reactions may involve partially covered areas of skin as well. The eruption caused by a topically applied sensitizer is limited to the area of application.

Clinical Diagnosis
The disease is diagnosed by the combination of dermatitis in a sun-exposed distribution and a history of concurrent exposure to a known or suspected photoallergic sensitizer. A high index of suspicion facilitates diagnosis.

Immunologic Diagnosis
Photopatch testing is a modification of the standard patch test. The suspected agent is applied in the standard fashion for patch testing, and then the site is exposed to artificial ultraviolet light or sunlight. A test site not exposed to light is used as a control. The appearance of an eczematous eruption at the light-exposed site is a positive test.

Differential Diagnosis
Certain chemicals and drugs produce dermatitis in sun-exposed areas of skin in all individuals, provided that sufficient amounts of the compound accumulate in the skin and that there is exposure to a particular wavelength of ultraviolet light. These are called phototoxic reactions and are not mediated immunologically. Differential diagnosis also includes ordinary contact dermatitis, sunburn, and other causes of photosensitivity.

Allergens
Some of the important drugs and chemicals that cause photoallergic and phototoxic contact dermatitis are listed in Table 28–3. Some drugs taken systemically produce photodermatitis.

Treatment
Avoidance of the sensitizing agent and sunlight and treatment with topical corticosteroids are usually sufficient. Systemic corticosteroids may be required in severe cases.

Table 28–3. Some topical causes of photoallergic and phototoxic reactions.

Photoallergic	Phototoxic
Drugs	Drugs
Sulfonamides	Sulfonamides
Phenothiazines	Phenothiazines
Soaps containing halogenated salicylanilides	Plant oils
	Psoralens
Sunscreen agents	Coal tar and its derivatives
p-Aminobenzoate esters	in dyes, perfumes, and other synthetics
Benzophenones	Acridine
Fragrances	Anthracene
	Phenanthrene

Prognosis

Occasionally the dermatitis will persist despite avoidance measures. The reason for this is unknown.

HYPERSENSITIVITY PNEUMONITIS

Major Immunologic Features

- Primary pathogenetic mechanism involves the effector T cell.
- Antibody precipitins are useful to establish exposure to the allergen.
- Allergens are frequently biologic organisms or their products.

General Considerations

Hypersensitivity pneumonitis (also known as extrinsic allergic alveolitis) has been known as an occupational disease for well over 200 years, but it was first recognized as an allergic disease just 30 years ago. The concept that it is a pulmonary Arthus reaction caused by immune complexes of inhaled allergen and precipitating IgG antibodies was then widely held. Recently, persuasive evidence from clinical, pathologic, epidemiologic, and experimental studies has shown that the disease is mediated predominantly by T lymphocyte (cellular) effector mechanisms. It shares some pathologic features with sarcoidosis and the pneumoconioses, but it differs from the former disease by having a recognized environmental cause and from the latter group of diseases by its immune responses to inhaled material. Hypersensitivity pneumonitis, like allergic asthma, is produced by inhaled allergens, and in fact there are allergens that can cause either disease. However, IgE antibodies play no known role in the pathogenesis of hypersensitivity pneumonitis.

A. Definition: Hypersensitivity pneumonitis is an allergic disease of the lung parenchyma with inflammation in the alveoli and interstitial spaces induced immunologically by acute or chronic inhalation of a wide variety of inhaled materials. The disease may present in an acute, subacute, or chronic form. It is not currently possible to ascribe all features of the illness to a single immunologic mechanism. There is evidence for several different immune pathways that operate separately or concurrently, but the most compelling mechanism of pathogenesis is allergen-specific cell-mediated hypersensitivity. Interstitial pneumonitis is the primary clinical manifestation for all forms of the disease.

B. Epidemiology: Cases have been reported worldwide. The disease is most frequently associated with occupational allergens, which determine its prevalence and geographic, age, and sex distribution. Males aged 30–50 years are therefore usually affected. Farmer's lung, the prototype and most widely reported form of hypersensitivity pneumonitis, is caused by thermophilic actinomycetes, usually from warm, moist, moldy hay, and therefore the disease predominates in wet regions and especially among dairy farmers. Several surveys suggest that 2–4% of farmers have been affected. Bird handler's disease (also known as bird fancier's lung, pigeon breeder's disease, and bird breeder's disease) has been diagnosed in 15–21% of exposed individuals. Humidifier lung disease occurs in 23–71% of those exposed to contaminated humidifiers. Many published reports identify a single case or a small epidemic in a workplace. Once recognized, elimination of the environmental source of the allergen eliminates the disease.

C. Allergens: Hundreds of sources of allergens have been reported to cause hypersensitivity pneumonitis, usually in single cases. Some of the more common ones are shown in Table 28–4. The exact allergenic molecule has been isolated only infrequently, but these include a variety of heterologous proteins and organic or inorganic compounds. In many cases the chemical identification has been made by serologic or skin testing in the affected patient. As explained below, precipitins and skin tests may be epiphenomena, so definitive identification of the allergen requires bronchial provocation testing.

The allergens come from a variety of environmental sources. The most common ones are microorganisms, especially bacteria and fungal spores, and animal products such as feathers and particles of dried excreta. The few industrial chemicals so far identified with this disease have been highly reactive ones, such as isocyanates and anhydrides. Many cases have been clearly associated with a product such as inhaled dust from a food or contaminated water without identification of the source, although microbial contamination is usually suspected.

To date most reported cases have been occupational, because these are more likely to be acute illnesses from high-dose exposure easily traced to the workplace by a history of an epidemic in a particular occupational site. The relatively few instances of disease caused by domestic exposure have been traced to thermophilic actinomycetes, fungi, mites, amebae, pet birds, and unknown organisms in contaminated water of home or automobile air conditioners, heaters, vaporizers, and evaporative air coolers. These tend to cause chronic and insidious pulmonary impairment. Physicians should be aware of this potential cause of "idiopathic" pulmonary fibrosis.

The allergen must be inhaled in a form, such as an aerosol or particle, that is capable of reaching the alveoli during normal respiration. Particulates, whether in the form of an organic dust or microorganism, must be less than 3 μm in diameter.

Many of the allergens associated with hypersensitivity pneumonitis have biologic properties, in addition to allergenicity, that may be important in causing disease. The thermophilic actinomycetes, which are classified in the same botanical order as *Mycobacterium tuberculosis,* are immunologic adjuvants for

Table 28–4. Allergens causing hypersensitivity pneumonitis.

Allergen	Source	Disease
Bacteria		
Thermophilic actinomycetes	Contaminated hay or grains	Farmer's lung
	Contaminated bagasse	Bagassosis
	Mushroom compost	Mushroom worker's lung
Bacillus subtilis	Contaminated walls	Domestic hypersensitivity pneumonitis
Streptomyces albus	Contaminated fertilizer	*Streptomyces* hypersensitivity pneumonitis
Fungi		
Aspergillus spp	Moldy barley	Malt worker's lung
	Moldy tobacco	Tobacco worker's lung
	Compost	Compost lung
Aureobasidium, Graphium spp	Redwood bark, sawdust	Sequoiosis
	Contaminated sauna water	Sauna worker's lung
	Contaminated humidifier	Humidifier lung
Cryptostroma corticale	Maple bark	Maple bark disease
Penicillium casei	Moldy cheese	Cheese worker's lung
Sacchoromonospora viridis	Dried grass	Thatched roof disease
Various undetermined puffball spores	Moldy dwellings	Domestic hypersensitivity pneumonitis
	Mold in cork dust	Suberosis
	Lycoperdon puffballs	Lycoperdonosis
Alternaria, Penicillium spp.	Wood pulp, dust	Woodworker's lung
Insects		
Sitophilus granarius (wheat weevil)	Infested flour	Wheat miller's lung
Organic chemicals		
Isocyanates	Various industries	Chemical worker's lung
Miscellaneous		
Pituitary snuff	Medication	Pituitary snuff taker's lung
Coffee bean protein	Coffee bean dust	Coffee worker's lung
Rat urine protein	Laboratory rats	Laboratory worker's lung
Animal fur protein	Animal pelts	Furrier's lung
Unknown	Contaminated tap water	Tap water hypersensitivity pneumonitis

both antibody synthesis and cell-mediated immunity. Many of the allergens can activate alveolar macrophages and the alternative complement pathway nonimmunologically. The role of these properties in disease pathogenesis is being actively investigated.

D. Pathology: The histopathology of hypersensitivity pneumonitis depends upon the stage of disease. Very few patients have been examined in the acute phase immediately after exposure. Such patients show involvement of centrilobular respiratory bronchioles, alveoli, and blood vessels with intense infiltration by granulocytes, monocytes, and plasma cells. There is Arthus-like vasculitis of alveolar capillaries. Some studies show bronchiolar destruction. There is alveolar-wall thickening, but without necrosis. Immunofluoresence studies show deposition of immunoglobulins, C3, and fibrin in and around affected blood vessels. Thus, any role of precipitating antibodies causing immune-complex deposition and complement-mediated Arthus-like vasculitis, alveolitis, and terminal bronchiolitis would be restricted to the early acute illness after allergen exposure.

The subacute phase, beginning within 3 weeks of exposure, is characterized by noncaseating granulomas in the interstitial spaces accompanied by lymphocytes and plasma cells with only occasional eosinophils and no vasculitis. Mild bronchiolitis obliterans in seen in 50% of cases.

Chronic disease is characterized by persistence of the subacute pathology. There are lymphocytes in alveolar walls, and interstitial fibrosis accompanies the granulomatous and mononuclear interstitial and alveolar inflammation. There is no eosinophilia, and immunofluorescence shows no immunoglobulin or complement deposits. Monoclonal antibody reagents reveal the presence of activated macrophages and T lymphocytes, predominantly CD8 cells.

The histopathology of hypersensitivity pneumonitis is not pathognomonic, with the possible exception of histiocytes with foamy cytoplasm surrounded by lymphocytes, which are seen in the chronic phase.

E. Pathogenesis: The allergic pathogenesis of hypersensitivity pneumonitis was first suspected in farmer's lung because of the granulomatous interstitial inflammation, a hallmark of T cell-mediated immunity. However, the discovery of precipitating antibodies to extracts of thermophilic actinomycetes in patient sera led to a persisting concept that this is an immune-complex disease, even after many studies showed that precipitins correlated with exposure to allergens and not necessarily to the presence of pulmonary disease. As explained above, an Arthus mechanism could be operative in the acute pneumonitis that occurs 4 hours after exposure and clears in 24 hours. However, the clinical manifestations, pathology, disease induced in animal models, epidemiologic data, and recent investigations of broncho-alveolar lavage samples all point to a complicated mechanism of disease involving specific cell-mediated immunity, immunoregulatory and immunogenetic factors, and nonspecific biologic effects of the inhaled material, but only a minor role, if any, for circulating antibodies. The disease is primarily a function of the local pulmonary mucosal cellular immune system, which is poorly reflected in peripheral-blood samples. The role of mucosal IgA has not been fully explored. Both IgA and IgG antibodies are present in bronchoalveolar lavage fluid in proportion to allergen exposure, but IgA and not IgG antibody titers are higher in patients than in exposed persons without disease.

Unlike IgE-mediated diseases, allergen exposure by inhalation must be either intensive and massive or prolonged. It has been calculated that a farmer working with moldy hay may inhale 750,000 fungal spores per minute.

In experimental disease in animals, inhalation of soluble antigens produces a very mild disease or an acute homorrhagic Arthus alveolitis analogous to human illness in workers exposed occupationally to high doses of trimellitic anhydride or isocyanate who develop high-titer circulating and alveolar-fluid antibodies and a restrictive infiltrative pulmonary disease with hemoptysis and anemia. On the other hand, the typical human hypersensitivity pneumonitis is best reproduced in animals by inhalation of particulate antigens that elicit alveolitis and interstitial granulomas, specific local and systemic cell-mediated hypersensitivity, activation of alveolar macrophages, local lymphokine production in alveolar fluid, and precipitins. Allergen inhalation challenge responses can be passively transferred by sensitized lymphocytes, and the disease can be inhibited with corticosteroids, with antimacrophage serum, and by neonatal thymectomy, all of which are consistent with cellular hypersensitivity.

Experiments in mice shed some light on the development and variability of the human disease. By using high- and low-responder strains, it has been shown that the disease is associated with a deficiency in allergen-specific suppressor T lymphocytes in the lung. The deficiency is determined by a dominant gene or genes linked to the immunoglobulin V_H haplotype but not to H-2 (analogous to human HLA) genes. Repeated exposure to the allergen causes a phenomenon of desensitization, with disappearance of infiltrates, refractoriness to disease by other, unrelated allergens, and cell-mediated anergy in some animals but not others. The anergic state is caused by an allergen-nonspecific suppressor macrophage, whose presence is controlled by a single recessive gene. Animals lacking this gene have sustained granulomatous disease and have failed to develop anergy. These intriguing experiments stress the role of genetic factors of immunoregulation that probably also control sus-

ceptibility to and expressions of the disease in humans.

Many of the allergens identified with this disease have intrinsic biologic effects that may be important in pathogenesis. These include adjuvant properties causing nonspecific stimulation of the immune system, activation of macrophages, and nonimmunologic activation of the alternative complement pathway.

Clinical Features

A. Symptoms: Clinical patterns are wide-ranging, but they may be classified into acute, subacute, and chronic forms. Acute reactions are single or multiple episodes of dyspnea, cough, malaise, fever, chills, and chest pain. Each episode begins 4–8 hours after a high-dose allergen exposure and clears within 24 hours. Weight loss and hemoptysis are rare. Subacute disease begins insidioiusly over a period of weeks, resulting in cough, dyspnea, and weight loss. The cough is initially dry and later productive. Dyspnea may become progressively profound, and there may be cyanosis. Chronic disease occurs from low-dose continuous exposure, as in the case of hypersensitivity to a single bird in the home. Fatigue and weight loss may be the first indication of illness. Gradual progressive dyspnea may be overlooked or denied until it is noticed at rest.

B. Signs: During acute reactions, the temperature is elevated to as high as 39.5 °C. The patient appears acutely ill, with tachypnea and tachycardia. There are bilateral crackling rales, especially at the lung bases, and occasional rhonchi and wheezes, but the lungs may be clear. In chronic disease, breath sounds are diminished and there may be a prolonged expiratory phase if an obstructive component is present.

C. Laboratory Findings: In acute disease there is usually slight leukocytosis without eosinophilia. The erythrocyte sedimentation rate is normal or mildly elevated. In chronic disease, serum immunoglobulin levels may be slightly increased and low-titer rheumatoid factor and antinuclear antibody may be present.

Pulmonary-function tests performed during the acute phase of the disease reveal a reversible restrictive pattern with reduced lung compliance and reduced diffusing capacity. Arterial blood gases show hypoxemia. The spirometric findings in chronic disease are those of irreversible restriction with or without an accompanying obstructive component due to bronchiolitis obliterans. In some patients there may be an additional element of bronchial hyperirritability.

Chest x-ray findings are highly variable. During an acute episode, the presence of multiple bilateral small nodules sparing the apices and bases is the typical pattern. This indicates the presence of interstitial inflammation and an alveolus-filling infiltrate. Less common findings are patchy pneumonia or a normal x-ray. In chronic disease a fibrotic linear pattern with or without nodules increases in intensity toward the periphery. There may be a loss of volume that is most marked in upper lobes, honeycombing, and cor pulmonale-induced cardiac enlargement. The disease does not cause pleural effusion or thickening, hilar adenopathy, calcification, cavitation, atelectasis, or coin lesions.

The classification described above should not obscure the fact that hypersensitivity pneumonitis is highly variable and that individual cases can be "atypical." Clinical manifestations depend upon the frequency, intensity, and chemical and physical properties of the allergen exposure, as well as on host factors. Clinical descriptions have been dominated by occupational syndromes such as farmer's lung, bagassosis, and bird handler's disease. Many unique case reports have been published with quaint names and unusual allergen sources, such as New Guinea thatched roof lung (contaminated thatch), paprika slicer's lung (*Mucor stalonifer*), Bible printer's lung (contaminated ink), and coptic lung (mummy cloth wrappings).

Clinical Diagnosis

The history is important, as in any allergic disease. Because of the variable nature of hypersensitivity pneumonitis and wide range of environmental sources for the allergens, the diagnosis requires a high degree of suspicion. Any patient with a history of recurrent pneumonia of uncertain etiology, "idiopathic" restrictive or fibrotic lung disease, or unexplained pulmonary abnormality on chest x-ray is a prime suspect. The environmental, especially occupational, history is essential for providing clues for possible causative allergens.

There are no pathognomonic signs from physical examination, routine laboratory tests, or chest x-rays. Even pulmonary-function testing may not show evidence of the restrictive abnormality between acute attacks of early disease. Lung biopsy is likewise not pathognomonic, since histopathology is similar to that of other interstitial diseases, but it is useful mainly to rule out other diagnoses.

Immunologic Diagnosis

Serum antibodies are not usually involved in disease pathogenesis, but their presence nevertheless will at least establish the fact of exposure. There are usually large quantities of precipitating antibodies, especially in early or acute disease, but they may disappear after a prolonged period of allergen avoidance. Ouchterlony analysis is usually adequate to detect precipitins (see Chapter 12), but occasionally the more sensitive radioimmunoassay, radioallergosorbent test (RAST), enzyme-linked immunosorbent assay (ELISA), and complement fixation test are necessary. Serum complement component levels are normal or occasionally increased with acute allergen exposure.

When precipitating antibodies are present in serum, an intradermal skin test will elicit a cutaneous Arthus reaction, characterized by localized diffuse edema and mild inflammation and erythema appearing at 4–6 hours and subsiding completely by 24 hours. Commercial test antigens are available for extracts of fungi and diluted avian serum. Many crude extracts of allergens known to cause this disease, eg, thermophilic actinomycetes, are too irritating for skin testing. The Arthus skin test, like the precipitin test, is an indication of exposure and is not by itself diagnostic of the disease.

Bronchial provocation testing with allergen extract currently has the highest sensitivity and specificity for diagnosis, but it is an experimental procedure because of technical limitations and danger. It must be done in a hospital with 24-hour monitoring. A reversible restrictive lung defect begins at 4–6 hours, peaks at 8 hours, and resolves by 24 hours. Although the timing of response is similar to a late-phase asthmatic response, the abnormality in pulmonary function is different (see Fig 24–3).

Examination of bronchoalveolar lavage fluid for humoral and cellular components has been reported to date for only a few cases of subacute disease. The procedure is still experimental, and the diagnostic usefulness is unknown.

A simpler alternative to bronchial provocation is "on-site" challenge to observe changes in symptoms, lung auscultation, pulmonary functions, and chest x-ray by trial exposure of the patient to the suspected environment (eg, home or work) after an adequate period of avoidance. If an acute reaction is provoked, the site must be investigated to uncover the causative allergen. Environmental assessment might require the specialized services of engineers, microbiologists, or others.

Differential Diagnosis

Pulmonary mycotoxicosis (atypical farmer's lung) is a recently described disorder caused by acute massive exposure to moldy silage. The disease is characterized by fever, chills, and coughing that last for several days to a week. There are diffuse infiltrations on chest x-ray and fungal organisms in alveoli and bronchioles, but no serum precipitins. The cause is unknown, but the illness is probably a toxic pneumonitis from a fungal product. Recurrent infectious pneumonias, other causes of interstitial lung disease, asthma, allergic bronchopulmonary aspergillosis, and pneumoconioses must also be differentiated from hypersensitivity pneumonitis.

Treatment

Systemic corticosteroid therapy is indicated for resolution of acute reactions and for terminating and reversing severe or progressive disease. The drug should not be used as an alternative to avoidance of the allergen, but it may be necessary to protect the patient by suppressing inflammation if the allergen source has not been identified. Inhaled corticosteroids are not indicated.

Complications

Respiratory failure and cor pulmonale may result from chronic disease. Bronchiolitis obliterans may lead to irreversible obstructive pulmonary disease. Death from respiratory failure is possible during any phase of the disease.

Prognosis

Prognosis for recovery is good in the acute or subacute stages once the cause has been identified and avoided. However, some patients with bird handler's disease have progressive pulmonary insufficiency even with complete avoidance of birds. On the other hand,

farmers can continue to have some exposure to thermophilic actinomycetes without progressive illness as long as the acute febrile symptomatic attacks are avoided.

Prevention

Avoidance is the only means of preventing this disease. Effective treatment therefore requires a specific immunologic diagnosis whenever possible, since the same allergen may be found in different environments (Table 28–4). The purpose of avoidance is prevention of irreversible lung disease.

Occupational preventive measures are obvious for the currently recognized causes. Proper workplace hygiene, filters and masks where appropriate, and other measures should be employed. Diseases caused by allergens in homes, automobiles, and offices are best prevented by physician awareness of the disease.

REFERENCES

Allergic Contact Dermatitis

Adams RM: *Occupational Skin Diseases,* 2nd ed. Grune & Stratton, 1989.

Fisher AA: Contact Dermatitis. 3rd ed. Lea & Febiger, 1986.

Huntley AC (editor): Allergic contact dermatitis. *Clin Rev Allergy* 1989;**7:**345. (Entire issue.)

Hypersensitivity Pneumonitis

Fink NJ: Hypersensitivity pneumonitis. *J Allergy Clin Immunol* 1984;**74:**1.

Novey HS (editor): Hypersensitivity pneumonitis. *Clin Rev Allergy* 1983;**1:**449. (Entire issue.)

Salvaggio JE: Hypersensitivity pneumonitis. *J Allergy Clin Immunol* 1987;**79:**558.

Salvaggio JE: Recent advances in pathogenesis of allergic alveolitis. *Clin Rev Allergy* 1990;**20:**137.

Drug Allergy

29

H. James Wedner, MD

Adverse reactions to therapeutic agents are a significant problem in the practice of medicine. The spectrum of adverse reactions to drugs comprises (1) side effects, toxic reactions, and drug interactions that are the result of unwanted pharmacologic properties of the therapeutic agent(s) in question; (2) idiosyncratic reactions, which occur in a variable proportion of the population and whose cause is unknown; and (3) immunologic reactions, which depend on the ability of the drug or its hydrolysis or biotransformation products to interact with the immune system and to invoke humoral or cellular immune mechanisms. Adverse reactions resulting from an immunologic mechanism make up a substantial portion of the spectrum. Although this chapter is concerned with reactions based on immunologic mechanisms, the entire spectrum of reactions must be kept in mind when approaching the problem of adverse reactions to drugs, because the clinical presentations of the reactions may be similar although the mechanisms differ. It is imperative that the underlying mechanism be established since the therapeutic approach will differ depending upon the type of reaction that has occurred.

Some texts define drug allergy as any reaction that results from an immune mechanism, whereas others limit the term to reactions mediated by IgE antibody directed against the drug or one of its metabolic products. This chapter discusses all immunologically mediated drug reactions and then concentrates on those resulting from IgE antibody-dependent release of mediators of anaphylaxis from sensitized mast cells and basophils and those caused by the nonimmunologic release of mediators from mast cells and basophils. The latter have been called "anaphylactoid" or "pseudoallergic" reactions. They are important since the symptoms of allergic and pseudoallergic reactions are identical.

IMMUNOLOGIC BASIS OF DRUG ALLERGY

General Considerations

Although the frequency of reactions to various drugs varies widely, it is probable that any drug is capable of inducing the production of humoral or cellular immune responses. In many cases, the resulting immune reaction is not detrimental. For example, a large proportion of individuals treated with intravenous penicillin develop IgG antibodies to penicillin or penicillin biotransformation products. In the vast majority of instances these antibodies do not result in either the appearance of a drug reaction or a decrease in the effectiveness of the drug. This is also true for patients treated with bovine or porcine insulin. Thus, the demonstration of antibodies or sensitized T cells directed against a drug does not indicate that this immune response will necessarily result in a drug reaction.

Drugs are capable of inducing allergic reactions by any of the hypersensitivity mechanisms that are discussed in Chapter 24, ie, IgE-mediated, cytotoxic-antibody-mediated, immune-complex-mediated, and T effector cell-mediated mechanisms. However, to induce these reactions, a drug must be immunogenic. Since most drugs are of low molecular weight, they are in and of themselves nonimmunogenic. Only when the drug is capable of interacting with tissue proteins and serving as a hapten will it induce an immune response. Some drugs, such as insulin or pituitary snuff (used as a source of antidiuretic hormone), are large polypeptides or proteins and therefore are capable of interacting with immunoreactive cells in their native state. A few relatively low-molecular-weight drugs such as polymyxin appear to be immunogenic without tissue conjugation. Although the exact mechanism is currently unknown, immunogenicity is probably related to the ability of these drugs to form long-chain polymers.

Metabolic Biotransformation & Haptenation

Most haptenic drugs conjugate to tissue protein via a covalent bond. In rare cases the bond may be noncovalent but of sufficient affinity for the drug-protein complex to remain intact during antigens processing and presentation. For this reason the ability of any drug to induce an immune response depends upon the tissue reactivity of that drug. Thus, drugs that easily form covalent bonds will be more immunogenic than those which are relatively unreactive. It is not necessary, however, that the native drug be highly reactive, since its hydrolysis or biotransformation products may serve as the haptens. For this reason, a thorough knowledge of the biotransformation products of a drug is critical in the evaluation of drug allergies, but, unfortunately, these products are not known for most drugs. This limits the ability to predict the immunogenicity of a given drug and, as discussed below, the ability to test for the presence of a drug allergy.

Early studies of patients with known allergy to penicillin demonstrated that only a small percentage of these patients reacted to penicillin G; the majority reacted to the penicilloyl moiety, which is generated by the cleavage of the β-lactam ring, and others reacted to the penilloate group generated by the cleavage of the 5-membered thiazolidine ring (Fig 29–1). This led to the development of accurate methods for detecting allergy to penicillin and other β-lactam drugs, as discussed below. Similarly, only a small percentage of patients allergic to sulfonamides react by skin tests to the native drug, so skin testing is not an accurate predictor of allergic reactivity for this class of drugs. On the other hand, Prausnitz-Küstner passive transfer of serum from sulfonamide-allergic patients to nonallergic individuals results in a wheal-and-flare at the site of the injection when the recipient ingests the drug. This suggests that metabolism of the drug results in a reactive molecule which, on conjugation to circulating proteins, is capable of interacting with and activating the locally sensitized mast cells.

The immune response generated by certain drugs that are highly tissue reactive may be directed neither to the drug or its metabolic by-products nor to the host tissue but rather to a new antigenic determinant, which is the result of the combination of the drug with a specific tissue protein. This is the mechanism of thrombocytopenia following the ingestion of quinine, an antimalarial drug. In this case, the patient produces an IgG antibody with specificity for quinine, which is bound to the surface of the platelet. The quinine-platelet interaction has generated a new antigenic determinant that does not cross-react with other blood cells or tissues. The exact immunologic mechanisms of most other tissue-specific drug reactions are currently unknown.

Finally, the interaction between a drug and a tissue protein or other tissue component may alter the tissue protein at a site distant from the actual binding of the drug to the protein. This now altered tissue protein can then be recognized as foreign by the immune system and can serve as an immunogen for either humoral or cell-mediated immune responses. This mechanism is of some importance, since the antibodies or cytotoxic T cells generated may be capable of recognizing not only the altered protein but also the protein in its native state. This is the mechanism of some types of drug-induced autoimmunity. A good example of this phenomenon is the systemic lupus erythematosus syndrome associated with the drug hydralazine. Some of these reactions may then persist long after the drug has been withdrawn. The various modes of hapten-carrier interaction in drug allergy are illustrated in Fig 29–2.

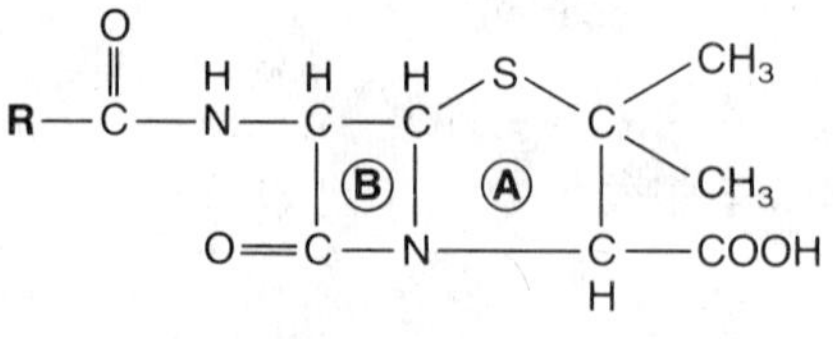

penicillin

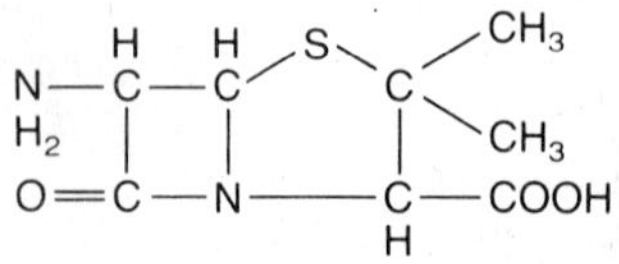

6-aminopenicillanic acid

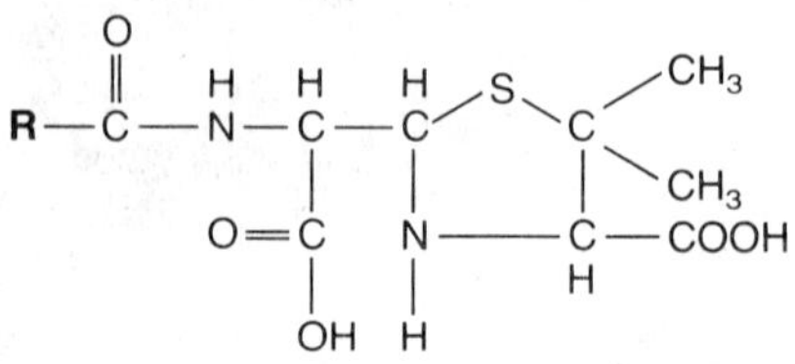

penicilloic acid

Figure 29–1. Penicillin and 2 allergenic biotransformation products. **A:** Thiazolidine ring; **B:** β-lactam ring.

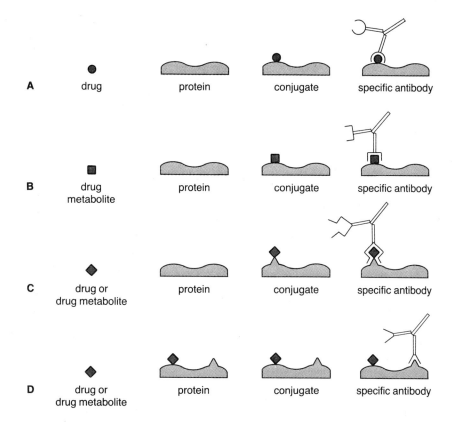

Figure 29–2. The interaction of a drug with tissue protein may result in antibodies (shown) or T cells directed against various determinants. **A:** The specific antibodies are directed against the native molecule. **B:** The antibodies are directed against a hydrolysis or biotransformation product of the drug. **C:** The antibodies are directed against a new determinant formed by the interaction of the drug or drug metabolite and the protein. **D:** Conjugation of the drug or its metabolites results in a conformational change in the tissue protein, which is then recognized as foreign by the immune system.

Other Factors in Drug Allergenicity

The type of immune response that will be generated by a given drug depends upon (1) the chemical nature of the drug, (2) the route of presentation (ingestion, injection, or application to the skin), and (3) the genetic makeup of the individual. Certain drugs produce a humoral immune response, whereas others more commonly induce T cell immunity. This difference most probably results from differences in tissue reactivity of the drug.

The site of presentation of the drug markedly influences both the ability of the drug to induce an adverse immunologic reaction and the type of reaction. In general, drugs are far more likely to induce an immune reaction when they are given parenterally (subcutaneously, intramuscularly, or intravenously) than when given orally or applied to the skin. For example, IgE and IgG antibodies to penicillin or its derivatives are produced in a greater proportion of individuals treated intravenously than in those treated orally with comparable doses of the drug.

The route of presentation may also determine the type of immune response (antibody or T cell) associated with a given drug. For example, antihistaminic drugs are rarely allergenic when given by the oral or parenteral route but frequently induce T cell sensitization when applied topically to the skin, causing allergic contact dermatitis.

The prevalence of allergic reactions to drugs is greater in acquired immune deficiency syndrome (AIDS) than in other diseases, presumably because of HIV-induced immune dysregulation. This is especially so for trimethoprim-sulfamethoxazole and other sulfonamides and their congeners. The spectrum of reactions covers a wide variety of allergic manifestations, including fever, rash, anaphylaxis, Stevens-Johnson syndrome, toxic epidermal necrolysis, and hematologic and hepatic disturbances.

Clinical Manifestations

An adverse reaction to a drug can be considered to be allergic if (1) the patient has antibodies or sensitized T cells with specificity for the drug, a drug metabolite, or a drug-tissue conjugate, and (2) the chemical features of the reaction are consistent with recognized immunologically induced inflammation (see Chapter 24). In some instances the adverse reaction closely follows the introduction of a drug and the reaction appears to be immunologic, but extensive immunologic studies fail to demonstrate drug-specific antibodies or T cells. This might be explained by failure to identify the appropriate antigen. Drug fever may be an example of this phenomenon. A number of drugs are commonly associated with episodic or persistent fever, which remits upon withdrawal of the drug and recurs promptly when the drug is readministered. Although it has long been suspected that drug fever is an immunologic phenomenon, studies to date have failed to provide a convincing immunologic mechanism.

As noted above, any type of hypersensitivity reaction may cause drug allergy. In some cases, the type of immune response determines the location of reaction. For example, the vast majority of reactions that are T cell-mediated produce dermatitis. Repeated application of the drug to the skin will induce a T cell response and cause allergic contact dermatitis localized to areas of skin in contact with the drug. Ingestion or injection of the drug generally causes a diffuse eczematoid dermatitis or, less commonly, erythema multiforme of either the minor or major (Stevens-Johnson syndrome) type, toxic epidermal necrolysis, or, in rare cases, erythema nodosum.

The manifestation of drug allergy mediated by antibody depends to a great extent on the type of antibody. Reactions attributed to IgE antibodies include pruritus, urticaria, angioedema, and systemic anaphylaxis. IgG antibodies to drugs result in cytotoxicity or immune-complex deposition with complement-mediated inflammation. These may be tissue-specific, as discussed above, or they may be generalized, with multiple organ involvement, eg, in patients with serum sickness.

DIAGNOSIS OF DRUG ALLERGY

Ideally, the diagnosis of drug allergy is made by in vivo or in vitro testing with the drug or its reactive metabolites. For this reason, the most important aspect of the diagnostic evaluation is an accurate and comprehensive history, with special attention to 3 areas: the nature of the symptoms, the drug history, and the temporal relationship between the institution of drug therapy and the onset of the reaction.

Nature of Symptoms

The nature of the symptoms helps to differentiate immunologic reactions from toxic or idiosyncratic reactions. Isolated gastrointestinal complaints following the institution of antibiotic therapy, pain at the site of drug injection, headache associated with nitroglycerin therapy, or fever and malaise following an influenza inoculation are all predictable side effects that do not have an immunologic basis. The nature of the reaction must be placed in the context of other disease that might have similar symptoms. For example, patients with systemic lupus erythematosus often present with symptoms resembling those of an allergic drug reaction. On the other hand, allergic drug reactions may stimulate other illnesses.

Drug History

Knowledge of the drugs that the patient has taken in the past and whether any of these drugs has been associated with an adverse reaction may reveal that a current allergic response is caused by the same or similar class of drug that caused a previous allergic reaction. On the other hand, the fact that a patient has taken a drug in the past without difficulty suggests that other causes for the patient's illness should be explored, but it does not rule out a newly developed drug sensitivity.

The history may be all the more difficult when patients are taking multiple medications; more often than not, this is the case. It has been estimated that the average patient on an internal-medicine ward is being treated with 10 separate medications, and in the outpatient setting it is not unusual to find patients on 5 or more medications. It is therefore very important that all of these medications be accurately defined. For inpatients this is best done by using a thorough chart review. For outpatients it is best to recommend that they bring all of their medications with them or, if this is not possible, that they bring a list of all their medications.

As noted above, certain drugs are frequently associated with allergic reactions, whereas reactions to others are very uncommon. For example, allergic reactions to digitalis glycosides are extremely rare, whereas reactions to some antibiotics are very common. Thus, in a patient taking both of these classes of drugs, it is far more likely that the antibiotic, rather than the cardiac glycoside, is the cause of the problem.

Temporal Relationship

The temporal relationship between the institution of drug therapy and the onset of the reaction is important. Immunologic reactions may occur at different times following drug therapy. IgE antibody reactions to drugs generally start within 30–60 minutes following administration of the drug. Allergic contact dermatitis is expected to have a latency period averaging 48–72 hours following application of the drug. The latency period in serum sickness is usually 7 days. In contrast to a reaction in a patient sensitized during a prior course of the drug, sensitization and reaction to a current drug course will cause a longer latency period for appearance of an adverse reaction. Thus, one might see the onset of symptoms of an IgE reaction 7–14 days following the introduction of the drug. It is unlikely but not impossible for a patient who has been on a drug for a long period to develop a de novo sensitization to that drug. It is also unlikely for a patient to develop a reaction to a drug after therapy with that agent has been discontinued, but this might occur with the use of depot medications, which are released into the body over a long period.

In Vivo Tests

It is sometimes possible to confirm a suspected allergic drug reaction by using in vivo testing.

A. Patch or Skin Tests: In vivo testing includes prick or intradermal skin testing for IgE sensitivity, patch testing for delayed-type hypersensitivity, and provocative-dose challenges. The wheal-and-erythema skin test cannot be used to diagnose IgE-mediated allergy to drugs that nonspecifically release the mediators of anaphylaxis from mast cells. A list of such drugs is found in Chapter 26.

When performing skin tests for IgE-mediated drug allergy or patch tests for allergic contact dermatitis, the immunogenic form of the drug (native drug or metabolite) must be used. In addition, for patch testing, the drug in question must not be irritating, as sufficient irritation can produce a false-positive result.

B. Provocative Tests: The provocative-dose challenge is a method whereby the patient is given increasing doses of the drug, beginning with small doses and increasing to the full therapeutic dose, and is observed for signs of an allergic response, at which point the drug is withdrawn. It must be remembered that the use of challenge testing is not without danger. It is reserved for instances when no alternative therapy is available (see p 377) and when the benefit of the drug far outweighs the potential harm. These tests must be performed only where adequate facilities and personnel are available to treat acute medical emergencies.

In Vitro Tests

These are designed to identify either the antibody that is reacting with a drug hapten or the drug determinant that can stimulate sensitized T cells. For IgE antibody-mediated reaction, the radioallergosorbent test (RAST) or enzyme-linked immunosorbent assay (ELISA) is applicable when the antigenic determinant is known and available. As noted above, the lack of knowledge of the true immunogen for most drugs has limited this type of testing. A RAST is available for detecting IgE antibodies to the penicilloyl determinant, and recently an ELISA for identifying allergy to the sulfonamide group has been developed. Tests of IgG or IgM antibodies are available for only a limited number of allergenic drugs.

For suspected cell-mediated reaction to drugs, lymphocyte activation assays have been used (see Chapter 13). These test the ability of the drug or a drug-protein conjugate to induce the proliferation of T lymphocytes. Lymphocyte activation analysis is

relatively simple to perform; however, the 3–5 days necessary to complete the test and the need for appropriate cell culture facilities have limited its use in practice.

TREATMENT OF DRUG ALLERGY

Since there are only a few drugs for which accurate in vivo or in vitro testing is available, a suspected drug reaction must be treated without such confirmation. There are 3 steps that can be taken. First, any drug necessary for the care of the patient is discontinued. Second, for drugs that cannot be eliminated, an alternative drug with similar pharmacologic properties but a different chemical structure should be substituted. Finally, in cases when no alternative drug is available and the allergic reaction is mild and not life-threatening, it may be possible to continue the drug and treat the patient symptomatically. If possible, the drug should be discontinued temporarily for a short time to confirm that it was the cause of the reaction.

PENICILLIN ALLERGY

Penicillin and the other β-lactam antibiotics are a frequent cause of all types of immunologic drug reactions including IgE-mediated anaphylaxis and urticaria, serum sickness, T cell-mediated contact dermatitis, and antibody-mediated cytolysis. However, by far the most common and potentially dangerous penicillin reactions are those resulting from the production of specific IgE. As a group, the β-lactam antibiotics are the most common cause of IgE-mediated allergic reactions to drugs. This class of drugs includes the penicillins, the cephalosporins, the cephamycins, the penems, and the monobactams (Fig 29–3). The penicillins have a β-lactam ring conjugated to a 5-membered thiazolidine ring. They differ from the cephalosporins in that the latter class has a 6-membered rather than a 5-membered sulfur-containing ring. The cephamycins are similar to the cephalosporins but have a methoxy group attached to the β-lactam ring. Penems are a large class that resemble the penicillins, with the exception that the 5-membered ring contains a carbon or oxygen in place of the sulfur. Finally, the monobactams are the only class of drug that do not have a second ring conjugated to the β-lactam ring.

Skin Testing

Specific skin test reagents are available to evaluate patients with suspected penicillin allergy. Skin testing with penicillin G is effective in demonstrating allergic reactivity in only a small percentage of patients. However, conjugation of penicillin to protein

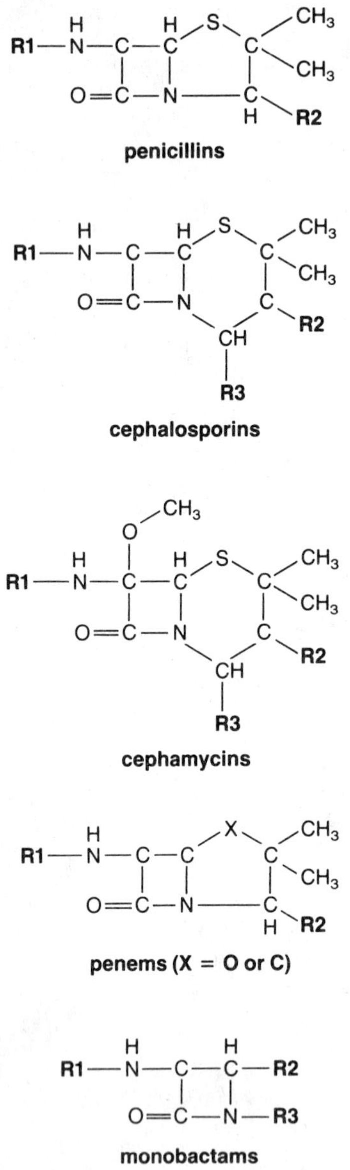

Figure 29–3. Core structures of the 5 groups of β-lactam antibiotics. R1, R2, R3, side chains; X, oxygen atom or CH$_2$ in penems.

following cleavage of the β-lactam ring has provided a skin test reagent that shows a positive correlation with clinical allergic sensitivity in more than 75% of all penicillin-allergic individuals, and so the penicilloyl group has been termed the "major determinant." Fewer patients react with penicilloic acid (7%) and with penicillin G (6%). These 2 molecules are presumed to conjugate to tissue proteins in the skin, thereby providing determinants other than the penicilloyl group. They are called the "minor determinants." In practice, penicilloyl-polylysine is used to

test for the major determinant since polylysine is a relatively nonimmunogenic molecule. This reagent is available commercially. The minor determinants, however, are not yet available commercially, although methods for their production and use have been published.

There are a number of protocols for skin testing in cases of suspected penicillin allergy. In one protocol, penicillin G and penicilloic acid are prepared at a concentration of 3.3 mg/mL and diluted 1:100 and 1:10,000. Penicilloyl-polylysine is used at a concentration of 6×10^{-5} mol/L. Skin prick or scratch testing is performed first with the most dilute concentration and then with the more concentrated solution if there is no reaction to the first test. If the scratch test is negative, intradermal testing is performed in a similar fashion. A positive skin test is defined as one in which the wheal-and-flare is greater than in a saline control performed at the same time. The patient is considered to be allergic to penicillin if there is a positive skin test to any of the reagents at any dilution.

The penicillin skin test has proven to be highly predictive. In one study with more than 1500 skin tests, only a single patient with negative skin tests had an acute anaphylactic reaction when given penicillin in full therapeutic doses. Patients who have a positive skin test are at risk for a systemic allergic reaction; in several studies the reaction rate was more than 25%. Thus, patients who are skin test positive will need to be desensitized before full therapeutic doses of this drug can be used.

A number of factors have been shown to correlate with skin test positivity to penicillin. For example, 100% of patients who reported a previous anaphylactic reaction to penicillin were skin test positive and 75% of patients with serum sickness had positive tests. In our studies, more than 40% of patients with other symptoms of an immunologic response to penicillin were skin test positive, although other studies have reported a significantly lower percentage. Skin test positivity correlates with the time course of the reaction during penicillin therapy. Immediate reactions in previously sensitized patients and reactions appearing 7–10 days after the institution of drug therapy in previously unsensitized patients are associated with the highest percentage of positive skin tests.

The time elapsed since the reported allergic reaction is also critical. Skin tests may be negative for several days or weeks after a systemic reaction before becoming positive. The tests remain positive over the next several years and then gradually decline, so that by 10 years following a reaction, fewer than 10% of history-positive patients are still skin test positive. This demonstrates that although drug-induced IgE may persist over a relatively long period, the IgE levels will eventually decline in the absence of further antigenic stimulation.

Patients who present a history of penicillin allergy

but are skin test negative can be given penicillin in full therapeutic doses with no greater risk of reaction than those without a history of penicillin allergy. Several studies have demonstrated that patients with a positive history and negative skin tests who are treated with oral penicillin or its analogs are rarely resensitized, and therefore skin testing following therapy is not necessary. In contrast, patients who receive high-dose intravenous penicillin are frequently (70%) resensitized and therefore should be retested at 6–8 weeks following the cessation of therapy.

It has been estimated that at least 250 patients in the USA die each year from anaphylactic reactions to parenteral penicillin. By contrast, there are only 6 reported cases of anaphylactic deaths from oral penicillin, and the number of reported nonfatal anaphylactic reactions from oral penicillin is less than 100. For this reason, we have chosen to use the oral route for penicillin desensitization.

Desensitization to Penicillin

The desensitization procedure is reserved for patients with a history of penicillin allergy and in whom the skin test is positive or cannot be performed. There should be no alternative antibiotic available, and the infection should be serious enough to risk the dangers of anaphylaxis from the treatment. If the patient meets these criteria, one of several protocols can be used. In one protocol, the patient is given increasing doses of oral phenoxymethyl penicillin beginning at 100 units and progressing until 400,000–800,000 U (250–500 mg) has been given. The drug is then given intravenously. This procedure has been performed in more than 100 patients, and in only 2 instances has it failed because of unacceptable reactions. In about one-third of patients there is minor skin reaction, but these reactions have not precluded achieving desensitization.

Others have preferred to use an intravenous desensitization. This method, in general, has a higher reaction rate but is effective, particularly when no oral form of the drug is available. Until recently this has been the case for patients sensitive to the third-generation cephalosporins (see below). Oral preparations of the third-generation cephalosporins should be used for desensitization when available.

Cross-Reactions with Other β-Lactams

The chemistry of penicillin metabolites has been studied, and the chemical structure of the allergenic epitopes is now established. Similar studies have not been carried out for the related antibiotics. Therefore, cross-reactivity of anti-penicillin IgE antibodies with the other β-lactam antibiotics has been evaluated only by in vitro tests such as RAST or ELISA inhibition or by clinical studies. Although many of the data are speculative, some generalizations can be made. Natural or semisynthetic penicillins tend to cross-react with one another. In addition, the cross-reactivity between penicillin and the first-generation cephalosporins appears to be relatively high (greater than 50%), particularly in patients with extreme sensitivity. The cross-reactivity between penicillin and the second- and third-generation cephalosporins is significantly lower than for the first-generation drugs. However, there is some cross-reactivity, and there are reports of at least 3 anaphylactic deaths resulting from the use of every second- and third-generation cephalosporin available in the USA. Only the monobactams appear to lack cross-reactivity with penicillin.

The problem of cross-reactivity is further complicated by the fact that some patients have IgE antibodies not to the β-lactam ring but rather to side-chain determinants. For these individuals, who may also have anti-β-lactam IgE as well, the cross-reactivity will depend on the similarity of the side chain. For example, aztreonam and ceftazidime contain the same side chain. Similarly, piperacillin and cephapyrizone contain identical side chains.

SULFONAMIDE ALLERGY

The sulfonamide drugs cause acute allergic reactions in a significant percentage of patients. This class of drugs is used for a variety of therapeutic uses; it includes the sulfonamide antibiotics such as sulfisoxazole and sulfamethoxazole, the diuretics furosemide and hydrochlorothiazide, and the angiotensin-converting enzyme (ACE) inhibitor captopril. The frequency of cross-reactivity among members of this class of drugs is not known. Patients sensitized to one sulfonamide may or may not react when treated with other sulfonamides. Skin testing is unreliable in confirming or rejecting the clinical history of an allergic reaction. Therefore, patients with a history of sensitivity to one member of this class should avoid all sulfonamide drugs. Alternative antibiotics are readily available: ethacrinic acid can be substituted for furosemide, and enalapril and alternative ACE inhibitors or another class of antihypertensive drug can be used to replace captopril.

Recently, an ELISA has been developed that uses sulfonamide conjugated with human serum albumin as antigen, but the test has yet to be studied in a sufficient number of patients to be used with confidence for diagnosis of sulfonamide allergy.

Experience with desensitization is very limited, and severe immediate reactions have been reported, so its use should be considered only in the very rare situations where a sulfonamide antibiotic is the only effective treatment for a life-threatening disease. Sulfonamides can cause severe skin reactions such as Stevens-Johnson syndrome. These are not amenable to desensitization. Thus, the potential danger from the administration of sulfonamides to sensitive individuals is significantly greater than for penicillin.

On the basis of a number of anecdotal reports, desensitization by oral administration of the drug is frequently successful for sulfa allergy in patients with AIDS.

INSULIN ALLERGY

Insulin is a frequent cause of allergic reactions. Both IgG and IgE antibodies may be induced by therapeutic insulin, but these antibodies may or may not cause allergic reactions. However, several syndromes are related to anti-insulin antibodies. Insulin allergic reactions may be local or systemic, and their onset can be either immediate or delayed. The immediate local reaction is mediated by IgE antibodies. It generally consists of local swelling and erythema, and, in contrast to other IgE-mediated reactions, it is often painful rather than pruritic. However, the delayed local reaction that occurs 4–12 hours following injection is an Arthus reaction resulting from IgG anti-insulin antibodies. Immediate and delayed systemic reaction are both IgE mediated.

The relationship of clinical cross-reactivity and the amino acid sequences of insulins from different animal species is not clear. Patients may be sensitized to either bovine insulin, which differs from human insulin by 3 amino acids in the α chain, or to porcine insulin, which differs from human insulin by a single amino acid in the β chain (Fig 29–4). Some patients are sensitized to proinsulin, which contaminates many insulin preparations. However, many patients sensitive to insulin will react not only to the bovine and porcine varieties but also to human insulin. This is a true cross-reactivity, because insulin-sensitive patients who are treated with recombinant human insulin will also react. Patients treated exclusively with recombinant human insulin, however, do not develop either IgE or IgG antibodies.

Treatment of patients with local reactions to insulin is largely symptomatic. The use of oral antihistamines or concomitant injection of the antihistamine with the insulin is effective in most cases. For very severe local reactions, insulin can be injected with corticosteroids (dexamethasone is preferred because it is compatible with most insulin preparations); however, the dose of corticosteroid must be relatively low (0.75 mg of dexamethasone or equivalent) to avoid steroid-induced gluconeogenesis.

For immediate systemic reactions, single-component (beef, pork, or human) insulin should be tried first. If the patient reacts to all of these, skin testing with beef, pork, and human insulin, followed by rapid desensitization, generally to human insulin, will usually be effective. It is preferable to have the patient discontinue insulin for several days prior to the desensitization if possible.

Most studies have demonstrated that there is a rapid decline in the anti-insulin IgE levels in desensitized patients. The mechanism for this decline is not known. However, patients who undergo desensitization to insulin must be cautioned that there should not be lapses in therapy, because this may lead to reappearance of IgE antibodies and allergic reaction when insulin therapy is resumed.

Patients with high levels of anti-insulin IgG antibodies are usually insulin resistant. The treatment of

species	amino acid sequence variations		
	A-chain position		B-chain position
	8	9	10	30
human	Thr-Ser-Ile		Thr
pig, dog, sperm whale	Thr-Ser-Ile		Ala
cattle, goat	Ala-Ser-Val		Ala

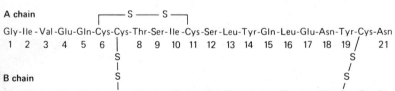

Figure 29–4. Covalent structure and variations of human and animal insulins. (Reproduced, with permission, from Ganong WF: *Review of Medical Physiology,* 14th ed. Appleton & Lange, 1989.)

insulin resistance is beyond the scope of this chapter, and the reader is referred to standard texts.

PSEUDOALLERGIC REACTIONS

Many drugs can induce the release of mediators of anaphylaxis from mast cells or circulating basophils by nonimmunologic means. Although IgE production is not involved, the symptoms of anaphylactic and anaphylactoid reactions are identical (see Chapter 26). Many of these drugs are capable of causing significant reactions in a certain portion of the treated population.

Radiocontrast media, particularly the ionic forms, are perhaps the best examples of drugs that cause pseudoallergic reactions. Other common drugs include aspirin and other nonsteroidal anti-inflammatory drugs (NSAID), curare and its derivatives, the opiate analgesics, and some local anesthetics. The reason for the susceptibility of only a portion of the treated population to nonimmunologic urticaria and anaphylactoid reactions to these drugs is not known. Several strategies have been developed for safe administration of drugs that cause pseudoallergic reactions. For patients who have previously reacted to radiocontrast media, pretreatment with H_1 and H_2 receptor-blocking antihistamines and corticosteroids has proven highly effective. Patients with sensitivity to aspirin or other NSAID are best treated by avoiding these drugs; however, oral "desensitization" to aspirin successfully prevents reactions to aspirin and other NSAID.

CONCLUSIONS

Immunologically mediated drug hypersensitivity makes up a significant portion of the overall spectrum of adverse reactions to drugs. The variety of immune responses to drugs accounts for the spectrum of drug allergy. Although the proportion of treated patients who will react to a given drug or class of drugs varies widely, it is most likely that any drug is capable of inducing an adverse immunologic reaction, and so any drug must be considered a possible cause of an individual patient's reaction.

The majority of drugs are considered to be haptens and therefore must conjugate to tissue protein in vivo to be immunogenic. Unfortunately, the actual immunogen is not known for most drugs. This has made the development of accurate in vivo or in vitro tests difficult. Thus, for most drug classes, an accurate clinical history is the only diagnostic test for suspecting a particular drug as the cause of a patient's reaction. When the history suggests a candidate, its effect can then be confirmed by testing. When testing is not possible, drug withdrawal and, if necessary, rechallenge will confirm the patient's sensitivity.

It is only in a minority of situations that continuation of or reintroduction of the drug will be necessary. In this case, pretreatment protocols, provocative challenge, and drug desensitization procedures are available. However, the best treatment for drug allergy is the use of a different drug with similar pharmacologic properties but different chemical (ie, antigenic) structure.

REFERENCES

Adverse reactions to radiocontrast media. *Invest Radiol* 1980;**15(Suppl 6):**S1. (Entire issue.)

Bayard PJ, Berger TG, Jacobson MA: Drug hypersensitivity reactions and human immunodeficiency virus disease. *J Acquired Immune Defic Syndr* 1992;**5:**1237.

Carrington DM, Earl HS, Sullivan TJ: Studies of human IgE to a sulfonamide determinant. *J Allergy Clin Immunol* 1987;**79:**442.

Evans R III, Kim K, Mahr TA: Current concepts in allergy: Drug reactions. *Curr Probl Pediatr* 1991;**21:**185.

Hansbrough JR, Wedner HJ, Chaplin DD: Anaphylaxis to intravenous furosemide. *J Allergy Clin Immunol* 1987;**80:**538.

Levine BB, Zolov DM: Prediction of penicillin allergy by immunological tests. *J Allergy* 1969;**43:**231.

Parker CW et al: Hypersensitivity to penicillenic acid derivatives in human beings with penicillin allergy. *J Exp Med* 1982;**115:**821.

Ring J: Pseudoallergic reactions. In: *Allergy: Theory and Practice,* 2nd ed. Korenblat PE, Wedner HJ (editors). Grune & Stratton, 1989.

Sullivan TJ et al: Desensitization of patients allergic to penicillin by orally administered beta-lactam antibiotics. *J Allergy Clin Immunol* 1982;**69:**275.

Sullivan TJ et al: Skin testing to detect penicillin allergy. *J Allergy Clin Immunol* 1981;**68:**171.

Volz MA, Nelson HS: Drug allergy. Best diagnostic and treatment approaches. *Postgrad Med* 1990;**87:**137.

Wedner HJ: Adverse reactions to drugs. Pages 640–646 in: *Current Pediatric Therapy,* 12th ed. Gellis SS, Kagan BM (editors). WB Saunders, 1986.

Wedner HJ: Protocols for penicillin desensitization. Appendix A, p 423 in: *Allergy: Theory and Practice.* Korenblat PE, Wedner HJ (editors). Grune & Stratton, 1984.

Weiss ME: Drug allergy. *Med Clin North Am* 1992;**76:**857.

30

Mechanisms of Disordered Immune Regulation

Alfred D. Steinberg, MD

Advances in basic and clinical immunology have shed light on mechanisms of disordered immune regulation underlying many immune-mediated diseases. For example, erythroblastosis fetalis has been traced to a mother's immune response to her fetus's paternally derived erythrocyte antigens. Initiating events in the bewildering disorder hereditary angioedema (once called angioneurotic edema) have been associated with a deficiency in a single inhibitor of several systems including the active form of the first component of complement, kallikrein, and Hageman factor; the resulting activation leads to increased permeability and edema. However, for many immune-mediated diseases, especially the so-called autoimmune diseases, the processes are still incompletely understood.

Autoimmune diseases are characterized by autoimmune phenomena, the most easily identifiable being production of antibodies reactive with self antigens. However, it is becoming clear that self-reactivity is a feature of normal immunity. Therefore, it is useful to try to separate normal from abnormal self-reactivity in considering autoimmune processes (Table 30–1). A related issue is the potential induction of autoimmune phenomena by foreign versus self antigens. Although autoantibodies may react with a self antigen, the inducer of those autoantibodies may or may not be the self antigen. Many studies have been devoted to foreign antigens that cross-react with self determinants as candidates for inducers of autoantibodies.

It is difficult to fulfill Koch's postulates when considering the etiology of various immune-mediated diseases. First, the often multifactorial pathogenetic processes provide substantial complexity. Second, genetic factors often play important roles as primary or secondary requirements for the immune phenomena, making transfer to a genetically different host very difficult.

DISEASE MECHANISMS

Normal versus Disease-Associated Autoreactivity

Normal immune reactivity involves self-recognition (Table 30–1). For example, interactions between the T cell and the antigen-presenting cell require binding of surface molecules on one cell to complementary surface molecules on the other cell. The same is true of interactions between migrating lymphocytes and determinants on endothelial cells. Another type of self-self interaction is called idiotypy. Here the immune system recognizes unique determinants that make up the variable regions of the B or T cell antigen receptor. For example, there is often recognition of the unique determinants on the immunoglobulin molecule that serves as the B cell antigen receptor or the comparable determinants on the secreted immunoglobulin. The result of such recognition may be an immune response (humoral or cellular) directed at those unique determinants. Antibody that recognizes unique determinants on another antibody molecule is called anti-idiotype antibody. It is thought that such idiotypic immunity is a normal component of the immune system and that some such idiotypic responses are immunoregulatory.

As a result of the vast array of normal autoimmune reactivity, it is sometimes difficult to relate autoimmune reactivity to disease pathogenesis. Examples of pathogenic disease-associated autoreactivity include the anti-cardiac immune responses of acute rheumatic fever (induced by cross-reactivity with antigenic determinants of certain streptococcal strains) and antibodies reactive with native DNA in patients with the nephritis of systemic lupus erythematosus (inducer incompletely understood). On the other hand, antibodies reactive with tRNA synthetases in polymyositis, Scl-70 in progressive systemic sclerosis, or Sm in lupus are not obviously pathogenic, although they may serve as diagnostic markers.

Autoimmune responses that give rise to disease act

Table 30–1. Normal and disease-associated autoimmunity.

Normal autoimmunity
Interaction of CD4 T cells with class II MHC determinants on antigen-presenting cells
Interaction of CD8 T cells with class I MHC determinants on antigen-presenting cells
Anti-idiotype antibodies
Anti-idiotypic T cells
Cell-cell interactions mediated by interaction of adhesion molecule with ligand
Interactions between lymphocytes and endothelial cells
Disease-associated autoimmunity
An epiphenomenon that may be a marker of a disorder but not cause disease
Pathogenic autoimmunity—important factors:
Quantity of the response (how much antibody, how great a T cell response, how much of a cytokine produced)
Qualitative factors (antibody affinity, isotype, fine specificity)
Genetic basis (multiple genetic factors may contribute)
Genes allowing susceptibility
Augmenting factors
Environmental contributors (infectious agents, chemicals, foods, UV light, etc)

through the same limited number of effector mechanisms that operate in immunity and allergy. These include anaphylactic, cytotoxic, antigen-antibody complex-mediated, and cell-mediated. Although a single effector mechanism may appear to dominate the induction of disease, many diseases are mediated by several effector modes. The ultimate magnitude of the disorder may be related not only to the vigor and persistence of the initiating immune reactions but also to the magnitude and chronicity of the effector processes.

Loss of Self-Tolerance

If autoimmune diseases represent quantitative or qualitative abnormalities in self-reactivity, it would seem logical to view autoimmune diseases as disorders resulting from defects in self-tolerance. Tolerance to self has long been viewed as occurring in the thymus early in life. However, recent studies have emphasized additional mechanisms of tolerance at the peripheral level. Thus, self-reactive T cells are deleted in the thymus; in addition, self-reactive T cells may be deleted in the periphery; finally, self-reactive T cells may be present but hypofunctioning (tolerant or anergic) in the periphery.

The mechanisms of deletion of self-reactive T cells are becoming better understood. It is thought that in the thymus there is positive selection of thymocytes followed by negative selection of self-reactive cells. The negative selection may lead to death of cells by a process of programmed cell death **(apoptosis).** This mechanism may also occur in the periphery. Finally, self-reactive cells escaping to the periphery may be tolerized by a nonstimulatory interaction with self antigen. A defect in any of these processes could allow

persistence or expansion of self-reactive cells sufficient to give rise to disease.

Antigen-presenting cells carry peptides bound to MHC-encoded molecules. Many of these peptides are derived from self antigens and serve to maintain tolerance to self. Although presentation of self-antigenic peptides in the absence of stimulatory signals may serve to inhibit autoimmune responses, their presentation in the presence of other stimulatory signals may favor autoreactivity. In addition, peptides from foreign antigens compete with these self peptides for presentation to lymphocytes. In certain infectious or parasitic diseases, such as tuberculosis, leprosy, trypanosomiasis, and mycoplasma infection, autoimmune phenomena are noted. These organisms interfere with normal immune tolerance, probably by several mechanisms.

The mechanisms that result in self-tolerance are incompletely understood. B cells capable of producing autoantibodies circulate in normal individuals. This includes B cells able to produce anti-thyroid antibodies and anti-DNA. Activation mechanisms that bypass T cell regulation could activate such cells to produce distinctive autoantibodies. For example, endotoxin released from intestinal bacteria or cytokines produced as a result of specific immune responses could potentially contribute to such B cell activation. However, under usual circumstances, most pathogenic autoantibodies appear to result from T cell stimulation of B cells that are able to produce autoantibodies.

Even with regard to the T cell compartment, it is likely that the enormous array of antigenic determinants of a given person represents a substantial fraction of determinants on foreign organisms. Should reactivity to all such determinants be eliminated, a person might be unduly susceptible to foreign organisms through failure to mount an appropriate immune response. Therefore, some balance occurs between deletion of T cells reactive with certain specificities and preservation of T cells that may react with self determinants. For example, recent studies have uncovered T cell reactivity to pancreatic islet cells in normal animals without necessarily leading to diabetes. A small increase in immunity or activation of otherwise dormant cells could result in pathogenic autoimmunity.

A relatively innocuous insult could initiate such a reaction. For example, a viral infection of the thyroid gland could lead to expression of class II MHC molecules that initiate presentation of antigen to infiltrating T cells so as to activate organ-specific immunity, and many positive feedback aspects of immunity serve to perpetuate such reactions. Individual variability in such perpetuating factors may determine which individuals have transient autoimmune reactions in contrast to those who progress to destruction of the organ involved.

It recently has been found that the islets of

Langerhans express an antigenic determinant which shares immune reactivity with a bovine protein found in milk. Therefore it is possible that an immune response directed at milk proteins includes a cross-reactive response to the islets and leads to islet destruction and type I diabetes. The extent to which various diseases result from specific foreign immunization as a mechanism of breaking self-tolerance remains to be determined.

The above serves to illustrate the delicate balance between protective immunity and autoimmunity. Females manifest greater autoimmunity than do males, probably because of the tendency of androgens to suppress immunity and of estrogens to augment immunity. These effects may be both direct and through the hypothalamic-pituitary axis.

Cross-Reactivity & Molecular Mimicry

It has long been held that one possible mechanism of induction of autoimmunity might be immunization with an antigen that cross-reacts with a self antigen. That is, one or more antigenic determinants on the foreign antigen would induce an immune response that would simultaneously be directed against a self antigen by virtue of the similar structures of the foreign antigen and self antigen. Such an immune response could be humoral or cell-mediated. For example, the human immune response to group A β-hemolytic streptococci includes a component that is directed at self antigens in the heart and, if sufficiently vigorous, can lead to acute rheumatic fever.

In addition to cross-reactivity, in which the antigenic determinants are similar but not identical, recent studies have demonstrated areas of identity between viruses and self antigens. This has been called **molecular mimicry.** For example, there are many instances in which a sequence of 5 amino acids has been found in common between a given foreign antigen and a self antigen. Even longer homologous stretches have been found between self antigens and retroviral proteins, bacterial proteins, herpesvirus glycoprotein, and others. The molecular mimicry observed has been proposed as the cause of the autoimmune disease characterized by an immune response against the relevant self antigen. Such a construction would be plausible if molecular mimicry were an extremely improbable event.

What is the probability of molecular mimicry? One can provide a gross estimate of the chance that a sequence of 5 amino acids on a human protein and a foreign protein might be identical on a random basis. For the estimate we will assume that (1) the average protein has 300 amino acids, (2) the 20 amino acids are distributed randomly and independently, and (3) the primary structure is critical to cross-reactivity. A 5-amino-acid sequence has a probability of $1/20^5$, or 3×10^{-7}. If there are 300 amino acids per protein, there are almost 300 possible pentapeptides in each of the human and foreign proteins. Therefore, we have to multiply 3×10^{-7} by 300 for the foreign protein and again by 300 for the self protein, which gives 3×10^{-2}. Thus, such calculations give approximately a 3% chance that a foreign and a human protein, each 300 amino acids long, will have a pentapeptide in common.

Many pentapeptides may not be readily accessible to the immune system in the 3-dimensional configuration of the native protein or the intracellular location of the protein. Moreover, many pentapeptides of self antigens may not be immunogenic because the relevant T cell specificities have not developed, possibly because of deletion in the thymus. Even if immunogenic, the pentapeptides might induce low-affinity antibody, which is not pathogenic. On the other hand, an immunogenic carrier, to which T cell clones have not been deleted in the thymus, which induces a vigorous immune response to a self pentapeptide adjacent to the carrier might be particularly pathogenic.

Since there are approximately 20,000 human genes capable of producing a protein, many potential 5-amino-acid sequences might share identical sequences with foreign proteins. In fact, a priori, it is highly probable that for any foreign protein there is a 5-amino-acid sequence of identity in some human (self) protein. Similarly, for every self protein, there is a strong probability that some foreign protein will have a 5-amino-acid sequence in common with it. Therefore, molecular mimicry should be the rule rather than the exception. However, demonstrating that a 5-amino-acid sequence is important in autoimmunity is another more difficult issue.

In addition to cross-reactivity and molecular mimicry as pathogenetic factors in the induction of disease, immunogenic foreign antigens could combine with self antigens and thereby induce an immune response to the self antigen. For example, virus-encoded antigens expressed on mammalian cell surfaces could act as carriers for self antigens adjacent to them on the cell membrane. In such a concept, the self antigen would appear as a hapten to which an immune response could not be induced without an immunogenic carrier.

Idiotypy

Idiotypy constitutes a normal self-self interaction (Table 30–1). Idiotypy in B cells consists of a set of B cells with receptors that recognize unique epitopes on antibodies produced by other B cells. Similarly, T cells have receptors able to recognize epitopes on other T cells or on antibody molecules. As a result, such idiotypic B cells or T cells can be activated by self antigens. It has been postulated that some degree of idiotypic response plays a role in normal immune regulatory processes. It is also possible that perturbation of the idiotype networks gives rise to pathogenic immune responses. Moreover, idiotypic interactions could serve as amplification systems for autoimmunity rather than as down-regulatory forces, in a manner similar to the induction of immunity by anti-idiotypic antibody simulating the role of antigen.

It is possible that the molecular mimicry described above acts in concert with idiotypy as a possible mechanism of autoimmunity. Many viruses utilize normal host receptors for their attachment to and entry into host cells. Therefore, the invading virus must contain a structure homologous with and presumably antigenically cross-reactive with a normal ligand for that receptor. If the host makes an immune response to that part of the foreign agent, it will be making an immune response resembling an autoimmune response to the normal ligand. In addition, the production of antibody to the normal ligand can trigger an anti-idiotype response to that antibody; such an anti-idiotype might represent an antibody reactive with the receptor itself. In such a manner, a virus or other microorganism that utilizes a receptor might be able to induce an autoimmune response to that receptor. This mechanism may be important in the induction of such antireceptor disorders as myasthenia gravis, anti-insulin receptor antibody syndrome, and Graves' disease. More generally, anti-idiotype autoantibodies could easily be the natural consequence of a normal immune response. If the external agent that induced such a response persisted, the stimulus to autoantibody production also would be maintained. If the stimulus were intermittent, the resulting autoimmune response also might be stimulated intermittently. The same reasoning would hold for T cell idiotypy.

Superantigens

Certain antigens, especially certain specific bacterial products, are able to interact with and stimulate families of T cells with a particular β chain of their receptors for antigen. This interaction is facilitated by the ability of the superantigen to interact with particular T cell receptor β chains outside of the usual antigen groove. As a result of such stimulation of very large numbers of T cells, there is an outpouring of cytokines and major perturbation of the immune system. Antigens that are able to interact with all of the T cells bearing a particular β chain are called superantigens. One such superantigen from a *Staphylococcus aureus* toxin is responsible for the toxic shock syndrome.

Following T cell stimulation, many of the T cells interacting with the particular superantigen undergo apoptosis. As a result, there is a marked diminution in numbers of the family of T cells bearing that particular β chain. Moreover, a given superantigen may be able to interact with a few β chain families and lead to subsequent deletion of members of all of those particular families.

Recent studies indicate that endogenous superantigens can derive not only from bacteria but also from viruses, especially retroviruses. Endogenous retroviral sequences, encoded by genes in the mammalian genome (once derived from retroviral infection of germ cells and then incorporated into the genetic material), can be transcribed and translated, leading to proteins that can act as superantigens. Present from early in life, such endogenous superantigens interact with specific β chain families of T cells and may be responsible for molding the T cell repertoire by inducing deletion of those T cells. Thus, both endogenous and exogenous superantigens may contribute to an individual's T cell repertoire.

One could imagine that bacterial stimulation of the immune system could lead to both specific immunity, including cross-reactive autoimmunity, and nonspecific immune stimulation through outpouring of cytokines. Normal deletion of the superantigen-reactive cells prevents expansion of many self-reactive cells, minimizes the duration of cytokine production, and brings the system back into balance. However, a defect in the ability of the T cells to undergo apoptosis might, instead, lead to continued production by the T cells of stimulatory cytokines and expansion of self-reactive T cells.

Recent studies suggest that MRL-*lpr/lpr* mice, which spontaneously develop features of systemic lupus erythematosus, Sjögren's syndrome, and rheumatoid arthritis, have such a defect in apoptosis. The *lpr* mutation represents a defect in the *fas* gene on mouse chromosome 19. The fas antigen, encoded by the *fas* gene, plays a critical role in apoptosis, which normally leads to peripheral T cell deletion following superantigen stimulation. By virtue of their genetic defect, *lpr/lpr* mice fail to normally express the fas antigen and thereby have impaired peripheral deletion of superantigen-stimulated and self-reactive T cells. The defect in apoptosis is thought to be responsible for the marked T cell expansion characteristic of these mice as well as the autoimmune phenotypes. More modest defects in responses to superantigens undoubtedly could contribute to other autoimmune disorders.

LESSONS FROM EXPERIMENTAL ANIMALS

Experimental tolerance is a well-established mechanism for preventing immunity to specific foreign antigens. For example, immunity to heterologous gamma globulins administered in an immunogenic form can be prevented by treatment with deaggregated gamma globulin before the immunogenic form is administered. This form of tolerance can be prevented by providing a B cell stimulus (eg, bacterial lipopolysaccharide) at the time of the deaggregated gamma globulin injection.

Interleukin-1 (IL-1), which is induced by agents that interfere with tolerance, probably plays a critical role in preventing tolerance. Impaired experimental tolerance and loss of self tolerance are features of mouse strains predisposed to systemic autoimmunnity. Increased production of stimulatory cytokines most probably leads to both the defective tolerance and the heightened immunity that characterize murine systemic lupus erythematosus.

In multifactorial organ-specific as well as generalized autoimmune diseases, increased immunity and decreased suppression, which is often antigen nonspecific, are among the predisposing factors. These nonspecific factors, however, do not negate a role for specifically sensitized T cells that recognize a critical self epitope, or the important role of cognate cellular interactions in tolerance induction and immunity. Antigen-specific defects in either tolerance or immunity also play critical roles in such disorders.

Rheumatoid Arthritis

The multifactorial pathogenesis of autoimmune disease (Table 30–1) is illustrated by the example of experimental rheumatoid arthritis in swine (Table 30–2). If the cause of arthritis in group 5 was unknown, identification of single causes, such as *Erysipelothrix, Mycoplasma,* trauma to the joints as a result of walking on cement floors, or a genetic basis of disease would be correct but only partially so, since the disease in full expression is multifactorial. The data suggest that genetic factors, at least 2 infectious agents, and other environmental factors (cement floors) all contribute to the disease experienced by group 5.

Other Organ-Specific Diseases and a Possible Role for Class II MHC Expression

Most autoimmune diseases preferentially affect a single tissue or organ system. As a result, the details of pathogenesis depend on the particular immune responses involved in the individual disorder. Organ-specific autoimmune diseases may be primarily cell-mediated or antibody-mediated; however, several different mechanisms may contribute to glandular destruction. In many cases, immunity to specific receptors probably is induced by anti-idiotypic effects (see above) or molecular mimicry (see above). For other diseases, a genetic predisposition to specific immunity may be critical. Table 30–3 summarizes the etio-

Table 30–2. Multifactorial etiology of rheumatoid arthritis-like disease in swine.

Factor	Arthritis
Swine of the wrong type (wrong genes) regardless of other manipulations	Trivial
Erysipelothrix insidiosa	Mild
Mycoplasma hyorhinis	Mild
2 + 3 (housed on dirt)	Moderate
2 + 3 (housed on cement)	Severe

Table 30–3. Etiologic factors from animal models of autoimmune disease.

Genetic susceptibility
Initial infection
Perpetuation
Severity of reaction
Initial insult(s)
Virus, bacterium, mycoplasma, etc (more than one may contribute to disease)
Factors allowing perpetuation
Impaired immune regulation
Excessive inflammatory response
Impaired degradation or clearance of foreign antigens
Trauma

logic factors gleaned from many studies of animal models of autoimmune diseases as they may apply to human disease.

It is established that antigen presentation to T cells occurs in the context of self major histocompatibility complex (MHC) molecules. As a result, aberrant expression of MHC molecules on tissues normally expressing very little MHC could lead to the "presentation" of self determinants in association with the aberrantly expressed MHC. Such a process might, for example, be induced by an infection that induces the MHC or by interferon production as a result of either viral or immune effects. It is likely that such MHC expression represents a mechanism producing secondary inflammation of certain endocrine organs in an autoimmune process.

It has become apparent that the central nervous system bears important analogies to the rest of the body in terms of MHC expression and interferon effects. For example, astrocytes can be induced by interferon to express MHC molecules and present antigens to T cells. As a result, viral infections of the central nervous system can induce immune and potentially autoimmune central nervous system effects. Consistent with such a view, interferon exacerbates multiple sclerosis and increases the immune response to myelin basic protein.

One aspect that has not yet been stressed is the possibility that an immune deficiency, either global or restricted, predisposes to autoimmune disease. Individuals who fail to clear infections of specific or varied types may develop chronic inflammatory diseases. For example, many individuals with hypogammaglobulinemia or with complement deficiencies develop rheumatic diseases. Patients with ankylosing spondylitis may be predisposed to disease because the HLA-B27 gene they carry allows an immune response to a common antigenic determinant shared by the HLA-B27 antigen and certain bacteria. Alternatively, this molecular mimicry could allow persistence of certain bacteria by virtue of self-tolerance to HLA-B27 and a failure of cross-reactive immune responses against the bacteria.

Systemic Lupus Erythematosus

Systemic lupus erythematosus (SLE) differs from many other autoimmune diseases in the relative organ nonspecificity of the disorder. Patients with SLE produce large amounts of antibodies reactive with epitopes on a variety of nuclear, cytoplasmic, and cell surface antigens. Although it is a complex disease, SLE provides a number of insights into autoimmune pathogenesis. Several different factors appear capable of predisposing to disease: genetic factors that increase humoral immunity, impaired clearance of immune complexes, defective immune regulation, and exogenous agents that stimulate humoral immunity. Thus, a decreased number of receptors for immune complexes on erythrocytes predisposes to impaired clearance of immune complexes and their increased deposition in tissues. Relatively unusual antibodies may underlie specific pathologic events. For example, antibodies reactive with platelet phospholipids may predispose to in situ thromboses and hence induce pulmonary infarcts or strokes.

In SLE, autoantibody production may be antigen-driven and T cell-dependent. On the other hand, SLE often is characterized by polyclonal B cell activation. Patients have marked increases in numbers of activated and immunoglobulin-producing circulating B cells and increased numbers of B cells producing anti-hapten antibodies (Table 30–4).

Studies on murine lupus show that a substantial portion of the immune systems of both normal strains and strains predisposed to autoimmunity are devoted to autoantibody production: approximately 1% to anti-DNA and another 1% to anti-T cell antibodies. The increase in numbers of autoantibody-producing cells early in the life of mice with lupus results not from a skewing of the B cell repertoire toward autoantibody production but from an increase in total numbers of immunoglobulin-secreting cells, of which autoantibody-producing cells are a relatively constant fraction. This polyclonal B cell activation is fertile soil for autoimmune disease to arise. Later in life, T cell-dependent responses become progressively more important in the induction of autoantibody synthesis. The polyclonal expansion precedes antigen-specific responses. The same sequence probably holds for some humans with SLE. Polyclonal ac-

Table 30–4. Impaired tolerance, B cells, T cells, and systemic lupus erythematosus

In lupus, there are defects in both self-tolerance and experimental tolerance:
1. Lupus is characterized by excess B cell activation
2. Some antigens are presented to T cells by B cells
3. Resting B cells present antigen to T cells with down-regulation of the T cell
4. Activated B cells present antigen to T cells with stimulation
5. Since activated B cells stimulate memory T cells, this causes a positive feedback loop (initially slow, later a crescendo)

Thus, excess B cell activation plus antigen presentation by the activated B cells of self antigen or antigen cross-reactive with self breaks tolerance and leads to autoimmunity. Disease occurs if the autoimmune responses are pathogenic.

tivation may interfere with development or maintenance of self tolerance and hence may predispose to production of pathogenic autoantibodies. Moreover, a switch to active SLE is associated with a switch from IgM to IgG autoantibody production, substituting a long-lived isotype for a much shorter-lived one. Therefore, even without any change in total numbers of immunoglobulin-secreting cells, there would be a substantial increase in serum autoantibody.

CONCLUSIONS

From the foregoing it might seem surprising that everyone does not have autoimmune diseases. In fact, we all have many autoantibodies. The difference between health and disease may be only a 10–20-fold difference in the quantity of certain immune responses. There are many mechanisms by which normal immune regulatory processes can go awry. Autoimmune diseases result when there is a disruption of such normal processes to a sufficient extent to bring about pathogenic autoimmunity.

Diseases that we recognize as single entities may, in fact, be syndromes with different underlying mechanisms by which the common disorder arises. Specific appropriate therapy for such individuals requires an understanding of the specific underlying mechanisms.

REFERENCES

General

Fuchs EJ, Matxinger P: B cells turn off virgin but not memory T cells. *Science* 1992;**258:**1156.

Kawabe Y, Ochi A: Programmed cell death and extrathymic reduction of Vbeta8+ CD4+ T cells in mice tolerant to *Staphylococcus aureus* enterotoxin B. *Nature* 1991;**349:**245.

Marrack P, Kappler J: The staphylococcal enterotoxins and their relatives. *Science* 1990;**248:**705.

Smith HR, Steinberg AD: Autoimmunity—a perspective. *Annu Rev Immunol* 1983;**1:**175.

Watanabe-Fukunga R et al: Lymphoproliferation disorder in mice explained by defects in Fas antigen that mediates apoptosis. *Nature* 1992;**356:**314.

Webb S, Morris C, Sprent C: Extrathymic tolerance of mature T cells: Clonal elimination as a consequence of immunity. *Cell* 1990;**63**:1249.

Molecular Mimicry

Beck S, Barrell BG: Human cytomegalovirus encodes a glycoprotein homologous to MHC class-I antigens. *Nature* 1988;**331**:269.

Dale JB, Beachey EH: Protective antigenic determinant of streptococcal M protein shared with sarcolemmal membrane protein of human heart. *J Exp Med* 1982;**156**:1165.

Krisher K, Cunningham MW: Myosin: A link between streptococci and heart. *Science* 1985;**227**:413.

Oldstone MBA: Molecular mimicry and autoimmune disease. *Cell* 1987;**50**:819.

Query CC, Keene JD: A human autoimmune protein associated with U1 RNA contains a region of homology that is cross-reactive with retroviral p30-gag antigen. *Cell* 1987;**51**:211.

Idiotypy & Autoimmunity

Gaulton EN, Greene MI: Idiotypic mimicry of biological receptors. *Annu Rev Immunol* 1986;**4**:253.

Plotz PH: Autoantibodies are anti-idiotypic antibodies to antiviral antibodies. *Lancet* 1983;**2**:824.

Powell TJ et al: Induction of effective immunity to Moloney murine sarcoma virus using monoclonal anti-idiotypic antibody as immunogen. *J Immunol* 1989;**142**:1318.

Loss of Immunologic Tolerance

Kappler JW, Roehm N, Marrack P: T cell tolerance by clonal elimination in the thymus. *Cell* 1987;**49**:273.

Kappler JW et al: Self-tolerance eliminates T cells specific for Mls-modified products of the major histocompatibility complex. *Nature* 1988;**332**:35.

Kisielow P et al: Tolerance in T-cell receptor transgenic mice involves deletion of nonmature CD4+8+ thymocytes. *Nature* 1988;**333**:742.

MacDonald H et al: T-cell receptor Vbeta8 use predicts reactivity and tolerance to Mls^a-encoded antigens. *Nature* 1988;**332**:40.

Weigle WO et al: The effect of lipopolysaccharide desensitization on the regulation of in vivo induction of immunologic tolerance and antibody production and in vitro release of IL-1. *J Immunol* 1989;**142**:1107.

Role of MHC-II (Ia) Expression

Traugott U, Lebon P: Interferon-gamma and Ia antigens are present on astrocytes in active chronic multiple sclerosis lesions. *J Neuroimmunol* 1988;**84**:257.

Wong GHW et al: Inducible expression of H-2 and Ia antigens on brain cells. *Nature* 1984;**310**:688.

Systemic Lupus Erythematosus

Blaese RM, Grayson J, Steinberg AD: Elevated immunoglobulin secreting cells in the blood of patients with active systemic lupus erythematosus: Correlation of laboratory and clinical assessment of disease activity. *Am J Med* 1980;**69**:345.

Budman DR et al: Increased spontaneous activity of antibody-forming cells in the peripheral blood of patients with active systemic lupus erythematosus. *Arthritis Rheum* 1977;**20**:829.

Gmelig-Meyling F, Dawisha S, Steinberg AD: Assessment of *in vivo* frequency of mutated T cells in patients with systemic lupus erythematosus. *J Exp Med* 1992;**175**:297.

Klinman DM, Eisenberg RA, Steinberg AD: Development of the autoimmune B cell repertoire in MRL-*lpr/lpr* mice. *J Immunol* 1990;**144**:506.

Steinberg AD et al: Theoretical and experimental approaches to generalized autoimmunity. *Immunol Rev* 1980;**118**:129.

Steinberg AD et al: Systemic lupus erythematosus. (edited transcript of Combined Staff Conference, February 27, 1991) *Ann Intern Med* 1991;**115**:548.

Rheumatic Diseases

31

Kenneth H. Fye, MD, & Kenneth E. Sack, MD

Many of the major rheumatologic disorders are autoimmune in nature. Therefore, a thorough understanding of the mechanisms of the immune response is essential to an understanding of these diseases. Of particular importance is information in Chapter 30 which describes mechanisms of disordered immune regulation. This chapter will discuss the rheumatologic diseases with proved or hypothesized immunologic pathogenesis.

SYSTEMIC LUPUS ERYTHEMATOSUS (SLE)

Major Immunologic Features

- Antinuclear antibodies are present.
- Anti-double-stranded DNA and anti-Sm antibodies are present.
- Serum complement levels are depressed.
- Immunoglobulin and complement are deposited along glomerular basement membrane and at the dermal-epidermal junction.
- Numerous other autoantibodies are present.

General Considerations

Osler described the systemic manifestations of systemic lupus erythematosus (SLE) in 1895. Prior to that time, lupus was considered to be a disfiguring but nonfatal skin disease. It is now known to be a chronic systemic inflammatory disease that follows a course of alternating exacerbations and remissions. Involvement of multiple organ systems characteristically occurs during periods of disease activity. The cause of SLE is not known. The disease affects predominantly females (4:1 over males) of childbearing age; however, the age at onset ranges from 2 to 90 years. It is more prevalent among nonwhites (particularly blacks) than whites.

Immunologic Pathogenesis

The discovery of the lupus erythematosus (LE) cell phenomenon (see Immunologic Diagnosis, below) marked the start of the modern era of research into the pathogenesis of SLE. This initial clinical observation led to the finding of multiple antinuclear factors, including antibodies to DNA, in the sera of patients with SLE. Further studies of renal eluates from patients with SLE established the importance of DNA-containing immune complexes in the causation of lupus glomerulonephritis. Reduced serum complement and the presence of antibodies to double-stranded (ds) DNA are hallmarks of active SLE, distinguishing this entity from other lupus variants. It is not known whether viral or host DNA is the immunogen for anti-DNA antibody formation.

Autoantibodies directed against numerous non-nucleic acid antigens also occur in patients with SLE. Many of these autoantibodies fix complement and thereby damage target tissues. For instance, the hemolytic anemia and thrombocytopenia characteristic of SLE are often caused by antierythrocyte and antiplatelet antibodies. Other autoantibodies, such as nonspecific anticytoplasmic antibodies, are probably of no pathogenetic significance. Lymphocytotoxic antibodies (with predominant specificity for T lymphocytes) occur in many patients with SLE. Family studies have demonstrated a genetic susceptibility to the development of SLE. Autoantibody formation in SLE is in part genetically determined; eg, patients with HLA-DR2 are more likely to produce anti-ds-DNA antibodies, those with HLA-DR3 produce anti-SS-A and anti-SS-B antibodies (Table 31–1), and those with HLA-DR4 and HLA-DR5 produce anti-Sm and anti-RNP antibodies.

Autoantibody formation is partially prevented through the action of regulatory T lymphocytes called suppressor T cells. Although the mechanism of suppression is unknown, such suppressor T cells probably play an important role in immunologic tolerance and self-nonself discrimination. A defect in suppressor T cell activity has also been observed in human beings with SLE; however, this defect may be

Table 31–1. Antinuclear antibodies.

Pattern	Antigen	Associated Diseases
Peripheral	Double-stranded DNA	SLE
Homogeneous	DNA-histone complex	SLE, occasionally other connective tissue disease
Speckled	SM (Smith antigen)	SLE
	RNP (ribonucleoprotein)	Mixed connective tissue disease, SLE, Sjögren's syndrome, scleroderma, polymyositis
	SS-A (Ro)	Sjögren's syndrome, SLE
	SS-B (La)	Sjögren's syndrome, SLE
	Jo-1	Polydermatomyositis
	Scl-70	Scleroderma
	Centromere	Limited scleroderma
	RANA (rheumatoid-associated nuclear antigen) (nuclear antigen induced by EBV)	Rheumatoid arthritis
Nucleolar	Nucleolus-specific RNA	Scleroderma
	PM-Scl	Polymyositis

due to anti-T cell antibody activity and may not represent a primary suppressor T cell deficiency.

SLE, like many rheumatic disorders, occurs predominantly in women. Studies have demonstrated that estrogens enhance anti-DNA antibody formation and increase the severity of renal disease in animal models. Androgens have an opposite effect on both anti-DNA antibody production and renal disease.

Pathology

There are numerous characteristic pathologic changes in SLE:

(1) The verrucous endocarditis of Libman-Sacks consists of ovoid vegetations, 1–4 mm in diameter, which form along the base of the valve and, rarely, on the chordae tendineae and papillary muscles.

(2) A peculiar periarterial concentric fibrosis results in the so-called "onion skin" lesion seen in the spleen.

(3) A pathognomonic finding in SLE, the "hematoxylin body," consists of a homogeneous globular mass of nuclear material that stains bluish purple with hematoxylin. Hematoxylin bodies occur in the heart, kidneys, lungs, spleen, lymph nodes, and serous and synovial membranes. It should be emphasized that patients with fulminant SLE involving the central nervous system, skin, muscles, joints, and kidneys may not have any distinctive pathologic abnormalities at autopsy.

Clinical Features

A. Symptoms and Signs: SLE presents no single characteristic clinical pattern. The onset can be acute or insidious. Constitutional symptoms include fever, weight loss, malaise, and lethargy. Every organ system may become involved.

1. Joints and muscles–Polyarthralgia or arthritis is the most common manifestation of SLE (90%). The arthritis is symmetric and can involve almost any joint. It may resemble rheumatoid arthritis, but bony erosions and severe deformity are unusual.

Avascular necrosis of bone is common in SLE. The femoral head is most frequently affected, but other bones may also be involved. Corticosteroids, which are major therapeutic agents in SLE, may play a role in the pathogenesis of this complication. Myalgias, with or without frank myositis, are common.

2. Skin–The most common skin lesion is an erythematous rash involving areas of the body chronically exposed to ultraviolet light. A few patients with SLE develop the classic "butterfly" rash. In some patients with systemic disease, discoid lupus erythematosus occurs. The rash may resolve without sequelae or may result in scar formation, atrophy, and hypo- or hyperpigmentation. A nonscarring skin lesion termed subacute cutaneous lupus erythematosus occurs predominantly in patients with anti-SS-A antibodies. In addition, bullae, patches of purpura, urticaria, angioneurotic edema, patches of vitiligo, subcutaneous nodules, and thickening of the skin may be seen. Vasculitic lesions, ranging from palpable purpura to digital infarction, are common. Alopecia, which may be diffuse, patchy, or circumscribed, is also common. Mucosal ulcerations, involving both oral and genital mucosa, occur in about 15% of cases.

3. Polyserositis–Pleurisy, with chest pain and dyspnea, is a frequent complication of SLE. Although one-third of cases have pleural fluid, massive effusion is rare. Pericarditis is the commonest form of cardiac involvement and can be the first manifestation of SLE. The pericarditis is usually benign, leading only to mild chest discomfort and a pericardial friction rub, but severe pericarditis with tamponade can occur. Peritonitis alone is extremely rare, although 5–10% of patients with pleuritis and pericarditis have concomitant peritonitis. Manifestations of peritonitis include abdominal pain, anorexia, nausea and vomiting, and, rarely, ascites.

4. Kidneys–Renal involvement is a frequent and serious feature of SLE. Seventy-five percent of patients have nephritis at autopsy. The study of renal tissue by light microscopy, immunofluorescence, and electron microscopy has revealed 5 histologic lesions associated with rather distinctive clinical features. (1) Mesangial glomerulonephritis manifests as hypercellularity and the deposition of immune complexes in the mesangium. This is a benign form of lupus nephritis. (2) In focal glomerulonephritis, segmental proliferation occurs in less than 50% of glomeruli. Immune complexes are found in the mesangium and in the subendothelium of the glomerular capillary. Focal glomerulonephritis is often a benign process, but it may progress to a diffuse proliferative lesion. (3) Diffuse proliferative glomerulonephritis is characterized by extensive cellular proliferation in more than 50% of glomeruli. Immunofluorescence reveals subendothelial deposits of immune complexes. This process frequently leads to renal failure. (4) In membranous glomerulonephritis, glomerular cellularity is normal but the capillary basement membrane is thickened. Immune complexes occur mainly in subepithelial and intramembranous areas. This lesion may be associated with the development of renal failure. (5) Sclerosing glomerulonephritis is defined by an increase in mesangial matrix glomerulosclerosis, capsular adhesions, fibrous crescents, interstitial fibrosis with tubular atrophy, and vascular sclerosis. This lesion portends a poor prognosis and is not responsive to drugs.

It must be emphasized that a benign renal lesion may evolve into a more serious one.

Systemic hypertension is a common finding in acute or chronic lupus nephritis and may contribute to renal dysfunction.

5. Lungs–Pleuritic chest pain occurs in about 50% of patients with SLE. Pleural effusions are less common, are typically unilateral, and resolve quickly with treatment. Clinically apparent lupus pneumonitis is unusual. When a pulmonary infiltrate develops in a patient with SLE, particularly one being treated with corticosteroids or immunosuppressive drugs, infection must be the first diagnostic consideration. Restrictive interstitial lung disease is the commonest form of parenchymal involvement. It may be asymptomatic and detectable only by pulmonary function tests. The chest x-ray is usually normal but may show "platelike" atelectasis or interstitial fibrosis with "honeycombing." Other pulmonary manifestations include pulmonary hypertension, alveolar hemorrhage, pneumothorax, hemothorax, and vasculitis.

6. Heart–Clinically apparent myocarditis occurs rarely in SLE but when present may result in congestive heart failure with tachycardia, gallop rhythm, and cardiomegaly. Arrhythmias are unusual and are considered a preterminal event. The verrucous endocarditis of SLE, with the characteristic Libman-Sacks vegetations, is usually asymptomatic and diagnosed only at autopsy. Thickening of the aortic valve cusps with resultant aortic insufficiency can occur. Coronary artery disease, possibly related to corticosteroid therapy, is commonly recognized.

7. Nervous system–Disturbances of mentation and aberrant behavior, such as psychosis or depression, are the commonest manifestations of central nervous system involvement. Convulsions, cranial nerve palsies, aseptic meningitis, migraine headache, peripheral neuritis, and cerebrovascular accidents may also occur.

8. Eyes–Ocular involvement is present in 20–25% of patients. The characteristic retinal finding (the cytoid body) is a fluffy white exudative lesion caused by focal degeneration of the nerve fiber layer of the retina secondary to retinal vasculitis. Scleritis is also a manifestation of ocular vasculitis. Corneal ulceration occurs in conjunction with Sjögren's syndrome (see below).

9. Gastrointestinal system–Gastrointestinal ulceration due to vasculitis can occur in SLE. Manifestations include abdominal pain, diarrhea, and hemorrhage. Pancreatitis, cholecystitis, and acute and chronic hepatitis may be seen.

10. Hematopoietic system–See Laboratory Findings, below.

11. Vascular system–Small-vessel vasculitis commonly occurs in active SLE. Cutaneous manifestations of small-vessel disease include splinter hemorrhages, periungual occlusions, finger pulp infarctions, and atrophic ulcers. Small-vessel vasculitis may also cause a "stocking-glove" peripheral neuropathy. Medium-vessel arteritis, involving arteries 0.5–1 mm in diameter, also occurs in SLE. Manifestations range from bowel infarction to mononeuritis multiplex to cerebrovascular accidents. Hypercoagulation leading to arterial and venous occlusive disease is seen in patients with antiphospholipid antibodies (see below). Raynaud's phenomenon occurs in 15% of patients with SLE.

12. Sjögren's syndrome–Five to 10% of patients with SLE develop the sicca complex (keratoconjunctivitis sicca, xerostomia).

13. Drug-induced lupuslike syndrome–Certain drugs may provoke a lupuslike picture in susceptible individuals. The most commonly implicated drugs are hydralazine and procainamide, but quinidine, chlorpromazine, methyldopa, isoniazid, and phenytoin are also known to produce this syndrome. Typical manifestations of drug-induced lupus are arthralgias, arthritis, rash, fever, and pleurisy. Nephritis and central nervous system involvement are rare. The disease usually remits when the offending drug is discontinued. The antinuclear antibodies typical of drug-induced lupus are anti-histone and anti-single-stranded DNA.

B. Laboratory Findings: Anemia is the most common hematologic finding in SLE. Eighty percent of patients present with a normochromic, normocytic anemia due to marrow suppression. A few develop Coombs-positive hemolytic anemia. Leukopenia and thrombocytopenia are common. Urinalysis may show hematuria, proteinuria, and erythrocyte and leukocyte casts. The sedimentation rate is typically high in active SLE. Serologic abnormalities are described in the section on immunologic diagnosis (below). The synovial fluid in SLE is yellow and clear, with a low viscosity. The leukocyte count does not exceed 4000/µL, most of which are lymphocytes. The pleural effusion of SLE is a transudate with a predominance of lymphocytes and a total leukocyte count of no more than 3000/µL. A hemorrhagic pleural effusion is very rare. In central nervous system lupus, the cerebrospinal fluid protein concentration is sometimes elevated, and there is occasionally a mild lymphocytosis.

C. X-Ray Findings: Chest-x-ray may reveal cardiomegaly (due to either pericarditis or myocarditis), pleural effusion, platelike atelectasis, or interstitial fibrosis with a "honeycomb" appearance. Joint x-rays may show soft tissue swelling and mild osteopenia but rarely show erosions.

Immunologic Diagnosis

A. Proteins and Complement: Most patients with SLE (80%) present with elevated α_2- and γ-globulins. Hypoalbuminemia is occasionally present. The serum complement is frequently reduced in the presence of active disease because of increased utilization due to immune complex formation, reduced synthesis, or a combination of both factors. Several complement components, including C3 and C4, and total hemolytic complement activity are decreased during disease activity. The serum of patients with active SLE occasionally contains circulating cryoglobulin consisting of IgM/IgG aggregates and complement.

B. Autoantibodies:

1. LE cell phenomenon—This phenomenon was first described in the bone marrow of patients with SLE. It reflects the presence of IgG antibody to deoxyribonucleoprotein. However, this relatively cumbersome and insensitive technique is only of historic interest.

2. Antinuclear antibodies (ANA)—Immunoglobulins of all classes may form antinuclear antibodies. The indirect immunofluorescence technique was introduced in 1957. Six different morphologic patterns of immunofluorescent staining have been described, 4 of which have clinical significance (Fig 31–1 and Table 31–1).

a. The "homogeneous" ("diffuse" or "solid") pattern is the morphologic expression of antihistone antibodies and occurs in patients with systemic or drug-induced lupus erythematosus. In this pattern, the nucleus shows diffuse and uniform staining.

b. The "peripheral" ("shaggy" or "outline") pattern is the morphologic expression of anti-ds-DNA antibodies. The outline pattern is best seen when human leukocytes are used as substrate. It is characteristic of active SLE.

c. The "speckled" pattern reflects the presence of antibodies directed against non-DNA nuclear constituents. The anti-ENA (extractable nuclear antigen) assay detects antibodies against 2 saline-extractable

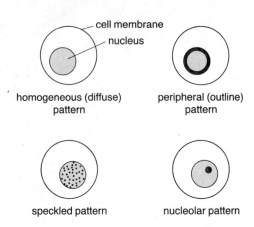

Figure 31–1. Patterns of immunofluorescent staining for antinuclear antibodies.

nuclear antigens, the Sm (Smith) antigen and RNP (ribonucleoprotein) antigen. Antibodies against the Sm antigen are characteristic of SLE. High titers of anti-RNP antibodies are the hallmark of mixed connective tissue disease, but low-titer anti-RNP antibodies may occur in SLE. Other antinuclear antibodies have been described in Sjögren's syndrome, rheumatoid arthritis, scleroderma, CREST syndrome, and polymyositis-dermatomyositis.

d. The "nucleolar" pattern is caused by the homogeneous staining of the nucleolus. It has been suggested that this antigen may be the ribosomal precursor of ribonucleoprotein. This pattern is most often associated with scleroderma or polymyositis-dermatomyositis.

A positive ANA test must be interpreted with caution because (1) the serum of a patient with any rheumatic disease may contain many autoantibodies to different nuclear constituents, so that a "homogeneous" pattern may obscure a "speckled" or "nucleolar" pattern; (2) different antibodies in the serum can be present in different titers, so that by diluting the serum one can change the pattern observed; (3) the stability of the different antigens is different and can be changed by fixation or denaturation; and (4) the pattern observed appears to be influenced by the types of tissues or cells used as substrate for the test.

The ANA determination is occasionally positive in normal individuals, in patients with various chronic diseases, and in the aged. However, high titers are most often associated with SLE. Absence of ANA is strong evidence against a diagnosis of SLE.

3. Anti-DNA antibodies and immune complexes—Three major types of anti-DNA antibodies can be found in the sera of lupus patients: (1) anti-single-stranded or "denatured" DNA (ss-DNA); (2) anti-double-stranded or "native" DNA (ds-DNA); and (3) antibodies that react to both ss-DNA and ds-DNA. These antibodies may be either IgG or IgM immunoglobulins. High titers of anti-ds-DNA antibodies are essentially seen only in SLE. In contrast, anti-ss-DNA antibodies are not specific and can be found in other autoimmune diseases, eg, rheumatoid arthritis, chronic active hepatitis, primary biliary cirrhosis, and drug-induced lupus. Antibodies to DNA can be quantitatively measured by RIA or ELISA techniques (see Chapter 12). Complement-fixing and high-avidity anti-ds-DNA antibodies may be associated with the development of renal disease. The amount of antibody correlates well with disease activity, and the antibody titer frequently decreases when patients enter remission.

Circulating immune complexes are present in the sera of patients with active disease. However, different assay techniques are required to detect complexes of different sizes, and there is controversy about how closely the level of soluble circulating immune complexes correlates with disease activity.

4. Antierythrocyte antibodies–These antibodies belong to the IgG, IgA, and IgM classes and can be detected by the direct Coombs test. The prevalence of these antibodies among SLE patients ranges from 10 to 65%. Hemolytic anemia does occasionally occur and, when present, is associated with a complement-fixing warm antierythrocyte antibody.

5. Circulating anticoagulants and antiplatelet antibodies–Antiphospholipid antibodies, called lupus anticoagulants, develop in 10–15% of patients with SLE. These antibodies are often associated with a false-positive VDRL and possess activity against cardiolipin. Although these anticoagulants prolong the partial thromboplastin and prothrombin times, hemorrhagic complications are rare. Paradoxic thrombotic states may develop owing to actions of antiphospholipid antibodies on platelets, vascular endothelial cells, or erythrocytes. Patients with antiphospholipid antibodies are at increased risk for thrombotic events, and women with these antibodies are subject to recurrent spontaneous abortions. Specific anti-factor VIII antibodies have also been described. These antibodies are potent anticoagulants and may be associated with bleeding. Antiplatelet antibodies are found in 75–80% of patients with SLE. These antibodies inhibit neither clot retraction nor thromboplastin generation in normal blood. They probably induce thrombocytopenia by direct effects on platelet surface membrane.

6. False-positive serologic test for syphilis–A false-positive VDRL test is seen in 10–20% of patients with SLE. The serologic test for syphilis can be considered an autoimmune reaction, because the antigen is a phospholipid present in many human organs (see above).

7. Rheumatoid factors–Almost 30% of patients with SLE have a positive latex fixation test for rheumatoid factors.

8. Anticytoplasmic antibodies–Numerous anticytoplasmic antibodies (antimitochondrial, anti-ribosomal, antilysosomal) have been found in patients with SLE. These antibodies are not organ- or species-specific. Antiribosomal antibodies are found in the sera of 25–50% of patients. The major antigenic determinant is ribosomal RNA. Antimitochondrial antibodies are more common in other diseases (eg, primary biliary cirrhosis) than in SLE.

C. Tissue Immunofluorescence

1. Kidneys–Irregular or granular accumulation of immunoglobulin and complement occurs along the glomerular basement membrane and in the mesangium in patients with lupus nephritis. On electron microscopy, these deposits are seen in subepithelial, subendothelial, and mesangial sites.

2. Skin–Almost 90% of patients with SLE have immunoglobulin and complement deposition in the dermal-epidermal junction of skin that is *not* involved with an active lupus rash. The immunoglobulins are IgG or IgM and appear as a brightly staining homogeneous or granular band. Patients with discoid lupus erythematosus show deposition of immunoglobulin and complement only in involved skin.

Differential Diagnosis

The diagnosis of SLE in patients with classic multisystem involvement and a positive ANA test is not difficult. However, the onset of the disease can be vague and insidious and can therefore present a perplexing diagnostic problem. The polyarthritis of SLE is often similar to that seen in viral infections, infective endocarditis, mixed connective tissue disease, rheumatoid arthritis, and rheumatic fever. When Raynaud's phenomenon is the predominant complaint, progressive systemic sclerosis should be considered. SLE can present with a myositis similar to that of polymyositis-dermatomyositis. The clinical constellation of arthritis, alopecia, and a positive VDRL suggests secondary syphilis. Felty's syndrome (thrombocytopenia, leukopenia, splenomegaly in patients with rheumatoid arthritis) can simulate SLE. Takayasu's disease should be considered in a young woman who presents with arthralgias, fever, and asymmetric pulses. The diagnosis of SLE can be facilitated by finding anti-ds-DNA or anti-Sm antibodies.

Some patients with discoid lupus erythematosus may develop leukopenia, thrombocytopenia, hypergammaglobulinemia, a positive ANA, and an elevated sedimentation rate. Ten percent of patients with discoid lupus erythematosus have mild systemic symptoms. The frequent presence of anti-ds-RNA in discoid lupus erythematosus suggests that SLE and discoid lupus erythematosus are part of a single disease spectrum.

Treatment

The efficacy of the drugs used in the treatment of SLE is difficult to evaluate, since spontaneous remissions do occur. There are few controlled studies, because it is difficult to withhold therapy in the face of the life-threatening disease that can develop in fulminant SLE. Depending on the severity of the disease, no treatment, minimal treatment (aspirin, antimalarials), or intensive treatment (corticosteroids, cytotoxic drugs) may be required.

When arthritis is the predominant symptom and other organ systems are not significantly involved, high-dose aspirin or another fast-acting nonsteroidal anti-inflammatory drug may suffice to relieve symptoms. When the skin or mucosa is predominantly involved, antimalarials (hydroxychloroquine or chloroquine) and topical corticosteroids are very beneficial. Because high-dosage antimalarial therapy may be associated with irreversible retinal toxicity, these drugs should be used judiciously and in low doses.

Systemic corticosteroids in severe SLE can suppress disease activity and prolong life. The mode of action is unknown, but the immunosuppressive and anti-inflammatory properties of these agents presumably play a significant role in their therapeutic efficacy. High-dosage corticosteroid treatment (eg, prednisone, 1 mg/kg/d orally) decreases immunoglobulin levels and autoantibody titers and suppresses immune responses. High-dosage corticosteroid therapy is recommended in acute fulminant lupus, acute lupus nephritis, acute central nervous system lupus, acute autoimmune hemolytic anemia, and thrombocytopenic purpura. One or more courses of "pulse" therapy (ie, 15 mg/kg/d intravenously for 3 days) may be effective in patients with recalcitrant disease. The course of corticosteroid therapy should be monitored by the clinical response and meticulous follow-up of laboratory and immunologic parameters—complete blood count with reticulocyte and platelet counts, urinalysis, anti-ds-DNA titer, and complement levels.

If the clinical and immunologic status of the patient fails to improve or if serious side effects of corticosteroid therapy develop, immunosuppressive therapy with cytotoxic agents such as cyclophosphamide, chlorambucil, or azathioprine is indicated. Intravenous "pulse" therapy with cyclophosphamide is a practical and effective means of treating lupus nephritis. Because of serious complications (cancer, marrow suppression, infection, and liver and gastrointestinal toxicity), immunosuppressive agents should be used with discretion.

Complications & Prognosis

SLE may run a very mild course confined to one or a few organs, or it may be a fulminant fatal disease. Renal failure and central nervous system lupus were the leading causes of death until the corticosteroids and cytotoxic agents came into widespread use. Since then, the complications of therapy, including atherosclerosis, infection, and cancer, have become common causes of death. The 5-year survival rate of patients with SLE has markedly improved over the past decade and now approaches 80–90%.

RHEUMATOID ARTHRITIS

Major Immunologic Features
■ Monomeric and pentameric IgM, IgA, and IgG rheumatoid factors exist in serum and synovial fluid.
■ Vasculitis and synovitis are present.

General Considerations
Rheumatoid arthritis is a chronic, recurrent, systemic inflammatory disease primarily involving the joints. It affects 1–3% of people in the USA, with a female to male ratio of 3:1. Constitutional symptoms include malaise, fever, and weight loss. The disease characteristically begins in the small joints of the hands and feet and progresses in a centripetal and symmetric fashion. Elderly patients may present with more proximal large-joint involvement. Deformities are common. Extra-articular manifestations are characteristic of the rheumatoid process and often cause significant morbidity. Extra-articular manifestations include vasculitis, atrophy of the skin and muscle, subcutaneous nodules, lymphadenopathy, splenomegaly, and leukopenia.

Immunologic Pathogenesis
The cause of the unusual immune responses and subsequent inflammation in rheumatoid arthritis is unknown. Approximately 70% of patients with rheumatoid arthritis carry the HLA-DR4 haplotype. This haplotype has 11 different variants. Certain HLA-DR alleles determine susceptibility and also the severity of the disease. It is possible that these and perhaps other genetic determinants impart susceptibility to an unidentified environmental factor, such as a virus, that initiates the disease process. Although no virus particles have ever been identified, theoretically an antigenic stimulus leads to the appearance of an abnormal IgG that results in the production of rheumatoid factor and the eventual development of rheumatoid disease (Fig 31–2).

Whatever the primary stimulus, synovial lymphocytes produce IgG that is recognized as foreign and stimulates an immune response within the joint, with production of IgG, monomeric IgM, and pentameric IgM anti-immunoglobulins, ie, rheumatoid factors. The presence of IgG aggregates or IgG-rheumatoid factor complexes results in activation of the complement system via the classic pathway. Breakdown products of complement accumulate within the joint and amplify the activation of complement by stimulation of the alternative (properdin) system. Activation of the complement system results in a number of inflammatory phenomena, including histamine release, the production of factors chemotactic for PMN and

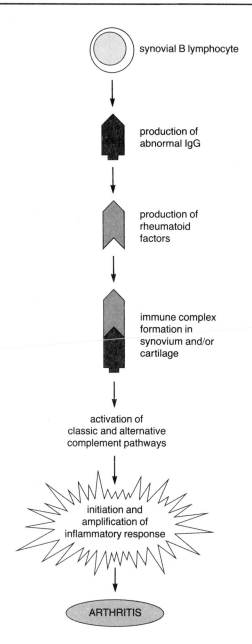

synovial B lymphocyte

production of
abnormal IgG

production of
rheumatoid
factors

immune complex
formation in
synovium and/or
cartilage

activation of
classic and alternative
complement pathways

initiation and
amplification of
inflammatory response

ARTHRITIS

Figure 31–2. Hypothetical immunopathogenesis in rheumatoid arthritis.

includes perivascular collections of helper T cells and interstitial collections of suppressor T cells, B lymphocytes, lymphoblasts, plasma cells, and macrophages. The immunologic interaction of these cells leads to the liberation of cytokines responsible for the accumulation of macrophages within the inflammatory synovium and to continued immunoglobulin and rheumatoid factor synthesis. Immune complexes in articular cartilage attract inflammatory cells, which damage cartilage by releasing proteases and collagenase.

Rheumatoid factor may play a role in the causation of extra-articular disease. Patients with rheumatoid vasculitis have high titers of monomeric and pentameric IgM, IgA, and IgG rheumatoid factors. Antigen-antibody complexes infused into experimental animals in the presence of IgM rheumatoid factor induce necrotizing vasculitis. Theoretically, immune complexes initiate vascular inflammation by the activation of complement. Pulmonary involvement is associated with the deposition of 11S and 15S protein complexes containing aggregates of IgG in the walls of pulmonary vessels and alveoli. 19S IgM rheumatoid factor has also been detected in arterioles and alveolar walls adjacent to cavitary nodules. Rheumatoid factors do not initiate the inflammatory process that causes rheumatoid disease, but they probably perpetuate and amplify that process.

Clinical Features

A. Symptoms and Signs:

1. Onset–The usual age at onset is 20–40 years. In most cases the disease presents with joint manifestations; however, some patients first develop extra-articular manifestations, including fatigue, weakness, weight loss, mild fever, and anorexia.

2. Articular manifestations–Patients experience stiffness and joint pain, which are generally worse in the morning and improve throughout the day. These symptoms are accompanied by signs of articular inflammation, including swelling, warmth, erythema, and tenderness on palpation. The arthritis is symmetric, involving the small joints of the hands and feet, ie, the proximal interphalangeals, metacarpophalangeals, wrists, and subtalars. Large joints (knees, hips, elbows, ankles, shoulders) commonly become involved later in the course of the disease, although in some patients large-joint involvement predominates. The cervical spine may be involved; the thoracic and lumbosacral spine is usually spared.

Periarticular inflammation is common, with tendonitis and tenosynovitis resulting in weakening of tendons, ligaments, and supporting structures. Joint pain leads to muscle spasm, limitation of motion, and, in advanced cases, muscle contractions and ankylosis with permanent joint deformity. The most characteristic deformities in the hand are ulnar deviation of the fingers, the "boutonnière" deformity (flexion of the proximal interphalangeal joints and

mononuclear cells, and membrane damage with cell lysis (see Chapter 10). There is a marked influx of leukocytes into the synovial space. Prostaglandins and leukotrienes produced by inflammatory cells are thought to play a major role in mediation of the inflammatory process. In addition, activated lysosomes and enzymes released into the synovial space by leukocytes further amplify the inflammatory and proliferative response of the synovium. The mononuclear infiltrate characteristically seen within the synovium hyperextension of the distal interphalangeal joints resulting from volar slippage of the lateral bands of the superficial extensor tendons), and the "swan neck" deformity (hyperextension of the proximal interphalangeal joints and flexion of the distal interphalangeal joints resulting from contractures of intrinsic hand muscles).

3. Extra-articular manifestations—From 20 to 25% of patients (particularly those with severe disease) have subcutaneous or subperiosteal nodules, so-called rheumatoid nodules. Rheumatoid nodules consist of an irregularly shaped central zone of fibrinoid necrosis surrounded by a margin of large mononuclear cells with an outer zone of granulation tissue containing plasma cells and lymphocytes. They are thought to be a late stage in the evolution of a vasculitic process, probably induced by the deposition of circulating immune complexes. These are usually present over bony eminences, with the most common sites of nodule formation being the olecranon bursa and the extensor surface of the forearm. Nodules are firm, nontender, round or oval masses that can be movable or fixed. They may be found in the myocardium, pericardium, heart valves, pleura, lungs, sclera, dura mater, spleen, larynx, and synovial tissues.

Lung involvement includes pleurisy, interstitial lymphocytic pneumonitis or fibrosis, and Caplan's syndrome (development of large nodules in the lung parenchyma of patients with rheumatoid arthritis who also have pneumoconiosis). The manifestations of rheumatoid cardiac disease include pericarditis, myocarditis, valvular insufficiency, and conduction disturbances.

Several types of vasculitis occur in rheumatoid arthritis. The most common type is a small-vessel obliterative vasculitis that leads to peripheral neuropathy. Less common is a subacute vasculitis associated with ischemic ulceration of the skin. The rarest form of rheumatoid vasculitis is a necrotizing vasculitis of medium and large vessels indistinguishable from polyarteritis nodosa. The major neurologic abnormalities in rheumatoid arthritis involve peripheral nerves. In addition to the peripheral neuropathy associated with vasculitis, there are a number of entrapment syndromes due to impingement by periarticular inflammatory tissue or amyloid on nerves passing through tight fascial planes. The carpal tunnel syndrome is a well-known complication of wrist disease; however, entrapment can also occur at the elbow, knee, and ankle. Destruction of the transverse ligament of the odontoid can result in atlantoaxial subluxation with cord or nerve root impingement.

Sjögren's syndrome (keratoconjunctivitis sicca and xerostomia) occurs in up to 30% of patients. Myositis with lymphocytic infiltration of involved muscle is rare. Ocular involvement ranges from benign inflammation of the surface of the sclera (episcleritis) to severe inflammation of the sclera, with nodule formation. Scleronodular disease can lead to weakening and thinning of the sclera (scleromalacia). A catastrophic but rare complication of scleromalacia is perforation of the eye with extrusion of vitreous (scleromalacia perforans).

4. Felty's syndrome—Felty's syndrome is the association of rheumatoid arthritis, splenomegaly, and neutropenia. Possible mechanisms of the hematologic abnormalities seen in these patients include anti-stem cell antibodies, antigranulocyte antibodies, and splenic sequestration of immune complex-coated polymorphonuclear leukocytes. The syndrome almost always develops in patients with high rheumatoid factor titers and rheumatoid nodules, although the arthritis itself is frequently inactive. Other features of hypersplenism and lymphadenopathy may also be present. These patients are at increased risk of developing bacterial infections.

B. Laboratory Findings: A normochromic, normocytic anemia and thrombocytosis are common among patients with active disease. The sedimentation rate is elevated, and the degree of elevation correlates roughly with disease activity.

The synovial fluid is more inflammatory than that seen in degenerative osteoarthritis or SLE. The leukocyte count is usually 5000–20,000/μL (rarely higher than 50,000/μL). Two-thirds of the cells are PMN that discharge lysosomal enzymes into the synovial fluid, presumably leading to depolymerization of synovial hyaluronate, decreased viscosity, and a poor mucin clot. The glucose level may be low or normal.

The rheumatoid pleural effusion is an exudate containing less than 5000 mononuclear or polymorphonuclear leukocytes per microliter. Protein exceeds 3g/dL, and glucose is often reduced below 20 mg/dL. Rheumatoid factors can be detected, and complement levels are usually low.

C. X-Ray Findings: The first detectable x-ray abnormalities are soft tissue swelling and juxtaarticular demineralization. The destruction of articular cartilage leads to joint space narrowing. Bony erosions develop at the junction of the synovial membrane and the bone just adjacent to articular cartilage. Destruction of the cartilage and laxity of ligaments lead to maladjustment and subluxation of articular surfaces. Spondylitis is usually limited to the cervical spine and may lead to osteoporosis, joint space narrowing, erosions, and, finally, subluxation of the involved articulations.

Immunologic Diagnosis

The most important serologic finding is the elevated rheumatoid factor titer, present in over 75% of patients. Rheumatoid factors are immunoglobulins with specificity for the Fc fragment of IgG. Most laboratory techniques detect pentameric IgM rheumatoid factor, but rheumatoid factor properties are also seen in monomeric IgM, IgG, and IgA. Pentameric

IgM rheumatoid factor may combine with IgG molecules to form a soluble circulating high-molecular-weight immunoglobulin complex in the serum.

In rheumatoid arthritis, serum protein electrophoresis may show increased α_2-globulin, polyclonal hypergammaglobulinemia, and hypoalbuminemia. Cryoprecipitates composed of immunoglobulins are often seen in rheumatoid vasculitis. Serum complement levels are usually normal but may be low in the presence of active vasculitis. Many patients have antinuclear antibodies.

Several tests are available in the laboratory to detect rheumatoid factor. The latex fixation test is a commonly used method for detection of rheumatoid factor. Aggregated γ-globulin (Cohn fraction II) is adsorbed onto latex particles, which then agglutinate in the presence of rheumatoid factor. The latex fixation test is not specific but is very sensitive, resulting in a high incidence of false-positive results. The sensitized sheep erythrocyte test (Rose-Waaler test) depends on specific antibody binding and is more specific than the latex fixation assay. Sheep erythrocytes are coated with rabbit antibody against sheep erythrocytes. The sensitized sheep erythrocytes then agglutinate in the presence of rheumatoid factor. Newer techniques, capable of detecting rheumatoid factor of all classes, include RIA, indirect immunofluorescence, ELISA, and laser nephelometry.

It is important to emphasize that a negative rheumatoid factor by routine laboratory procedures does not exclude the diagnosis of rheumatoid arthritis. The so-called seronegative patient may have IgG, IgA or monomeric IgM rheumatoid factors. Conversely, rheumatoid factors are not unique to rheumatoid arthritis. Rheumatoid factor is also present in patients with SLE (30%), in a high percentage (90%) of patients with Sjögren's syndrome, and less often in patients with scleroderma or polymyositis. Positive agglutination reactions with the latex test also occur in patients with a number of chronic inflammatory conditions including chronic active hepatitis, kala-azar, sarcoidosis, neoplasia, and syphilis. The sensitized sheep erythrocyte test is usually negative in these conditions. In some chronic infectious diseases such as leprosy and tuberculosis, both the latex and the sensitized sheep erythrocyte tests may be positive. In subacute bacterial endocarditis, both tests may be positive during active disease and revert to negative as patients improve. The transient appearance of rheumatoid factor has been noted following vaccinations in military recruits. Epidemiologic studies have shown that a small number of normal people also have rheumatoid factors. A large proportion of the elderly have a positive latex test, though the sensitized sheep erythrocyte test is generally negative.

Differential Diagnosis

In the patient with classic articular changes, bony erosions of the small joints of the hands and feet, and a positive rheumatoid factor, the diagnosis of rheumatoid arthritis is not difficult. Early in the disease, or when extra-articular manifestations dominate the clinical picture, other rheumatic diseases (including SLE, Reiter's syndrome, gout, psoriatic arthritis, degenerative osteoarthritis, and the peripheral arthritis of chronic inflammatory bowel disease) or infectious processes may mimic rheumatoid arthritis. Patients with SLE can be distinguished by their characteristic skin lesions, renal disease, and diagnostic serologic abnormalities. Reiter's syndrome occurs predominantly in young men, generally affects joints of the lower extremity in an asymmetric fashion, and is often associated with urethritis and conjunctivitis. Gouty arthritis is usually an acute monoarthritis with negatively birefringent sodium urate crystals present within the white cells of inflammatory synovial fluid. Psoriatic arthritis is usually asymmetric and often involves distal interphalangeal joints. Degenerative arthritis is characterized by Heberden's nodes, lack of symmetric joint involvement, and involvement of the distal interphalangeal joints. The peripheral arthritis of bowel disease usually occurs in large weight-bearing joints and is often associated with bowel symptoms. The polyarthritis associated with rubella vaccination, parvovirus infection, HB-sAg antigenemia, sarcoidosis, and infectious mononucleosis can mimic early rheumatoid arthritis.

Treatment

A. Physical Therapy: A rational program of physical therapy is vital in the management of patients with rheumatoid arthritis. Such a program should consist of an appropriate balance of rest and exercise and the judicious use of heat or cold therapy. The patient may require complete or intermittent bed rest on a regular basis to combat inflammation or fatigue. In addition, specific joints may have to be put at rest through the use of braces, splints, or crutches. An exercise program emphasizing active range-of-motion movements helps to maintain strength and mobility. Heat or cold is valuable in alleviating muscle spasm, stiffness, and pain. Many patients need a hot shower or bath to loosen up in the morning, and others cannot perform their exercises adequately without prior heat treatment. Heating pads or paraffin baths are often used to apply heat to specific joints. In some patients ice massage is more effective than heat. Physical and occupational therapists provide valuable help in devising an appropriate physical therapy program.

B. Drug Treatment:

1. Salicylates–Aspirin is the mainstay of medical therapy of rheumatoid arthritis. Although its exact mechanism of action is uncertain, it effectively inhibits the production of prostaglandins, thereby reducing inflammation. The doses used to attain therapeutic levels (ie, 20–30 mg/dL) range from 3.6 to 6.5 g per day in divided doses. High-dosage aspirin therapy is associated with numerous side effects. Tinnitus—with or without hearing loss—is reversible with a decrease in dosage. Gastric distress is common but can be partly alleviated by using antacids, histamine H_2 receptor blockers, sucralfate, or misoprostol (prostaglandin E_1) and by encouraging patients to take their aspirin with meals. Although any of these modalities may alleviate gastrointestinal symptoms in the individual patient, only misoprostol has been shown to decrease gastritis and gastric ulcer formation in patients on anti-inflammatory levels of aspirin or other nonsteroidal anti-inflammatory drugs. Some patients can avoid gastric irritation by using enteric-coated aspirin. Microscopic blood loss from the gastrointestinal tract is common and is not an indication for stopping aspirin therapy. Since aspirin does decrease platelet adhesiveness, its use should be avoided in patients about to have surgery, those with a bleeding diathesis, or those receiving coumarin anticoagulants.

2. Other nonsteroidal drugs—Several other nonsteroidal anti-inflammatory agents such as fenoprofen, ibuprofen, naproxen, sulindac, tolmetin, mefenamic acid, ketoprofen, diclofenac, carprofen, indomethacin, piroxicam, etodolac, and nabumatone are useful in patients with rheumatoid arthritis. Combining 2 or more nonsteroidal anti-inflammatory agents provides little or no additional benefit over maximum doses of single agents and may increase gastrointestinal toxicity.

3. Antimalarial Drugs—Many rheumatologists advocate the use of antimalarial drugs for prolonged periods in patients with severe disease. Their mechanism of action is unclear, but they appear to affect monocyte function. The antimalarial drugs act slowly, often requiring 1–6 months of treatment for maximum therapeutic benefit. The preparation most often used is hydroxychloroquine, 200–600 mg/d. Toxic side effects include skin rashes, nausea and vomiting, myopathy, and both corneal and retinal damage. Eye toxicity is rare at the low doses used in rheumatoid arthritis, but patients should have ophthalmologic examinations every 4–6 months while on antimalarial therapy.

4. Gold salt therapy—Although associated with a high incidence of toxic side effects, parenteral gold salt therapy is of significant benefit to some patients. Gold shots have to be administered every week for up to 20 weeks and then monthly for as long as the patient has active disease. Toxic side effects occur in 40% of patients and include dermatitis, photosensitivity, stomatitis, thrombocytopenia, agranulocytosis, hepatitis, aplastic anemia, peripheral neuropathy, nephritis with nephrotic syndrome, ulcerative enterocolitis, pneumonitis, and keratitis.

An oral gold salt preparation, auranofin, is available. Side effects, although similar to those of parenteral gold salt preparations, may occur less frequently. Diarrhea, however, is more common. The usual dose is 3 mg twice daily. As with parenteral gold preparations, it may take 3–6 months to achieve therapeutic benefit.

5. Penicillamine—Penicillamine has been used in the treatment of rheumatoid arthritis. Like gold, penicillamine is a slow-acting nonsteroidal anti-inflammatory agent, and it may take up to 6 months for a therapeutic response to become apparent. The incidence of drug toxicity is similar to that of parenteral gold. Toxic side effects include rash, loss of sense of taste, nausea and vomiting, anorexia, proteinuria, agranulocytosis, aplastic anemia, and thrombocytopenia. Less commonly, myasthenia, myositis, Goodpasture's syndrome, pemphigus, bronchiolitis, and a lupuslike syndrome may be seen.

6. Corticosteroids—Intermittent intra-articular injection of corticosteroids is useful for the patient with only a few symptomatic joints. Relief may last for months. However, multiple intra-articular corticosteroid injections in weight-bearing joints should be avoided, since they may lead to degenerative arthritis. Low-dose systemic corticosteroids may be indicated in patients who do not respond to NSAIDs or other remittive therapy. The usual dose is 5–10 mg of prednisone daily. Withdrawal from corticosteroids should be gradual, since clinical exacerbation of arthritis or steroid withdrawal syndrome may occur. Long-term systemic corticosteroid treatment results in hyperadrenocorticism and disruption of the pituitary-adrenal axis. Manifestations of corticosteroid toxicity include weight gain, moon facies, ecchymoses, hirsutism, diabetes mellitus, hypertension, osteoporosis, avascular necrosis of bone, cataracts, myopathy, mental disturbances, activation of tuberculosis, and infections.

7. Immunosuppressive agents—The antimetabolite methotrexate can produce dramatic improvement in patients with severe disease. Methotrexate has largely replaced gold and penicillamine in the treatment of rheumatoid arthritis. Side effects include marrow suppression, liver toxicity, oral ulcers, and teratogenesis. Alkylating agents (eg, chlorambucil, cyclophosphamide) and purine analogs (eg, mercaptopurine, azathioprine) have also been used in the treatment of rheumatoid arthritis. However, these drugs are associated with major toxic side effects including an increased incidence of neoplasm and infection. They should, therefore, be used with great caution.

C. Orthopedic Surgery: Surgery is often an essential part of the general management of the patient with rheumatoid arthritis to correct or compensate for joint damage. Arthroplasty is employed to maintain or improve joint motion. Arthrodesis can be used to correct deformity and alleviate pain, but it results in loss of motion. Early synovectomy might prevent joint damage or tendon rupture and will decrease pain and inflammation in a given joint, but the synovium often grows back and symptoms return.

Complications & Prognosis

Several clinical patterns of rheumatoid arthritis are apparent. Spontaneous remission may occur, usually within 2 years after the onset òf the disease. Some patients have brief episodes of acute arthritis with longer periods of low-grade activity or remission. Rare patients will have sustained progression of active disease resulting in deformity and death. The development of classic disease within 1 year of the onset of symptoms, an age of less than 30 years at onset of disease, and the presence of rheumatoid nodules and high titers of rheumatoid factor are unfavorable prognostic factors.

Follow-up of patients after 10–15 years shows that 50% are stationary or improved, 70% are capable of full-time employment, and 10% are completely incapacitated. Death from vasculitis or atlantoaxial subluxation is rare. Fatalities are more often associated with sepsis or the complications of therapy.

JUVENILE ARTHRITIS

Major Immunologic Features

■ Overt or "hidden" rheumatoid factors exist.
■ Antinuclear antibodies may occur.

General Considerations

Juvenile arthritis consists of a group of disorders that occur in individuals under 16 years of age. The incidence of the disease peaks in boys at age 2 and again at age 9, whereas in girls it peaks between 1 and 3 years of age. Juvenile arthritis may present as a systemic illness (Still's disease), as a seronegative pauci- or polyarthritis, or as a seropositive polyarthritis identical to adult rheumatoid arthritis. The outlook for girls with pauciarticular disease is excellent, whereas boys with pauciarticular disease may eventually develop ankylosing spondylitis. Although upper respiratory infections and trauma have both been implicated as precipitating factors, the roles of infection, trauma, and heredity in the pathogenesis of the disease are unclear.

Immunologic Pathogenesis

The basic immunopathogenic mechanisms in juvenile arthritis are unknown. However, both humoral and cellular defects occur in these patients. Diffuse hypergammaglobulinemia, involving IgG, IgA, and IgM, is present. Rheumatoid factors of all immunoglobulin classes have been detected. Approximately 10% of children with juvenile arthritis have a positive latex fixation test for IgM rheumatoid factor. The sera from some patients with negative latex fixation tests may actually contain IgM rheumatoid factors. Two major theories have been offered in an attempt to explain the presence of these "hidden" rheumatoid factors in juvenile arthritis. First, IgM rheumatoid factor may bind avidly to native IgG in the patient's serum and therefore may not be able to bind IgG coating the latex particles. Second, an abnormal IgG may be present that preferentially binds IgM, thereby blocking latex fixation. Cold-reacting (4 °C) pentameric IgM rheumatoid factors (cryoglobulins) are associated with severe disease.

Serum components of both the classic and alternative (properdin) complement systems are elevated, although this elevation is less in patients who have rheumatoid factors or severe disease. Elevation of serum complement may reflect a secondary overcompensation in response to increased consumption, or possibly a general increase in protein synthesis. Studies of the metabolism of complement actually demonstrate hypercatabolism. The depression of complement in synovial fluid is probably secondary to complement activation by immune complexes, similar to that seen in rheumatoid arthritis.

Preliminary studies suggest that patients with juvenile arthritis possess certain HLA tissue types with greater than expected frequencies. Thus, patients with early-onset pauciarticular disease tend to be HLA-DR5- or HLA-DR8-positive, while those with late-onset pauciarticular disease tend to be HLA-B27-positive. Patients with rheumatoid factor-positive polyarticular disease tend to be HLA-D4-positive, and those with systemic disease tend to be HLA-DR5-positive.

Clinical Features

A. Symptoms and Signs:

1. Onset–

a. Twenty percent of children, usually under age 4, present with high, spiking fever, an evanescent rash, polyserositis, hepatosplenomegaly, and lymphadenopathy (Still's disease).

b. Forty percent of patients present with polyarthritis (more than 4 joints involved during the first 6 months of illness), sometimes accompanied by low-grade fever and malaise. In 25% of this group, the onset is in late childhood and is associated with rheumatoid factor.

c. Forty percent of patients present with pauciarticular (involvement of 4 or fewer joints) disease and few systemic manifestations. Slightly more than 50% of these patients are young girls with antinuclear antibodies, who are particularly likely to develop iridocyclitis.

2. Joint manifestations–Even in the presence of severe arthritis, young children may not complain of pain but may instead limit the use of an extremity. The knees, wrists, ankles, and neck are common sites of initial involvement. Early involvement of the hip is extremely rare in young children with pauciarticular disease. Older children occasionally develop symmetric involvement in the small joints of the hands (metacarpophalangeal, proximal interphalangeal, and distal interphalangeal) similar to that seen in adults. In seronegative patients, the metacarpophalangeal

joints may be spared. With severe hand involvement, children are more likely to develop radial rather than ulnar deviation. Involvement of the feet may lead to hallux valgus or to hammer toe deformity. Achillobursitis and achillotendinitis may cause tender, swollen heels. Older boys with pauciarticular disease commonly develop ankylosing spondylitis.

3. Systemic manifestations–Fever, often with a high evening spike, is characteristic of Still's disease. Anorexia, weight loss, and malaise are common. Most children with Still's disease develop an evanescent, salmon-colored maculopapular rash that coincides with periods of high fever. Occasional patients manifest cardiac involvement. Pericarditis occurs commonly but rarely leads to dysfunction or constriction. Myocarditis is an unusual manifestation of the cardiac disease, but, when present, can lead to heart failure.

Cases of acute pneumonitis or pleuritis have been described, but chronic rheumatoid lung disease is rarely seen in patients with juvenile arthritis.

Iridocyclitis occurs most commonly in young girls with pauciarticular disease and can precede articular involvement. It typically runs an insidious course and often persists even when joint disease becomes quiescent. Iridocyclitis is best monitored by frequent slit lamp examinations, at least through puberty.

Lymphadenopathy and hepatosplenomegaly are associated with severe systemic disease and are uncommon in patients with chiefly articular manifestations.

Subcutaneous nodules occur in children with polyarticular disease, usually in association with a positive test for rheumatoid factor.

Rarely, Still's disease occurs in adults. Characteristic manifestations include high spiking fevers, evanescent rash, arthritis, and elevated leukocyte count and hepatic enzyme levels.

4. Complications–The major complication of juvenile arthritis is impairment of growth and development secondary to early epiphyseal closure. This is particularly common in the mandible, causing micrognathia, and in the metacarpals and metatarsals, leading to abnormally small fingers and toes. The extent of growth impairment usually correlates positively with the severity and duration of disease but may also reflect the growth-inhibiting effects of steroids. Children in whom arthritis begins before age 5 occasionally undergo increased growth of an affected extremity. Vasculitis and encephalitis are occasionally observed in patients with juvenile arthritis. Secondary amyloidosis occurs rarely.

B. Laboratory Findings: Mild leukocytosis (15,000–20,000/μL) is the rule, but some patients develop leukopenia. A normochromic microcytic anemia, an elevated erythrocyte sedimentation rate, and an abnormal C-reactive protein occur commonly. Because an elevated ASO titer is so frequently encountered, this test cannot be used to differentiate juvenile arthritis from rheumatic fever. Positive tests for rheumatoid factor occur in older children with polyarticular disease, while antinuclear antibodies are found both in patients with polyarticular disease and in young patients with pauciarticular disease. A positive ANA almost never occurs in Still's disease. Serum protein electrophoresis shows an increase in acute-phase reactants (α-globulins) and a polyclonal increase of γ-globulin. The synovial fluid in active juvenile rheumatoid arthritis is exudative, with a leukocyte count of 5000–20,000/μL (mostly neutrophils), a poor mucin clot, and decreased glucose compared to serum glucose. Mononuclear cells may predominate in the synovial fluid of patients with pauciarticular disease.

C. X-Ray Findings: Radiographic changes early in the disease include juxta-articular demineralization, periosteal bone accretion, premature closure of the epiphyses, cervical zygapophyseal fusion (particularly at C2–3), osseous overgrowth of the interphalangeal joints, and erosion and narrowing of the joint space. Carpal arthritis with ankylosis is seen as a late manifestation of Still's disease.

Immunologic Diagnosis

Currently, the diagnosis of juvenile arthritis is based on clinical criteria. Although certain abnormalities of immunoglobulins, complement, and cellular immunity are compatible with the diagnosis of juvenile arthritis, no specific immunologic test is diagnostic.

Differential Diagnosis

The diagnosis of juvenile arthritis is extremely difficult, since the disease can present with nonspecific constitutional signs and symptoms in the absence of arthritis. Other causes of fever, particularly infections and cancer, must be considered. Leukemia can present in childhood with fever, lymphadenopathy, and joint pains. Rheumatic fever closely resembles juvenile arthritis, particularly early in the disease, but the patient with juvenile arthritis tends to have higher spiking fevers, lymphadenopathy and hepatosplenomegaly in the absence of carditis, and a more refractory, long-lasting arthritis. Rheumatic fever patients are more likely to have evidence of recent streptococcal infection, including elevated titers of antihyaluronidase, antistreptokinase, and antistreptodornase antibodies. In addition, patients with rheumatic fever tend to have a less intense leukocytosis and respond more dramatically to low doses of aspirin. An expanding skin lesion followed in weeks or months by arthritis suggests the diagnosis of Lyme disease, an inflammatory arthropathy caused by the spirochete *Borrelia burgdorferi*. Rheumatic diseases that may begin in childhood, such as SLE or dermatomyositis, can be differentiated by their different clinical course, different organ system involvement, and characteristic serologic abnormalities.

When juvenile arthritis presents primarily with arthritis, examination of synovial fluid is of paramount importance in excluding infection.

Treatment

The major goals of therapy are to relieve pain, prevent contractures and deformities, and promote normal physical and emotional development. These goals are best achieved by a comprehensive program of physical, medical, and, when necessary, surgical therapy.

A. Physical Therapy: Exercise promotes muscle strength, encourages growth, and prevents deformity. The goal in children is to maintain mobility. The tricycle is always preferable to the wheelchair! As in the treatment of adult rheumatoid arthritis, rest can be an important part of physical therapy. Complete rest is indicated during severe exacerbations and may be necessary for short afternoon periods on a routine basis. Specific joints can be put at rest by the use of splints, collars, and braces that support the joint and help prevent deformity. Judicious use of heat will decrease pain and muscle spasm and is particularly useful before exercising.

B. Drug Treatment:

1. Aspirin–The disease responds to aspirin at a dosage level of 90–130 mg/kg/d given in 4–6 divided doses. Tinnitus and decreased hearing are poor indicators of aspirin toxicity in children. Irritability, drowsiness, or intermittent periods of hyperpnea are early signs of salicylate intoxication. Therefore, it is essential to monitor blood salicylate levels during aspirin therapy. Acidosis and ketosis may develop in infants. Respiratory alkalosis, due to primary stimulation of the respiratory center, occurs in older children.

2. Remittive agents–Children with refractory arthritis may benefit from injectable or oral gold, antimalarials, penicillamine, or methotrexate.

3. Corticosteroids–Intra-articular corticosteroid injections are useful in pauciarticular disease. Systemic corticosteroids are reserved for patients with myocarditis, vasculitis, refractory iridocyclitis, or Still's disease that is unresponsive to aspirin therapy. Patients with iridocyclitis may require prolonged corticosteroid therapy. In children, the major toxic effects of corticosteroid therapy include subcapsular cataract formation, vertebral osteoporosis and collapse, infection, premature skeletal maturation with diminished growth, and pseudotumor cerebri with intracranial hypertension.

C. Surgical Treatment: The aims of surgery in juvenile arthritis are to relieve pain and maintain or improve joint function. Synovectomy may diminish pain due to chronic synovitis, but long-term effectiveness is questionable. Synovectomy for severe extensor tenosynovitis of the hand may prevent tendon rupture. Tendon release procedures help relieve joint contractures. Hip replacement is of benefit in selected cases but should be delayed as long as possible, since in some children hip cartilage may regenerate with continued weight-bearing.

Complications & Prognosis

Seventy percent of patients experience a spontaneous and permanent remission by adulthood. Patients with Still's disease tend to have several recurrences per year. Patients presenting with oligoarthritic disease, particularly if they are female, tend to remain oligoarthritic, while those presenting with polyarthritis remain polyarthritic. Rarely, the disease persists into adulthood. This usually occurs in children with symmetric polyarthritis similar to that seen in adults. Sometimes a patient with juvenile arthritis in apparent remission develops rheumatoid arthritis as an adult. In an occasional unfortunate case, the disease is relentless and crippling. Small-joint involvement, positive serum rheumatoid factor, and onset in later childhood all portend a poor prognosis.

SJÖGREN'S SYNDROME

Major Immunologic Features

- Lymphocytes and plasma cells infiltrate involved tissues.
- There are rheumatoid factors and antinuclear antibodies.
- There are autoantibodies against salivary duct antigens.

General Considerations

Sjögren's syndrome is a chronic inflammatory disease of unknown cause characterized by diminished lacrimal and salivary gland secretion resulting in keratoconjunctivitis sicca and xerostomia. There is dryness of the eyes, mouth, nose, trachea, bronchi, vagina, and skin. In half of patients, the disease occurs as a primary pathologic entity (primary Sjögren's syndrome). In the other half, it occurs in association with rheumatoid arthritis or other connective tissue disorders. Ninety percent of patients with Sjögren's syndrome are female. Although the mean age at onset is 50 years, the disease does occur in children.

Immunologic Pathogenesis

It has been hypothesized that patients with Sjögren's syndrome have an abnormal immunologic response to one or more unidentified antigens, perhaps viral antigens or virus-altered autoantigens. This abnormal response is characterized by excessive B cell and plasma cell activity, manifested by polyclonal hypergammaglobulinemia and the production of rheumatoid factors, antinuclear antibodies, cryoglobulins, and anti-salivary duct antibodies. Immunofluorescence studies have shown both B and T helper lymphocytes and plasma cells infiltrating involved tissues. Large quantities of IgM and IgG are synthesized by these infiltrating lymphocytes. In patients with coexisting macroglobulinemia, monoclonal IgM may be synthesized in the salivary glands. Excessive B cell activity could be due either to a primary B cell defect or to defective T lymphocyte regulation, since there is evidence of decreased suppressor T cell function in patients with Sjögren's syndrome.

Pathology

Histologically, there is lymphocytic infiltrate in exocrine glands of the respiratory, gastrointestinal, and vaginal tracts as well as glands of the ocular and oral mucosa. Histologic demonstration of lymphocytic infiltration in a biopsy specimen taken from the minor labial salivary glands is the most specific and sensitive single diagnostic test for Sjögren's syndrome.

Clinical Features

A. Symptoms and Signs:

1. Oral–Dryness of the mouth is usually the most distressing symptom and is often associated with burning discomfort and difficulty in chewing and swallowing dry foods. Polyuria and nocturia develop as the patient drinks increasing amounts of water in an effort to relieve these symptoms. The oral mucous membranes are dry and erythematous, and the tongue becomes fissured and ulcerated. Severe dental caries is often present. Half of patients have intermittent parotid gland enlargement with rapid fluctuations in the size of the gland. The parotid gland in Sjögren's syndrome is firm, in contrast to the soft parotid enlargement characteristic of diabetes mellitus or alcohol abuse. Glossitis and angular cheilitis are manifestations of oral candidiasis in Sjögren's syndrome.

2. Ocular–The major ocular finding is keratoconjunctivitis sicca. Symptoms include burning, itching, decreased tearing, ocular accumulation of thick mucoid material during the night, photophobia, pain, and a "gritty" or "sandy" sensation in the eyes. Decreased tearing is demonstrated by an abnormal Schirmer test. Slit lamp examination reveals punctate rose bengal or fluorescein staining of the conjunctiva and cornea, strands of corneal debris, and a shortened tear film break-up time. Severe ocular involvement may lead to corneal ulceration, vascularization with opacification, or perforation.

3. Miscellaneous–Dryness of the nose, posterior oropharynx, larynx, and respiratory tract may lead to epistaxis, dysphonia, recurrent otitis media, tracheobronchitis, or pneumonia. The vaginal mucosa is also dry, and women with the disease commonly complain of dyspareunia. Active synovitis is a common finding, particularly in patients who also have rheumatoid arthritis. Twenty percent of patients with primary Sjögren's syndrome complain of Raynaud's phenomenon. Ten percent of patients have extraglandular lymphocytic infiltrates, particularly in the kidneys, lungs, lymph nodes, and muscles. A few such patients develop lymphoma.

B. Laboratory Findings: Anemia, leukopenia, and an elevated erythrocyte sedimentation rate are common features. Parotid salivary flow is less than the normal 5 mL/10 min/gland. Secretory sialography with radiopaque dye demonstrates glandular disorganization. Salivary scintigraphy with Tc99m pertechnetate reveals decreased parotid secretory function.

Immunologic Diagnosis

No immunologic test is diagnostic for Sjögren's syndrome. However, a myriad of nonspecific immunologic abnormalities occur in these patients.

A. Humoral Abnormalities: Hypergammaglobulinemia is seen in half of patients. Although serum protein electrophoresis usually shows a polyclonal hypergammaglobulinemia, occasional patients develop a monoclonal IgM paraproteinemia, usually of the kappa type. Patients who develop lymphoma sometimes become severely hypogammaglobulinemic and show disappearance of autoantibodies. Rheumatoid factors can be detected by the latex fixation test in 90% of patients with Sjögren's syndrome. ANA in a speckled or homogeneous pattern is present in 70% of patients. Many of these antinuclear antibodies are directed against acid-extractable nuclear antigens. Antibodies against one such antigen, termed SS-B, are relatively specific for patients with primary Sjögren's syndrome. Antibodies against a second acid-extractable nuclear antigen, SS-A, may be found in Sjögren's syndrome alone or in Sjögren's syndrome associated with SLE. Patients with Sjögren's syndrome and rheumatoid arthritis have neither anti-SS-A nor anti-SS-B antibodies. Autoantibodies against salivary duct antigens have been detected in 50% of patients with Sjögren's syndrome associated with rheumatoid arthritis.

B. Cellular Abnormalities: Thirty percent of patients with Sjögren's syndrome have decreased lymphocyte responses to mitogenic stimulation. A few patients also have decreased numbers of circulating T lymphocytes in the peripheral blood (see Immunologic Pathogenesis, above).

C. HLA Associations: HLA typing studies suggest a genetic predisposition to the development of Sjögren's syndrome. The prevalence of HLA-B8, -DR3, -DR2, and, most markedly, -DRw52 is significantly increased in patients with primary Sjögren's syndrome. HLA-DR3, -DQ1, and -DQ2, but not -DRw52, are associated with polyclonal hypergammaglobulinemia and high titers of anti-SSA antibodies.

Differential Diagnosis

The diagnosis of Sjögren's syndrome can be made on the basis of 2 of the 3 classic manifestations of xerostomia, keratoconjunctivitis sicca, and rheumatoid arthritis. However, the varied and multisystemic nature of the disease may obscure the diagnosis. Any patient with a rheumatic disease—eg, SLE, rheumatoid arthritis, or scleroderma—should be observed for Sjögren's syndrome; likewise, any patient with Sjögren's syndrome should be assessed for the possibility of other rheumatic diseases. Other causes of bilateral parotid swelling include nutritional deficiencies, endocrine disorders, sarcoidosis, drug reactions, infections (including HIV), amyloid, and obesity. Parotid gland cancer must always be considered in a patient with unilateral parotid swelling.

Treatment

A. Symptomatic Measures:

1. Oral–Patients must be urged to maintain fastidious oral hygiene, with regular use of fluoride toothpaste and mouthwashes and with regular dental examinations. Frequent sips of water and the use of sugarless gum or candy to stimulate salivary secretion are sometimes helpful in relieving xerostomia. Many patients find aerosolized preparations of artificial saliva helpful. A bedroom humidifier will help decrease nocturnal xerostomia and nasal dryness. The most effective treatment for oral candidiasis in Sjögren's syndrome is the oral use of nystatin lozenges.

2. Ocular–Artificial tears alleviate ocular symptoms and protect against ocular complications. Shielded glasses offer protection against the drying effects of wind. Therapy for refractory ocular complications includes mucolytic agents, punctal occlusion, soft contact lenses, and partial tarsorrhaphy.

3. Other–Dryness of the skin can be treated with moisturizing skin creams or oils. Vaginal and nasal dryness is often relieved with sterile, water-miscible lubricants.

B. Systemic Measures: Sjögren's syndrome can usually be controlled with symptomatic therapy. Nonsteroidal anti-inflammatory drugs are useful in the treatment of the nonerosive arthritis of Sjögren's syndrome. Corticosteroids or immunosuppressive agents may be useful in treating patients with severe or life-threatening disease, such as lymphoma, Waldenström's macroglobulinemia, or massive lymphocytic infiltration of vital organs.

Complications & Prognosis

In the vast majority of patients, significant lymphoproliferation is confined to salivary, lacrimal, and other mucosal glandular tissue, resulting in a benign chronic course of xerostomia and xerophthalmia. Rarely, patients develop significant extraglandular lymphoid infiltration or neoplasia.

Splenomegaly, leukopenia, and vasculitis with leg ulcers may occur. Hypergammaglobulinemic purpura, often associated with renal tubular acidosis, has been described and may be a presenting complaint.

Five percent of patients with Sjögren's syndrome develop chronic autoimmune thyroiditis. Other associations include primary biliary cirrhosis, chronic active hepatitis, gastric achlorhydria, pancreatitis, renal and pulmonary lymphocytic infiltration, cryoglobulinemia with glomerulonephritis, hyperviscosity syndrome, and adult celiac disease. Neuromuscular complications include polymyositis, peripheral or cranial (particularly trigeminal) neuropathy, and cerebral vasculitis. Rarely, patients with Sjögren's syndrome develop lymphoma, immunoblastic sarcoma, or Waldenström's macroglobulinemia. The lymphoma is often a monoclonal B cell neoplasm containing intracellular IgM-κ immunoglobulin.

PROGRESSIVE SYSTEMIC SCLEROSIS

Major Immunologic Features

- Antinuclear antibodies with a speckled or nucleolar pattern occur.
- Anticentromere antibodies occur in 75% of patients.
- Antibodies against an acid-extractable nuclear antigen occur.

General Considerations

Progressive systemic sclerosis is a disease of unknown cause characterized by abnormally increased collagen deposition in the skin. The course is usually slowly progressive and chronically disabling, but it can be rapidly progressive and fatal because of involvement of internal organs. It commonly begins in the third or fourth decade of life. Children are occasionally affected. The prevalence of the disease is 4–12.5 cases per million population. Women are affected twice as often as men. There is no racial predisposition.

Immunologic Pathogenesis

The association of progressive systemic sclerosis with Sjögren's syndrome and, less often, with thyroiditis or primary biliary cirrhosis—and the serologic abnormalities seen in the majority of cases (presence of ANA, rheumatoid factor, polyclonal hypergammaglobulinemia)—are suggestive of an immunologic aberration in these patients. At present, there is scanty evidence for a humoral mechanism in the pathogenesis of the disease, although a serum factor toxic to vascular endothelium has been identified. Humoral factors may stimulate increased collagen production by fibroblasts. Immunoglobulins have not been found at the dermal-epidermal junction in scleroderma, although examination of the fibrinoid lesions seen in the walls of renal arterioles has revealed the presence of immunoglobulins and complement. There is new evidence that T cell-directed autoimmune events perturb vascular endothelium, leading to fibroblast activation and fibrosis.

Pathology

Biopsy of clinically involved skin reveals thinning of the epidermis with loss of the rete pegs, atrophy of the dermal appendages, hyalinization and fibrosis of arterioles, and a striking increase of compact collagen fibers in the reticular dermis.

Synovial findings range from an acute lymphocytic infiltration to diffuse fibrosis with relatively little inflammation.

The histologic changes seen in muscles include interstitial and perivascular inflammatory infiltration followed by fibrosis and myofibrillar necrosis, atrophy, and degeneration.

In patients with renal involvement, the histologic appearance of the kidney is similar to that of malignant hypertensive nephropathy, with intimal proliferation of the interlobular arteries and fibrinoid changes in the intima and media of more distal interlobular arteries and of afferent arterioles.

There is increased collagen deposition in the lamina propria, submucosa, and muscularis of the gastrointestinal tract. Small-vessel changes similar to those that occur in the skin may also result. With loss of normal smooth muscle, the large bowel is subject to development of the characteristic wide-mouthed diverticula and to infiltration of air into the wall of the intestine (pneumatosis cystoides intestinalis).

Clinical Features

A. Symptoms and Signs:

1. Onset–Raynaud's phenomenon heralds the onset of the disease in at least 90% of patients. Progressive systemic sclerosis frequently begins with skin changes, but in one-third of patients polyarthralgias and polyarthritis are the first manifestations. Skin involvement may be limited to the hands, forearms, feet, or face or may be more diffuse with extensive truncal involvement. Initial visceral involvement without skin manifestations is very unusual.

2. Skin abnormalities–There are 3 stages in the clinical evolution of scleroderma. In the edematous phase, symmetric nonpitting edema is present in the hands and, rarely, in the feet. The edema can progress to the forearms, arms, upper anterior chest, abdomen, back, and face. In the sclerotic phase, the skin is tight, smooth, and waxy and seems bound down to underlying structures. Skin folds and wrinkles disappear. The hands are involved in most patients, with painful, slowly healing ulcerations of the fingertips in half of those cases. The face appears stretched and masklike, with thin lips and a "pinched" nose. Pigmentary changes and telangiectases are frequent at this stage. The skin changes may stabilize for prolonged periods and then either progress to the third (atrophic) stage or soften and return to normal. It should be emphasized that not all patients pass through all the stages. Subcutaneous calcifications, usually in the fingertips (calcinosis circumscripta), occur more often in women than in men. The calcifications vary in size from tiny deposits to large masses and may develop over bony prominences throughout the body.

3. Joints and muscles–Articular complaints are very common and may begin at any time during the course of the disease. The arthralgias, stiffness, and frank arthritis seen in progressive systemic sclerosis may be difficult to distinguish from those of rheumatoid arthritis, particularly in the early stages of the disease. Involved joints include the metacarpophalangeals, proximal interphalangeals, wrists, elbows, knees, ankles, and small joints of the feet. Flexion contractures caused by changes in the skin or joints are common. Muscle involvement is usually mild but may be clinically indistinguishable from that of polymyositis, with muscle weakness, tenderness, and pain of proximal muscles of the upper and lower extremities.

4. Lungs–The lungs are frequently involved in progressive systemic sclerosis, either clinically or at autopsy. A low diffusion capacity is the earliest detectable abnormality, preceding alterations in ventilation or clinical and radiologic evidence of disease. Dyspnea on exertion is the most frequently reported symptom. Orthopnea, paroxysmal nocturnal dyspnea, chronic cough, hemoptysis, chest pain, and hoarseness are also manifestations of pulmonary involvement. Pleurisy (with associated pleural friction rub) can also occur. Pulmonary fibrosis may occur early in the disease in patients with diffuse truncal involvement but occurs later in disease, often in association with pulmonary hypertension, in patients with limited scleroderma. Patients with diffuse pulmonary involvement have intimal proliferation of small and medium-sized pulmonary arteries and arterioles and may have an intense bronchiolar epithelial proliferation.

5. Heart–Because of the frequency of pulmonary fibrosis, cor pulmonale is the commonest cardiac finding. Myocardial fibrosis, leading to digitalis-resistant left-sided heart failure, carries a poor prognosis. Cardiac arrhythmias and conduction disturbances are common manifestations of myocardial fibrosis. Pericarditis is usually asymptomatic and is found incidentally at autopsy. Although 40% of patients have pericardial effusion by electrocardiography, tamponade is extremely rare.

6. Kidneys–Renal involvement is an uncommon but life-threatening development in patients with diffuse disease. Although renal insufficiency may follow an indolent course, it frequently presents as rapidly progressive oliguric renal failure with or without malignant hypertension.

7. Gastrointestinal tract–The gastrointestinal tract is commonly affected. The esophagus is the most frequent site of involvement, with dysphagia or symptoms of reflux esophagitis occurring in 80% of patients. Gastric and small bowel involvement presents with cramping, bloating, and diarrhea alternating with constipation. Hypomotility of the gastrointestinal tract with bacterial overgrowth may result in malabsorption. Colonic scleroderma is associated with chronic constipation.

8. Sjögren's syndrome–Sicca syndrome is seen in 5–7% of patients.

9. Uncommon clinical manifestations–Biliary cirrhosis or mononeuropathy, either cranial or peripheral, may rarely be associated with progressive systemic sclerosis.

10. Mixed connective tissue disease–Mixed connective tissue disease is a syndrome with features of scleroderma, rheumatoid arthritis, SLE, and polymyositis-dermatomyositis. The manifestations of the disease include arthritis, Raynaud's phenomenon, scleroderma of the fingers, muscle weakness and tenderness, interstitial lung disease, and a skin rash resembling either dermatomyositis or SLE. These patients have a high-titer speckled pattern of ANA and antibody to the ribonuclease-sensitive component of extractable nuclear antigen (eg, RNP). Renal disease is unusual in these patients. The disease appears to respond to moderate doses of corticosteroids.

B. Laboratory Findings: The normochromic normocytic anemia of chronic inflammatory disease is occasionally seen in progressive systemic sclerosis. Microangiopathic anemia can also occur. An elevated erythrocyte sedimentation rate and polyclonal hypergammaglobulinemia are common. A positive speckled or nucleolar pattern ANA is frequently encountered.

C. X-Ray Findings:

1. Bones–Thickening of the periarticular soft tissues and juxta-articular osteoporosis are seen in involved joints. Absorption of the terminal phalanges is often associated with soft tissue atrophy and subcutaneous calcinosis.

2. Chest–Characteristically, a diffuse increase in interstitial markings is seen in the lower lung fields of patients with moderate to severe pulmonary involvement. "Honeycombing," nodular densities, and disseminated pulmonary calcifications may also occur.

3. Gastrointestinal tract–Upper gastrointestinal series often reveal decreased or absent esophageal peristaltic activity, even in patients without symptoms of dysphagia. Long-standing disease leads to marked dilation of the lower two-thirds of the esophagus. Gastrointestinal reflux is present in the majority of cases, and ulcers or strictures of the lower esophagus due to peptic esophagitis are commonplace. With gastrointestinal involvement, barium is often retained in the second and third portions of the duodenum. Intestinal loops become dilated and atonic, with irregular flocculation and hypersegmentation.

The barium enema may reveal large, wide-mouthed diverticula along the antimesenteric border of the colon.

4. Renal arteriography–Marked changes are seen on renal arteriography in patients with scleroderma kidney. Irregular arterial narrowing, tortuosity of the interlobular arterioles, persistence of the arterial phase, and absence of a nephrogram phase are typical findings.

Immunologic Diagnosis

Polyclonal hypergammaglobulinemia is a frequent serologic abnormality in progressive systemic sclerosis. The fluorescent ANA test shows a speckled or nucleolar pattern in 70% of cases. Thirty percent of patients with diffuse truncal involvement have antibodies against topoisomerase (anti-Scl-70 antibodies). Seventy-five percent of patients have anti-centromere antibodies.

Differential Diagnosis

When classic skin changes and Raynaud's phenomenon are associated with characteristic visceral complaints, the diagnosis is obvious. In patients presenting with visceral or arthritic complaints and no skin changes, the diagnosis is difficult. In many cases, only the presence or absence of antibodies to ribonuclease-sensitive extractable nuclear antigen (RNP) makes it possible to differentiate scleroderma from mixed connective tissue disease. Patients with eosinophilic fasciitis present with marked thickening of the skin similar to that seen in the edematous phase of scleroderma. However, in eosinophilic fasciitis Raynaud's phenomenon and visceral involvement are rare and fibrosis and inflammatory cell infiltration are seen in the deep facial layers, whereas in scleroderma the fibrosis occurs predominantly in the dermis. The differential diagnosis also includes scleromyxedema, polyvinyl chloride toxicity, L-tryptophan-induced eosinophilia myalgia syndrome, carcinoid syndrome, phenylketonuria, porphyria cutanea tarda, amyloidosis, Werner's syndrome, and progeria.

Treatment

There is no cure for progressive systemic sclerosis. Sympathectomy has resulted in only transient relief of vascular symptoms, but vasodilating agents, particularly calcium channel-blockers, have provided relief for patients with severe Raynaud's phenomenon. Corticosteroids have no effect on the visceral progression of the disease, though they are beneficial in scleroderma with myositis and in mixed connective tissue disease. Colchicine has limited efficacy in treatment of the cutaneous manifestations of the disease. Penicillamine is often effective in the treatment of cutaneous scleroderma, and evidence suggests that it may be of benefit in slowing the progression of visceral disease.

Patients should avoid exposure to cold and should wear gloves to protect their hands. Tobacco should be avoided. Skin ulcers require careful antiseptic care. Cor pulmonale and left-sided heart failure may be treated with diuretics and digitalization, although the response is often poor. Antibiotics may be beneficial in decreasing intestinal bacterial overgrowth that leads to malabsorption.

Hypertensive crisis in renal disease associated with progressive systemic sclerosis is very difficult to control even with potent hypotensive agents. Angiotensin-converting enzyme inhibitors may be of benefit in treating the renal disease associated with scleroderma. The arthritis can usually be controlled with aspirin and other fast-acting nonsteroidal anti-inflammatory drugs. Skin lubricants can alleviate dryness and cracking.

Complications & Prognosis

Spontaneous remissions occur, but the usual course of the disease is one of relentless progression from dermal to visceral involvement. Involvement of the heart, lungs, or kidneys is associated with a high mortality rate. Aspiration pneumonia resulting from esophageal dysfunction is a complication in advanced disease.

Although the prognosis for any given patient is extremely variable, the overall 5-year survival rate for progressive systemic sclerosis is approximately 40%.

POLYMYOSITIS-DERMATOMYOSITIS

Major Immunologic Features

- There is lymphocytic and plasma cell infiltration of involved muscle.
- Antibodies to the nuclear antigens Jo-1, PM-Scl, and RNP are present.

General Considerations

Polymyositis-dermatomyositis is an acute or chronic inflammatory disease of muscle and skin that may occur at any age. Women are affected twice as commonly as men. There is no racial preponderance. The incidence of the disease is one per 200,000 population.

Polymyositis-dermatomyositis can be subclas-sified into 5 categories: (1) idiopathic polymyositis, (2) idiopathic dermatomyositis, (3) polymyositis-dermatomyositis associated with cancer, (4) childhood polymyositis-dermatomyositis, and (5) polymyositis-dermatomyositis associated with other rheumatic diseases (Sjögren's syndrome, SLE, progressive systemic sclerosis, mixed connective tissue disease).

Immunologic Pathogenesis

Although the precise pathogenetic mechanisms are unknown, evidence suggests that autoimmunity plays a role in disease causation. Experimental polymyositis has been induced in rats and guinea pigs by the injection of allogeneic muscle tissue in Freund's complete adjuvant. Polymyositis-dermatomyositis may coexist with other autoimmune diseases.

A. Humoral Factors: Polyclonal hypergammaglobulinemia is common in patients with polymyositis-dermatomyositis, and rheumatoid factors and antinuclear antibodies occur in 20% of cases. In children, focal deposits of complement, IgG, and IgM have been seen in vessel walls of involved skin and muscle. Some patients with polymyositis-dermatomyositis have been shown to produce antibodies both against a component of the extractable nuclear antigen and against purified human skeletal muscle myoglobin.

B. Cellular Factors: Cellular immunity may play a role in the pathogenesis of polymyositis-dermatomyositis. Lymphocytes from patients with polymyositis-dermatomyositis, after incubation with normal autologous muscle, produce a lymphokine that is toxic to monolayers of human fetal muscle cells. The lymphocytes in the muscle infiltrate of patients with polymyositis-dermatomyositis produce this lymphotoxin upon simple incubation of involved muscle. Thus, the lymphocytes of patients with polymyositis-dermatomyositis may respond to their own muscle antigens as if they were foreign (Fig 31–3). It is not known whether this is a primary defect in antigen recognition by the lymphocytes or whether these muscle antigens are cross-reactive with an unidentified foreign antigen. Polymyositis has been induced

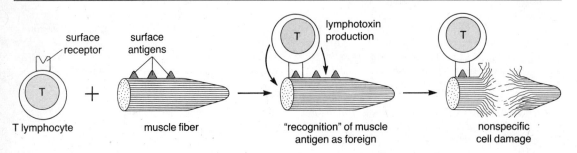

Figure 31–3. Defective "recognition" in polymyositis.

surface receptor / surface antigens

T lymphocyte

muscle fiber

lymphotoxin production

"recognition" of muscle antigen as foreign

nonspecific cell damage

in rats and guinea pigs by the transfer of sensitized lymphoid cells.

Pathology

Biopsy of involved muscles is diagnostic in only 50–80% of cases. Therefore, a normal muscle biopsy does not rule out the diagnosis of polymyositis-dermatomyositis in a patient with a characteristic clinical picture, muscle enzyme elevations, and an abnormal electromyogram. The histologic findings in acute and subacute polymyositis-dermatomyositis include (1) focal or extensive primary degeneration of muscle fibers, (2) signs of muscle regeneration (fiber basophilia, central nuclei), (3) necrosis of muscle fibers, and (4) a focal or diffuse lymphocytic infiltration. Chronic myositis leads to a marked variation in the cross-sectional diameter of muscle fibers and a variable degree of interstitial fibrosis.

Clinical Features

A. Symptoms and Signs:

1. Onset–Although the symptoms may begin abruptly, the onset of the disease is usually insidious.

2. Muscle involvement–The commonest manifestation is weakness of involved striated muscle. The proximal muscles of the extremities are most often affected, usually progressing from the lower to the upper limbs. The distal musculature is involved in only 25% of patients. Weakness of the cervical muscles with inability to raise the head and weakness of the posterior pharyngeal muscles with dysphagia and dysphonia are also seen. Facial and extraocular muscle involvement is unusual. Muscle pain, tenderness, and edema also occur.

3. Skin involvement–The characteristic rash of dermatomyositis, present in approximately 40% of patients, consists of raised, smooth or scaling, dusky red plaques over bony prominences of the hands, elbows, knees, and ankles. An erythematous telangiectatic rash may appear over the face and sun-exposed areas. Less commonly seen is the pathognomonic "heliotrope" rash of the face (a dusky, lilac suffusion of the upper eyelids). One-fourth of patients have various dermatologic manifestations ranging from skin thickening to scaling eruptions to erythroderma.

4. Cancer–Some patients with polymyositis-dermatomyositis are found to have a concomitant malignant tumor. In patients older than 40 years, the association between polymyositis-dermatomyositis and cancer appears to be more common. Removal of the tumor may result in a dramatic improvement in the polymyositis-dermatomyositis.

5. Miscellaneous features–A mild transitory arthritis is not unusual. Sjögren's syndrome occurs in 5–7% of cases. In children, vasculitis may result in gastrointestinal ulceration with abdominal pain, hematemesis, and melena. Patients with severe muscle disease are particularly susceptible to the development of interstitial pneumonia and pulmonary fibrosis. Raynaud's phenomenon occurs occasionally.

B. Laboratory Findings: An elevated erythrocyte sedimentation rate and a mild anemia are very common. Half of patients have elevated α_2- and γ-globulins on serum protein electrophoresis. Myoglobinemia and myoglobinuria are often seen. Up to 20% of patients with acute polymyositis have nonspecific T wave abnormalities on the ECG.

1. Muscle enzymes–When muscle cells are injured, a number of muscle enzymes, including glutamic-oxaloacetic transaminase, creatine phosphokinase, and aldolase, are released into the blood. The serum enzyme elevation reflects the severity of muscle damage as well as the amount of muscle mass involved.

2. Urinary creatine–Creatine is normally produced in the liver and transported via the circulatory system to the musculature. After attaching to receptor sites on the muscle cell surface, it is carried into the cell, where it is converted to creatinine. Polymyositis-dermatomyositis and other myopathies lead to a decrease in the number of cell surface receptors, causing an increase in circulating creatine that is quickly cleared by the kidneys. An increase in the urine creatine concentration is the most sensitive laboratory test for muscle damage and is a valuable indicator of disease activity. It is the first detectable laboratory abnormality in relapse of disease.

3. Electromyography–When involved muscles are examined, 70–80% of patients will demonstrate myopathic changes on electromyography. These changes are nonspecific but can point to the diagnosis of myositis. They include (1) spontaneous "sawtooth" fibrillatory potentials and irritability on insertion of the test needle; (2) complex polyphasic potentials, often of short duration and low amplitude; and (3) salvos of repetitive high-frequency action potentials (pseudomyotonia).

Immunologic Diagnosis

The diagnosis must be based on the nonimmunologic clinical and laboratory data discussed above. However, antibodies to the nuclear antigen histidyl-sRNA synthetase (Jo-1) occur in a substantial number of patients with polymyositis, particularly those with pulmonary involvement. Antibodies to PM-Scl (a nucleolar antigen) are more common in patients with polymyositis and scleroderma. Anti-RNP antibodies occur most frequently in patients with myositis as a component of mixed connective tissue disease.

Differential Diagnosis

At least 3 of the following criteria must be present for a definite diagnosis of polymyositis: (1) weakness of the shoulder or pelvic girdle, (2) biopsy evidence of myositis, (3) elevation of muscle enzymes, and

(4) electromyographic findings of myopathy. Typical skin changes must also be present for a definite diagnosis of dermatomyositis. A number of diseases can affect muscles and lead to clinical and laboratory abnormalities that are identical to those seen in polymyositis-dermatomyositis. The diagnostic criteria outlined above cannot be strictly applied in patients with infection (including HIV), sarcoidosis, muscular dystrophy, SLE, progressive systemic sclerosis, mixed connective tissue disease, drug-induced myopathy (alcohol, clofibrate), rhabdomyolysis, and various metabolic and endocrine disorders (McArdle's syndrome, hyperthyroidism, myxedema, acid maltase deficiency, carnitine palmityl transferase deficiency, and AMP deaminase deficiency). In addition, various neuropathies and muscular dystrophies can mimic inflammatory myopathy. A diligent search for occult cancers should be made in any patient who develops polymyositis-dermatomyositis as an adult.

Treatment

A. Corticosteroids: Prednisone, 60–80 mg orally daily, will usually decrease muscle inflammation and improve strength. The dose is tapered slowly, with clinical and laboratory monitoring. Creatinuria is the most sensitive index of disease activity and is often the first indication of relapse as corticosteroid dosage is reduced. However, assessment of muscle strength and determination of serum enzyme levels are usually sufficient indicators of disease activity. Some patients require chronic prednisone therapy (5–20 mg daily) to control the disease.

B. Cytotoxic Agents: Methotrexate and azathioprine have each been used with success in patients who do not respond to corticosteroids or who develop severe complications of corticosteroid therapy.

Complications & Prognosis

Polymyositis-dermatomyositis is a chronic disease characterized by spontaneous remissions and exacerbations. Most patients respond to corticosteroid therapy. Patients with severe muscle atrophy show little response to either corticosteroid or other immunosuppressive therapy. When the disease is associated with cancer, the prognosis depends on the response to tumor therapy.

BEHÇET'S DISEASE

Behçet's disease is a chronic recurrent inflammatory disease affecting adults of both sexes. The major manifestations of the disease are aphthous stomatitis, iritis, and genital ulcers. Other findings include vasculitis (particularly of the skin), pulmonary artery aneurysms, arthritis, meningomyelitis, enterocolitis, erythema nodosum, thrombophlebitis, and epididymitis. The differential diagnosis includes viral (herpes simplex) or chlamydial (inclusion conjunctivitis, lymphogranuloma venereum) infections, Reiter's syndrome, inflammatory bowel disease, Stevens-Johnson syndrome, oral pemphigus, and SLE. A pustular lesion appearing after needle puncture of the skin is highly suggestive of Behçet's disease.

Genetic and environmental factors probably play a role in pathogenesis. Some studies show an increased prevalence of HLA-B5 and HLA-B51 in Behçet's disease. There is also evidence suggesting that a virus may play a role in disease causation. Antibodies against various human mucosal antigens have been detected, and indirect immunofluorescence has demonstrated vascular deposition of immunoglobulins as well as circulating anticytoplasmic antibodies. There is a decrease in circulating helper T lymphocytes and an increase in gamma-delta T cells and natural killer cells. Furthermore, lymphocytes and plasma cells are prominent in the perivascular infiltrate of Behçet's vasculitis. Amyloidosis may develop in these patients.

Local corticosteroids are useful in the treatment of mild ocular and oral disease. Systemic corticosteroids are helpful in the treatment of systemic manifestations, but chlorambucil is thought to be the most useful agent for treating ocular disease. Unproved remedies include whole-blood transfusions, transfer factor, levamisole, colchicine, cyclosporin, and thalidomide.

ANKYLOSING SPONDYLITIS

Ankylosing spondylitis is a chronic progressive inflammatory disorder involving the sacroiliac joints, spine, and large peripheral joints. Ninety percent of cases occur in males, with the usual age at onset being the second or third decade of life.

The disease begins with the insidious onset of low back pain and stiffness, usually worse in the morning. Symptoms of the acute disease include pain and tenderness in the sacroiliac joints and spasm of the paravertebral muscles. Findings in advanced disease include ankylosis of the sacroiliac joints and spine, with loss of lumbar lordosis, marked dorsocervical kyphosis, and decreased chest expansion. Peripheral arthritis, when present, usually involves the shoulder or hips. Twenty-five percent of patients also have iritis or iridocyclitis. Carditis with or without aortitis occurs in 10% of patients and in a few who develop insufficiency of the aortic valves. Rare complications include pericarditis and pulmonary fibrosis.

Patients with ankylosing spondylitis are seronegative for rheumatoid factor. Hypergammaglobulinemia and ANA are not seen in ankylosing spondylitis, but an elevated erythrocyte sedimentation rate and a mild anemia are common during active disease. Electrocardiographic abnormalities, such as atrioventricular block, left or right bundle branch block, and left ventricular hypertrophy reflect cardiac involvement. X-rays of the sacroiliac joints reveal osteoporosis and erosions early in the disease and sclerosis with fusion in advanced disease. Calcification of the anterior longitudinal ligament of the spine and squaring of the vertebrae are seen on lateral x-rays of the spine. Ossification of the outer margins of the intervertebral disk (syndesmophyte formation) may lead to fusion of the spine.

On pathologic examination, these patients have a chronic proliferative synovitis very similar to that of rheumatoid arthritis. The characteristic skeletal change in advanced disease is ossification of the sacroiliac joints and interspinous and capsular ligaments. Pathologic cardiac findings include focal inflammation and fibrous thickening of the aortic wall and the base of the valve cusps.

The physical findings in patients with severe osteoarthritis of the spine may resemble those of patients with end-stage ankylosing spondylitis. However, degenerative osteoarthritis begins much later in life, does not extensively involve the sacroiliac joints, and is characterized radiographically by osteophytes rather than syndesmophytes. The differentiation of ankylosing spondylitis from other diseases associated with sacroiliitis and spondylitis, such as psoriatic arthritis, Reiter's syndrome, regional enteritis, and ulcerative colitis, depends upon the presence or absence of the clinical and radiologic characteristics of those diseases. The flowing ossification of the spine that occurs in patients with diffuse idiopathy skeletal hyperostosis (DISH) typically involves only one side of the vertebral bodies and spares the annulus fibrosis.

The basic pathogenesis of ankylosing spondylitis is unknown. There is a strong genetic predisposition to ankylosing spondylitis. Several members of the same family are often involved, and twin concordance for ankylosing spondylitis has been described. Furthermore, 90% of patients with ankylosing spondylitis have HLA-B27, compared with about 8% in the white US population.

The treatment of ankylosing spondylitis consists of giving anti-inflammatory agents to decrease acute inflammation and relieve pain and of instituting physical therapy to maintain muscle strength and flexibility. Therapy is designed to maintain a position of function even if ossification and ankylosis progress. Posturing exercises (lying flat for periods during the day, sleeping without a pillow, breathing exercises), the judicious use of local heat, and job modification are all part of a rational physical therapy program. Total hip replacement may offer considerable relief to patients with ankylosis of the hips, although recurrent ankylosis is sometimes a problem.

REITER'S SYNDROME

Reiter's syndrome is clinically defined as a triad consisting of arthritis, urethritis, and conjunctivitis. However, the arthritis is frequently accompanied by only one of the other characteristic manifestations. Although Reiter's syndrome usually affects men, it may also occur in women and children. The arthritis is recurrent or chronic, migratory, asymmetric, and polyarticular, involving primarily joints of the lower extremity. Fever, malaise, and weight loss occur commonly with episodes of acute arthritis. Characteristically, patients have an asymptomatic urethritis. The conjunctivitis is mild, but 20–50% of patients develop iritis. Balanitis circinata, painless oral ulcerations, and keratoderma blennorrhagicum (thick keratotic lesions of the palms and soles) are mucocutaneus manifestations. Complications include spondylitis and carditis.

Most patients have a mild leukocytosis. The urethral discharge is purulent, and smear and culture are negative for *Neisseria gonorrhoeae.* Synovial fluid is sterile, with a leukocyte count of 2000–50,000/μL, mostly PMN. The classic radiographic finding is fluffy periosteal proliferation of the heels, ankles, metatarsals, phalanges, knees, and elbows. Bony erosions may be seen in severe cases but rarely, if ever, occur in upper extremities.

Major diseases in the differential diagnosis include gonococcal arthritis, psoriatic arthritis, ankylosing spondylitis, Lyme arthritis, and the arthritis of inflammatory bowel disease. Patients with psoriatic arthritis occasionally develop urethritis or conjunctivitis. The differentiation of psoriatic arthritis and Reiter's syndrome is difficult to make on the basis of the skin lesion, since keratoderma blennorrhagicum is histologically indistinguishable from pustular psoriasis. Reiter's syndrome can be differentiated from ankylosing spondylitis by the presence of the urethritis and conjunctivitis, the prominent involvement of distal joints, and the presence of asymmetric radiologic changes in the sacroiliac joints and spine.

In Reiter's syndrome, the arthritis is thought to be an immunologic response to infection elsewhere in the body. Predisposing infectious agents include shigellae, salmonellae, gonococci, mycoplasmas, chlamydiae, yersiniae, and campylobacters. The manifestations of Reiter's syndrome appear to be more severe in AIDS. Eighty percent of patients with Reiter's syndrome have HLA-B27. It is not known whether this antigenic marker imparts an increased susceptibility to environmental or infectious agents or is associated with an unusual immune response gene.

Nonsteroidal agents may be used to control acute inflammation. Immunosuppressive drugs, such as methotrexate or azathioprine, may be necessary in treatment of patients with recalcitrant disease. Although the acute attack usually subsides in a few months, recurrences are common and some patients develop a chronic deforming arthritis.

PSORIATIC ARTHRITIS

Psoriatic arthritis is a chronic, recurrent, asymmetric, erosive polyarthritis that occurs in about 25% of patients with psoriasis. The onset of the arthritis may be acute or insidious and is usually preceded by skin disease. It characteristically involves the distal interphalangeal joints of the fingers and toes and may involve the hips, sacroiliac joints, and spine. Distal interphalangeal joint disease is frequently accompanied by nail pitting or onycholysis secondary to psoriasis of the nail matrix or nail bed. Constitutional signs and symptoms, such as fever and fatigue, may occur. Severe erosive disease may lead to marked deformity of the hands and feet (arthritis mutilans), and marked vertebral involvement can result in ankylosis of the spine.

An elevated erythrocyte sedimentation rate and a mild anemia are common. Hyperuricemia is occasionally seen in patients with severe skin disease. Serum immunoglobulin levels are normal, and rheumatoid factor is absent. Synovial fluid examination reveals a leukocyte count of 5000–40,000/μL, mostly PMN. Characteristic x-ray findings include "pencil cup" erosions, fluffy periosteal proliferation, and bony ankylosis of peripheral joints. Sacroiliac changes, including erosions, sclerosis, and ankylosis similar to that in Reiter's syndrome, occur in 10–30% of patients.

The major diseases that must be differentiated from psoriatic arthritis include rheumatoid arthritis, ankylosing spondylitis, and Reiter's syndrome. Psoriatic arthritis is differentiated from rheumatoid arthritis by the absence of rheumatoid factor and subcutaneous nodules, the involvement of distal interphalangeals, the characteristic x-ray findings of psoriatic arthritis, and the presence of psoriasis. The occurrence involvement of distal interphalangeals, and differences in the radiologic appearance of the spine help differentiate psoriatic arthritis from ankylosing spondylitis. The differentiation of psoriatic arthritis from Reiter's syndrome is particularly difficult, because both diseases are associated with HLA-B27 and involve the sacroiliac joints and spine and because keratoderma blennorrhagicum is histologically indistinguishable from pustular psoriasis. A helpful clinical distinction is the greater likelihood of upper extremity involvement in psoriatic arthritis.

The cause of psoriasis and psoriatic arthritis is unknown. Genetic factors appear to play a role in disease causation. Psoriasis and rheumatic diseases are found in family members of approximately 15% of patients. Patients with psoriasis and peripheral arthritis have an increased prevalence of haplotypes HLA-DR4, DR7, B13, B17, B38 and B39. Forty-five percent of patients with psoriasis and spondylitis have HLA-B27. Evidence for an immunopathogenesis in psoriatic arthritis includes the presence of antibodies directed against skin antigens and of activated T cells in skin and synovium.

Skin and arthritic manifestations require therapy. Topical corticosteroids, coal tar and ultraviolet light, or immunosuppressive drugs can be used to treat the skin disease. Treatment of arthritis is similar to that of rheumatoid arthritis.

RELAPSING POLYCHONDRITIS

Relapsing polychondritis is a rare disease characterized by recurrent episodes of inflammatory necrosis involving cartilaginous tissues of the ears, nose, upper respiratory tract, and peripheral joints. It often begins abruptly with swollen, painful, erythematous lesions of the nose or ears, usually associated with fever. Destruction of supporting cartilaginous tissues leaves patients with characteristic "floppy ear" and "saddle nose" deformities and can lead to collapse of the trachea. The commonest cause of death in these patients is airway obstruction. Recurrent episcleritis, anterior inflammatory ocular disease, auditory and vestibular defects, systemic vasculitis, necrotizing glomerulitis, vasculitis, and arthritis are other manifestations of relapsing polychondritis. Aortic insufficiency due to destruction and dilatation of the aortic valve ring occurs rarely.

Laboratory abnormalities include an elevated erythrocyte sedimentation rate, increased serum immunoglobulins, a false-positive VDRL, and mild anemia. Pathologic examination reveals infiltration of the cartilage-connective tissue interface with lymphocytes, plasma cells, and PMN. As the lesion evolves, the cartilage loses its basophilic stippling and stains more acidophilic. Eventually, the cartilage becomes completely replaced by fibrous tissue.

The pathogenesis of this disease is unknown. However, there is some evidence that autoimmune phenomena play a role. Immunofluorescence has revealed the presence of immune complexes at the fibrocartilaginous junction. Antibodies to human cartilage and to type II collagen are frequently present but also occur in other rheumatic diseases. Electron microscopy reveals electron-dense deposits of lysosomal origin in involved cartilage. In some patients with relapsing polychondritis, cartilage antigen will induce lymphocyte activation and lymphocyte production of migration inhibitory factor (MIF).

Corticosteroids, dapsone, colchicine, nonsteroidal anti-inflammatory drugs, and cytotoxic agents have been used with success in the treatment of relapsing polychondritis.

RELAPSING PANNICULITIS
(Weber-Christian Disease)

Relapsing panniculitis is a rare syndrome characterized by recurrent episodes of discrete nodular inflammation and nonsuppurative necrosis of subcutaneous fat. Most patients are women. Painful, erythematous nodules usually appear over the lower extremities but may involve the face, trunk, and upper limbs and progress to local atrophy and fibrosis. Occasionally, they may undergo necrosis, with the discharge of a fatty fluid. Constitutional signs, including fever, usually accompany an acute episode. Histologically, one sees edema, mononuclear cell infiltration, fat necrosis, perivascular inflammatory cuffing, and endothelial proliferation. The differential diagnosis includes superficial thrombophlebitis, polyarteritis nodosa, necrotizing vasculitis, erythema induratum, erythema nodosum, and factitious disease.

The cause of relapsing panniculitis is not known, and in fact the syndrome may be simply a nonspecific response to any one of a number of inciting factors, including trauma, cold, exposure to toxic chemicals, and infection. It has been seen in patients with SLE, rheumatoid arthritis, diabetes mellitus, sarcoidosis, tuberculosis, withdrawal from corticosteroid therapy, acute and chronic pancreatitis, pancreatic carcinoma, and α_1-antitrypsin deficiency. An autoimmune mechanism is suggested by the presence of hypocomplementemia, circulating immune complexes, and the association of relapsing panniculitis with several autoimmune diseases. The only autoantibodies demonstrated to date are circulating leukoagglutinins.

Acute episodes respond to corticosteroid therapy. Prostaglandin inhibitors, antimalarial drugs, and immunosuppressive drugs have been used to treat severe disease.

HEREDITARY COMPLEMENT DEFICIENCIES & COLLAGEN VASCULAR DISEASES

Complement deficiency is seen in one in a million normal adults and is associated with various rheumatoid diseases. C2 deficiency is the most common hereditary complement deficiency (see Chapters 10 and 23).

Deficiencies of C1r, C1s, C2, C4, C5, C6, C7, C8, and C1 esterase have all been associated with lupuslike syndromes. Hereditary complement deficiency could lead to an increased susceptibility to infectious agents, which may then stimulate the autoimmunity. Lack of complement could impair clearance of immune complexes. Alternatively, a neighboring gene predisposing to autoimmune phenomena could be inherited along with the defective gene for complement production.

HYPOGAMMAGLOBULINEMIA & ARTHRITIS

Hypogammaglobulinemia is an acquired or congenital disorder that may involve all or any one of the specific classes of immunoglobulin (see Chapter 24). Hypogammaglobulinemia is associated with infections, chronic inflammatory bowel disease, sarcoidosis, SLE, scleroderma, Sjögren's syndrome, polymyositis-dermatomyositis, and cancer. Patients with classic adult and juvenile rheumatoid arthritis may develop hypogammaglobulinemia.

Hypogammaglobulinemia patients may develop a seronegative, symmetric arthritis, with morning stiffness, occasional nodule formation, and radiographic evidence of demineralization and joint space narrowing. Bony erosions are rarely seen. Biopsy of the synovium reveals chronic inflammatory changes without plasma cells. Despite the reduction of serum immunoglobulins, immunoglobulin may be detected in the inflammatory synovial fluid. Total hemolytic complement is commonly depressed in the synovial fluid, suggesting immune complex formation.

The mono- or pauciarticular arthritis seen in hypogammaglobulinemia may be caused by mycoplasma or enterovirus infection.

Hypogammaglobulinemic arthritis may improve after the administration of gamma globulin.

REFERENCES

Systemic Lupus Erythematosus

Balow JE et al: Lupus nephritis. *Ann Intern Med* 1987; **106**:79.

Budman D, Steinberg A: Hematologic aspects of systemic lupus erythematosus: Current comments. *Ann Intern Med* 1977;**86**:220.

Dubois EL: Antimalarials in the management of discoid and systemic lupus erythematosus. *Semin Arthritis Rheum* 1978;**8**:35.

Fritzler MJ: Antinuclear antibodies in the investigation of rheumatic diseases. *Bull Rheum Dis* 1985; **35(6)**:1.

Haupt H et al: The lung in systemic lupus erythematosus: Analysis of the pathologic changes in 120 patients. *Am J Med* 1981;**71**:791.

Hochberg M: Systemic lupus erythematosus. *Rheum Dis Clin N Am* 1990;**16**:617.

Hughes GRV, Harris NN, Gharavi AE: The anticardiolipin syndrome. *J Rheumatol* 1986;**13**:486.

Levin RE et al: A comparison of the sensitivity of the 1971 and 1982 American Rheumatism Association criteria for the classification of systemic lupus erythematosus. *Arthritis Rheum* 1984;**27**:530.

Mandell BF: Cardiovascular involvement in systemic

lupus erythematosus. *Semin Arthritis Rheum* 1987; **17:**126.

McCluskey R: The value of renal biopsy in lupus nephritis. *Arthritis Rheum* 1982;**25:**867.

McCune WJ, Golbus J: Neuropsychiatric lupus. *Rheum Dis Clin N Am* 1988;**14:**149.

Steinberg A et al: Systemic lupus erythematosus: Insights from animal models. *Ann Intern Med* 1984; **100:**714.

Tan EM et al: 1982 Revised criteria for the classification of systemic lupus erythematosus. *Arthritis Rheum* 1982;**25:**1271.

Urman JD, Rothfield NF: Corticosteroid treatment in systemic lupus erythematosus: Survival studies. *JAMA* 1977;**238:**2272.

Wilson J et al: Mode of inheritance of essential C3b receptors on erythrocytes of patients with systemic lupus erythematosus. *N Engl J Med* 1982;**307:**981.

Zwaifler N, Bluestein H: The pathogenesis of central nervous system manifestations of systemic lupus erythematosus. *Arthritis Rheum* 1982;**25:**862.

Rheumatoid Arthritis

Arnett FC et al: The American Rheumatism Association 1987 revised criteria for the classification of rheumatoid arthritis. *Arthritis Rheum* 1988;**31:**315.

Boens M, Ramsden M: Long acting drug combinations in RA: A formal overview. *J Rheumatol* 1991;**18:**316.

Hurd ER: Extra-articular manifestations of rheumatoid arthritis. *Semin Arthritis Rheum* 1979;**8:**151.

Kremer JM, Lee JK: A long-term prospective study of the use of methotrexate in rheumatoid arthritis. *Arthritis Rheum* 1988;**31:**577.

Scott D et al: Systemic rheumatoid vasculitis: A clinical and laboratory study of 50 cases. *Medicine* 1981; **60:**288.

Sharp JT et al: The progression of erosion and joint space narrowing in rheumatoid arthritis during the first twenty-five years of disease. *Arthritis Rheum* 1991;**34:**660.

Van Zeben D et al: Association of HLA-DR4 with a more progressive disease course in patients with rheumatoid arthritis. *Arthritis Rheum* 1991;**48:**822.

Zvaifler N: New perspectives on the pathogenesis of rheumatoid arthritis. *Am J Med* 1988;**85(Suppl 4A):**12.

Juvenile Arthritis

Cassidy J et al: A study of classification criteria for a diagnosis of juvenile rheumatoid arthritis. *Arthritis Rheum* 1986;**29:**274.

Fink C: Treatment of juvenile arthritis. *Bull Rheum Dis* 1982;**32:**21.

Howard JF, Sigsbee A, Glass DN: HLA genetics and inherited predisposition to JRA. *J Rheumatol* 1985;**12:**7.

Schaller JG, Wedgwood RJ: Juvenile rheumatoid arthritis: A review. *Pediatrics* 1972;**50:**940.

Singsen BH: Rheumatic diseases of childhood. *Rheum Dis Clin N Am* 1990;**16:**581.

Sjögren's Syndrome

Alexander E et al: Sjögren's syndrome: Association of anti-Ro (SSA) antibodies with vasculitis, hematologic abnormalities, and serologic hyperactivity. *Ann Intern Med* 1983;**98:**155.

Arnett FC, Bias WB, Reveille JD: Genetic studies in Sjögren's syndrome and systemic lupus erythematosus. *J Autoimmun* 1989;**2:**403.

Daniels T: Labial salivary gland biopsy in Sjögren's syndrome: Assessment as a diagnostic criterion in 362 suspected cases. *Arthritis Rheum* 1984;**27:**147.

Fox R et al: Primary Sjögren's syndrome: Clinical and immunopathologic features. *Semin Arthritis Rheum* 1984;**14:**77.

Fox R et al: Sjögren's syndrome. Proposed criteria for classification. *Arthritis Rheum* 1986;**29:**577.

Progressive Systemic Sclerosis

Barnett A et al: A survival study of patients with scleroderma over 30 years (1953–1983): The value of a simple cutaneous classification in the early stages of disease. *J Rheumatol* 1988;**15:**276.

Nimelstein S et al: Mixed connective tissue disease: A subsequent evaluation of the original 25 patients. *Medicine* 1980;**59:**239.

Rocco V, Hurd E: Scleroderma and sclerodermalike disorders. *Semin Arthritis Rheum* 1986:**16:**22.

Rodnan GP: When is scleroderma not scleroderma? *Bull Rheum Dis* 1981;**31:**7.

Steen VD: Systemic sclerosis. *Rheum Dis Clin N Am* 1990;**16:**641.

Subcommittee for Scleroderma Criteria of the American Rheumatism Association Diagnostic and Therapeutic Criteria Committee: Preliminary criteria for the classification of systemic sclerosis (scleroderma). *Arthritis Rheum* 1980;**23:**581.

Polymyositis-Dermatomyositis

Benbasset J et al: Prognostic factors in polymyositis/dermatomyositis: A computer-assisted analysis of ninety-two cases. *Arthritis Rheum* 1985;**28:**249.

Bunch TW: Prednisone and azathioprine for polymyositis: Long-term follow-up. *Arthritis Rheum* 1981;**24:**45.

Hochberg M et al: Adult onset polymyositis/dermatomyositis: An analysis of clinical and laboratory features and survival in 76 patients with a review of the literature. *Semin Arthritis Rheum* 1986; **15:**168.

Targoff IN: Immune mechanisms in myositis. *Curr Opin Rheumatol* 1990;**2:**882.

Behçet's Disease

James D: "Silk route disease" (Behçet's disease). *West J Med* 1988;**148:**433.

O'Duffy J: Vasculitis in Behçet's disease. *Rheum Dis Clin N Am* 1990;**16:**423.

Shimizu T et al: Behçet's disease (Behçet's syndrome). *Semin Arthritis Rheum* 1979;**8:**223.

Ankylosing Spondylitis

Ahearn J, Hochberg M: Epidemiology and genetics of ankylosing spondylitis. *J Rheumatol* 1988;**15:**22.

Calin A et al: Ankylosing spondylitis—an analytical review of 1500 patients: The changing pattern of disease. *J Rheumatol* 1988;**15:**1234.

Khan MA: An overview of clinical spectrum and heterogeneity of spondyloarthropathies. *Rheum Dis Clin N Am* 1992;**18**:1.

Reiter's Syndrome

Aho K et al: Reactive arthritis. *Clin Rheum Dis* 1985; **11**:25.

Calin A, Fries J: An "experimental" epidemic of Reiter's syndrome revisited: Follow-up evidence on genetic and environmental factors. *Ann Intern Med* 1976; **84**:564.

Gaston JSH: How does HLA-B27 confer susceptibility to inflammatory arthritis? *Clin Exp Immunol* 1990; **82**:1.

Keat AC, Knight SC: Do synovial cells indicate the cause of reactive arthritis? *J Rheumatol* 1990; **17**: 1257.

Neuwelt C et al: Reiter's syndrome: A male and female disease. *J Rheum* 1982;**9**:268.

Psoriatic Arthritis

Gladman D: Psoriatic arthritis: Recent advances in pathogenesis and treatment. *Rheum Dis Clin N Am* 1992;**18**:247.

Polychondritis

McAdam LP et al: Relapsing polychondritis: Prospective study of 23 patients and a review of the literature. *Medicine* 1976;**55**:193.

Michet CJ et al: Relapsing polychondritis. Survival and predictive role of early disease manifestations. *Ann Intern Med* 1986;**104**:74.

Panniculitis

Panush R et al: Weber-Christian disease: Analysis of 15 cases and review of the literature. *Medicine* 1985; **64**:181.

Hereditary Complement Deficiency

Atkinson JA: Complement deficiency: Predisposing factor to autoimmune syndromes. *Am J Med* 1988; **85(Suppl 6a)**:45.

Frank M: Complement in the pathophysiology of human disease. *N Engl J Med* 1987;**316**:1525.

Moore T, Weiss T: Mediators of inflammation. *Semin Arthritis Rheum* 1985;**14**:247.

Hypogammaglobulinemia & Arthritis

Grayzel AI et al: Chronic polyarthritis associated with hypogammaglobulinemia: A study of two patients. *Arthritis Rheum* 1977;**20**:887.

Lederman HM, Winkelstein JA: X-linked agammaglobulinemia: An analysis of 96 patients. *Medicine* 1985;**64**:145.

Webster ADB et al: Polyarthritis in adults with hypogammaglobulinemia and its rapid response to immunoglobulin treatment. *Br Med J* 1976;**1**:1314.

32

Endocrine Diseases

James R. Baker, Jr, MD

In the 30 years since the first demonstration of the immune basis for thyroiditis, autoimmune disease has been identified as a major cause of dysfunction of all endocrine organs. It is now apparent that such diverse disorders as idiopathic Addison's disease, insulin-dependent diabetes mellitus, (IDDM) and the polyglandular endocrinopathy syndromes all have an autoimmune pathogenesis. Although primary therapy for these disorders remains the replacement of hormones deficient as a result of the destruction of endocrine organs, research is now being conducted into the genesis of the autoimmune process itself. It is hoped that through this research treatments could be developed to abort the autoimmune process before the gland is destroyed, thereby allowing normal endocrine function to continue.

MECHANISM OF DEVELOPMENT OF AUTOIMMUNE ENDOCRINE DISEASE

Endocrine disease has become a favored model for the study of autoimmune pathogenesis. Two possible factors in the development of human autoimmunity have been identified specifically through the study of endocrine disorders. The first is the discovery of aberrant expression of class II human leukocyte antigens (HLA) (see Chapter 5) on the surface of target cells in autoimmune disease (Fig 32–1). It is postulated that autoimmunity begins with an inflammatory process, possibly of infectious origin, in an endocrine organ. The inflammatory cells in the gland produce gamma interferon and other cytokines, which induce the aberrant de novo expression of class II HLA molecules on endocrine cell membranes. After expression of class II major histocompatibility complex (MHC) molecules, endocrine cells may function as antigen-presenting cells for their own cellular proteins, which are recognized by autoreactive T and B cells. This leads to enzymatic and oxidative destruction of endocrine cells, which further releases cellular proteins for processing by antigen-presenting cells, propagating the autoimmune response. Either abnormalities in the presentation of antigen owing to allogenic specificities in class II MHC or inappropriate recognition of the class II HLA-antigen complex as a result of their inherited differences in the T cell antigen receptor structure can then cause these autoantigens to be recognized as foreign in a genetically susceptible host.

Another potentially important factor in the genesis of autoimmunity is antigen cross-reactivity. The mechanism by which an immune response to a pathogen or an environmental or dietary protein might lead to a cross-reactive response to an autoantigen is not fully understood. However, several examples are now documented for Graves' disease and IDDM (Figure 32–2), and it is apparent that this cross-reactivity may occur at either the T or B cell level.

ORGAN-SPECIFIC AUTOANTIBODIES

The presence of organ-specific autoantibodies is often utilized as an adjunct to the diagnosis and occasionally the management of some autoimmune disorders. Table 32–1, showing the relative sensitivity and specificity of autoantibodies in different diseases, should be referred to during study of this chapter.

One of the other hallmarks of autoimmune endocrine diseases is the presence of organ-specific autoantibodies in the sera of affected patients.

Organ-specific antibodies are defined by several methods, including their binding to tissue as determined by immunohistologic staining and the binding of specific proteins, lipids, carbohydrates, and hormones in immunoassays. In addition, autoantibody activity is defined by the inhibition of hormone binding to receptor or through physiologic alterations of organ and cells physiology in vitro. However, there

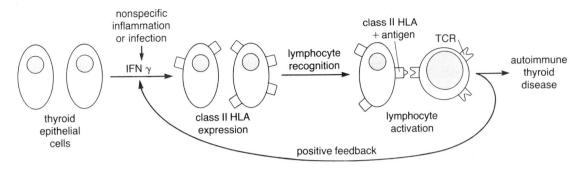

Figure 32–1. Initiation of autoimmunity through class II HLA expression. The expression of class II HLA results in lymphocyte activation, which causes the production of more lymphokines. These cause feedback stimulation of HLA expression and produce cytotoxic cells, which can destroy epithelial cells.

are difficulties in the use of these autoantibodies in diagnosis and evaluation of autoimmune diseases. There are often inconsistencies in the way many of the bioassays are conducted, leading to variability in sensitivity of autoantibody results. Also, in immunoassays for antibodies to ill-defined antigens, differences in the antigen preparation can cause variable results.

Often, even well-characterized autoantibodies are not specific for an associated autoimmune disorder. This raises concern about the pathogenic role of the autoantibody in the autoimmune disorder. A good example of this is the presence of antithyroglobulin antibodies in healthy relatives of patients with autoim-

mune thyroid disease and in some healthy elderly individuals. In contrast, some antibodies found in only a small proportion of patients with autoimmune disease, such as insulin receptor antibodies, correlate well with disease activity in those patients (Table 32–1). Thus, it is always important to evaluate autoantibody findings in the context of the patient's clinical situation.

THYROID AUTOIMMUNE DISEASES

CHRONIC THYROIDITIS (Hashimoto's Thyroiditis)

Major Immunologic Features
- There is lymphocytic infiltration of the thyroid gland.
- Antibodies to thyroid antigens are present.
- There is cellular sensitization to thyroid antigens.

General Considerations
Hashimoto's thyroiditis is an inflammatory disorder of unknown etiology, which results in progressive destruction of the thyroid gland. It is found most commonly in middle-aged and elderly females, but it also occurs in other age groups, including children, in whom it may cause goiter. Although it is distributed throughout the world without racial or ethnic restriction, it occurs more commonly in families where another member has an autoimmune thyroid disease. It is observed in conjunction with Graves' disease in a form of autoimmune-overlap syndrome. In addition, it is associated with other autoimmune disorders such as systemic lupus erythematosus (SLE), chronic active hepatitis, dermatitis herpetiformis, and scleroderma. Although no formal mode of inheritance is

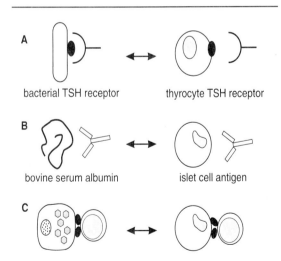

Figure 32–2. Proposed examples of molecular mimicry in the pathogenesis of autoimmune endocrine disease. **A:** Cross-reactive antibodies to bacterial TSH receptors and thyroid cell TSH receptors in Graves' disease. **B:** Cross-reactivity of antibodies to bovine serum albumin and an islet antigen in IDDM. **C:** Cross-recognition of coxsackie virus peptides and glutamic acid decarboxylase (GAD).

Table 32–1. Specificity and sensitivity of autoantibodies.

Autoantigen/Autoantibody	Associated Autoimmune Disease	Percentage of Patients Having Autoantibody (Sensitivity)	Specificity for Disorder
Thyroid peroxidase (microsomal antigen)	Hashimoto's thyroiditis	80–95	High
	Graves' disease	50–80	Low
	Subacute thyroiditis	30–50	Moderate
	Idiopathic hypothyroidism	50–80	Moderate
Thyroglobulin	Hashimoto's thyroiditis	40–70	Moderate
	Graves' disease	20–40	Low
	Subacute thyroiditis	10–30	Moderate
	Idiopathic hypothyroidism	10–30	Low
Thyroid-stimulating immunoglobulin (TSI)	Graves' disease	50–90	High
	Hashimoto's thyroiditis	10–20	Low
	Idiopathic hypothyroidism	0–5	ND[1]
Thyroid growth-stimulating immunoglobulin (TGSI)	Graves' disease	20–50	Moderate
	Hashimoto's thyroiditis	0–5	ND
	Idiopathic hypothyroidism	0–5	ND
Thyrotropin binding-inhibitory immunoglobulin (TBII)	Graves' disease	50–80	High
	Hashimoto's thyroiditis	5–10	Low
	Idiopathic hypothyroidism	10–20	Moderate
Anti-islet cell antibodies	IDDM	35–80	High
Glutamic acid decarboxylase	IDDM	50–80	High
Anti-insulin antibodies	IDDM	20–60	Low
	Insulin resistance	0–2	High
Antibodies to insulin receptors	IDDM	5–10	Low
	Type B insulin resistance	90–100	High
Antibodies to adrenal cortex	Addison's disease	30–60	High
21-Hydroxylase	Addison's disease	60–80	High

[1]ND, not determined.

recognized, there have been reported associations with several class II HLA antigens, including DR4 and DR5. However, these associations are not consistent among different ethnic populations.

Pathology

The hallmark of Hashimoto's thyroiditis is lymphocytic infiltration that almost completely replaces the normal glandular architecture of the thyroid (Fig 32–3). Plasma cells and macrophages abound, whereas scattered through this infiltrate are dying thyroid cells with acidophilic granules called Askenasze cells. Formations of germinal centers often give the impression that the thyroid gland is being converted into a lymph node. Lymphocytes infiltrating the thyroid are mainly B cells and CD4 T cells, although CD8 cytotoxic T cells have been cloned from Hashimoto's glands.

Clinical Features

Hashimoto's thyroiditis is primarily associated with symptoms of altered thyroid function. Early in the course of the disease the patient is usually euthyroid but may experience clinical hyperthyroidism due to the inflammatory breakdown of thyroid follicles with release of thyroid hormones. In contrast, late in the disease the patient is often hypothyroid be-

cause of progressive destruction of the thyroid gland. The most common eventual outcome of Hashimoto's disease is hypothyroidism.

A consistent physical sign seen in Hashimoto's disease is an enlarged thyroid gland. The goiter is often large and "rubbery" and may feel nodular, similar to its condition in other goitrous diseases. Often, lymph nodes surrounding the gland become enlarged. Rarely, patients will show symptoms of generalized vasculitis with urticaria and nephritis, and this has been associated with the presence of circulating immune complexes.

General laboratory findings are not helpful in making the diagnosis and relate primarily to the thyroid status of the patient. Patients with hyperthyroidism are differentiated from those with Graves' disease by the demonstration of patchy or decreased uptake on a radioiodine scan of the thyroid.

Immunologic Diagnosis

The hallmark of the diagnosis of Hashimoto's disease is the presence of circulating autoantibodies to thyroglobulin and thyroid microsomal antigen (now known to be the enzyme thyroid peroxidase). These antibodies were first detected by immunofluorescence (Fig 32–4), but they are now measured by agglutination assays or ELISA (see Chapter 12). They

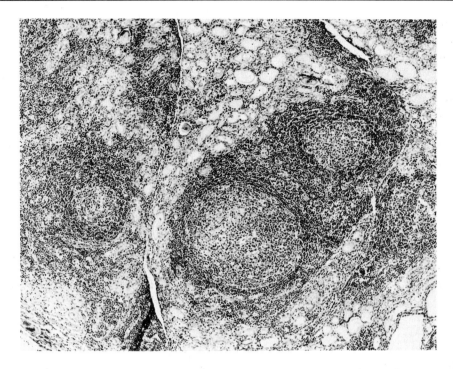

Figure 32–3. Pathology of Hashimoto's thyroiditis. Note the germinal centers and the lack of normal thyroid architecture. (Original magnification × 100.)

are present in the serum of more than 90% of Hashimoto's disease patients, with antimicrosomal antibodies being more common and of higher titer than antithyroglobulin antibodies. In patients without serum antibodies, autoantibody production may be localized to the intrathyroidal lymphocytes and plasma cells. Of interest, the immune responses to both thyroglobulin and thyroid peroxidase are heterogeneous, with several areas of each molecule conferring immunogenicity.

Other thyroid antibodies are often present in Hashimoto's disease patients, including antibodies that displace TSH from its receptor on thyroid cells and others that stimulate thyroid cells to produce hormones. Other important thyroid antigens stimulate the production of autoantibodies, since multiple unidentified protein bands are recognized by sera from patients with Hashimoto's thyroiditis in Western blots of thyroid membranes. In addition, lymphocytes of these patients proliferate in response to thyroid antigens.

Differential Diagnosis

One must differentiate Hashimoto's disease from other forms of goiter. This is usually done by using clinical criteria with the help of antithyroid antibody titers. On occasion, the rapid enlargement of one lobe of the thyroid gland will be confused with thyroid cancer or thyroid lymphoma, which are observed with an increased incidence in Hashimoto's glands. In these cases, needle biopsy of the nodule may be helpful, whereas computed tomograms or magnetic resonance images of the neck can be used to evaluate cervical adenopathy.

Treatment

Treatment of Hashimoto's disease usually consists of thyroid hormone replacement for hypothyroidism. If the patient has a symptomatic goiter, doses of thyroid hormone that suppress TSH secretion can often decrease the size of the gland. Rarely, thyroidectomy will be necessary for an unusually large or painful gland.

Prognosis

While the prognosis of Hashimoto's disease is excellent, serial thyroid function tests, especially TSH levels, are necessary to monitor the requirement for thyroid hormone replacement.

TRANSIENT THYROIDITIS SYNDROMES

Major Immunologic Features

- There is "giant cell" infiltration of the thyroid.
- There is transient production of antithyroid antibodies.

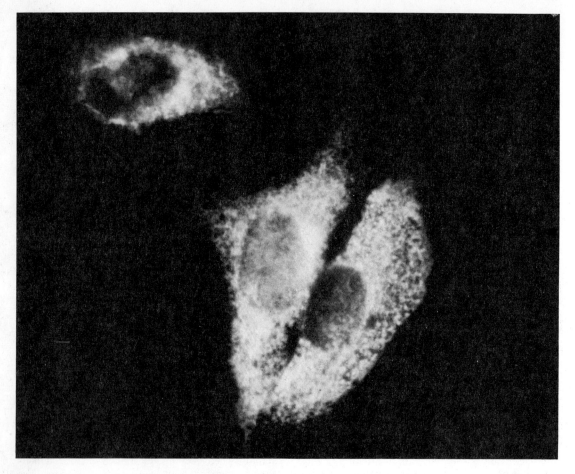

Figure 32–4. Immunofluorescent staining of a cultured human thyroid cell by antithyroglobulin antibodies showing the distribution of the antigen. (Original magnification × 400.) (Courtesy of Donald Sellitti.)

General Considerations

Several heterogeneous, self-limited thyroiditis syndromes have been described that have in common a transient immune activity against the thyroid. The 2 most common are subacute (de Quervain's) thyroiditis and postpartum thyroiditis. Subacute thyroiditis is possibly caused by a viral infection of the thyroid gland. It has a seasonal and geographic distribution common to infections with mumps virus, coxsackie virus, and echo virus. Patients with this disorder usually have an acute phase of thyroiditis in which the gland may be painful and antithyroid antibodies may be present. At this time, patients are thyrotoxic, with an elevated serum T4 and decreased radioiodine uptake. Progressive euthyroid and hypothyroid periods of 4–8 weeks may follow before thyroid functions finally normalize.

Similar in clinical course, postpartum thyroiditis is a common disorder that usually presents within 3 months of delivery. Patients may be either hypo- or hyperthyroid, and a significant percentage develop chronic thyroid dysfunction. Of interest, patients who have this disorder often have recurrent courses with subsequent pregnancies.

Postpartum thyroiditis occurs in about 5–8% of pregnant women and, unlike subacute thyroiditis, is not thought to be related to a viral infection of the thyroid. Supporting this are the presence of antithyroid antibodies preceding the onset of clinical disease and an association with HLA-DR3 and -DR5 haplotypes.

Pathology

Although the lymphocytic infiltrate seen in subacute thyroiditis is similar to that in Hashimoto's disease, 2 findings in subacute thyroiditis are distinctive. First, giant cells with a small center of thyroid colloid can be seen (this is known as colloidophagy) and the follicular infiltration tends to progress to form granulomas. These findings are not seen in postpartum thyroiditis, however.

Clinical Features

Subacute thyroiditis and postpartum disease have in common the clinical presentation of rapidly enlarging thyroid gland and signs of thyroid dysfunction. Subacute thyroiditis has a much more acute course than postpartum disease and is more commonly associated with pain and tenderness in the area of the gland. Postpartum thyroiditis and other types of transient thyroiditis without pain or other symptoms are sometimes termed "silent" thyroiditis.

Subacute thyroiditis is also accompanied by an elevated erythrocyte sedimentation rate. Both syndromes can cause "low-uptake" toxicosis, in that they can produce elevated serum levels of thyroid hormones in the face of low to normal levels of radioactive iodine uptake.

Immunologic Diagnosis

Antibodies to thyroglobulin and thyroid microsomes (peroxidase enzyme) are present acutely in both syndromes; however, they tend to be transient and of low titer in subacute thyroiditis. Thyroid-stimulating antibodies have also been demonstrated in a few patients with postpartum disease.

Treatment & Prognosis

In most cases thyroid function returns to normal within several months in both disorders. Patients with subacute thyroiditis who have especially painful glands may be treated with anti-inflammatory drugs. Postpartum patients who are clinically hypothyroid can benefit from thyroid hormone replacement. There is some evidence that the persistence of antithyroid antibodies identifies patients who will have protracted hypo- or hyperthyroidism. This finding offers a means for monitoring patients for eventual therapy with thyroid hormone or antithyroid drugs.

GRAVES' DISEASE

Major Immunologic Features

- Antibodies against thyroid antigens are present that stimulate thyroid cell function and displace TSH binding.
- There is class II HLA expression on the surface of thyroid cells.
- There is associated autoimmune ophthalmopathy and dermopathy.

General Considerations

Graves' disease is an autoimmune disorder of unknown etiology, which presents as thyrotoxicosis with a diffuse goiter. It is unique among autoimmune disorders since it is probably caused by autoantibodies that actually stimulate thyroid cellular activity. In addition, patients with Graves' disease often have as-

sociated phenomena of ophthalmopathy and a proliferative dermopathy, which appear to be autoimmune in nature. The endocrine, skin, and eye disorders are most commonly seen in combination. However, they can exist separately and often have different clinical courses even when they coexist in the same patient.

Graves' disease is most common in the third and fourth decades of life and has a marked female predominance of 7:1. Unlike Hashimoto's disease, it rarely occurs in children but often occurs in individuals past the fifth decade of life. It is a relatively common disorder, occurring in 0.1–0.5% of the general population.

Graves' disease was among the first autoimmune disorders noted to have an association with HLA haplotypes. There is a strong association with DR3 and several DQβ genotypes in whites and with Bw35 and Bw46 in Asians. Also, the disease tends to occur in families and is associated with the same HLA and Gm haplotypes in affected kindred. The disease seems to be associated with a type of "autoimmune susceptibility" in some families, since other family members often have autoimmune disorders such as Hashimoto's disease and antibodies to gastric parietal cells and intrinsic factor.

Pathology

Thyroid glands from patients with Graves' disease present a uniformly enlarged and diffuse goiter. Microscopic analysis reveals small thyroid follicles with hyperplastic epithelium, but little colloid. Although there is often a lymphocytic and plasma cell infiltrate, it is much less intense and does not have the associated destruction of normal tissue seen in Hashimoto's disease. These findings resolve in patients treated with antithyroid drugs.

Immunofluorescence analysis indicates that a high proportion of thyroid cells express HLA-DR antigens on their surface. In addition, analysis of the lymphocyte subsets in the gland reveals both CD4 and CD8 T cells and B cells.

Clinical Features

Graves' disease typically presents with diffuse goiter and thyrotoxicosis. The signs of hyperthyroidism are heat intolerance, hand tremor, nervousness, irritability, warm moist skin, weight loss, muscle reflex changes, hyperdynamic cardiovascular status with tachycardia, hyperdefecation, and changes in mental status. The exception to this is in the elderly, in whom apathetic hyperthyroidism may present with tachycardia as the sole clinical manifestation. Patients with accompanying ophthalmopathy may have proptosis, lid lag, and a characteristic "stare." Dermopathy usually presents as a swelling in the pretibial area (myxedema), and in the feet, face, or hands.

Laboratory findings are those of hyperthyroidism,

with elevated levels of total and free T3 and T4. TSH levels in this disease are low or undetectable because the stimulation of the thyroid gland is exogenous rather than from the pituitary axis and the elevated levels of the thyroid hormones cause a feedback inhibition of pituitary TSH secretion.

The thyroid gland in patients with Graves' disease always shows an increased uptake of radioactive iodine. A diffuse homogeneous uptake on a radio isotopic scan of the thyroid is almost pathognomonic of Graves' disease.

Immunologic Diagnosis

The immunologic diagnosis of Graves' disease rests on the identification of antithyroid antibodies with the ability to alter thyroid cell function. These antibodies tend to fall into 3 categories (Fig 32–5): (1) antibodies that stimulate the production of cAMP (thyroid-stimulating immunoglobulins [TSI]), (2) antibodies causing proliferation of thyroid cells as measured by the incorporation of [3H]thymidine into their DNA (thyroid growth-stimulating immunoglobulins [TGSI]), and (3) antibodies that displace the binding of TSH from its receptor (thyroid binding-inhibitory immunoglobulins [TBII]). Although these antibodies have been found in several other disorders, especially Hashimoto's thyroiditis, their presence in the appropriate clinical setting is virtually pathognomonic of Graves' disease. In addition, monitoring the function of these antibodies may, in some cases, correlate with the clinical course of the disease and its response to antithyroid drugs.

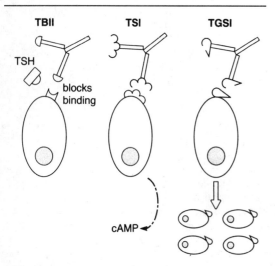

Figure 32–5. The 3 classes of antithyroid antibodies associated with Graves' disease. TBII antibodies block binding of TSH to its receptor, whereas TSI antibodies stimulate the production of cAMP and TGSI antibodies cause proliferation of thyroid cells. Whether these 3 antibodies bind to a single antigen, separate antigens, or separate epitopes on a single antigen is still unknown.

Initial efforts to measure the activity of TSI involved injecting IgG fractions from patients with Graves' disease into animals and measuring thyroid activity. This test has been replaced by the Fisher rat thyroid line 5 (FRTL-5). These cells are grown in culture with IgG from patients with Graves' disease, and the effect on cell function (either the production of cAMP or the incorporation of [3H]thymidine) is measured. The ability of the IgG to displace TSH from its receptor is still measured as described more than 15 years ago. The test involves the incubation of IgG with porcine thyroid membranes and radiolabeled TSH. The amount of TSH bound to the membrane is then calculated and compared with the amount bound in the presence of control IgG or unlabeled TSH. This results in a "percent displacement" of radiolabeled TSH, which gives a relative activity of the IgG. The recent identification and sequencing of the TSH receptor should allow classification of the specific function of these autoantibodies.

Recently, studies with recombinant TSH receptor protein have tried to identify specific sites in the receptor bound by autoantibodies. These studies are inconclusive but suggest that there are several sites in the external domain of the receptor to which autoantibodies bind. This suggests that the autoantibody response to the TSH receptor in Graves' disease is complex and heterogeneous.

Differential Diagnosis

The differential diagnosis of Graves' disease involves exclusion of other thyroid disorders with hyperthyroidism such as Hashimoto's disease, pituitary tumors, or thyroid adenomas. Most of these can be ruled out by determining that the thyroid gland has a diffuse increase in iodine uptake. The presence of ophthalmopathy and dermopathy also supports the diagnosis of Graves' disease.

Treatment

The initial treatment of Graves' disease involves the inhibition of symptomatic β-adrenergic hyperstimulation with β-adrenergic blocking agents. Therapy with drugs to inhibit thyroid cell function is also given soon after diagnosis. These drugs, propylthiouracil and methimazole, offer several advantages in the treatment of Graves' disease. They not only inhibit the production of thyroid hormones, relieving hyperthyroidism, but also decrease the size and vascularity of the goiter, making it more amenable to definitive therapy with surgery or radioactive iodine. Of interest, these drugs may also interrupt the perpetuation of the underlying autoimmune process, possibly through the resolution of the hyperthyroidism, as thyroid hormones appear to have nonspecific immunostimulatory activities in vitro.

Recently, it has been shown that administering suppressive doses of thyroid hormone in conjunction with anti-thyroid drugs may lead to long-term remission of Graves' disease. The mechanism of this effect is unknown, but may be the result of suppression of thyrocyte autoantigen expression.

Definitive therapy for Graves' disease involves the destruction of the thyroid gland, either by ^{131}I or by complete surgical removal of the gland. Although personal preference and experience often dictate which therapy is used, surgery has been the therapy of choice in women of childbearing age because of the potential risks of radiation to the gonads and fetus. Recent studies do not show risk to the ovaries, however, and radioiodine is becoming increasingly popular in premenopausal women once pregnancy is ruled out.

Prognosis & Complications

The prognosis for most patients is very good once their thyroid function is controlled. The most serious problems in Graves' disease often come from the associated ophthalmopathy and dermopathy, which in some cases do not respond to treatments that normalize thyroid function. Treatment with corticosteroids will provide relief in some cases, but occasionally the ophthalmopathy progresses to a point that vision is threatened. At that point, radiotherapy or surgical decompression of the orbit is often required. More aggressive treatment protocols with immunosuppressive drugs such as cyclosporine have shown some success in reversing the autoimmune process in these patients.

PRIMARY HYPOTHYROIDISM

Major Immunologic Features
- There is lymphocytic infiltration of the thyroid gland.
- Antithyroid antibodies can be present.

General Considerations

Primary hypothyroidism, or thyroid atrophy, is the most common cause of hypothyroidism (other than iatrogenic ablation) in adults. Much like the other autoimmune thyroid diseases, it is more common in women than men and occurs most often from age 40 to 60 years. The atrophy probably results from asymptomatic or unrecognized thyroiditis with resulting progressive destruction of the gland. However, some data suggest that some of these cases are related to antibodies which block TSH binding to its receptor, thereby inhibiting the trophic effect of the hormone. Thyroid atrophy also occurs as part of the polyglandular syndromes (see below).

Pathology

The thyroid is markedly atrophic and often fibrotic. In some cases there is residual lymphocytic infiltration.

Clinical Features

Although most patients demonstrate the usual findings of hypothyroidism and a small, impalpable thyroid gland, some present with palpable fibrosis in the area of the thyroid gland. Laboratory findings include elevated TSH levels with low (or low normal) levels of circulating thyroid hormones. TSH response to thyrotropin-releasing hormone (TRH) administration is often exaggerated, indicating an increased state of activation of the pituitary axis.

Immunologic Diagnosis

Antithyroid antibodies are found in a high proportion of patients (> 80%), but they are not necessary for the diagnosis. No other specific immunologic tests are available.

Treatment & Prognosis

Treatment consists of thyroid hormone replacement. Most patients do well with this therapy. However, replacement is required throughout the rest of the patient's life.

DISORDERS OF THE ENDOCRINE PANCREAS

INSULIN-DEPENDENT DIABETES MELLITUS (IDDM or Type I diabetes)

Major Immunologic Features
- There is monocytic and lymphocytic infiltration of the islets of Langerhans.
- There are antibodies against multiple antigens of islet beta cells.
- There is HLA-DR expression on the beta cells.
- There is some evidence for partial responses to immunosuppressive therapy.

General Considerations

IDDM is a disorder in which the destruction of the insulin-producing beta cells of the pancreatic islets of Langerhans results in a deficiency of insulin. This is in contrast to the defect in type II diabetes mellitus, in which resistance of target organs to the effects of insulin is present. Although IDDM has only recently been associated with an immune pathogenesis, it is now clear that there is an autoimmune cause in essentially all patients with this disorder. The postulated sequence of events leading to islet cell destruction is similar to the scheme outlined in Fig 32–1. After an initiating event such as a viral infection, an inflammatory response to beta cells of the islets results. This inflammation is characterized by HLA-DR expression on the beta cells and lymphocytic infiltration of the islets. Subsequently, either a persistent stimulation of the immune system or a defect in immune regulation allows the propagation of the autoimmune response in a genetically predisposed individual. This causes destruction of the beta cells and leads to insulin deficiency.

The hypothesis that a viral infection is the initial insult leading to the development of IDDM in humans is unproven. There is, however, much evidence in favor of this hypothesis including reports of the development of IDDM following infections with viruses such as mumps virus, cytomegalovirus, influenza virus, and rubella virus, as well as a direct relationship between viral infection and diabetes in experimental animals. Mumps virus, coxsackie virus types B3 and B4, and reovirus type 3 can infect and destroy human islet cells in vitro. In addition, evidence now suggests amino acid sequence similarities between coxsackie virus proteins and the islet cell autoantigen, glutamic acid decarboxylase. As yet, however, there is no direct causal link between the common occurrence of infections with these viruses and the rare event of developing autoimmune diabetes mellitus. It seems that the heterogeneous genetic susceptibility to development of autoimmunity is what has made identification of a specific environmental cause difficult.

Epidemiologic studies support the concept of a genetic susceptibility to develop IDDM. Seen almost entirely in individuals under the age of 30 years, it has a peak age of onset between 10 and 14 years. It occurs predominantly in whites and has a prevalence of approximately 0.25% in both the USA and Europe. Unlike most other autoimmune disorders, males are more commonly affected than females, by a small margin. The incidence of this disorder has increased slightly over the past 50 years. There are also seasonal fluctuations.

The genetics of type I diabetes mellitus have come under intense study recently. It is well documented that more than 90% of patients have HLA-DR3, -DR4, or both and that there is a negative association with HLA-DR2. An additive risk occurs when both HLA-DR3 and -DR4 are present. However, few individuals who have the HLA-DR3 and -DR4 haplotypes develop IDDM. This paradox may be partially explained by the association of the MHC antigens with particular DQβ genotypes. It has been noted that unique substitutions of amino acids at critical positions in this DQβ-chain may be related to susceptibility to diabetes. One substitution (an uncharged amino acid for Asp at position 57) was noted in animals genetically susceptible to diabetes. While this substitution does not perfectly identify humans at risk for this disease, it does indicate the potential importance of MHC antigens in diabetes.

Pathology

Patients show evidence of lymphocytic infiltration in the pancreatic islets even before evidence of glucose intolerance is noted. This inflammatory lesion progresses to cause specific destruction of the beta cells with atrophy and scarring of the islets. The other endocrine cells in the islets usually remain functional.

Immunofluorescence staining of the islet inflammation reveals several interesting findings. First, there is HLA-DR expression on the beta cells, as well as on the infiltrating lymphocytes. The majority of these lymphocytes stain positively with monoclonal antibodies for CD8, indicating a cytotoxic/suppressor phenotype. Antibody-producing cells are also seen, and antibody and complement components are present on the surface of the beta cells.

Clinical Features

The signs and symptoms are well known and are beyond the scope of this chapter. Unlike type II disease, there is a true insulin deficiency in type I diabetes mellitus, which leaves the patient prone to greater fluctuations in blood glucose concentration and to subsequent ketosis.

The laboratory diagnosis still rests on the documentation of elevated blood glucose concentrations. A fasting blood glucose level greater than 140 mg/dL in the appropriate clinical setting is diagnostic for diabetes. If the fasting glucose concentration is normal, the use of a glucose tolerance test may be helpful, but this is controversial. The level of hemoglobin A1c is helpful primarily in monitoring the ongoing control of blood glucose concentrations in patients on therapy.

Immunologic Diagnosis

Presently, no immunologic test is useful clinically. Antibodies to both islet cell cytoplasm and membranes can be identified by using immunofluorescence; however, these antibodies are not helpful in determining whether a susceptible individual will develop the disease. In the future, genetic analysis of HLA polymorphism or antibodies against a specific pancreatic antigen may serve this purpose. In this regard, the recent description that antibodies to glutamic acid decarboxylase precede the development of clinical glucose intolerance may suggest that the immune response to this enzyme will be a useful marker to monitor.

Treatment

Treatment of diabetes requires normalization of blood glucose concentrations by using oral hypoglycemic drugs or insulin injections. Most patients with IDDM require insulin, and the availability of human insulin may allow better therapy for some patients with insulin antibodies. Segmental pancreas or islet cell transplantation may offer a more physiologic form of insulin replacement in the future.

There have now been many trials of immunosuppressive therapy to attempt to reverse the inflammatory process that causes islet cell destruction (Fig 32–5). Although most of these trials were started a short time after the development of glucose intolerance, there have been some (Table 32–2) successful increases in C peptide levels and clinical improvement in blood glucose control, obviating a need for insulin injections. All of these drugs have potentially severe toxicity and require larger-scale clinical trials before they go into general use.

ADRENAL INSUFFICIENCY (Addison's Disease)

Major Immunologic Features
- Circulating antibodies against adrenal cells are present.
- Complement is fixed on the surface of adrenal cells.
- It is associated with other autoimmune diseases.

General Considerations
Since the decline of tuberculosis, idiopathic Addison's disease is the most common form of adrenal insufficiency, accounting for 70–80% of all cases. The prevalence is relatively low, only 40–50 cases per million, and it tends to affect young individuals in their third or fourth decade. The female-to-male ratio is lower than that seen in other autoimmune disorders, only 1.8:1. It can present as an isolated disorder or in combination with other autoimmune diseases. It is most commonly seen as part of a polyglandular syndrome (see below), which accounts for up to 40% of the cases of this disease. The disease is associated with HLA-DR 3/4 in a manner similar to type I diabetes mellitus, except when part of a polyglandular syndrome.

Pathology
Grossly, adrenal glands from patients with idiopathic Addison's disease show progressive scarring and atrophy. Microscopic examination often reveals a lymphocytic infiltrate early in the course of the disease, and immunofluorescence shows antibody and complement fixed to cortical cells.

Clinical Features
Idiopathic Addison's disease is usually slowly progressive, with the development of clinical manifestations such as salt wasting, hypotension, anorexia, malaise, and hyperpigmentation occurring so gradually that they can easily be undetected. Serum levels of adrenocorticotropic hormone (ACTH) are often elevated long before clinical disease develops. The finding of small, noncalcified adrenal glands on x-ray or computed tomography of the abdomen helps to differentiate this disorder from adrenal insufficiency secondary to carcinoma (primary or metastatic) and tuberculosis. The laboratory diagnosis rests on the lack of a cortisol (and possibly aldosterone) response to ACTH administration.

Immunologic Diagnosis
Serum antibodies against adrenal cortical cells are demonstrable by immunofluorescence in up to 80% of cases.

Treatment
Treatment consists of corticosteroid hormone replacement and, when needed, replacement of mineralocorticoid hormones. No trials of immunosuppressive therapy have been published.

LYMPHOCYTIC ADENOHYPOPHYSITIS

Lymphocytic adenohypophysitis is a rare disorder characterized by the rapid development of hypopituitarism without evidence of pituitary adenoma. It occurs most often in women during or after pregnancy. Although the incidence of this disorder is unknown, the finding of antibodies against pituitary cells in 18% of patients with Sheehan's syndrome suggests that at least some of these patients may have had an autoimmune basis for their hypopituitarism. It also occurs as part of a polyglandular syndrome (as discussed below), in which it has been associated with isolated deficiencies of gonadotropic hormones.

Table 32–2. Immunotherapy trials in type I diabetes mellitus.

Drug	C Peptide Increase Period	Insulin Therapy-Free Period
Prednisone	24 mo	Transient
Alpha interferon	None	None
Prednisone, antithymocyte globulin, and azathioprine	12 mo	3–26 mo
Cyclosporin	> 12 mo	12 mo (25% of subjects)

PREMATURE OVARIAN FAILURE

Evidence is accumulating that some individuals may have an autoimmune basis for premature gonadal failure. There have been several cases in which autoimmune oophoritis is associated with other autoimmune endocrine diseases, especially adrenal insufficiency. This is especially true in polyglandular syndromes.

IDIOPATHIC HYPOPARATHYROIDISM

This is another uncommon disorder seen primarily in polyglandular autoimmune syndromes. Although antibodies against parathyroid tissue commonly occur in the polyglandular syndromes, their presence does not correlate with overt hypoparathyroidism. It has been reported that antibodies from patients with this disorder cause complement-mediated cytolysis of parathyroid cells, suggesting that a subset of antibodies may have pathogenic significance.

AUTOIMMUNE POLYGLANDULAR SYNDROMES

Major Immunologic Features
- There are circulating antibodies against multiple endocrine organs.
- There is evidence of HLA-DR expression on affected cells.
- There is genetic susceptibility to autoimmunity.

General Considerations
Polyglandular syndromes are groupings of multiple endocrine dysfunctions of autoimmune origin in a genetically susceptible individual. There were initially many versions of these syndromes identified by multiple eponyms; however, recently a classification scheme for these disorders has been developed (Table 32–3).

A. Type I Syndrome: The type I syndrome is a disorder that occurs in childhood, usually before the age of 10 years, with a slight female predominance. It was previously known as mucocutaneous candidiasis endocrinopathy. The most common association is between candidiasis and hypoparathyroidism (> 70% of cases), but 40–70% of patients also go on to develop adrenal insufficiency. With the exception of gonadal failure, which occurs in approximately 40% of patients, the other autoimmune endocrine disorders are less common in the type I syndrome. There is, however, an association with chronic active hepatitis (10–15% of cases), alopecia areata, malabsorption, and pernicious anemia.

The pathogenesis of this disorder is unknown, but the problems with chronic fungal infection suggest a defect in cell-mediated immunity. Autoantibodies

Table 32–3. Classification of polyglandular syndromes.

Syndrome	Major Criteria	Minor Criteria
Type I	Candidiasis Adrenal failure Hypoparathyroidism	Gonadal failure Alopecia Malabsorption Chronic hepatitis
Type II	Adrenal failure Thyroid disease IDDM	Gonadal failure Vitiligo Nonendocrine autoimmune disease
Type III[1]	Thyroid disease	a. IDDM b. Gastric disease c. Nonendocrine autoimmune disease

[1]Type III is composed of thyroid disease plus only one of a, b, or c.

against cells from most affected organs are also seen in a large percentage of patients.

Although type I polyglandular syndrome occurs sporadically, it is more commonly seen as a familial disorder with inheritance suggestive of an autosomal recessive trait. It has not, however, been associated with a particular HLA haplotype.

B. Type II Syndrome: Type II polyglandular syndrome was originally known as Schmidt's syndrome. It tends to occur most often between the ages of 20 and 30 years and has a 2:1 female predominance. It is a rare disorder, with a prevalence of 20 per million. It is characterized by the presence of a second, autoimmune disorder (usually diabetes or thyroid disease or both) with idiopathic Addison's disease. Gonadal failure occurs in a smaller percentage of cases, and nonendocrine autoimmune disorders have been occasionally noted.

Although at least half the cases of type II polyglandular syndrome are familial, the mode of inheritance is unknown. Both autosomal dominant and recessive patterns have been suggested, and there is also a high frequency of HLA-DR3 in these patients. Autoantibodies against cells of the affected organs are present in the majority of patients, and there have also been reports of alterations in cell-mediated immunity.

C. Type III Syndrome: Type III polyglandular syndrome is the least well characterized but probably the most common of the disorders. It is defined by the presence of autoimmune thyroid disease with another autoimmune disorder. This syndrome is composed of at least 3 clinical entities. The first is the association of diabetes mellitus with autoimmune thyroid disease. The second is the association of autoimmunity against gastric components such as parietal cells or intrinsic factor in association with autoimmune thyroid disease. The association of any other organ-specific autoimmune disorder, such as myasthenia gravis, with autoimmune thyroid disease comprises the third component. Patients with type III polyglandular syndrome, by definition, do not have Addison's disease.

The cause of type III polyglandular syndrome is unclear, but it tends to primarily involve female patients (7:1 female predominance) who have HLA-DR3-associated autoimmune disease. Again, organ-specific autoantibodies are present in the sera of patients with this disorder.

D. Other Considerations: The pathology, symptoms, and treatment of patients with the polyglandular syndromes are the same as for the individual autoimmune disorders, with a few important exceptions. Patients with type I polyglandular syndrome should have their candidiasis treated with ketoconazole. This not only provides symptomatic relief but also may help resolve some of the defects in cell-mediated immunity. In addition, all patients with the polyglandular syndromes should be monitored for the development of other autoimmune disorders associated with their syndrome. This will prevent missing disorders such as Addison's disease, which may develop later in the course of the syndrome.

REFERENCES

General

Bach JF: Antireceptor or antihormone autoimmunity and its relationship with the idiotype network. *Adv Nephrol* 1987;**16**:25.

Bigazzi PE: Autoimmunity in diabetes mellitus and polyendocrine syndromes: Current concepts of pathogenesis and etiology. *Immunol Ser* 1990;**52**:295.

Buse JB, Eisenbarth GS: Autoimmune endocrine disease. *Vitam Horm* 1985;**42**:253.

Chaplin DD, Kemp ME: The major histocompatibility complex and autoimmunity. *Year Immunol* 1986–87;**3**:179.

De Baets MH: Autoimmune endocrine diseases. *Year Immunol* 1986;**2**:289.

Patrick CC: Organ-specific autoimmune diseases. *Immunol Ser* 1990;**50**:435.

Pujol-Borrell R et al: Inappropriate major histocompatibility complex class II expression by thyroid follicular cells in thyroid autoimmune disease and by pancreatic beta cells in type I diabetes. *Mol Biol Med* 1986;**3**:159.

Thyroid Diseases

Baker JR Jr et al: Seronegative Hashimoto thyroiditis with thyroid autoantibody production localized to the thyroid. *Ann Intern Med* 1988;**108**:26.

Bottazzo GF, Doniach D: Autoimmune thyroid disease. *Annu Rev Med* 1986;**37**:353.

Burman KD, Baker JR Jr: Immune mechanisms in Graves' disease. *Endocr Rev* 1985;**6**:183.

Jacobson DH, Gorman CA: Endocrine ophthalmopathy: Current ideas concerning etiology, pathogenesis and treatment. *Endocr Rev* 1984;**5**:200.

Kosugi S et al: Identification of separate determinants on the thyrotropin receptor reactive with Graves' thyroid-stimulating antibodies and with thyroid-stimulating blocking antibodies in idiopathic myxedema: These determinants have no homologous sequence on gonadotropin receptors. *Mol Endocrinol* 1992;**6(2)**:168.

Nagayama Y, Rapoport B: The thyrotropin receptor 25 years after its discovery: New insight after its molecular cloning. *Mol Endocrinol* 1992;**6(2)**:145.

Weetmen AP, McGregor AM: Autoimmune thyroid disease: Developments in our understanding. *Endocr Rev* 1984;**5**:309.

Insulin-Dependent Diabetes Mellitus

Baekkeskov S et al: Identification of the 64K autoantigen in insulin-dependent diabetes as the GABA-synthesizing enzyme glutamic acid decarboxylase. *Nature* 1990;**347**:151.

Baisch JM et al: Analysis of HLA-DQ genotypes and susceptibility in insulin-dependent diabetes mellitus. *N Engl J Med* 1990;**322**:1836.

Karjalainen J et al: A bovine albumin peptide as a possible trigger of insulin-dependent diabetes mellitus. *N Engl J Med* 1992;**327**:302.

Lernmark A et al: Islet-specific immune mechanisms. *Diabetes Metab Rev* 1987;**3**:959.

Riley WJ et al: A prospective study of the development of diabetes in relatives of patients with insulin-dependent diabetes. *N Engl J Med* 1990;**323**:1167.

Skyler JS: Immune intervention studies in insulin-dependent diabetes mellitus. *Diabetes Metab Rev* 1987;**3**:1017.

Todd JA: Genetic control of autoimmunity in type I diabetes. *Immunol Today* 1990;**11**:122.

Addison's Disease

Betterle C et al: Complement-fixing adrenal autoantibodies as a marker for predicting onset of idiopathic Addison's disease. *Lancet* 1983;**1**:1238.

Burke CW: Adrenocortical insufficiency. *Clin Endocrinol Metab* 1985;**14**:947.

Latinne D et al: Addison's disease: Immunological aspects. *Tissue Antigens* 1987;**30**:23.

Scheithauer BW, Kovacs K, Randall RV: The pituitary gland in untreated Addison's disease. A histologic and immunocytologic study of 18 adenohypophyses. *Arch Pathol Lab Med* 1983;**107**:484.

Vita JA et al: Clinical clues to the cause of Addison's disease. *Am J Med* 1985;**78**:461.

Weetman AP et al: HLA associations with autoimmune Addison's disease. *Tissue Antigens* 1991;**38**:31.

Winqvist O, Karlsson FA, Kampe O: 21-Hydroxylase, a major autoantigen in idiopathic Addison's disease. *Lancet* 1992;**339**:1559.

Lymphocytic Adenohypophysitis & Hypoparathyroidism

Brandi ML et al: Antibodies cytotoxic to bovine parathyroid cells in autoimmune hypoparathyroidism. *Proc Natl Acad Sci USA* 1986;**83**:8366.

Guay AT et al: Lymphocytic hypophysitis in a man. *J Clin Endocrinol Metab* 1987;**64:**631.

Homberg JC: Hypoparathyroidism, ovarian insufficiency and adrenal insufficiency of autoimmune origin. *Rev Prat* 1986;**36:**3505.

McDermott MW et al: Lymphocytic adenohypophysitis. *Can J Neurol Sci* 1988;**15:**38.

Polyglandular Syndromes

Ahonen P: Autoimmune polyendocrinopathy candidosis ectodermal dystrophy (APECED): Autosomal recessive inheritance. *Clin Genet* 1985;**27:**535.

Appleboom TM, Flowers FP: Ketoconazole in the treatment of chronic mucocutaneous candidiasis secondary to autoimmune polyendocrinopathy candidiasis syndrome. *Cutis* 1982;**30:**71.

Brun JM: Juvenile autoimmune polyendocrinopathy. *Horm Res* 1982;**16:**308.

Leshin M: Polyglandular autoimmune syndromes. *Am J Med Sci* 1985;**290:**77.

Neufeld M, MacLaren NK, Blizzard RM: Autoimmune polyglandular syndromes. *Pediatr Ann* 1980;**9:**154.

Hematologic Diseases

33

J. Vivian Wells, MD, FRACP, FRCPA, & James P. Isbister, FRACP, FRCPA

There are many areas in hematology that are significantly affected by immunologic processes. An important group of disorders—the autoimmune hemolytic anemias, autoimmune neutropenias, and immune thrombocytopenias—are characterized by immunologic destruction of circulating blood cells. Even hematopoietic precursor cells in the bone marrow may be destroyed or suppressed by immunologic mechanisms, as seen in pure erythrocyte aplasia and some cases of aplastic anemia. Another large group of hematologic disorders—the plasma cell dyscrasias, lymphatic leukemias, and lymphomas—represent abnormal proliferations of primary cells of the immune system (see Chapter 45).

This chapter will be devoted primarily to hematologic disorders in which immunologic cells or mechanisms play a major role. The chapter discusses immunologic disorders of leukocytes, erythrocytes, and coagulation.

LEUKOCYTE DISORDERS

LEUKOPENIA

Leukopenia is defined as a reduction in the number of circulating leukocytes below 4000/μL. Granulocytopenia may be caused either by decreased granulocyte production by the bone marrow or by increased granulocyte utilization or destruction. Decreased granulocyte production occurs in aplastic anemia, leukemia, and other diseases marked by bone marrow infiltration; many drugs also cause leukopenia by this mechanism. Increased granulocyte utilization or destruction occurs in hypersplenism, autoimmune neutropenia, and some forms of drug-induced leukopenia. The major causes of leukopenia are listed in Table 33–1.

1. AUTOIMMUNE NEUTROPENIA

Autoimmune neutropenia may occur as an isolated disorder or secondary to an underlying autoimmune disease. These patients may be asymptomatic or may have recurrent infections. Antigranulocyte antibodies have been detected by a variety of procedures, including the utilization of anti-immunoglobulin antisera with fluorescence or antiglobulin consumption techniques, functional assays, and cytotoxicity assays. The presence of leukoagglutinins does not correlate well with leukopenia. Bone marrow function is relatively normal in autoimmune neutropenia, with myeloid hyperplasia and a shift to the left in maturation, presumably in response to increased peripheral granulocyte destruction. The autoantibody may also suppress bone marrow myeloid cell growth in vitro and in vivo.

Autoimmune neutropenia may also be seen in systemic lupus erythematosus (SLE), Felty's syndrome (rheumatoid arthritis, splenomegaly, and severe neutropenia), and other autoimmune disorders. Immune neutropenia in these disorders may be caused by adsorption of immune complexes onto the neutrophil membrane with premature cell destruction rather than by an antibody directed at specific neutrophil antigens. Some patients with Felty's syndrome also appear to have depressed granulocyte production by the bone marrow, probably also on an immunologic basis.

2. CYCLIC NEUTROPENIA

These patients have a 3–6 week cycle, which includes a period of neutropenia lasting 4–10 days. Patients may be asymptomatic, but many show a pattern

Table 33–1. The major causes of leukopenia.

Infections
  Viral—rubella
  Bacterial—typhoid fever, miliary tuberculosis, brucellosis
  Rickettsial
Therapy
  Ionizing radiation
  Cytotoxic drugs
  Drugs
    Selective neutropenia
    Agranulocytosis
    Aplastic anemia
Hematologic diseases
  Megaloblastic anemia
  Acute leukemia
  Myelodysplasia
  Aplastic anemia
  Multiple myeloma
  Paroxysmal nocturnal hemoglobinuria
  Leukoerythroblastic anemia
    Metastatic carcinoma
Autoimmune neutropenia
  Hypersplenism
  SLE
  Felty's syndrome
Chronic idiopathic neutropenia
Cyclic neutropenia
Miscellaneous
  Anaphylaxis
  Hypopituitarism

of recurrent fever, pharyngitis, recurrent aphthous stomatitis, lymphadenopathy, and infections during the period of neutropenia. The treatment of choice for symptomatic patients is granulocyte colony-stimulating factor (G-CSF; see below).

3. DRUG-INDUCED IMMUNE NEUTROPENIA

Although most drugs produce neutropenia by bone marrow suppression, some may cause neutropenia by the attachment of drug-antibody immune complexes to the surface of the granulocytes, with premature cell destruction. This "innocent-bystander" mechanism is known to occur in drug-induced immune hemolytic anemia and thrombocytopenia. Cephalothin causes granulocytopenia in approximately 0.1% of patients given the drug, probably by this mechanism.

4. AGRANULOCYTOSIS

Agranulocytosis is characterized by the total absence of granulocytes and granulocyte precursors from the peripheral blood and bone marrow. This most often results from exposure of the patient to certain drugs, eg, aminopyrine, dipyrone, and phenylbutazone. Patients with agranulocytosis usually present with infections—often serious, life-threatening ones. Prior to the antibiotic era, agranulo-

cytosis was almost invariably fatal. Patients now usually recover with intensive antibiotic treatment and granulocyte transfusions when necessary. Unlike drug-induced aplastic anemia, agranulocytosis usually resolves spontaneously within a few days to a few weeks after discontinuing the offending drug.

Although antigranulocyte antibodies or leukocyte drug-dependent antibodies generally have not been demonstrated in agranulocytosis, there is circumstantial evidence that immunologic damage to peripheral blood and bone marrow granulocytic cells is the mechanism of cell destruction, at least in some cases. Such patients often develop agranulocytosis after taking the responsible drug for weeks or months. If they recover from the agranulocytosis after the drug is discontinued and later are rechallenged with a small test dose of the same drug, acute agranulocytosis occurs immediately, associated with the acute onset of fever, chills, and hypocomplementemia.

5. MANAGEMENT OF NEUTROPENIA

The first step in the management of a patient with neutropenia is identification of any underlying disease or drugs that may be responsible for the neutropenia.

The offending drug should be withdrawn, unless it is "essential" treatment eg, antitumor cytotoxic chemotherapy, antiretroviral therapy in HIV-infected patients, or recombinant alpha interferon in hairy cell leukemia. Underlying diseases such as SLE should be treated appropriately, and generally no specific treatment is required for the neutropenia, which tends to resolve as the underlying disease goes into remission or is controlled. On occasion, patients with autoimmune neutropenia have required treatment with corticosteroids, immunosuppressive drugs, or splenectomy.

The major advance in the management of cytopenias has been the therapeutic use of cytokines/hemolymphopoietic growth factors.

Cytokines are bioactive cell secretions, which function as hormones for immune and other cells. The growth factors function as growth regulators, and more than 14 such factors have been identified and their genes cloned, including erythropoietin, the colony-stimulating factors, and the interleukins. A few are now used in clinical practice (see Chapter 9), but their use is still restricted in many ways. Many ongoing clinical trials are assessing the role of cytokines in treating various diseases. Table 33–2 lists the major cytokines currently in clinical use or suggested for further studies.

For the management of neutropenia, cytokine therapy has been used in the following clinical settings:

(1) Chronic neutropenia/cyclic neutropenia: G-CSF is now the treatment of choice.

(2) Autoimmune neutropenia: G-CSF is considered for symptomatic patients not responding to corticosteroid therapy.

Table 33–2. Cytokines/hemolymphopoietic growth factors with clinical applications.

Cytokine	Major Biologic Effects	Clinical Applications[1]
Erythropoietin	Erythrocyte production	Anemia of end-stage renal disease Zidovudine anemia in AIDS patients
Granulocyte colony-stimulating factor (G-CSF)	Granulocyte lineage and differentiation Early myeloid stem cell action Neutrophil phagocytosis increase Release of neutrophils from bone marrow	Neutropenia Aplastic anemia Transplantation
Granulocyte-monocyte colony-stimulating factor (GM-CSF)	Granulocyte, macrophage, and megakaryocyte proliferation and differentiation Enhancement of neutrophil functions	Neutropenia Aplastic anemia Transplantation
Colony-stimulating factor-1 (CSF-1)	Macrophage-monocyte proliferation and differentiation (lesser for granulocytes) Stimulation of macrophage activities	Neutropenia (Cancer)
Interleukin-2 (IL-2)	Growth induction for T cells Activation of cytotoxic T cells Enhancement of NK function	(AIDS) (Cancer)
Interleukin-3 (IL-3)	Stimulation of proliferation and differentiation of granulocyte, macrophage, mast cell, megakaryocyte, early myeloid stem cell, and T and B cell lineages.	Neutropenia Aplastic anemia Transplantation
Interleukin-6 (IL-6)	Stimulation of B cell differentiation and IgG secretion Synergy with IL-3 for stimulation of early myeloid stem cells Stimulation of platelet production	(Aplastic anemia) (Transplantation)

[1]Items in parentheses indicate conditions that have been tested but not proven.

(3) Drug-associated neutropenia: GM-CSF has been used in HIV-infected patients who developed significant neutropenia after treatment with the antiretroviral agent zidovudine. Its role in this setting is still unproven.

(4) Neutropenia associated with hairy cell leukemia: G-CSF is effective in this setting.

(5) Cytotoxic chemotherapy: Neutropenia is virtually inevitable following full-dose multidrug cytotoxic therapy. Several trials have studied G-CSF and GM-CSF to determine whether they prevent or modify the severity of the neutropenia and permit complete treatment courses at full dosage. Encouraging but variable results have been reported, but it is likely that a combination of cytokines will prove to be the best approach.

(6) Transplantation: There are 2 possible uses in transplantation medicine. The first is to use cytokines to increase the neutrophil count in patients who have neutropenia posttransplant. The second is to use the cytokines in nonneutropenic patients to purge the bone marrow prior to autologous bone marrow transplantation. The latter is still under study.

(7) Aplastic anemia: GM-CSF, G-CSF, and IL-3 have all produced increases in neutrophil counts in such patients, but only while the drug is continued and with no effect on red cell and platelet counts. Their current use in this setting is therefore limited, mainly to support patients pending bone marrow transplantation for severe aplastic anemia.

The side effects of G-CSF are few, mainly axial bone pain during intravenous, (but not subcutaneous) therapy and splenomegaly with long-term treatment. GM-CSF has a wider range of side effects, including fever and, at higher doses, capillary leak (fluid retention) syndrome, pericarditis, and pleuritis.

It is clear that cytokine/growth factor therapy will increase in the future, especially with the development of combination therapy for multilineage effects (eg, IL-3 and G-CSF or GM-CSF).

ERYTHROCYTE DISORDERS

The erythrocyte disorders in which immune processes play an important role are the immune hemolytic anemias, paroxysmal nocturnal hemoglobinuria, and aplastic anemia and related disorders.

IMMUNE HEMOLYTIC ANEMIAS

The immune hemolytic disorders are classified in Table 33–3. The classification is based on the behavioral characteristics of antibodies involved and

Table 33–3. Classification of immune hemolytic anemias.

Autoimmune hemolytic anemias
A. Warm-antibody types
   1. Idiopathic warm autoimmune hemolytic anemia (AIHA)
   2. Secondary warm autoimmune hemolytic anemias
      a. SLE and other autoimmune disorders
      b. Chronic lymphocytic leukemia, lymphomas, etc
      c. Hepatitis and other viral infections
B. Cold-antibody types
   1. Idiopathic cold agglutinin syndrome
   2. Secondary cold agglutinin syndrome
      a. *Mycoplasma pneumoniae* infection; infectious mononucleosis and other viral infections
      b. Chronic lymphocytic leukemia, lymphomas, etc
   3. Paroxysmal cold hemoglobinuria
      a. Idiopathic
      b. Syphilis, viral infections

Drug-induced immune hemolytic anemias
   1. Drug absorption mechanism
   2. Membrane modification mechanism
   3. Immune complex mechanism

Partial list of drugs:

Aminosalicylic acid (PAS)	Methyldopa
Antihistamines	Penicillin
Carbromal	Phenacetin
Cephalothin	Pyramidon
Chlorinated hydrocarbons	Quinidine
Chlorpromazine	Quinine
Dipyrone	Rifampin
Insulin	Stibophen
Isoniazid	Sulfonamides
Levodopa	Sulfonylureas
Mefenamic acid	Tetracyclines
Melphalan	

Alloantibody-induced immune hemolytic anemias
A. Hemolytic transfusion reactions
B. Hemolytic disease of the newborn
C. Allograft-associated anemias

whether there is a demonstrable underlying disease. The clinical picture may be one of an acute self-limiting hemolytic disorder but is more often chronic. Since correct identification of the type of antibody is essential to correct diagnosis in patients with suspected immune hemolytic anemia, the immunologic laboratory investigation of such patients will be discussed before the individual diseases.

Immunologic Laboratory Investigations

There are 2 groups of immunologic tests necessary to properly investigate patients with suspected immune hemolytic anemias: (1) tests to detect and characterize antibodies involved in the hemolytic process, and (2) tests to aid in diagnosis of possible underlying disease processes. Tests that define underlying disorders include detection of anti-DNA antibodies and antinuclear antibody (ANA) in SLE, rheumatoid factors in rheumatoid arthritis, and monoclonal B cells in chronic lymphocytic leukemia.

The serologic tests used to characterize antibodies in serum and on erythrocytes are basic blood-banking procedures, with the addition of monospecific anti-

sera to identify specific proteins on erythrocytes and titration techniques to precisely quantitate antibody activity. Laboratory evaluation of such patients can be considered in terms of a series of questions: (1) Are the erythrocytes of the patient coated with immunoglobulin, complement components, or both? (2) How heavily are the erythrocytes sensitized? (3) What antibodies are eluted from the erythrocytes? (4) What antibodies are present in the serum?

Routine screening is performed by means of the direct antiglobulin (Coombs) test by tube or slide agglutination (see Chapter 15) using antisera with broad specificity. Subsequent evaluation requires testing the red cells with dilutions of monospecific antisera, especially antisera to IgG and C3. The autoantibody is examined at different temperatures to see whether the temperature of maximal activity identifies it as a "warm" or "cold" antibody.

False-negative and false-positive results can be obtained in direct antiglobulin tests. Approximately 20% of all patients with immune hemolytic anemias will have a negative or only weakly positive direct antiglobulin test unless the antiserum contains adequate titers of antibodies to complement components, especially C3. A positive direct antiglobulin test may be seen in situations other than autoantibodies on erythrocytes and does not necessarily mean autoimmune hemolytic anemia. Causes of such reactions include: (1) antibody formation against drugs rather than intrinsic erythrocyte antigens (see below); (2) damage to the erythrocyte membrane due to infection or cephalosporins, leading to nonimmunologic binding of proteins; (3) in vitro complement sensitization of erythrocytes by low-titer cold antibodies (present in many normal individuals) in clotted blood samples stored at 4 °C prior to separation; (4) delayed transfusion reactions; and (5) unknown mechanisms. The above reactions are generally weak and can be differentiated by clinical and detailed serologic studies.

Serologic investigations of the patient's serum and erythrocyte eluates should then answer another series of questions: (1) Are antibodies present? (2) Do they act as agglutinins, hemolysins, or incomplete antibodies? (3) What is their thermal range of activity? (4) What is their specificity?

The patient's serum is tested both undiluted and with fresh added complement against untreated and enzyme-treated pools of erythrocytes. Enzyme treatment enhances the sensitivity of the Ii system or abolishes activity in the case of the Pr system. The tests are run at both 37 and 20 °C and examined at 1 hour for agglutination and lysis. Cold agglutinin titration at 4 °C is also performed. Erythrocyte eluate is similarly tested.

Specialized tests may be performed to detect antibodies to drugs (eg, penicillin) in cases of drug-induced immune hemolytic anemia.

The specificity of the antibodies is tested at different temperatures with a panel of erythrocytes of different Rh genotypes and with cells of different types in the Ii blood group system (see below).

The results of the serologic investigations are then correlated with clinical and other laboratory investigations to establish a definitive diagnosis.

1. WARM AUTOIMMUNE HEMOLYTIC ANEMIA

Major Immunologic Features
- There is a positive direct antiglobulin (Coombs) test.
- Associated lymphoreticular cancer or autoimmune disease may be present.
- Splenomegaly is common.

General Considerations
Warm-antibody autoimmune hemolytic anemia is the most common type of immune hemolytic anemia. It may be either idiopathic or secondary to chronic lymphocytic leukemia, lymphomas, SLE or other autoimmune disorders or infections (Table 33–3). The idiopathic form may follow overt or subclinical viral infection.

Clinical Features
A. Symptoms and Signs: Patients usually present with symptoms of anemia and hemolysis. There may also be manifestations of an underlying disease, eg, lymphadenopathy, hepatosplenomegaly, or manifestations of autoimmune disease.

B. Laboratory Findings: Normochromic normocytic or slightly macrocytic anemia is usually present; spherocytosis is common, and nucleated erythrocytes may occasionally be found in the peripheral blood. Leukocytosis and thrombocytosis are often present, but occasionally (especially in SLE) leukopenia and thrombocytopenia are seen. There is usually a moderate to marked reticulocytosis. The bone marrow shows marked erythroid hyperplasia with plentiful iron stores. There is an increase in the serum level of indirect (unconjugated) bilirubin. Stool and urinary urobilinogen may be greatly increased. Transfused blood has a shortened survival time.

Immunologic Diagnosis
The results of the serologic tests discussed above are summarized in Table 33–4. The most common pattern is IgG and complement on erythrocytes, with IgG in the eluate. The eluate generally has no activity if the erythrocytes are sensitized only with complement.

Warm hemolysins active against enzyme-treated erythrocytes occur in 24% of sera, but warm serum agglutinins or hemolysins against untreated erythrocytes are rare. The indirect antiglobulin test (see Chapter 15) is positive at 37 °C in approximately 50–60% of patients' sera tested with untreated erythrocytes but in 90% of serum samples tested with enzyme-treated erythrocytes. This warm antibody is usually IgG but rarely may be IgM, IgA, or both.

The specificity of antibodies in warm antibody autoimmune hemolytic anemia is very complex, but the main specificity is directed against determinants in the Rh complex (see below).

Table 33–4. Summary of serologic findings in patients with autoimmune hemolytic anemia.[1]

| Disease Group | Erythrocytes | | | Serum | | |
	Direct Antiglobulin Test	Eluate	Immunoglobulin Type	Serologic Characteristics	Specificity
Warm antibody type	IgG 30% IgG + complement 50% Complement 20%	IgG IgG No activity	IgG (rarely also IgA or IgM)	Positive indirect antiglobulin test 50% Agglutination of enzyme-treated erythrocytes 90% Hemolysis of enzyme-treated erythrocytes 24% Agglutination of untreated erythrocytes (20 °C) 20% Agglutination or hemolysis of untreated erythrocytes (37 °C) Very rare	Rh system (often with a "nonspecific" component)
Cold agglutinin syndrome	Complement	No activity	IgM (rarely IgA)	High-titer cold agglutinin (usually 1:1000 at 4 °C) up to 32 °C; monoclonal IgM in chronic disease	Anti-I usually (can be anti-i or anti-Pr)
Paroxysmal cold hemoglobinuria (very rare)	Complement	No activity	IgG	Potent hemolysin also agglutinates normal cells. Biphasic (usually sensitizes cells in cold up to 15 °C and hemolyzes them at 37 °C)	Anti-P blood group

[1]Modified from Petz LD, Garratty G: Laboratory correlations in immune hemolytic anemias. Page 139 in: *Laboratory Diagnosis of Immunologic Disorders.* Vyas GN, Stites DP, Brecher G (editors). Grune & Stratton, 1975.

Differential Diagnosis

Congenital nonspherocytic hemolytic anemia, hereditary spherocytosis, and hemoglobinopathies can usually be differentiated by the family history, routine hematologic tests, hemoglobin electrophoresis, and a negative direct antiglobulin test.

Treatment

A. General Measures: Treatment of the primary disease is necessary. Blood transfusions may be necessary for life-threatening anemia but should be avoided when possible, since the transfused cells are rapidly destroyed. Careful serologic studies are needed to minimize the risks of serious hemolytic transfusion reactions, and successful cross-matching can be difficult or impossible in this situation. Alloantibodies are common and are difficult to detect.

B. Specific Measures: Hemolysis can be controlled with high doses of corticosteroids in most patients (40–120 mg of prednisone per day). The steroids are fairly rapidly tapered and then slowly reduced until the clinical state, hemoglobin level, and reticulocyte count indicate the appropriate maintenance dose. Occasionally it is possible to gradually withdraw steroids completely. Regular monitoring is necessary since relapses often occur in patients in remission.

Monitoring generally includes serologic studies, eg, direct and indirect antiglobulin tests, and these may show improvement with reduced amounts of IgG and complement on erythrocytes and lower antibody titers or a negative antibody test. However, there is no consistent correlation between clinical response and serologic tests; prednisone often induces clinical remissions in patients with warm-antibody autoimmune hemolytic anemia despite persistently positive direct antiglobulin tests.

If prednisone therapy fails or if unacceptable side effects occur, splenectomy is usually performed. Splenectomy is the treatment of choice if hemolysis persists after 2–3 months of corticosteroids and 60% respond to this procedure. ^{51}Cr-labeled erythrocyte survival studies can be used to identify abnormal splenic erythrocyte sequestration prior to splenectomy; however, clinical remissions may occur after splenectomy even when abnormal splenic sequestration cannot be documented. Continued significant hemolysis or late relapse sometimes occurs after splenectomy and requires therapy with steroids with or without other immunosuppressive agents.

Other immunosuppressive drugs include oral azathioprine (1.0–1.5 mg/kg/d for at least 3 months), cyclophosphamide at low dosage (1.0–1.5 mg/kg/d), or cyclosporin.

Prognosis

The prognosis of idiopathic warm-antibody autoimmune hemolytic anemia is fairly good; however, relapses are not infrequent, and death sometimes occurs. The prognosis of secondary warm autoimmune hemolytic anemia is determined by the underlying disease, eg, SLE or lymphoma.

2. COLD-AGGLUTININ SYNDROMES

These diseases may be primary or may be secondary to infection or lymphoma (Table 33–3). The infections include mycoplasmal pneumonia and infectious mononucleosis and other viral infections.

The clinical features are often those of the underlying disease. Cold-reactive symptoms such as Raynaud's phenomenon, livedo reticularis, or vascular purpura are seen in some patients. Hemolysis is generally mild but occasionally severe, especially in cases secondary to lymphoreticular cancer. The onset may be acute in cases secondary to infection. The idiopathic form is generally gradual in onset and runs a chronic and usually benign course in older patients.

These diseases usually are characterized by very high serum titers of agglutinating IgM antibodies which react optimally in the cold. These patients have cold-agglutinin titers in the thousands or millions, whereas normal individuals may have low-titer IgM cold agglutinins, and patients with chronic parasitic infections and most patients with *Ancylostoma* infection have titers up to 1:500. The presence of hemolysis is determined by the thermal range of the cold agglutinin. The high-titer, narrow-thermal-range antibodies will cause acral ischemic symptoms. Some, however, may have a low titer but a thermal range reacting up to 37 °C. The specificity of the IgM is generally anti-I in the Ii system, but occasionally it is anti-i or anti-Pr (Table 33–4). In chronic idiopathic cases or cases associated with lymphoreticular malignancy, the cold agglutinin is generally a monoclonal IgM-κ paraprotein. The direct antiglobulin test is always positive using antiserum to C3.

Treatment consists of keeping the patient warm and waiting for spontaneous resolution in acute cases. Chronic cases sometimes respond to chlorambucil or cyclophosphamide in low doses. Corticosteroids and splenectomy are probably not helpful, unless an underlying lymphoma is present.

The prognosis is generally good except for patients with severe underlying disease such as malignant lymphoma.

3. DRUG-INDUCED IMMUNE HEMOLYTIC ANEMIA

Many cases of immune hemolytic anemia have been reported in association with drug administration; the most common examples are included in Table 33–3. There are 3 stages in the investigation of a patient with suspected drug-induced hemolytic anemia: a history of intake of the drug, confirmation of hemolysis, and serologic tests. Detailed serologic tests are necessary, since different drugs produce hemolysis by different mechanisms. The immunopathologic mechanisms and clinical and laboratory features are summarized in Table 33–5. The mechanisms are classified as immune complex formation, hapten adsorption, nonspecific adsorption, and other, unknown mechanisms.

(1) Immune-complex formation: Circulating preformed immune complexes between the drug and antibody to the drug sensitize the erythrocyte ("innocent-bystander" phenomenon). Quinine in low doses is a typical example. There is great variability in clinical features and serologic findings.

(2) Drug (hapten) adsorption: The drug acts as a hapten in that it is bound to the erythrocyte membrane and stimulates the production of a high titer of antidrug antibodies.

(3) Nonspecific adsorption: The drug affects the erythrocytes so that various nonimmunologic proteins are adsorbed onto erythrocytes and give a positive Coombs test. This does not result generally in marked hemolysis.

(4) Unknown mechanisms: This type is exemplified by the positive Coombs test that develops within 3 months in 20% of patients treated with methyldopa. The IgG that coats erythrocytes in these patients does not have antibody activity against the drug, and the drug is not required in in vitro tests.

The hemolysis may be acute and severe, but only rarely is blood transfusion required. The main treatment is to stop the offending drug and monitor the patient to be sure the hemolysis disappears. The prognosis is therefore excellent.

4. PAROXYSMAL COLD HEMOGLOBINURIA

This rare disease may be transient or chronic and constitutes 10% of the cold autoimmune hemolytic anemias. It may occur as a primary idiopathic disease or secondary to syphilis or viral infection. It is characterized clinically by signs of hemolysis and hemoglobinuria following local or general exposure to cold. Symptoms may include combinations of fatigue, pallor, aching and pain in the back, legs, or abdomen, chills and fever, and the passing of dark brown urine. The symptoms may appear from within a few minutes to a few hours after exposure to cold.

The disease is characterized by the presence of the classic biphasic Donath-Landsteiner antibody. This polyclonal IgG antibody sensitizes erythrocytes in the cold (usually below 15 °C), so that complement components are detected on the erythrocytes by the direct antiglobulin test after rewarming. Heavily sen-

Table 33–5. Summary of immunopathologic mechanisms and clinical and laboratory features in drug-induced immune hemolytic disorders.[1]

Mechanism	Drugs	Clinical Findings	Serologic Evaluation	
			Direct Antiglobulin Test	Antibody Characterization
Immune complex formation (drug + antidrug antibody)	Quinine, quinidine, phenacetin	History of small doses of drugs. Acute intravascular hemolysis and renal failure. Thrombocytopenia occasionally found.	Complement (IgG occasionally also present).	Drug + patient's serum + enzyme-treated erythrocytes → Hemolysis, agglutination, or sensitization. Antibody often complement-fixing IgM. Eluate generally nonreactive.
Drug adsorption to erythrocyte membrane (combination with high-titer serum antibodies to drug)	Penicillins, cephalosporins	History of large doses of drugs. Other allergic features may be absent. Usually subacute extravascular hemolysis.	IgG (strongly positive if hemolysis occurs). Rarely, weak complement sensitization also present.	Drug-coated erythrocytes + serum → Agglutination or sensitization (rarely hemolysis). High-titer antibody. Eluate reacts only with antibiotic-coated erythrocytes.
Membrane modification (nonimmunologic adsorption of proteins to erythrocytes)	Cephalosporins	Hemolytic anemia rare.	Positive with reagents with antibodies to a variety of serum proteins.	Drug-coated erythrocytes + serum → Sensitization to antiglobulin antisera in low titer.
Unknown	Methyldopa	Gradual onset of hemolytic anemia. Common.	IgG (strongly positive if hemolysis occurs).	Antibody sensitizes normal erythrocytes without drug. Antibody in serum and eluate identical to warm antibody. No in vitro tests demonstrate relationship to drug.

[1]Adapted from Garratty G, Petz LD: Drug-induced immune hemolytic anemia. *Am J Med* 1975:**58:**398.

sitized cells are hemolyzed when warmed to 37 °C. The antibody has specificity for the P antigen.

Acute attacks are treated symptomatically, and postinfectious cases generally resolve spontaneously, but transfusion is often necessary.

5. HEMOLYTIC DISEASE OF THE NEWBORN

Immunologic Pathogenesis

During pregnancy, very small amounts of fetal blood leak into the maternal circulation, especially during the last trimester but usually does not trigger antibody formation in the mother. During delivery, when the placenta is detached, bleeding of cord blood into the mother's circulation can elicit an immune response to fetal erythrocyte alloantigens.

Hemolytic disease of the newborn results from the mother's antibodies crossing the placenta and destroying fetal erythrocytes. This leads to hemolytic anemia and hydrops in the newborn infant. Hyperbilirubinemia occurs as a postnatal complication.

The first child is seldom affected by the hemolytic disease, but the chances for alloimmunization increase with each incompatible pregnancy. The primary stimulus for immunization can also be a previous incompatible blood transfusion or abortion.

Formation of Rh antibodies is the most common form of alloimmunization to give rise to clinically important disease. Antibodies to blood groups A and B (see Chapter 15) may also cause hemolysis of fetal cells if IgG maternal antibodies cross the placenta. In these cases, the mother usually belongs to group O and the baby to group A. In fact, ABO immunization during pregnancy occurs more often than Rh immunization, but it seldom results in serious problems. If the fetus secretes soluble A or B substances, the maternal antibodies become neutralized before they cause damage to erythrocytes, since A or B substances are also present on other tissues, including the placental endothelium.

Clinical Features

The most frequent signs in the newborn are anemia and rapidly developing jaundice, usually within the first 24 hours (in contrast to the physiologic icterus that occurs later). The infant's response to the anemia is marked reticulocytosis and erythroblastosis. As bilirubin accumulates in the plasma, it may cross the blood-brain barrier and cause damage to the nervous system (kernicterus). Severe alloimmunization causes fetal hydrops, and the fetus may die in utero. In these cases, if the father is homozygous for the relevant blood group, the prognosis is very poor for future babies.

Immunologic Diagnosis

Since the cause of the disease is antibody on erythrocyte membrane, the direct Coombs test is usually positive. In ABO incompatibility, it is often negative. The reason for this is somewhat unclear, but the relatively small amount of IgG antibody and the adsorption by other tissues may result in so few antibody molecules on the erythrocyte surface that the conventional Coombs method is not able to detect them. Thus, a negative direct Coombs test does not rule out an immunologic cause for neonatal icterus. If antibodies are not found in the mother's serum, however, immune hemolysis is unlikely.

Alloimmunization should be detected during pregnancy. In many countries, all Rh-negative women are screened for the presence of blood group antibodies during pregnancy. As the number of D immunizations decreases, the relative proportion of immunizations to other blood groups has increased. Consequently, antibody screening should not be restricted to Rh-negative women. No reliable screening test is available for ABO disease, although several assays for detection of clinically important IgG anti-A or anti-B have been used.

When unexpected antibodies are found in the mother's serum, the father's blood groups should be determined. If the father is negative for the relevant blood group, there is no risk; if he is heterozygous, the baby has only a 50% chance of being affected. Increasing antibody titer or a history of previously ill children increases suspicion that the fetus can be affected, and amniocentesis is done to determine the concentration of bile pigments and possibly antibodies in the amniotic fluid. With these procedures and with ultrasound examination, the presence and seriousness of the hemolytic disease can be assessed. Detectable amounts of antibodies sometimes develop in the serum so late in the pregnancy that they remain unnoticed until the time of delivery. Alloimunization should always be suspected if the bilirubin level starts rising rapidly in an anemic newborn infant.

Treatment & Prevention

Treatment is started during the last trimester of pregnancy if amniocentesis and antibody determinations indicate that the fetus has serious disease. Compatible blood is injected into the abdominal cavity of the fetus and is rapidly absorbed into the circulation. Direct intravascular transfusion may be achieved by fetoscopy as early as 18 weeks, but only in specialized centers. The blood should be free of viable leukocytes to avoid the risk of subsequent graft-versus-host disease. Intrauterine transfusions may help the fetus to survive until mature enough to live outside the uterus. The last weeks of pregnancy are the most critical time for the fetus. Careful monitoring of clinical data by the obstetrician and neonatologist may prompt a decision to deliver the affected baby prior to term.

Immediately after delivery, the infant's blood group is determined and the cord cells are tested by the direct Coombs technique. If the baby is affected, exchange transfusions are usually needed, although in mild cases phototherapy with ultraviolet light or close supervision of bilirubin levels may be sufficient.

Women who have antibodies to the fetal erythrocytes should deliver in hospitals experienced in exchange transfusion. Despite modern advances in the treatment of hemolytic disease of the newborn, the mortality rate in severe intrauterine cases remains high.

Over 90% of Rh-negative women having Rh-positive offspring do not form anti-D antibodies. The immunization of the rest can be prevented by giving the mother 100 µg of concentrated anti-D (Rh₀) immunoglobulin within 72 hours of delivery if she does not have any preexisting anti-D antibodies. Since it is not possible to predict who will make antibodies, all Rh-negative women with an Rh-positive baby must be given prophylaxis. Since Rh antigens are detectable in an embryo a few weeks postconception, anti-D immunoglobulin should also be given to Rh-negative women who have aborted.

The mechanism of inhibition of antibody synthesis is unclear, but rapid destruction and clearance of Rh-positive cells from the circulation seem to play a role. In experimental conditions, Rh-positive cells coated with blood group antibodies other than anti-D are quickly destroyed and anti-D antibodies are not formed. Mothers with anti-A or anti-B antibodies reacting with fetal cells produce Rh antibodies less often than in ABO-compatible pregnancies.

Systematically applied anti-D prophylaxis has reduced the number of immunized women from about 7–8% to a little over 1% if measured by the number of Rh-negative women with antibodies after 2 consecutive Rh-positive babies. Several reasons have been suggested for the few failures: immunization early during the pregnancy (not starting at the time of delivery); abnormally large volume of fetal blood leaking into the maternal circulation with insufficient anti-D immunoglobulin; and unusual sensitivity of the maternal immune system to the antigen D.

PAROXYSMAL NOCTURNAL HEMOGLOBINURIA

This rare disease covers a wide spectrum of clinical presentations. It can occur in adults as a chronic hemolytic anemia with acute exacerbations. It may follow other hematologic disorders such as idiopathic or drug-induced bone marrow aplasia and may terminate in acute myelogenous leukemia. The intravascular hemolysis causes intermittent hemoglobinemia and hemoglobinuria. This activity fluctuates throughout the day, but the classic nocturnal timing of hemoglobinuria is seen in only 25% of cases. Venous thrombosis is a recognized complication.

The diagnosis is suggested by the findings of inter-mittent or chronic intravascular hemolysis, iron deficiency, hemosiderinuria, a low leukocyte alkaline phosphatase value, and frequently pancytopenia. The diagnosis of paroxysmal nocturnal hemoglobinuria is confirmed by any of the following tests: the acid hemolysis (Ham) test, the sugar water test, and the inulin test. These tests detect the abnormal clones with the 2 presently known abnormalities in paroxysmal nocturnal hemoglobinuria, ie, the exquisite sensitivity of paroxysmal nocturnal hemoglobinuria erythrocytes to complement lysis and the abnormally low acetylcholinesterase activity in the erythrocyte membrane.

Although the actual cause is unknown, several abnormalities have been defined on the various abnormal red cells (types I, II, and III). There is excessive binding of C3 molecules on the red cell membrane, partly from increased C3-convertase activity in the alternative pathway, partly from absent or reduced decay-accelerating factor, partly from deficiency of other factors that bind through a phosphatidylinositol linkage, and possibly from other factors.

The end result is that cells from such patients are more easily destroyed by complement than are normal cells. Patients' cells are lysed by approximately 4% of the amount of complement required to lyse normal erythrocytes.

Treatment is mainly symptomatic but otherwise unsatisfactory. Transfusions are often required, and reactions are not infrequent. Androgens may be useful if there is underlying bone marrow hypoplasia. Corticosteroids and splenectomy are probably not useful. Rarely, bone marrow transplantation may be possible.

APLASTIC ANEMIA & RELATED DISORDERS

Some cases of aplastic anemia and related disorders may be immunologic in origin.

Pure Erythrocyte Aplasia

This rare form of anemia is characterized by a marked reduction or absence of bone marrow erythroblasts and blood reticulocytes, with normal granulopoiesis and thrombopoiesis. It occurs as an acquired disorder in adults, either in an idiopathic form or associated with thymoma (in 30–50% of cases), lymphoma, other tumors, or certain drugs. Patients usually present with progressive anemia requiring transfusion support. Bone marrow examination confirms the diagnosis. Thymoma is present in a small number of patients. Other immunologic abnormalities, such as hypogammaglobulinemia, monoclonal gammopathy, autoimmune hemolytic anemia, myasthenia gravis, and features of SLE may be seen in patients with pure erythrocyte aplasia.

Many patients with pure erythrocyte aplasia, with

or without thymoma, have serum antibodies that react with bone marrow erythroblasts. These IgG antibodies have been demonstrated by immunofluorescence microscopy, with staining of nuclei of bone marrow erythroblasts. These antibodies fix complement and are specifically cytotoxic for erythroblasts. Plasma from patients with pure erythrocyte aplasia suppresses in vitro erythropoiesis by normal bone marrow, while bone marrow from patients with pure erythrocyte aplasia shows normal erythropoiesis when cultured in vitro in normal plasma. This plasma factor suppressing erythropoiesis in pure erythrocyte aplasia is an IgG antibody.

Patients with pure erythrocyte aplasia usually require total erythrocyte transfusion support. Patients with thymomas should have these tumors removed; this will produce a remission in about 30% of these patients. Patients with idiopathic pure erythrocyte aplasia and those who do not respond to thymectomy should be treated with intravenous gamma globulin (IVGG) if they do not have parvovirus infection, since some patients respond well to IVGG. If not, the next step is immunosuppressive drugs. Corticosteroids are usually used first, but few patients respond, and most are subsequently treated with cyclophosphamide plus prednisone. This combination produces remissions in 30–50% of patients, but relapses may occur when drugs are discontinued. Splenectomy has also been advocated for refractory patients with pure erythrocyte aplasia, as has plasma exchange.

Diamond-Blackfan Syndrome

This disorder, also known as congenital hypoplastic anemia, represents the congenital form of pure erythrocyte aplasia seen in infants. Anemia is usually noted in the first year of life but may occur later. These patients must be distinguished from patients with transient erythroblastopenia of infancy and childhood, which is a less serious, self-limited disorder.

There is heterogeneity in this syndrome in its clinical features, and, although it is familial, no single genetic mode of transmission has been confirmed.

The abnormality appears to be mainly in early erythroid stem cells since erythropoietin is normal. Recent studies have suggested that responses may be obtained with GM-CSF and IL-3, and a reduction in transfusion requirements is obtained with these agents.

Aplastic Anemia

Aplastic anemia is defined as pancytopenia due to bone marrow aplasia. Patients with severe aplastic anemia have no hematopoietic precursor cells present in their bone marrow and must be supported with erythrocyte and platelet transfusions and antibiotics.

In the past, aplastic anemia was usually associated with exposure to toxic drugs or chemicals (benzene, chloramphenicol, arsenicals, gold, anticonvulsants, etc). Recent series, however, indicate that most patients have no such exposure and no other associated illness, so that they are classified as having idiopathic aplastic anemia. Such patients should be tested for HIV infection.

Lymphocytes from the bone marrow of about one-third of patients with aplastic anemia suppress the growth of or kill granulocyte colonies from normal bone marrow in vitro. When these abnormal suppressor lymphocytes are separated from the marrow granulocytic stem cells or killed with a specific cytotoxic antilymphocyte serum, increased granulocyte colony formation occurs. Other investigators found that peripheral blood lymphocytes from patients with aplastic anemia may suppress erythropoiesis of normal bone marrow when cultured in vitro.

Problems in management exist with continuing transfusion support; even with optimal supportive care, severe aplastic anemia rarely undergoes spontaneous remission, and there is a 75–90% mortality rate. Trials have confirmed the efficacy of antilymphocyte globulin (ALG) in selected patients, with response in approximately 50% of patients. Treatment with high doses of androgens may benefit some patients, but few patients with severe aplasia respond. Treatment with GM-CSF, G-CSF, IL-3, or CSF-1 is only a short-term measure. Bone marrow transplantation produces longterm remissions in 50–80% of patients with severe aplastic anemia, and early bone marrow transplantation is currently considered the treatment of choice for patients with a histocompatible matched donor.

Aplastic anemia, therefore, may result from different defects involving the stem cells, the hematopoietic environment, cytokines/hemolymphopoietic growth factors, or suppressor cells. Characterization of the nature of the defects would permit more rational management of patients with aplastic anemia, since those patients with evidence of increased suppressor cell activity would be considered for treatment with immunosuppressive drugs or antithymocyte globulin (ATG) and those with obvious stem cell defects would be considered for early bone marrow transplantation.

PLATELET DISORDERS

Thrombocytopenia may be caused by decreased platelet production, increased platelet destruction, or abnormal platelet pooling. Immunologic thrombocytopenias, the subject of this section, are caused by increased platelet destruction, usually following platelet sensitization with antibody. Thrombocytopenias from decreased platelet production (aplastic anemia, leukemias, etc) have already been discussed with regard to immunologic features. Thrombocytopenia due to abnormal platelet pooling in an enlarged spleen (hypersplenism) is generally not associated with immunologic abnormalities.

Immunologic Mechanisms of Platelet Destruction

Several immunologic mechanisms of platelet damage leading to thrombocytopenia have been described. Platelet autoantibodies sensitize circulating platelets in idiopathic thrombocytopenic purpura and related disorders, leading to premature destruction of these cells in the spleen and generally involving Fc receptors on macrophages and other parts of the monocyte-machrophage system (see following section). Platelet alloantibodies may develop after multiple transfusions with blood products, or maternal sensitization can occur during pregnancies. Such platelet alloantibodies are becoming a major problem in long-term platelet support for patients with bone marrow failure. Alloantibodies may cause shortened platelet survival after transfusion or produce immediate platelet lysis with severe fever and chill reactions. Shortened platelet survival appears to be mediated by non-complement-dependent IgG or IgM antibodies similar to autoantibodies seen in idiopathic thrombocytopenic purpura. Platelet lysis, on the other hand, appears to be mediated by complement-dependent cytotoxic antibodies. These alloantibodies are directed primarily at HLA antigens, but non-HLA platelet antigens may also be involved. Alloantibody-dependent lymphocyte-mediated cytotoxicity has also been described in some patients. Neonatal thrombocytopenia due to passive transfer of maternal alloantibody or autoantibody is fortunately rare but may be life-threatening when it occurs.

Other immunologic mechanisms of platelet destruction include development of antibodies to drugs or other antigenic substances (haptens) absorbed to the platelet membrane and adsorption of preformed antigen-antibody complexes onto the platelet membrane, with rapid removal of these sensitized cells from the circulation ("innocent-bystander" phenomenon). The reactions are often complement-dependent. These mechanisms occur in drug-induced immune thrombocytopenia, in some infections, especially HIV, and in autoimmune disorders such as SLE. It has been suggested that cell-mediated immunity, ie, lymphocyte activation, may alone be able to cause platelet damage and thrombocytopenia. Lymphocyte activation has been observed in response to autologous platelets in some patients with idiopathic thrombocytopenic purpura. Whether this represents a true cellular immune response or whether the lymphocytes are reacting to immune complexes or otherwise altered platelets remains uncertain. Finally, it is known that bacterial endotoxin can cause thrombocytopenia directly, usually involving activation of the complement system. Antibodies are not required for this reaction.

Table 33–6 shows a classification of immunologic thrombocytopenias that are discussed in more detail in the following section.

IDIOPATHIC THROMBOCYTOPENIC PURPURA

Major Immunologic Features

- Antiplatelet antibodies are demonstrable on platelets and in serum.
- Platelet survival is shortened.
- There is a therapeutic response to prednisone and splenectomy.

General Considerations

Idiopathic thrombocytopenic purpura is an autoimmune disorder characterized by increased platelet destruction by antiplatelet autoantibody. IgG autoantibodies sensitize the circulating platelets, leading to accelerated removal of these cells by the macrophages of the spleen and at times the liver and other components of the monocyte-macrophage system. Although there is a compensatory increase in platelet production by the bone marrow (total platelet

Table 33–6. Classification of immune thrombocytopenias.

Idiopathic (autoimmune) thrombocytopenic purpura (ITP)
Secondary autoimmune thrombocytopenias
SLE and other autoimmune disorders
Chronic lymphocytic leukemia, lymphomas, some nonlymphoid malignancies
HIV infection
Infectious mononucleosis and some other infections
Drug-induced immune thrombocytopenias (partial list of drugs)

Acetazolamide	Imipramine
Allymid	Meprobamate
Aminosalicylic acid (PAS)	Methyldopa
Antazoline	Novobiocin
Apronalide	Phenolphthalein
Aspirin	Phenytoin
Carbamazepine	Quinidine
Cephalothin	Quinine
Chlorothiazide	Rifampin
Digitoxin	Spironolactone
Factor VIII concentrate	Stibophen
Heparin	Sulfamethazine
Hydrochlorothiazide	Thioguanine

Posttransfusion purpura
Thrombotic thrombocytopenic purpura (TTP)
Neonatal immune thrombocytopenias
Due to autoantibodies (ITP)
Due to alloantibodies (maternal sensitization)
Due to alloantibodies (destruction of transfused platelets)
Sensitization from previous transfusions
Maternal sensitization during pregnancies

turnover may be 10–20 times the normal rate), thrombocytopenia occurs, and, depending on the severity, gives rise to the 2 typical clinical features of the disease: purpura and bleeding.

Idiopathic thrombocytopenic purpura most often occurs in otherwise healthy children and young adults. Childhood idiopathic thrombocytopenic purpura often occurs within a few weeks following a viral infection, suggesting possible cross-immunization between viral and platelet antigens, or adsorption of immune complexes, or a hapten mechanism. Adult idiopathic thrombocytopenic purpura is less often associated with a preceding infection. An identical form of autoimmune thrombocytopenia can also be associated with SLE, chronic lymphocytic leukemia, lymphomas, nonlymphoid cancers, infectious mononucleosis, and other viral and bacterial infections. Certain drugs can also cause immune thrombocytopenia, and these can produce a clinical picture that is indistinguishable from idiopathic thrombocytopenic purpura.

Although adult and childhood idiopathic thrombocytopenic purpura appear to have similar basic pathophysiologic features, there are significant differences in their course and therefore their treatment. The features of idiopathic thrombocytopenic purpura in children and adults are compared in Table 33–7. Most children have spontaneous remissions within a few weeks to a few months, and splenectomy is rarely necessary. Adult patients, on the other hand, rarely have spontaneous remissions and usually require splenectomy within the first few months after diagnosis. Idiopathic thrombocytopenic purpura has been described in many AIDS patients, and HIV-associated immune thrombocytopenic purpura is recognized more frequently in patients infected with HIV who have not yet had an AIDS-associated disease.

Immunologic Diagnosis

Harrington and coworkers first showed in 1951 that the plasma from patients with idiopathic thrombocytopenic purpura caused thrombocytopenia when transfused into normal human recipients. Techniques to detect antiplatelet antibodies are shown in Table 33–8. Immuno-injury techniques (platelet factor 3 release, ^{14}C-serotonin release) detect antiplatelet anti-

Table 33–7. Idiopathic thrombocytopenic purpura in children and adults

Parameter	Children	Adults
Peak age incidence (yr)	2–6	20–30
Sex incidence (M:F)	1:1	1:3
Clinical onset	Acute	Gradual
Antecedent infection	Common	Uncommon
Average duration of disease	1 mo	Months to years
Spontaneous remission	90%	10–20%
Presenting platelet count	$< 20 \times 10^9$/L	$(30–50) \times 10^9$/L

Table 33–8. Tests for platelet autoantibodies in idiopathic thrombocytopenic purpura (ITP).

Method	Percent Positive
Standard immunologic tests (agglutination, complement fixation, etc)	0
Transfusion of plasma from patients with ITP into normal donors	63–75
Platelet factor 3 release	65–70
^{14}C-serotonin release	60
Lymphocyte activation by autologous platelets	70
Lymphocyte activation by platelet-antibody immune complexes	90 +
Phagocytosis of platelet-antibody immune complexes by granulocytes	90 +
Measurement of platelet-associated IgG by competitive binding assays	90 +
Radiolabeled Coombs antiglobulin test	90 +
Fluorescein-labeled Coombs antiglobulin	90 +
Enzyme-linked immunosorbent assay (ELISA)	90 +

bodies in the serum of 60–70% of adult patients with idiopathic thrombocytopenic purpura. Other methods to show positive results in almost all patients with idiopathic thrombocytopenic purpura include methods to detect platelet-autoantibody complexes by lymphocyte activation or ingestion by granulocytes, or competitive binding assays or antiglobulin tests for the measurement of antiplatelet antibodies on the platelet surface.

Platelet Kinetics

^{51}Cr-platelet kinetic studies show that all patients with idiopathic thrombocytopenic purpura and other types of autoimmune thrombocytopenia have markedly shortened platelet survival times ($t_{1/2}$ 0.1–30 hours; normal $t_{1/2}$ 100–120 hours) and have normal or only slightly subnormal platelet recoveries at t_0 (40–80%; normal 60–80%). About 75% of patients have splenic platelet sequestration, and 25% have both splenic and hepatic sequestration. Patients with thrombocytopenia due to an enlarged splenic platelet pool can be easily distinguished from patients with autoimmune thrombocytopenia by these kinetic methods. Both groups had an 85–90% complete remission rate at 2 years' follow-up postsplenectomy.

Clinical Features

A. Symptoms and Signs: The onset may be acute, with sudden development of petechiae, ecchymoses, epistaxis, and gingival, gastrointestinal, or genitourinary tract bleeding. More commonly, the disease is gradual in onset and chronic in course. Often, however, chronic idiopathic thrombocytopenic purpura is slowly progressive or suddenly becomes acute.

B. Laboratory Findings: The platelet count is usually less than 20,000–30,000/μL in acute cases and 30,000–100,000/μL in chronic cases. There may be moderate anemia due to blood loss and iron deficiency. The leukocyte count is normal or slightly increased but may be low in SLE. Platelets are often larger than normal on peripheral blood smear, and no immature leukocytes are present. The bone marrow shows normal or increased numbers of megakaryocytes and is otherwise normal. The megakaryocytes may be normal or immature in appearance but at times are larger than normal with increased numbers of nuclei.

Differential Diagnosis

All causes of thrombocytopenia must be considered when evaluating a patient with suspected idiopathic thrombocytopenic purpura (Table 33–9). Patients with idiopathic thrombocytopenic purpura characteristically feel and look well, and all physical and laboratory findings are normal except for thrombocytopenia and the associated purpura and possible bleeding. Patients with "consumptive" thrombocytopenias, on the other hand, tend to be acutely ill, often with fever and evidence of multisystem disease, especially renal disease. These patients generally have microangiopathic hemolytic anemia, the fragmented erythrocytes being a critical diagnostic finding on the peripheral blood smear. Abnormalities of clotting function are also often present. Patients with acute leukemia, aplastic anemia, and other serious bone marrow disorders are also often acutely ill, and bone marrow examination is diagnostic. Patients with hypersplenism sufficient to cause thrombocytopenia usually have an easily palpable spleen; hypersplenism alone rarely causes a platelet count of less than 50,000/μL.

Secondary causes of autoimmune thrombo-

Table 33–9. Differential diagnosis of thrombocytopenic purpuras.

Thrombocytopenias due to increased platelet destruction
Immune thrombocytopenias
  Idiopathic thrombocytopenic purpura
  Secondary autoimmune thrombocytopenias
  Drug-induced immune thrombocytopenias
  Posttransfusion purpura
  Neonatal immune thrombocytopenias
  Thrombocytopenia due to use of factor VIII concentrate
  HIV infection
Consumptive thrombocytopenias
  Thrombotic thrombocytopenic purpura
  Hemolytic-uremic syndrome
  Disseminated intravascular coagulation
  Vasculitis
  Sepsis
Hypersplenism
Thrombocytopenias due to decreased platelet production
Bone marrow suppression by drugs, alcohol, toxins, infections
Aplastic anemia
Leukemias and other bone marrow cancers
Megaloblastic anemia
Refractory anemias, preleukemia, hematopoietic dysplasia

cytopenia, such as HIV infection and SLE, must be ruled out by appropriate laboratory tests. If a patient with apparent idiopathic thrombocytopenic purpura has been taking any suspicious drugs, the possibility of drug-induced thrombocytopenia must be considered. In some areas, HIV-associated disease is now the most common cause of thrombocytopenic purpura, especially in males between 20 and 50 years of age. Testing for antibodies to HIV is an essential part of the assessment of idiopathic thrombocytopenic purpura.

Treatment

Management of patients with idiopathic thrombocytopenic purpura is based mainly on clinical features and progress.

If the patient is asymptomatic and the platelet count remains over 30,000/μL, observation is the preferred approach.

Children with mild or moderately severe idiopathic thrombocytopenic purpura should be observed without therapy. In children who require active treatment, IVGG is the treatment of choice. A 5-day course of 400 mg/kg/d is given. Responses occur in 75% in 1–4 days, but many patients respond for only a short time, and repeat courses may be necessary.

Splenectomy is the treatment of choice for adult patients with idiopathic thrombocytopenic purpura who have persistent symptomatic thrombocytopenia. Corticosteroids (prednisone, 1–2 mg/kg/d) are usually able to increase the platelet count temporarily but probably do not alter the course of the underlying disease, and most patients relapse when steroid use is tapered or discontinued. Adults rarely have spontaneous remissions. Splenectomy is therefore usually necessary in adults with idiopathic thrombocytopenic purpura within the first few months after diagnosis. Large doses of steroids over long periods should be avoided in these patients, since 75–90% will have prolonged complete remissions following splenectomy. Immunosuppressive therapy with cytotoxic drugs should generally not be used until the patient has had the benefit of splenectomy; this is particularly true for younger patients, since these drugs may cause serious late adverse effects.

Vincristine seems to be a valuable agent in patients with autoimmune thrombocytopenia who do not respond to splenectomy, who relapse after an initial response to splenectomy, or in whom the risk of splenectomy is unacceptable. A significant increase in platelet count occurs in 70–80% of patients with refractory autoimmune thrombocytopenia treated with vincristine. Vincristine appears to be more effective, less toxic, and better tolerated than cyclophosphamide or other standard immunosuppressive drugs. Its mechanism of action in increasing the platelet count in autoimmune thrombocytopenia remains uncertain; it appears to work by a different mechanism from other immunosuppressive drugs. IVGG may be used as a short-term measure in adults prior to splenec-tomy, if corticosteriod has failed to maintain a satis-factory platelet count at an acceptable dose. IVGG is also used in patients with HIV-associated immune thrombocytopenic purpura, prior to splenectomy, where one would prefer not to use long-term immu-nosuppressive and cytotoxic therapy. Zidovudine (AZT) is effective in raising platelet counts in pa-tients with HIV-associated immune thrombocytope-nic purpura.

Corticosteroids may be given when severe throm-bocytopenia and bleeding occur in children, although the platelet count does not respond as consistently to steroids in children as in adults. Splenectomy should be considered in children only when severe throm-bocytopenia persists for 3–6 months, since most chil-dren will have had a spontaneous remission by that time. The postsplenectomy state is much more likely to predispose to serious or overwhelming infection in young children than in adults. Immunosuppressive drugs should generally not be used in children.

DRUG-INDUCED IMMUNE THROMBOCYTOPENIAS

The principal drugs that may cause immune throm-bocytopenic purpura are listed in Table 33–6. The best-studied example was the sedative apronalide (Sedormid) (no longer in use); the drugs most com-monly used in clinical practice that can produce im-mune thrombocytopenic purpura are sulfonamides, thiazide diuretics, chlorpropamide, quinidine, hepa-rin, and gold. A syndrome resembling acute drug-in-duced immune thrombocytopenia has also been ob-served in heroin addicts, although the mechanism of this kind of thrombocytopenia has not been proved. Further reports have confirmed the increasing fre-quency of the heparin-induced thrombosis thrombo-cytopenia syndrome. This unusual combination in-cludes clinical features of hemorrhagic tendencies due to development of thrombocytopenia in patients treated with heparin for thrombosis. It appears that the heparin-dependent IgG-class antibody induces thromboxane synthesis and aggregation of the plate-lets.

There is a variable period of sensitization after ini-tial exposure to the drug, but subsequent drug reexposure is rapidly followed by thrombocytopenia. Patients therefore usually give a history of having taken the drug in the past for at least several weeks if this is their first exposure. A very small plasma con-centration of the drug and very small amounts of an-tibody may induce severe thrombocytopenia. The drug itself generally shows only weak and reversible binding to the platelet; the thrombocytopenia in most cases appears to be caused by adsorption of the drug-antibody complexes to the platelet membrane with complement activation.

Treatment consists mainly of withdrawal of the of-fending drug (or all drugs) and monitoring for return of normal platelet counts, generally within 7–10 days. Thrombocytopenia may persist if the drug is excreted slowly. When a patient who is taking a num-ber of suspicious drugs is first seen, it is often impos-sible to tell whether the patient has drug-induced immune thrombocytopenia or idiopathic thrombocy-topenic purpura. In vitro tests can now be used in some centers to confirm drug-antibody reactions in-volving platelets. In vivo drug challenges of sensi-tized patients for confirmation of drug-induced im-mune thrombocytopenia should be avoided, since they are too hazardous.

POSTTRANSFUSION PURPURA

There are 2 types of posttransfusion purpura. The first is due to dilution and occurs during massive blood replacement, as in the treatment of hemorrhage and shock. Further bleeding from the dilutional thrombocytopenia may complicate clinical manage-ment. The second type, which is due to alloantibod-ies, is an acute severe thrombocytopenic state appear-ing about 1 week after transfusion of a blood product. It occurs almost exclusively in women. It is mediated by an alloantibody, usually directed against the plate-let Pl^{A1} antigen. Platelets both with and without the Pl^{A1} antigen are destroyed.

The diagnosis is suspected when acute thrombo-cytopenia occurs 7–10 days after blood transfusion. Coagulation studies are normal, and the bone marrow shows abundant megakaryocytes. The anti-Pl^{A1} anti-body is detected in the plasma.

Gradual recovery from posttransfusion purpura usually occurs in 1–6 weeks. Corticosteroids do not appear to alter the course of the disease. Massive ex-change transfusions have been associated with more rapid recovery, but severe transfusion reactions often occur. Aggressive plasma exchange has also been shown to be effective without the risks of severe transfusion reactions.

COAGULATION DISORDERS

HEMOPHILIA & VON WILLEBRAND'S DISEASE

Classic hemophilia and von Willebrand's disease are both congenital bleeding disorders caused by ab-normalities of the factor VIII molecule complex. He-mophilia is an X-linked disorder characterized by se-vere deficiency of factor VIII procoagulant activity

(VIII:C), which is measured in clotting assays. Von Willebrand's disease is an autosomally inherited disorder also characterized by a deficiency of VIII:C, but it is also associated with defective platelet function, resulting in a prolonged bleeding time. The abnormal platelet function in von Willebrand's disease is due to a deficiency of factor VIII-related protein (VIIIR), which is also known as von Willebrand factor (vWF). vWF activity is measured by testing the ability of plasma to support platelet agglutination by the antibiotic ristocetin or ristocetin cofactor (VIIIR:RC) activity.

The gene for factor VIII is located near the tip of the long arm of the X chromosome (Xq2.8/Ter). The large gene has approximately 186 kb with 27 exons. Defects in the hemophilia A gene include point mutations and partial deletions, so there is heterogeneity in defective factor VIII molecules.

Heterogeneous antibodies made to purified factor VIII are able to detect antigenic determinants on VIIIR (VIIIR:Ag). VIIIR:Ag has been found to be normal in patients with classic hemophilia, indicating that these patients have a normal amount of the basic factor VIII molecule but that they lack the portion of the molecule necessary for normal procoagulant activity. The heterologous antibodies therefore appear to recognize antigenic determinants distinct from the functional site responsible for procoagulant activity. Patients with von Willebrand's disease, on the other hand, have reduced levels of both VIII:C and VIIIR:Ag, indicating a true deficiency of factor VIII complex molecules. Measurement of VIII:C and VIIIR:Ag can therefore be used to differentiate between classic hemophilia and von Willebrand's disease and in most cases can differentiate between female carriers of hemophilia (heterozygotes) and normal individuals. Measurement of ristocetin cofactor (VIIIR:RC) can also be used to identify patients with von Willebrand's disease. Studies with antibodies have helped to clarify the relationships of the factor VIII complex.

Prenatal diagnosis is now possible for hemophilia A with a chorionic villus biopsy and restriction fragment length polymorphism methods or a polymerase chain searcher (PCR) assay.

Human antibodies to factor VIII, unlike heterologous antibodies, are usually directed at antigenic determinants at the functional procoagulant site of factor VIII (VIII:CAg), and these antibodies are capable of blocking factor VIII clotting activity. These antibodies sometimes develop in patients with severe hemophilia after they have been transfused with factor VIII-containing blood products and sometimes develop spontaneously in otherwise healthy individuals. When present in high titer, they cause a severe hemorrhagic disorder that is difficult to correct with factor VIII transfusions, since the transfused factor VIII is simply inactivated by the factor VIII antibodies (see next section).

Most hemophiliacs treated in the early 1980s with factor VIII concentrate have developed AIDS, and AIDS is now the most common cause of death in hemophiliacs. Centers switched from treating the hemophiliac with factor VIII concentrate from large donor pools back to using cryoprecipitate from a single donor. Infectivity can be abolished by heating the preparation.

It is hoped that in the future, recombinant engineered factor VIII will be available to overcome problems with supply, purity, and cross-infection.

CIRCULATING INHIBITORS OF COAGULATION

Abnormal bleeding is occasionally due to circulating inhibitors that block one or more plasma coagulation factors. These inhibitors, also called endogenous circulating anticoagulants, have in most cases been shown to be IgG antibodies. Inhibitors against factor VIII and against the prothrombin activator complex ("lupus inhibitor") occur most often, but inhibitors directed against factors V, IX, XIII, and vWF have also been reported. There are rare reports of human monoclonal proteins (especially IgM) with antibody activity directed against clotting components, eg, factor VIII, phospholipid. Inhibitors may appear abruptly and be associated with life-threatening hemorrhage or may be chronic and associated with little or no bleeding.

Factor VIII inhibitors develop in 15% of patients with classic hemophilia after they have been transfused with factor VIII-containing blood products; genetic factors appear to determine which patients develop inhibitors. Factor VIII inhibitors also occasionally occur spontaneously in women postpartum, in patients with autoimmune disorders such as SLE, and in older patients without demonstrable underlying disease. Rarely, the paraprotein in a monoclonal gammopathy has specific inhibitor activity against factor VIII or other clotting factors.

High-titer factor VIII inhibitors (antibodies) often cause serious bleeding and require aggressive treatment. Patients with serious bleeding can be given several times the calculated amount of factor VIII to saturate the inhibitor, provided the inhibitor titer is not too high. When bleeding cannot be stopped, even after giving large amounts of factor VIII, activated prothrombin complex concentrates should be given, since these will often stop the bleeding by providing activated clotting factors which bypass the factor VIII step. If this is unsuccessful, aggressive large-volume plasma exchange can be used to remove the inhibitor.

A recent study found that combination therapy with factor VIII, cyclophosphamide, vincristine, and prednisone (CVP) was highly effective in the eradication of factor VIII inhibitors in nonhemophiliacs, but not in hemophiliacs.

Anticardiolipin Antibody (Lupus Anticoagulant)

The lupus anticoagulant was so named because of its initial identification in association with SLE, but the term has turned out to be a slight misnomer. The lupus anticoagulant appears to be an IgG anticardiolipin antibody directed at phospholipid epitopes which explains false-positive syphilis serologic screening tests. Anticardiolipin antibody should be suspected in patients with a prolongation of the partial thromboplastin time, but it is associated only with classic SLE in a minority of patients and is not associated with an in vivo hemostatic defect. Paradoxi-

cally, the lupus anticoagulant is associated with a venous and arterial thrombotic tendency. A distinct syndrome has been identified in recent years, with recurrent arterial and venous thrombosis, recurrent abortion due to placental infarction, and thrombocytopenia. Venous thrombosis may occur in unusual sites, such as hepatic, renal, retinal, and mesenteric veins. Classic SLE serologic tests in this group of patients are often negative. Specialized tests are necessary to further categorize this unusual hemostatic defect.

Recently, circulating coagulation inhibitors similar to lupus anticoagulant were reported in AIDS patients with active opportunistic infections. The inhibitors tended to disappear with successful resolution of the infection.

REFERENCES

Leukopenias

Goldman JM: Granulocytes, monocytes, and their benign disorders. Chapter 11 in: *Postgraduate Haematology.* Hoffbrand AV, Lewis SM (editors). Heinemann, 1989.

Levine JD et al: Recombinant human granulocyte-macrophage colony-stimulating-factor ameliorates zidovudine-induced neutropenia in patients with acquired immunodeficiency syndrome (AIDS)/AIDS-related complex. *Blood* 1991;**78:**3148.

Lieschke GJ et al: Effects of bacterially synthesized recombinant human granulocyte-macrophage colony-stimulating factor in patients with advanced malignancy. *Ann Intern Med* 1989;**110:**357.

Minchinton RM, Waters AH: The occurrence and significance of neutrophil antibodies. *Br J Haematol* 1984;**56:**521.

Robinson BE, Quesenberry PJ: Hematopoietic growth factors: overview and clinical applications. *Am J Med Sci* 1990;**300:**163, 237, 311. (Three parts.)

Schaafsma et al: In vivo production of interleukin-5, granulocyte-macrophage colony-stimulating factor, and interleukin-6 during intravenous administration of high-dose interleukin-2 in cancer patients. *Blood* 1991;**178:**1981.

Takahashi K et al: Human recombinant granulocyte colony-stimulating factor for the treatment of autoimmune neutropenia. *Acta Haematol* 1991;**86:**95.

Verhoef G, Boogaerts M. In vivo administration of granulocyte-macrophage colony-stimulating factor enhances neutrophil function in patients with myelodysplastic syndromes. *Br J Haematol* 1991;**79:**177.

Erythrocyte Disorders

Beal RW, Isbister JP: *Blood Component Therapy in Clinical Practice,* Blackwell, 1985.

Bertrand Y et al: The successful treatment of two cases of severe aplastic anaemia with granulocyte colony-stimulating factor and cyclosporine A. *Br J Haematol* 1991;**79:**648.

Dunbar CE et al: Treatment of Diamond-Blackjan anaemia with haematopoietic growth factors, granulocyte-macrophage colony-stimulating factor and interleukin 3: Sustained remissions following IL-3. *Br J Haematol* 1991;**79:**316.

Engelfriet CP, Van Logham JJ, Von Dem Borne AEGK: *Immunohaematology.* Elsevier, 1984.

Eschbach JW et al: Recombinant human erythropoietin in anemic patients with end-stage renal disease. Results of a phase III multicenter clinical trial. *Ann Intern Med* 1989;**111:**992.

Finelli C et al: Steroid-resistant acquired pure red cell aplasia: A partial remission induced by recombinant human erythropoietin. *Br J Haematol* 1991;**79:**125.

Gordon-Smith EC, Hows J: Acquired haemolytic anaemias. Chapter 7 in: *Postgraduate Haematology.* Hoffbrand AV, Lewis SM (editors). Heinemann, 1989.

Klingemann HG et al: Bone marrow transplantation in patients aged 45 years and older. *Blood* 1986;**67:**770.

Marsh JCW et al: Survival after antilymphocyte globulin therapy for aplastic anemia depends on disease severity. *Blood* 1987;**70:**1046.

Petz LD, Garratty G: *Acquired Immune Hemolytic Anemias.* Churchill Livingstone, 1980.

Rosse WF, Parker CJ: Paroxysmal nocturnal hemoglobinuria. *Clin Hematol* 1985;**14:**105.

Sanders JE et al: Bone marrow transplantation experience for children with aplastic anemia. *Pediatrics* 1986;**77:**179.

Platelet Disorders

Bussel JB, Hilgartner MW: The use and mechanism of action of intravenous immunoglobulin in the treatment of immune haematologic disease. *Br J Haematol* 1984;**56:**1.

Cines DB et al: Platelet antibodies of the IgM class in immune thrombocytopenic purpura. *J Clin Invest* 1985;**75:**1183.

Firkin BG: *The Platelet and Its Disorders.* MTP Press, 1984.

Hardisty RM: Platelet disorders. Chapter 22 in: *Postgraduate Haematology.* Hoffbrand AV, Lewis SM (editors). Heinemann, 1989.

Karpatkin S, Nardi MA, Hymes KB: Immunologic thrombocytopenic purpura after heterosexual transmission of human immunodeficiency virus (HIV). *Ann Intern Med* 1988;**109:**190.

Kelton JG: The measurement of platelet-bound immunoglobulins: An overview of the methods and the biological relevance of platelet-associated IgG. *Prog Hematol* 1983;**13:**163.

Leaf AN et al: Thrombotic thrombocytopenic purpura associated with human immunodeficiency virus type 1 (HIV-1) infection. *Ann Intern Med* 1988;**109:**194.

Oksenhendler E et al: Zidovudine for thrombocytopenic purpura related to human immunodeficiency virus (HIV) infection. *Ann Intern Med* 1989;**110:**365.

Tomar A et al: Menstrual cyclic thrombocytopenia. *Br J Haematol* 1989;**71:**519.

Coagulation Disorders

Cohen AJ, Philips TM, Kessler CM: Circulating coagulation inhibitions in the acquired immunodeficiency syndrome. *Ann Intern Med* 1986;**104:**175.

Einstein BI: The polymerase chain reactions. A new method of using molecular genetics for medical diagnosis. *N Engl J Med* 1990;**332:**178.

Eyster ME at al: Long term follow-up of hemophiliacs with lymphocytopenia or thrombocytopenia. *Blood* 1985;**66:**1317.

Gastineau DA et al: Lupus anticoagulant: An analysis of the clinical and laboratory features of 219 cases. *Am J Hematol* 1985;**19:**265.

Kasper CK: Treatment of factor VIII inhibitors. *Prog Hemostasis Thromb* 1989;**9:**57.

Lian ECY, Larcada AF, Chiu AYZ: Combination immunosuppressive therapy after factor VIII infusion for acquired factor VIII inhibitor. *Ann Intern Med* 1989;**110:**774.

Lottenberg R, Kentro TB, Kitchens CS: Acquired hemophilia. A natural history study of 16 patients with factor VIII inhibitors receiving little or no therapy. *Arch Intern Med* 1987;**147:**1077.

Triplett DA, Brandt J: Laboratory identification of the lupus anticoagulant. *Br J Haematol* 1989;**73:**139.

Warkentin TE, Kelton JG. Heparin-induced thrombocytopenia. *Annu Rev Med* 1989;**40:**31.

White GC, Shoemaker CB. Factor VIII gene and hemophilia A. *Blood* 1989;**73:**1.

34   Cardiac & Vascular Diseases

Thomas R. Cupps, MD

CARDIAC DISEASES

A variety of immunologic diseases probably involve cardiac tissues without causing any clinically relevant effects; nevertheless, there are several recognized syndromes characterized by clinically significant immune-mediated damage of the pericardium, myocardium, and endocardium.

PERICARDIAL DISEASES

Relapsing Pericarditis

This is a disease of unknown cause, characterized by chronic recurrent episodes of pericardial inflammation. Other disease processes associated with pericarditis, including infection, neoplasm, and collagen vascular disease, should be actively excluded. Chest pain and shortness of breath with or without pericardial effusion make up the characteristic pattern during an episode of pericarditis. Complications including pericardial tamponade, hemopericardium, and constrictive pericarditis have been reported. Nonsteroidal anti-inflammatory drugs, such as aspirin and ibuprofen, constitute the initial form of treatment. Some patients with relapsing pericarditis develop a chronic pattern, which requires treatment with corticosteroids. A subset of these patients may become corticosteroid-dependent, requiring prolonged suppressive treatment. Pericardiectomy may be considered in patients who cannot be successfully treated medically.

An immunologic pathogenesis for this disease is presumed, largely on the basis of histopathology, which includes infiltration by acute and chronic inflammatory cells and fibrin deposition.

Postinfarction Syndrome & Postpericardiotomy Syndrome

Pericardial inflammation also occurs following damage to cardiac tissue after myocardial infarction, cardiac surgery, or trauma. Postinfarction (Dresseler's) syndrome is characterized by chest pain, profound malaise, fever, pericardial inflammation and effusion, leukocytosis with or without pleural effusion, pulmonary infiltrates, arthralgia, or transient arthritis that develops 2–3 weeks following surgical or traumatic opening of the pericardium. The presence of myocyte antibodies detected by immunofluorescence and rising titers of antiviral antibodies suggests that these syndromes may be associated with a concurrent or reactivated viral illness triggering the immunologic response that produces the characteristic clinical syndrome. Increasing titers of antibodies to coxsackie virus type B, cytomegalovirus, and adenovirus occur frequently. The response is therefore not limited to a particular type of virus. The postinfarction syndrome occurs in 3% or fewer of patients with myocardial infarction. The presence of a pericardial friction rub during the first several days postinfarction increases the likelihood of developing the syndrome. The postpericardiotomy syndrome occurs in approximately 25% of patients following surgical intervention or blunt trauma to the heart. Rare complications include pericardial tamponade and restrictive pericarditis. Nonsteroidal anti-inflammatory drugs will suppress the clinical symptoms in most cases. A brief course of corticosteroid therapy may be required in the more severe cases. These syndromes generally run a self-limited course lasting several weeks to several months.

MYOCARDIAL DISEASES

Autoimmune Myocarditis

This is a rare disease characterized by an aberrant immune response that damages myocardial tissue and is generally seen as part of a systemic autoimmune syndrome. Autoimmune myocarditis is associated most commonly with polymyositis/dermatomyositis and systemic lupus erythematosus (SLE) and less commonly with rheumatoid arthritis, scleroderma, mixed connective tissue disease, and sarcoidosis. Little is known about the etiology of autoimmune myocarditis. The presence of mononuclear cell infiltrates in the myocardium and the association with immunologically mediated diseases suggest an autoimmune pathogenesis. Autoimmune myocarditis may present with signs and symptoms of congestive heart failure, arrhythmias, or conduction abnormalities. Chest pain from an associated pericarditis may also be present. Findings on chest radiograph, echocardiogram, and electrocardiogram may reflect diffuse myocardial dysfunction and rhythm or conduction abnormalities. Other laboratory studies may suggest the diagnosis of an associated autoimmune disease. There is an increased occurrence of the anti-ribonucleoprotein (RNP) autoantibody in patients with SLE who develop autoimmune myocarditis. Autoimmune myocarditis generally responds rapidly and dramatically to corticosteroid therapy. The outlook is generally favorable, with the patients's prognosis being determined by the underlying disease.

Autoimmune myocarditis is differentiated clinically from viral myocarditis by its association with SLE, rheumatoid arthritis, myositis, and, less commonly, scleroderma. Favorable response to immunosuppressive and anti-inflammatory treatment is also a distinguishing feature. However, the histopathology of mononuclear cell infiltration in autoimmune and viral pericarditis is identical.

Dilated Cardiomyopathy

A subset of patients with dilated cardiomyopathy may have a component of myocarditis. This disease is associated with low cardiac output and ejection fraction, in contrast to the hypertrophic and restrictive forms of cardiomyopathy. Transvenous endomyocardial biopsy studies in patients with nonischemic dilated cardiomyopathy demonstrate a 15–25% prevalence of myocarditis. The clinical presentation, including signs and symptoms associated with congestive heart failure, rhythm, and conduction disturbances, is similar whether or not myocarditis is present. Treatment with immunosuppressive drugs including corticosteroids may result in a short-term improvement in myocardial function but does not appear to alter the long-term prognosis. The role of chronic immunosuppressive therapy in dilated cardiomyopathy remains to be defined. Treatment is directed at the underlying congestive heart failure. The prognosis is guarded and is associated with the cardiac functional status. Selected patients may be considered for cardiac transplantation.

ENDOMYOCARDIAL DISEASES

The association of eosinophilia with endomyocardial fibrosis is recognized in a number of clinical syndromes including **tropical endomyocardial fibrosis, Löffler's endomyocardial disease, eosinophilic leukemia,** and the **hypereosinophilic syndrome.** It has been suggested that these clinical entities may represent a spectrum of a single disease process. Morphologic abnormalities of eosinophils include decreased numbers of crystalloid granules, vacuolation, and hypersegmentation. Presumably, aberrant tissue invasion and inappropriate degranulation of the eosinophils result in the endomyocardial pathology, which involves both ventricles. Three stages of the disease are recognized: (1) an acute stage with infiltration of eosinophils and myocytolysis; (2) an intermediate thrombotic stage, in which a thickened endocardium is covered by thrombus; and (3) a fibrotic stage, in which dense fibrosis occurs in the endocardium and myocardium. An immunologic pathogenesis is presumed because of the eosinophilia. In these conditions there is a marked tendency for clot formation with fibrosis on resolution of the clots, and it is possible that the eosinophilia is secondary to this process.

The clinical presentation is that of a restrictive cardiomyopathy with a pattern of biventricular involvement. Emboli from intraventricular thrombi may be a prominent clinical component of the disease. Therapy is directed at the management of the cardiac dysfunction and thromboembolic complications. Treatment with prednisone and hydroxyurea may benefit patients with hypereosinophilic syndrome. Surgical intervention (endomyocardiectomy, thrombectomy, or valve replacement) may benefit carefully selected patients. Despite therapeutic intervention, the prognosis remains guarded.

VASCULAR DISEASES: THE VASCULITIDES

Vasculitis is defined as a clinicopathologic process characterized by inflammation and necrosis of blood vessels. The clinical spectrum ranges from a primary disease involving exclusively blood vessels to an involvement of vessels as a relatively insignificant component of another systemic disease. Because vasculitis can potentially involve any blood vessel, a complex and often confusing array of clinical syndromes results (Table 34–1). The vasculitides are a heterogeneous group of clinical syndromes, and therefore no single cause explains the pathophysiology of all of the inflammatory vessel diseases. The

Table 34–1. Classification of the vasculitides.

Systemic necrotizing vasculitis
  Polyarteritis nodosa
  Allergic angiitis and granulomatosis
  Overlap syndromes
  Associated diseases (connective-tissue diseases, hepatitis
    B, cytomegalovirus infection, hairy cell leukemia)

Small-vessel (hypersensitivity) vasculitis
  Henoch-Schönlein purpura
  Serum sickness
  Other drug-related vasculitides
  Vasculitis associated with food, foreign protein, or other
    exogenous antigens
  Vasculitis associated with a systemic disease (Table 34–2)
  Hypocomplementemic urticarial vasculitis
  Congenital deficiencies of the complement system
  Erythema elevatum diutinum

Behçet's disease

Wegener's granulomatosis

Arteritis of larger arteries
  Giant cell (temporal) arteritis
  Takayasu arteritis
  Large-artery arteritis-complicating diseases such as
    ankylosing spondylitis, Reiter's syndrome, and relapsing
    polychondritis
  Aortitis-associated syphilis

Thromboangiitis obliterans (Buerger's disease)

Isolated angiitis of the central nervous system

**Mucocutaneous lymph node syndrome (Kawasaki's
disease)**

Miscellaneous vasculitis syndromes

best-characterized mechanism is immune complex-mediated vasculitis. The elements necessary for the expression of this process include (1) soluble immune complexes larger than 19S formed in slight antigen excess, (2) increased vascular permeability with passive deposition of complexes in the vessel wall, (3) activation of complement with subsequent attraction of polymorphonuclear neutrophils (PMN) to the site of immune-complex deposition, and (4) release of inflammatory mediators and disruption of vascular integrity. Other potential mechanisms are less well established. Aberrant regulation of T cell, B cell, monocyte, fixed tissue macrophage, and endothelial cell function may be important in some of the vasculitides. In addition, soluble cytokines and the expression of cell surface adhesion molecules on leukocytes and blood vessels may play a role in the expression of vasculitis. With the exception of the small vessel (hypersensitivity) vasculitis, the vasculitides are relatively rare syndromes.

SMALL-VESSEL (HYPERSENSITIVITY) VASCULITIS

Major Immunologic Features

- Small vessels undergo inflammation.
- It is an immune complex-mediated process.

General Considerations

Small-vessel vasculitis, which includes a heterogenous group of clinical syndromes, is characterized by inflammation of arterioles, capillaries, and venules. The most commonly involved vessel is the venule, producing a venulitis. Skin involvement is characteristic of small-vessel vasculitis, although any organ system can be affected. Immune-complex deposition is an important mechanism in at least a subset of cases of small-vessel vasculitis. A variety of agents have been suggested as causal factors in hypersensitivity vasculitis; these include (1) microorganisms (bacteria, mycobacteria, viruses, and parasites), (2) foreign proteins (animal serum and monoclonal antibodies), (3) chemicals (insecticides, herbicides, and petroleum products), and (4) drugs (antibiotics, antihypertensives, antiarrhythmics, nonsteroidal anti-inflammatory drugs, antirheumatic drugs, and others). The chemicals and drugs are presumed to function as haptens, binding covalently to unknown host carrier molecules and thereby eliciting an immune response. Small-vessel vasculitis can also occur in association with a wide variety of systemic diseases. It most commonly occurs in the fifth decade of life, with a slight female predominance.

Pathology

The most common histologic pattern is a neutrophilic leukocyte infiltrate of the postcapillary venules with leukocytoclasis (presence of nuclear debris), fibrinoid necrosis, endothelial swelling, and disruption of vascular integrity (Fig 34–1). Patterns of mixed acute and chronic inflammatory infiltrates, as well as a chronic infiltrate composed predominantly of lymphocytes, are also recognized.

Clinical Features

A nonblanching palpable purpuric lesion (palpable purpura) is characteristic. Other associated skin findings include papular, petechial, and ulcerative lesions. The lesions tend to recur in crops varying in number from a few to more than a 100. Each crop resolves over 2–4 weeks. The lesions have a symmetric distribution and are most often found in dependent areas, particularly the distal lower extremities. Vasculitis produces pain, a burning sensation, or dependent edema in up to 40% of patients. Evidence of joint, kidney, lung, gastrointestinal, or peripheral nervous system involvement is present in the minority of cases.

Immunologic Diagnosis

No specific laboratory test is diagnostic for small-vessel vasculitis. The following tests may or may not be abnormal: sedimentation rate, cryoglobulins, immune complexes, rheumatoid factor, and serum complement levels. A biopsy of a newly developing skin lesion should establish the diagnosis.

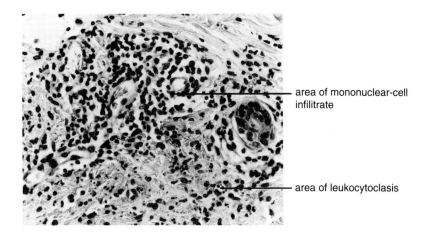

area of mononuclear-cell infilitrate

area of leukocytoclasis

Figure 34–1. Skin biopsy specimen from a patient with hypersensitivity vasculitis. A venulitis with a mixed cellular infiltrate is seen. A mononuclear-cell infiltrate around a venule is present in one area of the specimen, while a neutrophil infiltrate with early leukocytoclasis (presence of nuclear debris) is seen in an adjacent area. Hematoxylin and eosin stain. (Original magnification x 330.) (Reproduced, with permission, from Cupps TR, Fauci AS: The vasculitides. In: *Major Problems in Internal Medicine.* Vol 21. Smith LH [editor]. Saunders, 1981.)

Differential Diagnosis

Once the diagnosis of small-vessel vasculitis is established, the patient should be evaluated for evidence of visceral involvement or an associated underlying disease process.

Treatment

Treatment should be directed at eliminating any inciting agent or treating any underlying systemic disease. A brief course of corticosteroid therapy or period of bed rest may expedite the resolution of an acute flare. Lengthy regimens of high-dose or split-dose daily corticosteroid treatment should be avoided. Analgesics may be required for symptomatic relief.

Complications & Prognosis

With rare exceptions, small-vessel vasculitis does not progress to life-threatening complications. The disease may be self-limited or, less commonly, develop a chronic recurrent pattern.

SYNDROMES ASSOCIATED WITH SMALL-VESSEL VASCULITIS

Several subgroups of hypersensitivity vasculitis have distinctive clinicopathologic patterns and are considered separate syndromes. In clinical practice these subsets may overlap. In this section the unique features of Henoch-Schönlein purpura, Behçet's disease, urticarial vasculitis, and small-vessel vasculitis associated with systemic disease processes are reviewed.

1. HENOCH-SCHÖNLEIN PURPURA

This syndrome, a distinctive subset of the small-vessel vasculitides, is characterized by normal platelet count, purpuric skin lesions, arthralgias, colicky abdominal pain with bleeding, and renal disease. It is the systemic form of small-vessel vasculitis. Deposition of IgA containing immune complexes with activation of the alternative complement pathway may be an important pathophysiologic mechanism. The majority of patients have symptoms of an upper respiratory tract infection prior to the onset of their disease. Other suspected causes including drugs (antibiotics and thiazides), foods (milk, fish, eggs, rice, nuts, beans, and others), and immunizations may appear to precipitate the disease clinically. There is a slight male predominance. The peak age of onset is between the ages of 4 and 7 years, although the disease does occur in adults. The disease has a seasonal variation, with the peak incidence reported in spring. The histopathology is a diffuse leukocytoclastic vasculitis involving small vessels of any involved organ system. In the bowel, hemorrhage may occur in the submucosal surface or subserosal areas. The kidneys show focal or diffuse glomerulonephritis. The clinical manifestation varies with age. In children, symptoms localized to skin, gut, and joints predominate. In adults, the disease presents predominantly with skin findings, whereas initial complaints related to the gastrointestinal tract or joints are present in fewer than one-quarter of patients. The cutaneous lesion of Henoch-Schönlein purpura evolves through the following phases: (1) an initial small urticarial lesion that may be pruritic; (2) a pink maculopapular spot that develops over several hours; (3) maturation of this spot to a raised, darkened lesion; (4) progression the following day to a 0.5–2 cm maculopapular lesion which, in some cases, may become a confluent patch; and (5) final resolution in 2 weeks without scarring. Arthralgias without synovitis tend to follow a migratory pattern involving most commonly the large joints of the lower extremities. Abdominal symptoms including colicky pain, nausea, vomiting, and blood loss are present in the majority of patients. Life-threatening gastrointestinal tract problems such as major bleeding, bowel perforation, or intussusception are present in fewer than 5% of patients. The most common form of intussusception is ileoileal. The mean age of patients with this complication is 6 years, although intussusception has been reported in young adults. Clinically, the diagnosis of intussusception is suggested in a patient with a worsening clinical course, an unchanging abdominal mass, bright-red rectal bleeding, and the clinical pattern of complete bowel obstruction. Kidney involvement is characteristically very mild, although a few patients may develop progressive renal failure. Radiographic studies of the bowel may be useful in diagnosing an intussusception. IgA containing immune complexes may be present. These complexes, however, are not pathognomonic and are not detected by C1q assay, although the Raji cell assay may be positive. A skin biopsy will establish the vasculitic nature of the process, and immunofluorescence showing IgA deposition in vessel walls will further support the diagnosis of Henoch-Schönlein purpura.

The differential diagnosis for a patient presenting with rash, abdominal pain, and joint symptoms includes, in part, inflammatory bowel disease, *Yersinia* entercolitis, meningococcemia, Rocky Mountain spotted fever, rheumatic fever, and viral infections. The disease usually resolves spontaneously after one or more recurrent episodes; consequently, the prognosis of even untreated patients is excellent. Therapy consists of supportive care and symptomatic relief. Timely surgical intervention may be required for the rare patients with life-threatening bowel complications. In the small number of patients with renal involvement with progressive functional impairment, corticosteroid therapy may be required.

2. BEHÇET'S DISEASE

Behçet's disease is characterized by recurrent episodes of oral ulcers, eye lesions, genital ulcers, thrombophlebitis, and other cutaneous lesions. The characteristic pathologic lesion is a venulitis, although vessels of any size in any organ system can be affected.

The primary lesion is a small-vessel vasculitis, presumably reflecting an antibody- or T cell-mediated response, although no antigenic epitope has yet been identified as a cause. Serum complement levels are normal, but circulating immune complexes may be present. There are studies showing complement deposition in lesions, but it is not known whether this is a primary or secondary event.

The oral lesions begin as raised erythematous areas with progression to shallow, punched-out lesions with yellow necrotic bases. These are discussed further in Chapter 35. The genital ulcers have similar appearance and follow a similar time course. Ocular involvement is mostly frequently observed in the anterior chamber, with iridocyclitis and hypopyon, which generally resolve without long-term complications. Involvement of the posterior structures is less frequent, but recurrent episodes over several years may lead to impaired vision. Renal, cardiovascular, and gastrointestinal tract involvement occurs in a minority of patients. In the absence of central nervous system or bowel involvement, the prognosis is good. No drug is uniformly successful in the treatment of Behçet's disease, but favorable results have been reported with indomethacin, colchicine, levamisole and corticosteroids. Azathioprine in combination with corticosteroids is effective in the treatment of ocular manifestations of Behçet's disease. The need for early aggressive therapy of central nervous system disease has been emphasized.

3. HYPOCOMPLEMENTEMIC URTICARIAL VASCULITIS

This disease is a clinicopathologic entity characterized by a reduction of the early complement components in serum, persistent urticaria, and a pattern of leukocytoclastic vasculitis. Characteristically, there is a selective depression of the C1q component of complement because of the binding of C1q by IgG molecules through the $F(ab)'_2$—not Fc—portion of the molecule. The clearance of C1q is increased. The primary clinical feature of this disease is a persistent urticarial eruption, with lesions lasting a day or longer. Additional findings may include angioedema with occasional laryngeal involvement, joint symptoms, abdominal distress, neurologic abnormalities, and glomerulonephritis. The characteristic complement profile is a depressed C1q level with near-normal C1r and C1s levels. Other complement components including C2, C3, and C4 may be depressed. The alternative pathway complement components are normal. Diseases such as SLE, urticaria-angioedema, and inherited partial C3 deficiency may present with a similar clinical pattern. Antihistamines, anti-inflammatory drugs (indomethacin), and immunosuppressive drugs have been tried, but their therapeutic efficacy has not been established.

4. SMALL-VESSEL VASCULITIS ASSOCIATED WITH SYSTEMIC DISEASES

Small-vessel vasculitis occurs in association with a wide variety of systemic diseases (Table 34–2). It generally resolves when the underlying disease process is adequately treated.

SYSTEMIC NECROTIZING VASCULITIS

Systemic necrotizing vasculitis is a category that includes polyarteritis nodosa, allergic angiitis and granulomatosis (Churg-Strauss syndrome), and overlap syndromes. These diseases have in common a multisystem necrotizing vasculitis of small and medium-sized muscular arteries.

1. POLYARTERITIS NODOSA

Major Immunologic Features
- There is necrotizing vasculitis of small- and medium-sized muscular arteries.
- Pulmonary involvement is uncommon.

General Considerations

Classic polyarteritis nodosa is a necrotizing vasculitis of small and medium-sized muscular arteries. Involvement of renal and visceral arteries with sparing of the pulmonary circulation is characteristic. Immune-complex deposition in involved arteries is considered to be the relevant pathophysiologic mechanism. In patients with polyarteritis nodosa in association with chronic hepatitis B virus infection, hepatitis B surface antigen, IgM, and complement components can be demonstrated in early vasculitic lesions. With more than 1000 cases reported, polyarteritis nodosa is considered an uncommon but not rare disease. The male-to-female ratio is 2.5:1. The mean age at onset is 45 years, although the disease occurs at both extremes of age.

Pathology

Involvement of the kidneys, heart, abdominal organs, and nervous system (both central and peripheral nervous systems) is characteristic. With the exception of the bronchial arteries, the pulmonary vessels are uninvolved. The vasculitic lesions are segmental and have a predilection for branching and bifurcating points of small- and medium-sized muscular arteries (Fig 34–2). Arterioles, venules, and veins are characteristically spared, and granuloma formation is rare. Destruction of the media and internal elastic lamina with aneurysm formation is characteristic. Endothelial proliferation, vessel wall degeneration with fibrinoid necrosis, thrombosis, ischemia, and infarction are present to various degrees. Lesions at all stages of evolution, including (1) the degenerative stage, (2) the acute inflammatory stage, (3) the chronic inflammatory stage, and (4) healing with scarring, may be present at any given time. Renal pathology includes the presence of vasculitis, hypertensive changes, and glomerulonephritis.

Immunologic Pathogenesis

Polyarteritis nodosa is associated with various infections, especially hepatitis B but also tuberculosis, streptococcal infections, and otitis media. Evidence

Table 34–2. Systemic diseases associated with small-vessel vasculitis.

Systemic vasculitides

Systemic necrotizing vasculitis of the polyarteritis nodosa group (particularly the Churg-Strauss syndrome and overlap syndromes), Wegener's granulomatosis, Behçet's disease, Henoch-Schölein purpura

Collagen vascular diseases

SLE, rheumatoid arthritis, Sjögren's syndrome, dermatomyositis, scleroderma, rheumatic fever, sarcoidosis, C2 deficiency, essential mixed cryoglobulinemia

Neoplasms

Lymphoproliferative neoplasms, carcinoma

Infections

Bacterial (endocarditis), viral, myobacterial, rickettsial

Miscellaneous syndromes

Chronic active hepatitis, inflammatory bowel disease, primary biliary cirrhosis, retroperitoneal fibrosis.
Goodpasture's syndrome, relapsing polychondritis, α-antitrypsin deficiency, celiac disease, and others

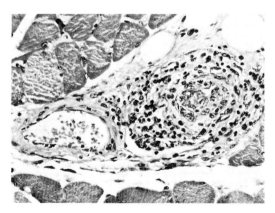

Figure 34–2. Muscle biopsy from a patient with classic polyarteritis nodosa. A necrotizing vasculitis of a small, muscular artery with a predominantly mononuclear-cell infiltrate is seen. The adjacent vein is not involved. Hematoxylin and eosin stain. (Original magnification x 330.) (Reproduced, with permission, from Cupps TR, Fauci AS: The vasculitides. In: *Major Problems in Internal Medicine.* Vol 21. Smith LH [editor]. Saunders, 1981).

for an exogenous antigen causing the vasculitis is strongest when hepatitis B virus is present. The surface antigen of the virus is present at higher concentrations in plasma than are other viral antigens. It is found in immune complexes, and it can also be detected in tissues. Immune complexes containing IgM antibody could bind to the surface antigen nonspecifically, so definite proof that the vasculitis is caused by a viral antigen-antibody immune complex is lacking.

Host factors predisposing to development of polyarteritis nodosa could include failure of the mononuclear phagocyte system to clear circulating complexes and defective immune regulation. To date, no human leukocyte antigen (HLA) association has been reported.

Clinical Features

Nonspecific signs and symptoms are common at the presentation of polyarteritis nodosa; these include weakness, abdominal pain, leg pain, neurologic symptoms, fever, and cough. The nonspecific nature of the presentation and the relatively uncommon occurrence of polyarteritis nodosa may contribute to the difficulty in establishing the diagnosis. Kidney involvement is common but tends to be asymptomatic. Arthritis, arthralgia, or myalgia occurs in more than half of the patients, as does hypertension. Diffuse renal vasculitis with secondary hyperreninemia appears to be an important cause of hypertension in patients with polyarteritis nodosa. The peripheral nervous system is involved in half of the cases. Several patterns of involvement are recognized. Mixed motor-sensory involvement with a pattern of mononeuritis multiplex suggests the diagnosis of vasculitis. There is clinical evidence for abdominal involvement in 45% of patients. Nausea, vomiting, and abdominal pain, which may suggest pancreatitis, are present. Less common manifestations of gastrointestinal tract disease include "intestinal angina" (postprandial abdominal pain, anorexia, and weight loss), malabsorption, and steatorrhea. Although rare, bowel infarction is a life-threatening complication, which requires rapid diagnosis and prompt surgical intervention.

Skin involvement is present in 40% of patients. The most common pattern is a maculopapular rash. In addition, subcutaneous painful nodules or livedo reticularis (a red to blue netlike mottling of the skin) can be seen. Clinical involvement of the heart is present in one-third of patients. Cardiac disease may be secondary to the hypertension, coronary vasculitis, or pericarditis. Central nervous system involvement including stroke, altered mental status, and seizures can be seen in one-quarter of patients. At autopsy there are changes secondary to hypertension as well as active vasculitis. Similarly, retinal vessel involvement from hypertension and vasculitis is recognized in patients with polyarteritis nodosa.

Abnormal laboratory studies include elevated erythrocyte sedimentation rate, leukocytosis, anemia, thrombocytosis, and cellular casts in the urinary sediment, indicating glomerular disease. Angiographic evaluation is important in establishing the diagnosis (Fig 34–3). Two abnormalities suggest the diagnosis of polyarteritis nodosa: (1) aneurysms (vascular dilatation with a circular appearance), and (2) changes in vessel caliber (these tend to have an asymmetric pattern). The aneurysms in a given individual tend to be similar in size, ranging most commonly between 1 and 5 mm. Angiography will establish the diagnosis of polyarteritis nodosa in approximately 80% of cases; consequently, a negative study does not totally exclude the diagnosis.

Immunologic Diagnosis

There may be immune complexes, cryoglobulins, rheumatoid factors, and reduced level of complement components. Antineutrophil cytoplasmic antibodies with a perinuclear pattern (p-ANCA) and specificity for myeloperoxidase are seen in some patients. The histologic diagnosis of systemic necrotizing vasculitis can be established from a variety of tissue sites. Biopsy specimens taken from symptomatic sites such

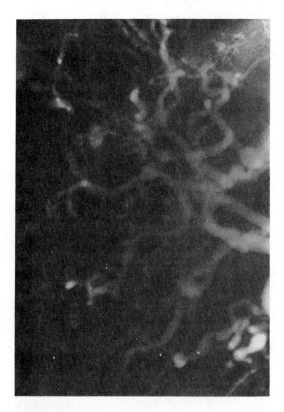

Figure 34–3. Hepatic angiogram from a patient with classic polyarteritis nodosa. Multiple saccular aneurysms and areas of symmetric narrowing are seen.

as skeletal muscle or nerves have a higher diagnostic yield than those from asymptomatic sites.

Differential Diagnosis

Because the initial signs and symptoms of polyarteritis nodosa are nonspecific, vasculitis should be considered in all patients with an undiagnosed systemic illness. At initial presentation many patients with polyarteritis nodosa are believed to have a neoplasm, infection, or other collagen vascular disease. The presence of an abnormal urinary sediment, recent onset of hypertension, or mononeuritis multiplex suggests the diagnostic possibility of vasculitis. A number of diseases occur in association with polyarteritis nodosa, including infections (hepatitis B virus infection, acute otitis media, endocarditis, and streptococcal infection), collagen vascular diseases (SLE, rheumatoid arthritis, Sjögren's syndrome, and others), and neoplasms (hairy cell leukemia).

Treatment

Although corticosteroids alone are generally recommended in the less fulminant cases of polyarteritis nodosa, cyclophosphamide is the treatment of choice in severe progressive polyarteritis nodosa. The drug is started in 2 mg/kg as a single daily oral dose, with monitoring of the leukocyte count to avoid a total leukocyte count of less than 3000 cells/mm^3. Prednisone (60 mg orally per day) is also started during the induction period of 10–14 days. After this induction period, a taper to an alternate-day schedule is initiated. The taper to alternate-day prednisone administration is generally completed in 2–3 months.

Complications & Prognosis

Cyclophosphamide will induce long-term clinical remissions in patients with systemic necrotizing vasculitis, including those who have been refractory to other treatment modalities. Meticulous control of hypertension is needed for several reasons. One reason is the potential for accelerated atherosclerosis in arteries damaged by the necrotizing vasculitis. Another major reason is that kidneys initially damaged by vasculitis or glomerulonephritis should be protected from the additional insult of poorly controlled blood pressure. Angiotensin-converting enzyme inhibitors may be particularly effective in this clinical setting.

2. ALLERGIC ANGIITIS & GRANULOMATOSIS (Churg-Strauss Syndrome)

Major Immunologic Features

- There is vasculitis of blood vessels of various type and sizes (including small- and medium-sized muscular arteries).
- Pulmonary involvement is common.

General Considerations

Allergic angiitis and granulomatosis is a rare disease characterized by a granulomatous vasculitis of multiple organ systems. Although vascular lesions identical to the pattern seen in polyarteritis nodosa may be present, this disease is unique for the following findings: (1) frequency of involvement of pulmonary vessels, (2) vasculitis of blood vessels of various types and sizes (small- and medium-sized muscular arteries, veins, and small vessels), (3) intra- and extravascular granuloma formation, (4) eosinophilic tissue infiltrates, and (5) association with severe asthma and peripheral eosinophilia. The pathophysiology of this syndrome appears to be similar to the pattern described for polyarteritis nodosa. There is a slight male predominance, and the mean age at the onset of disease is 44 years. In one series of patients with systemic necrotizing vasculitis, approximately 30% of patients had a clinical pattern of allergic angiitis and granulomatosis.

Pathology

In autopsy studies, the frequent involvement of the spleen and pulmonary vessels with sparing of central nervous system contrasts with the pattern seen in polyarteritis nodosa. In addition to the pattern of arteritis seen in polyarteritis nodosa, involvement of smaller vessels is commonly seen. Eosinophils and granulomata are seen in and around the vascular infiltrates. The veins are involved in approximately half of the patients, and small-vessel vasculitis is seen in the purpuric skin lesions.

Clinical Features

The clinical manifestation of allergic angiitis and granulomatosis is similar to the pattern seen in polyarteritis nodosa, except for the high frequency of pulmonary signs and symptoms. Asthma and transient pulmonary infiltrates are frequently noted. Symptoms related to the lungs generally precede the diagnosis of systemic vasculitis by 2 years, although the range is from 0 to 30 years. A short duration of pulmonary symptoms has been associated with a poorer prognosis. Peripheral-blood eosinophilia is seen in 85% of cases at some point in the course of the disease.

Immunologic Diagnosis

Elevation of IgE has been reported in allergic angiitis and granulomatosis. The p-ANCA test is positive in some patients. In addition to the peripheral biopsy sites described for polyarteritis nodosa, an open-lung biopsy may be useful to establish the diagnosis of necrotizing vasculitis.

Differential Diagnosis

In addition to the differential diagnosis discussed for polyarteritis nodosa, the diagnosis of allergic angiitis and granulomatosis should be considered in patients with bronchospasm and pulmonary infiltrates.

Treatment, Complications, & Prognosis

Treatment and prognosis are similar to those of polyarteritis nodosa. The bronchospasm may persist after successful treatment for the systemic vasculitis, and specific treatment of asthma may be required.

3. OVERLAP SYNDROMES

There are patients who share clinical and pathologic features characteristic of both polyarteritis nodosa and allergic angiitis and granulomatosis, as well as other vasculitic syndromes, but do not fit precisely into these strictly defined diagnostic categories. The presence of an overlap syndrome emphasizes that there is a continuum of disease manifestations in patients with systemic necrotizing vasculitis. The approach to the patients with overlap syndromes is similar to the one described for other systemic necrotizing vasculitides.

WEGENER'S GRANULOMATOSIS

Major Immunologic Features
- This is a necrotizing granulomatous vasculitis.
- There is focal segmental glomerulonephritis.
- There are antineutrophil cytoplasmic autoantibodies.

General Considerations

Wegener's granulomatosis is a clinicopathologic complex of a necrotizing, granulomatous vasculitis of the upper and lower respiratory tracts, glomerulonephritis, and variable degrees of small-vessel vasculitis. The cause is unknown. Because of the predominant involvement of the upper and lower respiratory tracts in this disease, it has been suggested that an infectious agent or an inhaled antigen may trigger an aberrant immune response. However, no such antigen or infectious agent has been identified as yet. There is a slight male predominance. The majority of cases begin in the fourth or fifth decade of life, although the disease has been described at both extremes of age.

Pathology

Wegener's granulomatosis is characterized by fibrinoid necrosis of predominantly small arteries and veins, with early infiltration of neutrophils followed by mononuclear cells. This is followed by healing with fibrosis. The vasculitis lesions occur at all stages of evolution. Granulomata are well-formed with plentiful multinucleated giant cells. Renal involvement is characterized by a focal segmental glomerulonephritis. Crescent formation can be seen in the

more severe cases. Renal vasculitis or granuloma formation is less frequent.

Clinical Features

The most common presenting complaints (present in 85% of patients) involve the upper respiratory tract and include sinusitis, nasal obstruction, otitis, hearing loss, and oropharyngeal symptoms. Lower respiratory tract symptoms occur in 35% of patients; these include cough, sputum production, dyspnea, pleuritic chest pain, and, less commonly, hemoptysis. Other presenting complaints include arthralgias, weight loss, and weakness. Wegener's granulomatosis can involve any organ system, but the lungs are involved in virtually all patients. Lung disease may be asymptomatic, but it can be seen radiographically. In addition to the presenting symptoms of cough and dyspnea, massive pulmonary hemorrhage can be seen, but it is rare. There is evidence of sinus involvement in 95% of patients; this can be complicated by a superimposed bacterial infection. Inflammatory lesions may involve any site in the upper airways. Destruction of the nasal septum results in the saddle nose deformity (Fig 34–4). A persistent sore throat is a frequent complaint. Shallow oral ulcerations with sharp margins occur. Renal involvement is generally

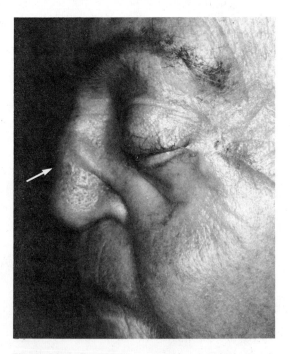

Figure 34–4. The saddle nose deformity of Wegener's granulomatosis (arrow) results from inflammation, scarring, and loss of height of the cartilaginous portion of the bridge of the nose. The bony portion (os nasale) is uninvolved. Note also the proptosis of the eye secondary to retro-orbital inflammation.

asymptomatic but can be documented in 80% of cases. Functional impairment may progress very rapidly in the absence of appropriate treatment. In contrast to patients with systemic necrotizing vasculitis, renal-vascular hypertension is not a significant clinical problem. Joint symptoms are present in more than half of the patients, but a deforming arthritis is not characteristically seen. Skin involvement including ulceration, vesicles, petechiae, and subcutaneous nodules occurs in almost half of the patients. The eyes are involved in 40% of patients. The most common abnormalities are proptosis secondary to a retroorbital inflammatory mass and inflammation of the anterior ocular structures (ie, conjunctivitis, episcleritis, scleritis, and corneoscleral ulceration). Vasculitis of the vessels in the optic nerve or retina occurs in 10% of cases. Cardiac involvement is reported in one-quarter of patients. The most common abnormality is pericarditis, but inflammation of other structures including the endocardium, the myocardium, and the coronary vessels has been reported. The nervous system is involved in one-quarter of patients. Different patterns of peripheral nerve involvement, including mononeuritis multiplex, are noted. Involvement of the central nervous system is less common but is a well-recognized complication.

Laboratory studies show leukocytosis, thrombocytosis, elevated sedimentation rate, and presence of C-reactive protein. An abnormal urinary sediment is present in 80% of patients. Hematuria, with or without cellular casts, and proteinuria make up the most common pattern. The most common pattern seen on a chest radiograph is multiple, nodular, bilateral cavitary infiltrates, although virtually any pattern has been described. Computed tomography of the chest may be more sensitive for identifying subtle lung lesions. Computed tomography of the orbits may be useful in diagnosing and monitoring retroorbital eye involvement.

Immunologic Diagnosis

Polyclonal elevations of IgG and IgA with normal levels of IgM is the characteristic pattern seen in active Wegener's granulomatosis. Elevation is variable. Circulating immune complexes can be detected in some patients. Antineutrophil cytoplasmic antibodies with a diffuse cytoplasmic pattern (c-ANCA) directed against proteinase 3 is present in most patients with active systemic disease. In some patients, the c-ANCA titer reflects disease activity. A definitive diagnosis of Wegener's granulomatosis is made by seeing the histologic pattern of granulomatous necrotizing vasculitis on a biopsy specimen. Open-lung biopsy has the highest diagnostic yield. Tissue taken from other sites has an approximately 10% yield in demonstrating the diagnostic pattern. Renal tissue will provide a histologic pattern that is consistent with the diagnosis of Wegener's granulomatosis.

Differential Diagnosis

Wegener's granulomatosis is included in the differential diagnosis of patients with chronic sinusitis or otitis media. Diseases that are associated with a pulmonary-renal syndrome (SLE, Goodpasture's syndrome, thrombotic thrombocytopenia purpura, etc) may be confused with Wegener's granulomatosis during the initial phases.

Treatment

Cyclophosphamide at 2 mg/kg orally as a single daily dose is the most effective form of treatment. After the initial induction period the total leukocyte count is monitored to adjust the dose of cyclophosphamide. Care should be taken to avoid lowering the leukocyte count below 3000 cells/mm^3. In addition, oral prednisone at 1 mg/kg/d is used. After 2 weeks of daily prednisone, a taper to an alternate-day regimen of prednisone is initiated; the taper is completed after 2–3 months. Treatment should continue until the patient is free of disease for 1 year before the drugs are discontinued; withdrawal should be gradual. Weekly oral methotrexate up to a dose of 20–25 mg/wk in combination with prednisone as outlined above may also be effective in selected patients with Wegener's granulomatosis.

Complications & Prognosis

Treatment with cyclophosphamide and prednisone will result in marked improvement in 90% of patients and in a complete remission in 75%. The incidence of relapse following discontinuation of therapy may approach 50%. Sinus damage by the disease may predispose to recurrent episodes of bacterial sinusitis. Obstruction from scarring of large airways can be seen in patients with severe endobronchial disease. The most common obstructed site is the subglottic region. Potential complications of cyclophosphamide therapy include hemorrhagic cystitis, bladder fibrosis, and, possibly, neoplasia.

GIANT CELL ARTERITIS

Major Immunologic Features
- This is a granulomatous panarteritis.
- It affects the elderly.
- Headache is common, but presenting symptoms are nonspecific.
- It is associated with polymyalgia rheumatica.

General Considerations

Giant cell arteritis (temporal arteritis) is a systemic panarteritis affecting any medium-sized or large artery. The disease predominantly affects the elderly, with clinical signs and symptoms resulting from vasculitis in branches of the carotid artery. Although studies suggest immune complex-mediated, antibody-mediated, and cell-mediated immune mechanisms, the precise cause is unknown. There is a slight female predominance, and the average age at onset of the disease is 70 years. More than 95% of cases occur in patients older than 50 years. The age-specific incidence per 100,000 population per year increases with age, rising from 1.7 in the sixth decade to 55.5 for patients older than 80 years.

Pathology

The disease is characterized by a panarteritis consisting of mononuclear cells, multinucleated giant cells, PMN, and eosinophils. The major site of involvement is the media, with smooth muscle necrosis and interruption of internal elastic membrane. The inflammatory lesions have a segmental pattern.

Clinical Features

The presenting signs and symptoms of giant cell arteritis have a nonspecific pattern. The most frequent presenting complaints of headache, malaise, and fatigue are common symptoms in an older population. Less-common presenting problems include jaw or extremity claudication, fever, arthralgias, chronic sore throat, and tender scalp nodules. Headache is the most common manifestation. The pain has a continuous, boring quality with intermittent exacerbations. Although the pain is most commonly located over the distribution of the temporal artery, radiation to the neck, face, jaw, or tongue occurs. Although abnormalities along the course of the temporal artery, including tenderness, absent pulse, and nodules, are seen in half of the patients (Fig 34–5), these findings appear later in the course of disease. Other findings include hair loss, erythema, and necrosis along the course of the temporal artery. Eye problems including visual impairment, blindness, amaurosis fugax, and diplopia, occur in more than one-third of patients. Although giant cell arteritis may present with sudden blindness, the majority of patients will have other symptoms for an average of 3.5 months prior to developing visual impairment. Because the loss of vision is the result of ischemic optic neuritis in the majority of cases, the funduscopic examination may be normal for several days after the onset of blindness.

Jaw claudication (pain brought on by chewing or talking and relieved by rest) occurs in one-third of patients and suggests the diagnosis of giant cell arteritis. Polymyalgia rheumatica, a syndrome characterized by proximal muscle pain, periarticular pain, and morning stiffness, occurs in approximately half of the patients with giant cell arteritis. Conversely, up to 50% of patients presenting with symptoms of polymyalgia rheumatica may have a positive temporal artery biopsy.

Laboratory abnormalities include a normochromic, normocytic anemia, elevated alkaline phosphatase, and mild elevation of hepatic transaminases.

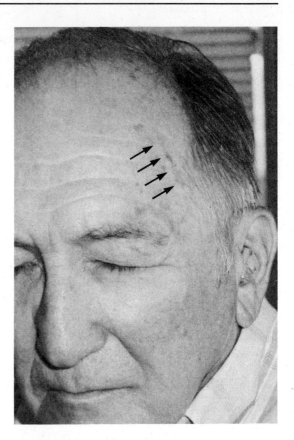

Figure 34–5. Giant cell arteritis involving the temporal artery (arrows) is shown. The temporal artery was swollen and tender. Biopsy of the contralateral temporal artery demonstrated the characteristic granulomatous panarteritis. The swelling and tenderness resolved following treatment with corticosteroids. (Courtesy of S. Ray Mitchell, Georgetown University Medical School, Washington, D.C.)

Immunologic Diagnosis

The sedimentation rate, total IgG, and acute-phase reactants are characteristically elevated. The diagnosis is established by finding the characteristic panarteritis on a temporal artery biopsy. Because of the segmental nature of the inflammation, the need for generous biopsy specimens and serial sectioning has been emphasized.

Differential Diagnosis

Because of the nonspecific nature of the majority of presenting symptoms, giant cell arteritis can be confused with a wide variety of disease processes including neoplasia, chronic infection, abnormal thyroid function, and other connective-tissue diseases.

Treatment

Prednisone at 40–60 mg/d orally is the initial treatment. As manifestations of the disease are suppressed, an attempt should be made to taper the dose of the drug. Although some patients may be adequately treated with 6 months of therapy, most will require a more prolonged course, for 1–2 years. Prednisone should be tapered to the minimum effective dose, generally in the range of 7.5–10 mg/d.

Complications & Prognosis

Corticosteroids are effective in suppressing the symptoms of giant cell arteritis and preventing visual impairment. In general, visual impairment is not reversible once present. Other than loss of vision, the major complication of this disease is the morbidity associated with prolonged corticosteroid use in an elderly population.

TAKAYASU ARTERITIS

Major Immunologic Features

- There is inflammation and stenosis of large and intermediate-sized arteries.
- There is frequent involvement of the aortic arch.

General Considerations

Takayasu arteritis is characterized by inflammation and stenosis of large and intermediate-sized arteries with frequent involvement of the aortic arch and its branches. There is a marked female predominance (about 9:1). The disease generally presents between the ages of 15 and 20 years. Although originally recognized in Asian women, Takayasu arteritis has a worldwide distribution.

Pathology

Takayasu arteritis is characterized by a panarteritis of large elastic arteries, with infiltration of all layers of the artery wall by mononuclear cells and giant cells. Other findings include intimal proliferation, fibrosis, disruption of elastic lamina, and vascularization of the media. Aneurysms, dissection, and hemorrhage are less common. In descending order of frequency, the following arteries are involved: subclavian artery (85%), descending aorta (58%), renal artery (56%), carotid artery (43%), ascending aorta (30%), abdominal aorta (20%), vertebral artery (17%), iliac artery (16%), innominate artery (15%), and pulmonary artery (15%).

Clinical Features

Two clinical stages, an initial inflammatory phase and a chronic occlusive phase, are recognized in Takayasu arteritis. The initial inflammatory phase occurs in 70% of patients and is characterized by a pattern of systemic inflammation including fever, night sweats, malaise, weakness, myalgias, and arthralgias. A migratory arthritis, episcleritis, iritis, and painful skin nodules are less common. A mean of 8 years (range, several months to several decades) may separate the initial inflammatory phase from clinical expression of the occlusive phase. Symptoms during the chronic phase reflect ischemia of the involved organ systems. Signs of vascular insufficiency are present in almost all patients. The pulse of the radial, ulnar, and carotid arteries is decreased or absent in 98% of patients. Bruits can be detected in 86% of patients. Symptoms of claudication or pain over the distribution of an artery occur in approximately one-third of patients. Central hypertension is present in half of the cases. Blood pressure determinations of the lower extremities more reliably reflect the true central blood pressure in the presence of severe aortic arch involvement. Sixty percent of patients experience difficulty in looking up, resulting in the characteristic "face-down" position. Patients assume this position to avoid transient decreases in visual acuity and narrowing of visual fields caused by a further decrement of compromised blood flow to the central nervous system. Ischemic changes to the retina and anterior structures of the eye are seen in a minority of patients. Cardiac symptoms are present in one-third of patients. Palpitations and congestive heart failure (right- and left-sided failure) secondary to hypertension are the most common manifestations. Less commonly, cardiac ischemia (secondary to coronary arteritis), aortic insufficiency, myocarditis, and pericarditis have been reported. Routine blood tests may show a mild anemia and leukocytosis.

Immunologic Diagnosis

The erythrocyte sedimentation rate is generally elevated. IgG, IgA, and IgM may be elevated, while the rheumatoid factor and antinuclear antibodies are generally negative. Arteriography is important in the diagnosis and management of Takayasu arteritis (Fig 34–6). Arteriographic abnormalities include symmetric narrowing to complete occlusion of large arteries with collateralization of flow. Aneurysms, including both saccular and fusiform patterns, can be seen. Other noninvasive tests to measure blood flow may be useful for serial follow-up evaluations.

Differential Diagnosis

Other causes of aortitis including syphilis, mycotic aneurysm, rheumatic fever, Reiter's syndrome, and ankylosing spondylitis should be excluded. Vascular occlusion secondary to emboli can also mimic Takayasu arteritis.

Treatment

Corticosteroids are usually effective in suppressing the inflammatory symptoms. The use of 30 mg of

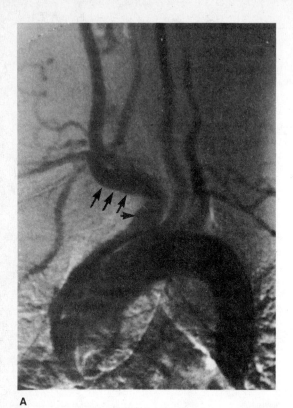

A

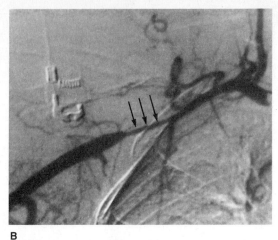

B

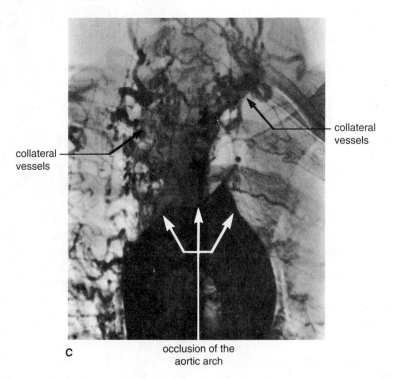

collateral vessels

collateral vessels

C

occlusion of the
aortic arch

Figure 34–6. Angiographic findings in Takayasu arteritis include saccular aneurysm of the brachiocephalic and common carotid arteries (arrows) (***A***), a prolonged segment of symmetric narrowing of the subclavian and axillary arteries (arrows) producing a "string sign" (***B***), and complete occlusion of the major aortic arch vessel (large arrow) with blood flow to the head established through collateral vessels (thin arrow) (***C***).

prednisone followed by a taper to a chronic maintenance therapy in the range of 5–10 mg/d has been
suggested. The use of a chronic maintenance regimen
may prevent the long-term vascular complications
and improve survival. Methotrexate or cyclophosphamide may be useful in treating patients who develop progressive occlusive disease despite corticosteroid therapy. Vascular surgery may prove useful in
selected cases.

Complications & Prognosis

In 2 large series a 10% mortality rate was
noted. The most common cause of death was congestive heart failure, and the second most common
was myocardial infarction. Less common causes of
death were renal failure and central nervous system
hemorrhage.

THROMBOANGIITIS OBLITERANS
(Buerger's Disease)

This syndrome is characterized by inflammatory
occlusive vascular disease of the intermediate to
small arteries and veins of the extremities. Three histopathologic phases of the disease are recognized: (1)
neutrophil infiltrate of the vessel wall associated with
microabscesses and thrombosis, (2) a subacute phase
with mononuclear cell and giant cell infiltrates, and
(3) a chronic phase with fibrosis and recanalization of
the thrombus. Although the disease predominantly
affects males younger than 40 years of age with a significant smoking history, an increasing incidence
among women has been noted. The most common
presenting symptoms are lower-extremity claudication or migratory thrombophlebitis. Less than 5% of
patients present with upper-extremity problems. During the course of the disease the majority of patients
will develop Raynaud's syndrome, and upper-extremity involvement will be seen in 90% of cases.
Systemic symptoms are characteristically absent.
Protection of ischemic tissue and cessation of tobacco use are imperative. Carefully selected patients
may benefit from surgical intervention. Morbidity
from tissue loss may be great, but survival is not affected.

Circulating immune complexes have been reported
by some investigators but not others. There are no diagnostic immunologic tests. It is not known whether
tobacco has a toxic or immunologic effect in this disease. However, the possibility of an immune pathogenesis is raised by the close resemblance of the histopathology in the early phase of the disease with that
of a hyperacute graft rejection.

OTHER VASCULITIC SYNDROMES

1. ISOLATED ANGIITIS OF THE CENTRAL NERVOUS SYSTEM

This is a distinct clinicopathologic entity characterized by vasculitis restricted to the vessels of the
central nervous system. The arteriole is the most
commonly affected vessel, although any size of vessel can be affected. The disease generally presents
with a pattern of higher-cortical dysfunction or severe headache and progresses to a pattern of multifocal neurologic deficits. Immunosuppressive therapy
is successful in inducing long-term clinical remissions.

2. ERYTHEMA NODOSUM

This is a clinical syndrome characterized by recurrent crops of painful nodular lesions (Fig 34–7) and is
generally associated with infection (mycobacterial,
fungal, or bacterial) or with sarcoidosis. The histopathology is characterized by acute and chronic inflammation of the dermis and subcutaneous tissue including a vasculitic component.

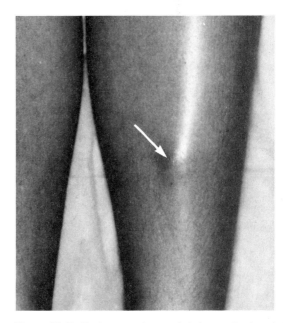

Figure 34–7. Erythema nodosum. A 2–3 cm raised, red
nodule in the characteristic pretibial distribution is shown
(arrow).

REFERENCES

General

Cupps TR, Fauci AS: The vasculitides. Vol 21 in: *Major Problems in Internal Medicine,* Smith LH (editor). Saunders, 1981.

American College of Rheumatology Subcommittee on Classification of Vasculitis: The American College of Rheumatology 1990 criteria for the classification of vasculitis. *Arthritis Rheum* 1990;**33**:1065.

Churg A, Churg J (editors): *Systemic Vasculitides.* Igaku-Shoin, 1991.

Hurst JW et al (editors): *The Heart: Arteries and Veins.* McGraw-Hill, 1990.

Pericardial Disease

Fowler NO: Recurrent pericarditis. *Cardiol Clin* 1990; **8**:.621.

Gregoratos G: Pericardial involvement in acute myocardial infarction. *Cardiol Clin* 1990;**8**:601.

Khan AH: The postcardiac injury syndromes. *Clin Cardiol* 1992;**15**:67.

Myocardial Disease

Dec GW Jr et al: Active myocarditis in the spectrum of acute dilated cardiomyopathies. Clinical features, histologic correlates, and clinical outcomes. *N Engl J Med* 1985;**312**:885.

Maze SS, Adolph RJ: Myocarditis: Unresolved issues in diagnosis and treatment. *Clin Cardiol* 1990;**13**:69.

Endomyocardial Disease

Chusid MJ et al: The hypereosinophilic syndrome: Analysis of fourteen cases with review of the literature. *Medicine* 1975;**54**:1.

Olsen EGJ, Spry CJF: The pathogenesis of Löffler's endomyocardial disease, and its relationship to endomyocardial fibrosis. Chap 12, pp 281–303, in: *Progress in Cardiology,* 8th ed. Yu PN, Goodwin JF (editors). Lea & Febiger, 1979.

Roberts WC, Liegler DG, Carbone PP: Endomyocardial disease and eosinophilia: A clinical and pathologic spectrum. *Am J Med* 1969;**46**:28.

Small-Vessel Vasculitis

Cupps TR, Fauci AS: Cutaneous vasculitis. Pages 136–140 in: *Current Therapy in Allergy and Immunology 1983–1984.* Lichtenstein LM, Fauci AS (editors). BC Decker, 1983.

Gibson LE: Cutaneous vasculitis: Approach to diagnosis and systemic associations. *Mayo Clin Proc* 1990; **65**:221.

Ilan Y, Naparstek Y: Schönlein-Henoch syndrome in adults and children. *Semin Arthritis Rheum* 1991; **21**(2):103.

Wisnieski JJ, Naff GB: Serum IgG antibodies to C1q in hypocomplementemic urticarial vasculitis syndrome. *Arthritis Rheum* 1989;**32**:1119.

Yazici H et al: A controlled trial of azathioprine in Behçet's syndrome. *N Engl J Med* 1990;**322**:322.

Systemic Necrotizing Vasculitis

Falk RJ and The Glomerular Disease Collaborative Network: Clinical course of anti-neutrophil cytoplasmic autoantibody-associated glomerulonephritis and systemic vasculitis. *Ann Intern Med* 1990;**113**:656.

Fauci AS et al: Cyclophophamide therapy of severe systemic necrotizing vasculitis. *N Engl J Med* 1979; **301**:235.

Lanham JG et al: Systemic vasculitis with asthma and eosinophilia: A clinical approach to the Churg-Strauss syndrome. *Medicine* 1984;**63**:65.

Travers RL et al: Polyarteritis nodosa: A clinical and angiographic analysis of 17 cases. *Semin Arthritis Rheum* 1979;**8**:184.

Wegener's Granulomatosis

Hoffman GS et al: Wegener granulomatosis: An analysis of 158 patients. *Ann Intern Med* 1992;**116**:488.

Hoffman GS et al: The treatment of Wegener's granulomatosis with glucocorticoids and methotrexate. *Arthritis Rheum* 1992;**35**:1322.

Nolle B et al: Anticytoplasmic autoantibodies: Their immunodiagnostic value in Wegener granulomatosis. *Ann Intern Med* 1989;**111**:28.

Temporal Arteritis

Hamilton CR Jr, Shelley WM, Tumulty PA: Giant cell arteritis: Including temporal arteritis and polymyalgia rheumatica. *Medicine* 1971;**50**:1.

Hunder GG: Giant cell (temporal) arteritis. *Rheum Dis Clin North Am* 1990;**16**:399.

Takayasu Arteritis

Fraga A et al: Takayasu's arteritis: Frequency of systemic manifestations (study of 22 patients) and favorable response to maintenance steroid therapy with adrenocorticosteroids (12 patients). *Arthritis Rheum* 1972;**15**:617.

Halls, S et al: Takayasu arteritis: A study of 32 North American patients. *Medicine* 1985;**64**:89.

Shelhamer JH et al: Takayasu's arteritis and its therapy. *Ann Intern Med* 1985;**103**:121.

Thromboangiitis Obliterans

Lie JT: Thromboangiitis obliterans (Buerger's disease) in women. *Medicine* 1986;**65**:65.

Shionoya S et al: Diagnosis, pathology, and treatment of Buerger's disease. *Surgery* 1974;**75**:695.

Other Syndromes

Cupps TR, Moore PM, Fauci AS: Isolated angiitis of the central nervous system: Prospective diagnostic and therapeutic experience. *Am J Med* 1983;**74**:97.

Gastrointestinal, Hepatobiliary, & Orodental Diseases

35

Stephen P. James, MD, Warren Strober, MD, & John S. Greenspan, BDS, PhD, FRCPath

As reviewed in Chapter 41, the gastrointestinal tract is normally a site of intense immunologic activity. The gastrointestinal lumen contains a complex mixture of harmless (and necessary) members of the bacterial flora, potential pathogens, and large quantities of complex macromolecules capable of eliciting immune responses. The mucosal immune system has evolved mechanisms to down-regulate immune responses to harmless flora and food antigens, while eliciting protective responses to pathogens. The diseases reviewed in this chapter are thought to be the result of aberrations of the mucosal immune response to harmless exogenous antigens or autoantigens, resulting in inappropriate injury to the host, or diseases such as hepatitis in which the immunologic host response to a pathologic agent is an important component of the disease process.

GASTROINTESTINAL DISEASES

Stephen P. James, MD, & Warren Strober, MD

GLUTEN-SENSITIVE ENTEROPATHY

Major Immunologic Features
- There is hypersensitivity to cereal grain proteins (gliadins).
- Antigliadin antibodies are present.
- The lamina propria is infiltrated with lymphocytes and plasma cells, associated with villous atrophy.
- It is associated with HLA-DR3 and -DR7.
- It may be associated with dermatitis herpetiformis.

General Considerations
Gluten-sensitive enteropathy (celiac sprue, nontropical sprue) is a disease of the small intestine that is characterized by villous atrophy and malabsorp-

tion. It is caused by hypersensitivity to cereal grain storage proteins (gluten or gliadin, a substance derived from gluten) found in wheat, barley, and oats. The disease is most common in whites and occurs only occasionally in African blacks and not in Asians. It is either limited to the intestine or associated with a vesicular skin disease, dermatitis herpetiformis.

Pathology
The inflammatory lesions are restricted to the small-intestinal mucosa, with the most severe changes being in the area most often in contact with ingested gluten, the proximal small intestine. Gliadin challenge studies show that the disease begins with subepithelial edema and thickening of the basement membrane followed by an influx of inflammatory cells. The latter initially consists of polymorphonuclear leukocytes, but these are soon replaced by lymphocytes and plasma cells. Although IgA plasma cells increase in number and continue to predominate, there is a disproportionate increase in IgG plasma cells; in contrast, few if any IgE plasma cells appear. These inflammatory changes are accompanied by shortening and eventual flattening of the villi and lengthening of the crypts; the latter is indicative of a marked increased in epithelial cell turnover (Fig 35–1). When dermatitis herpetiformis is present, the intestinal lesions are similar to (but usually milder than) those when it is absent, while the skin lesions consist of subepidermal collections of inflammatory cells near areas of fluid accumulation. A characteristic feature of the skin lesions is the presence of granular deposits of IgA and complement in both lesional and normal skin.

Immunologic Pathogenesis
Gluten-sensitive enteropathy is most probably due to a specific immunologic hyperreactivity to gliadin, which leads to the induction of gliadin-specific lymphocytes in the mucosa. Consistent with this hypoth-

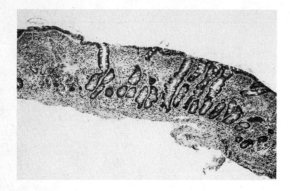

Figure 35–1. Gluten-sensitive enteropathy. Jejunal biopsy specimen shows complete loss of villi, elongation of crypts, and lymphocytic infiltrate in a severe case.

esis, patients have antibody responses to gliadin that are quantitatively and qualitatively distinct from those found in the other gastrointestinal tract diseases. They also have gliadin-specific T cell-mediated responses that are not seen in controls. Further evidence of an immunologic origin comes from organ culture studies that show that gliadin is not toxic by itself but instead requires the participation of an endogenous effector mechanism. In addition, 80–90% of patients both with and without dermatitis herpetiformis bear a particular complex of HLA antigens including HLA-B8, HLA-DR3, HLA-DR7, and certain DP and DQ locus antigens. This finding suggests that particular immune response genes are the basis of the inappropriate antigliadin immune responses that are presumably causing the disease.

Clinical Features

In gluten-sensitive enteropathy alone, the clinical course is dominated by gastrointestinal tract symptoms and malabsorption, whereas when dermatitis herpetiformis is present the course is dominated by a vesicular skin eruption and the intestinal disease is usually absent. The intestinal symptoms of gluten-sensitive enteropathy are highly variable and consist of weight loss, diarrhea, symptoms due to nutritional deficiencies, and growth failure in children. When dermatitis herpetiformis is present, the skin disease consists of a vesicular, intensely pruritic skin eruption on extensor and exposed surfaces. Typical laboratory findings in gluten-sensitive enteropathy include evidence of malabsorption: increased fecal fat, abnormal D-xylose absorption, vitamin deficiencies, anemia, and, in severe cases, biochemical evidence of osteomalacia and abnormal coagulation due to vitamin K deficiency. Intestinal contrast studies during active disease show dilatation and thickening of the proximal small bowel. The intestinal biopsy is the most important specific diagnostic test, particularly in association with gluten challenge studies.

Immunologic Diagnosis

The diagnosis of gluten-sensitive enteropathy is established by demonstrating villous atrophy in the small-bowel biopsy, which resolves with removal of gluten from the diet and which reappears with gluten challenge. Antigliadin antibodies are present in active disease, but their presence is not entirely specific, unless they are present in high titers and are of the IgA class. The presence of HLA-B8, -DR3, or -DR7 is supportive of the diagnosis but not pathognomonic.

Differential Diagnosis

The differential diagnosis includes all intestinal diseases causing malabsorption. However, small-bowel biopsy showing villous atrophy and inflammation considerably narrows the diagnostic possibilities to gluten-sensitive enteropathy, tropical sprue, hypogammaglobulinemia, and some forms of intestinal lymphoma.

Treatment

Treatment consists of lifelong elimination of gluten-containing foods from the diet. It is recommended that such treatment be instituted even in patients with mild disease because a major complication of gluten-sensitive enteropathy is an increased prevalence of small-bowel carcinoma and lymphoma, and it is thought that reduction of chronic inflammation by gluten restriction may diminish the risk of this complication. Nutritional supplements should be instituted as needed in patients with active disease. Very severe disease, particularly associated with severe villous atrophy and small-bowel ulceration, may respond to corticosteroids. When dermatitis herpetiformis is present, both the intestinal and skin lesions can also be treated with a gluten-free diet. However, more usually, diaminodiphenylsulfone (dapsone), an anti-inflammatory drug that provides good control of the skin lesions, is used.

Complications & Prognosis

Unrecognized and untreated gluten-sensitive enteropathy may lead to severe debility and death, but following treatment, patients usually return to normal health and have a normal life expectancy. As noted above, the incidence of intestinal carcinoma and lymphoma is increased. Recently it has been shown that intestinal lymphoma is most often a CD8 T cell lymphoma. Patients with long-standing intestinal changes may be relatively unresponsive to a gluten-free diet and may require corticosteroid therapy. Rarely, patients develop villous atrophy associated with severe intestinal ulceration (ulcerative iliojejunitis), a syndrome that in some instances becomes life-threatening.

NON-GLUTEN (NON-GLIADIN) HYPERSENSITIVITY

Major Immunologic Features
- There is IgE-mediated hypersensitivity or gluten-sensitive enteropathy-like hypersensitivities.
- There are ill-defined mucosal abnormalities marked by eosinophilic infiltration or villous atrophy of the mucosa.

General Considerations
Several conditions marked by hypersensitivity to food substances other than gluten (gliadin) also occur. These include IgE-mediated food allergy localized to the gastrointestinal tract, usually associated with nongastrointestinal allergic symptoms. The causative food substance in this case can induce an increase in mucosal IgE plasma cells and mast cell degranulation, which may lead to a severe protein-losing enteropathy. Treatment consists of eliminating the offending food from the diet (see Chapter 25).

A second type of hypersensitivity is due to food substances that induce a clinical picture nearly identical to that in gluten-sensitive enteropathy: villous atrophy and malabsorption developing days to weeks after exposure to the causative substance. This condition is more or less limited to young children and is most frequently caused by cow's milk protein; however, soy, egg, and wheat proteins have also been implicated. It frequently occurs after a gastrointestinal infection and resolves spontaneously after the age of 3 years. It may be due to immaturity of the mucosal immune system and hence an inability to develop immunologic tolerance to food antigens.

Finally, there is an ill-defined group of gastrointestinal tract hypersensitivity states marked by either eosinophilic infiltration of the bowel or villous atrophy and not definitely associated with a causative food or other agent. In some cases these conditions may be due to a self-perpetuating inflammation that was initiated by an inappropriate immune response, whereas in other cases it may be due to an autoimmune process.

CROHN'S DISEASE

Major Immunologic Feature
- There is transmural granulomatous inflammation of the bowel wall.

General Considerations
Crohn's disease (regional ileitis, granulomatous ileitis, or colitis) is a syndrome of unknown origin characterized by transmural inflammation of the bowel wall. It occurs worldwide, but is most common in persons of European origin. The prevalence ranges from 10 to 70 per 100,000, and it is much more common in industrialized countries. There is a slight female predominance. The disorder can begin at any age, but most typically begins between 15 and 30 years of age. There is a familial aggregation of cases but no clear mode of inheritance.

Pathology
Crohn's disease may involve any part of the alimentary tract from the mouth to the anus, although most patients fall into one of the typical patterns of the disease, having predominant involvement of the ileocolic, small-intestinal, or colonic/anorectal regions. The gross pathology of Crohn's disease is characterized by transmural inflammation of the bowel wall, often in a discontinuous fashion, with ulceration, strictures, and fistulae being typical findings. The histopathologic findings are those of a discontinuous granulomatous inflammatory process (true granulomas are found in about 60% of surgically resected specimens) (Fig 35–2), crypt abscesses, fissures, and aphthous ulcers. The inflammatory infiltrate is mixed, consisting of lymphocytes (both T and B cells), plasma cells, macrophages, and neutrophils. There is a disproportionate increase in IgM- and IgG-secreting plasma cells compared with IgA-secreting cells, but the latter are also increased. The number of T cells is increased, but a normal proportion of CD4 and CD8 cells is maintained.

Crohn's disease (like ulcerative colitis, below) is found primarily in industrialized countries, suggesting that one or more environmental factors are important in pathogenesis; however, no such factors have yet been identified. Infection with *Mycobacterium paratuberculosis* species has been suggested as a cause, but recent evidence makes it more likely that this organism is a commensal that does not have an etiologic role. Because of the failure to identify a specific causative infectious microorganism, it has been suggested that the disease has a primary immunologic basis. One leading possibility in this regard is that the mucosal inflammation in Crohn's disease is the result of abnormality of mucosal T cell regulation, which leads to an inappropriate mucosal im-

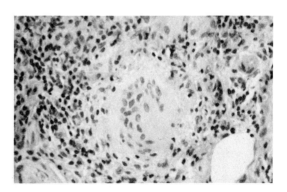

Figure 35–2. Crohn's disease. Rectal biopsy specimen shows mucosal granuloma.

mune response to ubiquitous intestinal antigens (see Chapter 15). In support of this concept are the facts that (1) the inflammatory lesion in Crohn's disease begins as a follicular collection of lymphocytes which resembles a normal (if inappropriate) immune response; (2) patients manifest excessive responses to oral antigen challenge; and (3) several immuno-regulatory defects have been identified, including the presence of circulating suppressor T cells and abnormal lymphokine secretory patterns in the mucosa. However, these data are not conclusive, and additional work is needed to establish an immunologic origin.

Clinical Features

Typical symptoms include abdominal pain, anorexia, weight loss, fever, diarrhea, perianal discomfort and discharge, and extraintestinal symptoms involving the skin, eyes, and joints. The manifestations vary somewhat according to the predominant pattern of intestinal involvement. Extraintestinal manifestations are not unusual and include arthritis, erythema nodosum, pyoderma gangrenosum, aphthous mouth ulcers, uveitis, anemia, urinary calculi, and sclerosing cholangitis. Typical laboratory abnormalities include anemia (chronic disease, iron deficiency, vitamin B_{12} deficiency, folate deficiency), leukocytosis, thrombocytosis, elevation of the erythrocyte sedimentation rate, hypoalbuminemia, electrolyte abnormalities (in severe diarrhea), and presence of occult blood in the stool. Many radiographic abnormalities may be present in small-bowel and colon contrast studies. These include aphthous ulceration, linear ulceration, edema, and thickening of the bowel wall (Fig 35–3), as well as strictures, fissures, fistulae, and mass lesions (inflammatory mass or abscess); the chronic inflammation also may lead to a characteristic "cobblestone" pattern. When the areas involved are accessible, endoscopy provides a direct method of evaluating disease activity and permits collection of biopsy material for pathologic confirmation as well as screening for colon carcinoma.

Immunologic Diagnosis

Multiple abnormalities of immune function have been described, but none has diagnostic specificity.

Differential Diagnosis

Diseases sometimes having an appearance similar to Crohn's disease are appendicitis, diverticulitis, intestinal neoplasia, and intestinal infections (*M tuberculosis, Chlamydia, Yersinia entercolitica, Campylobacter jejuni, Entamoeba histolytica, Cryptosporidium,* herpes simplex virus, cytomegalo-virus, *Salmonella,* and *Shigella*). A combination of stool cultures, intestinal biopsies, and clinical follow-up are usually sufficient to exclude these possibilities.

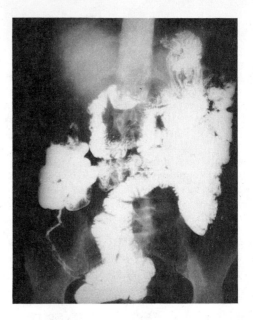

Figure 35–3. Crohn's disease. Small-bowel barium contrast x-ray shows marked narrowing of the terminal ileum as a result of transmural inflammation.

Treatment

The anti-inflammatory drug sulfasalazine and newer 5-aminosalicylic acid (5-ASA) agents are useful in treating mildly active colonic Crohn's disease and is commonly used in an attempt to maintain remission of disease, although a National Cooperative Crohn's Disease trial did not prove that such prophylaxis is effective. Metronidazole is similar in efficacy to sulfasalazine and appears to be particularly useful for perianal disease, although its side effects (seizures, peripheral neuropathy, disulfuram-like reaction to alcohol) may be significant. In more severe active disease, corticosteroids are effective in treating acute exacerbations and possibly in maintaining remission in some patients. There is no evidence, however, that corticosteroids prevent the progression of subclinical disease. Azathioprine and 6-mercaptopurine are used as steroid-sparing drugs in patients who require chronic corticosteroids and are not amenable to surgical therapy; in addition, it has been suggested but not proved that these drugs may have a role in long-term prophylaxis. There may be a long delay in the onset of action of these drugs (6 months). Antidiarrheal drugs provide symptomatic relief in some patients. Dietary management with elemental diets or total parental nutrition is useful for improving the nutritional status of patients and in inducing symptomatic improvement of acute disease, but diet alone does not induce sustained clinical remissions. Antibiotics are used in treating secondary small-bowel bacterial overgrowth and in treatment of pyogenic complications. Cyclosporin is currently under investigation in controlled trials; early, uncontrolled experience with this drug indicates that it produces improvement in some but not all patients with severe Crohn's disease. Finally, surgical treatment is necessary when the disease is not controlled medically and when various complications occur (see below).

Complications & Prognosis

Patients typically have recurrent episodes of active disease with periods of intervening quiescence. However, they often have low-grade symptoms even during periods of apparent disease inactivity, and the disease has high social and economic costs. Approximately two-thirds of patients require surgery at some time during their life for diseases not treatable with tolerable doses of steroids or for complications such as obstruction, abscess, fistula, hemorrhage, or megacolon. However, the disease is clearly not curable by surgical resection and recurs at a rate approaching 90% in very long-term follow-up. The mortality rate of Crohn's disease is approximately twice that in the general age-matched population, although most mortality occurs early in the course of the disease and there is only a small increase in mortality in patients with long-standing disease. The incidence of intestinal carcinoma is increased, but the frequency is much lower than that associated with ulcerative colitis.

ULCERATIVE COLITIS

Major Immunologic Features

- Colonic mucosa is chronically inflamed, with ulceration of the epithelial layer.
- Anticolon antibodies are present.
- ANCA is present in subgroups of patients.

General Considerations

Idiopathic ulcerative colitis is a disease of unknown origin characterized by chronic inflammation of the colonic mucosa. As with Crohn's disease, ulcerative colitis is found primarily in industrialized nations, although it does occur worldwide. The prevalence ranges from 37 to 80 per 100,000 with a slight female predominance. Although it was previously reported to be much more common in Jews, this finding was probably due to selection bias. There are two peaks of incidence: one in the third decade and one in the fifth decade. There is a significant familial association but no clear pattern of inheritance.

Pathology

Ulcerative colitis, in contrast to Crohn's disease, is limited to the colon and involves mainly the superficial layers of the bowel. In addition, the inflammation is continuous and is not associated with granulomas. Typically, the disease is found in the distal colon and rectosigmoid area, but it extends proximally to involve the entire colon in more severe cases. Gross pathologic findings include edema, increased mucosal friability, and frank ulceration. Histologic features are crypt abscesses consisting of accumulations of polymorphonuclear cells adjacent to crypts, necrosis of the epithelium, and surrounding accumulations of chronic inflammatory cells (Fig 35–4). Over time, there is distortion of the crypt architecture. Finally, in long-standing disease, epithelial-cell dysplasia and colonic carcinoma may be found.

As in Crohn's disease, the immunopathogenesis is uncertain. Autoantibodies reactive with mucin-associated antigens or with colonic epithelial-cell antigens have been identified in patients. These antibodies have in some cases been demonstrated to cross-react with bacterial cell wall antigens and have been identified in relatives of patients. Other studies have shown that lymphocytes from patients with ulcerative colitis can be cytotoxic for colonic epithelial cells; although not completely proven, this is probably due to arming of Fc receptor-bearing cytotoxic cells with anti-epithelial cell antibodies. These findings suggest that primary immunologic mechanisms, possibly involving an autoimmune component, are the basis of the disease. Overall, the disease mechanism appears to be similar but not identical to that underlying Crohn's disease.

Clinical Features

The clinical features are highly variable. The onset may be insidious or abrupt. Symptoms include diarrhea, tenesmus, and relapsing rectal bleeding. With fulminant involvement of the entire colon, toxic megacolon, a life-threatening emergency, may occur. Extraintestinal manifestations include arthritis, pyoderma gangrenosum, uveitis, and erythema nodosum. As mentioned above, colonic dysplasia and carcinoma may ensue in long-standing disease. Typical

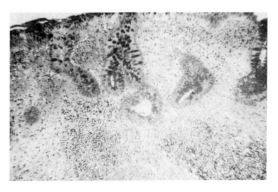

Figure 35–4. Ulcerative colitis. Rectal biopsy specimen shows distortion of crypts and lymphoid aggregates.

laboratory abnormalities include anemia (chronic disease, iron deficiency), leukocytosis, thrombocytosis, elevation of the erythrocyte sedimentation rate, electrolyte abnormalities (in severe diarrhea), and the presence of occult blood in stool. A barium enema study may demonstrate ulcerations and, in more severe disease, pseudopolyps. In chronic disease the colon may be shortened, narrowed, and tubular. Colonoscopy is useful for direct assessment of the degree and extent of inflammation, for biopsy confirmation of the diagnosis, and for screening for dysplasia and carcinoma.

Immunologic Diagnosis

No immunologic test is specific for the disease. Anti-colon epithelial-cell antibodies have been identified in research laboratories, but they have not been shown to be of diagnostic utility. Antineutrophil cytoplasmic antibodies (ANCA) have been identified in subgroups of patients, but their presence does not correlate with disease activity and is not specific for ulcerative colitis.

Differential Diagnosis

The differential diagnosis is similar to that listed above for Crohn's disease, with the addition of ischemic colitis, radiation-induced enteritis, and pseudomembranous colitis. It is occasionally difficult to distinguish between Crohn's disease of the colon and ulcerative colitis. Such differentiation is usually based on the fact that Crohn's disease, but not ulcerative colitis, is a discontinuous lesion and is associated with granulomatous inflammation.

Treatment

As in the case of Crohn's disease, sulfasalazine and related salicylate-containing drugs are effective in mild cases and corticosteroid drugs are effective in severe cases. Sulfasalazine is used to maintain remission, although with variable results. Topical administration of either salicylates or corticosteroids is effective in some patients, particularly those with disease limited to distal bowel, and is associated with decreased side effects compared with systemic use. Supportive measures such as administration of iron and antidiarrheal agents are sometimes indicated. Azathioprine and 6-mercaptopurine are sometimes used in refractory corticosteroid-dependent cases.

Complications & Prognosis

Ulcerative colitis patients usually respond to medical therapy and enjoy a reasonable quality of life without surgical intervention. However, patients with severe intractable disease or with megacolon may require colectomy. In contrast to Crohn's disease, surgery completely eliminates the disease. In patients who have the disease for longer than 2 decades, the incidence of colon carcinoma increases significantly, and so patients should be subjected to periodic screening examinations. Whether the presence of colonic dysplasia is an indication for prophylactic colectomy is controversial.

ALPHA HEAVY-CHAIN DISEASE

Major Immunologic Features
- The small intestine is infiltrated with malignant, α-chain-producing B cells.
- α-Heavy chain protein is present in serum.

General Considerations

The immunoproliferative intestinal diseases consist of a rare group of premalignant or malignant lymphomas that are limited mostly to the small bowel. The pathognomonic feature is infiltration of the bowel by aberrant B cells, which produce α-heavy chains. The diseases are usually found in underdeveloped countries, especially in the Middle East, and generally in young patients of low socioeconomic status. It has been suggested that the disease begins as a response to excessive antigenic stimulation as a result of infectious agents in the setting of malnutrition, since it may respond initially to antibiotic administration. The diffuse infiltration of the intestine is associated with villous flattening and malabsorption. Mucosal ulceration and small-bowel obstruction may occur with progression. The diagnosis is established by intestinal biopsy and the presence of α-heavy chain in the serum.

PERNICIOUS ANEMIA

Major Immunologic Features
- Anti-parietal cell antibodies are present.
- Anti-intrinsic factor antibodies are present.

General Considerations

Pernicious anemia is an autoimmune disease in which there is progressive destruction of the gastric fundic glands, leading to atrophic gastritis, achlorhydria, loss of production of intrinsic factor, and vitamin B_{12} malabsorption. The disease presents insidiously with megaloblastic anemia and rarely with neurologic complications due to vitamin B_{12} deficiency. Recognition and treatment of the disease prior to onset of neurologic symptoms is important to prevent irreversible neurologic damage. There is an increased familial incidence and an association with other autoimmune diseases, particularly those involving the thyroid and adrenal glands. Other associations include vitiligo, hypoparathyroidism, and common variable hypogammaglobulinemia. Most patients with pernicious anemia have anti-parietal cell antibodies, and the majority have anti-intrinsic factor antibodies. The fact that such antibodies are found with increased frequency in unaffected family members as well as in patients with other autoimmune diseases suggests that (1) the disease has a genetic component and (2) these antibodies do not cause disease by themselves. This fact, as well as other data, suggests that the disease is caused primarily by T cell-mediated immune damage to the stomach. Routine laboratory abnormalities in pernicious anemia include the presence of megaloblastic anemia, vitamin B_{12} deficiency, and increased serum gastrin. The diagnosis is confirmed by the demonstration of achlorhydria and an abnormal Shilling test, which corrects with addition of intrinsic factor. Treatment consists of vitamin B_{12} replacement. Patients with pernicious anemia have an increased incidence of gastric polyps and gastric carcinoma, and therefore attention to gastric symptoms and screening for occult blood in the stool are indicated.

WHIPPLE'S DISEASE

Major Immunologic Features
- There is massive infiltration of the lamina propria with periodic acid-Schiff-positive macrophages.
- There are secondary T cell abnormalities.

General Considerations
Whipple's disease is a rare infectious disease caused by the bacterium *Tropheryma whippelii*, which has not yet been cultured. Characteristic features include abdominal pain, diarrhea, weight loss,

and a variety of central nervous system manifestations. The diagnosis is established by intestinal biopsy, which discloses free-lying bacteria and the characteristic presence of large numbers of macrophages containing bacterial cell wall debris (periodic acid-Schiff-positive material) in the lamina propria. The infection is not limited to the gastrointestinal tract and can involve the heart, lungs, serosal surfaces, joints, and central nervous system. In the gastrointestinal tract, the cell infiltration leads to "clubbed" villi, lymphatic obstruction, malabsorption, and protein-losing enteropathy. These patients suffer progressive inanition. In addition, when lymphatic obstruction is severe, they may lose lymphocytes into the gastrointestinal tract, become lymphopenic, and develop a secondary T cell immunodeficiency. The cause of the disease is unclear, but it may be due to an inability to respond immunologically to particular bacterial antigens. In any case, the disease frequently responds to antibiotic therapy.

HEPATOBILIARY DISEASES

Stephen P. James, MD, & Warren Strober, MD

Several diseases of the liver and biliary tract have important immunologic features in pathogenesis. These include acute viral hepatitis (Table 35–1), chronic hepatitis, and primary sclerosing cholangitis.

Table 35–1. Viral and serologic characteristics of hepatitis.

| Type | Viral Markers | | Serologic Markers | |
	Antigen	Characteristics	Antibody	Characteristics
Hepatitis A	HAAg (hepatitis A antigen)	Found in stool during incubation and transiently during acute symptomatic phase.	IgM anti-HAV IgG anti-HAV	Acute hepatitis Long-lived antibody found during convalescence
Hepatitis B	HBsAg B surface antigen	Viral coat; present in acute and chronic phase.	Anti-HBe	Found during convalescence
	HBcAg	Core antigen found in nuclei of infected hepatocytes.	IgM anti-HBc IgG anti-HBc	Acute hepatitis High titer in chronic hepatitis
	HBeAg	Virus-encoded protein of unknown function; marker of active viral replication.	Anti-HBe	Found after resolution of active replication
	DNA polymerase (HBV DNA)	Found in serum during active replication.		
Hepatitis D	Delta antigen	Found primarily in hepatocyte nuclei and occasionally in serum during active infection.	Anti-delta	High titer in chronic infection
	HBV markers	Requires coinfection with HBV.		
Hepatitis C	HCV recombinant antigens	HCV mRNA in serum	Anti-HCV	Acute and chronic hepatitis
Hepatitis E			Anti-HEV	Acute and chronic hepatitis

HEPATITIS A

Major Immunologic Feature

■ There are antibodies to HAV (IgG antibodies are long-lived).

General Considerations

Hepatitis A is an acute liver infection caused by a small RNA picornavirus (hepatitis A virus, HAV). The virus may cause dramatic epidemics or appear sporadically. Transmission is virtually always by the fecal-oral route. During acute viral hepatitis, there is ballooning and acidophilic degeneration of hepatocytes and portal and periportal infiltration with mononuclear cells. In severe disease, there may be massive necrosis of the liver. HAV particles may be identified in the cytoplasm of infected hepatocytes. Young children with hepatitis A may be asymptomatic, whereas adults usually have nausea, vomiting, dark urine, abdominal pain, and fatigue. Hepatomegaly, abdominal tenderness, and jaundice are typical findings in symptomatic patients. HAV is one of the causes of fulminant hepatitis, which is associated with hepatic encephalopathy and a high mortality rate. Although a relapsing course may rarely occur, the disease usually resolves completely. Typical laboratory features include striking elevations of the serum aminotransferases.

It is thought that the mechanism of liver injury in hepatitis A is not due to the virus itself but rather to the immune response to viral antigens present on the surface of the hepatocytes. In this regard, cytolytic CD8 T cells, which specifically kill hepatitis A-infected target cells, have been shown to be present in the liver in hepatitis A patients. It is thought that variability in the outcome of acute hepatitis A infection, ie, mild versus fulminant disease, might be due in part to genetically controlled differences in the magnitude of the immune response to the virus.

Immunologic Diagnosis

The diagnosis is confirmed by the presence of IgM anti-HAV antibodies. IgG antibodies are long-lived and may persist for the life of the host, and their presence signifies immunity to infection.

Differential Diagnosis

The differential diagnosis of acute hepatocellular necrosis includes acute viral hepatitis from other viruses; toxic hepatitis due to drugs, chemicals, or physical agents; acute fatty liver associated with pregnancy; acute reactivation of chronic hepatitis; fulminant Wilson's disease; and Reye's syndrome.

Treatment

Hepatitis A usually resolves quickly, and there is no evidence of a long-lasting carrier state. Treatment is supportive. No vaccine currently exists, but prophylaxis for close contacts with immune serum globulin is indicated.

HEPATITIS B

Major Immunologic Features

■ In acute hepatitis there are HBsAg, HBeAg, and IgM anti-HBc in serum.
■ In acute hepatitis (convalescent phase) there is IgG anti-HBs in serum.
■ In chronic hepatitis (active viral replication phase) there are HBV DNA, DNA polymerase, HBsAg, HBeAg, and high-titer IgG anti-HBc in serum.
■ In chronic hepatitis (viral integration phase) there are HBsAg, anti-HBc, and anti-HBe in serum.
■ HBV is not cytopathic; immune mechanisms are thought to cause hepatocyte necrosis.

General Considerations

Hepatitis B virus (HBV) infection is a double-stranded DNA virus of worldwide distribution. The mode of transmission is parenteral or maternal-infant. Individuals at risk for infection include recipients of blood or blood products, drug addicts, dialysis patients, male homosexuals, some health care workers, and infants born to HBV-infected mothers. The risk of chronic infection is higher in infants, immunosuppressed patients, patients with lymphoid cancer, and children with Down's syndrome. Infection has many possible outcomes, including an acute asymptomatic infection or symptomatic hepatitis, a chronic carrier state with or without development of chronic or progressive liver disease, fulminant hepatitis, and hepatocellular carcinoma. Other syndromes associated with HBV include polyarteritis nodosa, aplastic anemia, glomerulonephritis, and essential mixed cryoglobulinemia.

Pathology

The histologic features of acute HBV infection include ballooning and eosinophilic degeneration of hepatocytes, the presence of focal areas of necrosis of hepatocytes, and lymphocytic infiltration of the parenchyma and portal areas. In more severe cases, extensive areas of necrosis of hepatocytes may be present in central and mid zones, which may lead to collapse of the reticulin framework, giving the pattern of "bridging necrosis." In chronic HBV infection, the pathologic findings are variable. In chronic carriers who are clinically well, there may be no histopathologic abnormalities. Alternatively, there may be variable degrees of hepatic inflammation ranging from scattered focal areas of hepatocyte necrosis and lymphocyte infiltration of portal tracts to more severe inflammation, resulting in disruption of the limiting plate between the portal tract and the parenchyma. The latter features are known as piecemeal necrosis. In addition, "ground-glass" hepatocytes, which contain large amounts of hepatitis B surface antigen (HBsAg), may be visible in hematoxylin-and-eosin-stained sections. Chronic type B hepatitis may progress to cirrhosis and hepatocellular carcinoma. Specific antibody staining for HBsAg or hepatitis B core antigen (HBcAg) in acute hepatitis B shows little detectable viral antigen in the liver. In chronic hepatitis, large amounts of HBsAg and (if viral replication is active) HBcAg may be found in hepatocytes.

There is no evidence that HBV is cytopathic, and thus it is thought that hepatocyte injury is mediated by the immune response against the virus. In this regard, evidence has been presented that lymphocytes derived from the liver or circulation of patients with hepatitis B infection are cytotoxic for autologous hepatocytes, but the specificity and mechanism of this cytotoxicity have not yet been completely defined.

Clinical Features

The symptoms of hepatitis B infection are highly variable. As many as half the cases of acute infection are anicteric, and patients have no symptoms or mild nonspecific symptoms of a viral illness. Symptoms described above for acute hepatitis A may occur in typical symptomatic cases. Acute hepatitis B is occasionally preceded by a serum sickness-like syndrome. Approximately 5–10% of patients develop chronic infection (lasting more than 6 months). They often have had a mild or asymptomatic acute infection. During the phase of active viral replication, nonspecific symptoms or symptoms of acute viral hepatitis may be present. With progressive chronic hepatitis, symptoms attributable to cirrhosis or hepatic decompensation may supervene.

Physical findings in acute hepatitis B infection are few. Icterus may be present, the liver may be enlarged and mildly tender, and splenomegaly is sometimes present. In chronic hepatitis B infection, there are often no physical abnormalities until chronic liver damage occurs; at that point, findings common to other chronic liver diseases are seen.

Laboratory findings of acute hepatitis B are similar to those of hepatitis A. In chronic hepatitis B, the serum aminotransferase levels are highly variable and may be normal. However, if significant liver damage is present, hypoalbuminemia and prolongation of the prothrombin time may occur.

Immunologic Diagnosis

Serum immunologic findings in hepatitis B infection are variable, depending on the length and clinical outcome of the infection (Fig 35–5). During acute infection, both HBsAg and IgM anti-HBc are present; in addition, HBV, DNA, and a viral protein antigen known as HBeAg make a transient appearance. With resolution of the acute infection, HBsAg disappears (usually after 1–6 months) and anti-HBsAg appears and persists for years. In chronic infection, the serum findings are variable and depend on the stage of the natural history of the infection. HBsAg is often present in very high titers, as is anti-HBc, but anti-HBs is absent. During the period of active viral replication, HBeAg, DNA polymerase, and HBV DNA are also present. Patients with asymptomatic chronic infection may have episodes of acute reactivation that correlate with the appearance of markers of active viral replication. Eventually, evidence of viral replication may disappear, and there is seroconversion to anti-HBe positivity.

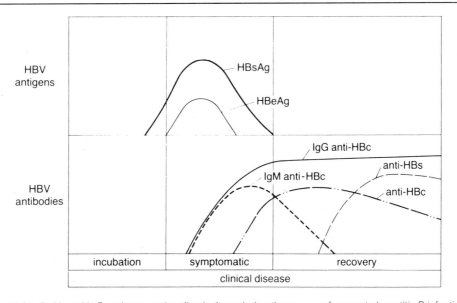

Figure 35–5. Hepatitis B antigens and antibody titers during the course of an acute hepatitis B infection.

Differential Diagnosis

The serologic diagnosis of acute and chronic hepatitis B infection is usually definitive. In the setting of chronic hepatitis B infection, an apparent relapse should prompt a search for other possible cases of liver disease including superimposed delta hepatitis (see below) or drug-induced hepatotoxicity.

Treatment

Acute hepatitis B usually resolves completely, and supportive care is needed only for severe hepatitis. Alpha interferon therapy may induce remission in some patients with chronic active hepatitis.

Prevention

Screening of blood products for hepatitis B virus has nearly eliminated blood products as a mode of transmission. Individuals at high risk of acquiring hepatitis B should be immunized with HBsAg vaccine, which is safe and confers long-lasting immunity in most individuals.

HEPATITIS D
(Delta Hepatitis)

Major Immunologic Features

- It is caused by a defective virus requiring the presence of HBV infection (hepatitis B markers present in serum).
- Anti-delta antibody is present in serum.

General Considerations

Hepatitis D is caused by a small defective (ie, unable to replicate in the absence of another virus) RNA virus (delta agent), which requires the presence of HBV for replication and production of infectious particles. The virus may be associated with acute or fulminant hepatitis due to coinfection with HBV, or it may cause a superimposed acute or chronic hepatitis in patients with chronic hepatitis B infection. The virus is found worldwide and has caused epidemics with high mortality rates. Transmission is primarily parenteral. Since inflammation is not a prominent feature, it is thought that the virus is directly cytopathic. Diagnosis is established by the presence of serum anti-delta antibody and consistent clinical features. There is no effective specific treatment; however, it may be prevented by immunization for hepatitis B, since this prevents the hepatitis B infection necessary for hepatitis D virus replication.

HEPATITIS C
(Non-A, Non-B Hepatitis)

Major Immunologic Features

- It presents as acute and chronic hepatitis similar to hepatitis B.

- There is a specific immunoassay for antibody to viral protein.

General Considerations

Shortly after the development of serologic tests for hepatitis B, it became clear that a significant proportion of patients with acute and chronic posttransfusion hepatitis did not have hepatitis B. A substantial literature subsequently evolved concerning this form of hepatitis, named non-A, and non-B. Hepatitis C virus was not identified until 1989, when Choo et al isolated a cDNA clone from the blood of a patient with non-A, non-B hepatitis and showed that patients with non-A, non-B hepatitis have serum antibodies reactive with synthetic proteins derived from the cDNA sequence. This led quickly to the routine screening of blood donors with an antibody assay, even before complete isolation of the virus.

Hepatitis C virus is an RNA virus that is a member of the Flavivirus group, which includes dengue and yellow fever viruses. Recent work has shown considerable heterogeneity of hepatitis C virus sequences, and these differences may cause differences in their pathogenicity. The distribution of the virus is worldwide and its frequency in blood donors is relatively uniform, ranging from 0.3 to 1.5%. The major known mode of transmission of the virus is by blood, and thus the risk groups for this viral infection include patients who have had blood transfusion, hemodialysis patients, recipients of blood products, intravenous drug abusers, and health care workers. A significant proportion of cases of sporadic, community-acquired hepatitis C virus infection are not associated with any known risk, and in these patients the mode of transmission is unknown. Unlike hepatitis B, vertical transmission from mother to infant does not occur at a significant frequency, probably because patients with chronic hepatitis C virus infection have very low levels of viremia. Furthermore, the risk of sexual transmission appears to be low. Screening of blood donors by using an assay that detects multiple different hepatitis C antigens has greatly diminished the risk of transmission of this disease by blood transfusion. However, since antibody-positivity does not appear immediately after infection, antibody screening cannot completely eliminate the risk of transmission by blood transfusion. The only definitive test for hepatitis C viremia is based on reverse transcription and polymerase chain reaction (PCR) amplification of viral sequences, which is currently available only as a research test.

Liver disease caused by hepatitis C virus has many similarities to hepatitis B. The infection frequently has an onset with a typical, acute hepatitislike illness as described above. Other presentations are possible, including fulminant hepatitis and subclinical infection. Chronic infection with chronic hepatitis is a common sequela of hepatitis C infection, occurring in about one-half of patients. The illness may be characterized by marked fluctuation in the serum transaminase levels. Progression to significant fibrosis and cirrhosis is also relatively common, occurring in about 10% of patients overall. It is now clear that some patients who had been classified as having autoimmune hepatitis in the past have evidence of hepatitis C virus infection (see below). Furthermore, many patients previously classified as having cryptogenic cirrhosis have evidence of hepatitis C virus infection. As with hepatitis B, there is a significant association of hepatocellular carcinoma with cirrhosis due to hepatitis C virus infection. Other syndromes are also associated with this infection, such as mixed cryoglobulinemia with glomerulonephritis.

Randomized controlled trials have demonstrated that some patients with chronic hepatitis C virus infection have beneficial response to long-term (26 weeks) treatment with alpha interferon. Because of the great expense, toxicity, and relatively low response rate, this therapy is generally limited to patients with evidence of significant disease, including persistently marked elevation of serum transaminase levels and liver biopsy abnormalities of chronic active hepatitis with bridging necrosis or cirrhosis and symptomatic cirrhosis. About one-half of patients have a beneficial response as indicated by a marked fall in transaminase levels and disappearance of viral RNA from serum; however only about one-fourth of patients have a sustained remission.

HEPATITIS E

Hepatitis E virus is an RNA virus that is a major cause of acute hepatitis resembling hepatitis A. The virus is a major cause of both sporadic and epidemic hepatitis in developing countries and is transmitted by the fecal-oral route. To date the only cases found in the United States have been found in travelers from areas where the infection is endemic. Hepatitis E has clinical features very similar to those of hepatitis A. It does not cause chronic hepatitis and is not associated with hepatocellular carcinoma. One interesting aspect of the disease that has not been explained is that there is a high fatality rate in pregnant women. Hepatitis E virus infection is associated with the appearance of serum antibodies that can be detected by ELISA. Hepatitis E viral RNA has been detected in stool by PCR assays. Preliminary studies have indicated that animals exposed to hepatitis E virus develop protective immunity, suggesting that the development of an effective vaccine is feasible.

AUTOIMMUNE CHRONIC ACTIVE HEPATITIS

Major Immunologic Features
- There are autoantibodies to smooth-muscle and liver membranes.
- There is polyclonal hypergammaglobulinemia.
- There is HLA-B8/DR3 association.
- There is destruction of hepatocytes associated with portal infiltration of lymphocytes.

General Considerations
Autoimmune hepatitis is a rare form of chronic hepatitis of unknown cause and is associated with various autoimmune phenomena. The disease usually affects women and is more common in individuals of northern European descent. The great majority of cases are sporadic. Of interest, there is a significant association with HLA-B8/DR3 as well as an association with the Gm allotype of IgG, termed "ax." For unknown reasons the incidence of the disease has been declining.

Pathology
The major histologic finding in the liver, one not specific to this disease and mentioned before in relation to hepatitis B infection, is piecemeal necrosis, in which there is necrosis of hepatocytes in the periportal region, disruption of the limiting plate of the portal tract, and local infiltration of lymphoid cells (Fig 35–6). The degree of piecemeal necrosis is variable, but in some patients it may lead to bridging necrosis and cirrhosis. The lymphoid cells infiltrating lesions of autoimmune hepatitis consist of plasma cells and CD4-positive T cells. There are immunoglobulin deposits on hepatocytes.

The mechanism of liver damage in autoimmune hepatitis is unknown. Although autoantibodies against the liver have been shown to be present, it is not clear that they play a role in liver damage. Lym-

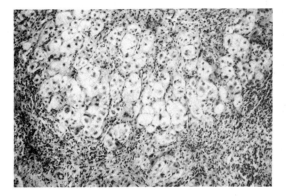

Figure 35–6. Chronic HBV infection. Liver biopsy specimen shows ballooning of hepatocytes and piecemeal necrosis typical of chronic active hepatitis.

phocyte-mediated killing of autologous hepatocytes has been demonstrated in vitro; however, the specificity and mechanism of this killing are uncertain.

Clinical Features

Typical symptoms of autoimmune hepatitis include easy fatigability, jaundice, dark urine, abdominal pain, anorexia, myalgia, delayed menarche, and amenorrhea. Late in the disease, symptoms attributable to progressive chronic liver disease may supervene. Abnormal physical findings include hepatomegaly, jaundice, splenomegaly, spider nevi, and cushingoid features. Common laboratory findings include elevation of serum aminotransferase levels and hypergammaglobulinemia.

Immunologic Diagnosis

There are no serologic features that are diagnostic of the disease. However, polyclonal hypergammaglobulinemia is typically found, and autoantibodies are common, particularly antinuclear antibodies and smooth-muscle antibodies. In addition, antibodies against liver membrane antigens are present. Antimitochondrial antibodies are usually absent and, when present, are found in low titer. Serologic markers of hepatitis viruses are absent. The presence of HLA-B8 supports the diagnosis.

Differential Diagnosis

Since there are no specific diagnostic tests, viral hepatitis and drug- or chemical-induced liver injury must be excluded as well as rare liver diseases such as Wilson's disease and other metabolic liver diseases such as α_1-antitrypsin deficiency. Primary biliary cirrhosis may have features that overlap those of autoimmune hepatitis, but this disease is associated with the presence of antimitochondrial antibodies (see below). Primary sclerosing cholangitis is occasionally misdiagnosed as autoimmune hepatitis, but this disease is associated with characteristic radiographic abnormalities of the biliary system.

Treatment

Unlike those with viral hepatitis, patients with severe autoimmune hepatitis respond favorably to corticosteroid treatment. This therapy may prevent or retard the development of cirrhosis and may improve survival.

PRIMARY BILIARY CIRRHOSIS

Major Immunologic Features
- Associated autoimmune syndromes are frequent.
- There is a high titer of antimitochondrial antibodies in most patients.
- Serum IgM with abnormal properties is elevated.

- There is lymphocytic infiltration and destruction of intrahepatic bile ducts.

General Considerations

Primary biliary cirrhosis is a chronic disease of unknown cause, primarily affecting middle-aged women. It is characterized by chronic intrahepatic cholestasis due to chronic inflammation and necrosis of intrahepatic bile ducts and progresses insidiously to biliary cirrhosis. Although syndromes resembling primary biliary cirrhosis may follow ingestion of drugs such as chlorpromazine or contraceptive steroids, no toxic or infectious agent has been identified. It has been suggested that primary biliary cirrhosis is an autoimmune disease because of the frequent association of other autoimmune syndromes, the presence of autoantibodies, and histologic features of the disease. Its prevalence has been estimated to be 2.3–14.4 per 100,000. The distribution of the disease is worldwide, without predilection for any racial or ethnic groups. The usual age at diagnosis is in the fifth and sixth decades, but age at onset varies widely from the third to the ninth decade. Ninety percent of patients are female. Familial aggregation has been reported but is rare; however, although there is no known HLA association, the incidence of immunologic abnormalities has been reported to be increased in family members.

Pathology

The histologic abnormalities in the liver have been divided into 4 stages, although they overlap, and more than one stage may be found in biopsies from the same patient. The earliest changes (stage I) are most specific and consist of localized areas of infiltration of intrahepatic bile ducts with lymphocytes and necrosis of biliary epithelial cells; these lesions may have granulomas in close proximity (Fig 35–7).

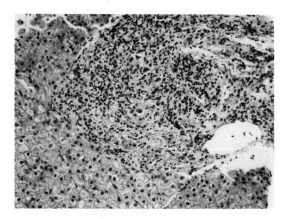

Figure 35–7. Primary biliary cirrhosis. Percutaneous liver biopsy specimen shows bile duct surrounded by dense lymphoid infiltrate typical of stage 1 disease.

In stage II there is proliferation of bile ductules, prominent infiltration of portal areas with lymphoid cells, and early portal fibrosis. Stage III is characterized by reduction of the inflammatory changes, paucity of bile ducts in the portal triads, and increased portal fibrosis. In stage IV, fibrosis is prominent in biliary cirrhosis and a marked increase in hepatic copper is found. Thus, the pathologic process is characterized by slowly progressive, spotty destruction of bile ducts, with associated inflammation and fibrosis and, ultimately, cirrhosis. Hepatocellular necrosis is not a prominent feature, although there are occasional cases of primary biliary cirrhosis-chronic active hepatitis overlap syndromes with piecemeal necrosis. Immunofluorescence shows predominantly IgM plasma cells in portal triads and deposition of IgM. CD4 T cells predominate in portal triads, but CD8 T cells have been observed in close proximity to damaged epithelial cells. HLA-DR antigen expression is increased on biliary epithelial cells, a finding associated with autoimmunity (see Chapter 30).

Although the mechanisms of liver injury in this disease are unknown, the presence of associated autoimmune syndromes and other features suggests that primary biliary cirrhosis is an autoimmune disease. Patients frequently have circulating immune complex-like materials, abnormalities of the complement cascade, and nearly always antimitochondrial antibodies. These antibodies have different specificities, the most prevalent being against the E2 component of pyruvate dehydrogenase, which is present on the inner mitochondrial membrane. In recent years, ample evidence of immunoregulator abnormalities have been found, and it is thought that these underlie the autoimmunity.

Clinical Features

The onset of symptoms is typically insidious, and as many as half of all patients are asymptomatic at diagnosis. Typical symptoms include pruritus, fatigue, increased skin pigmentation, arthralgias, and dryness of the mouth and eyes. Jaundice and gastrointestinal bleeding from varices are uncommon presentations. There may be no abnormalities on physical examination. Typical findings that occur with disease progression include hepatomegaly, splenomegaly, skin hyperpigmentation, excoriations, xanthomata, xanthelasma, spider telangiectasia, and, late in the disease, deep jaundice, petechiae, purpura, and signs of hepatic decompensation. In addition, symptoms or signs of the many associated autoimmune syndromes may be present. The most common include keratoconjunctivitis sicca, arthritis, hypothyroidism, scleroderma (CREST variant), Raynaud's phenomenon, and pulmonary alveolitis.

Common laboratory abnormalities include elevation of serum alkaline phosphatase and γ-glutamyl transpeptidase. Total bilirubin is normal early in the disease but increases progressively as the disease advances. Hypercholesterolemia is also common. Nonspecific laboratory changes of hepatic decompensation are found late in the disease. Cholangiography is normal early in the course of the disease but may reveal distortion of bile ducts due to cirrhosis late in the disease.

Immunologic Diagnosis

The nearly pathognomonic immunologic feature of primary biliary cirrhosis is the presence in high titer of non-species-specific, non-organ-specific antibodies against the inner-membrane components of mitochondria. Antimitochondrial antibodies are found in other autoimmune syndromes, but only in low titer. Less than 10% of primary biliary cirrhosis patients lack these antibodies. Many other autoantibodies are commonly found in patients but are not useful in diagnosis. Other immunologic abnormalities such as circulating immune complex-like materials, complement abnormalities, and abnormalities of lymphocyte function are not useful in diagnosis.

Differential Diagnosis

Chronic cholestasis may follow the administration of drugs such as chlorpromazine, but this does not lead to progressive loss of bile ducts, and it resolves following withdrawal of the drug. Hepatic sarcoidosis may closely mimic primary biliary cirrhosis, but mitochondrial antibodies are absent. Graft-versus-host disease may be found in patients with primary biliary cirrhosis, but in the former disease the basement membrane around bile ducts remain intact. Hepatic allograft rejection may also be associated with nonsuppurative destructive cholangitis.

Treatment

Medical treatment includes supportive treatment such as anion exchange resins to relieve pruritus and administration of lipid-soluble vitamins for nutritional deficiencies. Attempts to suppress the primary inflammatory process have been disappointing. Corticosteroids are considered to be contraindicated because of their tendency in uncontrolled studies to exacerbate metabolic bone disease, complicating the disease. Azathioprine and colchicine may improve survival marginally. D-Penicillamine does not increase survival and is associated with severe side effects. Cyclosporin has been used on an investigational basis but has not yet been proved to be efficacious. Treatment with ursodeoxycholic acid has been associated with improved clinical findings and chance of survival in some patients. The only treatment for end-stage disease is hepatic transplantation.

Complications & Prognosis

Progressive disease is often associated with metabolic bone disease and may lead to chronic hepatic decompensation. Survival from the time of diagnosis is highly variable; asymptomatic patients may have a normal life span. For symptomatic patients, survival from diagnosis is about 12 years. Patients with end-stage disease may be excellent candidates for transplantation, and the long-term prognosis in patients who survive the procedure is good.

PRIMARY SCLEROSING CHOLANGITIS

Major Immunologic Features
- There is chronic inflammation and fibrosis of intrahepatic and extrahepatic bile ducts.
- It is frequently associated with inflammatory bowel disease.

General Considerations
Primary sclerosing cholangitis is a disease of unknown origin characterized by inflammation and fibrosis of both intrahepatic and extrahepatic bile ducts. The disease occurs primarily in young men but may be found in children and older adults. It is often associated with chronic inflammatory bowel disease (usually ulcerative colitis). It is usually progressive and leads to biliary cirrhosis. In addition, it has a significant association with cholangio-carcinoma.

The symptoms are similar to those of other chronic cholestatic diseases and include fatigue, pruritus, hyperpigmentation, xanthelasma, and jaundice. Patients may have fever and abdominal pain associated with superimposed acute bacterial cholangitis. Symptoms of underlying inflammatory bowel disease may be prominent, mild, or absent. Extrahepatic manifestations (other than inflammatory bowel disease) are unusual. Laboratory findings are generally similar to those in primary biliary cirrhosis; however, it is distinct from the latter disease in that anti-mitochondrial antibodies are absent.

The most important laboratory test is cholangiography, which demonstrates tortuosity and areas of dilatation and stricture of either intrahepatic bile ducts, extrahepatic bile ducts, or both.

The liver biopsy is usually abnormal but is often not diagnostic; in fact, the abnormalities occasionally resemble those in primary biliary cirrhosis or autoimmune hepatitis. A characteristic feature that does occur is a fibrous-obliterative process in which segments of bile ducts are replaced by solid cords of connective tissue, leading to an "onion skin" appearance. The differential diagnosis includes biliary stricture secondary to stones, surgery, or neoplasia. Like primary biliary cirrhosis, treatment is supportive (eg, antibiotics for cholangitis), and the underlying disease has proved resistant to treatment with anti-inflammatory agents. Patients with localized areas of high-grade obstruction in large bile ducts may benefit from palliative surgical procedures to relieve obstruction. Patients with advanced diseases who have not had prior surgery may be excellent candidates for hepatic transplantation.

ORODENTAL DISEASES

John S. Greenspan, BDS, PhD, FRCPath

The mouth is the portal of entry for a variety of antigens, including numerous microorganisms, into the alimentary and respiratory systems. Normally, these antigens do not cause disease and are flushed away with swallowed saliva into the distal parts of the alimentary tract. The mucosal barrier, continual desquamation of oral epithelium, toothbrushing, and other forms of mouth cleaning mechanically protect the mouth. Immunologic defense mechanisms, particularly secretory IgA antibodies, probably prevent adherence of microorganisms to mucosal and tooth surfaces by aggregating them and possibly rendering them more susceptible to phagocytosis.

Several of the most important oral diseases, including caries, the common forms of gingival and periodontal disease, oral herpes simplex virus infections, candidal infections, and the oral manifestations of primary and secondary immunodeficiency, especially AIDS, are due to an imbalance between oral organisms and the host response. This imbalance results from hypersensitivity or immunologic deficiency. Alternatively, particularly in the case of dental caries and chronic inflammatory periodontal disease, specific pathogenic microorganisms may directly damage the tissues regardless of the status of the host response.

Another group of oral diseases in which immunologic factors have been implicated are those in which oral tissues are a target for autoimmune reactions. Manifestations may be confined to the mouth or may involve other systemic organs. Many are mucocutaneous diseases, several are rheumatoid diseases, and others involve mainly the gastrointestinal tract. The role of tumor immune mechanisms in oral homeostasis and the part that defects in these mechanisms play in the cause and pathogenesis of oral precancerous lesions and mucosal malignancy constitute a growing field of interest. Tumor immune mechanisms are probably important but must be considered in the context of other factors including oncogenic viruses and chemical carcinogens.

LOCAL ORAL DISEASES INVOLVING IMMUNOLOGIC MECHANISMS

1. INFLAMMATORY PERIODONTAL DISEASES: GINGIVITIS & PERIODONTITIS

Major Immunologic Features
- Bacterial dental plaque induces inflammation of tissues immediately surrounding the teeth.
- The local responses of the host are not effective in eliminating the bacteria, which continue to adhere to the tooth surfaces. Humoral and cellular immunity are both involved in these responses.
- Local responses include complement activation, infiltration of leukocytes, release of lysosomal enzymes and cytokines, and production of a serous gingival crevicular exudate.
- Inflammatory agents from the bacteria and immunopathologic reactions of the host result in gingivitis and periodontitis.

General Considerations

Inflammation of the supporting tissues of the teeth produces one of the most common forms of human diseases. Depending on its severity, the destructive process may involve both the gingiva (gingivitis) and the periodontal ligament and alveolar bone surrounding and supporting the teeth (periodontitis). Periodontitis may involve both the direct cytotoxic and proteolytic effects of dental plaque and the indirect pathologic consequences of the host immune response to the continued presence of bacterial plaque microorganisms (Fig 35–8).

Dental plaque consists of a mass of bacteria that adheres tenaciously to the tooth surfaces. In gingivitis, the plaque generates inflammation of the gingival tissue without affecting the underlying periodontal ligament and bone. In periodontitis, attachment between the gingiva and the involved teeth is lost, subgingival bacterial plaque forms on the root surfaces, and bone loss is clinically apparent (Fig 35–9 and 35–10). Elimination of the plaque usually stops the inflammatory process. In children with poor oral hygiene, gingivitis is common but periodontitis is rare.

The microflora of the dental plaque is complex, comprising many different strains of bacteria including gram-positive rods and cocci and gram-negative rods, cocci, and filamentous forms. In general, the healthy gingival crevice contains only a few gram-positive streptococcal and facultative *Actinomyces* species. As gingivitis develops, many more gram-negative organisms are found, including *Fusobacterium nucleatum, Bacteroides intermedius,* and *Haemophilus* species. Many motile rods and spirochetes are also seen. In advanced adult periodontitis, the organisms usually cultured are predominantly gram-negative anaerobic rods such as *Bacteroides gingivalis, B intermedius,* and *F nucleatum.* Furthermore, phase-contrast examination shows that as many as 50% of organisms from such lesions are motile rods and spirochetes. There is some indirect evidence for a relationship between particular forms of periodontal disease and specific microorganisms. Thus, elevated levels and increased frequency of serum antibodies to *Actinobacillus actinomycetemcomitans, Capnocytophaga* spp, and *Eikenella corrodens* are found in localized juvenile periodontitis (rapidly progressive periodontitis) (see below).

Immunologic Pathogenesis

A delicate balance exists between dental plaque organisms and the host response. In healthy individuals, the immunologic response provides a well-regulated specific defense against infiltration by plaque substances. The tissue-destructive mechanisms thought to be involved in periodontal disease include direct effects of plaque bacteria, polymorphonuclear-induced damage, neutrophil complement-mediated damage initiated by both antibody and the alternative pathway, and cell-mediated damage.

Clinically apparent gingivitis is probably the result of an exaggerated response to bacterial plaque. Individuals with mild gingivitis have, in addition to a continued polymorphonuclear infiltration, a gingival influx of a few T lymphocytes. However, those with prolonged severe gingivitis and severe periodontitis have an influx composed mainly of B lymphocytes and plasma cells, with resulting IgG antibody production. Most noteworthy in severe periodontal disease is the extremely low proportion of gingival plasma cells committed to IgG2 production, while serum levels of the other IgG subclasses are normal. The proportions of antibodies of IgG3, IgG1, or IgG4 subclasses with specific antibody activity for plaque antigens in the gingival tissues are unknown. This unusual local IgG subclass response may indicate a degree of nonspecific activation of B lymphocytes arriving in the inflamed area, possibly caused by a variety of mechanisms involving bacterial mitogens and proteases. The bacteria may also activate the alternative complement pathway. Associated with gingivitis is the generation of a serum exudate known as crevicular fluid, which flows from around the teeth and contacts the dental plaque. This exudate, like serum, contains functional complement components as well as low levels of specific antibodies to the various plaque antigens.

The onset of flow of crevicular fluid is an important stage in the progression of periodontal disease. Crevicular fluid complement is rapidly activated by a combination of effects. These include activation of the classic pathway by IgG and IgM antibodies to subgingival plaque antigens; activation of the alternative complement pathway by endotoxins and peptidoglycan from gram-negative and gram-positive mircoorganisms, respectively; and activation of complement components by host and bacterial proteolytic enzymes. Complement activation results first in the

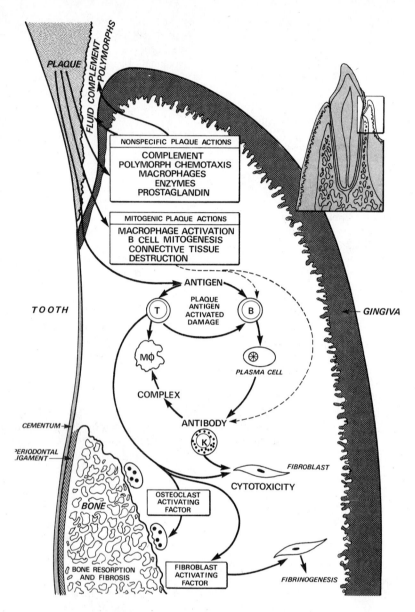

Figure 35–8. The pathogenesis of periodontal disease.

release of C3a and C5a, which cause additional edema and increase crevicular fluid flow, and subsequently in chemotactic attraction of polymorphonuclear leukocytes. Other chemotactic factors are produced directly by the plaque microorganisms. The release of proteolytic enzymes with collagenase and trypsinlike activities by host cells is believed to damage tissue and activate additional complement components and subsequent release of prostaglandin E. In vitro, prostaglandin E can induce bone resorption through its effect on osteoclasts.

Cell-mediated immunity may also play a role in the progression of periodontal disease. In some studies,

individuals with periodontal disease generally exhibit increased peripheral blood T lymphocyte reactivity to plaque antigens. Yet, for reasons unknown, in severe gingivitis and severe periodontitis the local T cell response to the plaque is conspicuously small. Bone destruction in periodontal disease may be mediated by lymphokines including osteoclast-activating factor as well as by parathyroid hormone and prostaglandins. Individuals with reduced immunologic capacity, notably primary immunodeficiency and immunodeficiency secondary to treatment associated with kidney transplantation, do not have more gingival and periodontal disease than do normal controls. However,

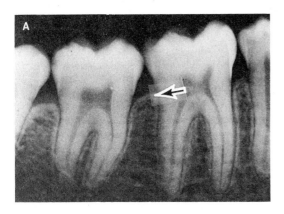
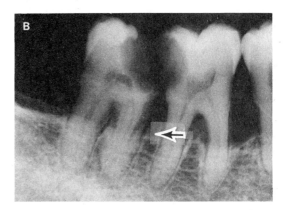

Figure 35–9. Radiographs of the lower molars of a 25-year-old man with a normal periodontium (**A**) and a 45-year-old man with advanced periodontitis and severe dental caries (**B**). In the patient with periodontitis, more than half of the supporting alveolar bone has been destroyed (arrows). (Courtesy of GC Armitage.)

severe periodontal disease is seen in association with HIV infection.

Immunologic Diagnosis

Lymphocytes from individuals with periodontal disease are more responsive to dental plaque antigens in vitro than are lymphocytes from normal individuals, but no clear relationships have been found between disease severity and serum or salivary antibody levels. At present, immunologic tests are not generally useful in the diagnosis of gingivitis and periodontitis. Most individuals with inflammatory periodontitis have gingivitis, but the clinical symptoms of the latter may be masked by fibrosis.

Treatment

Although gingivitis and periodontitis are apparently caused by dental bacterial plaque, there is a reluctance to treat this disease with antibiotics because elimination of one group of organisms by antibiotics may lead to the emergence of antibiotic-resistant strains. However, some clinicians use local application of tetracycline depending on the severity of the periodontal disease. Treatment may range from simply good routine oral hygiene to periodontal surgery. Reduction of plaque accumulation to an absolute minimum is essential for the arrest of gingivitis or the reduction of periodontal ligament destruction and bone loss. Topical antibacterial agents, notably chlorhexidine, are valuable for this purpose.

2. JUVENILE PERIODONTITIS

In a small percentage of the population, periodontal bone loss occurs very rapidly, sometimes within 2–5 years. In this condition—juvenile periodontitis, formerly known as periodontitis—conventional periodontal treatment is ineffective. There is a characteristic gram-negative anaerobic flora, different from

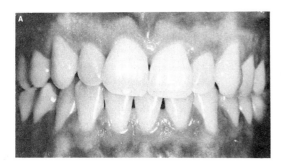
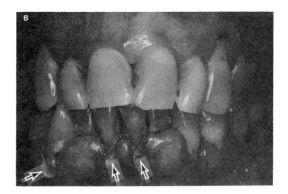

Figure 35–10. Clinical appearance of the anterior teeth and periodontal tissues of a 22-year-old man with healthy gingiva (**A**) and a 48-year-old man with advanced periodontitis (**B**). Note the heavy deposits of plaque and calculus (arrows) in the patient with periodontitis. Marked gingival inflammation is particularly noticeable around the lower anterior teeth. Most teeth have either pocket formation or extensive gingival recession. (Courtesy of GC Armitage.)

that in the more slowly progressive form of periodontitis. Short-term antibiotics are probably useful in these cases, but there is no evidence that the results of such treatment are permanent. Several reports suggest that defects in granulocyte or monocyte function may be involved.

RECURRENT APHTHOUS ULCERATION (Aphthous Stomatitis or RAU)

Major Immunologic Features

- Lymphocyte infiltration is present at the earliest stage of the lesion.
- Circulating antibodies to oral mucous membranes are present in some patients and may cross-react with oral organisms.
- Cellular immunity to the same antigens is reported.
- Circulating immune complexes are found in some patients.
- There is association with HLA-B12.
- Response to topical or systemic corticosteroids is favorable.

General Considerations

After caries and chronic periodontal disease, oral ulceration probably represents the most common lesion of the mouth. Although oral ulcers can be due to a large number of diseases, the most common form is recurrent aphthous ulceration (aphthous stomatitis) Fig 35–11. Recurrent oral ulcers usually occur alone but may be a local manifestation of Behçet's disease when accompanied by uveitis, genital ulcers, and perhaps lesions of other systems. Estimates of the prevalence of recurrent oral ulceration vary, but probably 20% of the population experience it. The condition may recur only once or twice a year or may be so frequent that a new set of ulcers overlaps a previous group. There is slight evidence of a familial incidence. Severe RAU can be seen in association with HIV infection. Emotional, hematologic, and nutritional factors may play a causative role, and an association has been suggested with changes in the hormone status during the menstrual cycle. Extensive searches for specific bacterial or viral causes have been unsuccessful. A possible role for herpes simplex virus type 1 has again been raised by the observation that part of the herpes simplex virus genome is present and transcribed in peripheral blood mononuclear cells of patients with recurrent aphthae and Behçet's disease. Additional evidence also indicates a possible role for *Streptococcus sanguis,* since this organism has been cultured from the ulcers and patients exhibit delayed hypersensitivity reactions to the organism and significant inhibition of leukocyte migration by antigens of this organism in vitro. However, the organism is a common commensal. One study has shown reduced lymphocyte transformation to *S sanguis* in patients compared with controls. A likely role for bacterial or viral agents in this disease is that of cross-reacting antigens, which elicit host responses to autologous oral mucous-membrane antigens.

Immunologic Pathogenesis

Patients have a raised level of circulating antibody to a saline extract of fetal oral mucous membrane. Slightly raised levels of the same antibody have been found in other ulcerative conditions, but in lower titers. The antibodies are of the agglutinating and complement-fusing types, suggesting that antibody cytotoxicity might be involved in the tissue destruction. However, some studies show poor correlation between the level of anti-mucous membrane antibody and clinical features of the disease. In addition, 2 other mechanisms could explain the presence of circulating autoantibodies of this type. The antibodies may cross-react with antigens of an organism present in the mouth, such as *S sanguis* or a virus, and oral mucous membrane epithelial cells. Alternatively, the antibodies may be a response to exposed tissue antigens from chronic ulcerations that had previously been protected from the immune system. Attempts to show that patient serum containing significant titers of this antibody has a direct cytotoxic effect against oral epithelial cells have been unsuccessful. Thus, it is unlikely that a cytotoxic anti-oral mucosal antibody is directly involved in the pathogenesis.

Interest in the role of cellular immunity in the pathogenesis of recurrent aphthous ulceration was aroused by the observation that the earliest histologic changes involve the presence of an infiltrate of lymphocytes. Other cells do not appear until a later stage. Furthermore, patients with recurrent oral ulceration have peripheral blood lymphocytes that are sensitized to oral mucous-membrane antigen. These 2 observations support the hypothesis that a cell-mediated hypersensitivity mechanism might be involved in the pathogenesis of the lesion. Lymphocytes from some patients with recurrent aphthous ulceration are cytotoxic to oral epithelial cells. The antigen eliciting the cytotoxic reaction has not been identified. It

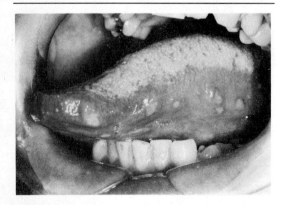

Figure 35–11. Recurrent aphthous ulcers.

might be one or more epithelial cell surface autoantigens, determinants cross-reacting with an infecting organism or organisms, or food or microbial antigens attached to oral epithelial cell surfaces or even by a hapten. Increased antibody-dependent cell-mediated cytotoxicity has been found, but the identity of the population of lymphocytes involved in these reactions is also unknown. Increased production of TNF by peripheral blood lymphocytes of patients with RAU has been observed. There is at present no acceptable hypothesis linking oral mucous membrane auto-antigens and effector mechanisms, although transient defects in immunoregulation have been postulated.

Patients with Behçet's disease and recurrent oral ulceration show elevated levels of serum C9 and of circulating soluble immune complexes. IgG and C3 have also been demonstrated in the basement membrane zone of the lesions. It is not clear whether these observations are clues to the immunologic pathogenesis of the disease or represent epiphenomena. There is also some evidence for an increased incidence of HLA-B12 in recurrent oral ulceration.

Treatment & Prognosis

Effective treatment depends on identification of any underlying systemic disease. In such cases, treatment of the systemic condition usually leads to cure of the oral ulceration. For the remaining group, uncomplicated by known systemic disease, several treatment forms are available. They are the use of topical corticosteroids, antibiotics, and immunostimulants. The most effective topical corticosteroids available are 0.1% triamcinolone in Orabase, 2.5-mg tablets of hydrocortisone sodium succinate, and 0.025% fluocinonide in Orabase. Some cases of major aphthous ulceration are sufficiently severe to warrant the use of systemic prednisone. Tetracycline mouth rinses have been used with some success in the herpetriform variety of recurrent aphthous ulceration. The treatment of Behçet's disease is discussed in Chapter 36.

ACQUIRED IMMUNODEFICIENCY SYNDROME (AIDS)

The oral mucosa is particularly hospitable to opportunistic pathogens. Thus, primary and recurrent herpes simplex virus, varicella-zoster virus, and several fungi, notably *Candida* species, are frequent features of primary cellular immunodeficiency syndromes (see Section IIIA). The same conditions, as well as a number of others, are seen in patients whose immune systems are compromised by chemotherapy, those receiving bone marrow transplants, patients with leukemia or lymphoma, and those with clinical expressions of HIV-induced immunosuppression.

The oral features of AIDS include Kaposi's sarcoma, non-Hodgkin lymphoma, and severe oral can-

didiasis (Fig 35–12), as well as persistent herpesvirus lesions (herpes simplex virus and varicella-zoster virus). Other conditions seen in AIDS and other HIV disease include severe periodontal disease, oral warts, and the recently described lesion known as oral hairy leukoplakia.

Hairy leukoplakia (Fig 35–13) is seen on the tongue in HIV-immunosuppressed patients. Ninety-nine percent of patients are HIV antibody-positive, and the majority of those tested carry the virus in blood lymphocytes. This lesion has characteristic histopathologic features suggestive of human papillomavirus, further evidence for the presence of which is provided by antigen staining. However, no human papillomavirus DNA is found by hybridization techniques. Instead, clear evidence for the presence of Epstein-Barr virus (EBV) comes from immunocytochemistry with monoclonal antibodies, from electron-microscopic morphology, and from DNA studies with EBV probes. Southern blot hybridization provides evidence for the presence of EBV DNA in complete linear virion form and in very high copy number. At the time of diagnosis of hairy leukoplakia, about 20% of patients have AIDS, but a very large number of those who are AIDS-free when first seen subsequently develop AIDS, with mean conversion rates at 48% at 16 months and 83% at 30 months, mostly with *Pneumocystis carinii* pneumonia.

Oral hairy leukoplakia is a significant indicator of HIV-induced immunosuppression and is highly predictive of the subsequent development of AIDS, although rare cases are seen in HIV-negative people, mostly in association with other forms of secondary immunodeficiency. It appears to be one of only 2 oral lesions specifically associated with HIV infection. It is the first form of oral leukoplakia consistently associated with a virus or viruses. The mechanism whereby HIV favors oral opportunistic infection presumably involves viral elimination of helper T cells and thus the loss of cell-mediated immunity to

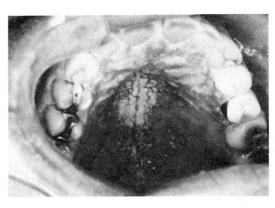

Figure 35–12. Pseudomembranous candidiasis in an HIV-positive man.

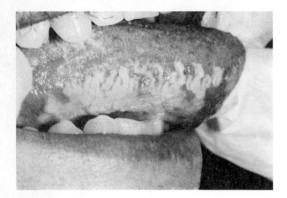

Figure 35–13. Hairy leukoplakia in an HIV-positive man.

herpesviruses and fungi as well as to other organisms. However, other mechanisms may also mediate the immune defect, including loss of Langerhans cells or their functions as well as polymorphonuclear cell and macrophage aberrations.

ORAL CANDIDIASIS

Major Immunologic Features

- There are many associated immunologic defects.
- It is the most significant oral indication of an underlying immunodeficiency.
- It is a prominent feature of HIV-induced immunodeficiency.

General Considerations

Oral candidiasis is the most common oral fungal disease. It may occur in acute or chronic form at any age. The disease may be a sign of life-threatening systemic disease or may be confined to a small part of the oral mucous membrane and have no general significance. *Candida* species are frequent oral commensals, and it has not yet been established whether candidiasis is predominantly of endogenous or exogenous origin.

Immunologic Pathogenesis

The immunologic features of generalized candidiasis are discussed in Chapters 20 and 49. A wide range of immunologic defects have been found, including defects in cytotoxicity to *Candida*, reduced lymphokine production, failure of anticandidal antibody response of one or more classes, generalized cytotoxicity defects, failure of lymphocyte activation to candidal antigen, absence of the delayed hypersensitivity skin test to *Candida* or to many antigens, and presence of an abnormal suppressor T cell population. However, immunologic defects alone do not explain the pathogenesis of candidiasis. High glucose levels in diabetics and low levels of serum iron transferrin and blood folate are also important factors. Granulocyte defects have been shown in some patients, as have defects in leukocyte myeloperoxidase. A few patients have been described in whom antibody production to *Candida* and other antigens was raised while cellular immune function was depressed.

Immunologic Diagnosis

The diagnosis of pseudomembranous candidiasis (thrush) is based on the clinical appearance and history. The immunologic approach is directed toward establishing the nature of the immunologic defect, if any. Although immunologic investigation of patients with oral candidiasis is still predominantly a research tool, it is likely that subtypes of patients will be identified and that specific immunologic treatment will be directed toward the correction of localized defects in cell-mediated immunity. The differential diagnosis of candidal leukoplakia from other white oral lesions involves smear, culture, and biopsy.

Treatment & Prognosis

Treatment of localized oral candidiasis consists of elimination of predisposing factors, when known, and administration of topical antifungal therapy. This may be prolonged in the treatment of chronic oral candidiasis. Systemic therapy is used in cases that are resistant to local measures and in generalized mucocutaneous candidiasis.

REFERENCES

GENERAL

Brown WR, Strober W: Immunological disease of the gastrointestinal tract. In: *Immunological Diseases,* Samter M et al (editors). Little, Brown, 1988.

James SP: Immunology of hepatobiliary diseases. In: *Immunological Diseases.* Samter M et al (editors). Little, Brown, 1988.

GASTROINTESTINAL DISEASES

Gluten-Sensitive Enteropathy

Kelly CP et al: Diagnosis and treatment of gluten-sensitive enteropathy. *Adv Intern Med* 1990:**35:**341.

O'Farrelly C, Gallagher RB: Intestinal gluten sensitivity: Snapshots of an unusual autoimmune-like disease. *Immunol Today* 1992:**13:**474.

Strober, W: Gluten-sensitive enteropathy: An abnormal immunologic response of the gastrointestinal tract to a dietary protein. In: *Gastrointestinal Immunity for the Clinician.* Kirsner JR, Shorter RG (editors). Grune & Stratton, 1985.

Crohn's Disease & Ulcerative Colitis

Curtis B, Schuman BM, Griffin JW Jr: Association of gluten-sensitive enteropathy and Crohn's colitis. *Am J Gastroenterol* 1992;**87**:1634.

Strober W, James S: The immunologic basis of inflammatory bowel disease. *J Clin Immunol* 1986;**6**:415.

Alpha Heavy-Chain Disease

Rambaud JC et al: Immunoproliferative small intestinal disease and "Mediterranean" lymphomas. *Springer Semin Immunopathol* 1990;**12**:239.

Seligman M: Immunochemical, clinical and pathological features of alpha-chain disease. *Arch Intern Med* 1975;**135**:78.

Pernicious Anemia

Kay MD: Immunological aspects of gastritis and pernicious anemia. *Beillieres Clin Gastroenterol* 1987; **1**:487.

HEPATOBILIARY DISEASES

Hepatitis

Czaja AJ: Natural history, clinical feature and treatment of autoimmune hepatitis. *Semin Liver Dis* 1984;**4**:1.

Dienstag JL: Non-A, non-B hepatitis: Recognition, epidemiology and clinical features. *Gastroenterology* 1983;**85**:439.

Hoofnagle JH: Chronic type B hepatitis. *Gastroenterology* 1983;**84**:422.

Kuo G et al: An assay for circulating antibodies to a major etiologic virus of human non-A, non-B hepatitis. *Science* 1989;**244**:362.

Rizzetto M et al: Hepatitis delta virus disease. *Prog Liver Dis* 1986;**7**:56.

Primary Biliary Cirrhosis

James SP et al: Primary biliary cirrhosis: A model autoimmune disease. *Ann Intern Med* 1983;**99**:500.

Primary Sclerosing Cholangitis

LaRusso NF et al: Primary sclerosing cholangitis. *N Engl J Med* 1984;**310**:899.

Choo et al: Isolation of a cDNA clone derived from a blood-borne non-A, non-B viral hepatitis genome. *Science* 1989;**244**:359.

Khuroo MS: Hepatitis E: The enterically transmitted non-A, non-B hepatitis. *Indian J Gastroenterol* 1991;**10**:96.

Misiani R et al: Hepatitis C virus infection in patients with essential mixed cryoglobulinemia. *Ann Intern Med* 1992;**117**:573.

Reyes GR et al: Isolation of a cDNA from the virus responsible for enterically transmitted non-A, non-B hepatitis. *Science* 1990;**247**:1335.

Tine F et al: Interferon for non-A, non-B chronic hepatitis: A meta-analysis of randomised clinical trials. *J Hepatol* 1991;**13**:192.

ORODENTAL DISEASES

Periodontal Disease

Boughman JA, Astemborski JA, Blitzer MG: Early onset periodontal disease: A genetics perspective. *Oral Biol Med* 1990;**1**:89–99.

Genco RJ: Host responses in periodontal diseases: Current concepts. *J Periodontol* 1992;**63**:338.

Page RC: The role of inflammatory mediators in the pathogenesis of periodontal disease. *J Periodont Res* 1991;**26**:230.

Ranney RR: Immunologic mechanisms of pathogenesis in periodontal diseases: An assessment. *J Periodont Res* 1991;**26**:243.

Socransky SS, Haffajee AD: Microbial mechanisms in the pathogenesis of destructive periodontal diseases: A critical assessment. *J Periodont Res* 1991;**26**:195.

Stiehm ER: New and old immunodeficiencies. *Pediatr Res* 1992;**33(Suppl)**:S2

Williams RC: Periodontal disease. *N Engl J Med* 1990;**322**:373.

Recurrent Aphthous Ulcers

MacPhail LA, Greenspan D, Greenspan JS: Recurrent aphthous ulcers in association with HIV infection: Diagnosis and treatment. *Oral Surg Oral Med Oral Pathol* 1992;**73**:283.

Nolan A et al: Recurrent aphthous ulceration: vitamin B1, B2, and B6 status an response to replacement therapy. *J Oral Pathol Med* 1991;**20**:389–391.

Taylor LJ et al: Increased production of tumour necrosis factor by peripheral blood leukocytes in patients with recurrent oral aphthous ulceration. *J Oral Pathol Med* 1992;**21**:21.

Verdickt GM et al: Expression of the CD54 (ICAM-1) and CD11a (LFA-1) adhesion molecules in oral mucosal inflammation. *J Oral Pathol Med* 1992;**21**:65–69.

AIDS & Candidiasis

Agabian N: Candidiasis and HIV infection. In: *Oral Manifestations of HIV Infection.* Greenspan JS, Greenspan D (editors). Quintessence, 1994.

Greenspan D et al: *AIDS and the Mouth: Diagnosis and Management of Oral Lesions.* Munksgaard, 1990.

Katz MH et al: Progression to AIDS in HIV-infected homosexual and bisexual men with hairy leukoplakia and oral candidiasis. *AIDS* 1992;**6**:95.

Miyasaki SH et al: The identification and tracking of *Candida albicans* isolates from oral lesions in HIV-seropositive individuals. *J Acquired Immune Defic Syndr* 1992;**5**:1039.

36

Renal Diseases

*Curtis B. Wilson, MD, Winson W. Tang, MD, Lili Feng, MD, Yiyang Xia, MD,
& David M. Ward, MB, ChB, FRCP*

Immunologically induced glomerulonephritis and tubulointerstitial nephritis are estimated to be responsible for nearly half of all instances of end-stage renal failure and its consequent mortality, morbidity, and expense. Nephritogenic antibody-antigen reactions most often lead directly or indirectly to glomerular or tubular immune deposits. The subsequent activation of humoral and cellular mediator systems produces foci of inflammation (Table 36–1). Recently, it has been shown experimentally that antibody-induced damage can be restricted to a single renal cell type when the surface antigens of that cell are involved. Immune activation of mediator systems, as postulated to occur in vasculitic injury associated with anti-neutrophil cytoplasmic antibodies (ANCA), must also be considered.

Immune deposits occur when nephritogenic antibodies react directly with antigens in the kidney. In humans, the major nephritogenic structural antigens are in the glomerular basement membrane (GBM). Antibodies may also react with nonrenal, often exogenous, antigens that have been "trapped" in the GBM by physiologic, immunologic, or physicochemical mechanisms such as the reaction of cationic molecules with the polyanionic glomerular capillary wall.

In contrast to the direct reaction of antibody with renal antigens, glomerular injury can occur when antibodies react with soluble antigens in the circulation to form immune complexes, which subsequently accumulate in the glomerulus. Immune-complex formation is a dynamic process with continual modification of the deposited immune complexes by ongoing interaction with additional antibodies, antigens, or immune complexes from the circulation. The local exchange with tissue-fixed immune complex results in some overlap between the direct and indirect mechanisms of glomerular immune deposit formation.

In renal biopsy tissue, antibodies reactive with the GBM have a characteristic linear configuration by immunofluorescence microscopy. In contrast, a granular pattern is much more common and can be due either to randomly deposited immune complexes or to antibodies directly reactive with fixed glomerular antigens that are distributed irregularly.

In glomerulonephritis, humoral mechanisms appear to dominate and there is much less evidence for a contribution by cellular immunity. A cellular immune response has been recognized in some forms of human glomerulonephritis. Sometimes T cells can be identified in nephritic glomeruli, and a role for T cells in some forms of experimental glomerulonephritis has been shown by cell transfer studies.

The glomerular (or tubular) injury caused by antibody reactions results in large part from the action of immunologic mediator systems. The most extensively studied of these are complement and neutrophils, representing the humoral and cellular mediator groups, respectively. Complement activation generates biologically active fragments that initiate vasoconstriction, platelet aggregation, immune adherence, opsonization, histamine release, and leukocyte chemotaxis. Complement products also can serve to solubilize immune-complex material and may affect handling of complexes via erythrocyte CR1 receptors. C5b–9, the membrane attack complex (MAC), is found in human glomerular immune deposits, and manipulative studies in experimental models indicate its contribution to injury in some situations. In addition to the chemotaxins, C3a and C5a, the MAC may promote leukocyte adhesion by increasing expression of P-selectin (CD62). The MAC can also enhance eicosanoid production as well as interleukin-1 (IL-1) and tumor necrosis factor (TNF), which in turn activate a cascade of cytokines including monocyte chemoattractant protein-1 (MCP-1) and IL-8. Other humoral mediators include the coagulation proteins. Coagulation can be induced by glomerular tissue factor, procoagulant activity of infiltrating macrophages, and platelet aggregation. The anticoagulant protein C with its cofactor protein S and activator thrombomodulin are found in the kidney along with

Table 36–1. Immunopathogenesis of humorally mediated renal disease classified by the solubility of the antigen.

Solubility	Mechanism	Antigen	Condition
Insoluble or tissue-fixed antigens	Antibodies react with structural components of the kidney.	GBM	Glomerulonephritis
		TBM	Tubulointerstitial nephritis
		Other glomerular wall antigens	Experimental glomerulonephritis
		Cell surface antigens	Experimental glomerulonephritis, tubulointerstitial nephritis
	Antibodies react with antigens trapped or "planted" in the glomerulus.	Mesangial accumulations, immune-complex components, lectins, cationic materials; possibly bacterial antigens, DNA.	Experimental glomerulonephritis. May contribute to human glomerulonephritis as well.
Soluble antigens	Antibodies react with antigens in the vascular compartment to form circulating immune complexes.	Exogenous antigens: drugs, products of infectious agents, etc.	Glomerulonephritis, tubulointerstitial nephritis, vasculitis
		Endogenous antigens: nuclear antigens, tumor antigens, etc.	
	Antibodies react with antigens in the extravascular fluid near the site of antigen release.	Tubular antigens	Experimental tubulointerstitial nephritis

protein C inhibitor. Abnormalities in fibrinolysis may occur in glomerular injury related to enhanced expression of plasminogen activator inhibitor-1, which inhibits the action of urokinase and tissue plasminogen activator. Fibrinolytic therapy may be beneficial in some models.

Recruitment of neutrophils includes chemotaxis by complement, platelet-activating factor (PAF), thrombin, platelet-derived growth factor (PDGF), IL-1, IL-8, and TNF. Molecules that promote neutrophil adhesion include P-selectin, E-selectin, and intracellular adhesion molecule-1 (ICAM-1), with its corresponding β_2 integrin (CD11a or CD11b/CD18). Neutrophils, as well as macrophages (which are also attracted to the site of injury), produce reactive oxygen species, nitric oxide, bioactive lipids, cytokines including IL-1 and TNF, proteinases, and growth factors. Platelets can also contribute factors including thrombospondin, thromboxane, PDGF, and platelet factor 4. PAF released from many cells associated with the inflammatory response has spasmogenic and vascular permeability properties.

Glomerular cells themselves can produce numerous mediator and adhesion molecules involved in the local inflammatory process. These include IL-1, IL-6, IL-8, TNF, MCP-1, PAF, colony-stimulating factor, endothelin, proteinases, and eicosanoids. The glomerular cells are also involved in the resolution of the injury, which, unfortunately, is often complicated by sclerosis and loss of function. The evolution of sclerosis is multifactorial and includes hemodynamic factors, lipid accumulation, and growth factor production. The growth factors, PDGF and transforming growth factor β, can lead to excessive production of extracellular matrix components including various collagens, proteoglycans, and laminin. Insufficiency or inhibition of proteinases responsible for degrading and remodeling the excess matrix may also contribute.

ANTI-GLOMERULAR BASEMENT MEMBRANE ANTIBODY-INDUCED GLOMERULONEPHRITIS

Major Immunologic Features
- Linear deposition of immunoglobulin and often of C3 occurs along the GBM.
- Anti-GBM antibodies are usually detectable in serum of radioimmunoassay (RIA), less often by indirect immunofluorescence techniques.

General Considerations
Anti-GBM antibodies can produce glomerulonephritis, Goodpasture's syndrome (glomerulonephritis and pulmonary hemorrhage), and, occasionally, idiopathic pulmonary hemosiderosis. The pathogenicity of these antibodies was demonstrated (1) by transfer to subhuman primates by using anti-GBM antibodies recovered from the serum of or eluted from the kidneys of affected patients and (2) by the observation of recurrence of anti-GBM antibody disease in renal transplants inadvertently placed in patients with residual circulating anti-GBM antibodies.

The nephritogenic GBM antigens appear to be in the noncollagenous carboxyl extension of the type IV procollagen molecule, a region termed NC1. This region of the type IV molecule is involved in intermolecular joining. The NC1 region of the $\alpha 3$ chain of type IV collagen carries a major reactive GBM epitope with limited reactivity to other type IV α chains or regions thereof. Of interest, anti-GBM antibodies do not react with the GBM from affected individuals in some kindreds of patients with hereditary nephritis (Alport's syndrome), a condition with GBM abnormalities. Transplantation of a normal kidney to such an individual lacking the reactive antigen may induce nephritogenic anti-GBM antibodies in the recipient. The genetic abnormalities of the $\alpha 5$ chain of type IV collagen associated with the different kindreds of Alport's syndrome and observed morphologic defects in GBM, characterized by structure, are being defined.

Little is known about the events responsible for the induction of spontaneous anti-GBM antibodies in humans. There is a suggested genetic association with HLA-DR2. Materials cross-reactive with the GBM have been identified in the urine of animals and humans. Mercuric chloride administered to rats produces a transient anti-GBM antibody response. Both hydrocarbon solvent inhalation and influenza A2 virus infections have been associated with anti-GBM antibody production and Goodpasture's syndrome in a few patients. The duration of the anti-GBM antibody response is self-limited, suggesting that the immunologic stimulus is also transient. Most affected individuals have only a single episode, although 2 or more episodes have been reported.

Less than 5% of human glomerulonephritis is caused by anti-GBM antibodies. There is a bimodal age distribution. Anti-GBM antibody-associated Goodpasture's syndrome is most commonly identified in males in the second to fourth decades of life; however, either sex can be involved, and children under 5 and adults over 70 can be affected. A second grouping of cases occurs in patients older than 50 years. Glomerulonephritis alone is more common in this group, and there is a female predominance.

Pathology

The renal pathology induced by anti-GBM antibodies is related to quantitative and temporal factors of antibody binding. Lesions may vary from mild focal proliferative glomerulonephritis to diffuse proliferative necrotizing glomerulonephritis with crescent formation. However, the latter is more common and may progress to glomerular destruction and hyalinization. The anti-GBM antibody deposits are not visualized by electron microscopy, in contrast to the electron-dense deposits of immune complexes. Tubulointerstitial nephritis in patients with anti-GBM antibody disease is caused by concomitant anti-tubular basement membrane (TBM) antibodies. The pulmonary pathology of Goodpasture's syndrome is intra-alveolar hemorrhage with hemosiderin-laden macrophages in alveoli and sputum.

Clinical Features

Half to two-thirds (depending on age and sex) of patients with anti-GBM antibody glomerulonephritis also have pulmonary hemorrhage and often respiratory impairment. This condition is referred to as Goodpasture's syndrome. The first symptoms may be either renal or pulmonary, occurring nearly simultaneously or separated by as much as 1 year. Episodes of pulmonary hemorrhage may occur at any time during anti-GBM antibody production. Alteration in the accessibility of the alveolar basement membrane antigen by such factors as fluid overload, toxin exposure (smoking, hydrocarbons), or infection may facilitate the binding of anti-GBM antibodies and precipitate the episodes of lung injury. In many patients, particularly those with Goodpasture's syndrome, influenzalike symptoms precede the onset of renal or pulmonary symptoms. Arthritis is an early complaint in fewer than 10% of patients, and central nervous system involvement may occur infrequently. Overall, about 75% of patients develop renal failure, necessitating dialysis, although the outlook is improving somewhat as a result of early diagnosis and more aggressive treatment. Milder forms of disease account for fewer than 10% of cases. Clinical presentations confined to the lung are rare. Nephrotic syndrome is unusual in anti-GBM antibody glomerulonephritis.

Immunologic Diagnosis

The diagnosis of anti-GBM antibody disease can be established by finding at least 2 of the following: (1) linear deposits of immunoglobulins along the GBM by immunofluorescence, (2) elution of anti-GBM antibody from renal tissue, and (3) detection of circulating anti-GBM antibody. By immunofluorescence, anti-GBM antibodies appear as linear deposits of IgG and infrequently IgA or IgM along the GBM (Fig. 36–1). Linear deposits of IgG are present along

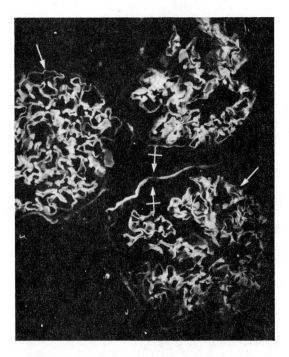

Figure 36–1. Smooth linear deposits of IgG (arrows) representing anti-GBM antibodies are seen outlining the GBM of 3 glomeruli from a young man with Goodpasture's syndrome. The antibody also had reactivity with Bowman's capsule (opposed hatched arrows). (Original magnification × 160.)

the TBM in about 70% of patients and may also be found along the alveolar basement membranes in some patients with pulmonary involvement; however, lung tissue is not as useful for detection of antibody as is kidney. Irregular glomerular IgM deposits may also be present. The linear glomerular deposits of immunoglobulins are accompanied by linear or irregular deposits of C3 in about two-thirds of kidneys from patients with linear IgG deposits. Fibrin may be striking in areas of extracapillary proliferation and crescent formation. When C3 is present, it is usually accompanied by deposits of other components of the classic complement pathway. Nonimmunologic linear accumulations of IgG are sometimes found in kidneys from patients with diabetes mellitus, in kidneys perfused in preparation for transplantation, and in some normal kidneys. These must be distinguished from linear anti-GBM antibody deposits; the latter can be eluted from the renal tissue.

Circulating anti-GBM antibodies are usually detected by indirect immunofluorescence or preferably by the more sensitive RIA. Almost all patients with confirmed anti-GBM antibody deposits have circulating anti-GBM antibodies detected by RIA in serum obtained early in the course of the disease.

Differential Diagnosis

Although anti-GBM antibodies are the classic cause of Goodpasture's syndrome and an important cause of crescentic glomerulonephritis, these clinical presentations are more commonly due to other immunologic mechanisms. "Pulmonary-renal" syndrome may also be related to immune-complex deposition, as in systemic lupus erythematosus (SLE), and to similar lesions with no or minimal immune deposits frequently associated with ANCA, as in Wegener's granulomatosis or polyarteritis (see below). Crescentic glomerulonephritis in the absence of pulmonary involvement has a similar spectrum of pathogeneses.

Treatment

There is no immunologically specific treatment. High-dose corticosteroids are generally helpful in the management of acute pulmonary hemorrhage in patients with anti-GBM antibody-associated Goodpasture's syndrome. To hasten the disappearance of antibodies, repeated and intensive plasmapheresis, in conjunction with immunosuppression, is usually performed. This appears useful if the combined therapy is instituted before irreversible renal damage has taken place, although data from controlled trials are limited.

Complications & Prognosis

The mean duration of the anti-GBM antibody response measured by sensitive RIA is about 15 months; it ranges from a few weeks to 5 years. Immunosuppression and plasmapheresis hasten the disappearance of the anti-GBM antibody. Nephrectomy has no immediate effect on the levels of circulating anti-GBM antibody but may speed its eventual disappearance. The ultimate outcome is influenced by the severity of disease at the initiation of therapy. Initial improvement is not sustained in all patients, so that long-term follow-up is needed. Circulating anti-GBM antibodies can transfer glomerulonephritis to a transplanted kidney, so transplantation should be postponed until circulating anti-GBM antibodies are absent or greatly reduced. Posttransplant immunosuppression may help suppress the recrudescence of the anti-GBM antibody response.

IMMUNE-COMPLEX GLOMERULONEPHRITIS

Major Immunologic Features

- Granular deposits of immunoglobulins and complement occur in glomeruli.
- Circulating immune complexes are detectable in some diseases but are of little diagnostic utility.

General Considerations

The demonstration by immunofluorescence of granular deposits of immunoglobulins in the glomerulus can usually be interpreted as evidence of immune complex-mediated glomerulonephritis. It must be kept in mind that the direct reaction of antibody with irregularly distributed fixed or "planted" antigens, as noted above, could be confused with immune-complex deposits by immunofluorescence; this stresses the need for identification of the antigen-antibody systems involved.

The glomerulus seems to be a uniquely susceptible site for immune-complex accumulation; this is probably related in part to its function as a filter with a fenestrated endothelial lining. Several factors may influence the tissue localization of immune complexes in terms of (1) the characteristics and quantity of immune complexes reaching the glomerulus and (2) local factors within the glomerulus itself. A number of factors influence the delivery of immune complexes to the glomerulus, including the blood flow or its alteration and the systemic clearance of immune complexes by the mononuclear phagocytic system. It has been demonstrated, for example, that patients with autoimmune disease and tissue deposition of immune complexes have defective Fc receptor-mediated phagocytic clearance.

The size of the circulating immune complex, which, in turn, is determined by the relative antigen/antibody ratio, the size, valence, and nature of the antigen, and the antibody class and affinity, also influences the fate of the immune complex. Great antigen excess produces small immune complexes that are not particularly nephritogenic. Great antibody excess produces large, often insoluble immune complexes, which are rapidly removed from the circulation by the mononuclear phagocytic system and are not available for vascular localization. Experimentally, large complexes in antibody excess that are delivered to the circulation leading to the kidney localize in vessels and mesangial areas but are rapidly removed, in contrast to those formed during a period when the antigen/antibody ratio is more closely balanced.

Local factors that affect immune-complex deposition in the glomerulus include permeability and electrical charge of the glomerular capillary wall and the composition of the immune complex. Vasoactive substances released as part of the immune response may enhance vascular permeability and immune-complex localization. The physicochemical properties of the antigen, antibody, and resultant immune complex have a bearing on their affinity for the highly charged glomerular capillary wall. Interchange with circulating antigens and antibodies appears to be particularly important. The size and composition of the immune complex are subject to modification with shifts in the relative concentration of either antigen or antibody. Once localization has begun, antigen, antibody, or immune complexes can interact at the site. The interchange of immune-complex components is influenced by such factors as the location, degree of inflammation, affinity of the antibody reaction, and physicochemical factors. Immune-complex cross-linking via secondary immune reactions with rheumatoid factors or anti-idiotypic antibodies could alter free interchange between the primary immune-complex reactants. Complement activation can solubilize the immune complex and could contribute to immune-complex lability.

Granular immunoglobulin deposits, presumably immune complexes, appear to be responsible for more than 75% of cases of human glomerulonephritis of various histologic types, clinical courses, and demographic presentation (Table 36–2). Immunogenetic factors may influence susceptibility to immune-complex disease with increasing numbers of associations between the HLA-DR system and glomerulonephritis being recognized (Table 36–2). It is not known how the actual gene products are involved in the generation of the disease. The ever-increasing number of antigen-antibody systems identified in immune-complex glomerulonephritis in humans can be divided into exogenous (or foreign) and endogenous (or self) antigens (Table 36–3). However, in most cases of presumed human immune-complex glomerulonephritis, the causative antigen-antibody systems are unknown and screening for antigens is difficult.

Pathology

Primary immune-complex glomerulonephritis (ie, glomerulonephritis in patients without identifiable systemic disease) is usually classified histologically (Table 36–2). The secondary forms of glomerulone-phritis (principally those associated with systemic diseases such as systemic lupus erythematosus (SLE), essential mixed cryoglobulinemia, Henoch-Schönlein purpura, and subacute infective endocarditis) are often of a proliferative type, although other histologic variants (noted above) occur. The main histologic patterns are described in Table 36–2 and Fig. 36–2. The immune-complex deposits are visualized as electron-dense deposits by electron microscopy and may appear in subepithelial, subendothelial, intramembranous, and mesangial locations (Table 36–2).

Clinical Features

Since immune-complex deposition in glomeruli can induce all histologic forms of glomerulonephritis, the clinical features vary widely depending on the type and severity of glomerulonephritis (Table 36–2). Proteinuria is almost always present and may be mild, moderate, or severe. Nephrotic syndrome occurs when urinary protein loss exceeds the body's capacity to completely replace it, after which serum oncotic pressure decreases and edema develops. Nephrotic syndrome most frequently accompanies membranous glomerulonephritis. Hematuria is more common in patients with proliferative or membrano-proliferative histologic findings. The presence of erythrocyte casts in the urinary sediment suggests an acute phase of glomerular inflammation. Acute nephritic syndrome frequently accompanies diffuse proliferative and membranoproliferative glomerulonephritis. It is characterized by hematuria, proteinuria, edema, hypertension, and a reduced glomerular filtration rate. Hypertension can be present from the outset of any of these diseases or may appear later if the nephritis progresses. The syndrome of rapidly progressive glomerulonephritis resembles that of acute glomerulonephritis except for the rapid progression (within weeks or a few months) toward end-stage renal failure.

Renal failure and chronic glomerulonephritis may follow any form of immune-complex glomerular injury, usually related to the particular histologic type (Table 36–2).

Immunologic Pathogenesis

The presumptive diagnosis of immune-complex glomerulonephritis is based on the finding in renal biopsy of granular deposits of immunoglobulin, usually accompanied by complement, in the glomeruli. IgG is the most common, with IgA or IgM occasionally predominating (Table 36–2). The glomerular immune-complex deposition may diffusely involve all capillary loops in membranous or diffuse proliferative glomerulonephritis (Fig. 36–3A). In focal glomerulonephritis the deposits tend to involve only segments of the glomerular capillary wall or mesangium, but they may be more widespread than expected from

Table 36–2. Morphologic, immunopathologic, serologic, and clinical features of the major histologic classifications of immune-complex glomerulonephritis.

Morphology of Glomeruli	Immunofluorescence of Glomeruli (Granular Pattern)	Immunology Laboratory Findings (Serology)	Clinical Presentation and Features
Glomerulonephritis types Diffuse proliferative glomerulonephritis, including poststreptococcal glomerulonephritis Diffuse hypercellularity, electron-dense deposits in the mesangia or along GBM. Poststreptococcal form: subepithelial "humps" by electron microscopy.	IgG and C3 scattered along GBM. Variable IgA and IgM. In poststreptococcal form, C3 may be present when immunoglobulin is minimal or absent.	Non-poststreptococcal forms: usually no abnormalities. Decreased C3, C4, and C1q, or presence of immune complex suggests underlying disease (eg, SLE or chronic infection). Poststreptococcal form: increased antistreptolysin O titer, decreased C3 (usually normal C4). Immune complexes and cryoglobulins may be present.	Non-poststreptococcal forms: microscopic hematuria and/or proteinuria, gross hematuria, hypertension. Onset and course variable. May progress to renal failure. Poststreptococcal form: acute nephritic syndrome, usually resolves, especially in children. Prevalence variable depending on serotype of streptococcus.
Diffuse proliferative crescent-forming glomerulonephritis Diffuse hypercellularity with extracapillary crescents. Electron microscopy as above.	Heavy fibrinogen-related antigen in areas of crescents. Immunoglobulin and complement as above.	Secondary forms: features of underlying disease as above. Idiopathic form: complement is normal or reduced. Variable immune-complex and cryoglobulin detection.	Rapidly progressive renal failure, even anuric or oliguric from onset. Microscopic or gross hematuria, erythrocyte casts in urine, proteinuria, nephrotic syndrome unusual. Uncommon; more common above age 50.
Focal proliferative glomerulonephritis, including mesangial IgA nephropathy Focal and segmental mesangial hypercellularity, with electron-dense deposits.	IgA often prominent, with or without C3 and IgG, sometimes IgM, in mesangial pattern (often segmental).	Variable increased serum IgA. Often immune complex of IgA class (less reactivity in usual immune-complex assays). IgA-fibronectin complexes often present in serum. Some association with HLA-Bw35 and -DR4.	Microscopic hematuria and/or proteinuria. Recurrent gross hematuria, may accompany intercurrent respiratory infections. Occasionally progresses to renal failure. Prevalent in young adults.
Membranous glomerulonephritis Thickening of GBM, little or no hypercellularity. Subepithelial spikes by silver stains, diffuse subepithelial electron-dense deposits.	IgG and C3 diffusely along the GBM. IgA and IgM unusual in idiopathic form.	Usually no abnormality in idiopathic form. (SLE form described below.)	Proteinuria, often nephrotic syndrome. Slow progression in one-third of cases. In older patients, may rarely be related to neoplasm. Common in adults; unusual before age 15.
Membranoproliferative glomerulonephritis Mesangial proliferation with interposition between endothelium and thickened GBM. At least 2 variants by electron microscopy: type I (subendothelial deposits) and type II (intramembranous dense deposits).	Type I: Heavy C3, some IgG, along GBM; occasional IgA or IgM. Type II: Heavy C3 along GBM. Immunoglobulin deposits uncommon.	Persistent low C3 in most type I and all type II. C4 usually normal. Nephritic factor often present, especially in type II.	Proteinuria, microscopic or gross hematuria, often nephrotic syndrome, often hypertension, usually progresses over several years to renal failure. Type I is somewhat uncommon. Type II is rare. Type II can be associated with partial lipodystrophy.

(continued)

Table 36–2. Morphologic, immunopathologic, serologic, and clinical features of the major histologic classifications of immune-complex glomerulonephritis. *(continued)*

Morphology of Glomeruli	Immunofluorescence of Glomeruli (Granular Pattern)	Immunology Laboratory Findings (Serology)	Clinical Presentation and Features
End-stage (chronic) glomerulonephritis Hyalinized glomeruli, extensive tubulointerstitial destruction. Electron microscopy occasionally detects features of original disease process.	Variable IgG, IgA, IgM, and C3 in least damaged glomeruli. C3 may persist in absence of immunogloublin deposits.	Abnormalities typical of original disease occasionally persist.	Renal failure, often hypertension, variable degree of proteinuria and/or hematuria. End stage of many morphologic forms of glomerulonephritis.
Systemic diseases with glomerulonephritis **Systemic lupus erythematosus** Classified into mesangial only, membranous glomerulonephritis, diffuse proliferative glomerulonephritis, and focal proliferative glomerulonephritis. Resemble lesions listed above. Some transitions from one type to another.	IgG, IgA, IgM (typically all three) and C3 (also C4 and C1q). Patterns of glomerular deposition in accord with morphologic type. Often prominent tubulointerstitial immune deposits.	ANA positive. Decreased C3, C4, and C1q; increased anti-DNA; circulating immune complexes, with or without cryoglobulins, especially in diffuse proliferative type; often fluctuating with changes in disease activity and can be normalized by immuno-suppressive treatment.	Only mild urinary abnormalities with minimal mesangial lesions. Proteinuria and microscopic hematuria, nephrotic syndrome in others; 10–50% progression to end-stage renal failure by 5 years, depending on morphologic type. Rapidly progressive course when crescentic glomerulonephritis. Lupus nephritis affects half or more of all patients with SLE.
Essential mixed cryoglobulinemia Usually proliferative glomerulonephritis (diffuse, occasionally focal or membranoproliferative).	IgG, IgM, C3 diffusely along the GBM; sometimes massive deposits in capillary lumens. Fibrinogen-related antigen variable.	Decreased C4, cryogloglobulins (especially IgMκ-IgG), rheumatoid factor.	Proteinuria, microscopic hematuria, acute nephritic episodes, hypertension, episodes of purpura. Progresses slowly to renal failure. Rare disease; affects females more than males.
Henoch-Schönlein purpura Focal or diffuse proliferative glomerulonephritis, sometimes crescentic.	IgA prominent, usually with IgG and C3, with or without IgM. Fibrinogen-related antigen frequently prominent.	Variable increased serum IgA. Often immune complex of IgA class (less reactivity in usual immune-complex assays). Some association with HLA-Bw35.	Microscopic hematuria, proteinuria, nephrotic syndrome, acute nephritic syndrome. Generally favorable outcome, but some cases progress to end-stage renal failure. Nephritis occurs in more than half of patients with Henoch-Schönlein purpura.

the focal nature of the histologic change, and in some patients the immune-complex deposition is confined to the mesangium (Fig. 36–3B).

Predominant IgA deposits are seen in patients with focal glomerulonephritis. The association has been so striking that the term "mesangial IgA nephropathy" has been coined to denote the condition. Circulating IgA-containing immune complexes can be detected in at least 60% of cases of IgA nephropathy, and the rapidity with which hematuria follows an infectious episode suggests that the immune complexes may be formed during antibody excess, possibly with preformed antibody to a common infectious microorganism in the oropharynx. The large, antibody-excess complexes would preferentially accumulate in the mesangium. Fifty percent of patients have raised serum IgA levels and evidence of abnormal regulation of IgA production in vitro, suggesting a primary immune abnormality. Many patients also have demonstrable circulating aggregates of IgA and fibronectin. Alternative explanations for the IgA accumulation have included IgA multimers and anti-mesangial antibodies. Occasionally, patients with similar clinical courses have predominantly IgM mesangial deposits.

Mesangial deposition of IgA, usually in a more diffuse pattern with C3 and fibrin, occurs in Henoch-Schönlein purpura. This is a systemic disease typified by arteriolar and venular lesions causing skin purpura, arthralgias, abdominal pain, intestinal hemor-

Table 36–3. Antigen-antibody systems known to cause or strongly suspected of causing immune-complex glomerulonephritis in humans.

Antigens	Clinical Condition
Exogenous or foreign antigens Iatrogenic agents	
Drugs, toxoids, foreign serum	Serum sickness, heroin nephropathy (?), gold nephropathy (?), etc
Infectious agents Bacterial: Nephritogenic streptococci, *Staphylococcus albus* and *S aureus*, *Corynebacterium bovis*, enterococci, *Streptococcus pneumoniae*, *Propionibacterium acnes*, *Klebsiella pneumoniae*, *Yersinia enterocolitica*, *Treponema pallidum*, *Salmonella typhi*, *Mycoplasma pneumoniae*	Poststreptococcal glomerulonephritis, infected ventriculoatrial shunts, endocarditis, pneumonia, yersiniasis, syphilis, typhoid fever, pneumonia
Parasitic: *Plasmodium malariae*, *Plasmodium falciparum*, *Schistosoma mansoni*, *Echinococcus granulosus*, *Toxoplasma gondii*	Malaria, schistosomiasis, toxoplasmosis, hydatid disease
Viral: Hepatitis B virus, retrovirus-related antigen, measles virus, Epstein-Barr virus, cytomegalovirus	Hepatitis, leukemia, subacute sclerosing panencephalitis, Burkitt's lymphoma, cytomegalovirus infection
Fungal: *Candida albicans*	Candidiasis
Perhaps others as yet undetermined	Endocarditis, leprosy, kala-azar, dengue, mumps, varicella, infectious mononucleosis, Guillain-Barré syndrome, AIDS (?)
Endogenous or self antigens Nuclear antigens	SLE
Immunoglobulin	Cryoglobulinemia
Tumor antigens	Neoplasms
Thyroglobulin	Thyroiditis

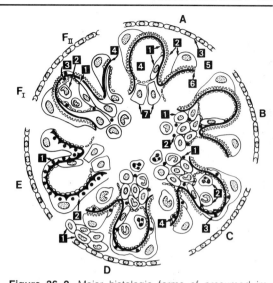

Figure 36–2. Major histologic forms of presumed immune-complex glomerulonephritis. ***A:*** *Normal glomerular anatomy.* 1, Glomerular endothelial cells, with fenestrated endothelium; 2, glomerular epithelial cells with specialized foot processes; 3, parietal epithelium lining Bowman's capsule; 4, glomerular capillary lumen; 5, urinary space; 6, GBM; 7, the glomerular mesangium, composed predominantly of smooth muscle-like mesangial cells and occasional mononuclear phagocytes. ***B:*** *Focal proliferative glomerulonephritis.* The lesion is characterized by focal (some glomeruli) and segmental (portions of glomeruli) mesangial hypercellularity (1). Immune deposits of immunoglobulin and C3 (2) are found in the mesangial area. IgA deposits predominate in IgA nephropathy. ***C:*** *Diffuse proliferative glomerulonephritis.* Extensive and widespread hypercellularity is present with infiltration of polymorphonuclear and mononuclear inflammatory cells (2). Immune deposits of immunoglobulin and C3 may be found in mesangial (1), subepithelial (3), or subendothelial (4) locations. In poststreptococcal proliferative glomerulonephritis, the subepithelial deposits have a characteristic humplike appearance in electron microscopy. ***D:*** *Diffuse proliferative glomerulonephritis with crescent formation.* In addition to the features of diffuse proliferative glomerulonephritis, macrophages and parietal epithelial cells accumulate in Bowman's space (1) in response to fibrin deposits, which accumulate in this area when severe glomerular capillary wall damage has occurred. The inflammation may be sufficiently intense to cause necrosis in the glomerular tuft. ***E:*** *Membranous glomerulonephritis.* This is typified by marked thickening of the GBM, the accumulation of immunoglobulin and C3 immune deposits in a subepithelial position (1), and a lack of glomerular hypercellularity. With time, GBM extensions or "spikes" (2) develop between the immune deposits and eventually engulf them. ***F$_I$/F$_{II}$:*** *Membranoproliferative glomerulonephritis.* Interposition of mesangial cells between the endothelium and the GBM (1) produces a "tram-track" appearance of the glomerular capillary wall. Mesangial hypercellularity and inflammatory cells are present (2). In type I, immune deposits of immunoglobulin and C3 are present predominantly in subendothelial positions (3). In type II, also called dense-deposit disease, the GBM is thickened and abnormally electron dense (4). Heavy C3 deposits are seen in the GBM and mesangial areas with little or no immunoglobulin.

rhage, and often a proliferative glomerulonephritis that rarely progresses to end-stage renal failure. It has been suggested that the disease may be triggered by infectious agents or drugs presented at mucosal surfaces and eliciting abnormal IgA responses. The role of food allergy is controversial.

Acute post-streptococcal glomerulonephritis is characterized by acute inflammatory changes due to immune deposits in a subepithelial location. These contain large amounts of C3 and smaller amounts of IgG. A streptococcal antigen that becomes trapped at this site is implicated; one proposed candidate is a streptococcal protein that may directly activate the alternative complement pathway.

In SLE, the immune-complex deposits may be widespread, involving glomeruli and, in 70% of instances, extraglomerular renal tissues as well. Indeed,

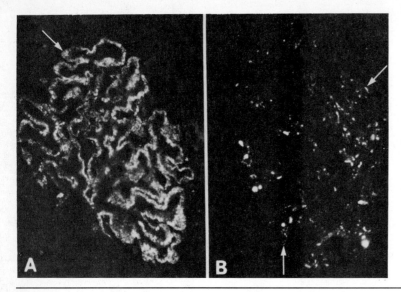

Figure 36–3. Granular deposits of IgG are seen in the glomeruli of patients with immune complex-induced glomerulonephritis. **A:** Heavy diffuse deposits (arrow) are present in a patient with membranous glomerulonephritis and nephrotic syndrome. **B:** Focal granular deposits (arrows), largely confined to the mesangium, are present in a patient with focal proliferative glomerulonephritis and mild proteinuria (Original magnification × 250.)

granular deposits of immunoglobulin and complement in TBM or peritubular capillaries should suggest the diagnosis of SLE. IgA and C1q deposits are prominent in kidneys of patients with SLE.

Immunologic Diagnosis

It is helpful to identify antigen-antibody systems in individuals with immune-complex glomerulonephritis. Serologic tests for common infectious etiologies should include streptococcal antibodies, hepatitis B antigen, hepatitis C antibodies, and human immunodeficiency virus (HIV) antibody. Antinuclear and anti-DNA antibodies should be sought, since SLE glomerulonephritis can occur without other overt organ involvement. The presence of ANCA, rheumatoid factors, or cryoglobulins may provide additional insight into the pathogenic process. However, in most cases serum antibody testing is unrevealing.

Serum complement levels may be helpful (Table 36–2). C3, C4, and total hemolytic complement (CH$_{50}$) are normal in the majority of cases of glomerulonephritis, but when abnormalities occur, they are of considerable diagnostic importance. Hypocomplementemia occurs frequently in certain forms of immune-complex glomerulonephritis, especially SLE, essential mixed cryoblobulinemia, and infection-associated glomerulonephritis (poststreptococcal, endocarditis, infected ventriculoatrial shunts, etc). It is also common in membranoproliferative glomerulonephritis, a group of diseases incorporating at least 2 varieties of nephritis with differing pathogenetic mechanisms: type I and type II membranoproliferative glomerulonephritis. Type I is an etiologically heterogeneous group with granular immune-complex deposits. Type II, or "dense-deposit" disease, is identified by electron-dense transformation of the GBM,

in which chemical analysis of the GBM suggests an increase in sialic acid-rich GBM glycoproteins, rather than the accumulation of a nonbasement membrane component.

A serum factor, termed nephritic factor, capable of activating the alternative complement pathway is present in many patients with membranoproliferative glomerulonephritis, particularly type II. Nephritic factor has been shown to be an immunoglobulin with immunoconglutinin properties, capable of reacting with activated components of the alternative complement pathway, specifically the bimolecular complex of C3b and activated factor B, stabilizing its C3 convertase activity.

Several sensitive methods for the detection of circulating immune complexes are available (see Chapter 12). In general, the immune-complex assays are positive when large amounts of circulating immune complexes are present in patients with SLE and with glomerulonephritis associated with other systemic immune-complex diseases.

Differential Diagnosis

The simultaneous presence of proteinuria (more than 1 g daily) and urinary casts almost invariably indicates a glomerular disease. The differential diagnosis is extensive and includes familial renal disease, hypertension, SLE, streptococcal infection, viral hepatitis, rheumatoid arthritis, and cryoglobulinemia.

Treatment

The most commonly used drugs are corticosteroids, cyclophosphamide, and azathioprine, and occasionally other "immunosuppressive" therapy used singly or in combination. Primary (idiopathic) membranous glomerulonephritis may respond somewhat to corticosteroids or regimens including chlorambucil, but the benefit is uncertain and the toxicity is of concern. Primary proliferative and membranoproliferative forms are usually quite unresponsive to immunosuppressive therapy. In contrast, patients with SLE nephritis often show considerable benefit from corticosteroid therapy, and in severe cases with diffuse proliferative histology, the addition of cyclophosphamide or azathioprine is often appropriate.

Ideally, management of immune-complex glomerulonephritis should either eradicate the source of antigen or inhibit production of the specific antibody. These approaches stress the need for identification of the antigen-antibody systems in each patient. For example, removal of antigen by treating *Treponema pallidum* infection has been beneficial to individuals with syphilitic immune-complex glomerulonephritis, as has removal of malignant tissue in immune-complex glomerulonephritis associated with neoplasia. The use of plasmapheresis and of specific immunoadsorbents to remove circulating antibodies, antigens, or immune complexes is under investigation.

Complications & Prognosis

The prognosis is extremely variable, depending on the histologic form of glomerulonephritis (Table 36–2). Generally, diffuse proliferative forms have worse prognoses than focal proliferative or nonproliferative forms. An exception is diffuse proliferative postinfectious glomerulonephritis, which usually remits in 90% of cases. Complications include progressive loss of glomerular filtration leading to renal failure and the eventual need for dialysis or kidney transplantation. Hypertension may occur with any form of immune-complex glomerulonephritis and is occasionally severe. Proteinuria of the degree found in the nephrotic syndrome may cause hypoalbuminemia (leading to edema or anasarca), depletion of the serum IgG level, and disturbed balance of coagulation factors manifesting as venous thrombosis, pulmonary embolism, or renal vein thrombosis.

Recurrence of some of the forms of glomerulonephritis in kidney transplants has been reported, especially with focal mesangial IgA nephropathy and type II membranoproliferative glomerulonephritis. However, because recurrence is infrequent in the former and slow in the latter, transplantation is not contraindicated.

TUBULOINTERSTITIAL NEPHRITIS

Major Immunologic Features

- There are extensive interstitial mononuclear cell infiltrates, predominantly T cells.
- In anti-TBM tubulointerstitial nephritis, linear deposits of immunoglobulin usually accompanied by complement are found along the TBM; circulating anti-TBM antibody may be detected.
- In immune-complex tubulointerstitial nephritis, granular deposits of immunoglobulin and complement are found in the TBM, interstitium, or peritubular capillaries; circulating immune complexes may be detected.
- In presumed cell-mediated tubulointerstitial nephritis, there is no detectable immunoglobulin along the TBM, and no anti-TBM antibody or immune complex is detected in the circulation.

Immune processes that lead to tubulointerstitial nephritis are similar to those described above for the glomerulus. These include anti-TBM antibodies, immune complexes, and cell-mediated immunity. Immune tubulointerstitial nephritis can accompany glomerulonephritis or occur as an independent event. Experimental models of anti-TBM antibody- and immune complex-induced tubulointerstitial nephritis have been developed, and similar processes have been identified in humans. Evidence exists that sensitized cells may transfer or contribute to tubulointerstitial nephritis in experimental models. Despite the conspicuous infiltration of interstitial mononuclear cells, including T cells, the pathogenetic role of cell-mediated immunity, other than in renal allografts, is not well established in humans.

General Considerations

Anti-TBM antibodies occur in about 70% of patients with anti-GBM glomerulonephritis and correlate with greater degrees of interstitial inflammation. Anti-TBM antibodies are occasionally found in drug-induced tubulointerstitial nephritis, in tubulointerstitial nephritis associated with immune complex-induced glomerulonephritis, in renal allografts, and rarely in primary tubulointerstitial nephritis.

In immune-complex tubulointerstitial nephritis, granular deposits of immunoglobulin and complement are found along the TBM, interstitium, or peritubular capillaries. These deposits are present in 50–70% of patients with SLE nephritis and infrequently in those with cryoglobulinemia, Sjögren's syndrome, membranoproliferative and rapidly progressive glomerulonephritis, and primary idiopathic tubulointerstitial nephritis. Tubulointerstitial immunoglobulin deposits may be present in the absence of glomerular immune-complex deposits and have occasionally been found in patients with SLE.

Mononuclear interstitial infiltrates without anti-TBM antibodies or immune complexes are the most common form of tubulointerstitial nephritis in humans. Frequently, the disease appears to be a hypersensitivity reaction to drugs, which may include a wide range of antibiotics, nonsteroidal anti-inflammatory drugs, and diuretics. Other situations in which mononuclear interstitial infiltrates may be prominent include acute allograft rejection, anti-GBM glomerulonephritis, pyelonephritis, sarcoidosis, Sjögren's syndrome, chronic active hepatitis, and idiopathic interstitial nephritis.

Pathology

Depending upon the duration, underlying causes, and severity of disease, renal pathology varies from focal to diffuse mononuclear interstitial infiltrates composed primarily of T lymphocytes and macrophages. Tubular lesions may range from minimal degeneration of the tubular epithelium to necrosis and atrophy. Polymorphonuclear leukocytes may be associated with necrotic tubules. As the inflammation advances, interstitial fibrosis and thickened TBM develop. Eosinophils may be prominent in drug hypersensitivity. The glomerulus is not involved unless there is an associated glomerulonephritis.

Clinical Features

The clinical course is usually that of renal functional impairment without urinary findings suggestive of glomerular disease. When anti-TBM antibody- and immune complex-induced tubulointerstitial nephritis is associated with glomerulonephritis, the features of the glomerulonephritis usually predominate. Evidence of tubular dysfunction manifesting as complete or partial Fanconi's syndrome

may occur. When anti-TBM antibodies occur in transplant recipients, their effects may be indistinguishable from those of cell-mediated immune rejection.

Drug-induced tubulointerstitial nephritis usually presents acutely with fever, rash, hematuria, azotemia, and eosinophilia associated with a course of drug therapy. Other features such as pyuria, eosinophiluria, mild proteinuria, flank pain, and arthralgia may also be present, together with an elevated serum IgE level. Progressive renal failure is the general rule unless the offending drug is discontinued.

Immunologic Diagnosis

To distinguish the immune mechanism responsible for the mononuclear infiltrate characteristic of tubulointerstitial nephritis, renal biopsy for immunopathologic studies is needed and should include determination of the phenotypes of the infiltrating cells. Linear deposits of immunoglobulin and complement are found along the TBM (Fig. 36–4A) in anti-TBM antibody-associated tubulointerstitial nephritis. As in anti-GBM antibody disease, the specificity should be confirmed by elution studies or detection of circulating anti-TBM antibodies. Rarely, anti-TBM antibodies have been found in drug-induced tubulointerstitial nephritis in which the drug or its metabolites can be detected bound to the TBM.

In immune-complex disease, the tubules, vessels, and interstitium should be carefully examined for im-

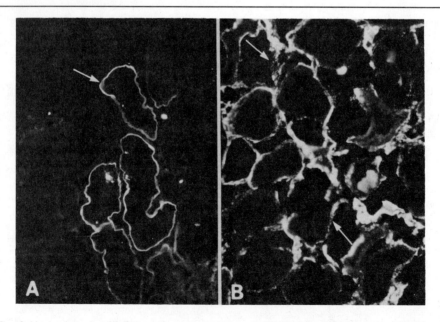

Figure 36–4. *A:* Linear deposits of IgG (arrow) are present along the TBM of focal renal tubules in the renal biopsy of a patient with anti-GBM glomerulonephritis. *B:* Diffuse granular deposits of IgG (arrows) are seen along the TBM of most renal tubules in the renal biopsy of a patient with SLE and immune-complex glomerulonephritis. (Original magnification ×250.)

munofluorescent deposits of immunoglobulin (Fig. 36–4B) and complement, which are often focal and less intense than are glomerular deposits. Prominent or widespread tubulointerstitial immunoglobulin deposits suggest SLE.

In presumed cell-mediated tubulointerstitial nephritis, no immunoglobulin deposits are found. T lymphocytes are the predominant cells, although a few B cells are also present. Monoclonal antibodies directed to T cell subsets identify both CD4 (helper/inducer) and CD8 (suppressor/cytotoxic) cells. However, the proportion of CD4 to CD8 cells appears to vary depending upon the underlying cause of disease. CD8 cells are the predominant phenotype found in drug-induced cases, whereas either CD4 or CD8 cells may be the major cells found in renal allograft rejection. The patient's reactivity to the drug can be tested by antibody measurement and lymphocyte proliferation (see Chapter 13).

Treatment

Tubulointerstitial nephritis associated with glomerulonephritis is treated as outlined in the previous sections. In cases of drug-induced tubulointerstitial nephritis, the offending drug should be discontinued immediately and replaced as needed with a structurally unrelated alternative drug. Corticosteroids may aid in quicker resolution of drug-induced tubulointerstitial nephritis.

MINIMAL-CHANGE NEPHROPATHY

General Considerations

Minimal-change nephropathy is the most common cause of nephrotic syndrome in children; however, it causes less than 10% of adult cases. No clear epidemiologic factor has been established. Abnormal T cell function or T cell products have been suggested as possible etiologic factors.

Pathology

Typically, no abnormalities are detected by light microscopy, and no immunoglobulin deposits are found by immunofluorescence. By electron microscopy, there is a diffuse effacement of the epithelial cell foot processes.

Clinical Features

Patients have nephrotic edema and selective proteinuria with no impairment of renal function, no hypertension, rare microscopic hematuria, and no hypocomplementemia; however, hypoproteinemia may be marked. The disease follows a naturally remitting and relapsing course. Repeated relapses in childhood are often followed by permanent remission in adolescence.

Treatment

Minimal-change nephropathy is particularly corticosteroid-sensitive, so that a rapid remission, in 2–8 weeks, on steroid therapy is considered diagnostic. Relapses may occur, and in these cases steroid treatment may be supplemented with immunosuppressive treatment.

FOCAL GLOMERULOSCLEROSIS

General Considerations

Focal glomerulosclerosis is another common cause of nephrotic syndrome in children and young adults. It is usually an idiopathic disease; however, a similar disease may develop in heroin abusers and in some patients with AIDS. Focal glomerulosclerosis may be difficult to distinguish from minimal-change nephropathy early in the course of the 2 diseases.

Pathology

The glomerular lesion is that of segmented hyalinosis and sclerosis. IgM, C3, and fibrin are present in small quantities in the hyalinized segments of glomeruli, although their immunopathogenic significance is unclear. AIDS nephropathy cases may have distinctive additional features such as tubuloreticular structures on electron microscopy of the glomeruli and microcyst formation in the renal tubulointerstitial regions.

Clinical Features

Nephrotic syndrome is common and may be associated with hypertension and microscopic hematuria and then progressive impairment of renal function. A large percentage of cases reach end-stage renal failure within 10 years. Patients with heroin or AIDS nephropathy typically progress even more quickly.

Treatment

Most focal glomerulosclerosis is corticosteroid-resistant, and there is little evidence that any other specific treatment alters the natural history of progression to renal failure. Nevertheless, some immunosuppressive regimens continue to be tried, with claims of success in some cases. Transplantation is not contraindicated, despite slow and inconsistent recurrence of the same histologic lesion in the transplant.

VASCULITIS

General Considerations

The vasculitides are syndromes with a spectrum of clinicopathologic features with the essential common component of vasculitis, an inflammatory reaction in vessel walls, leading to ischemia of the supplied tissues. Increasing evidence points to an immunologic pathogenesis of the vascular lesions, particularly the deposition of circulating immune complexes triggering the inflammatory process through humoral and cellular mediators. Several vasculitides involve the renal vessels and glomeruli. Of these, Henoch-Schönlein purpura has been discussed above. Polyarteritis nodosa, Wegener's granulomatosis, and some cases of crescentic glomerulonephritis without overt vasculitis are increasingly being recognized as a group of closely related entities in which a substantial subset of patients have circulating ANCA. In addition to being useful markers for the diagnosis and classification of these diseases, there is evidence that ANCA are directly involved in the pathogenesis of the vasculitic lesions.

Pathology

Vasculitis is diagnosed by the presence of segmental vasculitic lesions, with a perivascular inflammatory infiltrate, fibrinoid necrosis, and, in the extreme, aneurysm formation. The lesion may have evidence of coagulation, luminal obliteration, and downstream ischemia.

Polyarteritis nodosa is a necrotizing vasculitis of small and medium-sized muscular arteries with arteriolar and glomerular lesions (often segmental and focal), glomerular necrosis, and proliferative and crescentic glomerulonephritis. Lesions may be present at all stages of development. Wegener's granulomatosis is a necrotizing granulomatous angiitis involving arteries and veins. The renal lesion consists of a proliferative necrotizing glomerulonephritis with crescent formation and granulomatous angiitis.

Clinical Features

Polyarteritis nodosa is a multisystemic disease, and its prognosis is influenced by the degree of kidney involvement. Renovascular hypertension occurs in more than 50% of the cases, and end-stage renal failure is the common cause of death. Wegener's granulomatosis occurs equally in both sexes and often involves the upper respiratory tract, the lungs, and the kidneys.

Immunologic Diagnosis

The diagnosis is based on a combination of renal biopsy and other biopsy studies, angiographic demonstration of vasculitis or vascular aneurysms, and serologic tests for ANCA. ANCA are of various types with different specificities, and 2 major categories predominate. Those with cytoplasmic staining (C-ANCA) are often specific for proteinase-3 and are common in patients with Wegener's granulomatosis. ANCA whose staining is perinuclear in alcohol-fixed targets (P-ANCA) are often specific for myeloperoxidase and are common in patients with disease limited to the kidneys. However, there is a considerable overlap of antibody specificities and clinical syndromes; for instance, rapidly progressive glomerulonephritis is a common feature of both specificities, and alveolar capillaritis with lung hemorrhage may occur with either. Immunofluorescence microscopy of renal biopsy specimens in ANCA-positive cases typically reveals no or scant immune deposits, leading to the description "pauci-immune" to differentiate this from the more abundant immunoglobulin and complement deposits seen in "immune-complex" lesions.

Treatment

Therapy with corticosteroids and cyclophosphamide has been shown to be effective in Wegener's granulomatosis, even when acute renal failure is already advanced. This therapy may be less effective in polyarteritis nodosa, and plasmapheresis therapy has been recommended in resistant cases. ANCA-positive crescentic glomerulonephritis in the absence of systemic vasculitis appears also to respond to treatment with corticosteroids and cyclophosphamide. For cases of polyarteritis nodosa associated with hepatitis B virus, trials of antiviral agents associated with plasmapheresis have shown considerable promise.

REFERENCES

Balow JE, Austin HA III: Clinical aspects of immunologic glomerular diseases. Page 213 in: *Contemporary Issues in Nephrology.* Vol 18. Wilson CB, Brenner BM, Stein JH (editors). Churchill Livingstone, 1988.

Brentjens JR, Andres G: Interaction of antibodies with renal cell surface antigens. *Kidney Int* 1989;**35**:954.

Couser WG: Mediation of immune glomerular injury. *J Am Soc Nephrol* 1990;**1**:13.

Glassock RJ et al: Primary glomerular diseases. Page 1182 in: *The Kidney,* 4th ed. Brenner BM, Rector FC Jr (editors). Saunders, 1991.

Glassock RJ et al: Secondary glomerular diseases. Page 1280 in: *The Kidney,* 4th ed. Brenner BM, Rector FC Jr (editors). Saunders, 1991.

Jennette JC, Falk RJ: Disease associations and pathogenic role of antineutrophil cytoplasmic autoantibodies in vasculitis. *Curr Opin Rheumatol* 1992;**4**:9.

Karp SL et al: The nephritogenic immune response. *Curr Opin Immunol* 1991;**3**:906.

Kashgarian M, Sterzel RB: The pathobiology of the mesangium. *Kidney Int* 1992;**41**:524.

Kelly CJ et al: Immune recognition and response to the renal interstitium. *Kidney Int* 1991;**31**:518.

Main IW et al: T cells and macrophages and their role in renal injury. *Semin Nephrol* 1992;**12**:395.

Oliveira DB, Peters DK: Autoimmunity and the pathogenesis of glomerulonephritis. *Pediatr Nephrol* 1990; **4**:185.

Rovin BH, Schreiner GF: Cell-mediated immunity in glomerular disease. *Annu Rev Med* 1991;**42:**25.

van Es LA: Pathogenesis of IgA nephropathy. *Kidney Int* 1992;**41:**1720.

Wilson CB: Immune aspects of renal diseases. (*Primer on Allergic and Immunologic Diseases,* 3rd ed.) *JAMA* 1992;**268:**2904.

Wilson CB: Nephritogenic immune reactions involving glomerular basement membrane and other structural renal antigens. Page 555 in: *Textbook of Nephrology,* 2nd ed.

Massry SG, Glassock RJ (editors). Williams & Wilkins, 1989.

Wilson CB: Nephritogenic tubulointerstitial antigens. *Kidney Int* 1991;**39:**501.

Wilson CB: The renal response to immunological injury. Page 1062 in: *The Kidney,* 4th ed. Brenner BM, Rector FC Jr (editors). Saunders, 1991.

Wilson CB, Tang, WW: Immunological renal diseases. In: *Samter's Immunological Diseases,* 5th ed. Frank MM et al (editors). Little, Brown, in press.

Dermatologic Diseases

Sanford M. Goldstein, MD, & Bruce U. Wintroub, MD

Several diseases of the skin have been linked strongly to disordered immune regulation, or, more precisely, to autoimmunity. These diseases are characterized by blistering and by the presence of autoantibodies that bind to various cutaneous structures (Figs 37–1 and 37–2). The discovery of these autoantibodies has revolutionized the understanding and classification of these diseases. These antibodies also serve as specific and clinically important diagnostic markers. They have been used as reagents to help identify and characterize important proteins in the skin. In the clinical diagnosis and management of blistering disorders, skin biopsy for direct and indirect immunofluorescence is indispensable.

Allergic and infectious diseases of the skin are discussed in other chapters.

BULLOUS PEMPHIGOID

Major Immunologic Features
- There is linear deposition of IgG and C3 at the dermal-epidermal junction.
- Circulating IgG binds to the bullous pemphigoid antigen in the lamina lucida of the dermal-epidermal junction.
- There are immune complexes in blood and in skin lesions.

General Considerations
A. Definition: Bullous pemphigoid is characterized by tense, often pruritic blisters located on the flexor surfaces of the extremities, axilla, groin, and lower abdomen. There is characteristic deposition of IgG or C3 or both at the dermal-epidermal junction, without which the diagnosis is in question.

B. Etiology: In vivo and in vitro models suggest that the binding of IgG to bullous pemphigoid antigens (named for the disease) at the lamina lucida of the dermal-epidermal junction is an initiating event in the disease. Autoantibodies in bullous pemphigoid

recognize 2 distinct keratinocyte hemidesmosomal proteins named BP 230 (BPAG1) and BP 180 (BPAG2), which were recently cloned. BP 230 is a cytoplasmic protein, whereas BP 180 is a highly conserved transmembrane protein, whose clinically relevant epitopes map to a short region between an extracellular collagenous domain and the transmembrane domain. BP 230 and PB 180 map to chromosome 6 and 10, respectively. The primary stimulus for production of the autoantibody is unknown. The disease may be passively transferred to animals by injection of patient antibody. Immunohistochemical studies also demonstrate activation of the complement cascade through the classic and alternative complement pathways. Antibody and complement, in addition to mast cell activation in situ, appear to direct the influx of inflammatory cells, including eosinophils, into the area. The release of mediators from inflammatory cells, including proteolytic enzymes, may contribute to the characteristic separation of the epidermis from the dermis. The typical distribution of lesions on the body surface may be correlated with the regional distribution and concentration of the bullous pemphigoid antigen at those sites.

C. Prevalence: The prevalence is unknown. Bullous pemphigoid is an uncommon but not rare disease. There is no sex or race predominance. Although the disease has been identified in children, it is primarily a disease of individuals aged 60 years or older. There are no known patterns of inheritance, and no HLA associations have been found.

Pathology
Biopsy specimens (3–4 mm in diameter) are obtained from the edge of a fresh blister and should also contain perilesional skin. A subepidermal bulla is seen with fibrin, neutrophils, eosinophils, and lymphocytes within the blister cavity (Fig 37–3). The epidermis is intact and not necrotic. Biopsy of older lesions may give the false appearance of an intraepidermal blister if the epidermis has begun to re-

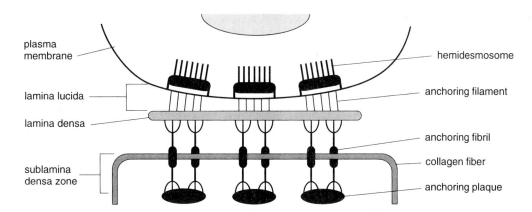

Figure 37–1. Schematic of epithelial basement membrane zone indicates major regions and structures. The lamina lucida is the electron-lucent region just below the keratinocyte plasma membrane and just above the electron-dense lamina densa. Skin incubated in 1 mol/L NaCl splits through the lamina lucida. (Reproduced and modified, with permission, from Gammon WR et al: Immunofluorescence on split skin for the detection and differentiation of basement membrane zone autoantibodies. *J Am Acad Dermatol* 1992;**27**:79.)

generate. The dermal infiltrate will vary depending on whether the base of the clinical lesion is grossly inflamed or normal, the former being characterized by an infiltrate in the papillary dermis similar to that seen in the blister cavity.

Clinical Features

A. Signs and Symptoms: The classic lesion of bullous pemphigoid is a tense blister with a diameter of 1 cm or more, appearing on a normal or erythematous base (Fig 37–4). The tenseness of the blisters in bullous diseases usually correlates with the thickness of the blister roof, which in bullous pemphigoid is full-thickness epidermis (Fig 37–3). The lesions may be very pruritic, but this is variable. Bullae are distributed over the extremities and trunk as noted above and may rupture and then heal. Smaller blisters, called vesicles, are sometimes seen in a clinical vari-

ant called vesicular pemphigoid. Blisters may remain localized to areas such as the lower legs in a variant termed localized pemphigoid. Occasionally, elderly patients present with perplexing and nonspecific papules, urticarial lesions, or widespread red and scaly areas. This presentation is sometimes called "pre-eruptive pemphigoid" and precedes the eruption of blisters. Recognizing these clinical variants will allow one to obtain a skin biopsy specimen for routine stains and direct immunofluorescence. Blisters may be found in the oral cavity in one-third of patients and, rarely, on other mucous membranes, including the esophagus, vagina, and anus.

B. Laboratory Findings: Peripheral eosinophilia and elevated serum IgE were present in 50% and 70% of patients, respectively, in one series. These tests are rarely clinically useful and are not routinely ordered.

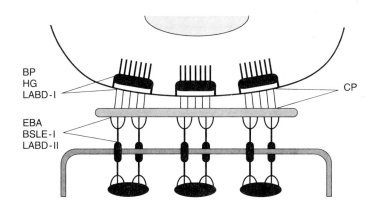

Figure 37–2. Schematic of the epithelial basement membrane zone shows ultrastructural binding sites of BMZ autoantibodies. BP, bullous pemphigoid; BSLE-I, bullous systemic lupus erythematosus type I; CP, cicatricial pemphigoid; EBA, epidermolysis bullosa acquisita; LABD, linear IgA bullous disease. (Reproduced and modified, with permission, from Gammon WR et al: Immunofluorescence on split skin for the detection and differentiation of basement membrane zone autoantibodies. *J Am Acad Dermatol* 1992;**27**:79.)

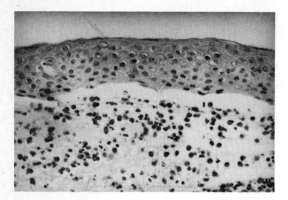

Figure 37–3. Histopathology of bullous pemphigoid. Note the full thickness of epidermis that makes up the blister roof. (Courtesy of Philip LeBoit.)

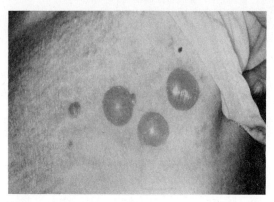

A

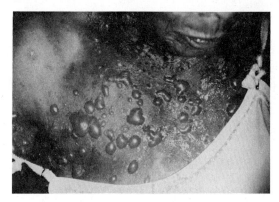

B

Figure 37–4. **A:** Tense blisters on a red base on the back of a patient with bullous pemphigoid. **B:** Multiple blisters on the chest of a patient. (Courtesy of Richard Odom.)

Immunologic Diagnosis

Punch biopsy specimens for immunofluorescence studies must be stored in liquid nitrogen or a special holding medium. Linear deposits of IgG are found at the dermal-epidermal junction in 50–90% of patients, and linear deposits of C3 are found at this junction in almost all patients, occasionally in the absence of immunoglobulin deposition (Fig 37–5). Other immunoglobulin classes and complement components are detected less commonly. Indirect immunofluorescence tests, identifying circulating IgG that binds to the dermal-epidermal junction of a target tissue such as monkey esophagus in vitro, are positive in 70% of cases. The direct immunofluorescence patterns of bullous pemphigoid, herpes gestationis, and epidermolysis bullosa acquisita are identical. Epidermolysis bullosa acquisita may be distinguished from the others by electron microscopy. Direct immunofluorescence is positive in only 25% of herpes gestationis cases. Unconfirmed electron microscopy studies suggest that the patterns of binding in bullous pemphigoid and herpes gestationis may be different, but this is not clinically applicable. Immunofluorescence, like all tests, requires clinical and pathologic correlation. An indirect immunofluorescence pattern in bullous pemphigoid may also be seen in epidermolysis bullosa acquisita and herpes gestationis, but they may be separated by using electron microscopy or a substrate split at the dermal-epidermal junction by using NaCl.

Differential Diagnosis

The differential diagnosis includes several diseases characterized by blistering. These may be definitively separated from bullous pemphigoid, most often on the basis of immunofluorescence tests and histopathology and less often by clinical features and natural course. In an elderly patient with tense blisters, the presence of a subepidermal blister on light microscopy and deposition of IgG or C3 or both on direct immunofluorescence confirm the diagnosis. However, the same features in a young woman who is pregnant or taking oral contraceptive drugs suggest herpes gestationis. Another diagnostic possibility is a bullous drug eruption, which may be similar histologically but has negative immunofluorescence studies. Bullous erythema multiforme often shows a few target or bull's-eye lesions with central blisters and will have distinct histologic and immunofluorescence findings. Other blistering diseases, such as cicatricial pemphigoid, dermatitis herpetiformis, pemphigus vulgaris, epidermolysis bullosa acquisita, and porphyria cutanea tarda, are readily distinguished from bullous pemphigoid on clinical grounds and laboratory findings. Localized vulvar pemphigoid has been misdiagnosed as sexual abuse in one girl.

Treatment

Treatment in the mildest and most localized cases consists of topical application of potent fluorinated steroids. In more generalized cases, in the absence of

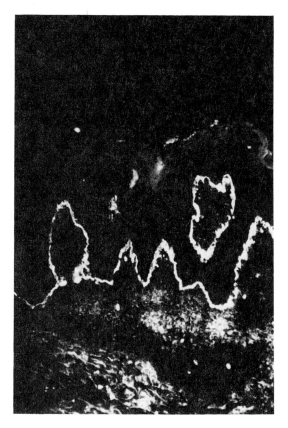

Figure 37–5. Linear deposition of IgG and C3 on direct immunofluorescence of lesional skin. (Courtesy of Richard Odom.)

contraindications, 60–100 mg of prednisone per day is administered until no new lesions are seen. The steroids may then be slowly tapered. Up to 50% of patients may experience a remission after total withdrawal of systemic therapy. Recently tetracycline or erythromycin in combination with niacinamide has been used. Although this regimen may be used alone as initial therapy, it appears to be somewhat slower and less effective in clearing the disease. Many clinicians use it concomitantly with corticosteroids or after the disease has been initially controlled with prednisone, to maintain remission during tapering of the prednisone. The use of azathioprine, cyclophosphamide, dapsone, high-dose pulse therapy with steroids, plasma exchange, or cyclosporin has been proposed, but is seldom required.

Prognosis

Bullous pemphigoid is usually a self-limited disease with a benign, if sometimes prolonged, course. Factors predictive of prognosis have been difficult to identify. Fatal complications may arise in the oldest and most debilitated of patients. The key to success-

ful management is adequate control of the disease while avoiding the complications of systemic corticosteroids. Patients with bullous pemphigoid were thought to have an increased prevalence of internal cancers, but data from several series have refuted this impression. It is possible, but unproven, that patients with negative indirect immunofluorescence tests ("seronegative") may be at increased risk for neoplasia. Because the disease typically affects older adults, concurrent internal cancers may be expected. Therefore a thorough history and physical examination is indicated in every case.

HERPES GESTATIONIS

Majolr Immunologic Features
- IgG and complement are deposited along the dermal-epidermal junction.
- Circulating IgG antibody to the herpes gestationis antigen is found in the basement membrane zone of skin. The IgG avidly binds complement.
- It is associated with HLA-DR3 and -DR4.

General Considerations
A. Definition: Herpes gestationis is characterized by extremely pruritic vesicles and bullae appearing during pregnancy. "Herpes" refers to the Greek word for "to creep," but this disease has no association with herpes simplex virus or varicella-zoster virus.

B. Etiology: The cause is unknown. The primary stimulus for antibody production is not known, but the antigen appears to be the same BP 180 (BPAG2) epidermal basement membrane hemidesmosomal protein that is the target epitope of bullous pemphigoid. The onset of herpes gestationis appears to require placental tissue, choriocarcinoma, or hydatiform moles; recurrences may be caused by exogenous estrogen alone. Antibodies bound to placental tissue in these patients are not cross-reactive with the skin. The antibody also reacts with the amnion epithelial basement membrane of second-trimester and full-term placentas, although the significance of this finding is unclear. Fixation of complement and activation of the classic complement pathway may be involved in the blistering seen clinically.

C. Prevalence: Herpes gestationis is rare, ranging from 1:3000–1:10,000 births in early studies to 1:50,000 births in recent series. There have been few reports of cases in blacks in the USA, and this may reflect the lower frequency of HLA-DR4 in this population. Between 61 and 83% of patients have the HLA-DR3 haplotype and 45% have both HLA-DR3 and -DR4, compared with 3% of women in the general population. However, the HLA type does not correlate with the duration, severity, or recurrence of disease or with antibody titer. Abnormal regulation of anti-HLA idiotype antibodies during pregnancy was demonstrated in one patient, but the prevalence and significance in this defect in immune regulation are not known.

Pathology

The classic picture on light microscopy of a subepidermal bulla with eosinophils in the blister cavity is seen in only a minority of cases. The papillary dermis shows edema and a mixed perivascular lymphohistiocytic infiltrate with eosinophils. Spongiosis (edema between epidermal cells), with or without eosinophils, liquefactive degeneration, or necrosis in the epidermis, may be present. Eosinophils are an important histologic feature when present (Fig 37–6A).

Clinical Features

A. Signs and Symptoms: The onset is usually in the second or third trimester; in 20% of cases it is in the first few days postpartum. Intense pruritus accompanies and at times precedes the eruption, which often begins around the umbilicus or on the extremities as hivelike plaques, blisters, or rings of vesicles at the edges of hivelike plaques (Figs 37–6B and 37–6C). The disease may worsen at delivery. It tends to recur with subsequent pregnancies and last for weeks to months postpartum, occasionally flaring with ovulation, menstruation, or use of oral contraceptives. Lactation may shorten the natural course of untreated postpartum skin disease. Barring secondary bacterial infection, the blisters heal without scarring.

B. Laboratory Findings: Routine investigations are not clinically useful. Peripheral eosinophilia may occur, with an elevated erythrocyte sedimentation rate. Serum complement concentrations are usually normal.

Immunologic Diagnosis

A skin biopsy specimen obtained at the edge of a fresh blister for direct immunofluorescence testing reveals deposition of C3 in virtually all cases. IgG is also found in 25% of biopsy specimens. Indirect immunofluorescence is usually negative. The pattern is identical to that seen in bullous pemphigoid.

Differential Diagnosis

The onset of pruritic, hivelike plaques with tense blisters in a pregnant woman requires punch biopsy specimens for light and immunofluorescence microscopy to confirm the diagnosis. The greatest confusion may exist in cases of herpes gestationis prior to the appearance of blisters, and one must rule out disorders causing pruritus and those causing hivelike rashes. There are reports of a large number of poorly defined pruritic cutaneous syndromes in pregnant women. One should also rule out atopic dermatitis, scabies, and dry skin. Hivelike or edematous plaques

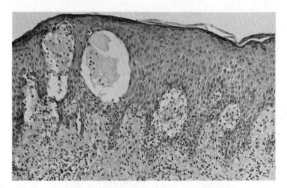

A

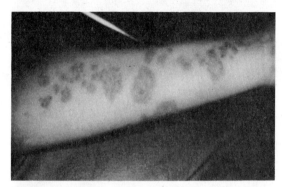

B

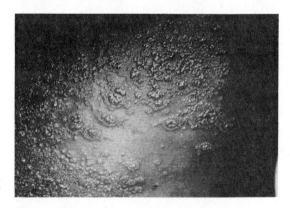

C

Figure 37–6. A: Histopathology of herpes gestationis showing early subepidermal blister formation. The teardrop-shaped vesicle at the left is characteristic of early herpes gestationis. (Courtesy of Philip LeBoit.) **B:** Hivelike and ringed lesions with vesicular edges on the arm of a patient with herpes gestationis. (Courtesy of Richard Odom.) **C:** Rings of vesicles at the edges of plaques in herpes gestationis. (Courtesy of Richard Odom.)

may be caused by pruritic urticarial papules and plaques of pregnancy (which, unlike herpes gestationis, typically spares the umbilicus), urticaria, and erythema multiforme, but these may be ruled out by skin biopsy.

Treatment

Treatment should be undertaken in consultation with the patient's obstetrician. Prednisone at 40–60 mg/d controls the disease in most cases within a week, but higher doses should be used in the event of a poor response. The steroid therapy is then slowly tapered over several weeks to a maintenance dose. Some patients improve spontaneously in the third trimester, but the condition flares at delivery. Cytotoxic immunosuppressive agents should be avoided during pregnancy. Antihistamines have little, if any, effectiveness. Dapsone has been used in the past, but its efficacy is questionable and its use in pregnancy is controversial.

Complications & Prognosis

Herpes gestationis tends to recur and appear earlier with subsequent pregnancies. There appears to be no increased risk of fetal or maternal complications, although retrospective data collected in some series suggest an increased number of low-birth-weight and premature infants and, possibly, stillbirths. Ten percent of newborns may exhibit transient mild cutaneous disease. Antibodies may remain detectable in the skin years after the disease has abated.

DERMATITIS HERPETIFORMIS

Major Immunologic Features

- Granular deposits of IgA and complement components are deposited at the dermal-epidermal junction in dermal papillae in lesional and normal-appearing skin.
- It is associated with HLA-B8, -DR3, and -DQw2.
- There is a critical sensitivity to dietary gluten.

General Considerations

Dermatitis herpetiformis is characterized by pruritic grouped papules, papulovesicles, and vesicles and the granular deposition of IgA in dermal papillae at the dermal-epidermal junction. The cause is unknown. The stimuli for production of IgA antibodies found on the skin, the antigen(s) to which they are bound, and cellular and biochemical causes of the clinical disease remain to be determined. The IgA antibody does not react with gluten or gliadin and may be found in clinically normal-appearing skin. Circulating IgA antibodies are found in only a very few patients. It is presumed that the primary stimulus for the disease occurs in the gastrointestinal tract. Patients with dermatitis herpetiformis also have circulating

IgA antiendomysial antibodies. In 21 patients on a gluten-free diet and 80 controls not on the diet, who all had bullous and other dermatologic or noncutaneous diseases, the sensitivity and specificity of these antibodies for dermatitis herpetiformis were 90 and 96%, respectively.

Prevalence estimates range from 10 to 39 persons per 100,000 in Scandinavia, but the rate is much lower in Japan. The rate may relate to the frequency of HLA types. Between 80 and 95% of patients with granular deposits of IgA in normal skin have the HLA-B8 haplotype, and up to 95% have HLA-DR3. More than 90% of patients may express the HLA antigen DQw2. The strongest HLA associations on a molecular level are with HLA-DQB1* 0201 and HLA-DQA1* 0501 and HLA-DR B1* 0301, as seen with gluten-sensitive enteropathy. The association with HLA-DP antigens is less strong than with HLA-DQw2 or HLA-DR3. HLA-B8 is also associated with "ordinary" gluten-sensitive enteropathy without skin lesions (see Chapter 35).

Pathology

The skin lesions optimal for biopsy are early papules or fresh, unbroken vesicles for light microscopy. Neutrophils are seen at the dermal papillary tips in early lesions that may evolve into subepidermal blisters. Eosinophils and a mild perivascular lymphohistiocytic infiltrate may be seen. Older vesicles and crusted lesions may yield nondiagnostic findings. For direct immunofluorescence tests, biopsy of normal-appearing perilesional skin is recommended.

Clinical Features

Grouped red papules, hivelike plaques, and vesicles are symmetrically distributed on the elbows and knees, upper back, buttocks, and posterior neck and scalp (Fig 37–7). This distribution may be quite helpful to the diagnosis. The lesions are pruritic or may burn or sting. When excoriated, they leave crusted areas.

There are no diagnostic laboratory findings. Endoscopy with biopsy or radiographic studies may detect signs seen in gluten-sensitive enteropathy, but this is neither clinically useful nor necessary for diagnosis or management. More than 70% of patients do not have symptomatic bowel disease. However, a majority have gastric atrophy or hypochlorhydria. Thyroid abnormalities may be more common in these patients.

Immunologic Diagnosis

Biopsy of normal-appearing perilesional skin will reveal granular deposits of polyclonal IgA along dermal papillae in all patients, and this defines the disease (Fig 37–8). IgA may not be found in lesional skin. C3 may also be found.

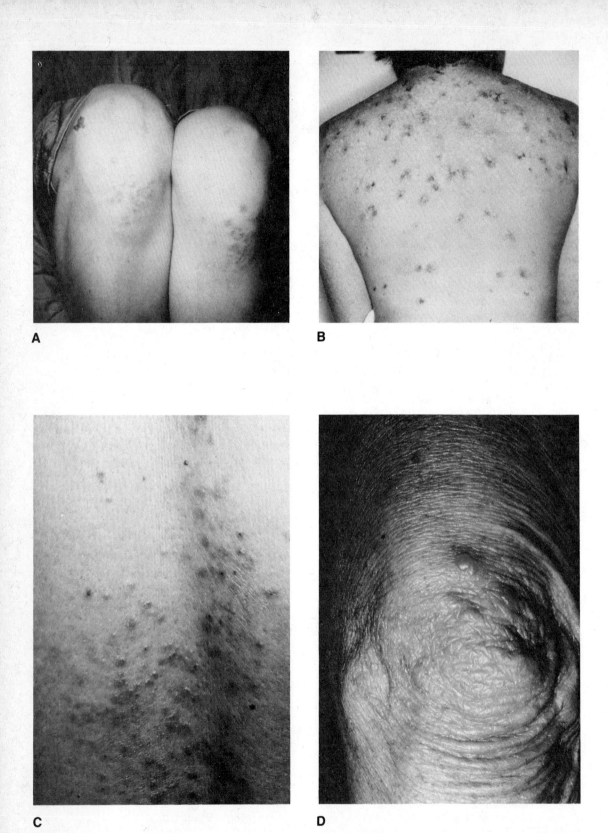

Figure 37–7. Dermatitis herpetiformis. **A** and **B:** Typical distribution of lesions on knees and upper back. (Courtesy of Richard Odom.) **C:** Papular lesions on the mid-back. (Courtesy of John Reeves.) **D:** Close-up view of papulovesicular lesions on elbow. (Courtesy of John Reeves.)

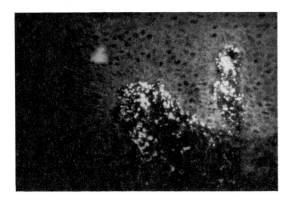

Figure 37–8. Direct immunofluorescence of perilesional skin demonstrates IgA deposition in dermal papillae in dermatitis herpetiformis. (Courtesy of Richard Odom.)

Differential Diagnosis

Vesicles may be seen in a variety of diseases, including varicella, herpes simplex, and herpes zoster. Cytologic smears and cultures, as well as their nongrouped or asymmetric distribution of lesions, distinguish these diseases from dermatitis herpetiformis. A clinically similar disease with different HLA associations, called linear IgA disease, is characterized by linear deposits of IgA in or below the lamina lucida of the basement membrane zone. Direct immunofluorescence can also rule out diseases such as bullous pemphigoid, herpes gestationis, and chronic bullous disease of childhood, all of which are usually clinically distinguishable as well.

Treatment

Strict avoidance of dietary gluten may control the disease entirely after 1–4 years or may lower the dosage of sulfones required by the vast majority of patients. Although gluten may not be the only dietary factor that plays a role in this disease, gluten avoidance by some patients has been shown to lead to a clearing of skin IgA deposits after more than a decade of dietary treatment. It is difficult to follow such a diet. Less than total avoidance may be helpful but will not be as effective. It may also be best to restrict gluten before initiating sulfone therapy. A glucose-6-phosphate dehydrogenase (G6PD) level must be determined for all patients prior to therapy with dapsone or sulfapyridine. Hemolysis may occur at high dapsone doses even in patients with normal G6PD levels. Dapsone at doses of 100–300 mg/d is usually beneficial. Patients on dapsone must be monitored for hemolysis and methemoglobinemia, as well as hepatic, renal, and neurologic complications of therapy.

Prognosis & Associated Diseases

Dermatitis herpetiformis is a chronic disease un-

less dietary avoidance of gluten is maintained. Even after clearing of lesions, reintroduction of gluten rapidly results in disease exacerbation. Lesions heal without scarring, although pigmentary changes may remain. There are reported associations of dermatitis herpetiformis with anti-gastric parietal cell antibodies, gastric hypochlorhydria or achlorhydria, antithyroid antibodies, IgA nephropathy, and, possibly, gastrointestinal lymphoma.

EPIDERMOLYSIS BULLOSA ACQUISITA

Major Immunologic Features

- IgG and, less frequently, IgA, IgM, C3, C1q, C4, factor B, and properdin are deposited at the basement membrane zone in the sublamina densa zone.
- Seventy-one percent of blacks and 100% of whites have been reported to have the HLA-DR2 haplotype in one series.

General Considerations

Epidermolysis bullosa acquisita is a blistering disease marked by skin fragility. It occurs on noninflamed skin over the distal extremities and heals with scarring. Immunoelectron microscopy detects linear immunoglobulin deposits in the sublamina dense zone of the dermal-epidermal junction. These may also be seen by immunofluorescence microscopy on the dermal side of skin separated at the dermal-epidermal junction after incubation in NaCl.

The cause is unknown. The epidermolysis bullosa acquisita antigen is the globular carboxyterminus of type VII procollagen, which is also synthesized by epidermal cells and fibroblasts in culture. Aggregates of type VII collagen form the anchoring fibrils that bind the epidermis and dermis together. Passive transfer experiments with human epidermolysis bullosa acquisita antibody in animals have not been successful. In vitro organ culture models of the disease indicate that epidermolysis bullosa acquisita antibody fixes complement and directs an influx of leukocytes into the skin, resulting in epidermal-dermal separation.

Pathology

There is a subepidermal blister. Other lesions, especially the dermal infiltrate, are variable and correlate with clinical features. Noninflammatory lesions may resemble porphyria cutanea tarda. Inflammatory lesions resemble bullous pemphigoid, but with a greater predominance of neutrophils.

Clinical Features

A. Signs and Symptoms: Epidermolysis bullosa acquisita is a disease of adult onset with 2 distinct presentations. The "classic presentation" involves acral skin fragility and blisters, which heal with scarring and milia. Alternatively, almost half of all patients have widespread vesicles and bullae on red or noninflamed bases; these are associated with pruritus, erosions, and erythematous plaques. These lesions may be accentuated in skin folds and flexural areas. This second presentation resembles bullous pemphigoid. Patients may also have combinations of both presentations during the evolution of their disease. Some patients also have nail changes, oral lesions, or a scarring process in the scalp, leading to hair loss. Epidermolysis bullosa acquisita may be significantly associated with inflammatory bowel disease, particularly Crohn's disease. Individual patients have been reported to have other systemic diseases such as thyroiditis, systemic lupus erythematosus (SLE), diabetes mellitus, or rheumatoid arthritis, but these associations are unclear.

B. Laboratory Findings: Routine tests are generally normal. Twenty-four-hour urine porphyrin levels are normal.

Immunologic Diagnosis

Direct immunofluorescence examination of perilesional skin demonstrates a broad linear band of IgG, C3, and, occasionally, other immune deposits at the dermal-epidermal junction. Immune deposits are not found within dermal blood vessels. This staining pattern is found in other conditions, especially bullous pemphigoid, so it is not pathognomonic for epidermolysis bullosa acquisita. However, 25–50% of patients have positive indirect immunofluorescence of the basement membrane zone below stratified squamous epithelium; the autoantibodies do not cross-react with the lungs and kidneys. When skin that has been split between the epidermis and dermis by incubation in a solution high in salt is used as the substrate for indirect-immunofluorescence tests, a characteristic staining of the area on the dermal side helps define epidermolysis bullosa acquisita. In the absence of positive indirect immunofluorescence, immunoelectron microscopy will localize the immune deposits to the sublamina densa fibrillar zone.

Differential Diagnosis

Family history and immunofluorescence tests will help rule out hereditary forms of epidermolysis bullosa. Noninflammatory lesions may clinically and histologically be confused with those of porphyria cutanea tarda, but determination of 24-hour urinary porphyrin excretion and the finding of immune deposits in dermal vessels should be diagnostic of porphyria cutanea tarda. Bullous pemphigoid may be similar clinically and histologically to one presentation of epidermolysis bullosa acquisita. However, immunoelectron microscopy, indirect immunofluorescence on split-skin substrates, the presence or absence of scarring and milia, and the response to treatment will distinguish between the two diseases. Bullous SLE may be indistinguishable from epider-

molysis bullosa acquisita clinically, histologically, by immunofluorescence testing, and by Western immunoblot analysis of patient sera against epidermolysis bullosa acquisita antigen. The distinction between patients with both epidermolysis bullosa acquisita and bullous SLE and those with bullous SLE alone is unclear, but patients with bullous SLE are said to respond more readily to dapsone, have less skin fragility, heal without scars and milia, and have a more granular staining pattern at the dermal-epidermal junction on direct immunofluorescence than patients with both epidermolysis bullosa acquisita and bullous SLE.

Treatment

Management is difficult, since patients respond poorly to topical and systemic corticosteroid therapy, even with the addition of dapsone and various immunosuppressive drugs. Initial studies with cyclosporin A have been promising. Currently, an initial trial of prednisone (2 mg/kg) with or without azathioprine has been recommended. Careful and gentle local measures to promote skin cleanliness, control infections, and minimize trauma are important.

Complications & Prognosis

Epidermolysis bullosa acquisita appears to be a chronic, nonremitting disease with great morbidity secondary to pain, scarring, and, ultimately, disfiguring skin lesions.

PEMPHIGUS VULGARIS & PEMPHIGUS FOLIACEUS

Major Immunologic Features

■ IgG is deposited in the intercellular regions in the epidermis.
■ Circulating IgG antibody binds to the intercellular regions of stratified squamous epithelium.

General Considerations

Pemphigus vulgaris and pemphigus foliaceus are described together because they are blistering diseases characterized by acantholysis and the deposition of intercellular autoantibodies. They may be distinguished clinically, histologically, and immunologically (Table 37–1). Other pemphigus variants, such as pemphigus erythematosus and pemphigus vegetans, will not be discussed.

Pemphigus vulgaris and pemphigus foliaceus are characterized by widespread blistering and denudation of skin and mucous membranes. They have a distinctive histologic picture demonstrating acantholysis (loss of cohesion) of epidermal cells and a typical pattern on direct immunofluorescence tests. The lesion is superficial in pemphigus foliaceus and deeper in pemphigus vulgaris. Untreated pemphigus vulgaris is uniformly fatal.

Table 37–1. Characteristic features of pemphigus vulgaris and pemphigus foliaceus.

Characteristics	Pemphigus Vulgaris	Pemphigus Foliaceus
Frequency	80% of patients with "pemphigus."	Uncommon.
Mucous membranes affected	Almost all.	Almost none.
Age at onset	Middle age.	Varies.
Ethnicity	Jewish, Mediterranean.	Less clear association.
Lesions	Large, flaccid bullae; crusts.	Small bullae, mostly crusts, arise on erythematous skin.
Course	Severe and fatal if untreated.	Causes morbidity, but chronic and less severe.
Histopathology	Acantholysis between and above basal cells.	Acantholysis superficially and in granular layer.
Immunofluorescence, direct and indirect	Identical.	Identical except occasionally more superficial in epidermis.

A. Etiology: The cause is unknown. The stimulus for antibody production is unknown, but the pemphigus antigen has been cloned and has significant homology with the cadherin family of Ca^{2+}-dependent cell adhesion molecules, which include desmoglein I. A mechanism of acantholysis in pemphigus vulgaris has been proposed. Because the addition of pemphigus antibody in high titer to skin in organ culture results in epidermal acantholysis that is blocked by serine protease inhibitors, it is postulated that the cross-linking of pemphigus antigen on epidermal cells by pemphigus antibody induces the secretion of a protease that results in the detachment of epidermal cells from each other. Evidence suggests that plasminogen activator is directly or indirectly involved in acantholysis, but the entire mechanism has not yet been elucidated. Addition of antibody and complement to such systems also results in epidermal separation, but complement is not necessary for acantholysis.

The sera of 50–75% of patients with pemphigus foliaceus precipitate desmoglein I, a major component of desmosomes and other desmosome-associated proteins. The epidemiology of pemphigus foliaceus in Brazil suggests an infectious vector in its transmission in that country, but such an agent(s) remains unidentified. Pemphigus has been reported to be associated with the administration of penicillamine and other drugs such as phenylbutazone, although the association with the latter is less clear. Immunoprecipitation and immunoblotting studies suggest that pemphigus vulgaris and pemphigus foliaceus sera do not cross-react with the same antigens.

B. Epidemiology: Pemphigus vulgaris occurs predominantly but not exclusively in persons of Jewish or Mediterranean ancestry. It may occur in all age groups, with an incidence of 0.5–3.2 cases per 100,000 per year, but it is more common in the fourth and fifth decades and is rare after age 60. A familial occurrence of pemphigus vulgaris, pemphigus veg-

etans, or pemphigus foliaceus has been reported in 25 families.

C. Genetics: HLA-A10 was first identified as being more commonly represented among patients with pemphigus vulgaris than in the general population. More recently it has been shown that 95% of pemphigus vulgaris patients are HLA-DR4/DQw3 or HLA-DRw6/DQw1 positive, and it is thought that pemphigus may segregate with the DQ alleles. In a series of 13 DQw1-positive patients with pemphigus vulgaris, all were identified as positive for an allele designated $PV6_\beta$ versus 1 of 13 DR/DQ-matched controls. This allele differs from the normal DQ_β allele in codon 57, where asparagine replaces valine or serine.

Pathology

Skin biopsy shows a suprabasal intraepidermal blister with loss of cohesion of keratinocytes (acantholysis) in pemphigus vulgaris (Fig 37–9). Pemphigus foliaceus demonstrates a superficial subcorneal or subgranular split.

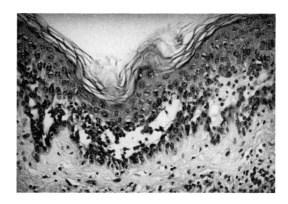

Figure 37–9. Histopathology of pemphigus vulgaris demonstrates intraepidermal blister formation with loss of cohesion of keratinocytes (acantholysis). (Courtesy of Philip LeBoit.)

Clinical Features

Pemphigus vulgaris is characterized by blisters that most commonly affect the scalp, chest, umbilicus, and body folds (Fig 37–10). In contrast to the lesions of bullous pemphigoid, these blisters are flaccid and fragile because the epidermal split occurs within the epidermis, resulting in a thinner roof (Fig 37–9). Lesions may easily rupture, and in some cases only crusts and no blisters are seen. Oral lesions may be the initial or, rarely, the only presentation of the disease. Nikolsky's sign (sloughing of the epidermis after lateral pressure with a cotton applicator or tongue blade) is positive in involved skin. Pemphigus foliaceus, with its more superficial histologic process of blistering, may show only scaly, crusted, and superficial erosions without frank blisters. Oral lesions are uncommon in pemphigus foliaceus. Routine laboratory tests are not helpful in diagnosis or management.

Immunologic Diagnosis

Direct immunofluorescence reveals the deposition of IgG in virtually all patients and complement components (mostly C3) in intercellular spaces in the skin, forming a honeycomb pattern (Fig 37–11), in 50% of patients. Complement components are depleted in pemphigus blister fluids. Between 80 and 90% of patients also have circulating IgG that stains the intercellular spaces of stratified squamous epithelium in target substrates such as monkey esophagus or human skin. Although it has been reported that pemphigus foliaceus sera stain the more superficial layers of the epidermis compared with pemphigus vulgaris sera, this seldom is seen in practice. Circulating pemphiguslike antibodies have been found in patients with burns, lepromatous leprosy, morbilliform rashes to penicillin, SLE, myasthenia gravis with thymoma or thymic hyperplasia, high titers of anti-A or anti-B isohemagglutinins, cutaneous *Trichophyton* infection, erythema multiforme, and cicatricial or bullous pemphigoid. Such antibodies are usually of low titer in the conditions, and the direct immunofluorescence is negative.

Differential Diagnosis

Several diseases may be confused with pemphigus vulgaris. The diagnosis depends on clinical suspicion when presented with a disease featuring blisters and crusting and biopsy with appropriate immunofluorescence studies. Oral lesions may be confused with aphthous ulcers or oral erythema multiforme. Scalp lesions may appear similar to impetigo. Occasionally pemphigus vulgaris will resemble other pemphigus variants, including pemphigus foliaceus and pemphigus erythematosus, but light microscopy is helpful in this situation. Other blistering eruptions (see above) are readily distinguished by clinical appearance (size, grouping, distribution, and tenseness of blisters), his-

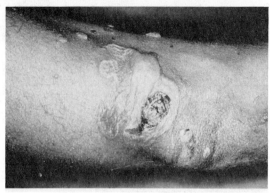

A

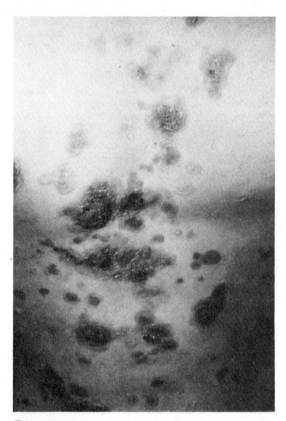

B

Figure 37–10. *A:* Flaccid blister on the elbow of a patient with pemphigus vulgaris (compare with the tense blister in bullous pemphigoid in Fig 37–4). *B:* Crusted and bullous lesions on the chest of a patient with pemphigus vulgaris. (Courtesy of Richard Odom.)

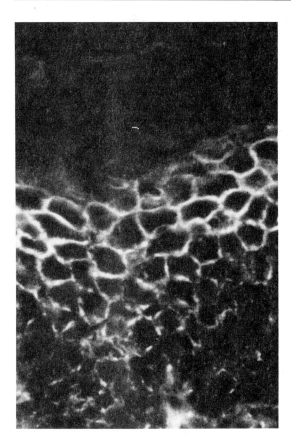

Figure 37–11. Direct immunofluorescence pattern of IgG deposition in pemphigus vulgaris. The immunoglobulins and complement components are deposited in intercellular regions in the epidermis forming a honeycomb pattern. (Courtesy of Denny Tuffanelli.)

topathology, and immunofluorescence pattern. Since pemphigus vulgaris and pemphigus foliaceus may be somewhat confused with widespread dermatitis or impetigo, the persistence in empirically treating a patient for these other diseases without a biopsy will often delay the correct diagnosis.

Recently, the clinically and immunologically distinct entity of paraneoplastic pemphigus has been described. Patients, mostly with lymphoreticular neoplasms, present with vesicles and bullae and with marked mucosal involvement and occasionally with erythema multiforme-like lesions. Skin biopsy specimens show acantholysis, but they also show keratinocyte necrosis and changes at the dermoepidermal junction. Direct immunofluorescence of perilesional skin demonstrates intercellular IgG and occasionally C3, as well as basement membrane immunoreactants. One autoantigen in this disease may be the desmosomal protein desmoplakin I.

Treatment

Successful treatment of pemphigus vulgaris is a delicate balance of control of this fatal disease and avoidance of fatal complications, especially sepsis, from therapeutic agents. There is much clinical experience, but there are no double-blind controlled studies to guide therapy. It is best to treat pemphigus vulgaris as early in its course as possible. There are several regimens tailored to inducing and then maintaining control of the disease. For treatment of pemphigus vulgaris, systemic corticosteroids beginning with prednisone, 80–120 mg/d in divided doses, alone or in combination with azathioprine, 50 mg 1–3 times daily is one regimen supported by much clinical experience. Lower doses of prednisone may be adequate in some cases of pemphigus foliaceus, but much higher doses of prednisone are sometimes required. Cyclophosphamide, methotrexate, and plasmapheresis have also been used in combination with corticosteroids. The experience with cyclosporin A has been limited and not always successful. The use of gold therapy in pemphigus vulgaris may be considered, but it has not been consistently effective. Plasmapheresis has been shown to be of benefit in pemphigus vulgaris and can reduce autoantibody levels by 83% within 3 weeks.

Prognosis & Associated Diseases

Pemphigus vulgaris is uniformly fatal if untreated. Many patients may be successfully maintained in remission for years. There are no statistics that permit estimates of average 5- or 10-year survival rates. The prognosis depends on adequate therapy to control the disease, with vigilant monitoring and avoidance of adverse side effects. Pemphigus vulgaris has been associated with myasthenia gravis and thymoma. Pemphigus foliaceus tends to be a chronic, relapsing disease, but it is less life-threatening. It, too, may be quite difficult to control.

LINEAR IgA BULLOUS DERMATOSIS

A subset of patients (10%) with vesicles and bullae appear to have a disease that falls between bullous pemphigoid and dermatitis herpetiformis. Like patients with bullous pemphigoid, they have larger bullae than seen in dermatitis herpetiformis, as well as linear deposits of immunoglobulin, usually IgA but sometimes IgG and C3 as well. Unlike patients with bullous pemphigoid, these patients respond to sulfones but not to corticosteroids, and deposits are at and below the lamina lucida. Other patients have small vesicles like those of dermatitis herpetiformis, but occasionally without the marked symmetry of dermatitis herpetiformis. However, unlike patients with dermatitis herpetiformis, histopathologically they show a linear bandlike infiltrate of polymorphonuclear neutrophils at the dermal-epidermal junction, in addition to papillary neutrophil microabscesses and linear deposits of IgA at the dermal-epidermal junction, in and below the lamina lucida. The disease is now called linear IgA bullous dermatosis. Patients present with vesicles and bullae that may clinically resemble bullous pemphigoid or dermatitis herpetiformis, or both. Oral lesions and ulcers may be minor findings or, rarely, the major manifestation of the disease. Direct immunofluorescence is positive for IgA and occasionally other immunoglobulins at and below the lamina lucida. Indirect immunofluorescence may be positive in some cases. Patients have a lower prevalence of HLA-B8 than those with dermatitis herpetiformis (ranging from a normal frequency up to 56% of patients versus 80–95% in dermatitis herpetiformis). They do not have jejunal changes of gluten-sensitive enteropathy, they lack the anti-endomysium antibodies seen in dermatitis herpetiformis and gluten-sensitive enteropathy, they do not benefit from a gluten-free diet, they respond to sulfones, and their disease tends to have a chronic course. An association between this disease and various hematologic malignancies has been suggested. The antigen(s) that binds the IgA has not been identified.

DISCOID LUPUS ERYTHEMATOSUS

Major Immunologic Features

- Immunoglobulins and complement components are deposited in lesional skin, particularly older established lesions.
- SLE occurs in some patients with discoid lesions.
- Low or negative antinuclear antibody levels, negative double-stranded and normal CH_{50} and C3 are found in patients without systemic disease.

General Considerations

Discoid lupus erythematosus lesions are round or irregular discrete skin lesions with follicular plugging, which tend to heal with scarring. They are seen in patients without SLE and occasionally in patients with SLE. The major reason for identifying discoid lesions in patients both with and without an established diagnosis of SLE is to treat such lesions aggressively so as to prevent or lessen their progression to disfiguring scarring. In patients presenting with discoid lesions, sufficient history, physical examination, and laboratory tests should be performed to exclude SLE and reassure patients and their families about their overall prognosis.

Pathology

Biopsy specimens of lesions with erythema, scale, and follicular plugging, stained with hematoxylin and eosin, are usually sufficient to make the diagnosis. In these cases direct immunofluorescence is not neces-

sary. In cases of old, "burned-out" discoid lupus erythematosus, or when the light-microscopic picture is nondiagnostic, direct immunofluorescence may be helpful when positive. However, false-positive direct immunofluorescence has occasionally been found in areas of the body that are continually exposed to the sun. Therefore, the diagnosis should not be established by any one particular test or finding, but by the constellation of findings. Specific histologic features include hyperkeratosis and follicular plugging, irregular epidermal atrophy and hyperplasia, and superficial and deep perivascular lymphocytic infiltrate. Immunofluorescence findings include a broad linear band of IgG at the dermal-epidermal junction. Histologic and immunopathologic differences appear to exist between patients with discoid lupus erythematosus and those with subacute cutaneous lupus erythematosus. The latter appears to be a more superficial inflammatory form of cutaneous lupus erythematosus with positive anti-Ro/SSA antibodies, photosensitivity, and annular or psoriasiform lesions.

Clinical Features

Discoid lupus erythematosus causes round or irregular, sharply bordered lesions characterized by erythema with or without the following: hyperpigmentation, scale, plugging of hair follicles with scaly debris, and telangiectasia. They are most common on the face and less common on the scalp and upper body. Extremity and trunk lesions are often seen with more widespread disease. The inner aspect of the pinna is a characteristic and relatively specific area to see the changes of discoid lupus erythematosus (Fig 37–12). Older lesions become scarred and are charac-

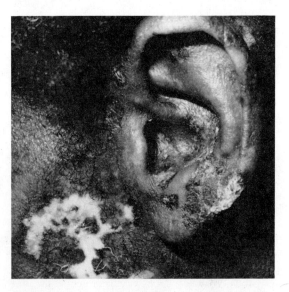

Figure 37–12. Active scaly areas and old depigmented scarred areas on the face and pinna in a patient with discoid lupus erythematosus.

terized by atrophy and decreased to absent pigmentation. Scalp lesions are characterized by follicular plugging, erythema, and loss of hair (Fig 37–13). Loss of hair may be temporary early in the lesion, but will become permanent when the follicle becomes scarred. Lesions may be tender or pruritic.

Differential Diagnosis

The differential diagnosis includes other red and scaly disorders, including psoriasis, seborrheic dermatitis, sarcoid, granuloma annulare, nummular dermatitis, tinea, sclerosing basal-cell carcinoma, and polymorphous light eruption. Scalp lesions may resemble lichen planopilaris, pseudopelade, and tinea infections *(Trichophyton tonsurans)*. Examination of the lesion, the rest of the body surface, and a fungal scraping or culture can often differentiate among these conditions.

Laboratory Findings

Since patients and their families will often be concerned or even confused about the possibility of SLE, initial workup should include biopsy, complete blood count, erythrocyte sedimentation rate, antinuclear antibody test, and urinalysis. If the antinuclear antibody test is positive, the physician may order anti-double-stranded DNA, CH_{50}, C3, and other tests appropriate for SLE. Up to two-thirds of discoid lupus erythematosus patients may have at least one mildly abnormal laboratory test without having SLE.

Treatment

Patients should be instructed to avoid sun exposure and to use sunscreens. Lesions on the face should be initially treated topically with high-potency fluorinated steroids, with close monitoring for steroid-induced skin atrophy. Resistant lesions and all scalp lesions may be treated with intralesional triamcinolone acetonide. Lesions should be treated until no activity (erythema) is present. If these modalities are not effective, an antimalarial drug such as hydroxychloroquine should be given for a 3-month trial after first obtaining an eye examination and G6PD level. Only 60% of patients with discoid lupus erythematosus benefit from antimalarial drugs. Further treatment requires consultation with a dermatologist or physi-

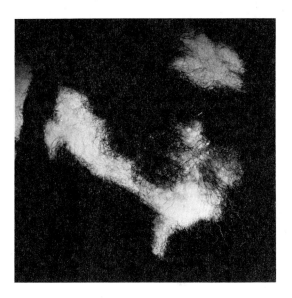

Figure 37–13. Scarring alopecia in patient with discoid lupus erythematosus lesions.

cian experienced with this entity. Most patients have a chronic course without developing SLE.

Prognosis

Discoid lupus erythematosus may be especially devastating in black patients, whose lesions may result in scarring with marked depigmentation and peripheral hyperpigmentation. On the scalp, permanent hair loss may result. From 5 to 10% of patients presenting only with discoid lupus erythematosus progress to SLE. Laboratory tests and clinical findings that suggest a greater likelihood of progression include a high-titer antinuclear antibody, low leukocyte count, anemia, low platelet count, false-positive VDRL, widespread lesions (generalized discoid lupus erythematosus), and, of course, signs and symptoms of SLE. There is some suggestion that SLE patients with discoid lupus erythematosus lesions may have a better overall prognosis than SLE patients without these lesions.

REFERENCES

Bullous Pemphigoid

Berk MA, Lorincz AL: The treatment of bullous pemphigoid with tetracycline and niacinamide: A preliminary report. *Arch Dermatol* 1986;**122:**670.

Giudice GJ et al: Cloning and primary structural analysis of the bullous pemphigoid autoantigen PB180. *J Invest Dermatol* 1992;**99:**243.

Goldstein SM, Wasserman IS, Wintroub BU: Mast cell and eosinophil mediated damage in bullous pemphigoid. In: *Immune Mechanisms in Cutaneous Disease.* Norris D (editor). Dekker, 1989.

Hopkinson SB et al: Cytoplasmic domain of the 180-kD bullous pemphigoid antigen, a hemidesmosomal component: Molecular and cell biologic characterization. *J Invest Dermatol* 1992;**99:**264.

Jordan RE, Kawana S, Fritz KA: Immunopathologic

mechanisms in pemphigus and bullous pemphigoid. *J Invest Dermatol.* 1985;**85(Suppl):**72.

Korman N: Bullous pemphigoid. *J Am Acad Dermatol* 1987;**16:**907.

Li K et al: Cloning of partial cDNA for mouse 180-kDa bullous pemphigoid antigen (BPAG2), a highly conserved collagenous protein of the cutaneous basement membrane zone. *J Invest Dermatol* 1992;**99:**258.

Sauramura D et al: Amino acid sequences deduced from cloned cDNAs predict biologically important peptide segments and protein domains. *J Biol Chem* 1991; **266:**17784.

Tivolet J, Barthelemy H: Bullous pemphigoid. *Semin Dermatol* 1988;**7:**91.

Venning VA, Wojnarowska F. Lack of predictive factors for the clinical course of bullous pemphigoid. *J Am Acad Dermatol* 1992;**26:**585.

Herpes Gestationis

Holmes RC, Black MM: The special dermatoses of pregnancy. *J Am Acad Dermatol* 1983;**8:**405.

Lawley TJ et al: Pruritic urticarial papules and plaques of pregnancy. *JAMA* 1979;**241:**1696.

Shornick JH: Herpes gestationis. *J Am Acad Dermatol* 1987;**17:**539.

Dermatitis Herpetiformis

Fronek Z et al: Molecular analysis of HLA-DP and DQ genes associated with dermatitis herpetiformis. *J Invest Dermatol* 1991;**97:**799.

Fry L: Fine points in the management of dermatitis herpetiformis. *Semin Dermatol* 1988;**7:**206.

Hall RP: The pathogenesis of dermatitis herpetiformis: Recent advances. *J Am Acad Dermatol* 1987;**16:**1129.

Kadunce DP et al: The effect of an essential diet with and without gluten on disease activity in dermatitis herpetiformis. *J Invest Dermatol* 1991;**97:**175.

Katz SI et al: HLA-B8 and dermatitis herpetiformis in patients with IgA deposits in skin. *Arch Dermatol* 1977;**113:**155.

Mazzola G et al: Immunoglobulin and HLA-DP genes contribute to the susceptibility to juvenile dermatitis herpetiformis. *Eur J Immunogenet* 1992;**19:**129.

Otley CC et al: DNA sequence analysis and restriction fragment length polymorphism (RFLP) typing of the HLA-DQ$_w$2 alleles associated with dermatitis herpetiformis. *J Invest Dermatol* 1991;**97:**318.

Peters MS, McEvory MT: IgA antiendomysial antibodies in dermatitis herpetiformis. *J Am Acad Dermatol* 1989;**21:**1225.

Epidermolysis Bullosa Acquisita

Crow LL et al: Clearing of epidermolysis bullosa acquisita on cyclosporine. *J Am Acad Dermatol* 1988;**19:**937.

Gammon WR et al: Differentiating anti-lamina lucida and anti-sublamina densa anti-BMZ antibodies by direct immunofluorescence on 1.0 M sodium chloride-separated skin. *J Invest Dermatol* 1984;**82:**139.

Roenigk HH Jr, Ryan JG, Bergfeld WF: Epidermolysis bullosa acquisita: Report of three cases and review of the literature. *Arch Dermatol* 1971;**103:**1.

Woodley DT et al: Epidermolysis bullosa acquisita antigen is the globular carboxyl terminus of type VII procollagen. *J Clin Invest* 1988;**81:**683.

Woodley DT et al: Review and update of epidermolysis bullosa. *Semin Dermatol* 1988;**7:**11.

Pemphigus Vulgaris & Foliaceus

Amagai M et al: Autoantibodies against a novel epithelial cadherin in pemphigus vulgaris, a disease of cell adhesion. *Cell* 1991;**67:**869.

Anhalt GJ et al: Paraneoplastic pemphigus. An autoimmune mucocutaneous disease associated with neoplasia. *N Engl J Med* 1990;**323:**1729.

Bystryn JC: Therapy of pemphigus. *Semin Dermatol* 1988;**7:**186.

Korman N: Pemphigus. *J Am Acad Dermatol* 1988; **18:**1219.

Peterson LL, Wuepper KD: Isolation and purification of a pemphigus antigen from human epidermis. *J Clin Invest* 1984;**17:**1113.

Rappersberger K et al: Immunomorphologic and biochemical identification of the pemphigus foliaceous autoantigen within desmosomes. *J Invest Dermatol* 1992;**99:**323.

Tan-Lim R, Bystryn J-C: Effects of plasmapheresis therapy on circulating levels of pemphigus antibodies. *J Am Acad Dermatol* 1990;**22:**35.

Discoid Lupus Erythematosus

David-Bajar KM et al: Clinical, histologic, and immunofluorescent distinction between subacute cutaneous lupus erythematosus and discoid lupus erythematosus. *J Invest Dermatol* 1992;**99:**251.

Prystowsky SD, Gilliam JN: Antinuclear antibody studies in chronic cutaneous discoid lupus erythematosus. *Arch Dermatol* 1977;**113:**183.

Prystowsky SD, Herndon JH, Gilliam JN: Chronic cutaneous lupus erythematosus (DLE)—a clinical and laboratory investigation of 80 patients. *Medicine* 1975;**55:**183.

Tuffanelli DC: Discoid lupus erythematosus. *Clin Rheum Dis* 1982;**8:**327.

Linear IgA Disease

McEvoy MT, Connolly SM: Linear IgA dermatosis: Association with malignancy. *J Am Acad Dermatol* 190;**22:**59.

Wilson BD et al: Linear IgA bullous dermatosis. *Int J Dermatol* 1985;**24:**569.

Neurologic Diseases

38

Hillel S. Panitch, MD, & Paul S. Fishman, MD, PhD

The role of immunologic mechanisms in diseases of the nervous system is the focus of increasing interest, and there have recently been major advances in the study of several of these conditions. In acute disseminated encephalomyelitis and acute inflammatory demyelinating polyneuropathy (Guillain-Barré syndrome), the host response to an infectious agent may trigger a direct autoaggressive assault on the nervous system. The pathogenesis of multiple sclerosis is less clear, but immunogenetic studies, defects of immunoregulation, and responses to immunomodulatory therapy suggest that the immune system is involved in the pathogenesis of the disease. In myasthenia gravis, an antibody response directed against the acetylcholine receptor directly inhibits neuromuscular transmission. In other conditions such as subacute sclerosing panencephalitis, paraneoplastic syndromes, amyotrophic lateral sclerosis, and certain chronic neuropathies, abnormal immune responses are known to occur; however, their significance is uncertain. In degenerative conditions such as Alzheimer's disease, the role of the immune system in pathogenesis is entirely conjectural.

DEMYELINATING DISEASES

The commonly accepted pathologic criteria for a demyelinating disease are destruction of myelin sheaths of nerve fibers with relative sparing of neurons and axons. Lesions are frequently perivascular in location and are accompanied by mononuclear inflammatory infiltrates, suggesting that immunologic mechanisms participate in their pathogenesis.

ACUTE DISSEMINATED ENCEPHALOMYELITIS

Major Immunologic Features
- It follows infectious diseases or immunizations.
- Inflammatory demyelination occurs in central nervous system white matter.
- There is cellular immunity to myelin basic protein.

General Considerations
Although acute disseminated encephalomyelitis is uncommon, it is important because of the widespread practice of vaccination for prevention of infectious diseases. The onset of clinical illness occurs several days to weeks following vaccination; in the case of natural viral infections, such as measles, rubella, varicella, mumps, and influenza, it can occur concomitantly with the illness (parainfectious) or after the acute phase (postinfectious). Except for measles, in which the incidence of acute disseminated encephalomyelitis is well defined and constant at 1:1000, reliable figures are not available. However, they are all much lower than the incidence following measles. The argument favoring an immunologic pathogenesis of this disorder is based on its similarity to experimental allergic encephalomyelitis, in which animals are immunized with extracts of brain tissue or specific myelin proteins, resulting in an autoimmune response mediated by T lymphocytes.

Pathology
Acute disseminated encephalomyelitis is marked by perivascular mononuclear cell infiltrates in white matter throughout the brain and spinal cord; polymorphonuclear leukocytes and microhemorrhages are seen in the most acute form of the disease. As the lesions age, they become sclerotic, with proliferation of astrocytes and formation of glial scars. The lesions are pathologically all of the same age, reflecting the monophasic nature of the illness.

Clinical Features

Systemic symptoms of fever, malaise, headache, myalgia, nausea, and vomiting generally precede neurologic symptoms by 24–48 hours. Neurologic symptoms and signs develop rapidly thereafter and include pain, paresthesias, motor weakness, spasticity, uncoordination, dysarthria, dysphagia, and respiratory distress. Seizures are common in severe cases and in the acute hemorrhagic form, and widespread brain lesions can lead to stupor and coma. A more restricted form of the same pathologic process may be confined to the spinal cord as acute transverse myelitis.

Immunologic Diagnosis

Cellular immunity to myelin basic protein can sometimes be demonstrated in acute disseminated encephalomyelitis by measuring the activation in vitro of peripheral blood or spinal fluid lymphocytes during the acute phase of the illness. Cerebrospinal fluid may be abnormal, with mild to moderate pleocytosis and elevated levels of IgG, but there is no evidence that this represents local immunoglobulin synthesis as occurs in multiple sclerosis.

Differential Diagnosis

Acute multiple sclerosis can be difficult to distinguish from acute disseminated encephalomyelitis. Fever and a preceding viral illness or vaccination favor the latter diagnosis. The vasculitis of systemic lupus erythematosus can effect the central nervous system, but neurologic symptoms generally accompany the systemic illness and tend to be more focal than in acute disseminated encephalomyelitis. Primary infections of the nervous system with herpes simplex virus or the arboviruses tend to involve gray as well as white matter, and they produce neuronal dysfunction such as seizures, stupor, and coma early in the illness. Direct isolation of viruses from cerebrospinal fluid and increasing serum antibody titers are helpful in differentiating viral encephalitides from acute disseminated encephalomyelitis. The subacute encephalitis of acquired immunodeficiency syndrome (AIDS) develops more slowly and is not usually associated with focal neurologic deficits. Toxoplasmosis of the central nervous system may be distinguished serologically. Computed tomography and magnetic resonance imaging may be useful in diagnosis; however, a diagnostic brain biopsy is sometimes necessary to exclude a treatable central nervous system infection.

Treatment

Although the course is unpredictable, high doses of corticosteroids given intravenously may be of value in treatment. The successful prevention of experimental allergic encephalomyelitis with immunosuppressive and immunomodulating agents offers hope that similar treatment may inhibit the attack of sensitized T lymphocytes on the nervous system in acute disseminated encephalomyelitis.

Complications & Prognosis

The mortality rate varies from 1 to 27%, with the highest rates reported in association with measles. Neurologic sequelae persist in 25–40% of survivors. The occasional occurrence of relapses blurs the distinction between this condition and multiple sclerosis in about 5% of cases.

MULTIPLE SCLEROSIS

Major Immunologic Features

- There is inflammatory demyelination in central nervous system white matter.
- There are alterations in immunoregulatory T cell function and cytokine production.
- There are oligoclonal immunoglobulins in cerebrospinal fluid.
- It responds to immunosuppressive and immunomodulating agents.

General Considerations

Multiple sclerosis is a chronic relapsing disease in which there are signs and symptoms of central nervous system involvement separated both in time and in location in the nervous system. Epidemiologic studies have uncovered important clues about multiple sclerosis, but the cause remains unknown. In high-risk areas the prevalence is 50–100 per 100,000 population, whereas in low-risk areas such as Africa and Japan the rate is less than 5 per 100,000. Individuals who migrate from high-risk to low-risk areas, or vice versa, after age 15 carry with them their native risk of acquiring the disease. In addition, the peak onset is at age 30, with few cases before age 15 or after age 55, suggesting that some critical event in determining the risk of acquiring multiple sclerosis occurs in adolescence. The risk of disease in a first-degree relative is 10–15 times higher than the risk in the general population, and the concordance rate in identical twins is at least 25%, indicating a strong genetic component. However, localized epidemics of multiple sclerosis have been described, most notably in the Faroe Islands, where the temporal clustering of cases suggests a transmissible cause. Studies of histocompatibility antigens have shown significant associations with HLA-A3 and HLA-B7 in northern European and North American populations and higher-level associations with HLA-DR2 and HLA-DQw1, which may be more closely linked to a multiple sclerosis susceptibility gene.

Numerous viruses have been implicated as possible etiologic agents, by the presence of specific antibodies in spinal fluid, identification of viral DNA or RNA in brain tissue or mononuclear cells, and, in some cases, actual viral isolation. However, none of these observations has been consistently confirmed. Numerous immunoregulatory defects have been identified, one of the best documented being abnormal suppressor T cell function in acute attacks and in the chronic progressive phase. Although decreases in the CD8 T cell subset are not consistently found, the defect may reside in a loss of CD4 suppressor-inducer cells identified by coexpression of the CD45RA surface antigen with CD4. In addition, there are excessive numbers of activated T cells in the blood and cerebrospinal fluid. These findings may be partially responsible for defective regulation of IgG synthesis within the nervous system. Monocytes and macrophages also appear to play important roles in multiple sclerosis, possibly related to their sensitivity to gamma interferon, which induces class II human leukocyte antigen (HLA) (HLA-DR, -DP, and -DQ) surface antigens and activates macrophages (Fig 38–1). Activated macrophages are prevalent in multiple sclerosis plaques, where they release proteinases and cytokines. The importance of gamma interferon as an immune activator was emphasized by a clinical trial in which patients treated with gamma interferon developed acute exacerbations. Minor viral infections often precipitate attacks; this effect may be mediated by gamma interferon or other cytokines. Within the central nervous system, gamma interferon induces class II antigens on astrocytes and microglia, enabling them to present antigens to T cells and to propagate the disease process. Unfortunately,

the specific antigen in question is unknown, but it is likely to be a major structural component of myelin such as basic protein or proteolipid protein. The autoimmune theory of multiple sclerosis is strengthened by its response to immunosuppressive drugs such as corticosteroids. Alpha and beta interferons, which inhibit the synthesis of gamma interferon and reverse some of its immunostimulatory effects, also seem to be effective in preventing exacerbations.

Pathology

The lesions of multiple sclerosis are confined to the central nervous system and primarily involve the white matter of the cerebrum, cerebellum, brain stem, and spinal cord. In the early stages they consist of perivascular infiltrates of T lymphocytes and macrophages. In older lesions, macrophage-mediated demyelination is further advanced and large numbers of reactive astrocytes are seen. These lesions or plaques appear to be of different ages and correlate with the appearance of clinical signs and symptoms at different times during the illness. Plasma cells within the plaques secrete oligoclonal IgG into the extracellular and cerebrospinal fluid. The similarities between the lesions of multiple sclerosis and the inflammatory demyelination seen in experimental allergic encephalomyelitis (particularly the relapsing form) suggest that cellular immune mechanisms are involved in the pathogenesis of multiple sclerosis.

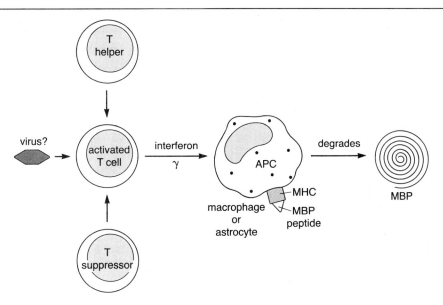

Figure 38–1. Interaction of T cells, cytokines, and antigen-presenting cells in multiple sclerosis. In this simplified representation, activated T cells proliferate, differentiate, enter the central nervous system, and secrete gamma interferon, which induces class II MHC antigens on macrophages and astrocytes. Activated macrophages attack and degrade myelin, take up myelin basic protein (MBP) peptides, and present them to other T cells, amplifying the immune response. Class II MHC containing astrocytes can also present MBP peptides. Suppressor T cells, which are functionally defective in multiple sclerosis patients, fail to regulate the immune response normally.

Clinical Features

Because multiple sclerosis plaques tend to involve many areas of the central nervous system, the symptoms and signs are extremely varied. The most common manifestations are motor weakness, paresthesias, impairment of visual acuity, and diplopia. Ataxia, urinary bladder dysfunction, impotence, spasticity, and mild to moderate cognitive impairment are also common. Symptoms may occur rapidly as acute exacerbations that develop over several days and persist for days to weeks with gradual recovery, or more slowly in the chronic progressive form of the disease. Exacerbations occur at varying intervals and tend to subside with less complete recovery of function and increasing disability as the disease progresses. Visual, auditory, and somatosensory evoked potentials are often abnormal and assist in diagnosis. However, the most important recent diagnostic advance has been the introduction of magnetic resonance imaging, which provides striking visualization of plaques in the cerebral white matter (Fig 38–2).

Immunologic Diagnosis

Despite the many immunologic abnormalities described above, there is no single diagnostic test for multiple sclerosis. Oligoclonal IgG bands are detectable in cerebrospinal fluid by electrophoresis or isoelectric focusing in more than 90% of patients (Fig 38–3). An elevated IgG index (ratio of cerebrospinal fluid to serum IgG corrected for albumin concentration in each compartment) indicates local IgG synthe-

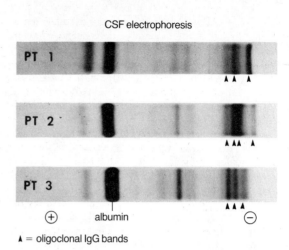

CSF electrophoresis

▲ = oligoclonal IgG bands

Figure 38–3. Oligoclonal bands in cerebrospinal fluid (CSF) specimen from a patient with subacute sclerosing parencephalitis. Cerebrospinal fluid electrophoresis pattern in agarose gel demonstrates the phenomenon of oligoclonal banding. In the gamma region (to the right), several dark, distinct bands are noted for all these patients. Similar abnormalities are noted in cerebrospinal fluid specimens from multiple sclerosis patients.

sis, but this can be found in other inflammatory diseases of the nervous system. Myelin basic protein may be detected by radioimmunoassay in the cerebrospinal fluid, but it is largely a reflection of myelin damage and can be seen in other conditions such as head trauma and stroke. Other immunologic findings such as HLA haplotypes, abnormal CD4/CD8 T cell ratios, reduced suppressor cell activity, activated T cells, and increased cytokine levels in cerebrospinal fluid are not specific or consistent enough to be useful in diagnosis.

Differential Diagnosis

Acute episodes of multiple sclerosis must be differentiated from structural lesions of the central nervous system such as brain and spinal cord tumors, spondylosis, or vascular malformations. A host of other medical conditions may produce signs, symptoms, spinal fluid findings, and, in some cases, magnetic resonance images that mimic those of multiple sclerosis, and they must be excluded by appropriate testing. These diseases include neurosyphilis, sarcoidosis, systemic lupus erythematosus, Sjögren's syndrome, vitamin B_{12} deficiency, and Lyme disease. Spinal and cerebellar disorders such as Friedreich's ataxia and olivopontocerebellar degeneration can mimic multiple sclerosis, but tend to be familial, chronically progressive, and associated with normal spinal fluid. Finally, tropical spastic paraparesis or HTLV-I-associated myelopathy should be considered. Some cases may be indistinguishable from mul-

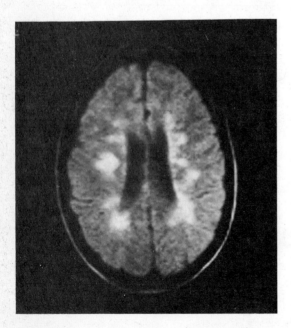

Figure 38–2. Magnetic resonance image of the brain of a multiple sclerosis patient, showing lesions (irregular white areas) in the white matter surrounding the lateral ventricles.

tiple sclerosis, but the diagnosis of HTLV-I-associated myelopathy may be made if antibody to HTLV-I is present.

Treatment

High doses of intravenous methylprednisolone given for 5–7 days have become the mainstay of therapy for severe acute exacerbations and may shorten their duration, particularly when optic neuritis is present, but the long-term benefits of such therapy are questionable. For less severe attacks, adrenocorticotropic hormone (ACTH) or oral prednisone may be used. Intensive immunosuppression with cyclophosphamide combined with ACTH was initially reported to arrest progression in some patients, but another more recent study showed no benefit.

The most striking advance in the therapy of multiple sclerosis in over 20 years occurred in 1993 with the publication of a multicenter placebo-controlled double-blind study showing that large doses of recombinant beta-1b interferon, given subcutaneously every other day for 3 years, significantly reduced exacerbation rates and the appearance of new or enlarging lesions on MR scans in patients with relapsing-remitting disease.

Copolymer I, a synthetic polypeptide that inhibits experimental allergic encephalomyelitis in animals, was effective in preventing exacerbations in a limited but well-controlled clinical trial, and a larger, more definitive study is in progress. A multicenter study of the effects of cyclosporin in patients with chronic progressive disease showed a statistically significant but biologically minimal effect on the clinical course of the disease. Targeted immunotherapy with monoclonal antibodies directed against subpopulations of activated T cells is in the preliminary stages of development. Other approaches include induction of oral tolerance to myelin antigens, vaccination with antigen-specific T cells, and vaccination with T cell receptor peptides derived from the variable region (Vβ) subtypes that recognize immunodominant epitopes of myelin basic protein. It remains to be seen which, if any, of these therapeutic modalities will survive testing in rigorously controlled double-blind clinical trials.

Complications & Prognosis

The prognosis of multiple sclerosis is difficult to predict because of its extremely variable nature. Benign cases in which patients function normally or with little neurologic deficit are not uncommon, while fulminant cases of acute multiple sclerosis can result in severe disability or death within a few years. Most patients fall between these extremes and continue to have exacerbations and remissions, or chronic progression, for many years. Despite substantial evidence for defective immunoregulation, patients with multiple sclerosis do not have increased susceptibility to other autoimmune disorders, infections, or neoplasms.

ACUTE INFLAMMATORY DEMYELINATING POLYNEUROPATHY (Guillain-Barré Syndrome)

Major Immunologic Features
- It commonly follows acute viral infections.
- There is inflammatory demyelination of peripheral nerves.
- There is cellular and humoral immunity to peripheral nerve antigens.

General Considerations

Acute inflammatory demyelinating polyneuropathy, like acute disseminated encephalomyelitis, frequently follows an infectious illness. Upper respiratory infections, exanthems, vaccinations, and viral illnesses such as infectious mononucleosis and hepatitis often precede acute inflammatory demyelinating polyneuropathy by 1–3 weeks. Increasing numbers of cases are being reported in patients with AIDS. The disease affects all age groups and is not related to sex, race, or genetic background. The annual incidence is approximately 2 per 100,000.

Pathology

Acute inflammatory demyelinating polyneuropathy is a multifocal demyelinating disease of the peripheral nervous system characterized by perivascular mononuclear-cell infiltrates with segmental demyelination in the areas of inflammation. In areas of most severe involvement, axonal destruction and wallerian degeneration occur. These lesions sometimes show infiltration of polymorphonuclear leukocytes as well as mononuclear cells early in the course of the disease.

Clinical Features

The onset is characterized by rapidly progressive weakness first of the lower extremities, then of the upper extremities, and finally of the facial, pharyngeal, and respiratory musculature. Weakness and paralysis are frequently preceded by paresthesias and numbness of the limbs, but objective sensory loss is mild and transient. The tendon reflexes are decreased or lost early in the illness, and nerve conduction in affected limbs in moderately to markedly slowed. Cerebrospinal fluid protein is increased in all cases but usually not during the first few days of the illness. The cerebrospinal fluid cell count is normal, except when the disease occurs in association with AIDS. The usual clinical course is one of rapid evolution of symptoms over 3 days to 3 weeks with improvement and return to normal function over 6–9 months. However, other patterns such as a more gradual onset, a prolonged period of complete paralysis, recovery with severe residual deficits, and a relapsing course have also been described.

Immunologic Diagnosis

In patients tested early in the course of their illness, high titers of complement-fixing antimyelin antibody of the IgM class have been detected. Clearance of this antibody from the serum often correlates with clinical improvement. Other antinerve and antimyelin antibodies have also been found, but it is uncertain whether these are pathogenic or simply reflect reactions secondary to nerve tissue destruction. Spontaneously transformed circulating lymphocytes have been described, as well as lymphocytes that respond to peripheral-nerve myelin proteins by proliferation or cytokine production. Both cellular and humoral immune responses are therefore thought to play roles in the pathogenesis of the disease.

Differential Diagnosis

Neuropathies associated with porphyria or heavy-metal poisoning can be excluded by appropriate blood or urine tests. Acute transverse myelitis or early spinal cord compression may resemble acute inflammatory demyelinating polyneuropathy, but increased reflexes and spasticity occur days to weeks after initial flaccidity, usually with bowel and bladder involvement. Vasculitides such as polyarteritis nodosa can produce peripheral neuropathies, but these tend to present with asymmetric multifocal involvement. Acute myasthenia gravis may resemble acute inflammatory demyelinating polyneuropathy, but is more likely to be associated with oculomotor weakness and generally responds to anticholinesterase drugs. Botulism and tick paralysis, uncommon diseases causing subacute generalized weakness through the effect of their associated toxins on the neuromuscular junction, can usually be distinguished by the clinical history and by neurophysiologic testing.

Treatment

Plasmapheresis, especially if begun as early as possible, is effective in shortening the course of the illness (Fig 38–4). Therapy with high doses of intravenous immunoglobulin was recently reported to be as effective as plasmapheresis and is now used as an alternative treatment, although its mechanism of action is very poorly understood. Intensive supportive care, including respiratory assistance, must be given

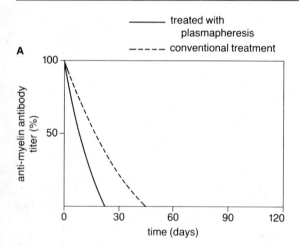

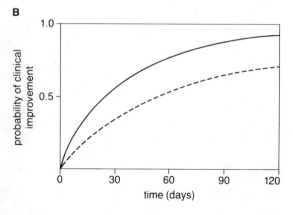

Figure 38–4. Effect of plasmapheresis on antimyelin antibody (**A**) and clinical recovery (**B**) in acute inflammatory demyelinating polyneuropathy (AIDP). Titers decline faster and recovery is more rapid and more nearly complete with plasma exchange, especially when performed during the first week of illness. (Panel A adapted from data provided by CL Koski; panel B adapted from Guillain-Barré Syndrome Study Group Clinical Trial, *Neurology* 1985;**35**:1096.)

as required. Corticosteroids tend to prolong the duration of illness and are therefore contraindicated, except in some cases of recurrent polyneuropathy.

Complications & Prognosis

Modern methods for assisting and maintaining respiration have resulted in a marked decrease in the mortality rate of acute inflammatory demyelinating polyneuropathy, which currently ranges from 1 to 5%. However, residual neurologic deficits, caused by irreversible axonal disruption and wallerian degeneration, occur in as many as 50% of patients. Respiratory muscle and pharyngeal weakness favor the development of infections, which may be life-threatening, and associated autonomic neuropathy may produce vasomotor instability and cardiac arrhythmias, resulting in sudden death despite adequate respiratory care.

CHRONIC DEMYELINATING POLYNEUROPATHIES

These are uncommon disorders that resemble acute inflammatory demyelinating polyneuropathy pathologically and physiologically but follow a more indolent and frequently relapsing course. Clinical manifestations include variable degrees of extremity weakness and sensory symptoms. Nerve conduction studies show profound slowing with conduction block. Cerebrospinal fluid protein is characteristically increased; deposits of immunoglobulin may be found in peripheral nerves; and complement-fixing antibody to myelin may be detected, suggesting an immune system-mediated process. Patients frequently respond to plasma exchange, intravenous immunoglobulin, long-term corticosteroid treatment (particularly in the relapsing type), or treatment with other immunosuppressive drugs.

Patients with multiple myeloma, Waldenström's macroglobulinemia, and primary systemic amyloidosis sometimes develop peripheral neuropathies in which the pathologic pattern is primarily axonal degeneration with secondary demyelination. The pathogenesis of these conditions has been largely unexplored. However, in patients with benign monoclonal gammopathy and peripheral neuropathy, the circulating paraproteins, usually of the IgM isotype, are monoclonal antibodies directed against the myelin-associated glycoprotein or other glycoprotein and glycolipid components of peripheral nerves. Evidence that these antibodies actually initiate demyelination is inconclusive. Nevertheless, plasma exchange and immunosuppression have produced remissions with reversal of conduction block and disappearance of the paraprotein from the serum in some cases. The role of immune cells has not been determined, although mononuclear cell infiltrates are often present in demyelinated areas of peripheral

nerve, and secretion of the IgM paraprotein is under T cell control. Another group of neurologic disorders, including a multifocal motor neuropathy with conduction block, has recently been described in association with high titers of circulating antibody to GM_1 ganglioside. Not only are these disorders immunologically interesting in their own right, but also they may serve as models for other more common immune mediated diseases of the peripheral and central nervous systems.

DISORDERS OF NEUROMUSCULAR TRANSMISSION

Myasthenia gravis and the myasthenic (Lambert-Eaton) syndrome are the neurologic diseases for which an autoimmune pathogenesis is best established.

MYASTHENIA GRAVIS

Major Immunologic Features

- It is commonly associated with thymic hyperplasia or thymoma.
- Pathogenic autoantibodies are directed against the acetylcholine receptor.
- It is often associated with other autoantibodies and autoimmune diseases.

General Considerations

Myasthenia gravis is a disease of unknown cause in which there is muscle weakness due to a disorder of neuromuscular transmission. The frequent occurrence of myasthenia gravis with thymomas, thymic hyperplasia, autoantibodies, and other autoimmune diseases strongly suggests that the immune system is involved in its pathogenesis. Anti-acetylcholine receptor antibody, which binds at the postsynaptic membrane of the neuromuscular junction, interrupts transmission by increasing endocytosis of acetylcholine receptors and forms immune complexes that bind complement, causing further destruction of the postsynaptic membrane (Fig 38–5). The prevalence of myasthenia gravis is 2–10 per 100,000. It occurs at all ages, but different subgroups are recognized. In patients with thymoma, in whom the onset is usually after age 40, there is no sex or HLA antigen association; in patients without thymoma and with onset before age 40, there is a female preponderance and association with HLA-A1, -B8, and -DR3; in patients without thymoma and with onset after age 40, there is a male preponderance and association with HLA-A3, -B7, and -DR2.

A

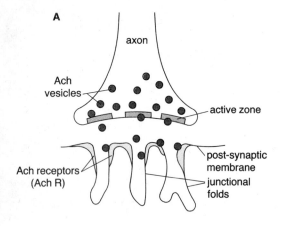

B

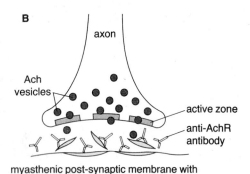

myasthenic post-synaptic membrane with loss of receptor sites and junctional folds

Figure 38–5. Normal (**A**) and myasthenic (**B**) neuromuscular junctions. At the normal junction, acetylcholine (Ach) is released from the nerve terminal and taken up by receptors on the complex folded postsynaptic membrane. In myasthenia gravis, anti-acetylcholine receptor (AchR) antibodies and immune complexes induce complement-mediated destruction of the membrane, with loss of normal folds and receptor sites.

Pathology

Scattered aggregates of lymphocytes are observed in the muscles. At the neuromuscular junction there is widening of the synaptic cleft and a marked abnormality of the postsynaptic membrane, with sparse, shallow postsynaptic folds. Eighty percent of patients have hyperplasia of lymphoid follicles with active germinal centers in the medulla of the thymus, whereas 10% have a thymoma (a locally invasive thymic neoplasm), and in the remaining 10% the thymus appears normal.

Clinical Features

Skeletal muscles are normal at rest but become increasingly weak with repetitive use. Weakness is often first noted in the extraocular muscles as diplopia or ptosis, while pharyngeal and facial weakness results in dysphagia and dysarthria. Skeletal-muscle

weakness is more often proximal than distal and causes difficulty in climbing stairs, rising from chairs, combing the hair, or even holding up the head. When respiratory muscles are weak, ventilatory assistance is sometimes necessary. Exacerbations can occur spontaneously but are often related to intercurrent infections, surgery, or emotional stress and may result in myasthenic crisis with severe bulbar and respiratory weakness. Except for muscle weakness and depressed reflexes, the neurologic examination is normal. Intravenous injection of edrophonium, a short-acting anticholinesterase, is useful in diagnosis, as it produces dramatic transient improvement of weakness by prolonging the availability of acetylcholine at the postsynaptic receptor.

Immunologic Diagnosis

Anti-acetylcholine receptor antibodies are found in 90% of myasthenia gravis patients and occasionally in thymoma patients without muscle weakness, but they may be absent in patients with purely ocular myasthenia. As they are found in no other neuromuscular disease, their presence in the appropriate clinical setting is diagnostic. Anti-striated-muscle antibodies are often detected in patients with an associated thymoma, but their pathogenic significance is unknown.

Differential Diagnosis

Myasthenia gravis can be differentiated from other myopathies on the basis of its response to anticholinesterase drugs. The various forms of periodic paralysis do not show the oculomotor involvement of myasthenia. The myasthenic (Lambert-Eaton) syndrome usually associated with small-cell carcinoma of the lung can be differentiated by electrodiagnostic studies and by lack of response to anticholinesterase agents. Botulism and tick paralysis can be diagnosed on the basis of the clinical history and electrophysiologic testing.

Treatment

Anticholinesterase drugs such as pyridostigmine and neostigmine are the mainstays of long-term therapy. Thymectomy is beneficial in the majority of cases, and all patients with myasthenia gravis except those with nondisabling ocular myasthenia should be considered for thymectomy. Dramatic improvement also occurs in severely ill patients treated with plasmapheresis, which removes anti-acetylcholine receptor antibodies from the circulation. Plasmapheresis is most effective when combined with corticosteroids and other immunosuppressive drugs to diminish the rapid increase in anti-receptor antibody that follows plasma exchange.

Complications & Prognosis

The course of myasthenia gravis prior to the widespread use of thymectomy, plasmapheresis, and corticosteroids was one of remission in 25% of cases and chronic persistent weakness with a 20–30% mortality rate in the remainder. Improvement or complete remission within 5 years can now be expected in up to 90% of patients undergoing thymectomy supplemented by the other treatment modalities. Potential hazards for the myasthenic patient include myasthenic crisis with respiratory impairment, cholinergic crisis with weakness caused by overdosage of anticholinesterase drugs, pulmonary infections resulting from respiratory insufficiency and pharyngeal weakness, and lowered resistance to invading organisms as a result of immunosuppressive therapy.

MYASTHENIC SYNDROME

This condition, also known as Lambert-Eaton syndrome, superficially resembles myasthenia gravis, but commonly spares ocular and bulbar muscles, affects proximal limb muscles, and is characterized by increasing strength with repeated muscle contraction. This phenomenon is reflected electrophysiologically in increased amplitude of motor unit action potentials evoked by rapid repetitive nerve stimulation. Myasthenic syndrome usually occurs as a remote effect of small-cell carcinoma of the lung; occasionally it is an isolated disorder. It is an autoimmune disease mediated by circulating IgG antibodies to components of the presynaptic membrane known as active zones, which function as calcium channels and are important in releasing acetylcholine at the nerve terminal. In cases associated with cancer, the antibodies are presumably directed against tumor cell antigens and cross-react with determinants in the active zones to down-regulate calcium channel activity. The disease can be experimentally transmitted to mice with serum IgG from affected patients and sometimes responds to treatment with plasmapheresis and immunosuppressive drugs.

IMMUNOLOGIC ABNORMALITIES IN OTHER NEUROLOGIC DISEASES

Immunologic findings have been described in several neurodegenerative disorders, but in only one, paraneoplastic cerebellar degeneration, has an autoimmune mechanism clearly been defined. The causes of Alzheimer's disease and amyotrophic lateral sclerosis are unknown, and the significance of immunologic abnormalities is speculative. In subacute sclerosing panencephalitis, progressive multifocal leukoencephalopathy, and Creutzfeldt-Jakob disease, transmissible agents are clearly involved and the role of the immune response is secondary or nonexistent.

PARANEOPLASTIC CEREBELLAR DEGENERATION

This is the best-described syndrome of neural degeneration occurring as an indirect effect of systemic cancer. Patients develop gait instability or ataxia and gross incoordination of their arms. If untreated, the condition can progress to disabling incoordination and unintelligible speech in a few months. Although such degeneration has been described in patients with a variety of cancers, it is strongly associated with carcinomas of the lung and ovary. In patients who present with nervous system disease, an occult tumor may be discovered only after prolonged investigation. Two features dominate the pathology of this condition: extensive loss of Purkinje cells (the major output neuron of the cerebellum) and proliferation of microglial cells. A patchy lymphocytic infiltrate may also be seen. Many patients have serum antibodies that bind to human cerebellum tissue slices. These antibodies are usually polyclonal IgG. Autoantibodies against 3 different nervous system antigens have been identified. Each is associated with a particular type of malignancy and a distinguishable clinical syndrome. Patients with antibodies against the cytoplasmic antigen termed Yo usually are women with ovarian or breast cancer and have the typical subacute cerebellar degeneration described above. Yo is highly expressed by both normal cerebellar neurons and ovarian cancer cells. An antinuclear antigen called Hu is strongly associated with small-cell carcinoma of the lung. Patients with this antibody frequently develop neuropathy and encephalopathy as well as cerebellar ataxia. Another neuronal nuclear antigen, called Ri, has been found in a few women with breast cancer together with an unusual syndrome of ataxia, myoclonus, and opsoclonus (irregular jerking eye movements). In antibody-mediated paraneoplastic disease, antibodies raised as a natural immune defense against tumor cells cross-react with a normal tissue component. Purkinje cells in vivo may extract antibody from the cerebrospinal fluid, leading to neuronal degeneration and death (Fig 38–6). Remission of the cerebellar disease may occasionally be seen after successful treatment of the underlying cancer. For clinical testing, detection of these antibodies in serum is recommended. However, these antibodies are usually detectable in the cerebrospinal fluid as well as the serum, and they seem to be produced by clones of lymphocytes residing within the central nervous system. Intrathecal production of the pathogenic antibody may explain the poor remission rate of this condition with either treatment of the malignancy or systemic immunosuppression.

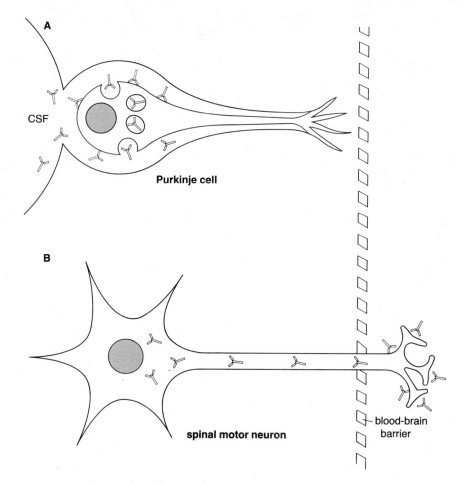

Figure 38–6. Uptake of antibodies by central nervous system neurons. **A:** Cerebellar Purkinje cell, a neuron that does not extend outside the blood-brain barrier. Antibody molecules diffuse from the cerebrospinal fluid (CSF) into the extracellular space, where they may bind to surface antigens and be taken up by endocytosis. **B:** Spinal motor neuron projecting to the neuromuscular junction outside the blood-brain barrier. Antibodies are taken up the nerve terminal and reach the cell body via retrograde axonal transport.

AMYOTROPHIC LATERAL SCLEROSIS

Amyotrophic lateral sclerosis causes progressive weakness, atrophy, and fasciculations due to degeneration of motor neurons of the spinal cord. Most patients also show degeneration of corticospinal upper motor neurons, resulting in spasticity, hyperreflexia, and poor control of voluntary movement. The disease progresses inexorably to death, usually within 3–5 years. Survival is poorest in patients who have wasting and weakness of the muscles of the pharynx, chest, and diaphragm, leading to aspiration pneumonia and respiratory failure. Commonly known as Lou Gehrig's disease, amyotrophic lateral sclerosis typically affects males after age 40. Although pathologic examination reveals neuronal loss and glial proliferation without inflammatory cells, an immunologic basis has been proposed for a subgroup of patients with a monoclonal IgM paraproteinemia. Recent work has identified the possible target antigens as glycolipids known as gangliosides, which are normal neural membrane components. Amyotrophic lateral sclerosis patients without paraproteinemia may also have increased antibody titers against gangliosides. Autoantibodies against other neuronal membrane and structural components such as neurofilaments have also been detected. Such circulating autoantibodies may either damage motor neurons directly or may be internalized at nerve terminals outside the blood-brain barrier and transported to the cell body, where they interfere with cellular metabolism (Fig 38–6). Immunoglobulins have been localized to motor neurons in tissue from patients with amyotrophic lateral sclerosis, but the significance of this observation is unclear since other plasma proteins can enter motor neurons by similar nonspecific mechanisms. Antibodies directed against calcium channels, similar to those found in the Lambert-Eaton myasthenic syndrome, have also been detected. Several immunosuppressive agents have been tested in patients with amyotrophic lateral sclerosis, but only cyclosporin has shown even a small effect on disease progression. A clinical trial of total lymphoid irradiation is currently in progress, although the significance of immune processes in pathogenesis remains unclear.

ALZHEIMER'S DISEASE

Alzheimer's disease was originally described as a presenile dementia. It is now clear that the same pathology occurs in patients older than 65 years and that it is the commonest cause of senile dementia. Memory and abstract reasoning are affected early in the course of the disease, which can eventually render patients unable to care for themselves. This makes Alzheimer's disease the single largest reason for nursing-home care. The disease is defined by its pathologic changes. Large neurons, particularly in the cortex and hippocampus, develop cytoplasmic filamentous abnormalities called "neurofibrillary tangles." Clusters of degenerating nerve terminals mixed with deposits of an amyloid-type protein form senile plaques, the other pathologic hallmark of Alzheimer's disease. Autoantibodies against neuronal antigens have been described, but their role in the pathogenesis of the disease is unclear, and they may represent only a secondary response to neuronal degeneration. The presence of amyloid protein in Alzheimer's disease was previously thought to suggest an immune-mediated process, since immunoglobulins can form amyloid deposits. The amyloid of Alzheimer's disease has now been characterized and is composed primarily of an abnormal cleavage product of a transmembrane protein, the A4 fragment of β-amyloid. Although this fragment may be derived from the brain, it is found in the circulation as well. The role of the immune system in the pathogenesis of Alzheimer's disease is currently unclear. Although inflammation is usually not seen, activation of macrophage-equivalent microglial cells has been described. Some investigators believe that amyloid deposition stimulates production of cytokines, which may potentiate the neurotoxicity of the amyloid protein.

SLOW & LATENT VIRUS INFECTIONS OF THE NERVOUS SYSTEM

Subacute Sclerosing Panencephalitis

This is a degenerative and demyelinating central nervous system disease of children that can occur several years after acute infection with measles virus. In countries where an active measles vaccination program has been implemented, the incidence of subacute sclerosing panencephalitis has declined dramatically, but it remains a serious pediatric neurologic problem in Central America, the Middle East, and other underdeveloped areas. Manifestations include personality change, dementia, seizures, and myoclonus, which progress rapidly to death in 12–18 months in most cases. Pathologically, there are intranuclear and cytoplasmic inclusion bodies that contain paramyxovirus nucleocapsids. Measles virus antigens can be demonstrated immunohistochemically, and measles virus may be recovered from infected brain tissue by cocultivation techniques. The persistence of the virus in the presence of high titers of antibody suggests an underlying defect in immunity. However, consistent defects in assays of cellular and humoral immunity cannot be identified. Measles virus strains isolated from patients with subacute sclerosing panencephalitis are indistinguishable from wild-type strains, but current evidence suggests that an abortive infection occurs and that mature virions are not produced. Incomplete expression or defective synthesis of particular measles virus proteins may be related to the high antibody titers in serum and cerebrospinal fluid. The accumulation of viral components in brain cells may alter cellular function, but infiltrates of mononuclear cells are also seen in lesions and may contribute to the pathogenic process. Treatment with the antiviral agent inosine pranobex (Isoprinosine), or with alpha interferon by intraventricular injection, has resulted in stabilization and even improvement in some cases.

PROGRESSIVE MULTIFOCAL LEUKOENCEPHALOPATHY

Progressive multifocal leukoencephalopathy is a rare disease of the central nervous system that presents with focal weakness, ataxia, spasticity, visual disturbances, aphasia, dementia, and rapid progression to coma and death within 6 months to 1 year. It occurs most frequently in adult patients with debilitating illnesses associated with some form of immunosuppression. These include lymphomas, leukemias, exogenous immunosuppression given to prevent transplant rejection, and AIDS. A papovavirus known as JC virus has been isolated from brain tissue and may be identified by immunohistochemical or in situ hybridization techniques in oligo-dendrocytes and astrocytes. Direct infection and destruction of oligodendrocytes causes the characteristic widespread demyelination. Inflammation is minimal or absent, and the cerebrospinal fluid is usually normal. JC virus is a ubiquitous human pathogen, and most normal adults have serum IgG antibodies, indicating prior exposure. The pathogenesis of progressive multifocal leukoencephalopathy is still not completely understood, but it is likely that generalized immunosuppression results in reactivation of a latent papovavirus infection, which selectively attacks oligodendrocytes and astrocytes to produce the clinical and pathologic findings of this disease.

REFERENCES

Acute Disseminated Encephalomyelitis

Johnson KP et al: Immune-mediated syndromes of the nervous system related to virus infections. Chap 20, pp 391–434, in: *Handbook of Clinical Neurology.* Vol 34. Vinken PJ, Bruyn GW (editors). North-Holland, 1978.

Johnson RT et al: Measles encephalomyelitis: Clinical and immunologic studies. *N Engl J Med* 1985; **310:**137.

Multiple Sclerosis

Beck J et al: Increased production of interferon gamma and tumor necrosis factor precedes clinical manifestation in multiple sclerosis: Do cytokines trigger off exacerbations? *Acta Neurol Scand* 1988;**78:**318.

Beck RW et al: A randomized, controlled trial of corticosteroids in the treatment of acute optic neuritis. *N Engl J Med* 1992;**326:**581.

IFNB Multiple Sclerosis Study Group: Interferon beta-1b is effective in relapsing-remitting multiple sclerosis. I. Clinical results of a multicenter, randomized, double-blind, placebo-controlled trial. *Neurology* 1993;**43:**655.

Martin R et al: Immunological aspects of demyelinating diseases. *Annu Rev Immunol* 1992;**10:**153.

Noronha A et al: Contrasting effects of alpha, beta, and gamma interferons on nonspecific suppressor function in multiple sclerosis. *Ann Neurol* 1992;**31:**103.

Ota K et al: T-cell recognition of an immunodominant myelin basic protein epitope in multiple sclerosis. *Nature* 1990;**346:**183.

Panitch HS: Interferons in multiple sclerosis. A review of the evidence. *Drugs* 1992;**44:**946.

Paty DW et al: Interferon beta-1b is effective in relapsing-remitting multiple sclerosis. II. MRI analysis results of a multicenter, randomized, double-blind, placebo-controlled trial. *Neurology* 1993;**43:**662.

Sharief MK et al: Association between tumor necrosis factor-α and disease progression in patients with multiple sclerosis. *N Engl J Med* 1991;**325:**467.

Acute Inflammatory Demyelinating Polyneuropathy

Ropper AH: The Guillain-Barré syndrome. *N Engl J Med* 1992;**326:**1130.

Van der Meché FGA et al: A randomized trial comparing intravenous immune globulin and plasma exchange in Guillain-Barré syndrome. *N Engl J Med* 1992; **326:**1123.

Vriesendorp FJ et al: Kinetics of anti-peripheral nerve myelin antibody in patients with Guillain-Barré syndrome treated and not treated with plasmapheresis. *Arch Neurol* 1991;**48:**858.

Chronic Demyelinating Polyneuropathies

Cornblath DR et al: Treatment of chronic inflammatory demyelinating polyneuropathy with intravenous immunoglobulin. *Ann Neurol* 1991;**30:**104.

Dyck PJ et al: Plasma exchange in polyneuropathy associated with monoclonal gammopathy of undetermined significance. *N Engl J Med* 1991;**325:**1482.

Mendell JR et al: Polyneuropathy and IgM monoclonal gammopathy: Studies on the pathogenetic role of anti-myelin-associated glycoprotein antibody. *Ann Neurol* 1985;**17:**243.

Pestronk A et al: A treatable multifocal motor neuropathy with antibodies to GM$_1$ ganglioside. *Ann Neurol* 1988;**24:**73.

Sadiq SA et al: The spectrum of neurologic disease associated with anti-GM$_1$ antibodies *Neurology* 1990; **40:**1067.

Myasthenia Gravis & Myasthenic Syndrome

Drachman DB et al: Functional activities of autoantibodies to acetylcholine receptors and the clinical severity of myasthenia gravis. *N Engl J Med* 1982;**307:**769.

Engel AG: Myasthenia gravis and myasthenic syndromes. *Ann Neurol* 1984;**16:**519.

Nagel A et al: Lambert-Eaton myasthenic syndrome IgG depletes presynaptic membrane active zone particles by antigenic modulation. *Ann Neurol* 1988;**24:**552.

Vincent A et al: Autoimmunity to the voltage-gated calcium channel underlies the Lambert-Eaton myasthenic syndrome. *Trends Neurosci* 1989;**12:**496.

Paraneoplastic Cerebellar Degeneration

Anderson NE, Rosenblum MK, Posner JB: Paraneoplastic cerebellar degeneration: Clinical-immunological correlations. *Ann Neurol* 1988;**24:**599.

Graus F et al: Plasmapheresis and antineoplastic treatment in CNS paraneoplastic syndrome with anti-neuronal antibodies. *Neurology* 1992;**42:**536.

Kalman J et al: Anti-Hu associated paraneoplastic encephalomyelitis/sensory neuropathy. A clinical study of 71 patients. *Medicine* 1992;**71:**59.

Peterson K et al: Paraneoplastic cerebellar degeneration: Clinical analysis of 55 anti-Yo antibody positive patients. *Neurology* 1992;**42:**1931.

Amyotrophic Lateral Sclerosis

Corbo M et al: Patterns of reactivity of human anti-GM1

antibodies with spinal cord and motor neurons. *Ann Neurol* 1992;**32:**487.

Rowland LP: Amyotrophic lateral sclerosis and autoimmunity. *N Engl J Med* 1992;**327:**1752.

Smith RG et al: Serum antibodies to L-type calcium channels in patients with amyotrophic lateral sclerosis. *N Engl J Med* 1992;**327:**1721.

Alzheimer's Disease

Selkoe D: Deciphering Alzheimer's disease: The pace quickens. *Trends Neurosci* 1987;**10:**181.

Yankner BA et al: Beta-amyloid and the pathogenesis of Alzheimer's disease. *N Engl J Med* 1991;**325:**1849.

Slow & Latent Virus Infections

Case Records of the Massachusetts General Hospital (case 45–1988): Progressive multifocal leukoencephalopathy. *N Engl J Med* 1988;**319:**1268.

Panitch HS et al: Subacute sclerosing panencephalitis: Remission after treatment with intraventricular interferon. *Neurology* 1986;**36:**562.

39

Eye Diseases

Mitchell H. Friedlaender, MD, & G. Richard O'Connor, MD

The eye is frequently considered to be a special target of immunologic disease processes, but proof of the causative role of these processes is lacking for all but a few disorders. In this sense, the immunopathology of the eye is much less clearly delineated than that of the kidney, the testis, or the thyroid gland. Because the eye is a highly vascularized organ and because the rather labile vessels of the conjunctiva are embedded in a nearly transparent medium, inflammatory eye disorders are more obvious (and often more painful) than those of other organs such as the thyroid or the kidney. The iris, ciliary body, and choroid are the most highly vascularized tissues of the eye. The similarity of the vascular supply of the uvea to that of the kidney and the choroid plexus of the brain has given rise to justified speculation concerning the selection of these 3 tissues, among others, as targets of immune complex diseases (eg, serum sickness).

Immunologic diseases of the eye can be grossly divided into 2 major categories: antibody-mediated and cell-mediated diseases. As is the case in other organs, there is ample opportunity for the interaction of these 2 systems in the eye.

ANTIBODY-MEDIATED DISEASES

Before it can be concluded that a disease of the eye is antibody-dependent, the following criteria must be satisfied: (1) There must be evidence of specific antibody in the patient's serum or plasma cells. (2) The antigen must be identified and, if feasible, characterized. (3) The same antigen must be shown to produce an immunologic response in the eye of an experimental animal, and the pathologic changes produced in the experimental animal must be similar to those observed in the human disease. (4) It must be possible to produce similar lesions in animals passively sensitized with serum from an affected animal upon challenge with the specific antigen.

Unless all of the above criteria are satisfied, the disease may be thought of as *possibly* antibody-dependent. In such circumstances, the disease can be regarded as antibody-mediated if only one of the following criteria is met: (1) if antibody to an antigen is present in higher quantities in the ocular fluids than in the serum (after adjustments have been made for the total amounts of immunoglobulins in each fluid); (2) if abnormal accumulations of plasma cells are present in the ocular lesion; (3) if abnormal accumulations of immunoglobulins are present at the site of the disease; (4) if complement is fixed by immunoglobulins at the site of the disease; (5) if an accumulation of eosinophils is present at the site of the disease; or (6) if the ocular disease is associated with an inflammatory disease elsewhere in the body for which antibody dependency has been proved or strongly suggested.

VERNAL CONJUNCTIVITIS & ATOPIC KERATOCONJUNCTIVITIS

These 2 diseases also belong to the group of atopiclike disorders. Both are characterized by itching and lacrimation of the eyes but are more chronic than hay fever conjunctivitis. Furthermore, both ultimately result in structural modifications of the lids and conjunctiva. The immunologic basis for these diseases is not delineated.

Vernal conjunctivitis characteristically affects children and adolescents; the incidence decreases sharply after the second decade of life. Like hay fever conjunctivitis, vernal conjunctivitis occurs only in the warm months of the year. Most of its victims live in hot, dry climates. The disease characteristically produces giant ("cobblestone") papillae of the tarsal conjunctiva (Fig 39–1). The keratinized epithelium from these papillae may abrade the underlying cor-

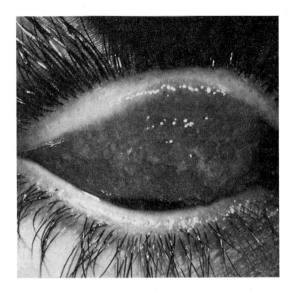

Figure 39–1. Giant papillae ("cobblestone") in the tarsal conjunctiva of a patient with vernal conjunctivitis.

nea, giving rise to complaints of foreign body sensations.

Atopic keratoconjunctivitis affects individuals of all ages and has no specific seasonal incidence. The skin of the lids has a characteristic dry, scaly appearance. The conjunctiva is pale and boggy. Both the conjunctiva and the cornea may develop scarring in the later stages of the disease. Atopic cataract has also been described. Staphylococcal blepharitis, manifested by scales and crusts on the lids, commonly complicates this disease.

RHEUMATOID DISEASES AFFECTING THE EYE

The diseases in this category vary greatly in their clinical manifestations depending upon the specific disease entity and the age of the patient. Uveitis and scleritis are the principal ocular manifestations of the rheumatoid diseases. **Juvenile rheumatoid arthritis** affects females more frequently than males and is commonly accompanied by iridocyclitis of one or both eyes. The onset is often insidious, the patient having few or no complaints and the eye remaining white. Extensive synechia formation, cataract, and secondary glaucoma may be far advanced before the parents notice that anything is wrong. The arthritis generally affects only one joint (eg, a knee) in cases with ocular involvement.

Ankylosing spondylitis affects males more frequently than females, and the onset is in the second to sixth decades. It may be accompanied by iridocyclitis of acute onset, often with fibrin in the anterior cham-

ber (Fig 39–2). Pain, redness, and photophobia are the initial complaints, and synechia formation is common.

Rheumatoid arthritis of adult onset may be accompanied by acute scleritis or episcleritis (Fig 39–3). The ciliary body and choroid, lying adjacent to the sclera, are often involved secondarily with the inflammation. Rarely, serous detachment of the retina results. The onset is usually in the third to fifth decade, and women are affected more frequently than men.

Reiter's disease affects men more frequently than women. The first attack of ocular inflammation usually consists of a self-limited papillary conjunctivitis. It follows, at a highly variable interval, the onset of nonspecific urethritis and the appearance of inflammation in one or more of the weight-bearing joints. Subsequent attacks of ocular inflammation may consist of acute iridocyclitis of one or both eyes, occasionally with hypopyon (Fig 39–4).

Immunologic Pathogenesis

Rheumatoid factor, an IgM autoantibody directed against the patient's own IgG, probably plays a major role in the pathogenesis of rheumatoid arthritis. The union of IgM antibody with IgG is followed by fixation of complement at the tissue site and the attraction of leukocytes and platelets to this area. An occlusive vasculitis resulting from this train of events is thought to be the cause of rheumatoid nodule formation in the sclera as well as elsewhere in the body. The occlusion of vessels supplying nutrients to the sclera is thought to be responsible for the "melting away" of the scleral collagen that is so characteristic of rheumatoid arthritis (Fig 39–5).

Although this explanation may suffice for rheumatoid arthritis, patients with the ocular complications of juvenile rheumatoid arthritis, ankylosing spondyli-

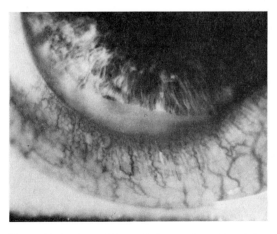

Figure 39–2. Acute iridocyclitis in a patient with ankylosing spondylitis. Note the fibrin clot in the anterior chamber.

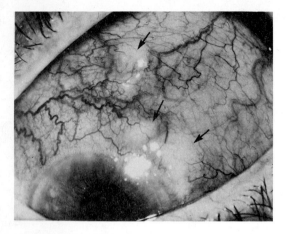

Figure 39–3. Scleral nodules in a patient with rheumatoid arthritis. (Courtesy of S Kimura.)

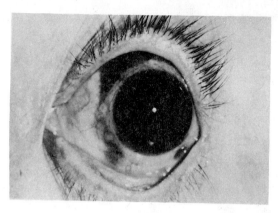

Figure 39–5. Scleral thinning in a patient with rheumatoid arthritis. Note the dark color of the underlying uvea.

tis, and Reiter's syndrome usually have negative tests for rheumatoid factor, so other explanations must be sought.

Outside the eyeball itself, the lacrimal gland has been shown to be under attack by circulating antibodies. Destruction of acinar cells within the gland and invasion of the lacrimal gland (as well as the salivary glands) by mononuclear cells result in decreased tear secretion. The combination of dry eyes (keratoconjunctivitis sicca), dry mouth (xerostomia), and rheumatoid arthritis (or other collagen vascular disease) is known as Sjögren's syndrome (see Chapter 31).

A growing body of evidence indicates that the immunogenetic background of certain patients accounts for the expression of their ocular inflammatory disease in specific ways. Analysis of the HLA antigen system shows that the incidence of HLA-B27 is significantly greater in patients with ankylosing spondylitis and Reiter's syndrome than could be expected by chance alone. It is not known how this molecule controls specific inflammatory responses.

Immunologic Diagnosis

Rheumatoid factor can be detected in the serum by a number of standard tests involving the agglutination of IgG-coated erythrocytes or latex particles. Unfortunately, the test for rheumatoid factor is not positive in the majority of isolated rheumatoid afflictions of the eye.

The HLA types of individuals suspected of having ankylosing spondylitis and related diseases can be determined by standard cytotoxicity tests with specific antisera. These tests are generally done in tissue typing centers where work on organ transplantation necessitates such studies. X-ray of the sacroiliac area is a valuable screening procedure that may show evidence of spondylitis prior to the onset of low back pain in patients with the characteristic form of iridocyclitis.

Treatment

Patients with uveitis associated with rheumatoid disease respond well to local instillations of corticosteroid drops (eg, dexamethasone 0.1%) or ointments. Orally administered corticosteroids must occasionally be resorted to for brief periods. Aspirin given orally in divided doses with meals is thought to reduce the frequency and blunt the severity of recurrent attacks. Atropine drops 1% are useful for the relief of photophobia during the acute attacks. Shorter-acting mydriatics such as phenylephrine 10% should be used in the subacute stages to prevent synechia formation. Corticosteroid-resistant cases, especially those causing progressive erosion of the sclera, have been treated successfully with immunosuppressive drugs such as chlorambucil. Hydroxychloroquine, an

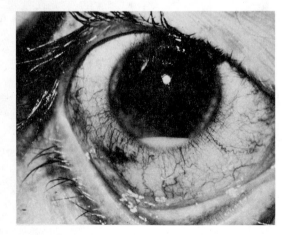

Figure 39–4. Acute iridocyclitis with hypopyon in a patient with Reiter's disease.

antimalarial drug, has been useful in the treatment of Sjögren's syndrome and other collagen-vascular diseases. Eye examinations at 6–12-month intervals are recommended, since deposits in the cornea and retina have been reported with high-dose Plaquenil therapy.

OTHER ANTIBODY-MEDIATED DISEASES

The following antibody-mediated diseases are infrequently seen by the practicing ophthalmologist.

Systemic lupus erythematosus (SLE), associated with the presence of circulating antibodies to DNA, produces an occlusive vasculitis of the nerve fiber layer of the retina. Such infarcts result in cytoid bodies or "cotton-wool" spots in the retina (Fig 39–6).

Pemphigus vulgaris produces painful intraepithelial bullae of the conjunctiva. It is associated with the presence of circulating antibodies to an intercellular antigen located between the deeper cells of the conjunctival epithelium.

Cicatricial pemphigoid is characterized by subepithelial bullae of the conjunctiva. In the chronic stages of this disease, cicatricial contraction of the conjunctiva may result in severe scarring of the cornea, dryness of the eyes, and, ultimately, blindness. Pemphigoid is associated with local deposits of tissue antibodies directed against one or more antigens located in the basement membrane of the epithelium.

Lens-induced uveitis is a rare condition that may be associated with circulating antibodies to lens proteins. It is seen in individuals whose lens capsules have become permeable to these proteins as a result of trauma or other disease. Interest in this field dates back to 1903, when Uhlenhuth first demonstrated the organ-specific nature of antibodies to the lens. Witmer showed in 1962 that antibody to lens tissue may be produced by lymphoid cells of the ciliary body.

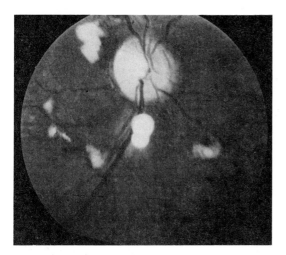

Figure 39–6. Cotton-wool spots in the retina of a patient with SLE.

CELL-MEDIATED DISEASES

This group of diseases appears to be associated with T-cell-mediated immunity (delayed hypersensitivity). Various structures of the eye are invaded by mononuclear cells, principally lymphocytes and macrophages, in response to one or more chronic antigenic stimuli. In chronic infections such as tuberculosis, leprosy, toxoplasmosis, and herpes simplex, the antigenic stimulus has clearly been identified as an infectious agent in the ocular tissue. Such infections are often associated with delayed skin test reactivity following the intradermal injection of an extract of the organism.

More intriguing but less well understood are the granulomatous diseases of the eye for which no infectious cause has been found. Such diseases are thought to represent cell-mediated, possibly autoimmune processes, but their origin remains obscure.

OCULAR SARCOIDOSIS

Ocular sarcoidosis is characterized by a panuveitis with occasional inflammatory involvement of the optic nerve and retinal blood vessels. It often presents as iridocyclitis of insidious onset. Less frequently, it occurs as acute iridocyclitis, with pain, photophobia, and redness of the eye. Large precipitates resembling drops of solidified mutton fat are seen on the corneal endothelium. The anterior chamber contains a good deal of protein and numerous cells, mostly lymphocytes. Nodules are often seen on the iris, both at the pupillary margin and in the substance of the iris stroma. The latter are often vascularized. Synechiae are commonly encountered, particularly in patients with dark skin. Severe cases ultimately involve the posterior segment of the eye. Coarse clumps of cells ("snowballs") are seen in the vitreous, and exudates resembling candle drippings may be seen along the course of the retinal vessels. Patchy infiltrations of the choroid or optic nerve may also be seen.

Infiltrations of the lacrimal gland and of the conjunctiva have been noted on occasion. When the latter are present, the diagnosis can easily be confirmed by biopsy of the small opaque nodules.

Immunologic Pathogenesis

Although many infectious or allergic causes of sarcoidosis have been suggested, none has been confirmed. Noncaseating granulomas are seen in the uvea, optic nerve, and adnexal structures of the eye as well as elsewhere in the body. The presence of macrophages and giant cells suggests that particulate matter is being phagocytized, but this material has not been identified.

Patients with sarcoidosis are usually anergic to extracts of the common microbial antigens such as those of mumps, *Trichophyton, Candida,* and *Mycobacterium tuberculosis.* As in other lymphoproliferative disorders such as Hodgkin's disease and chronic lymphocytic leukemia, suppression of T cell immunity impairs normal delayed hypersensitivity responses to common antigens. Meanwhile, circulating immunoglobulins are usually detectable in the serum at higher than normal levels.

Immunologic Diagnosis

The diagnosis is largely inferential. Negative skin tests to a battery of antigens to which the patient is known to have been exposed are highly suggestive, and the same is true of the elevation of serum immunoglobulins. Biopsy of a conjunctival nodule or scalene lymph node may provide positive histologic evidence of the disease. X-rays of the chest reveal hilar adenopathy in many cases. Elevated levels of serum lysozyme or serum angiotensin-converting enzyme may be detected. A gallium scan, utilizing gallium 67, may be useful in detecting clinically inapparent lesions.

Treatment

Sarcoid lesions of the eye respond well to corticosteroid therapy. Frequent instillations of prednisolone acetate 1% eye drops generally bring the anterior uveitis under control. Atropine drops should be prescribed in the acute phase of the disease for the relief of pain and photophobia; short-acting pupillary dilators such as phenylephrine should be given later to prevent synechia formation. Systemic corticosteroids are sometimes necessary to control severe attacks of anterior uveitis and are always necessary for the control of retinal vasculitis and optic neuritis. The latter condition often accompanies cerebral involvement and carries a grave prognosis.

SYMPATHETIC OPHTHALMIA & VOGT-KOYANAGI-HARADA SYNDROME

These 2 disorders are discussed together because they have certain common clinical features. Both are though to represent autoimmune phenomena affecting pigmented structures of the eye and skin, and both may give rise to meningeal symptoms.

Clinical Features

Sympathetic ophthalmia is an inflammation in the second eye after the other has been damaged by penetrating injury. In most cases, some portion of the uvea of the injured eye has been exposed to the atmosphere for at least 1 hour. The uninjured or "sympathizing" eye develops minor signs of anterior uveitis after a period ranging from 2 weeks to several years. Floating spots and loss of the power of accommodation are among the earliest symptoms. The disease may progress to severe iridocyclitis with pain and photophobia. Usually, however, the eye remains relatively quiet and painless while the inflammatory disease spreads around the entire uvea. Despite the presence of panuveitis, the retina usually remains uninvolved except for perivascular cuffing of the retinal vessels with inflammatory cells. Papilledema and secondary glaucoma may occur. The disease may be accompanied by vitiligo (patchy depigmentation of the skin) and poliosis (whitening) of the eyelashes.

Vogt-Koyanagi-Harada syndrome consists of inflammation of the uvea of one or both eyes characterized by acute iridocyclitis, patchy choroiditis, and serous detachment of the retina. It usually begins with an acute febrile episode with headaches, dysacusis, and occasionally vertigo. Patchy loss or whitening of the scalp hair is described in the first few months of the disease. Vitiligo and poliosis are commonly present but are not essential for the diagnosis. Although the initial iridocyclitis may subside quickly, the course of the posterior disease is often indolent, with longstanding serous detachment of the retina and significant visual impairment.

Immunologic Pathogenesis

In both sympathetic ophthalmia and Vogt-Koyanagi-Harada syndrome, delayed hypersensitivity to melanin-containing structures is thought to occur. Although a viral cause has been suggested for both disorders, there is no convincing evidence of an infectious origin. It is postulated that some insult, infectious or otherwise, alters the pigmented structures of the eye, skin, and hair in such a way as to provoke delayed hypersensitivity responses to them. Soluble materials from the outer segments of the photoreceptor layer of the retina have recently been incriminated as possible autoantigens. Patients with Vogt-Koyanagi-Harada syndrome are usually Asians, which suggests an immunogenetic predisposition to the disease.

Histologic sections of the traumatized eye from a patient with sympathetic ophthalmia may show uniform infiltration of most of the uvea by lymphocytes, epithelioid cells, and giant cells. The overlying retina is characteristically intact, but nests of epithelioid cells may protrude through the pigment epithelium of the retina, giving rise to **Dalen-Fuchs nodules.** The inflammation may destroy the architecture of the entire uvea, leaving an atrophic, shrunken globe.

Immunologic Diagnosis

Skin tests with soluble extracts of human or bovine uveal tissue are said to elicit delayed hypersensitivity responses in these patients. Several investigators have recently shown that cultured lymphocytes from patients with these 2 diseases undergo transformation to lymphoblasts in vitro when extracts of uvea or rod outer segments are added to the culture medium. Circulating antibodies to uveal antigens have been found in patients with these diseases, but such antibodies are to be found in any patient with long-standing uveitis, including those suffering from several infectious entities. The spinal fluid of patients with Vogt-Koyanagi-Harada syndrome may show increased numbers of mononuclear cells and elevated protein in the early stages.

Treatment

Mild cases of sympathetic ophthalmia may be treated satisfactorily with locally applied corticosteroid drops and pupillary dilators. The more severe or progressive cases require systemic corticosteroids, often in high doses, for months or years. An alternate-day regimen of oral corticosteroids is recommended for such patients in order to avoid adrenal suppression. The same applies to the treatment of patients with Vogt-Koyanagi-Harada syndrome. Occasionally, patients with long-standing progressive disease become resistant to corticosteroids or cannot take additional corticosteroid medication because of pathologic fractures, mental changes, or other reasons. Such patients may become candidates for immunosuppressive therapy. Chlorambucil and cyclophosphamide have been used successfully for both conditions. More recently, cyclosporin has shown promise in the treatment of corticosteroid-resistant uveitis.

OTHER CELL-MEDIATED DISEASES

Giant cell arteritis (temporal arteritis) (see Chapter 34) may have disastrous effects on the eyes, particularly in elderly individuals. The condition is manifested by pain in the temples and orbit, blurred vision, and scotomas. Examination of the fundus may reveal extensive occlusive retinal vasculitis and choroidal infarcts. Atrophy of the optic nerve head is a frequent complication. Such patients have an elevated erythrocyte sedimentation rate. Biopsy of the temporal artery reveals extensive infiltration of the vessel wall with giant cells and mononuclear cells.

Polyarteritis nodosa (see Chapter 34) can affect both the anterior and posterior segments of the eye. The corneas of such patients may show peripheral thinning and cellular infiltration. The retinal vessels reveal extensive necrotizing inflammation characterized by eosinophil, plasma cell, and lymphocyte infiltration.

Behçet's disease (see Chapter 31) has an uncertain place in the classification of immunologic disorders. It is characterized by recurrent iridocyclitis with hypopyon and occlusive vasculitis of the retinal vessels. Although it has many of the features of a delayed hypersensitivity disease, dramatic alterations of

serum complement levels at the very beginning of an attack suggest an immune complex disorder. Furthermore, high levels of circulating immune complexes have recently been detected in patients with this disease. Most patients with eye symptoms are positive for HLA-B5 (subtype B51).

Contact dermatitis (see Chapter 28) of the eyelids represents a significant though minor disease caused by delayed hypersensitivity. Atropine, perfumed cosmetics, materials contained in plastic spectacle frames, and other locally applied agents may act as the sensitizing hapten. The lower lid is more extensively involved than the upper lid when the sensitizing agent is applied in drop form. Periorbital involvement with erythematous, vesicular, pruritic lesions of the skin is characteristic.

Phlyctenular keratoconjunctivitis (Fig 39–7) represents a delayed hypersensitivity response to certain microbial antigens, principally those of *M tuberculosis*. It is characterized by acute pain and photophobia in the affected eye, and perforation of the peripheral cornea has been known to result. The disease responds rapidly to locally applied corticosteroids. Since the advent of chemotherapy for pulmonary tuberculosis, phlyctenulosis is much less of a problem than it was 30 years ago. It is still encountered occasionally, however, particularly among Native Americans and Alaskan Eskimos. Rarely, other pathogens such as *Staphylococcus aureus* and *Coccidioides immitis* have been implicated in phlyctenular disease.

Acquired Immunodeficiency Syndrome (AIDS) (see Chapter 52) is commonly associated with ocular disorders, seen mainly in homosexual men, intravenous drug abusers, and hemophiliacs. Cotton-wool exudates are the most common ocular sign. They have the same appearance as those seen in SLE (Fig

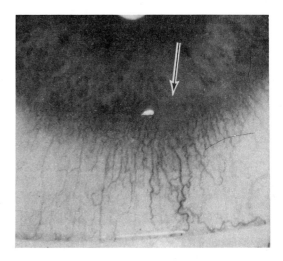

Figure 39–7. Phlyctenule (arrow) at the margin of the cornea. (Courtesy of P Thygeson.)

39–6), but it is not known whether the cotton-wool spots of AIDS have the same pathogenesis. As is the case with SLE, patients suffering from AIDS may have elevated serum immune complexes.

In addition to cotton-wool spots, AIDS patients may develop Kaposi's sarcoma of the conjunctiva or lids as well as chorioretinitis associated with any one of a number of different opportunistic pathogens such as cytomegalovirus, *Cryptococcus, Toxoplasma,* or *Candida.* These patients have a fundamental disorder of cell-mediated immunity reflected in reduced levels of CD4 cells and chronic infection by HIV. These patients often die of systemic opportunistic infections such as *Pneumocystis carinii* pneumonia or toxoplasmal encephalitis. Since cotton-wool spots are an early sign of AIDS, the ophthalmologist may be the first physician to alert the patient to the existence of this serious disorder.

CORNEAL GRAFT REACTIONS

General Considerations

Blindness due to opacity or distortion of the central portion of the cornea is a remediable disease (Fig 39–8). If all other structures of the eye are intact, a patient whose vision is impaired solely by corneal opacity can expect great improvement from a graft of clear cornea into the stroma, and a single-layered endothelium. Although the surface epithelium may be sloughed and later replaced by the recipient's epithelium, certain elements of the stroma and all of the donor's endothelium remain in place for the rest of

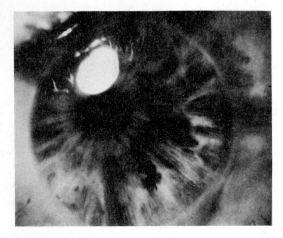

Figure 39–8. A cornea severely scarred by chronic atopic keratoconjunctivitis into which a central graft of clear cornea has been placed. Note how distinctly the iris landmarks are seen through the transparent graft.

the patient's life. This has been firmly established by sex chromosome markers in corneal cells when donor and recipient were of opposite sexes. The endothelium must remain healthy in order for the cornea to remain transparent, and an energy-dependent pump mechanism is required to keep the cornea from swelling with water. Since the recipient's endothelium is in most cases diseased, the central corneal endothelium must be replaced by healthy donor tissue.

A number of foreign elements exist in corneal grafts that might stimulate the immune system of the host to reject this tissue. In addition to those mentioned above, the corneal stroma is regularly perfused with IgG and serum albumin from the donor, although none—or only small amounts—of the other blood proteins are present. While these serum proteins of donor origin rapidly diffuse into the recipient stroma, these substances are theoretically immunogenic.

Although the ABO blood antigens have been shown to have no relationship to corneal graft rejection, the HLA antigen system probably plays a significant role in graft reactions. HLA incompatibility between donor and recipient has been shown by several authors to be significant in determining graft survival, particularly when the corneal bed is vascularized. It is known that most cells of the body possess these HLA antigens, including the endothelial cells of the corneal graft as well as certain stromal cells (keratocytes). The epithelium has been shown by Hall and others to possess a non-HLA antigen that diffuses into the anterior third of the stroma. Thus, while much foreign antigen may be eliminated by purposeful removal of the epithelium at the time of grafting, that amount of antigen which has already diffused into the stroma is automatically carried over into the recipient. Such antigens may be leached out by soaking the donor cornea in tissue culture for several weeks prior to engraftment.

Immunologic Pathogenesis

Both antibody and cellular mechanisms have been implicated in corneal graft reactions. It is likely that early graft rejections (within 2 weeks) are cell-mediated reactions. Cytotoxic lymphocytes have been found in the limbal area and stroma of affected individuals, and phase microscopy in vivo has revealed an actual attack on the grafted endothelial cells by these lymphocytes. Such lymphocytes generally move inward from the periphery of the cornea, making what is known as a "rejection line" as they move centrally. The donor cornea becomes edematous as the endothelium becomes compromised by an accumulation of lymphoid cells.

Late rejection of a corneal graft may occur several weeks to many months after implantation of donor tissue into the recipient eye. Such reactions may be antibody-mediated, since cytotoxic antibodies have been isolated from the serum of patients with a history of diseased area. Trauma, including chemical burns, is one of the most common causes of central corneal opacity. Others include scars from herpetic keratitis, endothelial cell dysfunction with chronic corneal edema (Fuchs' dystrophy), keratoconus, and opacities from previous graft failures. All of these conditions represent indications for penetrating corneal grafts, provided the patient's eye is no longer inflamed and the opacity has been allowed maximal time to undergo spontaneous resolution (usually 6–12 months). It is estimated that approximately 10,000 corneal grafts are performed in the USA annually. Of these, about 90% can be expected to produce a beneficial result.

The cornea was one of the first human tissues to be successfully grafted. The fact that recipients of corneal grafts generally tolerate them well can be attributed to (1) the absence of blood vessels or lymphatics in the normal cornea and (2) the lack of presensitization to tissue-specific antigens in most recipients. Reactions to corneal grafts do occur, however, particularly in individuals whose own corneas have been damaged by previous inflammatory disease. Such corneas may have developed both lymphatics and blood vessels, providing afferent and efferent channels for immunologic reactions in the engrafted cornea.

Although attempts have been made to transplant corneas from other species into human eyes (xenografts), particularly in countries where human material is not available for religious reasons, most corneal grafts have been taken from human eyes (allografts). Except in the case of identical twins, such grafts always represent the implantation of foreign tissue into a donor site; thus, the chance for a graft rejection due to an immune response to foreign antigens is virtually always present.

The cornea is a 3-layered structure composed of a surface epithelium, and oligocellular collagenous multiple graft reactions in vascularized corneal beds. These antibody reactions are complement-dependent and attract polymorphonuclear leukocytes, which may form dense rings in the cornea at the sites of maximum deposition of immune complexes. In experimental animals, similar reactions have been produced by corneal xenografts, but the intensity of the reaction can be markedly reduced either by decomplementing the animal or by reducing its leukocyte population through mechlorethamine therapy.

Treatment

The mainstay of the treatment of corneal graft reactions is corticosteroid therapy. This medication is generally given in the form of frequently applied eye drops (eg, prednisolone acetate 1%, hourly) until the clinical signs abate. These clinical signs consist of conjunctival hyperemia in the perilimbal region, a cloudy cornea, cells and protein in the anterior chamber, and keratic precipitates on the corneal endothelium. The earlier that treatment is applied, the more effective it is likely to be. Neglected cases may require systemic or periocular corticosteroids in addition to local eye drop therapy. Occasionally, vascularization and opacification of the cornea occur so rapidly that corticosteroid therapy is useless, but even the most hopeless-appearing graft reactions have occasionally been reversed by corticosteroid therapy. Topical corticosteroids are often used once or twice a day as prophylaxis against transplant rejection. More recently, topical cyclosporin eye drops have been used.

Patients known to have rejected many previous corneal grafts are managed somewhat differently, particularly if disease affects their only remaining eye. An attempt is made to find a close HLA match between donor and recipient. Pretreatment of the recipient with immunosuppressive agents such as azathioprine has also been resorted to in some cases. Although HLA testing of the recipient and the potential donor is indicated in cases of repeated corneal graft failure or in cases of severe corneal vascularization, such testing is not necessary or practicable in most cases requiring keratoplasty.

REFERENCES

Dugel PU, Rao NA: Ocular infections in acquired immunodeficiency syndrome. *Int Ophthalmol Clin* 1993;**33:**103.

Friedlaender MH: *Allergy and Immunology of the Eye,* 2nd ed. Raven, 1993.

Friedlacnder MH (editor): Ocular allergy. *Int Ophthalmol Clin* 1988;**28:**261.

Friedlaender MH, Tabbara KF (editors): Immunological ocular disease. *Int Ophthalmol Clin* 1985;**25:**1.

Kraus-Mackiw E, O'Connor GR (editors): *Uveitis: Pathophysiology and Therapy.* Thieme-Stratton, 1983.

Michelson JB, Nozik RA: *Surgical Treatment of Ocular Inflammatory Disease.* Lippincott, 1988.

O'Connor GR (editor): *Immunologic Diseases of the Mucous Membranes.* Masson, 1980.

O'Connor GR, Chandler JW (editors): *Advances in Immunology and Immunopathology of the Eye.* Masson, 1985.

Smith R, Nozik R: *Uveitis: A Clinical Approach to Diagnosis and Management.* Williams & Wilkins, 1983.

Smolin G, O'Connor GR: *Ocular Immunology.* Little, Brown, 1986.

Webb R, Friedlaender M: Immunology and uveitis. Pages 133–152 in: *Modern Management of Ocular Disease.* Spoor TC (editor). Slack, 1985.

Respiratory Diseases

John F. Fieselmann, MD, and Hal B. Richerson, MD

Respiratory diseases of putative disordered immune regulation include those caused by exaggerated inflammation to exogenous antigen (hypersensitivity or allergic response), immune response to self-antigen (autoimmunity), or the failure to mount a protective immune response to a harmful agent (immunodeficiency). **Hypersensitivity responses** to known antigens include hypersensitivity pneumonitis, allergic asthma (atopic and occupational), some examples of eosinophilic pneumonias (parasitic, drug-induced, and allergic bronchopulmonary aspergillosis), and other manifestations of drug-induced lung diseases. Most respiratory diseases attributed to disordered immune regulation are of unknown etiology, but their pathology appears to involve immunologic mechanisms. Examples include collagen-vascular diseases, granulomatous diseases, vasculitis syndromes, and idiopathic interstitial fibrosis. Respiratory diseases associated with **primary or secondary immunodeficiency** are caused by infectious agents: viral, bacterial, fungal, or parasitic.

The lung must cope with antigens, including infectious organisms, that reach it by way of inspired air, aspiration, and the circulation. The pulmonary immune system normally mounts a protective effector response against harmful agents and ignores those that are harmless. Protection is helped by nonspecific clearance mechanisms involving alveolar macrophages, ciliary action, secretions, and cough. In general, the combination of specific (immunologic) and nonspecific mechanisms protects the lung very well. Why the system fails and how it leads to disease in some individuals is not well understood for many of the conditions included in this chapter.

Several respiratory diseases of disordered immune regulation are fully discussed elsewhere in this volume. For completeness, they are mentioned at the end of this chapter with reference to the chapters where they are treated in full.

DRUG-INDUCED RESPIRATORY DISEASES

Drugs cause pulmonary adverse effects by several different mechanisms, although details of pathogenesis are lacking in most cases. Potential mechanisms include hypersensitivity, direct toxicity, production of free oxygen radicals, stimulation of collagen synthesis, and lipidosis induction. This section will primarily consider reactions involving proven or suspected immunologic mechanisms. Lists of common drugs are provided in Table 40–1.

Immunologic Mechanisms

Drug-induced hypersensitivity reactions involving the lungs may be associated with one or more types of immunologic response that damage host tissue. In the Gell and Coombs classification system, hypersensitivity responses may involve IgE antibodies (type I), cellular cytotoxicity (type II), antigen-antibody complexes (type III), or T cell-mediated hypersensitivity (type IV). Except for wheal-and-flare (immediate-type) skin tests in type I hypersensitivity, documentation of drug allergy by in vivo or in vitro testing has not been clinically useful. In the following section, selected drugs are discussed to illustrate prototypic manifestations of adverse pulmonary reactions.

Airway Involvement

Asthma may be caused by drugs eliciting IgE-mediated systemic anaphylaxis. This is commonly seen in response to beta-lactam antibiotics, foreign proteins, and exogenous hormones. Latex from surgical gloves or catheters is an increasing problem. Inhalation of psyllium (eg, Metamucil) dusts may induce asthma in a sensitized individual administering or otherwise handling the drug.

Aspirin and other nonsteroidal anti-inflammatory agents can cause sudden, severe bronchospasm. No evidence exists that IgE antibodies play a role; rather, shunting of the arachidonic pathway toward

Table 40–1. Drug-induced respiratory diseases that may involve immunologic mechanisms.

Structure Affected or Disease Induced	Drug[1]	Major Pulmonary Manifestations	Suspected Mechanism
Airways	ACE inhibitors Aspirin and other NSAIDs Sulfites Cisplatin, L-asparaginase D-Penicillamine Psyllium (inhaled)	Cough, asthma (rare) Asthma Bronchospasm Bronchospasm Bronchiolitis obliterans Asthma	Unknown Unknown Unknown Unknown Hypersensitivity IgE-mediated
Parenchyma	Anti-infectious agents Isoniazid Nitrofurantoin p-Aminosalicylic acid Penicillin Sulfonamides	Pulmonary infiltrates	Hypersensitivity
	Chemotherapeutic agents Azathioprine Methotrexate Procarbazine	Pulmonary infiltrates	Hypersensitivity
	Chemotherapeutic agents Azathioprine Bleomycin Busulfan Chlorambucil Cyclophosphamide Melphalan Mitomycin Nitrosoureas	Pulmonary fibrosis/pneumonitis	Unknown Oxidants? Toxic metabolites? Toxic metabolites? Toxic metabolites? Toxic metabolites? Toxic metabolites? Oxidants?
	Miscellaneous agents Carbamazepine Cromolyn Gold salts NSAIDs	Pulmonary infiltrates	Hypersensitivity
	Miscellaneous agents Amiodarone Diphenylhydantoin D-Penicillamine Methysergide Nitrofurantoin	Pulmonary fibrosis/pneumonitis	Toxic lipidosis? Free oxygen radicals?
Pleura	Chemotherapeutic agents Bleomycin, busulfan, methotrexate mitomycin, procarbazine Methysergide, ergonovine Bromocryptine Nitrofurantoin	Pleurisy and effusion	Unknown
Mediastinum	Diphenylhydantoin	Pseudolymphoma with adenopathy	Hypersensitivity
Lupus syndrome	Diphenylhydantoin Hydralazine Isoniazid Procainamide	Infiltrates, pleuritis, effusion	Hypersensitivity
Pseudo-Goodpasture's syndrome	D-Penicillamine	Pulmonary hemorrhage	Unknown

[1]Abbreviations: ACE, angiotension-converting enzyme; NSAID, nonsteroidal anti-inflammatory drug.

lipoxygenase products (leukotrienes C_4, D_4, and E_4) has been suggested as a possible mechanism. Asthma can also be provoked by the direct pharmacologic effects of drugs such as β-adrenergic blockers or an idiosyncratic effect of drugs such as angiotensin-converting enzyme (ACE) inhibitors.

Parenchymal Involvement

Parenchymal involvement induced by drugs includes diffuse, discrete, or interstitial infiltrates that may be associated with eosinophilia or with fibrosis. **Nitrofurantoin** may cause acute or, less commonly, chronic pulmonary disease. The acute form usually has a sudden onset of fever, cough, dyspnea, and occasionally pleurisy within 7–10 days of beginning medication. Crackles and wheezes may be heard, and eosinophilia is found in 20–30% of patients. Chest x-rays show an interstitial, alveolar, or mixed pattern most prominent at the bases. Patients usually improve rapidly after the drug is withdrawn. The uncommon chronic form begins after months to years of nitrofurantoin use and is manifested by an insidious onset of dyspnea on exertion, bibasilar crackles, and diffuse interstitial pneumonitis or fibrosis. Some resolution typically occurs on discontinuation of the drug, but the fibrosis may progress. Studies suggest an immunologic pathogenesis in the acute form and cumulative toxicity, perhaps from oxygen radicals, in the chronic form. **Amiodarone** pneumonitis occurs in 4–6% of patients taking this antiarrhythmic agent and results in death in about 25% of those affected. The risk of this complication is dose- and duration-related and is manifested by dyspnea and cough with x-ray findings of interstitial and alveolar infiltrates. Although hypersensitivity may play a role, the condition is associated with lipid accumulation in lung cells (lipidosis), which may be the cause of the inflammatory response. Withdrawing the drug early in the course of pulmonary involvement results in resolution in most patients. **Chemotherapeutic agents,** especially methotrexate, bischloroethylnitrosourea (BCNU), and bleomycin, are well known to cause adverse pulmonary responses. Methotrexate generates pulmonary complications in about 8% of patients, but there appears to be a threshold dose requirement of 20 mg/wk. The time interval before onset of symptoms may vary from days to years. The acute syndrome of fever, cough, dyspnea, and bilateral pulmonary infiltrates progresses over 1–2 weeks and then regresses whether or not methotrexate therapy is stopped. Acute lymphocytic leukemia of childhood seems to be a specific risk factor for the acute syndrome, and it results in death in 10% of those affected. BCNU, especially in higher doses, has been reported to cause pulmonary fibrosis in 20–30% of patients. The mechanism of injury is probably oxidant toxicity rather than an immunologic one. Bleomycin produces both acute and chronic pulmonary injury with inflammatory infiltrates and fibrosis. The chronic, but not the acute, form is dose-dependent, occurring in about 15% of patients receiving total doses that exceed 450 mg. Older age, previous irradiation, and oxygen therapy increase the risk. The chest x-ray most commonly shows lower-lobe linear or nodular densities.

Gold salts produce pneumonitis in fewer than 1% of patients; this condition occurs 1–26 months after institution of therapy. Eosinophilia and lymphokine production provide evidence favoring type I and IV hypersensitivity responses. **Sulfasalazine** has been reported to cause pulmonary infiltrates, eosinophilia, fibrosis, and bronchiolitis obliterans after months or years of therapy. Hypersensitivity is the most likely mechanism.

Pleura

Drugs causing inflammation of the pleura with or without other lung structures are listed in Table 40–1.

Pleuritis may also occur as a part of the lupus syndrome.

Mediastinum

Diphenylhydantoin may cause a pseudolymphoma affecting mediastinal as well as peripheral lymph nodes.

Lupus Syndrome

Procainamide and **hydralazine** are the most common agents that cause drug-induced systemic lupus erythematosus with pulmonary manifestations of pneumonitis or pleural effusions. **Isoniazid, D-penicillamine,** and **diphenylhydantoin** are less frequent lupus inducers. Features of the syndrome suggest hypersensitivity mechanisms that may involve an adjuvant effect or alteration of DNA nucleoproteins and subsequent autoantibody production.

Pseudo-Goodpasture's Syndrome

D-Penicillamine in high doses occasionally causes pseudo-Goodpasture's syndrome with abrupt onset of dyspnea, cough, hemoptysis, and hematuria, followed by increasing respiratory distress and renal failure. Intra-alveolar hemorrhage and fibrosis are seen histologically. In contrast to Goodpasture's syndrome, anti-basement membrane antibodies are not found.

EOSINOPHILIC PNEUMONIAS

Peripheral blood eosinophilia is commonly associated with atopic diseases, parasitic infestations, and some allergic drug reactions. There are many less common causes. When eosinophilia is present together with pulmonary infiltrates, however, the diagnostic possibilities are more limited and constitute the eosinophilic pneumonias or pulmonary infiltrates with eosinophilia (PIE) syndromes (Table 40–2). Although the etiology is usually unknown, hypersensitivity is suspected because similar syndromes result from hypersensitivity to drugs, parasites, and fungi. Affected patients usually have peripheral blood eosinophilia over 10%, or 500 eosinophils/mm^3, but some have eosinophilic pulmonary infiltrates without peripheral eosinophilia.

Many eosinophilic pneumonias are associated with asthma, and the presence or absence of asthma is useful in the differential diagnosis (Table 40–2).

Asthma essentially always occurs in and usually predates the onset of ABPA and allergic granulomatosis of Churg and Strauss, and it is often associated with Carrington's chronic eosinophilic pneumonia. The patient is always atopic in ABPA (with demonstrable IgE antibodies to *Aspergillus fumigatus*), often atopic in allergic granulomatosis of Churg-Strauss, but not atopic in Carrington's chronic eosinophilic pneumonia.

ABPA is fully discussed in Chapter 27.

Table 40–2. Eosinophilic pneumonias.

Disease Entity	Association with Asthma	Comments
Allergic bronchopulmonary aspergillosis	Essentially always (extrinsic asthma)	Complication of atopic asthma with evidence of IgE and IgG antibodies to *A fumigatus*.
Chronic idiopathic eosinophilic pneumonia (Carrington's)	Frequent (intrinsic asthma)	Subacute to chronic symptoms of cough, fever, dyspnea, sweats, and weight loss; classically peripheral infiltrates on radiogram.
Allergic granulomatosis (Churg-Strauss syndrome)	Essentially always	Multisystem vasculitis with fever, malaise, weight loss, pulmonary infiltrates, peripheral neuropathy, arthralgias, myalgias.
Acute simple idiopathic pulmonary eosinophilia (Loeffler's syndrome)	Occasional	Migratory or transient infiltrates on chest x-ray and minimal or no symptoms.
Acute eosinophilic pneumonia	None	Recently described noninfectious eosinophilic pneumonia with rapid progressive respiratory failure.
Eosinophilia-myalgia syndrome	None	Caused by dietary supplements of tryptophan (L-tryptophan); sometimes associated with pulmonary infiltrates.
Drug-induced eosinophilic pneumonia	None	Penicillins, sulfonamides, nitrofurantoin, isoniazid, and many others (see Table 40–3).
Parasite-induced eosinophilic pneumonia (including visceral larva migrans and tropical pulmonary eosinophilia)	Occasional	*Ascaris, Trichinella, Strongyloides, Dirofilaria, Wuchereria, Toxocara*, and others (see Table 40–3).
Hypereosinophilic syndrome	None	Eosinophilia > 1500/mm^3 for 6 months or more; characteristic organ involvement; absence of secondary cause.

Chronic Idiopathic Eosinophilic Pneumonia

This disease is often called Carrington's chronic eosinophilic pneumonia. Clinical manifestations include fever, night sweats, weight loss, and progressive dyspnea. Most patients are white women with a history of recent-onset nonatopic asthma. The classic x-ray shows widespread shadows in a peripheral distribution (Fig 40–1), described as the "photographic negative" of that produced by pulmonary edema, although localized nonsegmental transient or migratory infiltrates are also found. Chest computed tomography may reveal predominant peripheral airspace consolidation even when the x-ray does not. Glucocorticoid therapy produces prompt remission of this potentially fatal disease, but relapses are common after discontinuation of treatment.

Allergic Granulomatosis of Churg and Strauss

This disease typically begins with upper respiratory symptoms of rhinitis and sinusitis followed by asthma and marked peripheral blood eosinophilia, with concurrent or subsequent pulmonary infiltrates. This is followed by evidence of a systemic vasculitis that may involve the heart, skin, and peripheral nerves. The kidneys are spared or only mildly involved. Mononeuritis multiplex is common, but polyneuropathy also occurs. Treatment requires glucocorticoids in this previously fatal disease; in re-

sistant cases, immunosuppressants such as cyclophosphamide or azathioprine are needed.

Simple Idiopathic Pulmonary Eosinophilia (Loeffler's Syndrome)

This is the name that has been applied to a self-limited, relatively mild illness with transient or migratory pulmonary infiltrates and peripheral eosinophilia regardless of etiology. Current usage arguably applies the term Loeffler's syndrome to simple pulmonary eosinophilia of unknown cause; similar manifestations due to drugs or parasites are better classified under specific etiology.

The condition is expected to resolve within a month, so the patient with minimal symptoms does not require treatment.

Acute Eosinophilic Pneumonia

This is an acute form of eosinophilic lung disease considered to be distinct from previously described syndromes. It was first reported by two groups in 1989. Specific features include (1) acute febrile illness, (2) severe hypoxemia, (3) diffuse infiltrates on the chest x-ray, (4) over 25% eosinophils in bronchoalveolar lavage fluid, (5) no pulmonary or systemic infection, (6) no history of asthma or atopic illness, (7) prompt response to glucocorticoid therapy, and (8) complete resolution with no sequelae. Distinctive features are the rapid development of se-

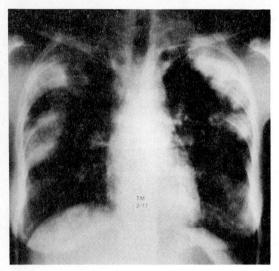

A

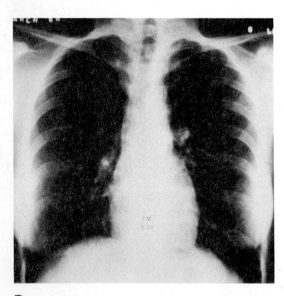

B

Figure 40–1. Chest x-ray of a patient with chronic idiopathic (Carrington's) eosinophilic pneumonia, showing peripheral distribution of infiltrates during the active phase of the disease **(A)** and resolution of the lesions within days of starting glucocorticoid therapy **(B).**

vere dyspnea and hypoxemia (PO$_2$ 46–58 mm Hg) within a few days of onset of an acute febrile illness in a previously healthy subject. Lung biopsy has shown diffuse alveolar edema, intra-alveolar and interstitial eosinophils, and no vasculitis.

Eosinophilia-Myalgia Syndrome

This syndrome is included here because it may present with pulmonary infiltrates and peripheral blood eosinophilia. The most notable clinical features are severe disabling myalgias, muscle weakness, skin rash, and soft tissue induration resembling scleroderma. This syndrome is associated with the ingestion of L-tryptophan (containing one or more contaminants) used in large doses as a dietary supplement.

Drug-Induced Eosinophilic Pneumonias

Pulmonary diseases induced by drugs and involving suspected immunologic mechanisms are described above. Those commonly associated with eosinophilic pneumonia are listed in Table 40–3. Nitrofurantoin may produce acute or chronic eosinophilic pneumonia, whereas most incriminated drugs produce acute syndromes beginning within a month of the institution of therapy. Treatment involves withdrawal of the drug with or without glucocorticoid therapy.

Parasite-Induced Eosinophilic Pneumonias

Eosinophilia is characteristic of all invasive helminthic infestations. Those that remain localized to the intestinal tract and cause minimal inflammatory lesions produce little if any eosinophilia; examples include oxyuriasis (pinworm) and trichuriasis (whip-

Table 40–3. Eosinophilic pneumonias secondary to drugs and parasites.

Drugs	
Ampicillin	Naproxen
Aspirin	Nickel
Arsenicals	Nitrofurantoin
Beclomethasone	Aminosalicylic acid
Bleomycin	Penicillamine
Carbamazepine	Penicillin
Chlorpromazine	Phenothiazine
Chlorpropamide	Propylthiourasil
Clofibrate	Phenylbutazone
Cromolyn	Streptomycin
Dilantin	Suflasalazine
Gold salts	Sulfonamide
Hydralazine	Tetracycline
Imipramine	Thiazide
Mephenesin	Tolazamide
Methotrexate	Tricyclic antidepressants
Methylphenidate	

Parasites
Ancyclostoma braziliense (hookworm)
Ancyclostoma duodenale (hookworm)
Ascaris species (roundworm)
Brugia malayi
Dirofilaria immitis (dog heartworm)
Fasciola hepatica (liver fluke)
Necator americanus (hookworm)
Schistosoma species (blood flukes)
Strongyloides stercoralis
Taenia saginata (beef tapeworm)
Toxocara canis (dog roundworm)
Toxocara cati (cat heartworm)
Trichinella spiralis
Trichuris trichiura (whipworm)
Wuchereria bancrofti

worm). Encystment of larval forms may be followed by disappearance of eosinophilia. Protozoan infestations (malaria, amebiasis, giardiasis, toxoplasmosis, leishmaniasis, trypanosomiasis) are not usually accompanied by eosinophilia. Thus, parasite-induced eosinophilic pneumonias are limited to tissue-invasive stages of helminthic parasites trafficking through the lung. Documented examples are listed in Table 40–3.

Visceral larva migrans most commonly affects young children and is caused by infection with the dog and cat ascarids, *Toxocara canis* and *T cati,* respectively; the raccoon ascarid *Bayliascaris procyonsis,* hookworm, and *Strongyloides stercoralis* are occasionally responsible. Clinical manifestations are due to free migration of larvae in the liver, lungs, brain, eyes, heart, and skeletal muscles, causing inflammation, eosinophilia, and, eventually, granuloma formation. Patients are often asymptomatic but may present with fever, hepatomegaly, splenomegaly, skin rash, and recurrent pneumonia.

Tropical pulmonary eosinophilia is associated with microfilarial infection (*Wuchereria bancrofti* and *Brugia malayi*) and is characterized by fever, weight loss, fatigue, dyspnea, wheezing, and cough, which are usually worse at night. The disease is seen mainly in India, Southeast Asia, and South Pacific islands. Treatment with diethylcarbamazine is usually successful, but progressive fibrosis has been reported following inadequate eradication of the organisms.

Hypereosinophilic Syndrome

Diagnostic criteria for this idiopathic condition include (1) persistent eosinophilia greater than 1500 eosinophils/mm^3 for longer than 6 months; (2) lack of other known causes of eosinophilia; (3) systemic involvement of the heart, liver, spleen, central nervous system, or lungs. Fever, weight loss, and anemia are common. The heart is frequently involved, with tricuspid valve abnormalities and biventricular restrictive and obliterative cardiomyopathy. Treatment is aimed at lowering the eosinophil count. Some patients progress with morphologic, cytologic, and karyotypic features of eosinophilic leukemia.

OCCUPATIONAL AND ENVIRONMENTAL LUNG DISEASES

Indoor air quality has become an increasingly important issue for workplace and home environments. For the most part, immune-mediated occupational and environmental diseases involving the lung are either asthma (Chapter 25) or hypersensitivity pneumonitis (Chapter 28). The environmental antigens associated with these disorders make up long and growing lists.

In addition to asthma and hypersensitivity pneumonitis, environmental exposures may result in non-immunologic disorders, such as the organic dust toxic syndrome (discussed above) or the sick building syndrome.

The **sick building syndrome** has symptoms of cough, irritation of the nose or throat, headache, fatigue, and difficulty concentrating. Investigations of outbreaks of these and other symptoms reported by workers in modern office buildings determine a specific cause, such as accumulation of toxic gases or contaminated humidification systems, in only about 25% of cases. Inadequate ventilation with outdoor air has also been reported.

SARCOIDOSIS

Major Immunologic Features

- T cell-mediated hypersensitivity to various skin test antigens is lost (anergy).
- T lymphocytes are activated, with cytokine release at foci of disease.
- There is CD4 lymphocytic alveolitis from a proliferation of local lymphocytes and chemotaxis of blood T-lymphocytes.
- There is granuloma formation.
- Polyclonal gammopathy is found.

General Considerations

Sarcoidosis is a multisystem granulomatous disease of unknown origin; it occurs most commonly in young adults. There appears to be a higher prevalence of this disease in the black population. It is characterized by a lymphocytic alveolitis and/or noncaseating granulomas involving multiple systems. Pulmonary manifestations occur in more than 90% of patients. Cutaneous, ocular, or hepatic manifestations are also common.

Immunologic Pathogenesis

The assumed inciting antigen of this disorder is unknown. Once the antigen is processed by monocytes or macrophages, however, a well-described cascade of immune-mediated events begins. The macrophage initially presents antigen to antigen-specific T lymphocytes, becomes activated, and produces interleukin-1. This in turn activates the CD4 lymphocyte to release interleukin-2, which results in the presence of a large number of T cells at the site of disease through 2 mechanisms: (1) chemotaxis (the attraction of T cells from the circulation to sites of granuloma formation) and (2) mitogenesis (the stimulation of T cells to proliferate at sites of granuloma formation). This compartmentalization of inflammatory cells in sites of disease results in peripheral blood lymphocytopenia and a CD4 lymphocyte-rich alveolitis. The activated T cells found at the periphery of the granuloma play an important role in the pathogenesis of this disorder by releasing a number of lymphokines. One of these, a monocyte chemotactic factor, attracts monocytes that are essential building blocks of the granuloma. Most components of the granuloma (macrophages, epithelioid cells, and multinucleated giant cells) are derived from blood monocytes. Other lymphokines activate macrophages and inhibit macrophage migration.

Activated T cells at sites of granuloma formation are probably responsible for the polyclonal gammopathy sometimes found in sarcoid. T cell-B cell interactions release B cell growth factor and B cell differentiation factor, which nonspecifically activate B cells to differentiate into immunoglobulin-secreting plasma cells.

Clinical Features

Acute sarcoidosis may present with fever, erythema nodosum, iritis, and polyarthritis; this combination of symptoms strongly suggests the presence of this disorder. Most often, however, patients note the insidious onset of fatigue, weight loss, malaise, weakness, anorexia, fever, sweats, nonproductive cough, and progressive exertional dyspnea. Patients may also be asymptomatic, diagnosed only by the presence of an abnormality on a routine chest x-ray. (Fig 40–2; Table 40–4). Pulmonary function studies may be normal or may reveal evidence of a restrictive lung disease characterized by loss of lung volume, decreased diffusing capacity, and exercise-induced hypoxemia. Up to 40% of patients have an obstructive ventilatory defect secondary to airway involvement.

Diagnosis

The diagnosis can be established by the following criteria: (1) a compatible clinical picture; (2) histologic evidence of a systemic granulomatous disease

Table 40–4. Chest radiography in sarcoidosis.

Type	Description
0	Normal
I	Bilateral hilar adenopathy alone
II	Hilar adenopathy and parenchymal abnormalities
III	Parenchymal abnormalities without hilar adenopathy

compatible with sarcoidosis; and (3) no evidence of exposure to an agent that is known to cause granulomatous disease. The disorder is also frequently associated with a peripheral-blood T lymphocytopenia, anergy to a panel of skin tests for cellular immunity, hypergammaglobulinemia, circulating immune complexes, increased serum angiotensin-converting enzyme activity, and increased numbers of macrophages and CD4 T cells in bronchoalveolar lavage fluid. These findings suggest but are not specific for sarcoidosis. The Kveim test, a cutaneous hypersensitivity test formerly used to diagnose sarcoidosis, is largely of historical interest owing to the unavailability of the antigen and to the availability of other diagnostic tests.

Differential Diagnosis

Sarcoidosis must be differentiated from a variety of granulomatous diseases, including various infectious diseases, hypersensitivity pneumonitis, berylliosis, drug reactions, and neoplasms such as lymphomas. Type III sarcoidosis must also be distinguished from the large number of other interstitial lung disorders.

Treatment & Prognosis

The overall prognosis is favorable, with the likelihood of spontaneous remission somewhat linked to the stage of the disease. Patients with a type 0 or I chest x-ray have a very good prognosis with a greater than 80% chance of spontaneous remission, whereas those with type II or III chest x-ray have a less favorable prognosis. Treatment with corticosteroids is normally reserved for symptomatic pulmonary disease; systemic involvement of the eyes, myocardium, and central nervous system; disfiguring skin lesions; and hypercalcemia.

IDIOPATHIC PULMONARY FIBROSIS

Major Immunologic Features

- Immune complexes can be found in the blood and in the lungs.
- Immune complexes may stimulate macrophages to release neutrophilic chemoattractants, oxidants, and growth signals for mesenchymal cells.
- T cells may direct lung B cells to produce "autoim-

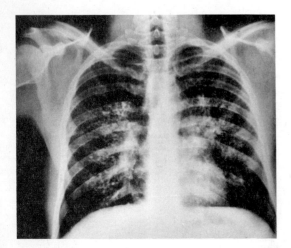

Figure 40–2. Chest x-ray of a patient with sarcoidosis (type II) showing bilateral hilar and parenchymal fibronodular infiltrates.

mune" antibodies and mediate cellular immune processes directed against lung parenchymal cells.

General Considerations

Although there is a rare familial form of the disease, idiopathic pulmonary fibrosis is, for the most part, an interstitial lung disease of unknown origin. Since the diagnosis is one of exclusion, a patient must have no history of exposure to environmental inorganic dusts or toxic fumes known to cause interstitial lung disease. This diagnosis also excludes underlying conditions such as sarcoidosis, eosinophilic granuloma, and collagen vascular disease. Pulmonary fibrosis secondary to lung infections and drugs are also excluded. Although some patients respond to treatment with corticosteroid or cytotoxic drug therapy, most patients die within 5 years.

Immunologic Pathogenesis

The trigger of this disorder is still unknown. It is known, however, that immune complexes are present in serum and in the lungs in the early, active phase of the disease. Although these immune complexes may trigger an inflammatory process in the lungs by activating the complement cascade, there is no evidence to date that this process actually occurs in the lungs. Immune complexes in the lungs, however, stimulate alveolar macrophages to release various factors that may play a role in the pathogenesis of this disorder. One such factor released by alveolar macrophages is leukotriene B_4 (LTB_4), a lipid chemotactic factor that attracts neutrophils and eosinophils. The alveolar macrophages also release oxidants, which injure the pulmonary epithelium, and a variety of growth factors for fibroblasts, which increase the numbers of fibroblasts in the lungs and hence leads to the deposition of collagen. These observations are consistent with the pathologic features of the disease: increased numbers of polymorphonuclear leukocytes and generalized fibrosis of the lung parenchyma.

Clinical Features

Although patients at any age can be affected by this disease, the average age at diagnosis is 60 years. The disease has an insidious onset, with patients often noting symptoms for weeks to months before seeking medical attention. The usual presenting symptoms are progressive dyspnea on exertion and a nonproductive cough. Constitutional symptoms such as fatigue, weight loss, malaise, and arthralgias are not uncommon. Physical examination reveals dry bibasilar crackles ("Velcro rales"), and there may be clubbing of the digits. In advanced cases, cyanosis and evidence of cor pulmonale may be present. The chest x-ray shows interstitial fibrosis predominantly in the basilar areas of the lungs. Honeycombing of the lungs occurs in later stages. Pulmonary-function testing shows a restrictive defect with decreases in lung volumes and diffusing capacity. Arterial blood gases show normal or slightly decreased oxygen tension, which may fall significantly with exertion.

Diagnosis

Because this is a diagnosis of exclusion, there are no definitive or specific confirmatory tests. Serologic abnormalities may include positive tests for antinuclear antibodies or rheumatoid factor, increased amounts of immunoglobulins, and circulating immune complexes. Various immunologic tests are used primarily to exclude the presence of other interstitial lung disorders. Pathologic abnormalities often reveal wide variability among patients. Even when several biopsy specimens are taken from an individual patient, pathologic heterogeneity is not uncommon, suggesting that lung injury can occur at different stages. The histologic pattern varies from an acute alveolitis with desquamation of type II pneumocytes and macrophages to an acellular stage with marked distortion of lung architecture and fibrosis. Some pathologists attempt to classify the alveolitis by the predominant cell type (eg, lymphocytic interstitial pneumonitis). Bronchoscopy with biopsy and lavage is often used to exclude other causes of chronic interstitial lung disease. Bronchoalveolar lavage reveals increased numbers of both alveolar macrophages and polymorphonuclear leukocytes; the most characteristic feature is an increased percentage of both neutrophils and eosinophils. Since the histology of bronchoscopically obtained specimens is often nonspecific, an open or transthoracic thoracoscopic lung biopsy is usually necessary to exclude other disorders (eg, granulomatous infections, sarcoidosis, or bronchiolitis with obstructive pneumonia) and select the patients most likely to respond to treatment.

Differential Diagnosis

The differential diagnosis includes a large number of interstitial lung diseases of both known and unknown origin (Table 40–5). The principal considerations, however, include sarcoidosis, hypersensitivity pneumonitis, interstitial lung disease associated with collagen vascular diseases, and interstitial lung disease associated with certain inorganic dust exposures.

Table 40–5. Differential diagnosis of idiopathic pulmonary fibrosis.

Aspiration pneumonia
Collagen vascular diseases
Drugs (antibiotics and chemotherapy)
Eosinophilic lung syndromes
Histiocytosis X
Hypersensitivity pneumonitis
Infections (mycobacterial, viral, or fungal)
Lymphocytic interstitial diseases
Noxious gases (eg, oxides of nitrogen)
Pneumoconioses
Radiation
Sarcoidosis

Treatment & Prognosis

Therapy is directed at suppressing active inflammation (alveolitis) and thus preventing further loss of function. High doses of corticosteroids may result in improvement and stabilization of pulmonary functions in approximately 20% of patients. Cytotoxic drugs have also been reported to benefit some patients. Unfortunately, despite treatment with corticosteroids or cytotoxic drugs, there is only a 50% survival at 5 years. Most recently, there has been some enthusiasm for single-lung transplantation in patients who respond poorly to medical trials. Supplemental oxygen, particularly during periods of exercise, allows for a more active lifestyle.

GOODPASTURE'S SYNDROME

Major Immunologic Features

- This syndrome is a type II cytotoxic antibody-mediated process.
- It is associated with circulating anti-glomerular basement membrane (anti-GBM) antibodies.
- There are linear deposits of immunoglobulin (principally IgG) and complement (C3) along the basement membrane of renal glomeruli and pulmonary alveoli.

General Considerations

Goodpasture's syndrome, a disease of unknown origin, is characterized by the triad of pulmonary hemorrhage, glomerulonephritis, and circulating antibody to basement membrane antigens. Intrapulmonary hemorrhage may be insignificant or may be severe and life-threatening. Renal involvement is commonly rapidly progressive, with oliguric renal failure occurring within weeks to months of the clinical onset of the disease. Without early treatment, permanent renal failure is the rule.

Immunologic Pathogenesis

In more than 90% of cases, circulating anti-GBM antibodies can be demonstrated early in the course of the disease. These antibodies are directed against renal tubular, renal glomerular, and pulmonary alveolar basement membranes. Immunofluorescence techniques can demonstrate that these tissues contain antibody deposited in a characteristic linear pattern, often accompanied by C3 deposition (see Fig 36–1). In a type II cytotoxic hypersensitivity reaction, antibody bound to basement membrane activates the complement cascade, resulting in the generation of chemotactic factors for various inflammatory cells. The inflammatory cells subsequently destroy the renal tubular, renal glomerular, and pulmonary alveolar basement membranes via the release of various reactive oxygen species and proteolytic enzymes. Recent studies demonstrate that the membrane antigenic site is probably a component of type IV collagen.

Clinical Features

Goodpasture's syndrome occurs predominantly in young males, often following a viral infection. Pulmonary manifestations include pulmonary hemorrhage with or without hemoptysis, dyspnea, weakness, fatigue, and cough. Recurrent pulmonary hemorrhage may result in iron deficiency anemia. The chest x-ray reveals diffuse or patchy opacities which have a confluent or acinar pattern. The pattern may change in intensity depending upon the degree of intra-alveolar hemorrhage (Fig 40–3). Bronchoalveolar lavage produces hemosiderin-laden macrophages with or without erythrocytes. Renal involvement is suggested by gross or microscopic hematuria and variable amounts of proteinuria, a decreased 24-hour urine creatinine clearance, and an increase in blood urea and serum creatinine.

Differential Diagnosis

Pulmonary hemorrhage with renal failure may be seen in Wegener's granulomatosis, systemic lupus erythematosus, polyarteritis nodosa, and renal vein thrombosis with pulmonary embolism. These disorders lack the constellation of clinical, pathologic, and immunologic features on which the diagnosis of Goodpasture's syndrome is based.

Treatment & Prognosis

Since the disorder may be rapidly fatal, it is imperative that it be diagnosed and treated promptly. Treatment is directed at removal of circulating anti-GBM antibody, modulation of the inflammatory response, and suppression of new antibody synthesis. This has been effectively orchestrated with plasma exchange to remove anti-GBM antibodies and immunosuppressive agents (corticosteroids and cytotoxic drugs) to

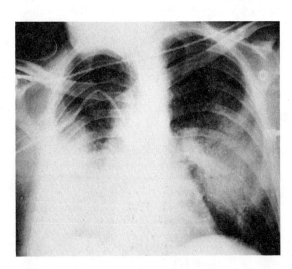

Figure 40–3. Chest x-ray of a patient with Goodpasture's syndrome, showing extensive bilateral pulmonary infiltrates typical of intra-alveolar hemorrhage.

suppress inflammation and new antibody formation. If instituted early in the course of the disease, this type of therapy may halt the progression of the disease and maintain renal function. A number of factors influence the response to treatment. The initial serum creatinine level and the percentage of crescents noted on the original renal biopsy are the best predictors of recovery: the prognosis for recovery is poor when the serum creatinine is >5 mg/dl and when crescents are present in >50% of glomeruli. Bacterial infections during the recovery period are often associated with relapse. For patients with end-stage renal disease, renal transplantation has been successful after the disappearance of the circulating anti-GBM antibodies. Unfortunately, involvement of the new kidney has occasionally been reported following renal transplantation. Mortality is associated with respiratory failure secondary to pulmonary hemorrhage, complications of renal failure, and infection.

PULMONARY VASCULITIS SYNDROMES

Granulomatous and nongranulomatous vasculitides of unknown etiology affecting the lung are listed in Table 40–6, along with conditions presenting as pulmonary-renal syndromes. Some are discussed fully elsewhere in this chapter or in other chapters.

Wegener's Granulomatosis

This is discussed in Chapter 34. The diagnosis and follow-up of disease activity in Wegener's granulomatosis has been facilitated by the discovery of antineutrophil cytoplasmic antibodies (ANCA), which are occasionally positive in other vasculitic syndromes.

Lymphomatoid Granulomatosis

This was described as a new entity in 1972 and has frequently been confused with Wegener's granulomatosis. Later studies recognized lymphomatoid granulomatosis, involving primarily the lungs, and **polymorphic reticulosis** (or lethal midline granuloma), involving primarily the nose and paranasal sinuses, as histopathologic entities. Both lymphomatoid granulomatosis and polymorphic reticulosis can involve other tissues including the skin, central nervous system, and abdominal organs, and both may result in malignant lymphoma. Radiation therapy is successful at treating localized disease.

Clinical manifestations of lymphomatoid granulomatosis include cough, fever, and dyspnea. Most patients are in early middle age, and men predominate. Pulmonary lesions are commonly in the lower lung fields bilaterally in a peripheral location without hilar adenopathy, and they tend to wax and wane. Skin lesions occur in one-half of the patients. Glomerulonephritis is absent, but nodular renal lesions occur. Nervous system involvement is common and may include central nervous system dysfunction and peripheral neuropathies. Treatment with cyclophosphamide and prednisone has been somewhat successful, but about 50% of patients die of malignant lymphoma.

Small-Vessel Vasculitides

These are discussed in Chapters 31 and 34. As a group, they usually present with cutaneous lesions. The lung is involved uncommonly, with the possible exception of essential mixed cryoglobulinemia that may present with interstitial pneumonitis and symptoms of asthma, hemoptysis, or pleuritis.

Collagen-Vascular Diseases

These diseases, including their effects on the lung, are discussed in Chapter 31.

PULMONARY MANIFESTATIONS OF IMMUNODEFICIENCY

Immunodeficiency diseases and disorders, including AIDS, are covered elsewhere in this volume (Chapters 19–23 and 52). These diseases increase the risk of specific pulmonary infections, depending largely on the type of defect in the immunocompromised host. Impaired antibody formation or complement deficiency predisposes patients to pneumonia caused by pyogenic organisms, chiefly *Streptococcus pneumoniae* and *Haemophilus influenzae*. Compromise of cellular immunity leads to increased risks for infections with mycobacteria and *Nocardia;* fungi such as *Pneumocystis carinii* (formerly classified as a protozoan), *Candida,* and agents of systemic mycoses; herpes viruses, vaccinia virus, and measles virus; and parasites including *Toxoplasma gondii* and *Strongyloides stercoralis.* Defects in granulocytes commonly result in staphylococcal abscesses that may involve the lung.

Table 40–6. Granulomatous and nongranulomatous vasculitis syndromes affecting the lung.

Granulomatosis-angiitis syndromes
  Wegener's granulomatosis
  Lymphomatoid granulomatosis
  Allergic granulomatosis of Churg and Strauss
  Sarcoidal vasculitis
Small-vessel vasculitis
  Leukocytoclastic angiitis
  Henoch-Schönlein purpura
  Essential mixed cryoglobulinemia
  Behcet's disease
  Collagen-vascular disease
Pulmonary-renal syndromes
  Goodpasture's syndrome
  Wegener's granulomatosis
  Lymphomatoid granulomatosis
  Allergic granulomatosis of Churg and Strauss
  Systemic lupus erythematosus
  Progressive systemic sclerosis (scleroderma)

LUNG TRANSPLANTATION

Major Immunologic Features
- Class II major histocompatibility complex (MHC) antigens are expressed on bronchiolar epithelium.
- Recipient's helper T lymphocytes are activated when chronic graft rejection occurs.

General Consideration
With the improvement in surgical techniques and a better understanding of the pathogenesis and treatment of rejection and infection, heart-lung transplantation and single-lung transplantation have become life-saving options for patients with end-stage pulmonary hypertension, cystic fibrosis, idiopathic pulmonary fibrosis, and selected cases of chronic obstructive pulmonary disease. The major threats to the success of these procedures have been related to reperfusion injury, airway anastomosis failure, hemorrhage, infection, and rejection. Chronic rejection causing airway obstruction secondary to obliterative bronchiolitis is now recognized as a significant complication in up to 50% of patients. Early recognition and treatment of chronic rejection and infection may improve long-term survival.

Immunologic Pathogenesis
Although initial triggers and subsequent immune mechanisms responsible for obliterative bronchiolitis are poorly understood, one hypothesis is that some inhaled stimulus (possibly viral) may induce HLA-DR antigens on bronchiolar epithelium. These class II MHC antigens would then be recognized by the patient's T lymphocytes as foreign, and their activation would subsequently mediate the rejection process. Substances such as gamma interferon, known to induce HLA-DR expression, may play an active role in this process. Pathologically, one sees the characteristic pattern of perivascular lymphocytic infiltrates and mucosal inflammation with lymphocytic bronchiolitis.

Clinical Features
The process of obliterative bronchiolitis secondary to chronic rejection takes a mean of 14 months to develop but can occur as early as 2 months posttransplant. Initial symptoms are bronchitic in nature, with cough and mucopurulent sputum production. Dyspnea follows within months. At this point a chest x-ray is normal in 60% of cases, but high-resolution computed tomography of the chest may reveal peribronchial infiltrates. Serial pulmonary function testing has proved valuable in detecting the onset of this process. Consistent, progressive reduction in vital capacity (VC), total lung capacity (TLC), and forced expiratory volume in 1 second (FEV_1) is the rule. The fall in flow rates is usually not responsive to bronchodilators. Hypoxemia and mild decrease in diffusion are common.

Diagnosis
It was initially hoped that serial bronchoalveolar lavage might predict early rejection by changes in the cellular and phenotypic analyses. Unfortunately, increasing cell counts, increased numbers of activated CD4 cells, and increased CD4/CD8 ratios have not proved to be sufficiently discriminating. The use of serial transbronchial biopsies is currently the best method for confirming early rejection, with sensitivities ranging from 70 to 84% and specificities of 100%. These bronchoscopic procedures have been successful in differentiating opportunistic infection from rejection.

Differential Diagnosis
The usual diagnostic dilemma centers on differentiating opportunistic infection from chronic rejection. This can be difficult since certain viruses (eg, cytomegalovirus) are known to play a role in acute and chronic rejection. Other causes of obliterative bronchiolitis include toxic injury from the oxides of nitrogen, hypersensitivity pneumonitis, lung injury secondary to collagen vascular diseases (particularly rheumatoid arthritis and Sjögren's syndrome), and small-airway involvement by various infections.

Treatment & Prognosis
During the early postoperative period, patients are treated prophylactically with cyclosporin, azathioprine, and antilymphocyte globulin to decrease the chance of rejection. Corticosteroids may be used briefly, although they are usually withheld to allow for anastomotic healing. Signs of rejection are treated with high-dose corticosteroids, cyclosporin, and azathioprine. Early treatment has significantly reduced the morbidity of airway obstruction and the mortality of respiratory failure.

ADULT RESPIRATORY DISTRESS SYNDROME

General Considerations
The adult respiratory distress syndrome (ARDS) is a form of acute lung injury characterized by noncardiogenic pulmonary edema from increased vascular permeability. It can occur in the setting of a wide variety of clinical conditions including sepsis, gastric acid aspiration, pancreatitis, trauma, fat emboli syndrome, and central nervous system insult.

Diagnosis
In the proper clinical setting, a diagnosis of ARDS is made when there are diffuse, bilateral infiltrates on chest x-ray (consistent with pulmonary edema), no

evidence of increased pulmonary capillary hydrostatic pressure (this usually requires placement of a pulmonary artery catheter), and refractory hypoxemia that cannot be corrected by high concentrations of oxygen. Despite recent improvements in supportive care, the mortality rate continues to remain as high as 60–70%. In most instances, mortality is not due solely to hypoxemia but instead results from the combined failure of multiple organ systems.

Immunologic Pathogenesis

The most common pathogenetic mechanism is the activation of the complement system with recruitment and sequestration of neutrophils in pulmonary interstitial capillaries. A number of cytokines released from macrophages may play a significant role in the recruitment of neutrophils. Tumor necrosis factor alpha (TNFα) is probably the most important cytokine to be synthesized in response to endotoxin. The actual amount of TNFα released is modulated by the metabolites of arachidonic acid (PGE$_2$). In the capillaries, neutrophils responding to these signals accumulate and release a number of toxic products including oxygen free radicals and proteases, which cause endothelial-cell damage, interstitial and intra-alveolar edema, hemorrhage, and fibrin deposition.

Treatment

A better understanding of the mediators of the inflammatory process has led to the development of a number of new therapeutic approaches for clinical trials. These treatments include receptor antagonists and monoclonal antibodies directed at specific mediators. These can potentially modulate the cascade of events associated with ARDS and reduce the mortality of this syndrome. At present, treatment of patients with adult respiratory distress syndrome is supportive.

ALLERGIC ASTHMA

Asthma has been classified as extrinsic or atopic asthma due to inhalation of common inhalant allergens (house dust mite, mold spores, pollens, animal danders), occupational asthma secondary to sensitization to a variety of allergens including simple chemicals acting as haptens, and idiopathic or intrinsic asthma of unknown cause. Asthma as an allergic disease is discussed in Chapter 25.

HYPERSENSITIVITY PNEUMONITIS

Hypersensitivity pneumonitis (extrinsic allergic alveolitis) is a pulmonary and constitutional illness that is due to an immunologic reaction to a variety of inhaled antigens. Diagnosis has often been confused with a condition called organic dust toxic syndrome that includes grain fever caused by inhalation of endotoxin, mycotoxins, or other agents. Sensitization is not required, and the lung may or may not be affected. These diseases are discussed in Chapter 28.

ALLERGIC BRONCHOPULMONARY ASPERGILLOSIS

Allergic bronchopulmonary aspergillosis (ABPA) usually presents as an eosinophilic pneumonia in patients with long-standing atopic asthma, is associated with allergy to *Aspergillus fumigatus* or occasionally other fungi, may complicate cystic fibrosis, and leads to proximal bronchiectasis and irreversible airways obstruction. It is discussed in Chapter 27.

REFERENCES

Drug-Induced Respiratory Diseases
Fulkerson WJ, Gockerman JP: Pulmonary disease induced by drugs. Pages 793–811 in: *Pulmonary Diseases and Disorders,* 2nd ed. AP Fishman (editor). McGraw-Hill, 1988.
Israel-Biet D, Labrune S, Huction GJ: Drug-induced lung disease: 1990 review. *Eur Respir J* 1991;**4**:465.
Rosenow EC III et al: Drug-induced pulmonary disease. *Chest* 1992;**102**:239.

Eosinophilic Pneumonias
Allen JN et al: Acute eosinophilic pneumonia as a reversible cause of noninfectious respiratory failure. *N Engl J Med* 1989;**321**:569.

Helfgott SM et al: Case records of the Massachusetts General Hospital (Case 18–1992). *N Engl J Med* 1992;**326**:1204.
Lopez M, Salvaggio JE: Eosinophilic pneumonias. *Immunol Allergy Clin N Am* 1992;**12**:349.
Mayock RL, Iozzo RV: The eosinophilic pneumonias. Pages 683–698 in: *Pulmonary Diseases and Disorders,* 2nd ed. AP Fishman (editor). McGraw Hill, 1988.

Occupational & Environmental Lung Diseases
Epler GR: Clinical overview of occupational lung disease. *Radiol Clin N Am* 1992;**30**:1121.
Kreiss K: The sick building syndrome in office build-

ings: a breath of fresh air (editorial). *N Engl J Med* 1993;**328:**877.

Grammer LC, Patterson R: Occupational immunologic lung disease. *Ann Allergy* 1987;**58:**151.

Reed CE: Hypersensitivity pneumonitis and occupational lung disease from inhaled endotoxin. *Immunol Allergy Clinics N Am* 1992;**12:**819.

Sarcoidosis

Semenzato G et al: Cellular immunity in sarcoidosis and hypersensitivity pneumonitis. Recent advances. *Chest* 1993;**103(Suppl):**139S.

Thomas PD, Hunninghake GW: Current concepts of the pathogenesis of sarcoid. *Am Rev Respir Dis* 1987; **135:**747.

Winterbauer RH, Hammar SP: Chap 5, pp 117–164 in: *Sarcoidosis and Idiopathic Pulmonary Fibrosis: A Review of Recent Events.* Yearbook Medical Publishers, 1986.

Idiopathic Pulmonary Fibrosis

Cherniack RM, Crystal RG, Kalria AR: Current concepts in idiopathic pulmonary fibrosis: A road map for the future. *Am Rev Respir Dis* 1991;**143:**680.

duBois RM: Idiopathic pulmonary fibrosis. *Annu Rev Med* 1993;**44:**441.

Goodpasture's Syndrome

Johnson JP et al: Therapy of anti-glomerular basement membrane antibody disease: Analysis of prognostic significance of clinical, pathologic and treatment factors. *Medicine* 1985;**64:**219.

Wilson CB, Dixon FJ: Antiglomerular basement membrane antibody-induced glomerulonephritis. *Kidney Int* 1973;**3:**74.

Granulomatosis-Vasculitis Syndromes

Buschman DL, Waldron JA Jr, King TE Jr: Churg-Strauss pulmonary vasculitis. High-resolution computed tomography scanning and pathologic findings. *Am Rev Respir Dis* 1993;**142:**458.

DeRemee RA, Weiland LH, McDonald TJ: Polymorphic reticulosis, lymphomatoid granulomatosis: Two diseases or one? *Mayo Clin Proc* 1978;**53:**634.

Fauci AS et al: Lymphomatoid granulomatosis: Prospective clinical and therapeutic experience over 10 years. *N Engl J Med* 1982;**306:**68.

Israel HL, Patchefsky AS, Saldana MJ: Wegener's granulomatosis, lymphomatoid granulomatosis, and benign lymphocytic angiitis and granulomatosis of lung. *Ann Intern Med* 1977;**87:**691.

Leavitt RY, Fauci AS: Pulmonary vasculitis. *Am Rev Respir Dis* 1986;**134:**149.

Nölle B et al: Anticytoplasmic autoantibodies: Their immunodiagnostic value in Wegener granulomatosis. *Ann Intern Med* 1989;**111:**28.

Strauss L, Lieberman KV, Churg J: Pulmonary vasculitis. Pages 1127–1156 in: *Pulmonary Diseases and Disorders,* 2nd ed. AP Fishman (editor). McGraw-Hill, 1988.

Lung Transplantation

Bierman MI et al: Critical care management of lung transplant recipients. *J Intensive Care Med* 1991; **6:**135.

Burke CM et al: Lung immunogenicity, rejection, and obliterative bronchiolitis. *Chest* 1987;**92:**547.

Acute Respiratory Distress Syndrome

Lewis JF, Jobe AH: Surfactant and the adult respiratory distress syndrome: State of the art. *Am Rev Respir Dis* 1993;**147:**218.

Repine JE: Scientific perspectives on adult respiratory distress syndrome. *Lancet* 1992;**339:**466.

MacNaughton PD, Evans TW: Management of adult respiratory distress syndrome. *Lancet* 1992;**339:**469.

Rinaldo JE, Christman JW: Mechanisms and mediators of the adult respiratory distress syndrome. *Clin Chest Med* 1990;**11:**621.

The Mucosal Immune System

41

Warren Strober, MD, and Stephen P. James, MD

The mycosal immune system is composed of the lymphoid tissues that are associated with the mucosal surfaces of the gastrointestinal, respiratory, and urogenital tracts. It has evolved under the influence of the complex and distinctive antigenic array present in mucosal areas and may be distinguished from the systemic (internal) immune system by a number of features. These include (1) a mucosa-related immunoglobulin, IgA; (2) a complement of T cells with mucosa-specific regulatory properties or effector capabilities; and (3) a mucosa-oriented cell traffic system for cells initially induced in the mucosal follicles to migrate to the diffuse mucosal lymphoid tissues underlying the epithelium. This last feature leads to the partial segregation of mucosal cells from systemic cells; thus, the mucosal immune system is a somewhat separate immunologic entity.

FUNCTIONS

The primary function of the mucosal immune system is to provide for host defense at mucosal surfaces. In this role it operates in concert with several nonimmunologic protective factors, including (1) a resident bacterial flora that inhibits the growth of potential pathogens; (2) mucosal motor activity (peristalsis and ciliary function) that maintains the flow of mucosal constituents, reducing the interaction of potential pathogens with epithelial cells; (3) substances such as gastric acid and intestinal bile salts that create a mucosal microenvironment unfavorable to the growth of pathogens; (4) mucus secretions (glycocalyx) that form a barrier between potential pathogens and the epithelial surfaces; and, finally, (5) substances such as lactoferrin, lactoperoxidase, and lysozyme that have inhibitory effects on one or another specific microorganism. Optimal host defense at the mucosal surface depends on both intact mucosal immune responses and nonimmunologic protective functions. Thus, antibiotic therapy that elimi-

nates normal flora may result in infection, despite the existence of an intact immune system; mucosal infections are common in congenital and acquired immunodeficiency states even in the presence of normal nonimmunologic protective factors.

A second but equally important function of the mucosal immune system is to prevent the entry of mucosal antigens and thus protect the systemic immune system from inappropriate antigenic exposure. This occurs both at the mucosal surface, by preventing the entry of potentially antigenic materials, and in the circulation, by providing for the clearance of mucosal antigens via a hepatic clearance system. In addition, the mucosal immune system contains regulatory T cells that down regulate systemic immune responses to antigens which breach the mucosal barrier. Abnormalities of this aspect of mucosal immune function may be important in the development of autoimmunity.

ANATOMY

The mucosal immune system is a quantitatively important part of the immune system. The human gastrointestinal tract contains as much lymphoid tissue as the spleen does. The system can be morphologically and functionally subdivided into 2 major parts: (1) organized tissues consisting of the mucosal follicles (also called gut-associated lymphoid tissues [GALT] and bronchus-associated lymphoid tissues [BALT]) and (2) a diffuse lymphoid tissue consisting of the widely distributed cells located in the mucosal lamina propria (see Fig 41–1 and Chapter 2). The former (or organized) tissues are "afferent" lymphoid areas, whcre antigens enter the system and induce immune responses, and the latter or diffuse tissues are "efferent" lymphoid areas, where antigens interact with differentiated cells and cause the secretion of antibodies by B cells or induce cytotoxic reactions by T cells. As mentioned above, the 2 parts of the mucosal

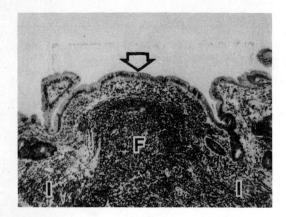

Figure 41–1. Histologic section of a human Peyer's patch lymphoid nodule from the terminal ileum. Antigens are taken up from the lumen through the follicle epithelium (arrow) for processing in the dome. The follicle (F) and its germinal center are composed largely of B cells. The interfollicular areas (I), composed of T cells, contain both high endothelial venules from which T lymphocytes enter follicles and lymphatics through which lymphocytes leave Peyer's patches. Magnification × 72. (Courtesy of Robert L. Owen.)

immune system are linked by a mucosal "homing" mechanism, so that sensitized cells from the lymphoid follicles travel to the diffuse lymphoid areas, where they can best interact with their inciting antigens. Finally, both the organized and the diffuse mucosal lymphoid areas are highly antigen-dependent; their numbers are remarkably reduced in germ-free states and expanded under conditions of increased antigenic stimulation.

Mucosal Lymphoid Aggregates

Mucosal lymphoid aggregates are morphologically different from those of the systemic lymphoid system. They receive antigen via the epithelium rather than through the lymphatic or blood circulation. More particularly, antigen enters through specialized epithelial cells called M cells (membranous cells) in the epithelium overlying the lymphoid aggregates (Fig 41–2).

A. M cells: M cells are flattened epithelial cells characterized by poorly developed brush borders, a thin glycocalyx, and a cytoplasm rich in pinocytotic vesicles, but they are virtually devoid of the proteolytic machinery found in absorptive epithelial cells. Antigen transport by M cells involves (1) initial binding to the M cell surface via as yet undefined binding sites, (2) uptake into pinocytotic vesicles, (3) vesicular transport across the cell body, and, finally, (4) release of material in an undegraded form into the subepithelial area. Such support is applicable to

widely disparate substances including particulates (viruses, bacteria, and protozoa) and soluble proteins. However, neither binding nor uptake is totally indiscriminate. For instance, there is some evidence that the transport of bacteria by M cells is inhibited by specific antibodies, which may interact with bacterial determinants necessary for binding to M cells. This fact may explain the lack of uptake of resident microorganisms into M cells. Furthermore, some organisms that bind to M cells are taken up, whereas others are not. The ability to be taken up by M cells may have an impact on the virulence of an organism. For example, viral binding to and uptake by M cells may be an obligate means of entry of the organism and therefore a positive virulence factor, whereas uptake leading to antibody formation and immune elimination of the organism has a negative impact on virulence.

B. Dome Cells: The area just below the epithelium of the lymphoid aggregate (the so-called dome area) is rich in cells bearing class II major histocompatibility complex (MHC) antigens (macrophages, dendritic cells, and B cells) and therefore is rich in cells capable of antigen presentation following exposure to antigens in vitro or via oral antigen feeding in vivo. For this reason, any lack of response following oral antigen administration is not due to a lack of antigen-presenting cells in mucosal lymphoid aggregates (see the discussion of oral unresponsiveness below). M cells do not bear class II MHC antigens and are therefore probably not involved in antigen presentation; on the other hand, absorptive epithelial cells, particularly in the presence of inflammation, do express class II MHC antigens and have been shown to have antigen-presenting function in vitro.

The dome areas also contain many T cells. Although most of these cells bear CD4, a number bear neither CD4 nor CD8. This latter population may correspond to the cells recently identified as contrasuppressor cells (see the discussion of IgA regulation below).

C. Follicles: Below the dome area is the follicular zone, which contains the germinal centers. B cells predominate in this region, although scattered T cells are also present. As in other germinal centers, the B cells are highly differentiated and bear surface IgD; however, unlike other germinal-center B cells, a large fraction (up to 40%) bear surface IgA. Thus, the lymphoid aggregates of the mucosal immune system form the site of IgA B cell development, but the mucosal follicle is conspicuous for the absence of the terminally differentiated IgA B cells (IgA plasma cells), presumably because such cells leave the follicle before differentiating into plasma cells. The interfollicular areas between and around the follicles are also rich in T cells; most of the small population of CD8 T cells in mucosal lymphoid aggregates are found in these areas.

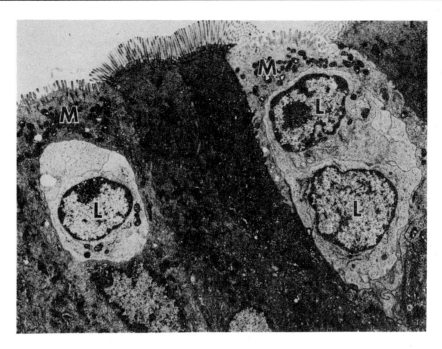

Figure 41–2. Transmission electron micrograph of the epithelium of a rat Peyer's patch lymphoid follicle. M cells (M) have short, irregularly shaped microvilli and surround intraepithelial lymphoid cells (L). Magnification × 6300. (Courtesy of Robert L. Owen.)

Diffuse Mucosal Lymphoid Tissue

The diffuse lymphoid tissues of the mucosal immune system consist of cell populations present in 2 separate compartments: the **intraepithelial lymphocyte (IEL) compartment** and the **lamina propria lymphocyte (LPL) compartment.**

A. Intraepithelial Lymphocytes: The IEL are, as the name implies, a population of cells lying above the basement membrane, among the epithelial cells. Although this population is numerically smaller than the lamina propria cell population, it is nonetheless considerable, there being 6–40 IEL/100 epithelial cells under normal conditions and a larger number in various inflammatory states. The IEL population is phenotypically heterogeneous, consisting for the most part of CD3 and CD2 T cells that are also predominately of the CD8 phenotype. Recently it has been shown that proliferation of human IEL can be induced by stimulation of these cells via the CD2 receptor but not the T cell receptor. The reason for such activation requirements is as yet unknown.

Studies with mice suggest that IEL have specialized immune effector functions, including natural killer (NK) cell activity, specific cell cytotoxicity, secretion of gamma interferon (IFN γ) with an increase in epithelial cell expression of class II MHC antigens, and expression of γ/δ T cell receptors.

B. Lamina Propria Lymphocytes: The lymphocyte population beneath the epithelial layer in the lamina propria, the LPL, is distinguished from the IEL population in being about equally divided between B cells and T cells. The B cell population is dominated by IgA B cells (and plasma cells), but IgM, IgG, and IgE B cells (and plasma cells) are also present (in descending order of frequency). In IgA deficiency, IgM rather than IgA cells are the predominant cells in the gastrointestinal mucosa and the number of IgG B cells is not increased; on the other hand, in various inflammatory diseases of the mucosa (eg, ulcerative colitis), the population of B cells producing each of the isotypes, particularly those producing IgG, is increased. In both normal and diseased mucosal tissue, the B cell population is composed of cells that display spontaneous immunoglobulin secretion in vitro.

The mucosal T cell population is composed of both CD4 and CD8 cells, with the former being twice as numerous as the latter, just as in peripheral blood. Recent evidence suggests that these cells have undergone prior activation. That is supported by the findings that lamina propria T cells contain IL-2 receptor (IL-2R) mRNA, have increased class II MHC and IL-2R expression, and have high expression of mRNA for IL-2 and IFN γ. Activated CD4 T cells act as helper cells in vitro; it is not surprising that the CD4 lamina propria T cells provide more help and less suppression than do the corresponding CD4 cells in other tissues. These findings and recent data that CD4 lamina propria T cells respond to specific antigens by secreting "helper" lymphokines rather than by proliferating have led to the concept that lamina propria T cells are a class of memory T cells.

Lamina Propria Macrophages

Cells with typical macrophage morphology are found in the diffuse mucosal areas throughout the mucosal immune system. In these areas they tend to be concentrated in the more superficial parts of the mucosa just below the epithelium. They may derive from the mucosal lymphoid aggregates (as do mucosal lymphocytes), because cells with monocyte morphology are found in the intestinal lymphatics that drain the intestinal tissue. A high proportion of lamina propria macrophages bear class II MHC and other surface markers associated with phagocytic cell activity, which suggests that they are in a more highly activated state than are the corresponding cells in other lymphoid areas. These cells probably are important in nonspecific host defense. In addition, they may produce cytokines (IL-1, IL-6) necessary for local B cell differentiation and other immune processes.

Lamina Propria NK & Lymphokine-Activated Killer (LAK) Cells

Cells bearing NK cell markers (CD16, CD56) are sparse in the lamina propria, and NK activity is difficult to demonstrate in LPL populations unless procedures to enrich for NK cells are used. On the other hand, definite, albeit low (as compared with the level in spleen or peripheral blood cells) NK activity is seen in primate and rodent LPL populations, which suggests that the lack of NK activity in human lamina propria is due in part to the fact that human habitats and habits are not conducive to stimulation of mucosal NK cells, even though the potential for such stimulation does exist. In contrast to cells having NK function, cells with lymphokine-activated killer (LAK) function are easily demonstrated among the LPL. LAK cells are either CD8 T cells for NK cells that manifest antigen-nonspecific cytotoxicity when exposed to IL-2. Because the lamina propria lacks cells with NK markers, the LAK activity in this population is likely to be mediated by T cells or other undefined cells. Finally, the LPL population contains CD8 T cells that can be activated by allogeneic cells, anti-CD3 antibody, and mitogens to manifest cytolytic or suppressor function; these cells probably originate from precursor cells induced in the mucosal aggregates, although some might arise locally. Cytotoxicity is mediated by CD57-negative cells in the lamina propria but by CD57-positive cells in blood, showing that mucosal cytolytic effector cell populations may sometimes be phenotypically different from corresponding populations in the systemic immune system.

Lamina Propria Mast Cells

The mucosal areas are rich in mast cell precursors, which rapidly differentiate into mature mast cells when they are appropriately stimulated. Through their release of mediators, mast cells constitute an important mechanism by which inflammatory cells rapidly enter mucosal tissues and participate in local host defense.

In humans, mast cells in mucosal tissue have relatively small amounts of histamine and tryptic protease, whereas those in connective tissue contain relatively large amounts of histamine and possess both tryptic and chymotryptic proteases. Differential mast cell development in these 2 tissues may depend on the types of cells and cytokines present in their local environments. In this regard, mast cell precursors differentiate into mucosal mast cells under the influence of lymphokines secreted by T cells such as IL-3, whereas connective-tissue mast cells appear to require these factors as well as a factor(s) produced by fibroblasts. This may account for the rapid appearance of mast cells in mucosal tissues infected with nematode parasites, since presumably the parasites can stimulate mucosal T cells to secrete lymphokines that cause differentiation of mast cell precursors into mucosal mast cells. Thus, the significance of the mucosal mast cell type to the mucosal immune system (and to the body as a whole) may lie in its unique capacity to rapidly expand in number under the influence of a T cell-derived signal.

IMMUNOGLOBULIN A

Structure & Function

The central role of IgA in the mucosal immune response is one of the distinguishing features of the mucosal immune system. This is based on the fact that IgA has a number of properties that allow it to function more efficiently than other immunoglobulins in the mucosal environment.

The biochemical structure, genetics, and synthesis of IgA are discussed in Chapter 6. The features of this immunoglobulin that relate to its function in mucosal immunity are discussed here.

IgA is quantitatively the most important of the immunoglobulins, having a synthetic rate exceeding that of all other immunoglobulins combined when secretory as well as circulating IgA is taken into account. In humans it is encoded by 2 genes that lie in the immunoglobulin region of the genome downstream of each of two blocks of γ and ϵ heavy-chain genes. The first IgA gene encodes IgA1, the predominant circulating IgA (ca 80% of the total), as well as a major component of the IgA in mucosal secretions. The second IgA gene encodes IgA2, the IgA that is particularly abundant in the secretions, especially those of the distal gastrointestinal tract (ca 60% of the total). IgA1 differs from IgA2 in being susceptible to cleavage in its hinge region by proteases secreted by a number of different bacteria. Such cleavage can lead to markedly reduced functional activity; however, given the fact that IgA2 is also present in the part of the mucosa where IgA protease-producing bacteria reside, such proteases probably have little effect on the host defense function of the IgA system as a whole. Another difference between IgA1 and IgA2 is that the latter occurs in 2 allotypic forms, IgA2(m1) and IgA2(m2), which, in turn, are distinguished from one another by the fact that IgA2(m1) lacks interchain (H-L) disulfide bonds.

IgA manifests 3 structural features that relate specifically to its role as the mucosal immunoglobulin (Fig 41–3).

A. IgG Polymerization: The IgA heavy chain, in common with the IgM heavy chain, has an extra cysteine residue-containing C-terminal domain. This domain permits IgA to interact with a bivalent (or multivalent) molecule, also produced by B cells, known as J (joining) chain to form IgA dimers and trimers. IgA polymerization is important to IgA function because polymerized IgA (pIgA) has an increased capacity to bind to and agglutinate antigens.

B. Secretory Component: Only dimerized IgA can react with secretory component (SC), a protein (MW 95,000) produced by epithelial cells. SC acts as a transport receptor for IgA and becomes part of the secreted IgA molecule (see discussion below). It renders the IgA molecule less susceptible to proteolytic digestion and more mucophilic, thus enhancing the ability of the IgA molecule to interact with potential pathogens and to prevent their attachment to the epithelial surface. In addition, the IgA hinge region contains a glycosylated, proline-rich region that is generally more resistant to proteolysis by mammalian proteases than is IgG. On this basis, IgA has greater survivability in the gastrointestinal lumen than IgG or other immunoglobulins have. Such survivability, as already mentioned, is enhanced by the presence of secretory component.

C. Fc Region Properties: The Fc domain of IgA is characterized by certain unique properties, both positive and negative. Unlike the IgM or IgG Fc region, the IgA Fc region does not react with components of either the classic or alternative complement pathway, except possibly when the IgA is highly polymerized or is in the form of an immune complex; even in the latter instance, it does not bind C3b and therefore does not recruit inflammatory cells and mediators. In addition, although IgA facilitates phagocytosis and other phagocytic cell functions in the presence of specific antigen, it actually down-regulates phagocytosis in the absence of the antigen.

These facts suggest that free IgA (ie, IgA not associated with antigen) has anti-inflammatory effects. This, of course, is a highly useful property in an area of the body that is replete with materials that can induce excessive inflammatory responses.

IgA has certain pro-inflammatory features as well. Its Fc region binds to lactoferrin and lactoperoxidase and thereby enhances the function of these nonspecific host defense elements. There is also evidence that IgA can interact via its Fc region with Fc receptors to mediate antibody-dependent cell-mediated cytotoxicity (ADCC) reactions.

Transport

As noted above, the capacity of dimeric IgA to bind to SC enhances its effectiveness as a mucosal immunoglobulin. More importantly, however, SC is the key factor in an IgA transport system in allowing the mucosal immune system to focus IgA at mucosal sites (Fig 41–4). The sequence of events occurring during IgA transport involves first the binding of polymeric IgA to SC (via a covalent interaction) on the basolateral surface of the epithelial cell (or hepatocyte, as noted below), followed by endocytosis of IgA into vesicles, movement of IgA-containing vesicles to the apical surface of the cell, and, finally, release of IgA-SC complexes into the mucosal lumen. This final step requires cleavage of the SC receptor molecule so that the receptor for IgA becomes part of the secreted IgA molecule. Cellular synthesis and translocation of SC is independent of the presence of IgA and usually exceeds the amount necessary for transport, leading to the secretion of free (unbound) SC.

IgA transport mediated by SC occurs in the epithelium of the digestive tract, the salivary glands, the bronchial mucosa, and the lactating mammary glands. It also occurs in the uterine epithelium, where it is regulated by the effects of estrogen on SC synthesis by uterine epithelial cells. IgA transport mediated by SC also takes place in the liver, in which case it results in secretion of IgA into the bile. This involves the biliary epithelial cells but not hepatocytes, as in rodents, implying that SC-mediated transport is less important in humans than in certain other species. However, lessened SC-mediated transport in humans in compensated for by other hepatic uptake mechanisms. In this regard, IgA1 can be internalized by hepatic cells via asialoglycoprotein receptors as well as by Fc receptors.

Hepatic uptake of IgA may be one mechanism by which IgA secreted into the circulation is redirected back to the mucosa in species with well-developed SC-mediated hepatic transport capabilities, possibly to clear the circulation of potentially damaging antigenic material that has penetrated the mucosal barrier and become bound to circulating IgA. This mechanism has, in fact, obtained limited support from experiments in animals, but further study is necessary to establish its validity in humans.

Immune Exclusion

The ability of IgA to undergo SC-mediated transport or other clearance mechanisms facilitates the

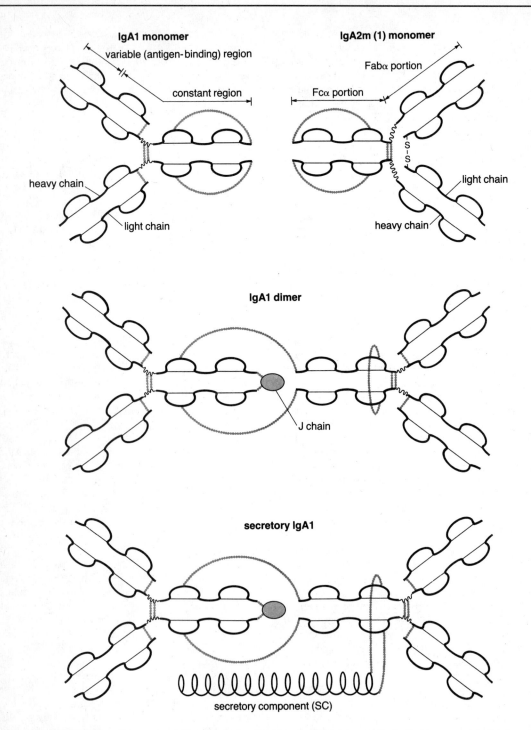

Figure 41–3. Diagrammatic representation of IgA structural forms. Hatched areas indicated immunoglobulin domains. Beads indicate disulfide bonds. In the actual IgA dimer and secretory IgA molecule, the J chain and secretory component molecules are intertwined with Cα heavy chains.

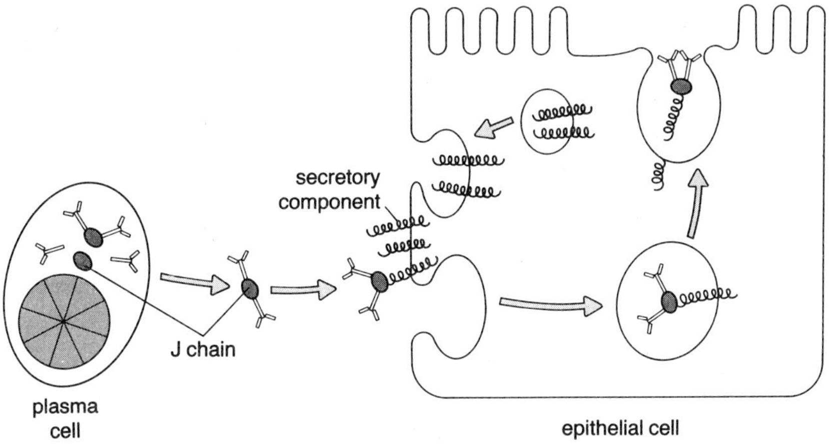

Figure 41–4. SC-mediated transport of IgA across the epithelial cell. Synthesis of SC (indicated as spirals) is independent of the transport process, and SC is released onto the luminal surface whether or not it is bound to IgA. Transport of IgA by this process does not result in its degradation.

process of immune exclusion, whereby the mucosal immune system prevents the entry of antigenic molecules that could potentially evoke harmful immune responses. First, IgA molecules delivered into the secretions by SC-mediated transport can bind to antigens at the mucosal surface and thus lead to their entrapment in the mucus layer and their degradation by proteases before they become bound to and taken up by epithelial cells. That IgA antibody is best suited to this function is shown by the fact that individuals with selective IgA deficiency (ie, those who have low IgA levels and normal IgM and IgG levels) show increased absorption of macromolecules and high levels of circulating immune complexes following ingestion of antigens. This may be the cause of the increase in autoimmunity associated with IgA deficiency. Second, there is good evidence in animals and some evidence in humans that injected antigens become bound to circulating IgA and are then cleared in the liver via SC-mediated transport. Thus, the mucosal immune system either prevents the entry of potentially harmful antigens to the circulation via the mucosa or facilitates their removal from the circulation. This has the effect of limiting the immune response to the antigens present in the mucosal area to the regulated response occurring in the mucosal immune system itself, as discussed below.

Secretory versus Circulating IgA

In recent years in vivo and in vitro studies of IgA synthesis and catabolism have allowed insights into the source of IgA present in various body compartments. The results of these studies show that in humans most circulating IgA is produced in the bone marrow and is in the form of IgA1 monomers, whereas secretory IgA is produced mainly at mucosal sites (either as IgA1 or IgA2 dimers or polymers).

Polymeric IgA (whether IgA1 or IgA2) is more rapidly catabolized then monomeric IgA because polymeric IgA is subject to additional clearance mechanisms such as SC-mediated transport and asialoglycoprotein receptor-mediated uptake. In rats and rabbits, polymeric IgA accounts for about half of the circulating IgA, although most IgA delivered into the circulation is polymeric IgA. This is explained by the fact that in these species SC-mediated transport in the liver is a quantitatively important process and thus polymeric IgA is more rapidly cleared than monomeric IgA. The importance of hepatic clearance of polymeric IgA in rats and rabbits is underscored by the observation that in these species (but not in humans) biliary obstruction leads to increased IgA levels.

The separate origin of mucosal and circulating IgA in humans has led Conley and Delacroix to suggest that the IgA system in humans is bipartite, ie, is composed of 2 relatively independent synthetic centers that are separately regulated. An alternative view more in keeping with the concept that the bone marrow is not an inductive site for IgA B cells is that the IgA1 B cells that produce IgA in the marrow originate in the mucosa and secondarily colonize the marrow to form a separate (but subordinate) locus of IgA-producing B cells. In any case, the monomeric IgA1 arising from the bone marrow in humans may provide a selective advantage in that such IgA may be better suited than other forms of IgA to mediate the clearance of mucosal antigens from the circulation (as discussed above). This is because a monomeric IgA1 molecule may form smaller, more nonpathogenic complexes with circulating antigens than polymeric IgA, yet retain the capacity to undergo removal via interaction with appropriate receptors in the liver.

PRODUCTION OF OTHER IMMUNOGLOBULINS IN THE MUCOSA

Immunoglobulins other than IgA also play a role in the mucosal immune system. Mucosal synthesis of IgM, which can be transported across the epithelial cell via the SC-mediated mechanism, is measurable and physiologically significant. Its capacity to act as a mucosal immunoglobulin is underscored by the fact that it usually replaces IgA adequately to produce mucosal immunity in individuals with selective IgA deficiency. Mucosal synthesis of IgG, on the other hand, is quite low in most mucosal areas, and IgG cannot be transported across the epithelium. Nevertheless, it does have a mucosal role. It is synthesized in substantial amounts in the distal pulmonary tract and is an important antibody class in pulmonary secretions, which it probably enters by passive diffusion. IgE is also synthesized in mucosal tissues, particularly during parasitic infection or during certain pathologic (allergic) states. However, there is no preferential localization of IgE B cells in the mucosa and the number of B cells synthesizing IgE is small, as it is in other tissues. Recent studies with rats suggest that the mucosa may be an important site for IgE B cells during neonatal development.

REGULATION OF IgA SYNTHESIS AT MUCOSAL SITES

Several factors are involved in the preferential synthesis of IgA in mucosal follicles rather than in other lymphoid areas. Cells derived from mucosal lymphoid aggregates (Peyer's patches), but not those from the spleen, have the capacity to induce secretory IgM (sIgM)-positive B cells to undergo isotype switching to sIgA-positive B cells in vitro. Cells

bringing about the isotype switching were identified as T cells, but it remains possible that other cells, including mucosal macrophages and stromal cells, also play a role (Fig 41–5). Although it is presumed that the switch cells produce an IgA-specific switch cytokine or lymphokine, such a material has yet to be identified. It is known, however, that neither IL-4 nor IL-5 can perform this function in the IgA system, unless perhaps they act in conjunction with other factors.

A second mechanism that accounts for the predominance of IgA B cells in the mucosal lymphoid aggregates involves the fact that B cells in mucosal areas come under the influence of post-isotype switch IgA-specific signals, ie, signals that favor terminal differentiation of IgA B cells (Fig 41–5). A class of T cells that bear Fc receptors specific for IgA (FcαR) and that enhance post-switch differentiation of sIgA-bearing B cells have been identified. It is thought that such cells act through the release of IgA-binding factors which act on sIgA-positive B cells. There is evidence that certain T cells secrete IL-5, which, along with other lymphokines such as IL-6, may have preferential effects on IgA B cell differentiation. Either of these types of T cells having effects on IgA B cell differentiation may be more abundant in mucosal areas than elsewhere and may therefore act in concert with switch cells to lead to preferential IgA B cell maturation in the mucosal follicles.

Other types of IgA class-specific regulatory cells have been reported. One such cell is the "contrasuppressor" T cell obtained from Peyer's patches. These cells appear to counteract the effects of suppressor T cells on IgA responses to a greater extent than they counteract the effects of suppressor T cells on IgG or IgM responses. There is also a suppressor T cell that bears IgA-specific Fc receptors and that down-regulates IgA responses in a class-specific

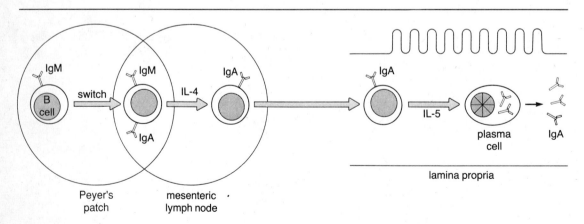

Figure 41–5. Regulation of the IgA response. This involves switching events on the mucosal follicle (Peyer's patch) and then a series of post-switch regulatory events in the mesenteric lymph node and lamina propria. The latter events are known to involve IL-4 and IL-5.

fashion. Cells of this type are induced in mice and humans bearing IgA plasmacytomas or myelomas, and in mice they mediate suppression of responses elicited by oral antigen administration. Thus, T cells bearing IgA-Fc receptors can act as both IgA-specific helper and suppressor cells and are, in this sense, analogous to cells having both positive and negative regulatory effects on IgE responses.

ORAL UNRESPONSIVENESS

The mucosal immune system responds negatively to the vast number of antigens from foods and normal bacterial flora in the mucosal environment. This unresponsiveness prevents the system from being overwhelmed by the antigens.

Oral unresponsiveness is more complete for antigens on the surface of erythrocytes, those associated with bacteria and viruses, and most protein antigens than it is for thymus-independent antigens and complex particulate antigens (including live viruses). This may explain why the mucosal system mounts immune responses to potential pathogens while remaining generally unresponsive to food antigens. Oral unresponsiveness is both B cell (antibody) and T cell mediated, but not necessarily to the same degree in all cases.

Adoptive transfer experiments with animals show that one cellular mechanism underlying oral unresponsiveness is the strong tendency for antigenic stimulation via mucosal follicles to induce **antigen-specific** suppressor T cells in Peyer's patches. However, it is not clear why suppressor circuits are initiated more readily in the mucosal system than elsewhere. The presence of **antigen-nonspecific** suppressor cells may be a second mechanism of oral unresponsiveness. Evidence for this comes from the observation that in animals that are genetically unresponsive to lipopolysaccharide (LPS; a B cell mitogen), oral responses to certain antigens are increased, suppressor T cell responses following oral challenge are reduced, and the phenomenon of oral unresponsiveness does not occur. Although the mechanism is unknown, it is significant that in the "normal" LPS-rich (B cell mitogen-rich) environment of the mucosa, antigen-nonspecific regulatory cells play an important role in down-regulating responses to specific antigens. A third possible mechanism is clonal inhibition (or clonal anergy) resulting from direct effects of antigens on B or T cells in mucosal follicles. Peyer's patches in sheep are sites of massive cell turnover and death; these cells may be undergoing negative clonal selection, just as they do in the thymus.

Abnormalities of oral unresponsiveness may relate to certain immunologic diseases. First, oral unresponsiveness appears to be decreased in several autoimmune mouse strains, which suggests that inappropriate reactivity to one or another antigen in the mucosal system may be a factor in the development of autoimmunity. This possibility gains credence from recent evidence that autoantibodies are structurally related to antibodies against simple antigenic determinants commonly present in the mucosal environment. Second, oral unresponsiveness is reduced in young children, resulting in hypersensitivity to certain oral antigens such as milk proteins. Third, genetically determined defects associated with oral unresponsiveness may form the basis of gluten-sensitive enteropathy or the inflammatory bowel diseases (see Chapter 35).

MUCOSAL HOMING

A characteristic feature of the mucosal immune system is the homing capability of cells developing in the mucosal follicles (Fig 41–6). As mentioned above, this mechanism acts to limit and focus the mucosal immune response to mucosal tissues. Studies of mucosal cell traffic show that B lymphoblasts arising in mesenteric or bronchial lymph nodes selectively localize to mucosal areas and that the majority (70–90%) of the localizing B cells are IgA B cells. T lymphoblasts from mesenteric node and thoracic duct lymph also localize to mucosal sites, both to the lamina propria and to the IEL compartment; however, compared with B cells, a smaller proportion of T cells arising in the mucosal follicles have this property. Small resting (or memory) B cells and T cells arising in the mucosal follicles also recirculate in the mucosal immune system.

Mucosal homing is not an antigen-trapping mechanism. Mucosal lymphoblasts migrate to antigen-free intestinal grafts in extraintestinal sites. Antigen challenge to an isolated area of mucosa results in the appearance of antigen-reactive cells in equal numbers at both exposed and nonexposed areas of mucosa, indicating that cell migration is not directed by antigen. After cells have migrated into the lamina propria, however, antigen does cause them to become sessile (fixed in tissue) and to proliferate. In fact, antigen-specific responses are enhanced at intestinal sites that have been previously exposed to antigen and reduced elsewhere in the intestine.

There is a growing body of data supporting the idea that mucosal homing is initiated by interactions between specific homing receptors on Peyer's patch-derived lymphocytes and ligands for such receptors on endothelial cells (addressins). These interactions are followed by cellular penetration of the endothelium and the entry of cells into mucosal tissue proper. Thus, the capacity of a Peyer's patch lymphocyte to home to the lamina propria can be explained by the

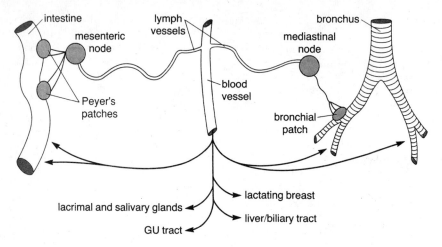

Figure 41–6. Cell traffic in the mucosal immune system. Cells originating in the mucosal follicles localize in subepithelial areas of many mucosal tissues. The ability to do so is governed by specific receptor-ligand interactions involving receptors on lymphoid cells and ligands on endothelial cells. GU tract, genitourinary tract.

selective induction of homing receptors on lymphocytes developing at this site.

BREAST MILK IMMUNOLOGY

The lactating breast is an important component of the mucosal traffic "loop" and ensures that mucosal immunoglobulins and cells are available to protect the neonate during a critical period of relative immunologic incompetence. The concentration of IgA in initial breast secretions (colostrum) is extremely high, averaging 50 mg/mL (versus 2.5 mg/mL in adult serum). However, it falls rapidly to serum levels after the first 4 days, in part owing to the dilutional effect of increased secretion volume. The IgA of breast milk originates from IgA B cells in breast tissue, which migrated there from gastrointestinal and respiratory mucosal follicles. Such migration is dependent on as yet unidentified changes in breast tissue brought about by the action of hormones. The locally synthesized IgA is then transported across the epithelium by an SC-mediated transport mechanism.

Human colostrum and milk are rich in antibodies to a variety of organisms. The beneficial effect of such antibodies may not be obvious in developed countries, but it is readily apparent in underdeveloped countries, where exposure to environmental pathogens is much greater. In addition to protecting the newborn from infection, breast milk antibodies may play a role in establishing the normal flora and in preventing the uptake of certain macromolecules. The latter effect may be relevant to the development of allergies, but this is not yet certain.

Breast milk secretion also contains a significant number of cells, and its ingestion results in the transfer of as many as 10^8 cells/d to the newborn. Most of the cells in breast milk are macrophages and granulocytes, but small numbers of B and T lymphocytes are also present. The macrophages are functionally active and contain ingested IgA; thus, they may be a vehicle for the delivery of IgA to critical areas. Although the T cells are present in small numbers, they are able to transfer specific immune reactivity; suggesting that these cells gain entry to the newborn circulation.

SUMMARY

The antigenic environment of the mucosa is a chaotic mix of virtually the entire antigenic universe, to which may be added potential mitogens that could further stimulate the mucosal system. In this situation it is essential that the relevant immune system be capable of discriminating between stimuli that have possible pathogenic import and those that are harmless and would merely engage the system in a fruitless and wasteful response. The mucosal immune system is shaped to fulfill this need. On the one hand, it has a highly focused response to stimuli, which produces antibodies that interact with and eliminate potential pathogens, without at the same time evoking undue inflammation. Such responses also help to prevent entry and to facilitate clearance of unwanted antigens. On the other hand, it also elaborates suppressor elements that interact with ubiquitous antigens and thus down-regulate responses both in the mucosal areas and in systemic lymphoid tissues. In pursuing these somewhat opposing goals, the mucosal immune system fulfills an important and critical "gatekeeper" function of the immune system, which ensures the integrity of the internal milieu.

REFERENCES

General

Mestecky J, McGhee J: Immunoglobulin A (IgA): Molecular and cellular interactions involved in IgA biosynthesis and immune response. *Adv Immunol* 1987;**40**:153.

Strober W, Brown WR: The mucosal immune system. In: *Immunological Diseases,* 4th ed. Samter M (editor). Little, Brown, 1988.

Antigen-Presenting Cells

Ermak TH, Owen RL: Differential distribution of lymphocytes and accessory cells in mouse Peyer's patches. *Anat Rec* 1986;**215**:144.

Richman LK, Graeff AS, Strober W: Antigen presentation by macrophage-enriched cells from the mouse Peyer's patch. *Cell Immunol* 1981;**62**:110.

M Cells

Sneller MC, Strober W: M cells and host defense. *J Infect Dis* 1986;**154**:737.

Intraepithelial Lymphocytes

Ernst PB, Befus AD, Bienenstock J: Leukocytes in the intestinal epithelium: An unusual immunological compartment. *Immunol Today* 1985;**6**:50.

Mucosal Mast Cells

Befus AD et al: Mast cells from the human intestinal lamina propria. *J Immunol* 1987;**138**:2604.

Irani AA et al: Two types of human mast cells that have distinct neutral protease compositions. *Proc Natl Acad Sci USA* 1986;**83**:4464.

Lamina Propria Lymphocytes

Fiocchi C et al: Modulation of intestinal immune reactivity by interleukin 2: Phenotypic and functional analysis of lymphokine-activated killer cells from human intestinal mucosa. *Dig Dis Sci* 1988;**33**:1305.

James SP et al: Intestinal lymphocyte populations and mechanisms of cell mediated immunity. *Immunol Allergy Clin N Am* 1988;**8**:369.

IgA Structure & Transport

Conley ME, Delacroix DL: Intravascular and mucosal immunoglobulin A: Two separate but related systems of immune defense? *Ann Intern Med* 1987;**106**:892.

Kilian J, Mestecky J, Russel MW: Defense mechanisms involving Fc-dependent functions of immunoglobulin A and their subversion by bacterial immunoglobulin A proteases. *Microbiol Rev* 1988;**52**:296.

Underdown BJ, Schiff JM: Immunoglobulin A: Strategic defense initiative at the mucosal surface. *Annu Rev Immunol* 1986;**4**:389.

Walker WA: Antigen handling by the small intestine. *Clin Gastroenterol* 1986;**15**:1.

Regulation of IgA Synthesis

Harriman GR et al: The role of IL-5 in IgA B cell differentiation. *J Immunol* 1988;**140**:3033.

Kawanishi H, Saltzman LE, Strober W: Mechanisms regulating IgA class-specific immunoglobulin production in murine gut-associated lymphoid tissues. *J Exp Med* 1983;**157**:433.

Kiyono H et al: Isotype-specific immunoregulation. IgA-binding factors produced by Fcα receptor-positive T cell hybridomas regulate IgA responses. *J Exp Med* 1985;**161**:731.

Oral Unresponsiveness

Mowat AM: The regulation of immune responses to dietary protein antigens. *Immunol Today* 1987;**8**:93.

Mucosal Cell Homing

Bienenstock J et al: Regulation of lymphoblast traffic and localization in mucosal tissues, with emphasis on IgA. *Fed Proc* 1983;**42**:3213.

Jalkanen S et al: Human lymphocyte and lymphoma homing receptors. *Annu Rev Med* 1987;**38**:467.

Breast Milk

Ogra PL, Losonsky GA, Fishaut M. Colostrum-derived immunity and maternal-neonatal interaction. *Ann NY Acad Sci* 1983;**409**:82.

42 Reproduction & the Immune System

Karen Palmore Beckerman, MD

Perhaps, then, the zoologist is right to think of placentation as one of the more easily understood innovations of vertebrate phylogeny. But as it happens, not all the problems of viviparity have been satisfactorily solved. The relationship between mother and foetus is still in some degree teleologically inept, and it will be argued that certain trends in the evolution of viviparity raise special immunological difficulties for the foetus. (P. B. Medawar, 1952)

This chapter will focus on basic principles of the immune response relevant to reproductive processes. Although many issues discussed here relate directly to contemporary immunology, most of the questions posed are far from new and, in fact, have remained essentially unanswered since they were first articulated by Medawar and his predecessors in the first half of this century.

The reader will be introduced to the field of reproductive biology by a brief overview of the anatomy and histology of the male and female genital tracts. Recent findings regarding genital mucosal immunity will be presented, followed by examination of the immune status of ovarian and testicular tissues, and, of course, of the remarkable immune privilege enjoyed by tissues of the fetus. Topics receiving significant attention in scientific and lay journals, such as immune causes of infertility and abortion, will be discussed critically.

Two areas of maternal-fetal medicine will be presented in some detail because of their critical clinical relevance and their importance to contemporary immunologic understanding of cellular interactions during gestation and parturition. The relatively well understood phenomenon of Rh isoimmunization and anti-Rh immunoglobulin prophylaxis will be examined first. Then we shall examine the perinatal transmission of human immunodeficiency virus (HIV) infection, which, although less completely understood, effectively illuminates neglected areas of investigation that have become indispensable to our understanding of the dynamics of maternal and fetal immune interactions.

REPRODUCTIVE TRACT ANATOMY & IMMUNITY

ANATOMY

Female

The mucosa of the vagina and outer portion of the uterine cervix (**ectocervix**) is made up of a highly vascularized submucosa and a superficial, non-keratinized, stratified squamous epithelium (Fig 42–1). This squamous epithelium abruptly changes to simple stratified columnar epithelium at the **transitional zone,** which marks the beginning of the inner portion of the cervix (**endocervix**), which is the site of hormonally regulated secretion of specialized mucus that facilitates sperm transport. The endocervix ends in the uterine cavity, whose lining is referred to as either **endometrium** (in the nonpregnant state) or **decidua** (during pregnancy). Depending on hormonal stimulation, the endometrium varies from 1 to 6 mm in thickness and is made of several glandular layers. The innermost layer, the **stratum functionale,** grows and thickens prior to and after ovulation. If pregnancy and implantation occur, it hypertrophies further to become the nutrient-rich, intensely glandular decidua; if pregnancy does not occur, it is shed at the time of menses.

The site of fertilization is the fallopian tube, a muscular membranous structure lined by a highly vascular mucosa (**endosalpinx**) that consists of ciliated and secretory cells. The endosalpinx is thrown into numerous branched, slender longitudinal folds and is ideally suited to the maintenance, nutrition, and transport of the conceptus during its 5-day journey to the uterus.

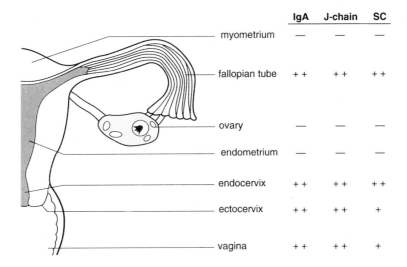

	IgA	J-chain	SC
myometrium	—	—	—
fallopian tube	+ +	+ +	+ +
ovary	—	—	—
endometrium	—	—	—
endocervix	+ +	+ +	+ +
ectocervix	+ +	+ +	+
vagina	+ +	+ +	+

Figure 42–1. The secretory immune system of the female genital tract. Immunofluorescence was used to analyze tissue from the uterus, fallopian tube, ovary endocervix, ectocervix, and vagina. Note that fallopian tube and endocervix are the only sites strongly positive for the presence of IgA, J-chain and secretory component (SC). –, negative; +, weakly positive; ++, strongly positive. (Reproduced, with permission, from Kutteh WH, McAllister D, Byrd W, Mestecky J: *Molecular Andrology* 1993;**4**:183.)

Male

The character of the penile urethral epithelium varies in different places. The most distal portion of the urethra lies in the glans penis and is termed the **fossa navicularis.** The urethral mucosa in this section is lined by stratified squamous epithelium. The remainder of the penile urethra (**pars cavernosa**) is composed of pseudostratified columnar epithelium. Both sections are surrounded by a highly vascular submucosa. Penile periurethral tissue contains many small, branched, tubular glands lined by columnar mucous secreting cells (**glands of Littré**), which can become chronically infected after urethritis. Nearer to the bladder, the urethra is lined by transitional epithelium characteristic of the bladder itself.

MUCOSAL IMMUNITY

The mucosa of the female genital tract is of central importance for protection against the spread of sexually transmitted diseases, including acquired immunodeficiency syndrome (AIDS). It is composed of immunologically reactive tissues capable of mounting local responses to foreign antigens in a manner similar to other immunologically active surfaces such as the respiratory and gastrointestinal tracts. Inductive sites for mucosal immunity of the reproductive tract consist of the cervix, vagina, large intestine, and rectum, as well as the obturator, iliac, and inguinal lymph nodes, which drain these structures. Immuno-globulin A (IgA)-containing plasma cells have been demonstrated in the lamina propria of the fallopian tube, endometrium, endocervix, and vagina, supporting an immune effector role for these structures. Unique distributions of Langerhans cells, CD4 and CD8 T lymphocytes, and plasma cells have been described in surgical specimens of the normal fallopian tube, cervix, and vulva.

The greatest number of intraepithelial and subepithelial lymphocytes is seen in the cervical transitional zone, suggesting that this site is an area of enhanced immune activity similar to other mucosal surfaces exposed to the external environment. As in the ileum, it appears that intraepithelial T cells of the fallopian tube and cervix are predominantly CD8 while subepithelial populations are CD4. The functional result of this tissue distribution is not entirely clear. However, taken together, these findings support an important inductive role for cervical and fallopian tube lymphoid tissues in host mucosal defenses.

Vaginal immunization results in the appearance of specific IgA and IgG in vaginal secretions and IgG in the uterine cavity. Nasopharyngeal and intramuscular immunization induces low-level secretion of IgG (but not IgA) in the vagina and uterus coincident with increasing serum IgG titers. It is generally agreed that cervical IgG is serum-derived whereas cervical IgA is locally produced. Along with the cyclical hormonal effects on mucosal integrity and mucous production, it is apparent that immunoglobulin levels in the cervix vary markedly during the menstrual cycle.

To date, although mucosal immunity has been well studied in the lower gastrointestinal tract, immune responses in the male genital mucosa have been less well characterized. It may be reasonable to assume that as the spread of sexually transmitted diseases is studied in further detail, similar mechanisms of mucosal immune defenses in the male will be described.

DEFENSE AGAINST PATHOGENS VERSUS TOLERANCE OF SPERM "INVASION"

Covering, as it does, more than 400 m² of mucosa, the mucosal immune system is the largest component of the host's immune apparatus and contains the majority of the body's antibody-producing plasma cells. Much as in gut-associated lymphoid tissues, resident populations of macrophages, Langerhans cells, dendritic cells, and T cells have been characterized in the superficial submucosa of the female genital tract. Antigens that reach the cervical or vaginal submucosa are thought to be phagocytosed by antigen-presenting cells (presumably the resident macrophages and Langerhans cells), which migrate to regional lymph nodes where processed antigen is presented. Once activated, T cells and B cells migrate to mucosal effector sites by specific binding to local post-capillary venule adhesion molecules. After arriving at mucosal tissues, B cells undergo clonal expansion as a result of activation by antigen, antigen-presenting cells, T cells, and cytokines to become IgA plasma cells. These cells contain J chain, and the IgA produced is largely polymeric. In addition, vaginal and cervical epithelium produces secretory component for transport of immunoglobulin into reproductive tract secretions.

Despite the regular, repetitive inoculation of millions of antigenically foreign spermatozoa in sexually active women, the immune system of the female reproductive tract is typically unresponsive to sperm antigens. Several factors may account for this. First, the ejaculate contains factors that inhibit immune responses. It is also thought that characteristics unique to female genital mucosal immunity must play an essential role in tolerance to sperm antigen. There is a 1–12% incidence of antisperm antibodies in fertile women, whereas sperm-reactive antibodies are formed in 75% of men engaged in oral-genital intercourse, suggesting that in the case of anti-sperm antibodies, at least, the inductive arm of mucosal immunity in the cervix and vagina is uniquely tolerant to sperm antigen.

THE TESTIS & THE OVARY

The Testis
The findings that germ cell antigens can behave more as foreign than as self and that in the male, hap-

loid germ cells do not develop until puberty, long after the fetal or neonatal period when self tolerance is established, led to the development of the theory that sperm autoantigens are sequestered behind a strong blood-testis barrier. Although tight junctional barriers exist between the supporting Sertoli cells that surround cells involved in spermatogenesis, the immune privilege enjoyed by male germ cells in the testis is not complete. The normal testis contains numerous class II major histocompatibility complex (MHC)-negative resident macrophages in the interstitial spaces between the seminiferous tubules. In the mouse, these cells can be induced to up-regulate their class II MHC expression, and early germ cells which lie outside the blood-testis barrier can be immunogenic to their host, as will be discussed below in the section on immune causes of infertility.

The Ovary
Unlike the testis, the ovary is clearly not a site of immune privilege. First, meiosis is not complete until just after the sperm penetrates the egg, so that haploid female gamete antigens have little opportunity to be expressed. Still, ovarian antigens can cause autoimmune disease, as discussed below. Within the ovary, resident macrophages are a major component of the interstitial ovarian compartment; there is an influx of leukocytes around the time of ovulation, and numerous macrophages are observed in the corpus luteum after follicular rupture. Macrophage secretory products have been shown to influence ovarian cells in vitro: tumor necrosis factor alpha (TNFα) inhibits steroid secretion by ovarian granulosa cells, whereas interleukin-1β (IL-1β) is cytotoxic to ovarian cell dispersates. Gonadotropin-dependent IL-1β gene expression has been identified in the human ovary prior to ovulation, along with expression of IL-1 receptor and an IL-1 receptor antagonist. Thus, ovulation can be thought of as an inflammatory-like reaction, with IL-1β as its centerpiece.

FERTILIZATION, IMPLANTATION, & THE IMMUNE RESPONSE TO FETAL TISSUES

SPERM-EGG FUSION

Fertilization is achieved following the successful completion of a complex sequence of events involving a spermatozoon and an egg. Although much of the cell biology of this process is well beyond the scope of this chapter, certain aspects of sperm-egg interactions deserve consideration. Fusion of gametes requires mutual, species-specific recognition of surface antigen and an initial adhesion step. Contact of gametes signals the **acrosome reaction,** whereby the covering of the head of the sperm is dissolved, activating enzyme systems that make it possible for the sperm to penetrate the cell mass (**cumulus oophorus**) and the thick, acellular mucopolysaccharide layer (**zona pellucida**) that surround the egg.

Complementary adhesion molecules have been characterized on the surface of mouse gametes. An 83,000-MW glycoprotein, murine zona pellucida 3 (mZP3), appears to act as a primary sperm receptor. Adhesion is carbohydrate mediated via serine-threonine O-linked oligosaccharides and results in initiation of the acrosome reaction. Another glycoprotein, mZP2, is involved in maintaining sperm binding to the ovum. On the acrosomal membrane of the head of the sperm, a putative 56,000-MW egg-binding protein has been identified as sp-56. It is assumed that homologous molecules regulate the early phases of fertilization in other mammals.

IMPLANTATION

After fertilization is completed and mitotic division is successfully initiated, it takes 6 days for the conceptus, surrounded by the zona pellucida, to traverse the fallopian tube and reach the uterus as an autonomous, cystic, embryonic cell mass known as the preimplantation **blastocyst.** Implantation of the blastocyst is regulated by complex interactions between peptide and steroid hormones that synchronize the preparation of the endometrium with development of the embryo. Progesterone secretion by the corpus luteum of the ovary is a critical component of these interactions and is necessary for decidual maintenance and development. Human chorionic gonadotropin (hCG) is secreted by the embryonic tissues by day 1 after implantation and is responsible for the conversion of the ovarian corpus luteum of the menstrual cycle to the corpus progesterone secreting luteum of pregnancy. Thus, the early conceptus is responsible for supporting the ovarian progesterone secretion that is necessary for its own survival. Besides maintenance of the decidua, progesterone, first of ovarian origin and later produced by the developing placenta itself, may play a significant immunosuppressive role at the maternal-fetal interface.

At the time of implantation, the endometrium and decidua contain numerous leukocytes, including T cells and macrophages. Their cytokine products may act as mediators of interactions between maternal and fetal tissues. Estrogen-dependent expression of epidermal growth factor (EGF) and its receptor have been identified in the mouse uterus, where it may regulate uterine angiogenesis and growth. The EGF receptor has been identified on the preimplantation blastocyst and in in vitro embryo cultures; EGF stimulates blastocyst development, suggesting a functional ligand-receptor interaction for EGF during preimplantation events. The colony-stimulating factor family of cytokines (GM-CSF, CSF-1, and IL-3) and the c-*fms* receptor for CSF-1 have been identified in murine placenta and decidua and in human placental cell lines. Recent data suggest that these cytokines modify blastocyst membrane properties in preparation for implantation. Indeed, the homozygous female CSF-1-deficient osteopetrotic mouse is infertile in matings with homozygous deficient males but can produce offspring in matings with heterozygous males.

Before implantation, the zona pellucida must be shed. It is not clear whether the source of enzymes needed for degradation of the zona pellucida is endometrial or embryonic, but it does appear that a burst of uterine expression of the cytokine leukemia inhibitory factor (LIF) is required for adhesion and implantation of the blastocyst into the endometrium. Female mice lacking a functional LIF gene are fertile, but their blastocysts fail to implant and develop. However, these conceptuses are quite viable and can be transferred to pseudopregnant wild-type controls, in which they implant and develop normally.

Other cytokines secreted by decidual T cells and macrophages can either facilitate or impede implantation events. In vitro studies show that IL-1β inhibits murine blastocyst attachment but enhances trophoblast outgrowth. Gamma interferon (IFN γ) inhibits trophoblast outgrowth and causes degenerative changes in these cells, suggesting that implantation events may be regulated by the types of cytokines present and the timing of their secretion relative to embryonic development.

TROPHOBLAST INVASION OF MATERNAL TISSUES (Fig. 42–2)

Human embryonic development (Fig 42–2) requires rapid access to the maternal circulation. **Cytotrophoblast** cells surrounding the embryonic tissues of the blastocyst quickly differentiate into invasive and noninvasive phenotypes. **Noninvasive cytotrophoblast** form "floating" villi, becoming polarized syncytial epithelial monolayers covering cores of fetal blood vessels. Columns of nonpolarized **invasive cytotrophoblast** cells which derive from "anchoring" villi that attach to the uterine wall first erode into endometrial stroma, then replace the endothelium and vascular smooth muscle of maternal spiral arterioles, establishing the maximally dilated **uteroplacental circulation**. This circulation is biologically unique; maternal blood enters the placenta through fetal trophoblast-lined maternal vessels and accomplishes the critical functions of gas and nutrient exchange for the developing embryo. Despite the fact that maternal blood is in continuous, direct contact with fetal villi, nutrient transport and elimination

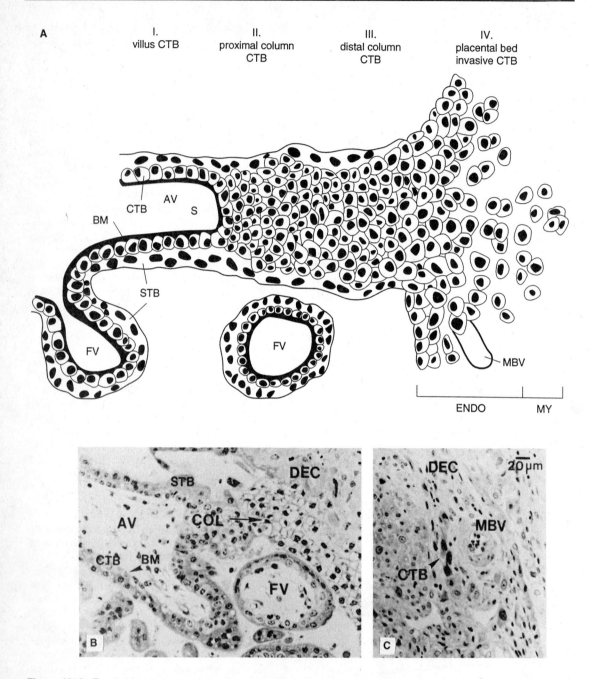

Figure 42–2. Trophoblast invasion at the maternal-fetal interface in the 10 week human placenta. **(A)** Diagram showing floating villi and an anchoring villus with an associated cell column invading endometrium and myometrium of the uterine wall. The spatial organization of this tissue recapitulates the differentiation of cytotrophoblast along the invasive pathway. Zone I contains floating villi where mononuclear cytotrophoblast stem cells fuse to form the overlying syncytiotrophoblast layer past which maternal blood will percolate throughout gestation as part of the utero-placental circulation. In an anchoring villus, cytotrophoblast form cell columns that connect the fetal and maternal compartments of the placenta (zones II and III). After shallow penetration of the uterine wall, columns spread laterally and break up into clusters of cells which penetrate endometrium (also called decidua) and myometrium layers of the pregnant uterus in zone IV. These invasive cytotrophoblast go on to invade and line maternal blood vessels, replacing endothelium and vascular smooth muscle in vessels of the inner one third of the uterine wall. **(B)** and **(C)** Sections of a 10 week human placental bed biopsy showing all stages of cytotrophoblast differentiation along the invasive pathway. FV, floating villi; AV, anchoring villus; ENDO, endometrium; MY, myometrium; CTB, cytotrophoblast; STB, syncytiotrophoblast; MBV, maternal blood vessel. (Reproduced, with permission, from Damsky CH, Fitzgerald ML, Fisher SJ: *Journal of Clinical Investigation* 1992;**89:**210.)

of waste across placental villi will continue for the remainder of the pregnancy unhindered by rejection or attack of antigenically distinct cells by the immune system of either the fetus or the mother.

THE PLACENTA AS AN IMMUNE ORGAN

The placenta is a unique, short-lived organ. While producing protein and steroid hormones that regulate physiologic activities of pregnancy, it also acts as the fetal lung, kidneys, intestine, and liver. Its function as a complex tissue of immunologic significance has received considerable attention in recent years.

Trophoblast

The multinuclear **syncytiotrophoblast** layer of the placenta (Fig 42–2) was traditionally thought to act as a sort of shield for the fetus by serving as a barrier to maternal immune effector mechanisms. This model alone, however, has not been sufficient to explain maternal tolerance of fetal tissues. The trophoblast secretes cytokines that have been primarily associated with mononuclear phagocytes, such as CSF-1 and its receptor, c-*fms*, IL-3, and GM-CSF. Like macrophages, the trophoblast expresses high levels of the LIF receptor (see above), is capable of phagocytosis and syncytium formation, and expresses FcR, CD4, and CD14. There has been one preliminary report of trophoblast expression of IL-10, and it appears from work done in a number of different experimental systems that the trophoblast is responsive to TNFα, IL-1, transforming growth factor beta (TGFβ), and IL-6. Taken together, these findings have led to speculation that the trophoblast could represent part of a network of macrophagelike tissues distributed throughout the body that share common cytokine pathways and other characteristics. Such a model itself may or may not yield meaningful clinical information in the near future; however, the introduction of concepts such as cytokine signaling and other dynamic interactions between maternal and fetal tissues will be critical to further advances in our understanding of trophoblast development and survival.

The Hofbauer Cell

This is a macrophagelike cell found within the fetal portion of the placenta (chorionic villus) in the stromal tissue that surrounds the fetal vessels of the villus core (Fig 42–3). It is present early in gestation and is probably of fetal origin. Early in pregnancy this cell may play a significant role in flow dynamics within the fetal villus, and later it is actively phagocytic; however, its function in placental development, phys-

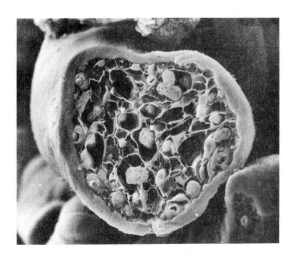

Figure 42–3. Scanning electron micrograph of a cross-fractured 10 week floating villus showing the villus core with its fetal vessels and numerous deep compartments formed by cytoplasmic processes of fixed stromal cells. Numerous Hofbauer cells are seen migrating between compartments. (Reproduced, with permission, from Castellucci M, Kaufmann P: *Placenta* 1982;**3**:269.

iology, and immunity has not been completely characterized.

Placental MHC Expression

It has become quite clear that trophoblast is distinct from all other cell types in its expression of MHC molecules. Trophoblast does not express class I or class II MHC either constitutively or in response to IFN γ, despite the presence of abundant receptors for IFN γ in placental tissues and despite demonstrable enhancement of RNA synthesis, production of renin, and transferrin receptor expression by first-trimester trophoblast culture in response to the cytokine. However, trophoblast does constitutively express the nonclassic class I HLA molecule HLA-G. The HLA-G gene was originally isolated from a human lymphoblastoid cell line, but it is not expressed on any human cell type except trophoblast, where it is expressed on the surface of extravillus cytotrophoblast and secreted in its soluble form. It is nonpolymorphic, is associated with β₂-microglobulin, and can interact with CD8. It is found in highest levels in the first trimester and is present in markedly decreased quantities in third-trimester trophoblast. No function has been identified for HLA-G in human tissues; however, the total absence of polymorphic HLA expression in trophoblast tissues in the presence of unique expression of nonpolymorphic HLA-G strongly suggests that this molecule plays a significant role in trophoblast invasion and interaction with maternal tissues.

IMMUNITY IN PREGNANCY

BACKGROUND: ALTERED SUSCEPTIBILITY TO INFECTION IN PREGNANCY

With the advent of antimicrobial therapy, many of the dangers posed by infection to maternal health have been obscured. It is difficult to imagine that the single most common indication for therapeutic abortion prior to the late 1950s was tuberculosis. Indeed, infections against which host defenses are primarily cell-mediated, such as diseases caused by viruses, intracellular bacteria, fungi, protozoa, and helminths, are more likely acquired or reactivated and are of greater virulence during pregnancy.

It is instructive to examine a few of the diseases to which pregnant women are more susceptible than those who are not pregnant. Until the 1960s, clinical poliomyelitis was 2–3 times more common and the incidence of residual paralysis was significantly higher in pregnant patients. Hepatitis A occurs more commonly with a more fulminant course in pregnancy: in Africa a 40% rate of coma with 33% mortality among pregnant women compared with an 8% rate of coma and no mortality in nonpregnant controls. The frequency and severity of hepatitis B probably increases greatly during the last trimester. In the 1957 epidemic of influenza A, 50% of women of childbearing age who died in New York City were pregnant, even though they accounted for only 7% of women in that age group.

Pregnant women are much more likely to suffer the serious sequelae of malaria, including cerebral malaria, blackwater fever, acute renal failure, disseminated intravascular coagulation, pulmonary edema, and splenic rupture. In addition, plasmodia have a special affinity for placental tissue: a 46% placental infestation rate has been reported in an affected population that had only 17% positive peripheral blood smears. Interestingly, resistance to malaria is promptly restored following parturition.

In areas where coccidiomycosis is endemic, it is a leading cause of maternal death. The risk of miliary tuberculosis is 3-fold higher in pregnancy, and leprosy is reported to progress rapidly in pregnant women. Infection with *Listeria monocytogenes* occurs in the immunocompromised. Humoral immunity plays a minimal role in defense against listeriosis, and up to one-third of cases are found in pregnant women, their fetuses, and neonates. Peripartum listeriosis generally starts with a flulike prodrome and progresses to acute chorioamnionitis, resulting in abortion or premature labor and delivery. Placental histology reveals chorioamnionitis, and fetal autopsy shows microorganisms in the fetal liver, lungs, amniotic fluid, and blood. After delivery and evacuation of infected uterine contents, maternal condition rapidly improves. Important findings in a murine model of placental listeriosis are discussed below.

PROPOSED MECHANISMS OF ALTERED IMMUNITY IN PREGNANCY

In pregnancy, B cell immunity is maintained at normal levels and serum immunoglobulin levels are unchanged. In addition, some manifestations of cell-mediated immunity, such as delayed hypersensitivity, skin reactions, skin allograft rejection, and in vitro responses to mitogen, are grossly unchanged. In the face of such impressive historical data on compromised host defenses during gestation, the exact role played by the gravid state in modulation of the immune response remains elusive.

Current discussions of immune responses during pregnancy generally embrace a theory of depression of selective aspects of cell-mediated immunity thought to be necessary for maternal accommodation to the so-called fetal allograft. Unfortunately, many of these discussions in the literature are highly speculative.

Local Immunosuppression at the Placenta and Adjacent Tissues

Experiments by Lu and Redline designed to study immunoregulatory mechanisms at the maternal-fetal interface during *L monocytogenes* infection in the pregnant mouse have yielded important information on cell-mediated immunity in pregnancy. Like the human, the adult mouse is able to mount an effective cell-mediated immune response to this intracellular parasite. During pregnancy, the maternal immune response in the liver and spleen was not impaired, even in the presence of overwhelming placental infection. In the placenta itself, large inflammatory infiltrates were identified in the maternal decidua; however, there was no inflammatory response in the fetal spongiotrophoblast and labyrinth layers of the murine placenta despite the presence of large numbers of bacteria. This led to the conclusion that local events at the maternal-fetal interface prevented an effective immune response and that the infected placenta might exert further detrimental effects by providing the bacteria a protected environment from which they could seed other maternal and fetal organs. Further work by this group has identified profound local deficits in macrophage function in the placenta, which cannot be accounted for by regional deficits in macrophage-activating cytokines or by immunosuppressive trophoblast products. These authors' speculation that mechanisms preventing optimal macrophage function in the murine placenta may have evolved not to make the fetoplacental unit susceptible to intracellular infections but to protect it from rejection by the maternal immune system is thought-provoking but as yet unproved.

Secretion of Placental Steroid Hormones

The placenta secretes high levels of estrogens and progesterone, which it synthesizes from maternal and fetal precursors, resulting in extremely high levels in the maternal placental circulation and causing a marked increase in maternal systemic hormone plasma levels. Levels of free and albumin-bound hydrocortisone of fetoplacental origin also increase.

Steroid hormones have been shown in vitro to depress different aspects of cell-mediated immunity in a variety of experimental models, including inhibition of graft rejection and suppression of lymphocyte activation of macrophages. Such experiments generally require high concentrations of hormones, in the 10–20 μM range, which is 20–50 times higher than levels found in maternal serum. It is conceivable, however, that such levels may be achieved in the placenta.

Secretion of Placental Proteins

hCG is produced by the trophoblast, increases in amount during the first trimester, and then decreases through the remainder of pregnancy. Inconsistent experimental data and recent work with purified hCG suggest there is minimal role for hCG alone in suppression of cell-mediated immunity in pregnancy. Alpha-fetoprotein (AFP) is secreted by the fetal liver into fetal serum and amniotic fluid in high levels during second trimester and then plateaus. Physiologic levels of AFP can depress proliferative T cell responses.

Intrinsically Decreased Lymphocyte Reactivity in Pregnancy

Although clinical evidence for depressed cellular immunity during pregnancy is indisputable, there is conflicting opinion regarding changes in T cell number, distribution, and reactivity during gestation. Some reports suggest a decrease in CD4 cells and others an increase in CD8 cells; cytotoxic activity of natural killer cells is said by others to be defective. Lymphocyte responsiveness to mitogens in vitro is moderately but significantly depressed in some studies but unchanged in others. Thymic involution, observed in other stressful conditions such as malnutrition and infection, has been observed in rodents during the latter half of gestation coincident with rising in plasma corticosteroid levels.

No consistent or significant changes in B cell immunity have been demonstrated during pregnancy.

Other Theories

There are many theories explaining decreased cell-mediated immunity in pregnancy. So-called IgG blocking antibodies of pregnancy have been implicated, along with other proteins (eg, the macroglobulin pregnancy associated α_2-glycoprotein), cell-associated pregnant serum factors, and altered balance between helper and suppressor T cells. To date, all such explanations of the status of cell-mediated immunity during pregnancy are incomplete. Further insight into placental physiology and immunology is needed before new hypotheses can be properly formulated and tested.

INFERTILITY & SPONTANEOUS ABORTION

Infertility and spontaneous abortion are perceived as increasing problems in the USA. Factors responsible include increased numbers of women of childbearing age, the routine availability of pregnancy diagnosis before the first missed menstrual period, and significant numbers of couples electing to delay childbearing until they are older. However, the actual rates of infertility and spontaneous abortion in the USA are not increasing. Nonetheless, the number of couples seeking medical advice and treatment for infertility is increasing rapidly, from 600,000 in 1968 to 1.6 million in 1986.

INFERTILITY

Infertility is the inability to establish pregnancy within a certain interval, usually 1 year. Primary infertility refers to a situation in which couples have never achieved a pregnancy, whereas secondary infertility refers to those who have. Documented causes of infertility include pelvic or tubal factors interfering with ovum transport, anovulation, abnormalities of the male reproductive system, and abnormal sperm-cervical mucus penetration. For 10% of couples undergoing evaluation, no etiology can be identified.

Immune Causes of Infertility

Antisperm antibodies have been studied since the early 1900s, when it was demonstrated that intraperitoneal injection of sperm into the female guinea pig induced antibody formation. Antisperm antibodies can be found in blood and lymphatic fluid (primarily IgG) and in local seminal or cervicovaginal secretions (primarily IgA) in both men and women. They can develop in the male following traumatic or inflammatory disruption of the blood-testis barrier. Vaginal inoculation is far less likely to result in development of antisperm antibodies than is oral-genital intercourse. Interest in this field springs from 2 different clinical areas: first, identification of a treatable cause of idiopathic infertility, and, second, development of a highly specific contraceptive method by vaccinating individuals "against" pregnancy by inoculation with sperm antigen.

Three types of assays have been used to detect antisperm antibodies: sperm agglutination assays, sperm immobilization assays, and assays that directly detect antibody. The source of sperm antigen used will determine whether antibodies of possible significance (eg, those directed against a sperm cell surface antigen) or of doubtful significance (eg, those directed against internal antigen) will be detected. Many assays do not measure or specifically identify IgA, the predominant class of antigen in mucosal secretions. Agglutination assays can be falsely positive owing to the presence of amorphous material in semen or to serum proteins. Immobilization assays may be affected by complement sources (guinea pig sera) that are toxic to sperm. Immunoglobulin-specific techniques such as enzyme-linked immunosorbent and immunofluorescence assays can be highly quantitative but cannot yield information about the location of an antibody on the sperm surface, whereas other tests such as immunobead and the mixed-antiglobulin reaction with erythrocytes can indicate the location of an antibody and can be used to evaluate the immunoglobulin isotype but do not provide quantitative information.

Depending on the assay used, antisperm antibodies are found in 1–12% of fertile women and 10–20% of women with unexplained infertility. In males, autoantibodies to sperm can be detected in both the seminal plasma and serum, and one-half of men undergoing vasectomy form antisperm antibodies following the procedure. Importantly, there are no data that document significant differences in the presence or titers of antisperm antibodies in fertile and infertile populations.

Autoimmune disease of the testis and ovary is a known cause of infertility in domestic animals and is a likely cause of some forms of human infertility. Granulomatous disease and immune complexes can be found in the testes of infertile men; they resemble changes seen in experimental autoimmune orchitis in mice. Ovarian autoantibodies and idiopathic oophoritis have been documented in women with premature ovarian failure. In addition, autoimmune orchitis and oophoritis have been identified as components of human polyendocrine and autoimmunity syndromes. Studies based on experimental autoimmune gonadal disease models have yielded new information on genetic control of organ-specific autoimmune disease and on antigen mimicry at the T cell receptor.

Experimental autoimmune oophoritis is induced 2 weeks following immunization of rats with bovine ovarian homogenate or immunization with synthetic peptide fragments of mZP3, the sperm receptor protein on the zona pellucida (see above). Disease is also induced 2 days after adoptive transfer of T cell lines and T cell clones derived from lymph node cells from immunized, diseased mice to normal untreated recipients. These lines and clones uniformly express CD4 and produce IL-2, TNF, and IFN γ on stimulation. Interestingly, 4 randomly positioned amino acids in the peptide nanomer ZP3 330–338 are critical for induction of disease and T cell response, whereas the poly-alanine peptide inserted with the critical mZP3 residues is fully capable of eliciting disease.

Experimental autoimmune orchitis in mice is under polygenic control involving *H-2-* and non-*H-2-* linked genes. Severe disease can be induced only by inoculation with homologous crude testis antigen and by adoptive transfer of T cell lines and clones derived from lymph nodes of immunized mice. Manipulations of the normal immune system can also cause autoimmune gonadal disease. For example, neonatal murine thymectomy performed between days 1 and 4 after birth can result in a variety of autoimmune sequelae including autoimmune disease of the testis, ovary, thyroid, prostate, and stomach, suggesting that the neonatal T cell repertoire is enriched with self-reactive T cells, and that such novel disease models may be powerful tools for examining and manipulating mechanisms of self-tolerance of a wide variety of potential autoantigens.

Immune Therapies for Infertility

Different therapies for the infertile couple with antisperm antibodies identified in either the male or the female have been used. **Condom therapy** has been advocated to reduce exposure to antigen in women with antisperm antibodies. Pregnancy rates following specified periods of condom use vary from 11 to 56%; however, most studies do not include proper control groups. In fact, one study has documented a 44% rate of spontaneous pregnancy in couples who rejected condom contraception as a means of achieving pregnancy. Attempts to **process semen or wash sperm** to reduce the amount of antibody present in the ejaculate has not improved pregnancy rates, and techniques to chemically dissociate antibodies from sperm result in irreversible loss of sperm motility.

There are reports of **intrauterine insemination** (to bypass antibody present in the cervical mucous), **corticosteroid therapy, in vitro fertilization,** and **gamete intrafallopian transfer** as successful therapies. Rare but serious and unpredictable complications, such as corticosteroid-induced aseptic necrosis of the femur or anaphylactic shock after intauterine insemination, can occur with these therapies, and none has been demonstrated effective in well-controlled, randomized trials. It would seem that the high spontaneous "cure" rate of this syndrome (ie, pregnancy without intervention), the difficulties involved in meaningful and standardized diagnostic evaluation of affected couples, and the large number of couples with unexplained infertility who might be subjected to these therapies would mandate such clinical trials in the near future. Until then, the detection of antisperm antibodies in couples with unexplained infertility can only be considered to be of unknown significance, and couples must be advised that prescribed treatments are of questionable benefit and carry the risk of serious complications.

RECURRENT SPONTANEOUS ABORTION

Background & Definitions

The occurrence of 3 or more spontaneous consecutive pregnancy losses defines this clinical syndrome. Given that a single clinically documented pregnancy carries a 15–20% chance of loss, some investigators believe that recurrent abortion is a chance phenomenon that occurs in 0.5% of the population, and most clinicians find that no cause can be found for the majority of repetitive losses. Others contend that an etiology can be found for losses in over 60% of affected couples. Fetal chromosomal abnormalities account for the largest share of repetitive losses, followed by uterine anatomic abnormalities, endometrial abnormalities, and hormonal abnormalities. Immunologic disorders may be associated with the large number of couples experiencing recurrent pregnancy loss for whom no specific cause is demonstrable. It is important to note that 70% of women with unexplained recurrent pregnancy loss will eventually carry a pregnancy successfully to term with no therapeutic intervention.

HLA Sharing

A large body of literature has appeared in the last decade invoking HLA homozygosity between parents as a cause of pregnancy loss. In theory, HLA sharing has been said to lead to decreased production of maternal "blocking" antibodies, which are said to appear in all successful pregnancies. These are postulated to be needed for suppression of the maternal immune response to allow survival of the fetal allograft. With limited studies to support such theories, some centers have advocated the immunization of women with paternal lymphocytes. Large, properly controlled clinical trials to study this treatment are lacking. Serious complications can result from this therapy and graft-versus-host-like reactions have been reported. A meta-analysis combining 4 randomized, controlled trials found not only that each trial dropped from analysis all women who received therapy and did not become pregnant but also that aggregate success rates for immunotherapy were 48% compared with 60% for no treatment.

Anti-Phospholipid Antibody Syndrome

The **anti-phospholipid antibody syndrome** was first described in the early 1950s in women who were noted to have prolonged bleeding times that were not correctable by addition of normal plasma, a history of hypercoagulability, a false-positive VDRL, and a history of recurrent pregnancy loss. Subsequently, the lupus anticoagulant and the anti-cardiolipin antibody were characterized as acquired antibodies, either IgG, IgA, or IgM, with specific activities against negatively charged phospholipids. These antibodies probably interfere with synthesis of the potent vasodilatory prostaglandin, prostacyclin, by endothelial cells, which theoretically would predispose to maternal thrombosis and placental infarction, resulting in placental insufficiency and pregnancy loss. For the lupus anticoagulant, diagnosis consists of prolongation of a phospholipid-dependent in vitro coagulation test, such as the partial thromboplastin time (PTT) or the Russell Viper Venom Time. Treatment has included prednisone (40–60 mg/d), low-dose aspirin (80 mg/d), and heparin therapies in various combinations. Recent data suggest that heparin or prednisone plus aspirin results in greater numbers of viable offspring than no treatment; however, the use of heparin or aspirin alone may have lower morbidity for both mother and fetus.

In normal obstetrical populations, one or other of these antibodies are seen in 2% of women tested; in referral populations of women with recurrent pregnancy loss, this figure may approach 15%. The anti-phospholipid antibody syndrome, however, must be viewed as quite rare. More importantly, the presence of anticardiolipin antibody is of no significance in women without a history of recurrent (at least 3) pregnancy losses, and the presence of the even rarer lupus anticoagulant is of unknown significance in women without clinical histories of recurrent thromboses and pregnancy losses. Even with such histories, patients must be advised that studies showing benefit of therapies have used largely historical controls (often the patients themselves) and are sometimes statistically seriously flawed.

Recurrent pregnancy loss and infertility are distressing problems that cause significant grief and suffering. Many couples presenting with these problems are panicked and desperate for a "cure." It is the duty of clinicians and scientists to thoroughly evaluate, educate, and protect these vulnerable individuals from empirical and potentially dangerous therapies whose benefits are largely unproved or have actually been disproved. For therapies that may still be of value, the need for properly performed prospective trials is clearly imperative.

ISOIMMUNIZATION

HISTORICAL BACKGROUND

Pathologic changes associated with **hydrops fetalis,** the syndrome of abnormal, sometimes massive collections of fluid in fetal tissues, were characterized in the late 19th century. In 1932 the critical observation was made by Diamond that this syndrome was associated with fetal anemia and large numbers of circulating immature red blood cells (**erythroblasts**), and thus the concept of **erythroblastosis fetalis** was introduced. Subsequent characterization of hemolytic disease of the fetus and newborn, the discovery of the rhesus (**Rh;** also referred to as **D** of the CDE blood group system) factor in 1940, and ultimately the development of effective maternal anti-Rh prophylaxis in the early 1960s represent one of the great medical triumphs of the 20th century. Today, the administration of anti-Rh immunoglobulin prophylaxis may seem routine; however, with the exception of immunization against infectious disease, no other immune therapy has had such a definitive and far-reaching impact on such a common and formerly devastating disorder.

PATHOPHYSIOLOGY OF ISOIMMUNE HYDROPS

The precise function of the Rh antigen is unknown. It is a polypeptide embedded in the lipid phase of the red blood cell membrane and may interact with a membrane ATPase, functioning as part of a cation or proton pump to control fluid and electrolyte fluxes across the cell membrane. Any individual who lacks a specific red cell antigen is capable of production of antibody to that antigen. To a variable degree, every pregnancy is associated with the passage of fetal blood cells into the maternal circulation, most notably at the time of delivery or after maternal trauma, ectopic pregnancy, abortion, or invasive diagnostic procedures such as amniocentesis and chorionic villus sampling. Of course, isoimmunization can also be the result of transfusion of Rh-positive blood into an Rh-negative individual. Once Rh-positive blood has entered the circulation, a primary immune response may occur and low levels of anti-Rh antibodies will be detected in maternal serum. Significantly, the fetus is at most only mildly affected during a primary isoimmunization. It is the Rh-positive products of subsequent gestations that are at risk for severe compromise from maternally produced antibody.

For incompletely understood reasons, an unimmunized Rh negative mother has only a 16% chance of becoming immunized against her Rh-positive fetus with any given pregnancy. Explanations that have been proposed include variable "antigenicity," insufficient transplacental passage of antigen, variable maternal response, and protection from isoimmunization by ABO blood type incompatibility (see below).

Anti-Rh IgG antibodies do not fix complement. Rather, intact Rh-positive cells are apparently sequestered in the maternal spleen and lymph nodes, where an anti-Rh immune response is generated or amplified, presumably initiated by processing and presentation of antigen by macrophages and other antigen-presenting cells (Fig. 42–4). Once primary sensitization has occurred, subsequent Rh-positive pregnancies elicit a much more potent secondary maternal immune response, and anti-Rh IgG gains access to the fetal circulation, where it binds to fetal red cells and is free in serum. Accelerated red blood cell destruction ensues, leading to various degrees of hemolysis and fetal anemia. Prolonged hemolysis results in erythroid hyperplasia of the bone marrow, extramedullary hematopoiesis in the fetal spleen and liver, and hydrops, which is characterized by various degrees of hepatomegaly, splenomegaly and placental edema. With severe hydrops, fatty degeneration, hemosiderin deposition and engorgement of hepatic canaliculi may also occur in the liver. Cardiac enlargement, pulmonary hemorrhage, and pleural and pericardial effusions may occur, in addition to massive ascites and subcutaneous edema, which result in severe dystocia. Hydrothorax can compromise neonatal respiratory status after birth.

The exact pathophysiology of progression from hemolysis and mild fetal anemia to the massively hydropic fetus still has not been fully characterized. Hydrops may result from high-output congestive heart failure secondary to profound anemia, portal and umbilical venous hypertension secondary to disruption of the hepatic parenchyma by extramedullary hematopoiesis, or decreased colloid osmotic pressure secondary to hepatic failure and disruption of capillary endothelial integrity owing to anemia and hypoxia. Hydropic fetuses may die in utero, whereas less severely affected infants can appear well at birth and develop hyperbilirubinemia shortly after birth as a result of loss of placental clearance of bilirubin from the fetal circulation. If untreated, this can lead to significant central nervous system damage, termed **kernicterus** in pathologic specimens.

ABO INCOMPATIBILITY

ABO hemolytic disease is more common and much milder than Rh disease. A and B antigens are frequently found in nature, and individuals lacking them on their red cells develop anti-A and anti-B antibodies early in life. Unlike anti-Rh, anti-A and anti-B bind complement. Transfusion of ABO-incompati-

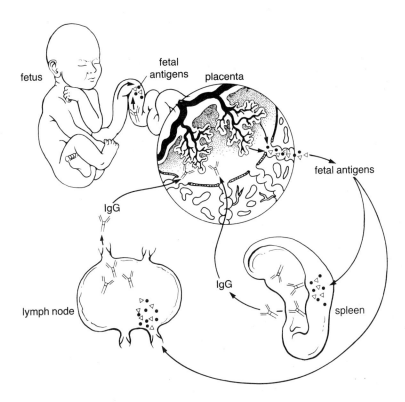

fetus

fetal antigens

placenta

fetal antigens

IgG

IgG

lymph node

spleen

Figure 42–4. Maternal immune activation by fetal antigen. Fetal antigen escapes from or across trophoblast tissues in the placenta, to be sequestered in the maternal spleen or lymph nodes where an immune response is generated. Only maternal IgG can cross the placenta and affect fetal tissues.

ble blood produces life-threatening intravascular hemolysis; however, ABO incompatibility of mother and fetus does not result in an increased rate of stillbirth, and ABO isoimmunization is considered a neonatal, not a fetal, problem. A firstborn can be affected, but, at worst, the disease results in moderate neonatal anemia and hyperbilirubinemia for which management is quite straightforward.

Although 20% of infants have ABO maternal blood group incompatibility, only 5% of these show overt signs of hemolytic disease. Individuals with group A or B blood types produce predominantly IgM anti-B or anti-A, which does not cross the placenta, whereas type O individuals produce predominantly IgG. Also, there are fewer antigenic sites on the fetal red cell than on the adult cell, and A and B antigens expressed in other tissues may compete with the fetal erythrocyte for binding of antibody.

Interestingly, ABO incompatibility reduces the risk of Rh isoimmunization from 10–16% to 1.5–2% after delivery of an Rh-positive fetus. This effect is most pronounced in pregnancies in which the mother is type O and the father is type A, B, or AB. Two mechanisms may be responsible for this. The number

of ABO-incompatible cells detectable following delivery in the maternal circulation is smaller than the number of cells of ABO-compatible fetuses, suggesting that there is increased clearance of ABO-incompatible cells from the circulation before they can be trapped in the spleen and lymph nodes, where an immune response would be initiated. Alternatively, maternal anti-ABO antibody may damage or alter fetal Rh antigen so that it is no longer immunogenic.

ANTI-Rh Ig PROPHYLAXIS

Use of Rh-Immune Globulin

The incidence of Rh isoimmunization has dramatically decreased in the USA since the introduction of passive immunization of Rh-negative women after delivery of Rh-positive infants by using anti-Rh immune globulin (also known by its trade name, Rhogam) (Fig 42–5). Because initial protocols calling for a single postpartum injection resulted in a low but significant incidence of prophylaxis failures, current recommendations are that anti-Rh immune globulin be administered to all pregnant Rh-negative

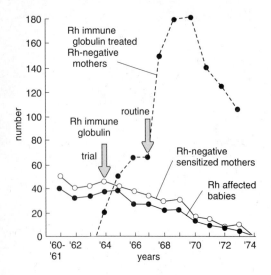

Figure 42–5. Incidence of Rh disease correlated with Rh immune globulin treatment during the years 1960 to 1974. A fairly constant number of sensitized mothers and affected infants was seen at the Columbia-Presbyterian Rh antepartum clinic prior to the first clinical trial with Rh immune globulin in 1964. Thereafter, a steady decline in the incidence of sensitization and hemolytic disease was seen annually. (Reproduced, with permission, from Freda VJ, Gorman JG, Pollack W, Bowe E: *New England Journal of Medicine* 1975;**292**:1014.

women at 28 weeks gestation and again postpartum, if the neonate is found to be Rh positive. In addition, prophylaxis is given at any time of pregnancy loss, ectopic pregnancy, maternal trauma, uterine bleeding, or other evidence of fetomaternal hemorrhage. Because platelets can express the Rh antigen, some authors recommend prophylactic treatment of Rh-negative women after platelet transfusion. Following these guidelines, Rh isoimmunization rates should approach zero.

Mechanism of Prophylaxis

Development of Rh isoimmunization prophylaxis in the 1960s was based on the well-recognized phenomenon of antibody-mediated immune suppression (AMIS), in which passively administered antibody was known to prevent active immunization by its specific antigen. Even today the mechanism of the AMIS response is not completely understood. Three general theories have been proposed: antigen deviation or diversion, competitive inhibition by antigen blocking, and central inhibition. The first 2 theories are unsatisfactory. Although studies of ^{51}Cr-labeled Rh-positive red cells infused into Rh-negative volunteers have shown that Rh-immune globulin increases clearance of Rh-positive cells, the antigen itself is not destroyed. Rather, the intact antibody-coated cells are

removed to the spleen or lymph nodes, where an immune response would normally be initiated. Antigen blocking cannot explain AMIS; first, less than 20% of available antigen is bound by Rh-immune globulin; and second, in murine models of immunization by sheep erythrocytes, $F(ab)'_2$ fragments, which bind avidly to sheep red blood cells, do not suppress the murine immune response, whereas whole antibody with an intact Fc region does.

Central inhibition may represent a plausible explanation for AMIS. Fetal red cells coated with anti-Rh are filtered out of the maternal circulation by the spleen and lymph nodes, where the increase in local concentration of complexes of anti-Rh antibody bound to Rh antigen is thought to suppress the primary immune response by interrupting helper T cell-mediated clonal expansion of Rh-specific B cells. Again, the Fc region appears to be required for AMIS; neither $F(ab)$ nor $F(ab)'_2$ fragments are effective. This model also is consistent with the observation that neither AMIS nor Rh-immune globulin prophylaxis inhibits secondary immune responses.

MANAGEMENT OF THE ISOIMMUNIZED PREGNANCY

Eradication of Rh disease will be achieved by prophylaxis, not by treatment of isoimmunization. Nevertheless, with the dramatically decreased but still significant occurrence of isoimmunization to the Rh antigen and, more importantly, to the comparatively rare "minor" or "atypical" erythrocyte antigens for which there is no prophylaxis, technological innovations in the fields of fetal diagnosis and treatment have become exceedingly important.

Screening maternal serum for erythrocyte antibodies is a cornerstone of modern prenatal care. When a low titer of anti-red cell antibody is first detected in the current pregnancy and remains stable, patients can simply be monitored. Even when titers are rising, if the involved antigen is not a proven cause of hemolytic disease of the newborn (such as anti-Lewis), no intervention is necessary. However, if titers of a potentially serious antibody (in addition to anti-Rh this includes the common atypical antibodies, ie, anti-E, anti-Kell, anti-c, anti-c+E, and anti-Fy^a) are detected in a second affected pregnancy or if markedly rising titers are detected in a first pregnancy, more aggressive intervention is warranted. Although diagnostic and treatment protocols are not yet standard, techniques available to most practitioners in major medical centers such as amniocentesis for ΔOD_{450} to detect hemoglobin and its breakdwon products in amniotic fluid (an indirect reflection of severity of disease and fetal anemia), sampling of umbilical cord blood in utero for fetal blood typing and direct fetal hematocrit, and fetal blood transfusion (either intra-peritoneally or intravascularly into the fetal umbilical vein) have revolutionized the treatment and prognosis of severely affected isoimmunized fetuses.

NEONATAL ALLOIMMUNE THROMBOCYTOPENIA

Platelet isoimmunization, most commonly against the Pl^A1 antigen, is a rare syndrome (less than 0.1% of births) and is analogous to Rh isoimmunization in that the mother forms IgG antibodies to antigen present in paternal and fetal platelets. These antibodies cross the placenta and result in increased platelet sequestration and destruction. Infants can be mildly affected, with only petechiae noted at birth; alternatively, severe hemorrhage (particularly intracranial) can lead to neonatal death.

Unlike Rh disease, the firstborn infant can be affected, suggesting that platelet antigen has greater access to the maternal circulation than red cell antigen. Postnatally, therapy is directed at treatment and prevention of hemorrhage. If a couple has previously had a severely affected infant, antenatal diagnostic fetal cord blood sampling may be performed. In utero therapy has been suggested for documented affected therapies. Although maternal corticosteroid therapy has no place here, maternal infusion of high-dose IgG may raise the fetal platelet count, and platelet transfusion into the umbilical vein has been reported. Because this syndrome is rare, the utility of these interventions has not yet been completely evaluated.

HIV INFECTION AND THE REPRODUCTIVE SYSTEM

HETEROSEXUAL TRANSMISSION OF HIV

AIDS was largely invisible as a disease among women until the late 1980s. Even now, most of the research on the disease has focused on adult males, whose source of infection was most likely to be homosexual contact or intravenous drug use. Until it became apparent that growing numbers of women were being infected sexually and that the overwhelming majority of these were of reproductive age and, when pregnant, were choosing to maintain their pregnancies, the reproductive health aspects of HIV infection and AIDS were not raised as a research priority.

Worldwide, heterosexual contact is by far the most common method of HIV transmission, despite the inefficiency of this mode of transmission. Whereas one

in 4 individuals exposed to *Neisseria gonorrheae* or hepatitis B virus will develop disease, it is estimated that for a single contact, the infectivity of HIV is 0.3%. Still, some individuals become infected after a single or few sexual contacts. Several cofactors have been found to increase the risk of acquiring disease through heterosexual contact. In the USA, male-to-female transmission is more efficient than female-to-male. It is generally agreed that compromise and alteration of vaginal mucosal immunity appear to have a significant impact on disease transmission. For example, postcoital bleeding, cervical ectopy (ie, migration of glandular endocervical epithelium from the endocervix to the ectocervix), lack of circumcision, genital ulcer disease, and infection with other sexually transmitted diseases have all been shown to be cofactors associated with HIV transmission. In addition, receptive anal intercourse increases the risk of male-to-female dissemination of disease.

Infectivity appears to vary among specific HIV strains, and the clinical stage of disease directly influences the amount of viral shedding in secretions. Susceptibility may be influenced by unique factors such as nutritional status, stage of menstrual cycle, or pregnancy. Both cell-associated and cell-free HIV are present in the cervicovaginal secretions and semen of asymptomatic individuals and AIDS patients. The fate of HIV-infected cells in ejaculate in the vagina is unknown. It is unlikely that infected cells can cross intact vaginal mucosa, and, because of low vaginal pH, normal vaginal flora, lysozyme, and proteases, latently infected cells in the ejaculate are unlikely to survive long enough to produce infectious virions, so that only cells producing infectious HIV particles at the time of infection itself are thought likely to contribute to sexual transmission.

The cellular targets of HIV during genital transmission are unknown. Since only a few CD4 T cells are present in the vaginal submucosa, the most likely targets are macrophages and Langerhans cells. Cervical biopsy specimens from HIV-infected women show no evidence of epithelial cell infection by HIV. CD4 positive class II MHC-bearing Langerhans cells and macrophages present in the vaginal mucosa may have a role in the sexual transmission of the virus (Fig 42–6). As antigen-presenting cells, they are well suited to disseminate virus from the mucosa to draining lymph nodes. In vitro, they have been shown to produce virus without exhibiting the cytopathic effects typical of T cell infection. Thus, it is likely that infection and initial viral replication occur in these local target cells and that the viruses then undergo further replication in draining lymph nodes before spreading to more distant lymphoid tissues. There has been considerable speculation regarding the association of tissue trauma with spread of disease. It is unlikely that the virus can gain direct entry into the bloodstream via breaks in the vaginal mucosa.

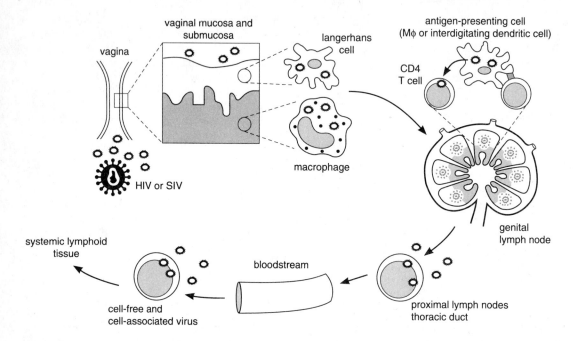

Figure 42–6. Viral dissemination during the genital transmission of HIV. This hypothetical model depicts viral contact with the genital mucosa and infection of target cells, presumably macrophages or Langerhans cell in the vaginal submucosa. Infected target cells move through lymphatic vessels to draining lymph nodes, enter the CD4 T cell rich lymph node paracortex and present processed antigen, thus initiating an immune response. Viral replication occurs in the lymph node. Cell-free and cell-associated virus then travel via efferent lymphatics to proximal lymph nodes and the thoracic duct into the bloodstream, ultimately resulting in systemic infection. (Reproduced, with permission, from Miller CH, McGhee JR, Gardner MB: *Laboratory Investigation* 1992;**68**:129.

Rather, it is more probable that blood cells (including CD4 T cells) escaping from the vasculature do not re-enter the bloodstream, but travel the same route as Langerhans cells and macrophages, through the lymphatics to draining lymph nodes. Trauma and infection are likely to be associated with increased numbers of CD4-positive target cells in genital tissues and thus increase the efficiency of HIV transmission; these conditions, however, are unlikely to alter the route of infection.

PERINATAL TRANSMISSION OF HIV

There is a wide variation in the rate of transmission of HIV from mother to infant. Diagnosis of HIV infection in the neonate is difficult since serologic studies are biased by the presence of maternally derived antibodies in neonatal serum. Prevalence studies of neonatal infection are based primarily on polymerase chain reaction (PCR) and virus culture studies and have yielded rates of 11–60% transmission in different parts of the world. For diagnosis in the individual

patient, it should be remembered that PCR is quite sensitive but can lack specificity whereas virus culture is time-consuming and difficult to perform routinely. Other methods to determine infection in the newborn that are currently being evaluated include serum IgA measurement and examination of antibody production in mitogen-stimulated newborn peripheral blood mononuclear cell cultures.

HIV can be transferred from mother to infant in utero or after delivery. Even though HIV has been isolated from umbilical cord blood, amniotic fluid, placenta, and other fetal tissues, there is considerable disagreement about the frequency of HIV infection of fetal tissues. Some find no virus in fetal tissues, whereas others report detection of HIV genomic sequences in 30% of second-trimester abortuses, virtually identical to newborn transmission rates, and conclude that most vertical transmission occurs early in gestation. On the other hand, the delay in the ability to isolate HIV from neonatal serum until after 1 month of life suggests that transmission is most likely to occur at parturition, secondary to maternal-fetal transfusion or fetal exposure to maternal secretions and blood during the delivery process. Cesarean section has not been shown to alter rates of transmission, but HIV infection has been transmitted via breast milk. Although this route of infection is considered rare, it has been particularly prominent in infants of mothers who are primarily infected postpartum.

The mechanism of in utero transmission of HIV is not understood. Transmission may correlate with absence of maternal antibody to the viral envelope, especially to the third variable region of gp120. Low maternal CD4 counts, viremia, and p25 antigenemia at the time of delivery have been reported to be predictive of transmission. Although HIV has been detected in fetal and placental tissues by in situ hybridization, PCR, and immunohistochemistry, identification of viral particles in highly purified primary trophoblast culture has not yet been reported. In vitro, however, trophoblast cultures and human choriocarcinoma cell lines have been successfully infected by virus or virus-infected cells. The CD4 receptor is identified in some cell populations studied; however, significant literature exists suggesting that trophoblast can become infected independently of the CD4-mediated pathway. Whatever the case, only low-level viral replication can be detected in these in vitro-infected cells.

Following transplacental transmission of HIV, the exact route and mechanism of disease induction in the fetus are not clear. After 16–20 weeks of gestation, mature T cells can be identified in fetal tissues, and CD4+ CD8+ positive T cell precursors are found even earlier. If early fetal infection occurs, it is unclear why entire T cell populations with $\alpha\beta$ receptors are not eliminated. Different authors speculate that infected T cell precursors could go on to differentiate while latently infected; alternatively, transmission may occur much later in pregnancy.

Whatever the mode of transmission, the incubation period for perinatally acquired infection is short. The majority of infected infants develop disease early in life and have a high mortality. For example, for infants in whom HIV is first diagnosed with *Pneumocystis carinii* pneumonia infection, median survival is 1 month; survival is somewhat longer with other initial presentations such as recurrent bacterial infections (50 months) and lobar interstitial pneumonia (72 months).

In developing countries, children make up 5–25% of HIV-infected populations. The vast majority of these pediatric infections are the result of vertical transmission of the virus. It is clear that intensive research is required for increased understanding of mechanisms of transplacental passage and pathogenesis of HIV infection in fetal tissues to identify methods of effectively blocking or interrupting perinatal disease transmission.

CONCLUSION

Medawar's 1952 observation that every well-documented, clinically significant example of immunization of the mother by fetal tissues has implicated antigen derived from either the red blood cell or platelet is still true today. Antigens responsible for the rapid and sometimes violent reactions provoked by grafting tissues from one individual to another remain relatively uninvolved in maternal and fetal interactions. Even with isoimmunization, the challenging question has become not how it occurs but why it does not occur more often. As with infectious processes, we know that this wrinkle, as it were, in the maternal immune response is located in inductive pathways: once immunized or isoimmunized, pregnancy does not modify a host's response to offending antigen. Precise characterization of the immunobiology of the maternal-fetal relationship properly begins with the detailed examination of the trophoblast and the tissues that it touches; further insight will be gained by attempts to understand interactions of these tissues in light of contemporary cellular and molecular immunologic models.

REFERENCES

General

Gill TJ, Wegmann TG, Nesbitt-Brown E (editors): *Immunoregulation and Fetal Survival.* Oxford University Press, 1987.

Grimes, DA: Technology follies: The uncritical acceptance of medical innovation. *JAMA* 1993;**269:**3030.

Medawar PB: Some immunological and endocrinological problems raised by the evolution of viviparity in vertebrates. *Symp Soc Exp Biol* 1953;**7:**320.

Strauss JF, Lyttle CR (editors): *Uterine and Embryonic Factors in Early Pregnancy.* Plenum Press, 1991.

Reproductive Tract Anatomy & Immunity

Bulmer D: The histochemistry of ovarian macrophages in the rat. *J Anat* 1964;**98:**313.

Hurwitz A et al: Human intraovarian interleukin-1 (IL-1): Highly compartmentalized and hormonally dependent regulation of the genes encoding IL-1, its receptor, and its receptor antagonist. *J Clin Invest* 1992;**89:**1746.

Kutteh WH et al: Secretory immune system of the female reproductive tract. I. Immunoglobulin and secretory component-containing cells. *Obstet Gynecol* 1988;**71:**56.

Kutteh WH et al: Secretory immune system of the female reproductive tract. II. Local immune system in normal and infected fallopian tube. *Fertil Steril* 1990;**54:**51.

Miller CH, McGhee JR, Gardner MB: Mucosal immunity, HIV transmission, and AIDS. *Lab Invest* 1992;**68:**129.

Yule TD, Mahi-Brown CA, Tung KSK: Role of testicular autoantigens and influence of lymphokines in testicular autoimmune disease. *J Reprod Immunol* 1990;**18:**89.

Fertilization, Implantation, & Immune Response to Fetal Tissues

Castellucci M, Kaufmann P: A three-dimensional study of the normal human placental villous core. II. Stromal architecture. *Placenta* 1982;**3:**269.

Damsky CH, Fitzgerald ML, Fisher SJ: Distribution patterns of extracellular matrix components and adhesion receptors are intricately modulated during first trimester cytotrophoblast differentiation along the invasive pathway, in vivo. *J Clin Invest* 1992;**89:**210.

Gilbert L, Robertson SA, Wegmann TG: The trophoblast as an integral component of a macrophage-cytokine network. *Immunol Cell Biol* 1993;**71:**49.

Paria BC, Dey SK: Preimplantation embryo development in vitro: cooperative interactions among embryos and role of growth factors. *Proc Natl Acad Sci USA* 1990;**87:**4756.

Saling PM: Mammalian sperm interaction with extracellular matrices of the egg. *Oxf Rev Reprod Biol* 1989;**11:**339.

Stewart CL et al: Blastocyst implantation depends on maternal expression of leukaemia inhibitory factor. *Nature* 1992;**359:**76.

Wassarman PM: Mouse gamete adhesion molecules. *Biol Reprod* 1992;**46:**186.

Immunity in Pregnancy

Castellucci M et al: Mitosis of the Hofbauer cell: Possible implications for a fetal macrophage. *Placenta* 1987;**8:**65.

Khayr WF, Cherubin CE, Bleck TP: Listeriosis: Review of a protean disease. *Infect Dis Clin Pract* 1992;**1:**291.

Lu CY et al: Pregnancy as a natural model of allograft tolerance. *Transplantation* 1989;**48:**848.

Redline RW, Lu CY: Specific defects in the anti-listerial immune response in discrete regions of the murine uterus and placenta account for susceptibility to infection. *J Immunol* 1988;**140:**3947.

Weinberg ED: Pregnancy-associated depression of cell mediated immunity. *Rev Infect Dis* 1984;**6:**814.

Infertility & Spontaneous Abortion

Fraser EJ, Grimes DA, Schulz KF: Immunization as therapy for recurrent spontaneous abortion: A review and meta-analysis. *Obstet Gynecol,* in press.

Haas GG: Immunologic Infertility. *Obstet Gynecol Clin North Am* 1987;**14:**1069.

Katz I et al: Cutaneous graft-versus-host-like reaction after paternal lymphocyte immunization for prevention of recurrent abortion. *Fertil Steril* 1992;**57:**927.

Kutteh WH, Carr BR: Recurrent Pregnancy Loss. Pages 559–570 in: *Textbook of Reproductive Medicine.* Carr BR, Blackwell RE (editors). Appleton & Lange, 1993.

Kutteh WH et al: Antisperm antibodies: Current knowledge and new horizons. *Mol Androl* 1993;**4:**183.

Luo YH et al: Antigen mimicry in autoimmune disease: Sharing of amino acid residues critical for pathogenic T cell activation. *J Clin Invest,* in press.

Mishell DR: Infertility. Pages 1189–1243 in: *Comprehensive Gynecology.* AL Herbst et al (editors). Mosby Year Book, 1992.

Tung KSK, Lu CY: Immunologic basis of reproductive failure. Pages 308–333 in: *Pathology of Reproductive Failure.* Kraus FT, Damjanov I, Kaufman N (editors). Williams & Wilkins, 1992.

Vazquez-Levin M et al: The effect of female antisperm antibodies on in vitro fertilization, early embryonic development, and pregnancy outcome. *Fertil Steril* 1991;**56:**84.

Isoimmunization

Branch DW, Scott JR: Isoimmunization in pregnancy. Pages 957–990 in: *Obstetrics: Normal and Problem Pregnancies.* Gabbe SG, Niebyl JR, Simpson JL (editors). Churchill Livingstone, 1991.

Cunningham FG, MacDonald PC, Gant NF: Hemolysis from isoimmunization. Pages 1004–1013 in: *Williams Obstetrics,* 19th ed. Appleton & Lange, 1993.

Freda VJ et al: Prevention of Rh hemolytic disease—ten years' clinical experience with Rh immune globulin. *N Engl Med* 1975;**292:**1014.

Pollack W: Recent understanding for the mechanism by which passively administered Rh antibody suppresses the immune response to Rh antigen in unimmunized Rh-negative women. *Clin Obstet Gynecol* 1982;**25:**255.

HIV Infection & the Reproductive System

Douglas GC, King BF: Maternal-fetal transmission of human immunodeficiency virus: A review of possible routes and cellular mechanisms of infection. *Clin Infect Dis* 1992;**15:**678.

Levy JA: Pathogenesis of human immunodeficiency virus infection. *Microbiol Rev* 1993;**57:**183.

Miller CH, McGhee JR, Gardner MB: Mucosal immunity, HIV transmission, and AIDS. *Lab Invest* 1992;**68:**129.

Mechanisms of Tumor Immunology 43

Philip D. Greenberg, MD

Tumor immunology is the study of (1) the antigenic properties of transformed cells, (2) the host immune responses to these tumor cells, (3) the immunologic consequences to the host of the growth of malignant cells, and (4) the means by which the immune system can be modulated to recognize tumor cells and promote tumor eradication. One potentially important function of the immune system is to provide protection from the outgrowth of malignant cells. This represents a formidable task because tumor cells have many similarities to normal cells, despite exhibiting abnormal propensities to proliferate, to spread throughout the host, and to interfere with normal organ functions. Thus, tumor cells present special problems to the host immune system beyond those presented by other self-replicating antigens such as bacteria, which can more easily be distinguished as foreign. Elucidating the processes that render a cancerous cell different from normal cells should aid in understanding how these transformed cells might be amenable to destruction and regulation by the immune system.

Normal cells have a variable capacity to proliferate and to express differentiated functions. These cell activities are tightly coordinated within an organ or tissue, so that the rate of cell loss due to the natural death of mature differentiated cells is equal to the rate of appearance of new cells from the less mature proliferating cell pool. If the stimulus for cell proliferation exceeds the requirement for cell replacement, as in some pathologic conditions, organ hypertrophy occurs with polyclonal expansion of cells from a pool that proliferates in response to growth signals. However, if the condition responsible for excess stimulation of cell growth is ablated, the rate of cell proliferation decreases and the organ hypertrophy resolves. In contrast to nonmalignant regulated polyclonal cell growth, an individual cell may undergo a transforming event and acquire the potential to produce daughter cells that proliferate independent of external growth signals. The autonomous growth of such

transformed cells of monoclonal origin represents the basis of malignant disease. Many of the properties of tumor cells are summarized in Table 43–1. The protean effects of cancer reflect in large part the unrestrained growth of tumor cells that locally invade and disrupt normal tissue as well as metastasize and grow in distant organs.

DEVELOPMENT OF TUMORS

The transformation of a normal cell to malignancy can result from a variety of different causes, the particular nature of which may help determine whether the immune system can control the outgrowth of the tumor cells. These transforming events may occur spontaneously by random mutations or gene rearrangements; alternatively, they may be induced by a chemical, physical, or viral carcinogen.

Tumors induced by chemical carcinogens were initially described in the 18th century, when chimney sweeps were observed to have an unusually high incidence of carcinoma of the scrotum. Polycyclic aromatic hydrocarbons in soot and tar have since been found to be a major class of carcinogens, and retention of tar in the wrinkles of the scrotum was apparently responsible for these tumors. In fact, painting tar on epithelial cells has become a useful experimental technique for inducing tumors in the laboratory. A second major class of carcinogens, the aromatic amines, was identified following the observation of a high frequency of bladder cancer among factory workers using aniline dyes. The mechanisms by which chemical carcinogens induce neoplastic transformation predominantly reflect the mutagenic activity of these compounds.

Evidence of tumor induction by physical carcinogens accrued rapidly following the discovery of x-rays and radioactivity in the late 19th century since many of the early radiologists developed skin cancer. The most dramatic evidence of radiation-induced car-

Table 43–1. Common properties of tumor cells.

1. Failure to respond to the regulatory signals responsible for normal growth and tissue repair.
2. Autonomous growth without an absolute requirement for exogenous growth signals.
3. Invasive growth through normal tissue boundaries.
4. Metastatic growth in distant organs following entry into blood and lymph channels.
5. Monoclonal origin, although genotypic and phenotypic heterogeneity may develop as tumor mass increases.
6. Differences in appearance and membrane antigenic display from nontransformed cells of the same tissue origin.

cinogenesis is in survivors of the atomic bomb explosions in Japan, who demonstrated an increased incidence of a wide range of tumors for more than 20 years after the nuclear holocaust. Such ionizing radiation directly injures cellular DNA, resulting in mutations, chromosomal breaks, and abnormal rearrangements. Another physical carcinogen, ultraviolet radiation, induces skin cancer on sun-exposed parts of the body, particularly in people with xeroderma pigmentosum, a disease in which there is a defective repair mechanism for UV induced damage to DNA.

Viral oncogenesis is of particular interest in tumor immunology because of the great likelihood that cells transformed by the introduction of viral genes will express new virus-associated antigens that can be recognized by the immune system. Oncogenic viruses can be subdivided into either DNA or RNA types, depending on the genetic information carried by the intact virus. Most cells infected by the potentially oncogenic DNA viruses, which include papovaviruses, herpesviruses, and adenoviruses, do not interfere with expression of viral genes and replication, which commonly result in cell lysis. However, infection of nonpermissive cells can result in integration of the viral DNA into the host genome and expression of only some of the viral genes, so that lytic virus particles are not formed. Transformation results either from direct triggering of host genes by the integrated viral DNA or from aberrant splicing of viral RNA messages by the host to produce new proteins that promote transformation. Although no DNA viruses with direct oncogenic potential have been isolated from human tumors, several cancers exhibit statistically significant linkage with particular viral infections. These include links between Epstein-Barr virus (EBV) infection and Burkitt's lymphoma, Hodgkin's disease and nasopharyngeal carcinoma, human papilloma virus and cervical carcinoma, and hepatitis B virus infection and primary liver cancers.

Oncogenic RNA viruses contain genes for a polymerase called **reverse transcriptase**, which permits the use of the viral RNA as a template for transcription of a DNA copy, which can be integrated into the host genome. Because this is a reversal of the normal DNA-to-RNA transcription of genetic information, these viruses are often referred to as **retroviruses.**

RNA tumor viruses were first discovered in chicken tumors and appear to be responsible for a large number of naturally occurring cancers in many species. Some of these viruses contain directly transforming oncogenes, whereas others must activate host genetic material. A class of human retroviruses, the human T cell leukemia viruses (HTLV), have been identified as responsible for certain T cell leukemias, particularly in cases occurring in a region of southern Japan where the infection is endemic. Many retroviruses, such as feline leukemia virus and HTLV, can spread horizontally from infected to normal hosts, and resistance to tumorigenesis appears to be partly dependent on the generation of an immune response to virus-associated antigens in exposed resistant hosts.

Advances in molecular biology have provided the tools to better understand the events involved in transformation. Analogues to many of the viral oncogenes have been identified in the normal cellular genome, and in vitro studies have demonstrated that activation of these cellular oncogenes can transform normal cells under appropriate conditions. The essential role of many of these cellular oncogenes in normal growth and development has been demonstrated, but the abnormal maintenance of these genes in a transcriptionally active state can result in transformation. This may occur by mutation, such as ones that interfere with regulation of transcription or of the activity of the protein; by a translocation that places the oncogene next to an active cellular gene, such as is observed in B cell tumors with the translocation of the c-*myc* oncogene next to an immunoglobulin V region gene; or by insertion of a promoter that enhances expression, such as may occur following integration of a slowly transforming retrovirus. Oncogenes code for a wide variety of products including membrane receptors, autocrine growth factors, and regulators of cell cycle progression and gene expression. The expression of at least some of these oncogene products, particularly those representing mutations of the normal protein, should render malignant cells sufficiently disparate from normal cells for detection by immunologic methods and potentially for elimination by immunologically directed attack.

ANTIGENS ON TUMOR CELLS

The field of tumor immunology is based in large part on the supposition that tumors express antigens which permit immunologic separation of malignant from normal cells. Problems in the past demonstrating the immunogenicity of tumor cells to the host of origin led to a great deal of skepticism about the concept that tumors express distinct antigens. However, more recent studies that have taken advantage of the advances in cellular and molecular immunology have convincingly demonstrated that many human tumors express antigens which can induce cellular and humoral responses in the host; they have also elucidated many of the reasons underlying the ineffective and often undetectable response in the primary host. The relevant tumor antigens fall into 2 major categories. **Unique tumor-specific antigens** are found only on tumor cells and therefore represent ideal targets for an immunologic attack. In contrast, **tumor-associated determinants** are found on tumor cells and also on some normal cells, but qualitative and quantitative differences in antigen expression permit the use of these antigens to distinguish tumor cells from normal cells.

A wide variety of cellular proteins have now been identified to function as tumor antigens. Although the expression of these antigens must reflect a transformation-related heritable change in the genetic material of the cells, there are many distinct molecular mechanisms that may result in the production of a tumor antigen. The most straightforward mechanism is a transforming event that results in the production of a new protein, such as would occur following infection with a potentially oncogenic virus such as EBV, HTLV, or human papillomavirus (HPV) and the introduction of new genetic material and subsequent expression of viral proteins. Similarly, point mutations or gene rearrangements affecting cellular oncogenes that promote the transformed phenotype, such as reported with *ras* and p53 in breast and colon cancer or bcr-*abl* in chronic myelogenous leukemia, could result in the expression of new epitopes potentially recognizable by the immune system. Unique tumor antigens could also result from the uncovering of normally nonexposed determinants, as observed with some of the complex branching glycolipid antigens in which deletion of a branch may expose a new antigenic determinant. Nonunique proteins that may nevertheless serve as tumor antigens can result from the aberrant expression of fetal or differentiation antigens, such as observed with the expression on human gastric carcinoma cells of ABO blood group antigens disparate from the host ABO blood type or of the MAGE antigens in human melanoma cells.

Unique Tumor Antigens

These are antigens that can be detected only on tumor cells and not on other host cells. The best-studied unique tumor antigens are the new antigens expressed on tumors induced in inbred mice by oncogenic viruses and chemical carcinogens. Identification of the presence of unique tumor antigens has been difficult with human tumors because of the inability to perform classic tumor transplantation studies, but it has become feasible owing to advances in molecular biology. Molecular techniques have now permitted the isolation of human retroviruses such as HTLV, the identification of viral proteins expressed in the tumor, and the demonstration that these unique viral antigens are potentially immunogenic. "Spontaneous" tumors, many of which may have actually been induced by exposure to environmental carcinogens, have no predictable antigenic markers and therefore have been harder to study. However, technologic advances have also occurred in lymphocytic isolation and culture and have made it possible to expand low-frequency antigen-reactive T cells and antibody-forming B cells from tumor-bearing hosts. These measures have permitted the identification of tumor-specific T cells and antibodies derived from tumor-draining lymph nodes of patients with melanoma, breast cancer, leukemia, lymphoma, and lung cancer, as well as from lymph nodes following immunization with human colon carcinoma cells in association with an immunoadjuvant. Such tumor-reactive immunologic reagents have been useful to screen expression libraries derived from tumor cells to characterize the target antigens.

The elucidation of the processing pathways for presentation of protein antigens in association with major histocompatibility complex (MHC) molecules to T cells has revolutionized our understanding of the potential origin of unique tumor-specific antigens. T cells recognize small peptides derived from intracellular degradation of proteins that are inserted into a peptide-binding cleft in the MHC molecule and are then transported with the MHC molecule to the cell surface (see Chapter 5). Therefore, any abnormal cellular protein, not just proteins detected on the membrane, is a potential immunogen. Thus, the presence in a tumor cell of a truncated or nonfunctional protein product of a mutated allele could result in the immunogenicity of that product. Moreover, these insights suggest that the difficulties that have been encountered in detecting unique antigens on human tumors with monoclonal antibodies are predictable; the results do not imply that these tumors do not express unique antigens but, rather, that the use of new molecular approaches that probe gene expression rather than surface phenotype would probably facilitate their identification.

Tumor-Associated Antigens

Although it may not be possible to detect unique tumor antigens on all tumors, many tumors display antigens that distinguish them from normal cells. These tumor-associated antigens may be expressed on some normal cells at particular stages of differentiation, but the quantitative expression and/or the composite expression in association with other lineage or differentiation markers can be useful for identifying transformed cells. The identification of tumor-associated antigens has progressed rapidly with the advent of technology for generating and screening monoclonal antibodies. These monoclonal antibody reagents have permitted the isolation and biochemical characterization of the antigens and have been invaluable diagnostically for distinction of transformed from nontransformed cells and for definition of the cell lineage of transformed cells.

The best-characterized human tumor-associated antigens are the oncofetal antigens. These antigens are expressed during embryogenesis but are absent or very difficult to detect in normal adult tissue. The prototype antigen is **carcinoembryonic antigen (CEA),** a glycoprotein found on fetal gut and human colon cancer cells but not on normal adult colon cells. Since CEA is shed from colon carcinoma cells and found in the serum, it was originally thought that the presence of this antigen in the serum could be used to screen patients for colon cancer. However, it soon became apparent that patients with inflammatory lesions involving cells of endodermal origin, such as colitis or pancreatitis, as well as patients with other tumors, such as pancreatic and breast cancer, also had elevated serum levels of CEA. Despite these limitations, monitoring the fall and rise of CEA levels in colon cancer patients undergoing therapy has proven useful for predicting tumor progression and responses to treatment. Moreover, studies in mice have suggested that antitumor T cell immunity can be elicited to tumors expressing CEA, and a human clinical trial in patients with colon cancer is currently evaluating whether a recombinant vaccinia virus vaccine expressing CEA can induce therapeutic T cell responses. Several other oncofetal antigens have been useful for diagnosing and monitoring human tumors. In particular, **alpha-fetoprotein,** an alpha-globulin normally secreted by fetal liver and yolk sac cells, is found in the serum of patients with liver and germinal cell tumors and can be used as a marker of disease status.

Differentiation and lineage-specific antigens, which are present on normal adult cells, may be aberrantly expressed on some tumor cells. For example, a T cell antigen, CD5, is commonly expressed on the malignant human B cells found in chronic lymphocytic leukemia, and an erythrocyte blood group antigen is frequently found on human stomach cancer cells. These inappropriately expressed antigens are very useful for identifying transformed cells, and their unexpected presence on tumor cells may ultimately aid in deciphering the regulation and function of such antigens on normally differentiated cells.

Many other tumor-associated antigens, which have unknown function but very limited tissue distribution on normal cells, have now been identified with monoclonal antibodies. Glycoprotein and glycolipid antigens isolated from malignant melanoma cells appear to be relatively specific for these tumors, although some expression on normal cells such as neuronal tissue has been detected. A glycoprotein found on human leukemia cells, called common acute lymphocytic leukemia antigen (CALLA or CD10), has been found to a minimal extent on other cells such as granulocytes and kidney cells. Many other similar examples exist, and the use of such antigenic markers for diagnostic and therapeutic purposes has great promise.

The recent successes in isolation and cloning of tumor-reactive T cells from cancer patients, coupled with expression cloning of tumor genes and/or analysis of mutated tumor cells, has made it possible to identify tumor-associated antigens that unequivocally can induce immune responses. In melanoma, T cell responses to at least 3 normal cellular proteins, including MAGE and tyrosinase, have been characterized. Immunogenic proteins have also been identified in breast cancer, lung cancer, and pancreatic cancer.

IMMUNOLOGIC EFFECTOR MECHANISMS POTENTIALLY OPERATIVE AGAINST TUMOR CELLS

Virtually all of the effector components of the immune system have the potential to contribute to the eradication of tumor cells. It is likely that each of these effector mechanisms plays a role in the control of tumor growth, but a particular mechanism may be more or less important, depending on the tumor and setting. Thus, immunologically specific effector responses are probably most important with highly immunogenic tumors, and nonspecific effector responses are presumably of greater significance with less immunogenic tumors.

T Cells

The T cell response is unquestionably the most important host response for the control of growth of antigenic tumor cells; it is responsible for both the direct killing of tumor cells and the activation of other components of the immune system. T cell immunity to tumors reflects the function of the two T cell subsets: class II-restricted T cells, which largely represent CD4 helper T (TH) cells that mediate their effect by the secretion of lymphokines to activate other effector cells and induce inflammatory responses, and class I-restricted T cells, which largely represent CD8 cytotoxic T (TC) cells that can also secrete lymphokines but mediate their effect mostly by direct lysis of tumor cells.

The precise contribution of each T cell subset and T cell function to the antitumor response appears quite variable, but tumor-specific T cells from each subset are capable of mediating tumor eradication and have been detected in the peripheral blood of individual patients and in the cells infiltrating human tumors. Because most tumor cells express class I but not class II MHC molecules, the TH cell subset cannot directly recognize these tumor cells. Therefore, most TH cell responses are dependent upon antigen-presenting cells such as macrophages to present the relevant tumor antigens in the context of class II molecules for activation. After antigen-specific triggering, these T cells secrete lymphokines that activate TC cells, macrophages, NK cells, and B cells and can produce other lymphokines, such as lymphotoxin or tumor necrosis factor (TNF), which may be directly lytic to tumor cells (see Chapter 9 and 11). In contrast to TH cells, the TC cell subset is capable of directly recognizing and killing tumor targets by disrupting the target membrane and nucleus. However, only a minor fraction of class I-restricted T cells are capable of providing helper functions, and thus effective TC cell responses are generally dependent on class II-restricted TH cell responses to provide the necessary helper factors to activate and promote the proliferation of TC cells.

B Cells & Antibody-Dependent Killing

A potential role for host antibody responses in human tumor immunity has been suggested by the occasional detection of tumor-reactive antibodies in the serum of patients. Moreover, recent studies in which hybridomas or B cell lines are formed from B cells derived from lymph nodes draining human tumors have suggested that human tumors may frequently elicit antibody responses to tumor-associated antigens. In addition to secreting antibodies that may contribute to the control of tumor growth, B cells with surface immunoglobulin reactive with tumor antigens may play a role in binding, processing, and presenting tumor antigens for induction of T cell responses to the tumor.

There are 2 major mechanisms by which antibodies may mediate tumor cell lysis. Complement-fixing antibodies bind to the tumor cell membrane and promote attachment of complement components that create pores in the membrane, resulting in cell disruption due to loss of osmotic and biochemical integrity. An alternative mechanism is antibody-dependent cell-mediated cytotoxicity (ADCC), in which antibodies, usually of the IgG class, form an intercellular bridge by binding via the variable region to a specific determinant on the target cell and via the FC region to effector cells expressing FC receptors. There are many potential effector cells that can mediate the lytic event, including natural killer (NK) and killer cells, macrophages, and granulocytes. ADCC is a more efficient in vitro lytic mechanism than is complement-mediated cytotoxicity, requiring fewer antibody molecules per cell to kill. Immunotherapy studies with monoclonal antibodies of different isotypes (and thus different capacities to fix complement or mediate ADCC) have also suggested that ADCC may be the more important in vivo effector mechanism.

Natural Killer (NK) Cells

NK cells can kill a wide range of tumor targets in vitro (see also Chapter 11). The mechanism by which NK cells preferentially recognize and lyse transformed rather than normal targets is not well-defined. However, recent studies have demonstrated that NK cells recognize target cells with diminished expression of self-class I MHC molecules. Down-regulation

or loss of class I molecule expression is commonly observed in virus-infected and many transformed cells and may partially explain the therapeutic activity reported with NK effector cells. Cytolysis by NK cells is mediated by the release of a cytotoxic factor(s) and the introduction of holes in the target cell membrane. The cytotoxic activity of NK cells can be augmented both in vitro and in vivo with the lymphokines interleukin-2 (IL-2) and interferon, and thus NK activity can be amplified by immune T cell responses. Recent studies have demonstrated that augmentation of NK activity in visceral organs enhances resistance to the growth of metastases. Therefore, NK cells may represent a first line of host defense against the growth of transformed cells at both the primary and metastatic sites, as well as providing an effector mechanism recruited by T cells (or the pharmacologic administration of cytokines) to supplement specific antitumor responses.

Additional cytotoxic effector cells that bear many similarities to but can be distinguished from classic NK cells have also been identified. Natural cytotoxic (NC) cells kill a somewhat different spectrum of tumor targets than do NK cells, are resistant to glucocorticoids, and respond to IL-3. Lymphokine-activated killer (LAK) cells can be induced by very high doses of IL-2, are phenotypically heterogeneous (including both NK and CD8T cells), and kill a much broader spectrum of tumor targets than do NK cells, but their role during physiologic antitumor responses remains to be elucidated.

Macrophages

Macrophages are important in tumor immunity as antigen-presenting cells to initiate the immune response and as potential effector cells to mediate tumor lysis. Resting macrophages are not cytolytic to tumor cells in vitro, but they can become cytolytic if activated with macrophage-activating factors (MAF). MAF are commonly secreted by T cells following antigen-specific stimulation, and therefore the participation of macrophages as effector cells may be dependent on T cell immunity. This is supported by studies showing that macrophages isolated from immunogenic tumors undergoing regression exhibit tumoricidal activity, whereas macrophages isolated from progressing or nonimmunogenic tumors generally show no cytotoxic activity. T cell lymphokines with MAF activity include gamma interferon, TNF, IL-4, and granulocyte-macrophage colony-stimulating factor (GM-CSF) (see Chapter 9).

The mechanisms by which macrophages recognize tumor cells and mediate lysis are not fully defined. As with NK cells, activated macrophages bind to and lyse transformed cells in marked preference to normal cells. Binding by activated macrophages is an energy-dependent process that is also dependent on trypsin-sensitive membrane structures. Several distinct mechanisms may be selectively elicited, depending on the MAF, by which macrophages can mediate lysis. These include intercellular transfer of lysosomal products, superoxide production, release of neutral proteases, and secretion of the monokine TNF.

POTENTIAL MECHANISMS BY WHICH TUMOR CELLS MAY ESCAPE FROM AN IMMUNE RESPONSE

The concept of host immune surveillance, with the immune system providing the function of surveying the body to recognize and destroy frequently developing immunogenic tumor cells, was formally proposed by Burnet. However, the failure to demonstrate an increased appearance of immunogenic tumors in immunodeficient hosts incapable of tumor rejection has modified current views of immune surveillance. Thus, effector populations, such as NK cells, rather than tumor antigen-specific immune responses are now believed to be important in the rejection of newly appearing tumor cells. It should be emphasized that antigen-specific responses may provide a surveillance function for the development of certain tumors, such as those induced by oncogenic DNA and RNA tumor viruses. Moreover, the failure of the immune system to prevent the emergence of other new tumors does not preclude the development of tumor-specific immune responses during the growth of established tumors. Indirect support for the presence of immunity to human tumors includes spontaneous regressions of tumors and regressions of metastatic lesions after removal of large primary tumors. Direct evidence of tumor-specific immunity has been provided by studies in which the use of in vitro technologies to selectively expand antigen-reactive T cells has permitted the detection in cancer patients of weak tumor-specific responses. Thus, it seems likely that even though the emergence of many tumors may reflect a failure of immune surveillance and the absence of an immune response during early tumor growth, a potentially detectable but unfortunately ineffective immune response may still be generated during progressive growth of the tumor. One important goal in tumor immunology is to determine why such responses are ineffective.

Many potential mechanisms permitting escape from immune destruction have been identified. Immunoselection of variant cells is suggested by analysis of the cells present in a tumor mass, which often reveals a heterogeneity with respect to morphology and surface phenotype. Some of these differences are cell cycle-dependent, but others result from random mutations due to genetic instability in the proliferating cell population. Regardless of the underlying reason, if some of these differences result in a reduction in the expression of a tumor antigen being recognized by the immune system, the cells derived from this clone may have a selective advantage. Moreover, as growth of such a tumor variant proceeds, it will be-

come the dominant population, which will make it increasingly difficult to identify that a host response to the tumor had been generated.

Antigenic modulation is similar to the immunoselection described above, in that an immune response to a tumor antigen results in the growth of antigen-negative cells. However, in this setting, antigen loss reflects only a phenotypic change in the tumor cell, and if the immune response is ablated, the antigen will be reexpressed. Antigenic modulation resulting from antibody responses has been extensively reported, but modulation from T cell responses has not yet been clearly identified.

As described in Chapter 5, the presentation of antigens by tumor cells for recognition by T cells requires the intracellular processing of proteins, with degradation to small 8–9-amino-acid peptides that are transported to the endoplasmic reticulum and then inserted into a cleft in the class I MHC molecule for subsequent transport to the cell surface. Recent studies show that some tumor cells have defective antigen-processing machinery, with the result that even highly immunogenic proteins cannot be presented to the immune system.

There are many mechanisms by which tumor cells can nonspecifically interfere with the expression of immunity in the host. Some tumor cells can release soluble factors that directly suppress immunologic reactivity. Perhaps the best-studied phenomenon is the inhibition of immune responses by macrophages obtained from hosts bearing progressive tumors. This appears to be mediated largely via the secretion of prostaglandins, and in vitro treatment of macrophages with the cyclooxygenase inhibitor indomethacin can overcome the inhibitory effects.

Patients with advanced cancer demonstrate increased susceptibility to opportunistic infections and exhibit global depression of T cell responses. Analysis of the T cell receptor signaling complex from T cells in such patients has demonstrated that this in part reflects the absence of a zeta chain in the T cell receptor. This defect, as well as the associated abnormal T cell function, is reversible, providing further support that tumor growth results in release of an immunosuppressive factor. Identification of such factor(s) could not only improve tumor immunity but also possibly provide insights into novel new immunoregulatory compounds.

The presence of tumor-specific suppressor T (Ts) cells may represent another reason for the difficulties in detecting tumor-specific immunity in cancer patients and for the impression that no response has been elicited. For example, even with many of the highly immunogenic animal tumors studied in the laboratory, the presence of Ts cells would prevent the detection of tumor-specific immunity in the host if the presence of immunity was not sought until the tumor had reached a stage comparable to that in which most cancer patients are studied.

The major obstacle to understanding the role of Ts cells in tumor immunity has been the difficulty in isolating and characterizing such cells. Despite this difficulty, the biologic phenomenon of antigen-specific T cell-mediated suppression has been unequivocally demonstrated in vivo, and future studies will have to elucidate the bases for these observations.

IMMUNOTHERAPY

Although the host immune system may often be inadequate for controlling tumor growth, the presence of identifiable tumor antigens on most tumor cells, the identification of a detectable but ineffective host response to many tumors, and an improved understanding of the mechanisms by which tumor cells evade immunity suggest that it may be possible to manipulate and amplify the immune system to promote tumor eradication. The recent technologic advances that permit isolation of lymphocyte subpopulations, identification and purification of tumor antigens, growth of selected antigen-specific T cells, amplification of immune responses with cytokines, and targeting of antibody-toxin conjugates to tumors have created a new potential and enthusiasm for the immunotherapy of tumors. Several distinct approaches to immunotherapy are being studied, and it seems likely that at least some of these approaches will soon be developed into important modalities for the treatment of tumors.

Immunization with Tumor Cells or Purified Antigens

Immunization of hosts bearing established progressing tumors with tumor cells or tumor antigen has generally been ineffective. This outcome may reflect in part the global immunoincompetence and suppressive state commonly detected in such individuals. Therefore, methods to modify the host-tumor relationship prior to immunization, such as by reduction of the tumor burden, in concert with methods to enhance the immunogenicity of tumor cells and tumor antigens are being explored. One approach has been to directly inject DNA encoding foreign MHC antigens into the tumor, with the hope that the expressed alloantigens will create an immunologic milieu that results in the induction of responses to both the alloantigens and tumor antigens. Studies in mice have been encouraging and have provided the rationale for a current human trial.

An alternative approach has been to isolate tumor cells from a biopsy specimen, introduce cytokine genes or genes encoding accessory molecules expressed by efficient antigen-presenting cells, and then use these gene-modified tumor cells to immunize the host. Studies in mice with genes encoding cytokine genes such as IL-2 and GM-CSF or costimulatory accessory molecules such as B7 have provided

provocative results—protective T cell responses to tumor cells previously perceived to be nonimmunogenic have been repeatedly detected. Approaches involving these methods are currently entering human trials.

The identification of tumor antigens shared by many tumors has provided another means of inducing antitumor responses, but studies in animal models have suggested that direct immunization with tumor proteins generally has limited or no apparent efficacy. Consequently, more immunogenic vectors are being evaluated. For example, the gene encoding CEA has been inserted into a recombinant vaccinia virus, and this highly immunogenic vaccine vector is being tested in colon cancer patients. A recently developed alternative has been to create a fusion protein in which the gene encoding the tumor protein is fused in frame with an immunostimulatory cytokine such as GM-CSF or IL-2. These approaches offer the potential of eventually developing both protective and therapeutic tumor vaccines.

Adoptive Cellular Immunotherapy

Animal models have been developed in which hosts bearing advanced tumors can be treated by the transfer of tumor-specific syngeneic T cells. These models, in which syngeneic donor T cells immune to the tumor are used, have served as prototypes of what might be achievable if the host immune response to an autochthonous tumor could be selectively amplified; they have been useful for elucidating the requirements for successful immunotherapy. Complete tumor elimination following adoptive therapy requires an extended period, and the cells transferred must therefore be capable of persisting in the host to be effective. Noncytolytic lymphokine-producing class II-restricted T_H cells, as well as directly lytic class I-restricted T_C cells, mediate antitumor effects in these models. Tumor-specific T cells expanded in vitro by culture with tumor and IL-2 are effective in adoptive therapy, and efficacy can be enhanced by infusing IL-2 after cell transfer, which has been shown to promote in vivo proliferation and survival of the transferred cultured T cells.

These studies are now being applied to the treatment of human cancers by isolating potentially tumor-reactive lymphocytes infiltrating solid tumors, expanding these cells in vitro by stimulation with tumor or IL-2 or both, and then reinfusing the cells into the patients. To enhance the efficacy of such therapy, IL-2 is being administered after transfer. Preliminary results have suggested that these T cells can localize to sites of tumor and can mediate a significant therapeutic effect, particularly with some tumors such as melanoma. Studies with cloned cytolytic T cells specific for human cytomegalovirus have demonstrated that transferred T cells can establish prolonged specific immunity in humans. These results suggest that with the continued development of methods to identify tumor antigens and to detect and expand the number of tumor-specific T cells from patients, specific adoptive therapy may become an important modality for the treatment of many tumors.

While the in vitro effects of increasing doses of IL-2 on the generation of tumor-specific T cells were being examined, it was observed that a cytolytic effector cell lacking antigen specificity but displaying a marked preference for transformed cells was induced. These LAK cells, generated only in the presence of exceptionally high, nonphysiologic doses of IL-2, have now been extensively characterized and studied both in vitro and in vivo. LAK cells are phenotypically heterogeneous, but the major effector cell appears to be a non-T cell most similar to an activated NK cell. Administration of cytolytic LAK cells, particularly in association with IL-2, has shown activity in the treatment of some human tumors. Although the efficacy of treatment with LAK cells and IL-2 appears to be limited by a lack of absolute specificity and toxicity to the host, there are many clinical settings, such as isolated pulmonary or liver metastases, in which it may be possible to use these effector cells to achieve a directed and potentially curative antitumor effect. Moreover, approaches are now being explored to improve the specificity of LAK cells. This can be accomplished by the introduction of genes encoding proteins such as TNF, which have antitumor activity, or by improving the likelihood that LAK cells will localize to tumors through the use of bifunctional antibodies, ie, hybrid or conjugated monoclonal antibodies that have 2 specificities, one for an antigen that resides on the LAK cell and permits attachment to the effector cell and one for an antigen that resides on the tumor and promotes specific targeting.

Administration of Monoclonal Antibodies

The development of the technology for generating monoclonal antibodies has converted the previously unpromising field of tumor serotherapy into a form of treatment with enormous potential. Studies with antibodies of different isotypes have demonstrated that ADCC rather than complement-mediated cytotoxicity is the major in vivo effector mechanism following infusion of antibody. However, despite occasional reports of exciting clinical results, a large number of biologic problems still need to be overcome for this modality to be generally effective. Antibodies and the necessary ADCC effector cells do not appear to penetrate large tumor masses effectively, and tumor escape mechanisms, such as modulation of the target antigen from the tumor cell surface and selection of antigen loss variants, may frequently interfere with monoclonal antibody therapy.

Several approaches are being studied to augment the therapeutic activity of monoclonal antibodies. The most promising involve conjugation of cytotoxic drugs, toxins, or radioisotopes to the antibody to deliver a lethal hit directly to the tumor without requiring the participation of host effector cells. Antibody, drug, or toxin conjugates may be particularly useful in settings in which the antigen is rapidly endocytosed. In contrast, radioisotopes may be useful with large tumors or in the presence of immunoselection, because radioisotopes kill by emitting ionizing radiation and thus do not need to fully penetrate the tumor to kill all cells and can kill antigen-negative tumor variants in the tumor mass if they are in the proximity of antibody-binding tumor cells. Most of the tumor-reactive monoclonal antibodies being used in clinical trials recognize tumor-associated rather than tumor-specific antigens and thus are likely to recognize some normal tissues. Consequently, administration of some antibodies or antibody conjugates may prove to be unacceptably toxic to the host. However, in many instances, such as if the antibody recognizes a determinant on normal B cells and causes a transient depression of B cell number, this toxicity may be acceptable if a significant antitumor effect can be achieved. Future studies will need to carefully define the distribution of normal antigens recognized by each antibody to be used in therapy and the potential toxic complications, but it seems safe to predict that sufficient monoclonal antibodies with appropriate characteristics will be identified to permit the treatment of a wide variety of human tumors.

REFERENCES

Anichini A et al: Melanoma cells and normal melanocytes share antigens recognized by HLA-A2-restricted cytotoxic T cell clones from melanoma patients. *J Exp Med* 1993;**177:**989.

Bishop JM: Molecular themes in oncogenesis. *Cell* 1991;**64:**235.

Boon T: Toward a genetic analysis of tumor rejection antigens. *Adv Cancer Res.* 1992;**58:**177.

Chen W et al: T-cell immunity to the joining region of p210BCR-ABL protein. *Proc Natl Acad Sci USA* 1992;**89:**1468.

Fearon ER et al: Interleukin-2 production by tumor cells bypasses T helper function in the generation of an antitumor response. *Cell* 1990;**60:**397.

Greenberg PD: Adoptive T cell therapy of tumors: mechanisms operative in the recognition and elimination of tumor cells. *Adv Immunol* 1991;**49:**281.

Grossbard ML et al: Monoclonal antibody-based therapies of leukemia and lymphoma. *Blood* 1992;**80:**863.

Jerome KR et al: Cytotoxic T-lymphocytes derived from patients with breast adenocarcinoma recognize an epitope present on the protein core of a mucin molecule preferentially expressed by malignant cells. *Cancer Res* 1991;**51**:2908.

Jung S, Schluesener HJ: Human T lymphocytes recognize a peptide of single point-mutated, oncogenic ras proteins. *J Exp Med* 1991;**173**:273.

Kantor J et al: Immunogenicity and safety of a recombinant vaccinia virus vaccine expressing the carcinoembryonic antigen gene in a nonhuman primate. *Cancer Res* 1992;**52**:6917.

Karre K: MHC gene control of the natural killer system at the level of the target and the host. *Semin Cancer Biol* 1991;**2**:295.

Klein G: Tumor antigens. *Annu Rev Microbiol* 1966; **20**:223.

Melief CJ: Tumor eradication by adoptive transfer of cytotoxic T lymphocytes. *Adv Cancer Res* 1992;**58**:143.

Mizoguchi H et al: Alterations in signal transduction molecules in T lymphocytes from tumor-bearing mice. *Science* 1992;**258**:1795.

Pardoll D: New strategies for active immunotherapy with genetically engineered tumor cells. *Curr Opin Immunol* 1992;**4**:619.

Restifo NP et al: Identification of human cancers deficient in antigen processing. *J Exp Med* 1993;**177**:265.

Riddell SR et al: Restoration of viral immunity in immunodeficient humans by the adoptive transfer of T cell clones. *Science* 1992;**257**:238.

Rosenberg SA et al: Use of tumor-infiltrating lymphocytes and interleukin-2 in the immunotherapy of patients with metastatic melanoma. A preliminary report. *N Engl J Med* 1988;**319**:1676.

Rosenberg SA: Prospective randomized trial of high-dose interleukin-2 alone or in conjunction with lymphokine-activated killer cells for the treatment of patients with advanced cancer. *J Natl Cancer Inst* 1993;**85**:622.

Tao MH, Levy R: Idiotype/granulocyte-macrophage colony-stimulating factor fusion protein as a vaccine for B-cell lymphoma. *Nature* 1993;**362**:755.

Townsend SE, Allison JP: Tumor rejection after direct co-stimulation of CD8+ T cells by B7-transfected melanoma cells. *Science* 1993;**259**:368.

Urban JL, Schreiber H: Tumor antigens. *Annu Rev Immunol* 1992;**10**:617.

van der Bruggen P et al: A gene encoding an antigen recognized by cytolytic T lymphocytes on a human melanoma. *Science* 1991;**254**:1643.

Vitetta ES, Thorpe PE: Immunotoxins containing ricin or its A chain. *Semin Cell Biol* 1991;**2**:47.

Waldmann TA: Monoclonal antibodies in diagnosis and therapy. *Science* 1991;**252**:1657.

44

Cancer in the Immunocompromised Host

John L. Ziegler, MD

In the late 1950s, Sir McFarlane Burnet and Lewis Thomas proposed that the immune system maintains vigil over both alien microorganisms and altered somatic cells. When discovered, these undesirables are selectively eliminated. The logic of "immune surveillance," defined more explicitly by Burnet in 1970, finds support in the defense systems of lower organisms, which must resist fusion, invasion, or destructive parasitism to survive. Plants and prokaryotes maintain their integrity through highly conserved cell surface recognition systems. Multicellular eukaryotes evolved a more complex "adoptive" defense system, one impressive feature of which is the ability to discriminate between self and nonself. Other cognate functions, such as immunologic memory, regulatory networks, and a large repertoire of attack strategies, make the mammalian immune system comparable to the brain in complexity and function. Throughout phylogeny, the role of the immune system in ensuring the autonomy of the host is a basic tenet of evolutionary survival.

IMMUNE SURVEILLANCE

Inferential support for immune surveillance against neoplasia in humans comes from a variety of clinical observations. Patients with congenital immune deficiencies and patients with organ transplants who receive immunosuppressive therapy develop an excess incidence of some forms of cancer. Rare instances of "spontaneous" regression of tumors are ascribed to immune mechanisms. More recently, the discovery of tumor-specific antigens (see Chapter 43) and the observation of tumor-directed immune responses by using autologous lymphocytes and lymphokines provide further evidence for tumor immunity.

Studies of transplantable and spontaneous tumors in animals also lend support to the notion of tumor-directed immunity. For example, surgical removal of a growing tumor in mice renders them resistant to subsequent inocula of the same, but not a different, tumor. Such experiments are more successful when using transplantable tumors rather than spontaneous, autochthonous tumors. Aside from evidence of specific tumor immunity mediated by antibody and T cells, tumor cells can be killed nonspecifically by activated macrophages and natural killer (NK) cells. Finally, examples of "blocking factors" that prevent an immune response are evident in tumor-bearing hosts.

Criteria for Intrinsic Defense

An intrinsic defense against the development of neoplasia might be advantageous to the host. To be successful, it must meet at least 4 conditions. First, the tumor should express unique antigens that are accessible to the immune system. Second, the host must have a competent immune system and attack the tumor antigen with an appropriate tumor-directed cytotoxic response. Third, there should be no suppressive or blocking influences to obstruct the immune response. Finally, the number of tumor cells should be small enough for the immune attack to locate and eliminate the tumor entirely.

Immunotherapy Research

The 1970s saw an era of empirical immunotherapy, based on the assumptions listed above. The main objects were to augment tumor cell antigenicity and to boost host immunity with various specific or nonspecific vaccines and stimulants. The results of these trials were disappointing, with only rare instances of clinical improvement. By the end of the decade, it was clear that most human tumors were at best only weakly antigenic. It was also obvious that immunotherapy was a "numbers game," with successful killing being dependent on a high lymphocyte-to-target cell ratio. Finally, successful therapeutic manipulation of the immune system demanded a much better appreciation of the intricacies of immunoregulation.

Advances in biotechnology have brought considerable enlightenment to the field of cancer immunology in the 1980s and 1990s. Antigens and separate cell populations can be defined by using monoclonal antibodies. The discovery, cloning, and production of purified growth factors permit experiments with high concentrations of purified lymphocytes. Advances in molecular genetics provide techniques to identify tumor clonality. Progress in understanding immunoregulation, mechanisms of immune diversity, and the interactions of the various cellular members of the immune system has opened new doors to pharmacologic and biologic manipulation of the immune response. Finally, the identification of proto-oncogenes and anti-oncogenes has enabled a better molecular genetic understanding of oncogenesis, including the potential to identify tumor-specific oncogene products.

IMMUNOCOMPROMISE & CANCER

This chapter will focus on the phenomenon of cancer in the immunocompromised human host. **Immunocompromise** is a preferable term to "immunodeficiency" or "immunosuppression." The latter terms imply that the immune system is binary and capable of swaying, like a seesaw, between a normal "replete" state and a suppressed "deficient" state. This is clearly oversimplified, given our knowledge of the contextual and integrated nature of immune responses. Immunocompromise should be defined as a state of functional unresponsiveness, due in some circumstances to depletion of specific immune compartments and in others to dysfunction induced by drugs, physical agents, infections, cancer, or autoimmunity.

Oncogenesis

Experimentally, 3 processes lead to neoplasia: initiation, promotion, and progression (Fig 44–1). **Initiation** involves the alteration of DNA by a chemical, physical, or biologic agent that confers malignant potential onto the cell genotype. "Initiated" cells appear histologically normal but are rendered constitutively susceptible to malignant transformation. **Promotion** is thought to be a process by which the expression of genetic information is altered in the cell. **Progression** is the clonal evolution of established tumors that accounts for heterogeneity and varied phenotypic manifestations such as invasiveness, drug resistance, and metastatic potential. Thus, cancer is the end stage of a multistep process that evolves over long periods. Its development and behavior in the intact host are driven internally by the renegade genetic program and influenced externally by microenvironmental factors such as hormonal milieu, vascular supply, and immunity.

Function & Dysfunction of Proto-Oncogenes & Anti-Oncogenes

Proto-oncogenes are highly conserved genetic sequences that control cell growth and differentiation. These genes code for growth factors, receptors, and regulatory proteins that govern cell proliferation. They are normally inactive unless required for embryogenesis, replenishment of replicating tissues, or response to injury. They act in concert, instructing cell growth and differentiation in an orderly fashion.

Proto-oncogenes may be damaged or dysregulated by a variety of insults that result in mutation or translocation to another site in the genome. These accidents, if unrepaired, may cause qualitative or quantitative dysfunction such that the protein products are abnormal in configuration or become overproduced, leading the cell to an autonomous proliferative state.

Studies of heritable cancers have disclosed another set of regulatory genes that are recessive oncogenes

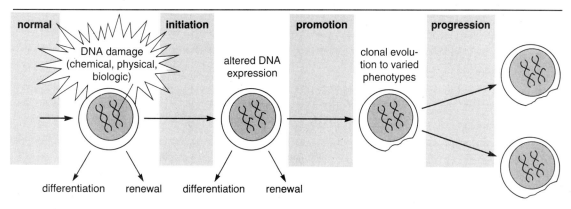

Figure 44–1. Pathogenesis of neoplasia. Normal cells have 2 choices upon division: differentiate or renew. When certain DNA mutations or chromosomal abnormalities occur, stem cells that are initiated may accumulate in a renewal cycle. These cells are more susceptible to a second genetic accident, and the chance of "promotion" to neoplastic transformation increases over time. As tumor develops, there is genetic drift in the cell renewal compartment, and clones of tumor cells "progress" in different phenotypic directions, producing tumor heterogeneity.

(eg, retinoblastoma [RB] gene). These genes act to encourage differentiation or retard cell proliferation, hence their designation as anti-oncogenes. A structural deletion or mutation of one of the alleles of these genes (either inherited in the germ line or produced by somatic mutation) results in a cell that is highly susceptible to malignant transformation. A subsequent genetic accident in the hemizygote disables any residual regulatory restraint and results in cancer. The phenomenon of "recessive oncogene mutation" is noted in many human cancers such as retinoblastoma, small cell carcinoma of the lung, and cancer of the breast and colon. Thus, oncogenesis is the result of cumulative genetic mishaps (Fig 44–2).

Epithelial versus Immune System Tumors

Two distinct phenomena must be distinguished in the relationship between cancer and compromised immunity. The first is the high incidence of tumors of the immune system in the immunocompromised host. The immune system itself is programmed for replication upon antigenic exposure, and lymphocyte proliferation might be expected to predispose the host to neoplasia of rapidly dividing cells. The second phenomenon is the emergence of an excess of epithelial neoplasms, particularly among patients who survive a prolonged immunosuppressed state. These tumors may result from a true failure of immune surveillance to detect and eliminate strongly antigenic transformed cells.

CONGENITAL IMMUNODEFICIENCY & NEOPLASIA

Table 44–1 indicates the risk of cancer in children with congenital immunodeficiencies. Most of these cancers are seen in 4 primary disorders: X-linked lymphoproliferative syndrome, Wiskott-Aldrich syndrome, ataxia-telangiectasia, and common variable immunodeficiency disease. Two-thirds of the patients were younger than 20 years of age when the tumors were diagnosed. True risk assessment is difficult to measure because the accurate prevalence of the congenital immunodeficiency is unknown. Mild forms of these disorders may be undiagnosed, and many patients with more severe forms may die before cancer develops.

In the X-linked lymphoproliferative syndrome (Duncan's syndrome) Epstein-Barr virus (EBV) infection of B lymphocytes causes progressive oligoclonal lymphoproliferation, leading to Burkitt-like non-Hodgkin lymphoma.

In the Wiskott-Aldrich syndrome, extranodal immunoblastic lymphoma occurs in up to 16% of patients. About half of these lymphomas are located in the brain, which may act as a "sanctuary" for lymphoproliferation. A role for an oncogenic virus (eg, papovavirus) has not been ruled out. In a minority of patients. Hodgkin's disease and acute myelocytic leukemia are also found.

In ataxia-telangiectasia, both Hodgkin's disease (the major subtype being lymphocyte depleted) and non-Hodgkin lymphoma occur, in a ratio of about 1:5. The latter cases are of histologic types associated with the 14q+ chromosomal abnormality characteristic of lymphocytes in patients with ataxia-telangiectasia. Patients with this disorder also manifest a defect in the repair of gamma radiation-induced DNA damage, possibly accounting for an excess of epithelial neoplasms (skin, ovarian, and stomach cancers) among older patients.

A small proportion of patients (2.5–8.5%, depending on survival) with common variable immunodeficiency develop non-Hodgkin lymphoma. In longer-surviving patients, an excess incidence of stomach cancer is also found.

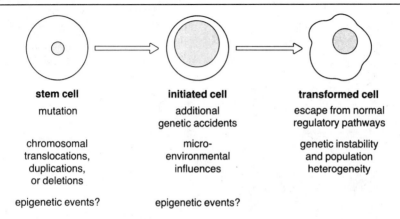

Figure 44–2. Molecular model of malignant transformation. Assuming that cancer is a disease of defective stem cells, there is consensus that the pathway to neoplasia involves multiple "hits" to stem cell DNA, such that the normal signals for self-renewal and differentiation become aberrant or misinterpreted. At the molecular level, these hits presumably alter the expression of regulatory proto-oncogenes that either stimulate or inhibit cell proliferation.

Table 44–1. Risk of cancer in congenital immunodeficiency syndromes.[1]

Syndrome	Immune Defect	Malignant Tumors[2]	Percent Risk Overall	Median Age of Onset (years)
X-linked immunodeficiency syndrome	Impaired B cell responses to EBV antigens.	NHL	35%	10
Wiskott-Aldrich syndrome	Complex, multicompartmental defects.	NHL, AML HD	15–37%	6
Ataxia-telangiectasia	Complex, multicompartmental defects; defective DNA repair after gamma irradiation.	ALL, NHL, HD, nerve, ovarian, skin, stomach cancers	12%	9
Common variable immunodeficiency	Cellular and humoral defects.	NHL, stomach cancer	8%	16

[1]These data are drawn from the University of Minnesota registry on Immunodeficiency and Cancer and from elsewhere in the literature.
[2]Abbreviations: NHL, Non-Hodgkin lymphoma; AML, acute myeloid leukemia; HD, Hodgkin's disease; ALL, acute lymphoblastic leukemia.

About 10% of lymphoid cancers recorded in patients with congenital immunodeficiency syndromes are unclassified as to histologic type. By histologic and biologic criteria, these lymphomas reside on the border between reactive hyperplasia and true malignancy. Oligoclonal "cancers" probably represent a transitional state in the pathway of B cell neoplasia.

CANCER IN ORGAN TRANSPLANT RECIPIENTS

Thanks to a meticulously maintained registry of organ transplant recipients (the Cincinnati Transplant Tumor Registry), epidemiologic data on cancer incidence in this population are both up-to-date and reliable. More than 95% of registry participants received renal transplants.

Recipients of organ allografts must receive drugs to suppress the immune response to alloantigens in order to avoid graft rejection. Over the past 3 decades, various forms of immune suppression have been used. The earlier "broad-spectrum" regimens included both corticosteroids and azathioprine. The introduction of cyclosporin in the 1970s has led to more effective T cell-specific immunosuppression.

Cancer trends in allograft recipients are reminiscent of the experience in patients with primary immunodeficiency syndromes. In general, there is a 3-fold increase of neoplasms in this population compared with age-matched controls. The average time from transplantation to development of all tumors is 60 months; for lymphomas it is 37 months, and for Kaposi's sarcoma, 23 months.

Skin Cancer

The most common tumors are carcinomas of the skin, which account for 1238 (38%) of 3251 transplant-associated cancers (from the Cincinnati registry). This represents a 4- to 21-fold increase over the expected skin cancer incidence. These tumors are also unusual in the overrepresentation of squamous cell carcinomas compared with the more common basal cell type and with melanomas. Skin cancers are diagnosed with higher frequency in younger persons, and carcinomas often develop at multiple sites. Another feature is the increased clinical aggressiveness of these tumors and a mortality rate of 6%. This rate can be compared with the very low (1–2%) mortality rate in the general population, most of which is attributed to malignant melanoma.

Immunologic control of skin cancer in humans is incompletely understood. Tumors caused by UV radiation in mice are antigenic in autochthonous hosts. Tumor-specific cytotoxic T cells are directed at the antigenic tumor cells. Diminished immunity has been attributed to increases in antigen-specific suppressor T cells that inhibit tumor cell rejection. It is also known that UV light can alter the expression of class I major histocompatibility complex (MHC) antigens in the skin. Specific T cells bearing γ/δ T cell receptors recognize these antigens. Perhaps a failure of this surveillance system in immunocompromised patients results in the emergence of excess skin cancers.

Anogenital Cancer

The second most common tumor in transplant recipients is carcinoma of the anogenital tract. Cervical carcinomas account for 16% of cancers (including 80% in situ lesions). Carcinoma of the vulva, perineum, scrotum, penis, and anus occurs in 3% of recipients with cancer. Taken together, anogenital tumors are increased more than 100-fold compared with the incidence in the age-matched general population.

A possible explanation for this excess is the association of anogenital neoplasia in general with human papillomavirus, especially with types 6, 11, 16, 18, 32, 35, and 37. Perhaps immunocompromise permits the activation of latent papillomavirus in anogenital tissues, and the resulting dysplastic epithelial lesions progress to neoplasia. Because these are virus-associated tumors, there may be some degree of immune surveillance in the immunocompetent host that is directed to virus-specific antigens on the epithelial cell surface. This response would normally identify and eliminate early papillomavirus-associated tumors. In an immunocompromised host, such immunity would be impaired and a higher frequency of tumors might result.

Non-Hodgkin Lymphoma

Non-Hodgkin lymphoma constitutes 14% of cancers in transplant recipients. The major histologic types were diffuse large cell and immunoblastic. The majority of tumors classified by modern immunologic techniques are of B cell origin; lymphomas of T cell origin account for 12%. As with lymphomas found in patients with primary immunodeficiencies, the majority are extranodal, with one-third involving the central nervous system. In addition, a small proportion of lymphomas are unclassified. In individual transplant series, these are oligoclonal and are associated with EBV. They may regress upon withdrawal of immunosuppressive therapy, treatment with antiviral agents, or infusion of anti-B cell monoclonal antibodies.

Kaposi's Sarcoma

Kaposi's sarcoma is 400–500 times overrepresented among transplant recipients compared with the general population. This rare and unusual tumor is of endothelial origin and occurs sporadically in Caucasian men of eastern European descent. A polymorphic variety is endemic in certain central African countries. Like non-Hodgkin lymphomas, this tumor may regress when immunosuppressive therapy is stopped. Although spontaneous Kaposi's sarcoma usually appears on the skin and runs a benign course, transplant-associated tumors tend to involve internal organs, and the mortality rate is 25%.

In a study of transplant recipients, no unusual epidemiologic features distinguished the subgroup with Kaposi's sarcoma, with the exception that one-third of the patients were women. Kaposi's sarcoma predominates among males, and women made of approximately one-third of the transplant series. Thus, the usual 9:1 male-to-female ratio became 2:1 in the transplant series.

There is an absence of data on cancer in appropriate control populations, such as organ graft recipients who are not immunosuppressed, or patients with organ failure who received immunosuppressive therapy but not allografts. A control group of otherwise healthy individuals who receive immunosuppressive treatment is obviously also lacking. Thus, the excess incidence of cancers in organ transplant recipients can be attributed to immunosuppression only by circumstantial inference, with some supporting evidence from experimental systems.

CANCER IN PATIENTS WITH AUTOIMMUNE DISORDERS

The true incidence of cancer in patients with autoimmune disorders is not known. Under certain conditions, chronic inflammation per se may predispose to neoplasia, possibly caused by the DNA-damaging effects of free radicals produced at the site. Because autoimmune disorders are treated with immunosuppressive drugs, the additional effect of immunosuppression over a "baseline" of cancer susceptibility cannot be ascertained.

Most series of cancer incidence in patients with any particular autoimmune disease are small. There is an increased risk of lymphoma in patients with celiac disease and Sjögren's syndrome. Patients with rheumatoid arthritis are not at increased cancer risk unless given long-term treatment with cyclophosphamide or chlorambucil. One large series that includes patients with many autoimmune disorders treated with immunosuppressive drugs disclosed a 12-fold increase of Hodgkin's disease, a 5-fold excess of squamous cell carcinoma of the skin, and a modest excess of other tumor types. Although limited in epidemiologic value, these series concur generally with the clinical experience in immunosuppressed organ transplant recipients.

SECOND TUMORS IN CANCER PATIENTS

Cancer patients, who are already partially immunocompromised by their tumors, may receive immunosuppressive anticancer therapy (ie, chemotherapy or radiotherapy or both) that worsens their immunocompromised state. Long-term follow-up of cancer survivors treated with cytotoxic drugs discloses a high incidence of second cancers. Most of these are acute leukemias of myeloid or monocytic origin and non-Hodgkin lymphomas. They occur an average of 4–6 years after treatment of the primary tumor. The most extensive follow-up has been performed in long-term survivors of Hodgkin's disease. Their overall risk of a second cancer is sixfold, with an actuarial risk of approximately 1% per year up to 10 years, after which a plateau is reached. Alkylating agents contribute to the risk of leukemia, whereas radiation therapy is associated with the development of solid tumors.

Interpretation of the epidemiologic data in these groups is confounded by the direct carcinogenic effects of the anticancer treatment, the extent and duration of immunocompromise, and the possibility of a neoplastic predisposition. In contrast to the cancers in patients with autoimmune disorders and transplant recipients, second cancers in surviving cancer patients appear more closely related to direct carcinogenic effects of therapy.

HUMAN IMMUNODEFICIENCY VIRUS (HIV) INFECTION & THE DEVELOPMENT OF CANCER

Immunopathogenesis of AIDS

A decade of intensive research has yet to define clearly the cause of progressive immune deficiency in persons infected with the human immunodeficiency virus type 1 (HIV). The pathogenesis of helper T (CD4) lymphocyte depletion appears to result from a complex and dynamic interaction between the host and the virus.

Early immunity to the virus gradually fails, and a phase of immune activation (during which there is nonspecific stimulation of B lymphocytes and cytotoxic-suppressor [CD8] T lymphocytes) gives way to a progressive lysis of B and T lymphocytes. This process may be mediated in part by an increasing viral burden and by acceleration of lymphocyte apoptosis (programmed cell death) induced by HIV and its protein products. The mimicry of the viral envelope gp120 to class II MHC antigens may induce a graft-versus-host response as well. Meanwhile, the virus itself is becoming more pathogenic and, in later stages of disease, takes on a virulent, syncytium-forming property. Viral replication is enhanced in a positive-feedback loop when infected lymphocytes become activated. The net result is an immune system at first diverted and later destroyed by HIV.

Kaposi's Sarcoma

Kaposi's sarcoma was the first clinical manifestation of AIDS to be recognized. Throughout the epidemic, this tumor has predominated in homosexual men, being present in 40% of new cases of AIDS in the early years of the epidemic but falling below 20% by the mid-1980s. Other risk groups in the USA and in Europe have a much lower prevalence of Kaposi's sarcoma. In Africa, where Kaposi's sarcoma is endemic, HIV-infected patients develop a widespread and aggressive form of the disease, with a much higher incidence in women than was encountered before the AIDS epidemic.

The epidemiology of Kaposi's sarcoma has suggested to some that it is caused by a sexually transmitted agent. In homosexual men, the tumor is most prevalent among those who practice oral-anal contact, implying a possible infectious route of the agent. Although a number of candidate viruses have been proposed, including human papillomavirus, none are unequivocally implicated.

Pathogenesis of AIDS-Associated Kaposi's Sarcoma

Recent experiments have advanced our understanding of the pathogenesis of Kaposi's sarcoma. The ability to grow Kaposi's sarcoma cells in vitro was enhanced by using conditioned media from a T lymphocyte line infected with another human retrovirus, HTLV-II. Such cell lines later became autonomous and were shown to produce a variety of autocrine growth factors, including a fibroblast growth factor (FGF)-like substance. Coincidentally, an oncogene has been found in Kaposi's sarcoma DNA that codes for a new member of the FGF family. On inoculation into nude mice, these cell lines induce an intense angiogenic reaction of mouse origin.

Other studies of the HIV *tat* gene in transgenic mice showed that some of the male mice developed endothelial tumors indistinguishable from Kaposi's sarcoma. *tat* is a gene that transactivates HIV transcription and is responsible for turning an HIV-infected cell into a veritable virion factory. *tat* is under the control of both cellular and viral regulatory genes and appears to "turn on" viral production when the cell is coinfected with another virus, stimulated antigenically, or subjected to certain lymphokines. Interestingly, the *tat-1* gene of HTLV-I is also oncogenic in transgenic mice, producing transplantable mesenchymal tumors. The predilection for tumors in male mice is not understood.

A current scheme to account for the pathogenesis of Kaposi's sarcoma in HIV-infected persons posits that the tumor is induced first by paracrine effects. HIV infection of local lymphocytes or macrophages induces production of cytokines, which in turn cause proliferation of endothelial and spindle cells. This is possibly assisted by local production of *tat* protein. These proliferating cells begin to produce autocrine growth factors (including a potent spindle cell inducer, oncostatin M), which expand the mesenchymal lesion and cause some degree of inflammatory infiltrate. Proliferation of spindle cells (mitogenesis) leads to transformation (mutagenesis), and the Kaposi's sarcoma lesion develops. Thus, Kaposi's sarcoma could be envisioned as a nonhealing wound, complete with angiogenesis, various mesenchymal properties, and a mild inflammatory infiltrate (Fig 44–3).

This theory helps explain the association of HIV with Kaposi's sarcoma combined with a total absence of the virus within the tumor. It fails to explain, however, the unusual epidemiology (prevalence in homosexual men, behavior as a sexually transmitted disease, paucity of tumors in women) or the eccentric anatomic distribution of tumors. Although some important molecular and physiologic insights have been provided, a number of unresolved problems remain.

Non-Hodgkin Lymphoma in HIV-Infected Persons

Soon after the initial reports of AIDS-associated opportunistic infections and Kaposi's sarcoma, non-Hodgkin lymphoma was found in homosexual men with AIDS. As the AIDS epidemic progressed, the incidence of lymphoma rose commensurately, predominating in the homosexual and intravenous drug-

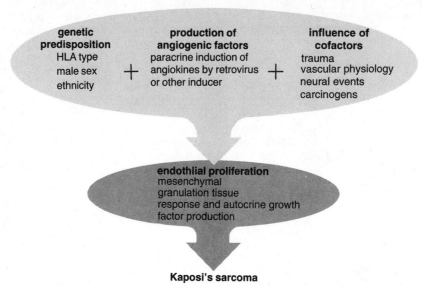

Figure 44–3. Suggested pathogenesis of Kaposi's sarcoma in immunocompromised patients. Kaposi's sarcoma is thought to begin as a vascular reaction to local angiokine production, which can be induced by a number of agents. The paracrine release of angiogenic factors (most probably those in the FGF family such as oncostatin) causes endothelial cell proliferation and spindle cell formation. Initially, these proliferative lesions may respond to regulatory restraints, probably mediated by the immune system. With time, however, the lesions become autonomous and produce their own sustaining growth factors. Yet to be explained in this pathway are the roles of genetic predisposition and local cofactors (see text).

abusing risk groups. As the survival of AIDS patients increases with improved therapy, a higher incidence of lymphoma is being reported. The majority of well-characterized lymphomas are of B cell origin, about evenly divided between intermediate-grade large cell, high-grade immunoblastic, and small non-cleaved cell types.

Clinically, the lymphomas are extranodal in distribution, with a high frequency of central nervous system and bone marrow involvement. In addition, homosexual men have an excess of oral and rectal tumors. All series report a poor response to treatment and a high mortality rate. The major determinants of poor prognosis are a prior AIDS diagnosis, low CD4 lymphocyte counts, presence of extranodal tumor, aggressive cytotoxic chemotherapy regimens, and poor clinical condition.

AIDS-associated lymphomas are clinically, pathologically, and biologically heterogeneous (Fig 44–4). One classification proposes 3 divisions. Central nervous system primary lymphomas are large-cell type, are monoclonal by immunoglobulin phenotyping, contain EBV genomes, and display c-*myc* oncogene rearrangements. Non-central nervous system (peripheral) lymphomas are of 2 types. One is polyclonal and lacks EBV or c-*myc* rearrangements. The other is monoclonal and may or may not contain EBV or c-*myc* rearrangements. On the basis of these findings, one is tempted to postulate that central nervous sys-

tem lymphomas are EBV-induced. Peripheral lymphomas contain polyclonal lymphoproliferations (some of which may be EBV-driven) that evolve over time into monoclonal tumors.

T Cell Lymphomas in HIV-Infected Persons

About 5% of the lymphomas associated with AIDS are of T cell origin. As with the B cell tumors, these lymphomas are heterogeneous, including T cell lymphoproliferative syndromes, cutaneous T cell lymphomas, lymphoblastic lymphoma, and T cell chronic lymphocytic leukemia. Thus far, only a single patient with a T cell lymphoproliferative syndrome has been shown to be dually infected with HIV-1 and HTLV-I. Because these 2 viruses may synergistically coinfect the same host, more T cell neoplasms may appear as the epidemic progresses, particularly among intravenous drug abusers who are at high risk for HIV-1 and HTLV-I coinfection.

Pathogenesis of AIDS-Associated Lymphoma

In a manner similar to the situation in immunosuppressed transplant recipients, AIDS-associated lymphoma is presumed to result from renegade growth of B cells, starting with polyclonal and progressing to oligoclonal proliferation. The latter condition may manifest clinically as malignant lymphoma, although most lymphomas are monoclonal by the time of clinical presentation.

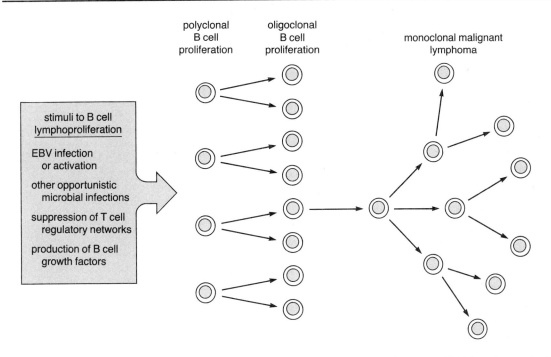

Figure 44–4. Suggested pathogenesis of B cell lymphoma in immunocompromised patients. Multiple pathways for B cell proliferation exist in the immunocompromised patient. These include direct viral activation (EBV) and indirect mitogenic stimuli from infecting microorganisms. In addition, the regulatory networks that normally hold B cell proliferation in check are impaired, and unrestrained B cell growth results. In this polyclonal population, the chances of autonomous growth of several clones increases over time, leading to oligoclonal and ultimately monoclonal lymphoma (see text).

Multiple factors conspire to stimulate polyclonal B cell proliferation in HIV-infected persons: HIV antigens, growth factors from T cells and macrophages, EBV infection, and antigenic stimulation from concomitant infections. Some investigators have described a "premalignant" condition of oligoclonal B cell hyperplasia and *c-myc* rearrangements followed by a stepwise progression to full-blown malignant lymphoma.

Aside from central nervous system lymphomas, a definitive role for EBV cannot be confirmed at this time, even though experimental *c-myc* transfection into virus-infected B cells will produce frank malignant lymphoma. Presumably, EBV is one of several stimuli that induce B cell proliferation. Other candidates include another retrovirus or DNA virus (either exogenous or B cell tropic), activation of another oncogene such as the *c-ras* oncogene, or induction of autocrine B cell growth factors in selected lymphocyte clones.

Hodgkin's Disease & Other Neoplasms in HIV-Infected Persons

Demographic surveys of cancer rates in HIV-epidemic regions have disclosed only an excess of Kaposi's sarcoma and non-Hodgkin lymphoma. Oncologists who care for HIV-infected persons with Hodgkin's disease report a more aggressive natural history, with a predilection for tumor sites in unusual locations such as the rectum and parotid gland. A majority of patients have advanced stages of disease, with noncontiguous anatomic spread. Most patients display the mixed-cellularity histopathologic subtype, but the tumors are depleted of CD4 lymphocytes. Because the highest frequency of Hodgkin's disease occurs in the age group predominantly affected by HIV, an absolute excess incidence cannot yet be inferred.

An increased incidence of anal carcinoma in homosexual men predated the AIDS epidemic, and, thus far, the incidence has not risen above the expected level. Careful surveillance of anogenital cancer in HIV-infected persons is important for 2 reasons. First, these tumors are associated with human papillomavirus, as noted above, and this virus is prevalent and active in AIDS patients, particularly in the risk groups who transmit the virus sexually. Second, studies of HIV-infected men and women disclose an increase of papillomavirus-induced epithelial dysplasia in the anogenital tract, indicating viral activity and a high frequency of premalignant lesions. As of 1993, invasive carcinoma of the uterine cervix has been added to the CDC AIDS defining criteria.

Other Cancers in HIV-Infected Persons

Scattered reports have appeared of other cancers in AIDS patients. However, overall there is no epidemiologic evidence of an increase over expected rates. Some reported cancers, such as acute leukemia and skin, testicular, lung, colon, and pancreatic cancers, are relatively common in the HIV are groups at risk. Because HIV infection leads to endogenous virus activation, one might expect an excess of virus-associated tumors such as hepatocellular carcinoma, anal and cervical cancer, and, possibly, nasopharyngeal carcinoma. Although this is theoretically possible, these tumors probably require cofactors that may or may not be present in HIV-infected individuals. Furthermore, these tumors generally have a very long incubation period before malignant transformation. Nevertheless, continued surveillance of HIV risk groups for increased cancer incidence is important.

CONCLUSIONS

This survey of neoplasia in immunocompromised patients permits several general inferences about oncogenesis and the immune system. The first is that neoplasia of compartments of the lymphoreticular system (eg, non-Hodgkin lymphomas from lymphocytes, Kaposi's sarcoma from endothelial cells) predominates in all immunocompromised states. A plausible explanation is dysregulation of the natural proliferative program of these cells, induced stepwise by paracrine or autocrine growth factors, viruses, and genetic accidents.

Second, if a general theory of immune surveillance were correct, we might predict an excess of non-hematopoietic cancers in immunocompromised individuals. These would represent "escape" of nascent tumor cells from the expected immune response. With few exceptions, these cancers are not encountered, and the exceptions can be accounted for by the presence of codeterminants in the persons at risk. For example, epithelial carcinomas in ataxia-telangiectasia may reflect defective DNA repair of radiation-induced damage. Anogenital carcinomas in immunosuppressed transplant patients may reflect activation of papillomavirus infection.

To date, the experimental and clinical literature supports isolated specific instances of immune surveillance but does not validate a general theory. Thus, certain virus-associated tumors are antigenic to their host and evoke a tumor-directed immune response. Animals immunized to virus-induced tumors will resist implantation and successfully reject small transplanted tumors. Conversely, animals made tolerant to the tumor at birth will accept tumor implants. In humans, virus-associated tumors, such as the EBV-associated African Burkitt's lymphoma, evoke immune responses to viral antigens expressed on the tumor cell. These tumor-directed responses may be responsible in part for spontaneous remissions and long-term survival of treated patients.

Certain human tumors seem to be antigenic to their host. A tumor-specific antigen has been found in patients with melanoma, and evidence of specific T cell responses to transitional carcinoma of the bladder, malignant glioma, and carcinomas of the skin is reported. Carcinoma of the kidney and malignant melanoma are particularly susceptible to nonspecific killing by activated NK cells. Other tumors express tumor-associated antigens of oncofetal origin, but these do not appear to evoke a protective immune response.

The majority of human cancers, however, are not strongly antigenic, presumably owing to such mechanisms as modification of histocompatibility antigens, cell surface glycosylation, or the production of blocking factors. Whatever the mechanism, the immune system fails to recognize most spontaneous tumors, not because of an immune defect, but because the tumors themselves are relatively nonantigenic.

REFERENCES

Beral V et al: AIDS-associated non-Hodgkin lymphoma. *Lancet* 1991;**337**:805.

Beral V et al: Kaposi's sarcoma among persons with AIDS: A sexually transmitted infection? *Lancet* 1990; **335**;123.

Beral V et al: Risk of Kaposi's sarcoma and sexual practices associated with fecal contact in homosexual or bisexual men with AIDS. *Lancet* 1992;**339**:632.

Burnet FM: Immunologic surveillance in neoplasia. *Transplant Rev* 1971;**7**:3.

Delli Bovi P et al: An oncogene isolated by transfection of Kaposi's sarcoma DNA encodes a growth factor that is a member of the FGF family. *Cell* 1987;**50**:729.

Ensoli B et al: AIDS-Kaposi's sarcoma-derived cells express cytokines with autocrine and paracrine growth effects. *Science* 1989;**243**:223.

Ensoli B et al: Pathogenesis of AIDS associated Kaposi's sarcoma. *Hematol Oncol Clin North Am* 1991;**5**:281.

Frizzera G et al: Lymphoreticular disorders in primary immunodeficiencies. *Cancer* 1980;**46**:692.

Hanto DW et al: Epstein Barr virus (EBV) induced polyclonal and monoclonal B-cell lymphoproliferative diseases occurring after renal transplantation. *Ann Surg* 1983; **198**:356.

Huang YQ et al: HPV-16 related sequences in Kaposi's sarcoma. *Lancet* 1992;**339**:515.

Kaplan LD et al: AIDS-related non-Hodgkin's lymphoma in San Francisco. *JAMA* 1989;**261**:719.

Kinlen LJ: Incidence of cancer in rheumatoid arthritis and other disorders after immunosuppressive treatment. *Ann Intern Med* 1985;**78 (Suppl):**44.

Knowles DM et al: Lymphoid neoplasia associated with the acquired immunodeficiency syndrome (AIDS). *Ann Intern Med* 1988;**108:**744.

Kremer KJ et al: Role of human immunodeficiency virus type 1 and other viruses in malignancies associated with acquired immunodeficiency syndrome. *J Natl Cancer Inst* 1990;**82:**1016.

Kripke ML: Immunoregulation of carcinogenesis: Past, present, and future. *J Natl Cancer Inst* 1988;**80:**722.

Lombardi I, Newcomb EW, Dalla-Favera R: Pathogenesis of Burkitt lymphoma: Expression on an activated c myc oncogene causes the tumorigenic conversion of EBV-infected human B lymphoblasts. *Cell* 1987; **49:**161.

Lymphoma in organ transplant recipients. (Editorial.) *Lancet* 1984;**1:**601.

Macmahon EME et al: Epstein-Barr virus in AIDS-related primary central nervous system lymphoma. *Lancet* 1991;**338:**1991.

Meeker T et al: Evidence for molecular subtypes of HIV-associated lymphomas: division into peripheral monoclonal, polyclonal and central nervous system lymphoma. *AIDS* 1991;**5:**669.

Nair BC et al: Identification of a major growth factor for AIDS-Kaposi's sarcoma cells as oncostatin M. *Science* 1992;**255:**1430.

Penn I: Tumors of immunocompromised patient. *Annu Rev Med* 1988;**39:**63.

Preston DS et al: Nonmelanoma cancers of the skin. *N Engl J Med* 1992;**327:**1649.

Purtilo DT: Opportunistic cancer in patients with immunodeficiency syndromes. *Arch Pathol Lab Med* 1987; **111:**1123.

Shiramizu B et al: Molecular and immunophenotypic characterization of AIDS-associated, Epstein-Barr virus-negative, polyclonal lymphoma. *J Clin Oncol* 1992;**10:**383.

Tucker MA et al: Risk of second cancers after treatment for Hodgkin's disease. *N Engl J Med* 1988;**318:**76.

Vogel J et al: The HIV tat gene induces dermal lesions resembling Kaposi's sarcoma in transgenic mice. *Nature* 1988;**335:**606.

Wahman A et al: The epidemiology of classic, African and immunosuppressed Kaposi's sarcoma. *Epidemiol Rev* 1991;**13:**178.

Ziegler JL, Dorfman RK (editors): *Kaposi's Sarcoma, Pathophysiology and Clinical Management.* Marcel Dekker, 1988.

45 Neoplasms of the Immune System

John W. Parker, MD, & Robert J. Lukes, MD

Lymphomas and leukemias involving lymphocytes, plasma cells, monocytes, and natural killer (NK) cells are neoplasms of the immune system. The effects of these neoplasms upon immune function result primarily from loss or malfunction of the neoplastic cells. With increasing knowledge of the specific functions and immunophenotypes of normal cells of the immune system and evidence that lymphomas and leukemias reflect clonal expansions of cells at different stages of normal cell differentiation, immunophenotyping has become useful in helping identify different types of lymphomas and leukemias. These tumors, which would not otherwise be detected by morphologic features alone, have different clinical behaviors and responses to therapy. Lymphomas and leukemias are frequently considered separate diseases, but most evidence indicates that they are essentially the same neoplasms, with different modes of onset, distribution, and spread.

CLASSIFICATION

Lymphomas and lymphocytic leukemias have traditionally been classified on the basis of morphologic and clinical features: leukemias as acute, subacute, or chronic, based on the onset and progression of disease, or according to morphologic characteristics as in the FAB (French-American-British) system, and lymphomas according to histologic features (Rappaport classification). Now that lymphoid neoplasms can be characterized immunologically as being of T or B lymphocyte origin, new, immunologically based classifications (Lukes-Collins and Kiel classifications) (Table 45–1) have been proposed. These recent classifications recognize lymphoid neoplasms as clonal expansions of single cells arrested at different stages of differentiation (Fig 45–1) and recognize that they can be identified as such by both morphology and immunophenotype.

A working formulation of non-Hodgkin lymphomas was developed in 1982 for clinical use (Table 45–1). This classification is based on a combination of histologic and clinical features that characterize lymphomas according to clinical behavior, ie, low-, intermediate-, and high-grade lymphomas. However, it does not distinguish between T and B lymphocytic neoplasms, thereby ignoring the importance of immunophenotypes in diagnosis, prognosis, and therapy.

GENERAL CONSIDERATIONS

Neoplasms of the immune system may present locally but are often widespread at the time of diagnosis, presumably because of the natural ability of the cells to circulate. Moreover, they frequently undergo changes in morphology and clinical behavior during the course of the disease; eg, well-differentiated cells transform into more rapidly proliferating, malignant cells. Some of these neoplasms are easily diagnosed from morphology on tissue sections or smears, but others are more subtle and require cytochemical, immunologic, ultrastructural, or karyotypic characterization for precise categorization. Even morphologically distinct cell types may be immunophenotypically heterogeneous and associated with differences in clinical behavior.

The morphologic appearance of neoplasms of immunopoietic cells is the result of several factors, including mixtures of neoplastic and normal cells, neoplastic and reactive cells at different stages of the cell cycle or transformation sequence, and differences in growth pattern. In early involvement of lymph nodes, the location of the lymphoma cells may help determine the cell of origin—B cell lymphomas arising in follicles and T cell neoplasms in the paracortical areas.

The clinical course of these neoplasms is related to the proportion of dividing and nondividing cells. Neoplasms such as chronic lymphocytic leukemia of

Table 45–1. Immunologically based lymphoma classifications and the "working formulation."[1]

Lukes-Collins Classification	Kiel Equivalent	Working Formulation
Undefined	**U Cell** Lymphoblastic, unclassified[2]	
B cell Small lymphocyte B-CLL Plasmacytoid lymphocyte Mantle zone lymphoma Parafollicular (monocytoid) B cell lymphoma Marginal zone lymphoma Hairy cell leukemia	**B cell** Lymphocytic, B-CLL Lymphoplasmacytic/-cytoid (LP immunocytoma)	ML,[3] small lymphocytic (CLL) ML, small lymphocytic plasmacytoid
Follicular center cell (FCC) types Small cleaved FCC Large cleaved FCC Small noncleaved FCC Burkitt Non-Burkitt Large noncleaved FCC Immunoblastic sarcoma of B cell type (IBS-B)	Centrocytic Centroblastic-centrocytic[4] B lymphoblastic Burkitt type others Centroblastic B immunoblastic	ML, follicular/diffuse, small cleaved ML, follicular/diffuse, large cell or mixed small cleaved and large cell ML, small noncleaved ML, Immunoblastic plasmacytoid
T cell Small lymphocyte T-CLL Convoluted lymphocyte Cerebriform lymphocyte Lymphoepitheliod lymphocyte Immunoblastic sarcoma (T-cell) including node-based T-cell lymphoma	**T cell** Lymphocytic, T-CLL T lymphoblastic (convoluted cell type and others) Lymphocytic, mycosis fungoides, and Sézary's syndrome [Lymphoepithelioid][4] T immunoblastic	ML, small lymphocyte ML, lymphoblastic convoluted or non-convoluted Mycosis fungoides ML, diffuse mixed and small and large cell with epithelioid cells ML, large cell, immunoblastic, clear cell, polymorphous

[1]Modified from Lukes RJ and Collins RD, *Tumors of the Hematopoietic System*, fascicle 28, AFIP, 1989.
[2]This category contains all lymphoblastic lymphomas that are immunologically undefined or cannot be typed for any of several reasons.
[3]ML, Malignant lymphoma.
[4]This category was not included in the Kiel classification, because at present many cases cannot be distinguished from Hodgkin's disease with a large number of T lymphocytes and very few Reed-Sternberg cells.

B cell type (B-CLL) are widespread but indolent, because of a predominant proportion of nondividing small lymphocytes. In contrast, Burkitt's lymphoma has a predominance of proliferating cells. The ability of an indolent process such as B-CLL to transform into a rapidly dividing immunoblastic lymphoma further illustrates the heterogeneity of these neoplasms. The stimuli or mechanisms for such transformations are largely unknown but, in some instances, appear to be the result of second mutational events. These transformations may be confusing diagnostically, but they are of extreme importance therapeutically. An additional complexity is the development of second, new neoplasms several years later, apparently the result of the chemotherapy or radiotherapy of the first neoplasm.

In summary, neoplasms of cells of the immune system are complex and may be difficult to diagnose. Nevertheless, recognition of morphologically distinct cell types and patterns of tissue involvement in conjunction with immunophenotyping, cytochemistry, karyotyping, and molecular biologic techniques make an orderly approach to diagnosis possible.

IMMUNOLOGIC FEATURES

The immunologic characteristics of neoplasms of the immune system reflect those of their cells of origin. Because each neoplasm is a clonal expansion of a normal immunopoietic cell type, and, because these clones may retain function, lose function, or malfunction, the immunologic end result varies considerably. Because most lymphocytic neoplasms are of the B cell type, the usual immunologic dysfunction relates to immunoglobulin production. T cell neoplasms may produce an excess of particular cytokines, but generally they are not functional.

B cell lymphoma or leukemia cells usually do not respond to antigens or mitogens with in vitro transformation or immunoglobulin production, but the addition of healthy helper T cells or removal of suppressor T cells may partially correct this deficit.

Serum Immunoglobulins

Monoclonal serum immunoglobulins are important features of multiple myeloma, Waldenström's macroglobulinemia, and, to a lesser degree, some B

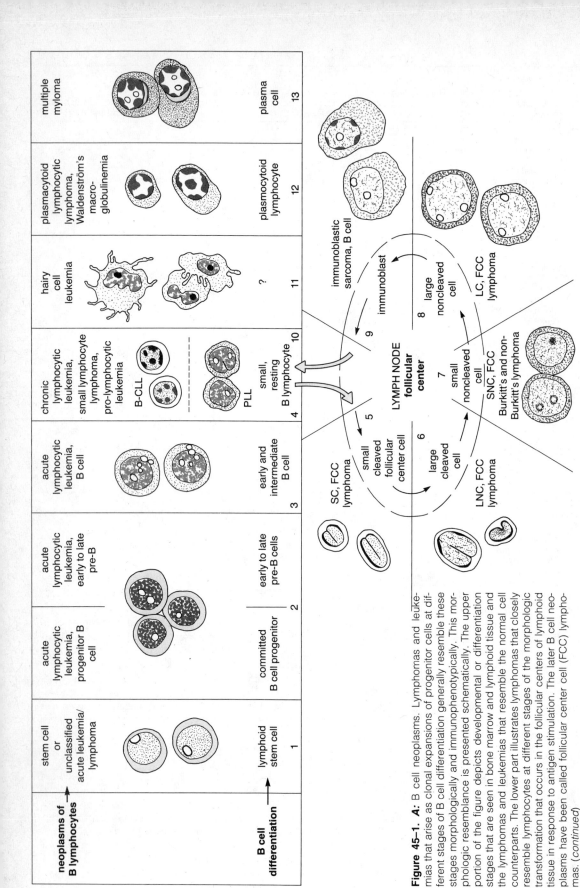

Figure 45–1. A: B cell neoplasms. Lymphomas and leukemias that arise as clonal expansions of progenitor cells at different stages of B cell differentiation generally resemble these stages morphologically and immunophenotypically. This morphologic resemblance is presented schematically. The upper portion of the figure depicts developmental or differentiation stages that are seen in bone marrow and lymphoid tissue and the lymphomas and leukemias that resemble the normal cell counterparts. The lower part illustrates lymphomas that closely resemble lymphocytes at different stages of the morphologic transformation that occurs in the follicular centers of lymphoid tissue in response to antigen stimulation. The later B cell neoplasms have been called follicular center cell (FCC) lymphomas. (*continued*)

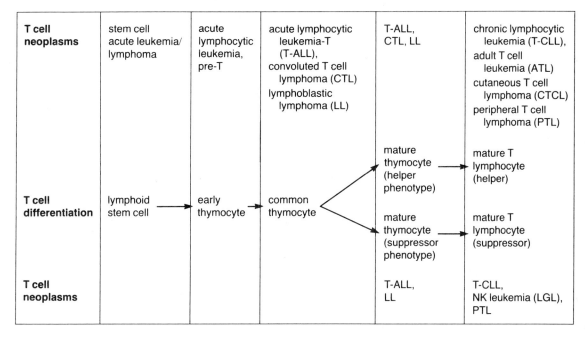

T cell neoplasms	stem cell acute leukemia/ lymphoma	acute lymphocytic leukemia, pre-T	acute lymphocytic leukemia-T (T-ALL), convoluted T cell lymphoma (CTL) lymphoblastic lymphoma (LL)	T-ALL, CTL, LL		chronic lymphocytic leukemia (T-CLL), adult T cell leukemia (ATL) cutaneous T cell lymphoma (CTCL) peripheral T cell lymphoma (PTL)
					mature thymocyte (helper phenotype)	mature T lymphocyte (helper)
T cell differentiation	lymphoid stem cell	early thymocyte	common thymocyte		mature thymocyte (suppressor phenotype)	mature T lymphocyte (suppressor)
T cell neoplasms				T-ALL, LL		T-CLL, NK leukemia (LGL), PTL

Figure 45–1. (cont'd). **B:** As with B cell lymphomas and leukemias, there is morphologic and immunophenotypic resemblance between specific T cell neoplasms and cells at different stages of differentiation in the T cell system. However, the cytologic differences between stages in development and different lymphomas and leukemias are not as distinctive as for B cells. In addition, the stages in and location of antigen induced lymphocyte transformation of T cells are not as clearly apparent as for B cells. Because of this, morphologic stages in development are not presented here. Nevertheless, certain T cell neoplasms are morphologically distinctive, eg, convoluted T cell lymphoma-leukemia and Sézary cell lymphoma-leukemia. Small T lymphocytes in lymphoid tissue undergo morphologic transformation in response to antigens and give rise to T immunoblasts. Immunoblastic sarcomas (lymphomas) which phenotype as T cells closely resemble antigen-induced transformed lymphocytes.

cell lymphomas and leukemias. Concordance between serum and monoclonal surface immunoglobulins is an important feature of B cell lymphomas and leukemias. Hypogammaglobulinemia in B-CLL or B cell lymphoma may occur in advanced disease and lead to serious bacterial infections.

Cellular Immunity

T cell dysfunction in T cell neoplasms may be manifested by delayed cutaneous anergy or defective in vitro responses to antigens and mitogens (see Chapter 13). Such indicators are most commonly, but not necessarily, seen in the late stages of disease. Infections with fungi, viruses, or opportunistic agents may be the clinical manifestation of T cell dysfunction.

Autoimmunity

Patients with a variety of autoimmune conditions (Sjögren's syndrome or Hashimoto's thyroiditis) are at a higher than normal risk for lymphomas. In turn, some patients with B cell lymphoma or leukemia may develop autoimmune hemolytic anemia, immune thrombocytopenia, or rheumatoid diseases. (See Chapters 30, 31, and 33.)

Immunophenotyping

Cells in smears or histologic sections can be diagnostically typed by immunofluorescence or enzyme immunocytochemistry with specific antibodies, particularly monoclonal antibodies. Similar studies can be performed on cell suspensions of blood, bone marrow, or lymphoid tissues by using flow cytometry (FCM) (see Chapter 13). Immunocytochemistry has the advantage of visualizing cells in situ, associating antigens with morphology. This is useful in heterogeneous displays of normal and neoplastic cells in smears or sections but has the disadvantages of background staining, interpretation ambiguities, small numbers of cells surveyed, and relative insensitivity in detecting small quantities of cell surface antigens. FCM has the disadvantage of not allowing visualization of the cells being analyzed, but it quantitatively and rapidly analyzes large numbers of cells, provides multiparameter analysis with 2 or more antibodies or other biologic probes on a cell-by-cell basis, and has exquisite sensitivity for detecting cellular antigens or receptors. This last characteristic is quite useful for detection of rare cells in blood, bone marrow, or lymphoid tissues in early staging or relapse of hematopoietic neoplasms.

There have been many immunophenotyping studies of lymphomas and leukemias (Tables 45–2 to 45–4). Some are based on the analysis of cell suspensions by FCM, and others are based on the analysis of cells in smears or histologic sections by using immunocytochemistry procedures, particularly immunoperoxidase staining. Both involve the use of monoclonal antibodies directed against so-called differentiation antigens.

Flow cytometers examine individual cells passing through a laser light beam simultaneously for size, nuclear irregularity, cytoplasmic granularity, and fluorochrome emission. Since multiple monoclonal antibodies, each labeled with a fluorochrome emitting a different color, and multiple color detectors are used, single cells can emit several colors and thus be characterized by multiple parameters.

As an example, a cell suspension prepared from a lymph node from a B cell lymphoma frequently shows 2 different populations based on cell size, nuclear shape, and cytoplasmic granularity (Fig 45–2). The large-cell population (LL) generally contains most of the lymphoma cells, and the small-cell population consists primarily of small normal lymphocytes (SL). These 2 populations can be examined separately by electronic gating. Presuming that the LL gate contains lymphoma cells and that all the cells have been exposed to a panel of antibodies that distinguish T and B lymphocytes, a dual-color phenotype can be determined by labeling one antibody with fluorescein isothiocyanate, which emits green, and the other with phycoerythrin, which emits orange-red (Fig 45–2). It is clear that the population of large cells is a homogeneous clone of B cells. The nonneoplastic small lymphocytes do not show this clonality, because they are primarily a mixture of normal or reactive T and B cells, with the B cells expressing combinations of heavy and light chains with both κ and λ present in a ratio of approximately 2.5:1 (eg, polyclonal or bitypic pattern). In addition, one of the antigens that is present on most of the lymphoma cells can be used to select the lymphoma cells for DNA analysis. Thus, clonality and DNA cell cycle analysis can be performed simultaneously, analyzing several thousand cells per second. Phenotyping results can be available within 2–3 hours of receipt of the specimen. Although surface antigens on viable cells are most commonly examined, intracytoplasmic and nuclear antigens can also be detected in properly fixed cells. The availability of new fluorochromes allows for the use of combinations of 3 antibodies and other probes in phenotyping, with further definition of neoplastic clones.

The immunocytochemical approach to immunophenotyping allows visualization of the morphology of the labeled cells, in situ, so that the architecture of the neoplasm is retained in histologic sections. Nuclear, cytoplasmic, and surface antigens are detected, although surface antigens of low density may be missed. This approach is somewhat slow, subjective, and semiquantitative, although automated image analysis resolves some of these problems and also allows for DNA analysis. Simultaneous multicolor analysis for more than one antigen per cell is generally not practical, and a complete panel of antibodies requires multiple sections, each stained for a different antigen.

DNA ANALYSIS

DNA cell cycle analysis by FCM has demonstrated a correlation of low-grade (favorable prognosis) and high-grade (unfavorable prognosis) lymphomas with the percentage of cells in S phase. High-grade lymphomas show evidence of increased proliferative rate because of an elevated proportion of cells in S phase or S phase plus G_2M. Aneuploidy is detected, by single-color FCM, in 50% or less of all lymphomas, but this percentage is higher in intermediate- and high-grade lymphomas. The percentage of cells in S phase appears to help discriminate between intermediate- and high-grade lymphomas even better than aneuploidy does.

When only the neoplastic cells of a lymphoma that also contains normal and reactive T and B lymphocytes and histiocytes are analyzed, by using an antibody which will identify the neoplastic cells, the sensitivity of detecting aneuploid populations is increased (Fig. 45–2). When only the cells bearing the restricted light chain of the B lymphoma cells are analyzed, the percentage of lymphomas that demonstrate aneuploidy increases to approximately 80%. Hyperdiploid B cell lymphomas tend to have higher S fractions and are intermediate- to high-grade lymphomas. Diploid lymphomas have low S fractions and are low-grade. Some may have 2 separate DNA clones, but both express the same light chain.

In acute lymphocytic leukemia (ALL) of childhood, aneuploidy is also relatively infrequent, but it is more frequent than in the nonlymphocytic leukemias. Changes in DNA content, as detected by FCM, correlate with changes in chromosome number, and stem lines can be detected with as few as 2 extra chromosomes.

Another use of FCM involves proliferation-associated nuclear antigens and DNA measurements. Such combinations help distinguish low-grade and high-grade lymphomas in both fresh and paraffin-embedded tissues.

Clonality

Lymphocytic neoplasms appear to be clonal expansions of cells at different stages of development, but 2 aspects tend to confuse the issue: the cells of origin may be stages in the normal sequence of T and B cell ontogeny and differentiation (Fig 45–1), or they may be stages in the normal T and B lymphocyte

Table 45–2. Immunophenotypes: B cell tumor antigens, receptors, and enzymes.

B Cell Neoplasms	TdT	HLA-DR	CD 19 (B4)[1]	CD 24 (BA-1)	Heavy Chain Gene[2,3]	Light Chain Gene[2,4]	CD 10[5] (CALLA)	CD 20 (B1)[1]	CIg	SIg	Monoclonal CIg/SIg Light Chain	CD21 (B2)	CD5 (T1)	Complement Receptor	FC Receptor	CD22 (HC-2)	PCA-1	Comments
Acute lymphocytic leukemia (non-T ALL)																		
Stem cell (non-classified) ALL	+	+	−	±[6]	G	G	−	−	−	−	−	−	−	−	−	−	−	
B progenitor cell ALL	+	+	−	±	G	G	−	−	−	−	−	−	−	−	−	−	−	
Early pre-B-ALL	+	+	+	±	R	G	+	−	−	−	−	−	−	−	−	−	−	
Mild pre-B-ALL 1	+	+	+	±	R	G/R	+	+	+μ	−	−	−	−	−	−	−	−	C ALL, FAB-L1, L2.
Mild pre-B-ALL 2	+	+	+	±	R	G/R	+	+	+μ	−	−	−	−	−	−	−	−	C ALL, FAB-L1, L2.
Late pre-B-ALL	+	+	+	±	R	G/R	+	+	+μ	−	−	+	−	−	−	−	−	
B-ALL	−	+	+	+	R	R	−	+	+μ	+	+	+	−	−	−	−	−	Small noncleaved FCC abdominal lymphoma frequent (Burkitt); FAB-L3.
Small lymphocytic leukemia or lymphoma (B-CLL)	−	+	±	+	R	R	−	±	+μ, μ/δ	+ Weak, μ, μ/δ	+	±	+	+	+	−	−	SIg Low intensity, CD5 common.
FCC lymphomas	−	+	±	±	R	R	±	±	+ μ, γ, or α	+ μ, γ, or α Strong	+	±	±	+	+	±	−	SIg strong, T101 ±.
Prolymphocytic leukemia	−	+	±	+	R	R	±	+	+	+ Strong	+	±	±	+	+		−	Differs from B-CLL because SIg strong; from hairy cell leukemia by no CD22.
Hairy cell leukemia	−	±	+	±	R	R	−	+	+, γ, or α	+ Strong μ, γ, or α	+	±	−	+	+	+	+	CD11(MO1), CD22(HC-2) monoclonal SIg and Ig gene rearrangement
Plasmacytoid lymphocytic lymphoma	−	+	+	+	R	R	−	+	+, γ, or α	±	+	−	−	+	+	±	+	Ig nuclear inclusions (Dutcher bodies)
Multiple myeloma	−	±	−	−	R	R	−	−	+, α, δ, ε, or μ	±	+	−	−	−	−	−	+	Ig cytoplasmic inclusions (Russell bodies)

[1] B cell differentiation antigens (B1, B2, and B4) tend to be present on all B cell neoplasms, particularly on differentiated ones; but the presence of each varies from one lymphoma to another.

[2] R, Rearranged immunoglobulin genes; G, germ line immunoglobulin genes. G/R, germ line or rearranged immunoglobulin genes.

[3] Immunoglobulin heavy chain gene rearrangement is seen in some patients with precursor T-ALL (10–20%), Hodgkin's disease (30–60%), immunoblastic lymphadenopathy (40%), and acute myelogenous leukemia (5%).

[4] Immunoglobulin κ gene rearrangement is seen in the Hodgkin's disease (30–60%) and immunoblastic lymphadenopathy (40%).

[5] CALLA present on pre-B cells, but also on FCC.

[6] ±, Expressed on some tumors of this type but not others.

Table 45–3. Immunophenotypes: T cell tumor antigens, receptors, and enzymes.

T Cell Neoplasms[1]	TdT	T Cell Receptor Gene Rearrangement		T9	T10	CD7 (Leu 9)	CD5 (Leu 1/ T1)	CD1 (T6)	CD2 (Leu 5/ T11)	CD3 (Leu 4/ T3)	CD4 (Leu3/ T4)	CD8 (Leu 2/ T8)	Comments
		β Chain	γ Chain[2]										
Early thymocyte (Pre-T-ALL)	+	+	+	+	+	+	+	–	±	–	–	–	
Common T thymocyte (T-ALL, CTL, LL)	+	+	...	–	+	+	+	+	+	±	±	±	
Late T thymocyte													
Helper differentiation (LL, T-ALL)	+	+	...	–	+	+	+	–	+	+	+	–	Phenotypic but not functional differentiation
Suppressor differentiation (T-ALL, LL)	+	+	...	–	+	+	+	–	+	+	–	+	
Mature T cell													
Helper differentiation (T-CLL, ATL, CTCL, PTL)	–	+	...	–	–	+	+	–	+	+	+	–	ATL phenotypes helper, but may show in vitro suppressor activity
Suppressor differentiation (T-CLL, T-gamma lymphoproliferative disorder [NK cell leukemia])	–	+	...	–	–	+	+	–	+	+	–	+	NK cell leukemia, Leu 7/HNK-1[+], CD57

[1]Abbreviations: LL, lymphoplastic lymphoma; CTL, convoluted T cell lymphoma; CTCL, cutaneous T cell lymphoma; PTL, peripheral T cell lymphoma.
[2]..., Unknown.

Table 45–4. Phenotypic markers useful for lymphomas and lymphocytic leukemias.

Designation[1]	Monoclonal Antibody	Description
TdT		Nuclear enzyme present in immature hematopoietic cells. Originally thought to be a marker for T cell neoplasms, but found in poorly differentiated lymphocytic neoplasms of either T or B cell type.
HLA-DR (Ia)		Class II HLA. Surface antigen found on most B lymphocytes, monocytes, and activated T lymphocytes; frequently present on neoplastic cells of non-T-ALL, granulocytic leukemia, B-CLL, and B cell lymphomas.
Fc receptor		Receptor for Fc portion of IgG molecule. May make SIg clonality determination difficult because of binding of plasma immunoglobulin to cells via this receptor.
SIg		Immunoglobulin on surface of B lymphocytes which is synthesized by cells and transferred to cell membrane. When only one light-chain type (κ or λ) is present on cells, indicates a clonally expanded population of neoplastic B cells. Monoclonal (restricted) light chain may be accompanied by one or 2 hyeavy chains (μ, γ, δ, or α).
CIg		Ig synthesized by B lymphocytes or plasma cells and present in cytoplasm. Restricted light and heavy chains (monoclonal) indicate neoplasm. CIg may be present in some B neoplastic cells when SIg is absent, particularly in plasmacytoid lymphocytic lymphomas and multiple myeloma.
B lymphocyte MAbs		
CD20	B1	Antigen present on essentially all B lymphocytes in blood, bone marrow, and lymphoid tissues. On most B lymphoma and B-CLL cells and about half of CALLA and ALLs. May be present in absence of SIg, and may be seen on some monocytes but not on plasma cells.
CD21	B2	On a subset of B lymphocytes in blood, bone marrow, and lymphoid tissues (mantle zone and FCC). Is lost before B1 in differentiation to plasma cells. Also found on dendritic reticulum cells. Present on cells of some B cell lymphomas and B-CLL. May be present in absence of SIg. Antigen recognized is complement receptor (C3d).
CD19	B4	On early or pre-B cells after expression of Ia antigen. Is lost before plasma cell differentiation. Present on cells of almost all non-T ALL cases (common ALL), most B cell lymphomas, and B-CLL and essentially all CGL blast crisis cells. May be present on lymphoma cells when B1 and SIG are absent or of low density. The suggested sequence of B cell differentiation, ie, (1) Ia+, (2)Ia+ B4+, (3) Ia+ B4+ CALLA+, (4) Ia+ B4+ CALLA+ B1+, (5) Ia+ B4+ CALLA+ B1+ CIg+, is reflected in different B cell neoplasms.
CD24	BA-1	On B lymphocytes, monocytes, granulocytes, and some B lymphoma cells.
CD22	HC-2/ Leu 14/ SHCL-1	Found on hairy cell leukemia cells and other B cells. Many help distinguish from prolymphocytic leukemia.
	PCA-1	On plasma cells and plasmacyotid lymphocytes, but also, weakly, on granulocytes, monocytes, and activated T cells. SIg may be absent, but CIg present. On cells of plasmacytoid lymphocytic lymphoma, multiple myeloma, plasma cell leukemia, and some hairy cell leukemias. Not on non-T-ALL, B-CLL, other B cell lymphomas, or T cell neoplasms. On some AML and CML cells.
CD10	J5/CALLA	Although a marker for non-T-ALL (common ALL), is also present on normal and activated early B or pre-B cells in bone marrow, lymph nodes (FCC), and blood. Found in about 80% of cases of non-T-ALL and some B and T cell lymphomas, including FCC lymphomas (small noncleaved, Burkitt's), and T lymphoblastic lymphoma, but also on blast cells in 40–50% of cases of CGL in blast crisis. Present on small percentage of cells in normal bone marrow (higher in reactive marrows) and on FCC in lymph nodes.
T lymphocytes and related cells		
CD1	T6	On common thymocytes and Langerhans cells of the skin but on 0–1% of peripheral T cells. Frequently seen on cells of convoluted T cell lymphoma or leukemia (lymphoblastic lymphoma) and small percentage of T-ALL cells. Not on differentiated T cell neoplasms.
CD2	T11/Leu 5	On more than 95% of T lymphocytes including all E rosetting T cells. On cells from T-ALL, T-CLL, T cell lymphomas including lymphoblastic lymphomas and cutaneous T cell lymphomas (mycosis fungoides/Sézary syndrome).
CD3	T3/Leu 4	Essentially all mature T cells and 20–30% of thymocytes. Part of T cell receptor. Antigen tends to be on same neoplastic T cells as CD2, but there are occasional discrepancies.
CD4	T4/Leu 3	On most thymocytes and 60% of blood lymphocytes. Defines helper/inducer T lymphocytes. On T-ALL cells and identifies the predominant subset in mycosis fungoides/Sézary syndrome, but also in may cases of Hodgkin's disease and some reactive or infectious conditions such as tuberculosis.

(*continued*)

Table 45–4. Phenotypic markers useful for lymphomas and lymphocytic leukemias (*continued*).

Designation[1]	Monoclonal Antibody	Description
CD8	T8/Leu 2	On 80% of thymocytes and 30–40% of blood lymphocytes. Suppressor/cytotoxic T lymphocytes. Found on cells in some cases of T-CLL, adult T cell lymphocytic leukemia, and T cell lymphomas.
CD5	T1/T101	Is a pan-T antigen, but also present on a small population of normal B cells in lymph nodes and tonsils and on medullary (high-density) and cortical (low-density) cortical thymocytes. On T-ALL, T lymphoblastic lymphoma cells, T-CLL, Sézary/mycosis fungoides cells. Also commonly on neoplastic cells of B-CLL and some B lymphoma cells. Useful in identifying a B cell neoplasm when other T cell markers or SIg are absent or of low intensity.
CD7	Leu 9	Pan-T cell antigen. On T-ALL cells and seen (rarely) in early acute myelogenous leukemia.
CD57	NKH-1/Leu 7	On LGLs (4–10% of mononuclear cells). Marker for NK cells. Found in NK cell leukemia (LGL leukemia, T-gamma lymphoproliferative disorder).
Activated or proliferating cells		
-	T9	On erythroid progenitors (antigen is transferrin receptor), but also on T cell precursors and activated/proliferating T and B lymphocytes. On convoluted T lymphoma or leukemia cells.
-	T10	On activated and proliferating T and B lymphocytes. Common on proliferating T and B cell lymphoma or leukemia cells.

[1]IUIS, WHO Committee on Human Leukocyte Differentiation Antigen Classification.

transformation process that occurs in response to antigens. Transformation results in increased numbers of effector cells, which give rise to cytokines (T) or antibodies (B). The morphology of cells at different stages in normal lymphocyte transformation closely resembles that of specific lymphoma cells. An example is the follicular center cell (FCC) lymphoma, in which normal stages of transformation occurring in germinal centers are identical to the predominant cells in each of the types of FCC lymphoma. Nevertheless, clonal expansion arising from single progenitor cells in either ontogeny or transformation can be recognized morphologically, cytochemically, and immunophenotypically.

Immunophenotypic clonality in B cell lymphomas is usually straightforward, in that the majority of cells express one (2 at the most) heavy chain and one light chain (κ or λ) on the surface or in the cytoplasm. Thus, there is evidence of "monoclonality" (Fig 45–3). With T cell lymphomas there is no such "gold standard" of monoclonality. Phenotypes using monoclonal antibodies against T cell differentiation antigens or receptors may be homogeneous. However, since there is no comparable standard for monoclonality and because homogeneous phenotypes (eg, CD2, CD3, and CD4 T cells) can reflect either neoplasia or reactive hyperplasia, T cell phenotypes lack the precision provided by surface or cytoplasmic immunoglobulin clonality. Although a monoclonal expansion of B cells may occur in benign reactive hyperplasia, it is rare and may actually be a harbinger of a developing neoplasm.

CYTOGENETICS

With modern methods, karyotypic abnormalities can be detected in almost all malignant neoplasms. These are somatic genetic changes, which are not present in normal cells. Generally, all of the cells of a tumor show the same or related chromosome abnormalities. This evidence strongly supports the notion that most neoplasms arise from a single altered cell with the somatic genetic changes providing a selective growth advantage for the progeny of the original "mutant" cell. However, although neoplasms represent clonal growth from a single cell of origin, they are frequently not homogeneous, since subpopulations evolve from the original clone because of the genetic instability of the neoplastic cells. Although distinguishing between primary and secondary chromosomal abnormalities may be difficult, it is clear that the appearance of late changes usually indicates evolution from indolence to aggressive behavior. Specific chromosomal changes associated with various types of tumors are particular rearrangements, gains, or losses of chromosomal segments. These changes probably point to sites in the genome where specific genes important in tumorigenesis are located.

Chromosomal changes are useful as adjunct diagnostic and prognostic tests in distinguishing lymphoid neoplasia from reactive hyperplasia, particularly if the former is clonal in nature. Specific abnormalities such as trisomy 12 or translocation involving chromosome 14 may help to identify the particular neoplasm and may be useful in monitoring remission, relapse, and clinical progression. Examples of specific karyotypic abnormalities in lymphomas

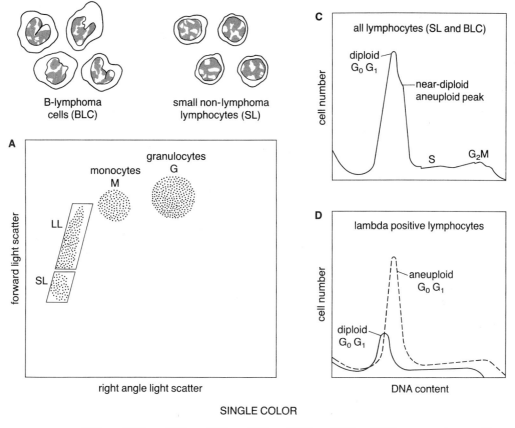

SINGLE COLOR

B	CD2 (T11)	CD3 (T3)	CD4 (T4)	CD8 (T8)	CD5 (T1)	CD21 (B1)	CD19 (B4)	CD10 (CALLA)	HLA-DR	SIg κ	SIg λ
% large lymphocytes	10	8	5	3	87	88	92	85	90	2	89
% small lymphocytes	60	55	40	15	58	32	28	12	22	30	12

DUAL COLOR

	B4+/CALLA+ (green) (red)	SIgλ+/B1+ (green) (red)
% large lymphocytes	86	84
% small lymphocytes	5	15

Figure 45–2. Immunophenotype and DNA cell cycle of a B cell lymphoma. By using FCM, a lymphoid cell suspension can be immunophenotyped with monoclonal antibodies and also analyzed for DNA content. If all of the lymphoid cells, including both the lymphoma cells (LL), which in this example are larger than the residual normal (smaller) T and B lymphocytes (SL), and small lymphocytes are analyzed together, the phenotype and true ploidy of the lymphoma cells may be obscured. However, with FCM the large lymphoma cells can be analyzed separately from the small normal lymphocytes because of light scatter differences. In this example (***top***), the immunophenotype of the lymphoma cells is distinctly monoclonal (CD5+, CD21+, CD19+, CD10+, HLA-DR+, SIg λ+), whereas the phenotype of the small lymphocytes is that of a mixture of normal T cells and polyclonal B cells. The lymphoma cells double mark for CD19 and CD10 and for SIgλ and CD21. When the total lymphocyte population is analyzed for DNA content, the DNA cell cycle histogram shows a small shoulder on the right downslope of the diploid G_0G_1 peak (***upper DNA histogram***). This can easily be missed as an aneuploid population. When the SIg λ+ population is analyzed separately, there is a well-defined near-diploid (hyper-diploid) population, which can be separated from the diploid population. The latter may represent a small number of normal lymphocytes or a diploid lymphoma stemline, or both. This capacity for multiparameter analysis with identification of subpopulations by size and configurational differences and immunophenotype makes FCM exceedingly useful clinically.

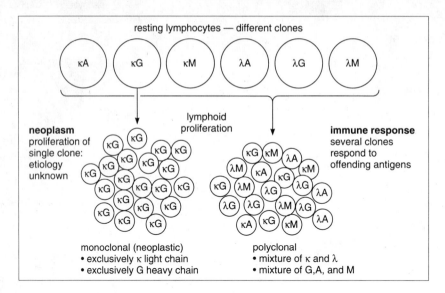

Figure 45–3. Monoclonal versus polyclonal proliferation of B lymphocytes. The monoclonal population contains one type of light and heavy chain in the example given (κ and G chains), whereas the polyclonal population consists of lymphocytes containing both κ and λ light chains and several different heavy chains. (Reproduced, with permission, from Chandrasoma P, Taylor CR: *Concise Pathology.* Appleton & Lange, 1991.)

and leukemias are represented in Table 45–5. Common chromosomal rearrangements involving translocation to the terminal portions of the long arm of chromosome 14 (band 14q32), with the donor chromosome being number 8, 11, or 18, have been observed in Burkitt's lymphoma and other non-Hodgkin lymphomas, as well as in multiple myeloma and B-CLL.

Cytogenetic information can help confirm a neoplastic or preneoplastic state, although the absence of a demonstrable karyotypic change does not rule out neoplasia. Certain nonrandom chromosomal abnormalities are so characteristic that they help establish a specific diagnosis [eg, the t(8;14) translocation of Burkitt's lymphoma; the trisomy 12 of B-CLL]. Prognostic value may also be provided as in ALL, in which the Ph-positive and t;11 subgroups have been shown to have a particularly poor prognosis, whereas cases with a normal karyotype or a chromosome count of 50–55 have a better than average prognosis.

Studies of Burkitt's lymphoma may explain the role of oncogenes in neoplasia and tumorigenesis. By a combination of cytogenetic and molecular genetic techniques, it has been demonstrated that translocations involving chromosomes 8 and 14, 8 and 22, or 2 and 8 result in a transcription of the active and rearranged immunoglobulin gene brought into juxtaposition with the so-called c-*myc* proto-oncogene, the human homolog of the retroviral v-*myc* oncogene. In the common t(8;14) translocation, the c-*myc* gene is translocated from its normal location on chromosome 8 to the immunoglobulin heavy chain locus on the long arm of chromosome 14 at band q32. In the other 2 translocations, 8 to 22 and 2 to 8, an immunoglobulin light chain locus is brought adjacent to c-*myc*. These rearrangements appear to bring the c-*myc* proto-oncogene under the influence of enhancers in or adjacent to the immunoglobulin loci, resulting in deregulation of expression of the *myc* gene and a presumed critical role in the altered growth of the neoplastic B cells. Studies in other patients have suggested that 2 new oncogenes on chromosomes 11 and 18 (*bcl-1* and *bcl-2*) may be activated in a manner similar to that of the c-*myc* gene in Burkitt's lymphoma.

Karyotypic studies indicating a clonal nature for T cell proliferations are less common, but occasionally they provide some prognostic or diagnostic information. Nonrandom karyotypic changes seem to be less frequent in T cell proliferations, but patterns are emerging. Some abnormalities are identical to those seen in B cell neoplasms (Table 45–5), including translocations to the terminal portion of the long arm of chromosome 14 (band q32) and deletions in the long arm of chromosome 6. In certain cases of T cell leukemia with a t(18;14) (q24;q11) translocation, a portion of the T cell receptor gene is brought into juxtaposition with the c-*myc* gene, with resultant deregulation similar to that seen in Burkitt's lymphoma involving the immunoglobulin genes.

Table 45–5. Common chromosomal translocation and other abnormalities in neoplasms.

Neoplasm	Translocation[1]
B cell neoplasms	
Burkitt's lymphoma	t(8;14) (q24;q32)
	t(8;22) (q24;q11)
	t(2;8) (p11;q24)
Multiple myeloma, B-CLL, small lymphocytic lymphoma, diffuse large cell lymphoma	t(11;14) (q13; q32)
B-CLL	t(2;14) (p11;q32)
	t(8;14) (q24;q11)
	t(14;17) (q32;q23)
Small cleaved FCC, diffuse and follicular large cell lymphoma	t(14;18) (q32;q21)
T cell neoplasms	
pre-T-ALL	t(11;14) (p13;q11)
T-CLL	t(14;14) (q11;q32)
	inv(14) (q11;q32)
ATL	inv(14) (q11;q32)
	t(9;21) (p24;q21)
	t(12;14) (q24;q11)
	del(6q)
Acute lymphocytic leukemia	
	Ph't(9,22) Philadelphia chromosome
	t(10;14) (q24–5;q11)
	t(8q–;14q+)
	t(8;14) (q24;q11)
	14 q +
	t(11;14) (p13;q11)
	t(11;14) (q23;q32)
	t(4;11) (q21;q23)
	t(4q–;11q+)

[1]t(8;14), Translocation from chromosome 8 to chromosome 14; (q24;q32), chromosome band q24 on chromosome 8 translocated to band q32 on chromosome 14.

MOLECULAR GENETICS

Many of the limitations of determining monoclonality of lymphoid neoplasms have been overcome by detection of rearrangements of DNA which assemble the antigen-specific receptor genes in B or T cells (see Chapters 7 and 8). The immunoglobulin and T cell receptor genes are composed of multiple, separated gene subsegments in their germ line or embryonic state. During development of the lymphoid system, this DNA recombination process assembles the components of the immunoglobulin genes in B cells and the T cell receptor genes in T cells. Much of what is known about these rearrangements was obtained from studies of lymphoid neoplasms. In turn, these studies have led to increased knowledge about the clonality, stage of development, and pathogenesis of leukemias and lymphomas.

Because there is a developmental order in the immunoglobulin and T cell receptor gene rearrangements during early B and T cell maturation, this information provides new means of categorizing neoplasms. Demonstration of phenotypic clonality of a presumed tumor has been largely limited to the demonstration of the exclusive presence of one immunoglobulin light chain (κ or λ) in B cell neoplasms. No comparable phenotypic marker of clonality has been available for T cell neoplasms. Normal or reactive B or T lymphocytes are polyclonal in origin and possess numerous immunoglobulin or T cell receptor gene rearrangements. A monoclonal neoplastic proliferation, however, represents the progeny of a single cell, so that all cells of the clone possess the same rearrangement. Therefore, it is possible to detect clonality for both B and T lymphocytes in a more sensitive manner then by immunophenotyping.

The developmental sequence of immunoglobulin and T cell receptor gene rearrangement has been derived from studies of fetal thymus and T- and B-ALL. So called non-T, non-B ALLs represent distinct stages of early B cell development, even though the cells lack expression of surface immunoglobulin. These tumors have a sequence of heavy-chain rearrangement before light chains and κ light chain before λ. In T-ALL the β T cell receptor genes are rearranged early in intrathymic ontogeny before the α T cell receptor genes. Most T-ALLs have a rearranged β chain gene and express the β T cell receptor, but only half are mature enough to express the α T cell receptor. More mature ALLs express a complete CD3-Ti receptor complex.

Although these immunoglobulin and T cell receptor gene rearrangements are used to determine the lineage of a particular neoplasm, there is not complete lineage fidelity, because there is normal crossover of both immunoglobulin and T cell receptor gene rearrangements into the opposite lymphocyte lineage. This infidelity may represent remnants of an early process occurring before absolute lineage commitment. However, by combining immunoglobulin gene and T cell receptor gene rearrangements with immunophenotyping, almost all leukemias and lymphomas can be assigned to the correct lineage. Some neoplasms that arise from very early, uncommitted progenitor cells and have only germ line DNA may not be classifiable by these techniques.

Lineage Infidelity versus Promiscuity

Leukemias and lymphomas are neoplasms that have a monoclonal origin and represent maturation arrests or uncoupling of proliferation and differentiation. Nevertheless, examples of lineage infidelity in which leukemic cells simultaneously express markers of 2 different cell lines (T and B lymphocytes or lymphoid and myeloid cells) exist. Some of these cases of so-called lineage infidelity may be explained by technical or other limitations. The first limitation is inadequate evaluation of monoclonal antibodies for cell specificity. Very few antigens are cell type- or lineage-restricted, but the lack of an extensive initial screening of normal cells with the antibodies has resulted in initially incorrect reports of specificity (eg, CD5 antigen is present on normal T cells but also on a subset of normal B cells and on B-CLL cells; CD4 antigen is present not only on T cells but also on monocytes). The second is that monoclonal antibodies are not monospecific. As with other antibodies, they are potentially able to cross-react with a variety of antigenic determinants because specificity is the result of the relative affinity of antibody-combining sites, so that antigen specificity is never absolute. In addition, they may bind by their Fc rather than Fab regions. The third is that before a particular leukemic cell type can be related to a normal progenitor cell population, the immunophenotype of the latter must be known. This knowledge is relatively complete for known major subsets of differentiated cells, but small subsets have been recognized only retrospectively from comparison with leukemic phenotypes (eg, CD5+ normal B cells recognized because of CD5+ B-CLL cells). Information about phenotypes of stem or early progenitor cells is incomplete.

Nevertheless, these technical problems do not explain all of the examples of apparent infidelity, such as examples of immunoglobulin gene rearrangement in T cell and myeloid leukemias or T cell receptor gene rearrangement or expression in non-T cell leukemias. A proposed explanation by Greaves is that early, multipotential, progenitor cells undergo simultaneous, incomplete gene rearrangements for immunoglobulin heavy chain, T cell receptor β gene, etc, so that if neoplastic clones arise from these cells, they may show similar mixed-gene rearrangements and expressions, not limited to immunoglobulin and T cell receptor. Greaves labeled this "lineage promiscuity," a transient phase of promiscuity of gene expression by bi- or multipotential progenitor cells, which may persist in leukemias and lymphomas arising from these precursor cells. Once cells are committed to a particular cell line, and this commitment may be influenced by external factors such as cytokines, they will express antigens, enzyme receptors, and other markers according to the lineage commitment, ie, lineage fidelity.

THERAPY

The therapy of neoplasms of the immune system is a combination of treating symptoms and signs (supportive) and administering cytotoxic therapy with multiple chemical agents (Table 45–6) in combination with radiation therapy and surgery. Most patients are treated on prescribed protocols, which vary somewhat from center to center and have different degrees of success depending on the type of neoplasm, the in-

Table 45–6. Multiple-agent chemotherapy for Hodgkin's lymphoma and the non-Hodgkin lymphomas.[1]

MOPP	Mechlorethamine (nitrogen mustard), Oncovin (vincristine), procarbazine, prednisone
C-MOPP	Cyclophosphamide, mechlorethamine, Oncovin, procarbazine, prednisone
COP	Cyclophosphamide, Oncovin, prednisone
CHOP	Cyclophosphamide, hydroxydaunorubicin, Oncovin, prednisone
BACOP	Bleomycin, Adriamycin (doxorubicin), cyclophosphamide, Oncovin, prednisone
ABVD	Adriamycin, bleomycin, vinblastine, dacarbazine

[1]Reproduced, with permission, from Chandrasoma P, Taylor CR: *Concise Pathology.* Appleton & Lange, 1991.
[2]All are given in spread doses and recycled at 4 weeks for 6 or more cycles, depending upon when (if) remission is achieved and upon patient tolerance.

volved organ(s), and degree of damage. Cytotoxic or other antitumor drugs in general affect DNA synthesis and are used in combination and in various delivery sequences to affect the maximum number of cells in S phase. The fact that proliferating cells are more vulnerable to cytotoxic therapy may explain why cure rates may be better with aggressive neoplasms than with low-grade ones. The latter may have an indolent, prolonged course in which remission may be readily induced but is often short-lived.

The selection of appropriate therapy is based on 2 major factors: cytologic/histologic type and extent of disease. The latter is determined by staging in Hodgkin's disease and the non-Hodgkin's lymphomas. The Ann Arbor Staging Classification for Hodgkin's disease defines 4 major stages (I–IV) extending from involvement of a single lymph node region (stage I) to disseminated involvement of distant extranodal organs (stage IV). Systemic symptoms such as fever, night sweats, and weight loss provide subcategories for the stages. Staging for non-Hodgkin's lymphomas is similar and utilizes history, physical examination, surgical and needle biopsies, x-rays including tomography, radioisotope scans, CT scans, and lymphangiograms. Because leukemias, by definition, involve bone marrow and peripheral blood, staging is not a factor but cell type is.

Radiation Therapy

Radiation therapy is more central to the therapy of Hodgkin's disease than of the non-Hodgkin lymphomas. It plays an important role in localized disease, may be the only treatment used for low-grade lymphomas, and may be used in conjunction with chemotherapy in intermediate- and high-grade lymphomas.

Chemotherapy

The alkylating agent chlorombucil has been used alone since 1955 to treat indolent lymphomas and CLL. However, it is toxic and may produce irreversible marrow suppression; it is also leukemogenic. Other drugs such as cyclophosphamide are also effective but are toxic. To increase effectiveness and reduce toxicity, combination chemotherapy was developed at the National Cancer Institute. The combinations listed in Table 45–6 and other third-generation programs are used in Hodgkin's disease and non-Hodgkin's lymphomas. The rationale for multiagent therapy is that drug-resistant cells arise spontaneously and acquired resistance to a drug results from genetic mutation. Thus exposure to several drugs may prevent the survival and proliferation of resistant cells. In addition, tumor cell death is related to dose intensity of drugs, so that a maximum dose of a maximum number of drugs over the shortest period should be most effective. This does not, however, avoid toxicity, and careful monitoring is required.

Bone Marrow Transplantation

Because of the ineffectiveness of radiation and chemotherapy in many patients with intermediate- and high-grade lymphomas or acute leukemias, a new therapeutic approach was needed. Autologous bone marrow transplantation (see Chapter 57) has extended survival in some patients, particularly children, but results have been spotty.

Eradication of lymphomas or leukemic cells with high-dose chemotherapy and total-body irradiation (purging) is followed by the introduction of marrow-replenishing "stem cells." Techniques for purification of these multipotential cells from autologous marrow or peripheral blood have steadily improved, so that repopulation of the hemopoietic system is increasingly effective.

Other Agents

2′-Deoxycoformycin (Pentostatin) is a purine analogue that is a potent inhibitor of adenosine deaminase. This drug has produced remission in some refractory lymphoid malignancies, particularly hairy cell leukemia, in which a brief course produces durable remission in 90% of patients. Although hairy cell leukemia is a B cell neoplasm, T cell lymphomas and leukemias are more responsive to this agent in general than are B cell neoplasms.

Recombinant alpha interferon has produced remissions in hairy cell leukemia and some low-grade lymphomas. Although remission may continue for as long as 3 years, it is generally shorter (median 8 months) and toxicity is common.

Monoclonal Antibody Therapy

In principle, treating neoplasms with highly specific monoclonal antibodies directed at lymphoma or leukemia antigens has great appeal. However, attempts to treat lymphoma and lymphocytic leukemia patients with monoclonal antibodies have had variable results. Generally, there has been relatively little initial effect, with only transient improvement in le-

sions, but there have also been relatively minor side effects, less than might have been expected since the antibodies are of mouse origin. Inherent problems of monoclonal antibody therapy exist because (1) potential modulation of the cell surface antigen may be induced by exposure to the antibody; (2) circulating shed tumor antigen may bind antibody and prevent it from reaching the tumor cells; and (3) the production of antimouse antibodies may lead to antibody neutralization or allergic reactions. These drawbacks to immunotherapy are also a factor when monoclonal antibodies are conjugated to chemical toxins or radioisotopes in order to direct them to the neoplastic cells. Nevertheless, monoclonal antibodies conjugated to radioisotopes for tumor imaging have been used with some success.

An initially exciting approach to therapy is the use of monoclonal antibodies directed against an individual patient's own tumor immunoglobulin idiotype. Because lymphoma cells from some patients express more than one idiotype, and these may change over time, the necessity for using more than one anti-idiotype antibody is clear. Encouraging recent studies have demonstrated that monoclonal antibodies made against one patient's immunoglobulin idiotype may also recognize immunoglobulin idiotypes from other patient's neoplasms.

Some problems yet unresolved include localization of monoclonal antibodies exclusively in the neoplasm, the response of the host to his or her own tumor antigens, antigenic heterogeneity, and tumor modulation. Therefore, the ultimate value of this approach cannot be completely assessed. It would appear that the major use of these antibodies may lie in radioimaging, bone marrow purging, and combined treatment in which they are used to eliminate small residual neoplastic cells after chemotherapy or radiotherapy.

LYMPHOCYTIC NEOPLASMS OF B CELL ORIGIN

B cell neoplasms are much more common than T cell neoplasms in the USA and Europe. They arise in all lymphoid areas of normal B cell production (Table 45–7) and in some nonlymphoid tissues. Diagnosis is usually straightforward because of monoclonal immunoglobulins in serum or urine and on the surface or cytoplasm of the cells and because of the distinctive morphologic features of the FCC and plasmacytoid types. Because the majority of these B cell neoplasms arise from the follicular centers of lymphoid tissues, many retain a follicular growth pattern. The variation in morphology and clinical expression

Table 45–7. Most common neoplasms of the immune system in different tissues.

Tissue	T Cell Neoplasm[1]	B Cell Neoplasm[1]	Mononuclear Phagocyte System[1]	Unknown[1]
Bone marrow	ALL	ALL, small lymphocytic (B-CLL) multiple my-eloma	ANLL	
Lymph nodes		SC FCC, LC FCC		Hodgkin's disease (LP, NS, MC)
Spleen		SC FCC, hairy cell leuke-mia	CML, ANLL	Hodgkin's disease (NS)
Thymus	HD, NS convoluted T-ALL			
Pharynx (Waldenström's myeloma)		SC FCC, LC FCC, LNC FCC		
Gonads		SNC FCC, IBS-B		
Lung		SC FCC, plasmacytoid		
Stomach and intestine		LNC FCC, IBS-B, plas-macytoid, SNC, LNC		
Skin	Cutaneous T cell lym-phoma (cerebriform), MF, Sézary, IBS-T, small T lymphocyte	Small B lymphocyte		
Conjunctiva		SC FCC, plasmacytoid		
Thyroid		LNC FCC, IBS-B, plas-macytoid		
Salivary gland		SC FCC		
Bone		SNC FCC (Burkitt's), ALL		
Central nervous system	T-ALL	IBS-B, SNC FCC		

[1]Abbreviations: convoluted T, convoluted T cell lymphoma or leukemia; ANLL, acute nonlymphocytic leukemia; SC, small cleaved; LC, large cleaved; LNC, large noncleaved; SNC, small noncleaved; CML, chronic myelogenous leukemia; MF, mycosis fungoides; LP, lymphocyte predominance; NS, nodular sclerosis; MC, mixed cellularity; LD, lymphocyte depletion.

reflects the varying predominance of different stages of the cell cycle and transformation from small lymphocytes to large proliferating (transformed) lymphocytes. In most instances, patients with B cell neoplasms are initially diagnosed with disease involving bone marrow or lymph nodes. When there is extensive bone marrow involvement, the cells frequently circulate in the peripheral blood and disseminate widely throughout lymphoid tissues. In B cell neoplasms such as multiple myeloma or plasmacytoid lymphocytic lymphomas, production of excessive quantities of immunoglobulins can be easily detected. Most patients with B cell neoplasms do not initially have splenomegaly or pancytopenia, and those who do usually have hairy cell leukemia.

Nonlymphoid tissue involvement by B cell lymphomas is common, particularly in the thyroid, gastrointestinal tract, salivary glands, and conjunctiva. Neoplasms of small lymphocytes and plasma cells can be morphologically identified, but less highly differentiated cells (pre-B-ALL) can be identified as B cells only by immunophenotyping. Small and transformed B lymphocytes cannot always be distinguished cytologically from small and transformed T lymphocytes, but they can be distinguished by immunophenotyping. Neoplasms such as small and large noncleaved FCC lymphomas and pre-B-ALL are predominantly actively dividing and show minimal differentiation. Cleaved FCC lymphomas, B-CLL, and hairy cell leukemia characteristically have few dividing cells and show minimal plasmacytic

differentiation. Multiple myeloma and plasmacytoid lymphocytic lymphomas are predominantly differentiated, with small proliferating populations. Immunoblastic sarcomas (lymphomas) of B cells (IBS-B) are composed primarily of transformed proliferating cells with various degrees of differentiation. The clinical features of B cell neoplasms relate to their proliferative rate, immunoglobulin production (hypo or hyper), and displacement of functioning cells in the bone marrow or other lymphoid tissues. Chromosomal abnormalities may also occur.

ACUTE LYMPHOCYTIC LEUKEMIA (ALL)

The etiology of acute leukemia in humans is still unknown, although implicating factors include RNA retroviruses, ionizing radiation, chemicals such as benzene, and genetic factors. Chromosomal abnormalities are detectable in some clinically healthy family members of patients with acute leukemia. Leukemic cells accumulate in bone marrow, blood, and other tissues, resulting in suppression of hematopoietic function with associated anemia, thrombocytopenia, and granulocytopenia. Infiltration of the central nervous system, liver, spleen, lungs, and other tissues adds to the expression and severity of the disease.

Improved understanding of the immunologic heterogeneity and biology of ALL has led to revisions in therapy. For example, the homing of normal T lymphocytes to tissues such as the central nervous system and testes has explained the frequent relapses involving these extramedullary sites in T-ALL and has shown the need for more focused and aggressive chemotherapy than is needed in "common ALL."

Common ALL or Pre-B-ALL

Most cases of ALL which are not T cell in origin fall into this group—the most common neoplasm of childhood. Onset is typically between the ages of 2 and 10 years; however, the disease may occur in individuals in their 30s and 40s. The incidence is higher in males than in females.

A. Clinical Features: Patients present with weakness, fatigue, bleeding, bruising, fever, chills, and infections. Bone and joint pain are common, and central nervous system symptoms due to increased intracranial pressure may be present. Pronounced leukocytosis, anemia, and thrombocytopenia are usual.

B. Pathology: This leukemia is characterized by massive marrow infiltration with blast cells, and massive marrow necrosis may be present. Hepatosplenomegaly and lymphadenopathy are common. Nuclei are round with fine nuclear chromatin and indistinct nucleoli. Relapses in the marrow are usually focal, but the testes may be involved.

C. Immunologic Features: Patients with acute leukemia may have decreased delayed hypersensitivity and variable immunoglobulin levels. Infections are common and life-threatening. Prognosis may relate in part to abnormalities in immune function as indicated by decreased lymphocyte responses to mitogens in vitro and depressed delayed hypersensitivity skin test reactions, both of which are reflections of poor cellular immunity. In both T and B cell acute leukemias, immune cell functions may be suppressed because of replacement of normal lymphocytes, an imbalance in regulatory cells, or production of immunosuppressive factors (Tables 45–2 and 45–4).

D. Differential Diagnosis: This includes granulocytic leukemia, other types of ALL, and metastatic neuroblastoma.

E. Therapy: Current multiagent therapy produces remission in 90–95% of childhood patients, with most achieving prolonged remission and apparent cure. Poor prognosis is associated with an onset at younger than 2 years or older than 10 years of age, leukocytosis in excess of 200,000/μL, and involvement of the central nervous system at diagnosis; black patients also have a poor prognosis.

B-ALL

A. Clinical Features: B-ALL is the least common and most aggressive form of ALL. Incidence is greater in males than in females. The median age of onset is 13 years, older than for common ALL of childhood. Extensive marrow involvement and leukemia in cases of small noncleaved FCC lymphoma, Burkitt's type, may be diagnosed as B-ALL. Marrow failure from infiltration and systemic symptoms is common. Lymphadenopathy, hepatosplenomegaly, bone involvement, neurologic abnormalities due to central nervous system infiltration, and abdominal masses are frequent. Circulating leukemia cells may account for 80% of leukocyte counts of 20,000–30,000/μL. Anemia, thrombocytopenia, and uricacidemia are common.

B. Pathology: In sections of involved tissues and in peripheral blood, blast cells are similar to those seen in other forms of ALL.

C. Immunologic Features: See Tables 45–2 and 45–4.

D. Differential Diagnosis: This includes small noncleaved FCC lymphoma (Burkitt's type), other types of ALL, and acute granulocytic leukemia.

E. Therapy: Combination chemotherapy (Table 45–6) may result in complete remission but is usually followed by rapid relapse, so survival is usually less than 6 months from diagnosis.

SMALL LYMPHOCYTIC LYMPHOMAS & LEUKEMIAS

A. Clinical Features: The onset is generally in elderly individuals (older than 55 years) and occurs more often in males than in females. Initial manifestations are lymphadenopathy or B-CLL. Patients may be initially asymptomatic or may present with fatigue, weakness, thrombocytopenia, hemolytic anemia, and hypogammaglobulinemia. Although most have disseminated disease at diagnosis, the course is usually indolent and prolonged, with survival for 7–10 years with no initial therapy and only conservative therapy thereafter. The staging of B-CLL correlates with survival: stage 0, lymphocytosis in blood and marrow; stage 1, lymphocytosis and lymphadenopathy; stage 2, lymphocytosis and hepatomegaly with or without splenomegaly; stage 3, lymphocytosis with anemia; stage 4, lymphocytosis with thrombocytopenia. Approximately 1% of patients transform to immunoblastic sarcoma of B cell type (Richter's syndrome), and aggressive terminal infection is common.

B. Pathology: There is diffuse involvement of superficial lymph nodes, bone marrow, spleen, liver, other tissues, and blood. Neoplastic cells are small, round lymphocytes with dense chromatin and scanty cytoplasm. Transformed lymphocytes and mitotic figures are seen in the pale, so-called proliferation centers.

C. Immunologic Features: See Tables 45–2 and 45–4.

D. Differential Diagnosis: This includes small cleaved FCC lymphoma, plasmacytoid lymphocytic lymphoma, small T cell lymphocytic lymphoma (T-CLL), hairy cell leukemia, and Hodgkin's disease.

E. Therapy: Because of the indolent course, aggressive multiagent therapy is contraindicated. Patients managed conservatively survive 7–10 years or more but require therapy when the leukemia transforms to a more aggressive cell type, eg, prolymphocytic leukemia or IBS-B.

PROLYMPHOCYTIC LEUKEMIA

Prolymphocytic leukemia is an uncommon variant of CLL. It differs from small cell CLL in that the leukemic cells are larger with more cytoplasm and a prominent nucleolus, and response to therapy is poor. Approximately two-thirds have the phenotype of B cells and one-third have that of T cells. Surface immunoglobulin staining is more intense than is seen in B-CLL, but the cells generally express HLA-DR, CD20, and CD19, as do B-CLL cells, but they do not form rosettes with mouse erythrocytes and are CD5 negative. Most cases of T prolymphocytic leukemia are CD4 positive but not CD8 positive. A small number of patients with B-CLL develop prolymphocytic leukemia after 1–5 years; this is followed by a more aggressive course.

FOLLICULAR CENTER CELL (FCC) LYMPHOMAS

These lymphomas usually arise from follicular centers in lymph nodes, spleen, tonsils, or intestines. They usually develop in superficial or retroperitoneal lymph nodes, but occasionally in other tissues such as thyroid or stomach. The predominant cell may be a dormant small lymphocyte (cleaved) or transformed lymphocyte (noncleaved). The majority of non-Hodgkin lymphomas are FCC in origin. However, histologically they may have a follicular or diffuse pattern, and they often change from follicular to diffuse over time. The indolent disease associated with the small cleaved type frequently changes to more rapidly proliferating aggressive disease. Although the cells all arise in the lymphoid follicles, there is a great range of expressions so that the different cell types closely resemble the stages in lymphocyte transformation that occur in the germinal centers of the follicles in response to antigen (Fig 45–1). Partial lymph node involvement occurs early in the disease, and the size and shape of the cells vary according to cell type or stage in transformation.

1. SMALL CLEAVED FCC LYMPHOMAS

A. Clinical Features: These lymphomas make up 20–30% of the lymphomas in the USA and most commonly occur in males 50–60 years of age. Asymptomatic peripheral lymphadenopathy is a common initial finding, and disseminated disease is usually present at diagnosis. However, the course is indolent, with survivals of 7–10 years with little or no therapy. About half of the cases progress to an aggressive noncleaved FCC lymphoma, which responds poorly to current therapy.

B. Pathology: A follicular growth pattern is seen in most cases, but there is interfollicular infiltration by the small cleaved cells, and perinodal extension is common. Lymph node, bone marrow, spleen, and hepatic portal areas are often involved, with occasional massive necrosis. Other tissue involvement is uncommon. Homogeneous infiltrates of small cells with irregular nuclear indentions, deep cleavage planes, and scanty cytoplasm are characteristic and distinctive.

C. Immunologic Features: See Tables 45–2 and 45–4.

D. Differential Diagnosis: This includes follicular hyperplasia, small lymphocytic lymphoma (T or B cell), plasmacytoid lymphocytic lymphoma, and large cleaved FCC lymphomas.

E. Therapy: Little or no therapy is necessary in asymptomatic individuals for 3–4 years, but after that time multiagent chemotherapy may be indicated as the disease progresses (Table 45–6).

2. LARGE CLEAVED FCC LYMPHOMAS

A. Clinical Features: These lymphomas account for approximately 5% of lymphoid neoplasms and 10% of FCC lymphomas in the USA. They are more common in males, and the mean age of onset is 50 years. There is peripheral and retroperitoneal lymphadenopathy, splenomegaly, hepatomegaly, and involvement of the gastrointestinal tract and bone marrow. Widely disseminated disease is common at diagnosis, and systemic symptoms are common. The disease is indolent or moderate in its rate of progression.

B. Pathology: There is follicular or diffuse involvement of peripheral, mesenteric, and retroperitoneal lymph nodes. Sclerosis is common is involved tissues, including extranodal masses. The nuclei vary widely in size and configuration but are frequently large and irregular with deep cleavage planes. They may be hyperlobated and may therefore be mistaken for Reed-Sternberg cells. The cytoplasm is indistinct but methyl green-pyronine (MGP)-positive, and there are occasional cases with cytoplasmic immunoglobulin inclusions. Small cleaved cells and reactive plasma cells are variably present.

C. Immunologic Features: See Tables 45–2 and 45–4.

D. Differential Diagnosis: This includes small cleaved FCC lymphoma, large noncleaved FCC lymphoma, Hodgkin's disease, nodular sclerosis, and metastatic carcinoma with sclerosis.

E. Therapy: Optimal therapy is yet to be determined, and the disease may be more indolent than was initially thought.

3. SMALL NONCLEAVED FCC LYMPHOMAS

Small noncleaved FCC lymphomas are characterized by rapidly enlarging lymph nodes or extradonal masses, and occasionally there is leukemia resembling B-ALL. Most show a diffuse pattern of involvement, and tumor masses obliterate the normal architecture of lymph nodes and other tissues. Necrosis may be pronounced. The cells are small transformed lymphocytes with variable nuclear size and many mitoses. A "starry-sky" appearance is present on microscopic examination in most cases, owing to large, pale "tingible-body" macrophages.

Burkitt Type
A. Clinical Features: This disease is endemic in equatorial Africa, but the incidence in the USA and Europe is low. The African disease is associated with Epstein-Barr virus (EBV) as a probable cause. These lymphomas are more common in males than females, with an average age at onset of 7 years. There is prominent, massive involvement of the jaw, ovaries, kidneys, liver, mesentery, and central nervous system.

Cases in the USA are not associated with EBV and arise in slightly older children (11 years), again more commonly in males than in females. Common involvement of the ileocecal region results in intussusception and obstruction. Peripheral lymph nodes, kidneys, ovaries, mesentery, bone marrow, and central nervous system are less frequently involved. Children older than 13 years at onset have a poorer prognosis than younger children.

B. Pathology: The lymphoma cells are uniform in size with small nuclei and MGP-positive cytoplasm containing lipid vacuoles.

C. Immunologic Features: See Tables 45–2 and 45–4.

D. Differential Diagnosis: This includes large noncleaved FCC lymphoma, immunoblastic sarcoma (B cell), convoluted T cell lymphoma and leukemia, granulocytic sarcoma, and carcinoma with "starry-sky" appearance.

E. Therapy: Response to cyclophosphamide therapy may be dramatic, but it depends on the size of the tumor and the age of the patient, with older children having a poorer prognosis.

Non-Burkitt Type
A. Clinical Features: This type makes up approximately 6% of lymphomas in the USA, with a median onset at 50 years of age (range, 10–70 years). Males and females are equally involved. There is peripheral lymphadenopathy and widespread disease in the great majority of cases, with bone marrow, central nervous system, gastrointestinal tract, and liver involvement. A B-ALL-like leukemia is seen occasionally.

B. Pathology: The non-Burkitt type is distinguished from the Burkitt type by its more variable nuclear size and shape. Large noncleaved cells are infrequently present.

C. Immunologic Features: See Tables 45–2 and 45–4.

D. Differential Diagnosis: This is the same as for the Burkitt type (above).

E. Therapy: Multiagent chemotherapy is generally ineffective, with a median survival time of approximately 1 year.

4. LARGE NONCLEAVED FCC LYMPHOMAS

A. Clinical Features: Approximately 6% of lymphoid neoplasms and 12% of FCC lymphomas in the USA are of this cell type. Males are more frequently affected than are females; the median age of onset is 54 years (range, 18–90 years). Three-quarters of the patients present with lymphadenopathy, pain, and systemic symptoms. The gastrointestinal tract, particularly the small intestine, is commonly involved. Fewer patients have central nervous system disease with masses or lymphomatous meningitis. Bone marrow involvement is relatively infrequent.

B. Pathology: Lymph nodes are diffusely involved in most cases, but there is extranodal involvement also. The cells are homogeneous with generally round nuclei, but occasional binuclear and multinuclear cells may be confused with Reed-Sternberg cells. Nuclei have fine dispersed chromatin, and nucleoli are prominent. MGP-positive cytoplasm is abundant.

C. Immunologic Features: See Tables 45–2 and 45–4.

D. Differential Diagnosis: This includes small noncleaved FCC lymphoma, large cleaved FCC lymphoma, immunoblastic sarcoma (B or T cell), granulocytic sarcoma, and carcinoma.

E. Therapy: Multiagent chemotherapy (bleomycin, doxorubicin, cyclophosphamide, vincristine, and prednisone) produces remission in approximately three-quarters of patients with disseminated disease. Complete response is generally followed by disease-free survival, but relapses may occur months or years later.

IMMUNOBLASTIC SARCOMA OF THE B CELL TYPE (IBS-B)

A. Clinical Features: This disease often arises from small lymphocytic neoplasms or from chronic immune disorders and accounts for 3–4% of lymphoid neoplasms in the USA. The onset is commonly in the fifth decade, with equal incidence in males and females. Approximately one-third of patients have a history of prior immune disease, such as congenital immune deficiency syndrome and autoimmune disease (Wiskott-Aldrich syndrome, X-linked immunoproliferative disease, acquired autoimmune disease, Sjögren's syndrome, rheumatoid arthritis, AIDS, immune deficiency related to organ transplant, and immunoblastic lymphadenopathy). Other patients have histories of other lymphocytic neoplasms, including B-CLL and plasmacytoid lymphoma. Initial presenting features include peripheral lymphadenopathy and, to a lesser extent, involvement of the gastrointestinal tract, lungs, and brain. Systemic symptoms, including fever, night sweats, and weight loss, are present in more than half of patients at the time of diagnosis. There is mild anemia and absolute lymphocytopenia, and some patients have bone marrow involvement. Occasional patients have monoclonal paraproteinemia or hypogammaglobulinemia.

B. Pathology: Involved organs show diffuse homogeneous populations of large transformed lymphocytes, plasmacytoid immunoblasts, and plasma cells. The cytoplasm is MGP-positive as a result of abundant RNA.

C. Immunologic Features: See Tables 45–2 and 45–4.

D. Differential Diagnosis: This includes immunoblastic sarcoma (T cell); large noncleaved FCC (diffuse), small noncleaved FCC (diffuse), and large cleaved FCC (diffuse) lymphomas; granulocytic sarcoma; carcinoma; and benign immunoblastic proliferations in abnormal immune responses.

E. Therapy: Multiagent chemotherapy produces complete remission in about half of all patients, but the overall median survival time is only about 2 years.

HAIRY CELL LEUKEMIA
(Leukemic Reticuloendotheliosis)

A. Clinical Features: Approximately 3% of lymphoid neoplasms in the USA and 2% of all leukemias are hairy cell leukemia. Four times as many males as females are affected. The disease is most common in the fifth decade, but the age range is 20–80 years. Commonly, patients present with marrow failure, granulocytopenia and infection, thrombocytopenia and bleeding, and anemia with weakness and fatigue. Splenomegaly occurs in most patients, with pain in the left upper quadrant, and hepatomegaly and lymphadenopathy are common. Occasionally, paraproteinemia and osteolytic lesions are seen. The course of disease varies from a slow, chronic progression to rapid deterioration. Median survival is 5–6 years, with patients most commonly dying from bacterial, fungal, or mycobacterial infec-

tions. Circulating hairy cells are not common, and marrow biopsy is used for diagnosis because marrow is difficult to aspirate in this disease.

B. Pathology: There is focal or diffuse involvement of the bone marrow, spleen (red pulp), lymph node (interfollicular), and liver. Cells in bone marrow, spleen, and other organs are larger than lymphocytes, with abundant eosinophilic or clear cytoplasm and oval or dumbbell-shaped nuclei containing fine, even chromatin. Nucleoli are not prominent, and mitotic figures are rare. These cells are closely packed in tissues, so that microvilli are not easily seen, although there is electronmicroscopic evidence of interdigitating cytoplasmic processes. Electron microscopy also demonstrates "ribosomal lamellar complexes." Hairy cells in peripheral blood are so called because of hairlike microvillar projections of the cytoplasm, but this feature is not always easily seen and is not specific for these cells. The most useful cytochemical marker is the presence of tartrate-resistant acid phosphatase in the cytoplasm.

C. Immunologic Features: See Tables 45–2 and 45–4.

D. Differential Diagnosis: This includes small lymphocytic lymphoma and leukemia (B or T cell), plasmacytoid lymphocytic lymphoma, multiple myeloma, and mast cell proliferations.

E. Therapy: Splenectomy may produce temporary remissions. Chemotherapy produces variable results, but excellent results have been obtained with 2'-deoxycoformycin.

PLASMACYTOID LYMPHOCYTIC LYMPHOMA

A. Clinical Features: Patients with plasmacytoid lymphocytic lymphoma may or may not have Waldenström's macroglobulinemia. The usual onset of this lymphoma is in the sixth to seventh decade, and males are slightly more commonly affected. Patients with Waldenström's macroglobulinemia show increased plasma viscosity and sometimes the hyperviscosity syndrome caused by an excess of monoclonal IgM. Clinical features include weakness, fatigue, malaise, anorexia, congestive heart failure, neurologic symptoms, and hematologic symptoms such as mucosal hemorrhage and anemia. There may be visual loss as a result of retinal hemorrhages and papilledema. Lymphadenopathy and hepatosplenomegaly are common. Unlike with multiple myeloma, bone lesions, pain, and renal failure are rare, although Bence Jones proteinuria occurs in some patients. Lung, skin, or conjunctival infiltrates may be present in patients with plasmacytoid lymphocytic lymphomas. Some of these patients may have no IgM paraproteinemia and no hyperviscosity syndrome but may have anemia, fever, night sweats, lymphadenopathy, and extranodal masses. The disease is relatively indolent, and survival for 3–7 years is common with non-aggressive therapy. Some patients may progress to IBS-B.

B. Pathology: Diffuse or focal involvement of lymph node, spleen, bone marrow, and other tissues is common. Small round lymphocytes and plasmacytoid cells with pyroninophylic, periodic acid–Schiff (PAS)-positive cytoplasm are characteristic. PAS-positive immunoglobulin inclusions may be seen in the nucleus (Dutcher bodies) or cytoplasm (Russell bodies). Pale pseudofollicles similar to those seen in B-CLL and plasmacytoid immunoblasts are typically present.

C. Immunologic Features: See Tables 45–2 and 45–4.

D. Differential Diagnosis: This includes small lymphocytic lymphoma (B-CLL), small cleaved FCC lymphoma (diffuse), and reactive lymphocytosis.

E. Therapy: Severe hyperviscosity may occur as a medical emergency, requiring prompt hydration and plasma exchange. The hyperviscosity is due to the high serum concentration of monoclonal IgM with polymer or aggregate formation and cryoprecipitation. Erythrocytes commonly form rouleaux. Plasmapheresis is effective in removing circulating IgM and offers immediate relief of the symptoms and signs of hyperviscosity. It may be performed on a maintenance schedule until chemotherapy is effective. Oral chlorambucil in low doses is given daily, but if there is no response, intermittent high-dose chlorambucil and prednisone may improve the average life expectancy.

PLASMA CELL NEOPLASMS & DYSCRASIAS

Neoplasms of plasma cells are considered neoplasms of the B lymphocytes system, since they appear to arise from plasmacytoid B lymphocytes. Because these cells are responsible for secreting immunoglobulins, malfunctions of this system result in the excessive production of abnormal immunoglobulins or portions of immunoglobulin molecules. The abnormal immunoglobulin is a product of a single clone of lymphoid cells (plasmacytoid lymphocytes or plasma cells) and is called a paraprotein or myeloma protein; the disease is referred to as a monoclonal gammopathy. These abnormal proteins have typical serum electrophoretic and immunoelectrophoretic patterns (see Chapter 12), and although they may be associated with neoplastic plasma cells, they may also be secondary to other conditions such as nonhematopoietic neoplasms, rheumatoid disorders, and chronic inflammation. Plasma cell dyscra-

sias therefore encompass a somewhat confusing spectrum of diseases in that there is evidence that patients may have paraproteins many years before the onset of clinical disease, with no progression to a neoplasm and no clinical evidence associated with the paraprotein. This period may be relatively short in multiple myeloma (2–3 years) or quite long in benign monoclonal gammopathy (25–30 years).

If the disease is suspected on clinical grounds, a complete clinical work-up includes routine laboratory tests, measurements for serum viscosity, radiologic examination, hematologic profile, and renal function tests. Specific immunologic laboratory tests should be performed. The most important of these are serum protein electrophoresis, immunoelectrophoresis, and immunofixation electrophoresis (see Chapter 12), which demonstrate diagnostic, quantifiable patterns of paraproteins. Because some patients may produce cryoglobulins, which precipitate at low temperatures, serum should be separated at 37°C. In immunoelectrophoresis, antibodies against the major heavy and light chains are used. One heavy-chain class and one light-chain type are usually detected (see Chapter 12). In almost all cases there will be an immunoelectrophoretic precipitin arc for κ and λ light chains similar in electrophoretic mobility to the heavy chain, except in "heavy-chain disease," in which κ and λ light chains are not present. Monoclonal κ or λ light chains are excreted in the urine of some patients with multiple myeloma and are designated Bence Jones protein. They may be detected by immunoelectrophoresis or immunofixation electrophoresis of concentrated urine.

MULTIPLE MYELOMA

A. Clinical Features: Diagnosis is based on finding large numbers of cytologically malignant plasma cells in the bone marrow, characteristic lytic bone lesions, and an associated serum or urine monoclonal protein. Approximately 80% of patients have a serum paraprotein and 50% have proteinuria. There are reduced levels of nonmyeloma immunoglobulins, and patients have recurrent infections, anemia, and, occasionally, renal failure or hypercalcemia. X-rays show characteristic punched-out lytic bone lesions throughout the skeleton in most patients. Generalized osteoporosis is also common, and spontaneous fractures occur.

Recurrent bacterial infections with pneumococci and gram-negative bacteria are common, particularly terminally. Hypercalcemia may be associated with vomiting, dehydration, uremia, and cardiac arrhythmias and requires rapid rehydration and other therapy. Multiple factors may cause renal failure, including precipitation of paraprotein in the tubules, amyloidosis, hypercalcemia, hyperuricemia, invasion of the kidneys by the neoplastic plasma cells, precipitation of cryoproteins, and, occasionally, the hyperviscosity syndrome and pyelonephritis. Renal disease is most frequent and severe in patients with Bence Jones proteinuria, possibly owing to the toxicity of Bence Jones proteins for renal tubular cells or precipitation at low pH.

Acute leukemia, usually monocytic or myelomonocytic, may occur 1–10 years after the diagnosis. Life expectancy following diagnosis of this acute leukemia is short (6 months). The leukemia may be the result of chemotherapy induced chromosomal abnormalities or it may represent a second neoplasm which arises as part of the natural history of the disease.

Plasma cell leukemia occurs in a few patients with neoplastic plasma cells in the peripheral blood. If it occurs early in the disease, it may be mistaken for ALL, acute myelogenous leukemia, or mast cell leukemia, but it is recognized by the paraprotein in blood and urine, the lytic bone lesions, the severe hypercalcemia, or renal failure. It may also be a terminal event in multiple myeloma.

B. Pathology: The bone marrow is usually infiltrated with nodules of myeloma cells, although diffuse involvement is occasionally seen. The cells are abnormal plasma cells with abundant MGP- and PAS-positive cytoplasm and nuclei with fine chromatin and single large nucleoli. Mitoses are rare, but patients may develop more aggressive disease such as IBS-B.

C. Immunologic Features: See Tables 45–2 and 45–4.

D. Differential Diagnosis: This includes metastatic cancer from breast, prostate, thyroid, and kidney, as well as other benign or malignant monoclonal gammopathies.

E. Therapy: Therapy is largely supportive, but local radiation therapy may relieve pain and reduce tumor masses. Extensive radiation of multiple sites may produce pancytopenia. About 70% of patients respond to cytotoxic chemotherapy, with increased median survival and improved quality of life. Melphalan, with or without prednisone, is the usual regimen, but cyclophosphamide is also used effectively and, although it has adverse side effects, is less toxic to bone marrow stem cells. Multiple drugs are also used in various combinations as initial therapy for certain patients and for patients in relapse.

SOLITARY PLASMACYTOMA

A solitary plasmacytoma may be found on routine x-ray or in patients who complain of bone pain or pressure on surrounding structures. The disease appears to represent an isolated malignant plasma cell neoplasm that can occur in bone or soft tissues. Bone and extramedullary plasmacytomas are probably different diseases. The former has a higher prevalence of

paraproteinemia and is associated with a poorer prognosis as a result of progression to multiple myeloma; it may be an early form of multiple myeloma. Extramedullary soft tissue plasmacytomas tend to have a more indolent course, usually show no paraprotein, and only occasionally progress to multiple myeloma. Treatment is generally by surgical excision or local radiotherapy.

AMYLOIDOSIS

Deposits of amyloid may be associated with plasma cell neoplasms and dyscrasias. Amyloid is a complex substance containing fragments of an immunoglobulin light chain, especially the V region. Antibodies directed against this light chain may react with Bence Jones proteins. A nonimmunoglobulin component has a molecular weight of approximately 8000, with 76 amino acids, and is of unknown origin. Another component is a glycoprotein related antigenically to an α_1 globulin present in small amounts in normal human plasma.

Amyloid may arise from (1) the catabolism by macrophages of antigen-antibody complexes; (2) synthesis in situ of whole immunoglobulins or of light chains with reduced solubility; (3) genetic deletions of the light chain gene, producing an anomolous protein with reduced solubility; of (4) separate synthesis of discrete regions of the light chain. Amyloid deposits may be detected in tissues by light microscopy as eosinophilic material on hematoxylin-eosin-stained sections. These deposits are birefringent with polarized light, and electron microscopy shows nonbranching fibrils, 8.5 nm wide and of various lengths. Special stains will selectively stain the material.

A suggested classification of amyloidosis is presented in Table 45–8.

HEAVY-CHAIN DISEASES

Patients with this rare disease complex have paraproteins of one of the 3 major types of heavy chain (γ, μ, or α) in blood and urine; α chain disease is the most common. Immunoelectrophoresis demonstrates that heavy chains, but not light chains, are present. There may be partial deletion of the Fc portion of the heavy chain, deletion in the hinge region, or a combination of the two.

α Chain Disease

Patients commonly present with a severe malabsorption syndrome accompanied by chronic diarrhea, steatorrhea, weight loss, and hypocalcemia. They may have lymphadenopathy. The small intestine is infiltrated with plasma cells, lymphocytes, and histiocytes; these may appear to be benign initially, but as

Table 45–8. Classification of amyloidosis.

	Clinical Type	Sites of Deposition
Familial	Amyloid polyneuropathy (Portuguese, dominant inheritance)	Peripheral nerves, viscera
	Familial Mediterranean fever (recessive)	Liver, spleen, kidneys, adrenals
Generalized	Primary	Tongue, heart, gut, skeletal and smooth muscles, nerves, skin, ligaments
	Associated with plasma cell dyscrasia	Liver, spleen, kidneys, adrenals
	Secondary (infection, inflammation)	Any site
Localized	Lichen amyloidosis	Skin
	Endocrine-related (eg, thyroid carcinoma)	Endocrine organ (thyroid)
Senile		Heart, brain

the disease progresses the plasmacytoid cells appear cytologically less mature and extend beyond the lamina propria. α chain disease is associated with abdominal lymphomas in patients living in the Mediterranean area, but the disease may occur in other geographic areas as well. Rare cases of involvement of the respiratory tract instead of the gastrointestinal tract have been reported.

γ Chain Disease

Some patients with this disease may die within weeks of onset, and others may survive for more than 20 years. Commonly, the patients have a lymphoproliferative disorder with hepatosplenomegaly, lymphadenopathy, and uvular and palatal edema. Infection is common and is the usual cause of death. The patients have recurrent fevers, anemia, leukopenia, and atypical circulating lymphocytes.

μ Chain Disease

IgM heavy chain disease is seen in patients with long-standing B-CLL with progressive hepatosplenomegaly.

BENIGN MONOCLONAL GAMMOPATHY

A small percentage of elderly people may have monoclonal serum or urine paraproteins without other evidence of neoplastic disease. Some may later develop multiple myeloma, but the majority do not. The presence of high and increasing serum levels of paraproteins, low serum levels of normal immunoglobulins, and significant amounts of Bence Jones protein in the serum and urine indicate an increased likelihood of developing multiple myeloma within a short period. Although patients with benign uncomplicated monoclonal gammopathy tend to remain asymptomatic, prolonged follow-up is necessary because some of them may develop multiple myeloma or other plasma cell neoplasms many years later.

CRYOGLOBULINEMIA

A variety of serum and plasma proteins precipitate at low temperature. Some of these are non-immunoglobulin cyroproteins such as cryofibrinogen, C-reactive protein-albumin complex, and heparin-precipitable protein. The cryoimmunoglobulins may precipitate at temperatures as high as 35°C, so that during collection of blood, the specimen must be maintained at 37°C to avoid loss of a cryoprecipitated globulin (see Chapter 12). The rate at which the cryoglobulins precipitate may vary from minutes to days. Therefore, detection of cryoglobulins requires observation of the serum at 4°C for at least 72 hours (see Chapter 12).

Small amounts of polyclonal serum cryoglobulin is normally present in healthy individuals. Three types of pathologic cryoglobulins have been identified: Type I (25%) includes IgM and occasionally IgG and rarely IgA or Bence Jones protein; type II (25%) includes mixed cryoglobulins with a monoclonal IgM or occasionally IgG or IgA complexed with autologous normal IgG; and type III (50%) includes mixtures of polyclonal IgM and IgG. Patients with monoclonal type I cryoglobulins usually suffer from the symptoms of their underlying disease (eg, multiple myeloma or Waldenström's macroglobulinemia). Patients with type II or III cryoglobulins may have immune complex disease with purpura, arthritis, and nephritis. These immune complexes often fix complement in vivo and in vitro.

Treatment is generally directed against the underlying disease, but avoidance of cold may be necessary to avoid vascular symptoms. Cytotoxic drugs directed against the plasmacytoid cells producing the globulins, with or without prednisone, sometimes produce remissions. Serious complications, such as vascular occlusion and hemorrhage, can be acutely treated by plasmapheresis.

BENIGN HYPERGAMMAGLOBULINEMIC PURPURA

This is a rare disease usually seen in young and middle-aged women. It is characterized by a dependent purpuric rash brought on by exercise or alcohol. Some of these patients have autoimmune disorders, particularly systemic lupus erythematosus or Sjögren's syndrome. The patients characteristically have a monoclonal IgG-κ paraprotein that acts as a rheumatoid factor, forming complexes with circulating IgG. Serum levels of IgA and IgM are normal or increased, and there are no findings of multiple myeloma. Treatment is directed at prevention and correction of the underlying autoimmune disorder. Severe symptoms may warrant plasmapheresis.

LYMPHOCYTIC NEOPLASMS OF T CELL ORIGIN

Evidence for the T cell origin of certain lymphomas and leukemias comes from their location in the thymus and paracortical areas of lymph nodes and from their immunophenotyping as T lymphocytes (Fig 45–1B; Tables 45–3, 45–4, 45–7, and 45–9). Approximately 20% of non-Hodgkin lymphomas and acute lymphocytic leukemias in the USA have T cell features. This is a complex group of diseases with marked biologic and clinical heterogeneity. Certain T cell lymphomas, including the cutaneous T cell lymphomas and convoluted T cell lymphoma, are distinct clinical and pathologic entities with defined diagnostic criteria and clinical expressions, but so-called peripheral or nodal T cell neoplasms are heterogeneous. Immunophenotypes of some T cell neoplasms may reflect fetal stages of T cell development, where others, such as the cutaneous T cell lymphomas and leukemias, have more differentiated phenotypes (Table 45–3). Still other T cell neoplasms have phenotypes that differ from those of known normal T cell populations and may reflect the neoplastic state of the affected T cells.

T cell lymphomas and leukemias usually arise in bone marrow, thymus, lymph nodes, or skin (Table 45–7). Clinical and pathologic distinction between the convoluted T cell lymphomas and the acute lymphoblastic leukemias of T cell type may be difficult, suggesting that they are essentially the same disease. T cell lymphomas arising in lymph nodes are usually diffuse but vary in histology and phenotype. They may be comparable to the FCC lymphomas and IBS-B, in which there are various predominant cell types and transitions to more primitive cells or differentiated cells. In B cell lymphomas, effector B cells (plasmacytoid lymphocytes) are easy to recognize, whereas in T cell neoplasms, dormant resting T cells cannot be distinguished from effector cells other than by functional assays.

A subset of T cell neoplasms involve primarily the skin. However, the diseases produced are frequently disseminated, with involvement of blood, lymph nodes, bone marrow, and viscera, and it appears that the neoplastic cells originate in lymphoid tissues and migrate from the blood to the skin. The neoplastic cells are characteristic because of their highly irregular (cerebriform) nuclei.

T cell neoplasms are generally more aggressive and grow more rapidly than their B cell counterparts. T-ALL and convoluted T cell lymphomas are quite aggressive, disseminating early and widely. The cutaneous T cell lymphomas frequently are initially indolent but later transform into aggressive immunoblastic sarcomas. The small T lymphocyte neoplasms (T-CLL) are more aggressive than their B cell counterparts. The more aggressive T cell neoplasms, particularly convoluted T cell lymphomas, are quite sensitive to chemotherapeutic agents, but therapeutically resistant relapses are common.

ACUTE LYMPHOCYTIC LEUKEMIA OF T CELL TYPE (T-ALL)

A. Clinical Features: This leukemia arises from bone marrow and constitutes approximately 20% of childhood ALL in the USA. Males are affected 2–3 times more frequently than females, and the median age at diagnosis is approximately 12 years. Clinical, pathologic, and immunologic features are similar to those of convoluted T cell lymphomas. Early symptoms and signs are of bone marrow failure with anemia, bleeding, thrombocytopenia, and infection. Mediastinal masses are present in about 50% of patients and produce the superior vena cava syndrome with pleural and pericardial effusions and cardiac decompensation. Central nervous system involvement, hepatosplenomegaly, peripheral lymphadenopathy, and marked leukocytosis are common; bone tenderness may be present; and serum terminal deoxyribonucleotidyl (TdT) transferase is elevated and present in the leukemic cells.

B. Pathology: Tissues show diffuse involvement by cells that typically contain irregular convoluted nuclei with granular, finely stippled nuclear chromatin. The cytoplasm is scant, and there is a wide range in nucleus and cell size. Focal cytoplasmic acid phosphatase activity and coarse granular or blocklike PAS positivity is present in about one-third of cases (Table 45–9).

C. Immunologic Features: See Tables 45–3 and 45–4.

D. Differential Diagnosis: This includes convoluted T cell lymphoma, common ALL, "stem cell"

Table 45–9. T cell lymphomas.[1,2]

Morphology	Lymphoma Type[2]	Morphologic Description	Important Clinical Features	Marker Results
	Lymphoblastic (convoluted T cell lymphoma); ALL T-cell type is related leukemia	Diffuse proliferation of "primitive" cells. Nuclear chromatin finely stippled, and nucleolus inconspicuous. Mitoses numerous. Some cells have convoluted or complexly folded nucleus.	Primarily a lymphoma-leukemia of children but may be of any age. Male predominance. Presentation usually in lymph nodes or mediastinum. Response to therapy poor. If present in blood or marrow, termed T-ALL. Prognosis worse than non-B, non-T-ALL.	Diagnostic cells mark with anti-T cell antibodies.
	Small lymphocytic lymphoma, T cells; CLL T cell type is related leukemia	Cells resemble small lymphocytes. Nuclei with compact chromatin. Rim of pale cytoplasm. Nuclei occasionally irregular in form.	May be leukemic resembling B cell CLL. Variant is common in Japan.	Diagnostic cells mark with anti-T cell antibodies. Often helper phenotype.
	Immunoblastic sarcoma; T cell	Admixture of small and transformed lymphocytes. Latter predominante. In sections they have pale, water-clear cytoplasm.	Less common than IBS-B from which it may be distinguished immunologically. Prognosis is poor.	Lymphoma cells mark with anti-T cell antibodies.
	Mycosis fungoides (MF) and Sézary cell	MF/Sézary cells have compact chromatin and few mitoses resembling normal small lymphocytes, except that they are larger and the nuclei often show complex folding.	MF and Sézary syndrome closely related. Affinity of cells for skin consistent with affinity of T cell for skin. MF may progress to involvement of nodes, spleen, and blood. Sézary involves blood ab initio.	Cells mark with anti-T cell antibodies. Frequently helper phenotype.
	Lymphoepithelioid cell lymphoma	Neoplastic T lymphocytes are admixed with reactive histiocytes. Sometimes confused with Hodgkin's disease.	Relatively rare. Intermediate grade of malignancy.	Lymphoid component marks as T cells.

[1]Modified from Lukes RJ et al: Immunologic approach to non-Hodgkin lymphomas and related leukemias. *Semin Hematol* 1978;**15:**322.
[2]Histologic type; related tumors having monoclonal serum proteins are discussed later with "myeloma."

leukemia, acute granulocytic leukemia, and neuroblastoma.

E. Therapy: Combination chemotherapy produces complete remission in most patients, and a significant number may achieve long-term disease-free survival; however, because of the predilection for central nervous system involvement, cranial irradiation and intrathecal chemotherapy are important.

CONVOLUTED T CELL LYMPHOMA

These lymphomas appear to be of thymic origin and usually are associated with mediastinal masses. Dissemination is frequent, as is development of a leukemic phase quite similar to T-ALL.

A. Clinical Features: This lymphoma makes up about 10% of all lymphoid neoplasms seen in the USA. It is typically a disease of teenagers and young adults and of males more often than females. A large mediastinal mass with associated symptoms requiring immediate therapy is common, as described for T-ALL above. However, it may present as leukemia with a lymphocytosis of greater than 100,000/μL associated with anemia and thrombocytopenia. Peripheral nodes and the central nervous system are commonly involved, the latter in the form of leukemic meningitis or masses. Other tissues may be involved.

B. Pathology: The cells that diffusely infiltrate the various tissues are characterized by nuclear irregularities or convolutions with scalloped nuclear borders or linear subdivisions. The chromatin is dispersed and granular, and nucleoli are inconspicuous. Cytoplasm is scant and typically contains prominent focal acid phosphatase activity. There is a high mitotic rate (Table 45–9).

C. Immunologic Features: See Tables 45–3 and 45–4.

D. Differential Diagnosis: This includes small noncleaved FCC lymphoma, T-ALL, and thymoma.

E. Therapy: Emergency radiation therapy is indicated for the mediastinal mass and results in rapid tumor regression. Relapse usually occurs. In the past, survival was approximately 1 year, but therapy comparable to that for childhood ALL with cranial irradiation and intrathecal chemotherapy has produced long-term disease-free survival in approximately half of all patients.

SMALL T LYMPHOCYTE NEOPLASMS

Adult T Cell Leukemia (ATL)

This disease is common in Japan and is endemic in the southwestern parts of that country. It also occurs in the Caribbean. ATL is associated with the human T cell leukemia virus type I (HTLV-I). Anti-HLTV-I antibodies are found in more than 90% of Japanese patients with ATL in regions where the disease is endemic, but 10–20% of healthy individuals also have antibodies. Antibodies have also been found in patients in the West Indies and, sporadically, in the USA. ATL occurs primarily in the fifth decade in Japan, although there is a wide age span. Males and females are affected equally. Lymphadenopathy, hepatomegaly, and splenomegaly are common, as are skin lesions. Leukocytosis ranges from 6000 to 480,000/μL. Marrow involvement is minor, but hypercalcemia is common. Response to therapy is poor, with a median survival of less than 1 year.

In the USA the age of onset is earlier than in Japan (mean, 33 years), and males are more commonly affected than females. Peripheral and retroperitoneal but not mediastinal lymphadenopathy is common. Other organs may be involved. Osteoporosis is accompanied by hypercalcemia, but parathormone levels are normal. Multiagent chemotherapy is generally unsuccessful, with a median survival of less than 1 year.

Prolymphocytic Leukemia of T Cell Type (T-PLL)

Elderly males are the most commonly affected by this disease. Splenomegaly is prominent, but hepatomegaly and peripheral lymphadenopathy are less common. CLL therapy is inadequate, as is splenic radiotherapy, with a median survival of less than 6 months.

T-CLL with Cytoplasmic Azurophilic Granules

A. Clinical Features: This is an indolent and protracted disease, with survivals of 10–20 years. Patients are generally in their mid-50s at diagnosis, although there is a wide age distribution. Splenomegaly may be prominent, but hepatomegaly, lymphadenopathy, and skin involvement are uncommon. A lymphocytosis of 50,000/μL or less is common, but neutropenia may result in recurrent infections. This is probably the same disease as large granular lymphocyte/natural killer (NK) cell leukemias (see below).

B. Pathology: The distinction between the more aggressive ATL and T-PLL, on the one hand, and T-CLL with azurophilic granules, on the other hand, is important. ATL cells have irregular (knotty or indented) nuclei. T-PLL cell nuclei have acidophilic chromatin and prominent nucleoli. The T-CLL cells with azurophilic granules are Downey-like cells with prominent azurophilic granules and basophilic nuclear chromatin. Although cytology helps distinguish among the 3 types, a diffuse tissue distribution may occur in all 3 types (Table 45–9).

C. Immunologic Features: See Tables 45–3 and 45–4.

D. Differential Diagnosis: This includes small B lymphocytic neoplasms, especially B-CLL.

E. Therapy: Therapy is the same minimal therapy used for B-CLL, and prolonged survival in the absence or limited use of specific therapy is common.

PERIPHERAL T CELL LYMPHOMAS

A. Clinical Features: Neoplasms in this heterogeneous group, which tend to involve lymph nodes, are relatively uncommon. The patients are generally adults presenting with regional or generalized lymphadenopathy, and frequently they have advanced disease at presentation. Retroperitoneal and mediastinal adenopathy is common.

B. Pathology: Involvement of tissues by the neoplastic cells is usually diffuse and uniform. Follicular centers are generally absent in involved lymph nodes. The cell infiltrates contain small and large lymphocytes with abundant clear cytoplasm, mixed with varying numbers of T immunoblasts. The small lymphocytes have irregular twisted nuclei with little cytoplasm, but in immunoblastic sarcoma of T cell type, transformed cells with indented irregular nuclei and conspicuous nucleoli are present. The cytoplasm of the immunoblasts is MGP-positive (Table 45–9).

C. Immunologic Features: See Tables 45–3 and 45–4.

D. Differential Diagnosis: This includes IBS-B, large noncleaved FCC lymphoma, and Hodgkin's disease (mixed cellularity).

E. Therapy: The remission rate with multiagent chemotherapy is low, and survival is usually less than 1 year.

LYMPHOEPITHELIOID LYMPHOCYTIC LYMPHOMA OF T CELL TYPE (Lennert's Lymphoma)

A. Clinical Features: This is a disease primarily of adult males, with cervical lymphadenopathy and tonsil involvement. It frequently evolves to IBS-T.

B. Pathology: Lymph nodes or tonsils are diffusely infiltrated with small lymphocytes having twisted irregular nuclei. There are clusters of epithelioid macrophages, which are distinct from the scattered individual epithelioid macrophages of the peripheral T cell lymphomas. There may be focal or multifocal immunoblasts. Skin and splenic white pulp are occasionally involved (Table 45–9).

C. Immunologic Features: See Tables 45–3 and 45–4.

D. Differential Diagnosis: This includes abnormal immune reactions, Hodgkin's disease (lymphocytic and histiocytic, diffuse), IBS-T, and immunoblastic lymphadenopathy.

E. Therapy: There is some question about whether this is a true lymphoma or a premalignant lymphocytic proliferation that may progress to IBS.

Therefore, therapy may be withheld until there is evidence of progression to IBS-T. Because there is a resemblance to Hodgkin's disease, some patients have been treated with Hodgkin's disease therapy.

CUTANEOUS T CELL LYMPHOMAS

These include cerebriform T cell lymphomas, mycosis fungoides, and Sézary syndrome.

A. Clinical Features: These neoplasms tend to be initially indolent but may evolve into widespread aggressive lymphomas. The disease occurs in middle age, with males affected more commonly than females. The first manifestation of disease is on the skin. In mycosis fungoides early skin involvement is nonspecific, but in time localized or generalized skin tumors develop. Peripheral and visceral lymphadenopathy and hepatosplenomegaly occur as the skin tumors develop. In the Sézary syndrome there is a generalized pruritic erythroderma with hyperpigmentation and exfoliation. Scaling and fissuring of the skin on the palms and soles are common. Even when the disease appears to be limited to the skin, the characteristic cerebriform cells present in the peripheral blood and lymph nodes provide evidence of more widespread disease.

B. Pathology: The skin is densely infiltrated with leukocytes and other cells, particularly in the epidermis. Characteristic clusters of cells in the epidermis are called Pautrier's abscesses. Lymph nodes may be diffusely infiltrated, but involvement is usually interfollicular and is mixed with the dermatopathic changes associated with skin disease. The predominant cell is usually small, with a "cerebriform" nuclear shape, so called because of extensive convolutions, which give the nuclei the 3-dimensional appearance of brain tissue. Larger dysplastic cells with condensed chromatin are also present, and although transformed T cells are not common in early disease, there may be a transformation in late disease to T immunoblasts. Mitoses are not common until the late, aggressive phase of the disease (Table 45–9).

C. Immunologic Features: See Tables 45–3 and 45–4.

D. Differential Diagnosis: This includes inflammatory reactive lymphocytoses of the skin and lymph nodes, small lymphocytic B neoplasms of the skin, other T cell lymphomas involving the skin, and psoriasiform dermatoses.

E. Therapy: During the first 5–10 years of disease, local skin therapy with superficial electron beam irradiation may be helpful for cosmetic improvement of the skin. However, the disease ultimately progresses. With advanced disease, multiagent chemotherapy may produce complete remissions, but survival averages only 1–2 years. Progression to an aggressive lymphoma of the skin or other tissues, which occurs in about 20% of patients, is associated with a poor prognosis.

HODGKIN'S DISEASE

Hodgkin's disease (lymphoma) comprises a group of neoplasms initially affecting lymph nodes and later involving the liver, spleen, bone marrow, and lungs, accounting for about one-third of all lymphomas. The neoplastic cells appear to be the Reed-Sternberg cells (Fig 45–4). Some are mononuclear, but the diagnostic Reed-Sternberg cells are binucleate with huge eosinophilic nuclear inclusions. Hodgkin's disease is quite heterogeneous, with different numbers of Reed-Sternberg cells and reacting lymphocytes and histiocytes in the different subtypes.

For many years the disease was considered to be infectious rather than neoplastic because of the clinical course and pathology. However, an infectious etiology has never been proven. It is now considered to be a neoplastic disease. The proliferating cells occasionally show aneuploidy and chromosomal abnormalities, indicating a clonal proliferation.

The pathologic diagnosis of Hodgkin's disease is made on the basis of a distinctive lymphoid tissue reaction, which in some ways resembles a cellular im-

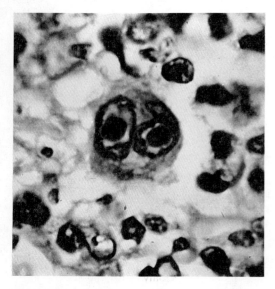

Figure 45–4. Hodgkin's lymphoma. High magnification of a classic Reed-Sternberg cell with 2 nuclei containing the typical nucleoli. (Reproduced, with permission, from Chandrasoma P, Taylor CR: *Concise Pathology.* Appleton & Lange, 1991.)

mune response, and the demonstration of the diagnostic Reed-Sternberg cells. Whether the apparent immunologic reaction is directed against T or B lymphocytes, macrophages, or the Reed-Sternberg cells is not clear. On occasion, the extraordinarily reactive lymphocytic component seen in Hodgkin's disease leads to confusion with non-Hodgkin lymphomas. The distinction between Hodgkin's disease and non-Hodgkin lymphoma may be artificial if the Reed-Sternberg cells ultimately prove to be of lymphocytic origin.

A. Clinical Features: There are different histologic and clinical types of Hodgkin's disease, but the most common clinical manifestation in all types is painless peripheral lymphadenopathy. Cervical and supraclavicular nodes are most commonly involved; axillary and inguinal node involvement is less common. Systemic symptoms are frequently prominent, particularly in older patients, and imply a worse prognosis. Pruritus and pain in enlarged lymph nodes following alcohol ingestion may occur but do not imply a poor prognosis. Extranodal presentation is not common; splenomegaly is present in less than 20% of patients. The progression of disease is predictable, spreading from initially involved lymph nodes to contiguous lymphoid tissues, either antegrade or retrograde. There is ultimate dissemination into parenchymal organs, with the liver and lungs most commonly involved. Bone marrow involvement is uncommon. Staging is by physical examination, laboratory analysis, chest x-ray, lymphangiogram, abdominal CT scan, and liver-spleen scan. The clinical stages determine specific treatment.

B. Pathology: The Rye classification divides the histopathology into 4 types: lymphocyte predominance, nodular sclerosis, mixed cellularity, and lymphocyte depletion (Table 45–10). The histopathologic differences appear to reflect the host response to the neoplastic Reed-Sternberg cells. The Reed-Sternberg cells vary in appearance in the different subtypes but are classically binucleated with huge inclusionlike nucleoli and pale cytoplasm (Fig 45–4). They are rarely seen in the lymphocyte-predominant type of disease but are often present in nodular sclerosis and in some cases of lymphocyte depletion. They are required for diagnosis in the mixed cellularity type because of the lack of other distinctive features. The lymphocyte-predominance, mixed-cellularity, and lymphocyte-depletion types are related, and progression from lymphocyte predominance to depletion occurs in individual patients. The nodular sclerosis type appears to be a different entity. In the lymphocyte-predominance type, the lymphocytosis may be diffuse or nodular, with the diffuse form being more likely to progress to lymphocyte depletion. Some patients initially present with the mixed-cellularity or lymphocyte-depletion type.

Because of this diversity, it is believed that Hodgkin's disease may represent several different

Table 45–10. RYE classification of Hodgkin's disease.

Histologic Subtype	Percentage of US Cases	Predominant Features	Prognosis
Lymphocyte predominance	10	Young adult males, stage 1 or 2 at diagnosis; few Reed-Sternberg cells, good lymphocyte host response, connective tissue bands minimal.	Excellent
Nodular sclerosis	60	Young females, stage 1 or 2 at diagnosis; predominant nodules due to wide bands or birefringent collgen, mediastinal mass, "lacunar" variants of Reed-Sternberg cells.	Excellent
Mixed cellularity	20	Majority with stage 3 or 4 at diagnosis; abdominal involvement common, lymphocytes, plasma cells, eosinophils mixed with Reed-Sternberg cells, diffuse involvement of nodes.	Good
Lymphocyte depletion	10	Older males, stage 3 or 4 at diagnosis; systemic symptoms, prolonged fever of unknown origin, abdominal and bone marrow involvement, numerous Reed-Sternberg cells, diffuse fibrosis, and few lymphocytes, indicating poor host response.	Relatively poor

clinical entities, particularly the lymphocyte-predominant type, which appears to be a B cell lymphoma.

C. Immunologic Features: Patients commonly have frequent bacterial infections (*Pneumococcus* or *Haemophilus influenzae*). This is related to an underlying secondary immunodeficiency involving defective phagocytosis and chemotaxis, as well as a decreased antibody response to certain antigens. However, immunoglobulin levels are normal or increased. Patients are also frequently anergic to delayed hypersensitivity skin test antigens, a T cell function, particularly when lymphocytopenia is severe.

The cellular origin of the diagnostic cell of Hodgkin's disease, the Reed-Sternberg cell, remains a mystery. Other cells (lymphocytes, histiocytes, eosinophils) appear to be reactive components of the lesions, whereas the Reed-Sternberg cell and its mononuclear variants are the true neoplastic cells. Evidence suggests derivation from B or T lymphocytes, histiocytes, interdigitating reticulum cells, or granulocytes. Recent immunoperoxidase staining with monoclonal antibodies shows staining patterns that do not answer the question other than to suggest an origin from the interdigitating reticulum cell or from an unrecognized cell precursor.

The lymphocytes in Hodgkin's disease show variable immunophenotypic patterns but are generally predominantly T cells and most frequently CD4 T cells. The latter may be so prominent in peripheral blood or lymph nodes as to suggest the neoplastic clonal expansion of CD4 T cells seen in mycosis fungoides and Sézary syndrome, but in Hodgkin's disease they are present because of reactive clonal expansion. Reed-Sternberg-like cells may also be seen in benign conditions such as infectious mononucleosis, other benign reactive states, and some non-Hodgkin lymphomas. Thus, they are diagnostic of Hodgkin's disease only in the appropriate histological setting.

D. Differential Diagnosis: Lymphocyte-predominance Hodgkin's disease may be confused with small cleaved FCC lymphomas, toxoplasmosis, and other reactive lymphocytoses. Nodular sclerosis may resemble nodular mixed-cellularity or lymphocyte-depletion Hodgkin's disease, or metastatic carcinoma. The differential diagnosis of mixed-cellularity Hodgkin's disease includes the other types of Hodgkin's disease, immunoblastic lymphadenopathy, lymphoepithelial lymphocytic lymphomas, granulomotous reactions, nodal T cell lymphomas, and reactive lymph node hyperplasia. The lymphocyte-depletion type of Hodgkin's disease must be differentiated from the changes seen in lymph nodes from patients receiving chemotherapy and immune-deficient states including advanced AIDS. In some cases of lymphocyte depletion, lymph nodes may be replaced by pleomorphic Reed-Sternberg cells, so that the pathology suggests IBS-T, IBS-B, or other pleomorphic neoplasms including carcinomas.

E. Therapy: The clinical prognosis is excellent for the lymphocyte-predominance and nodular sclerosis types of Hodgkin's disease, good for the mixed-cellularity type, and relatively poor for the lymphocyte-depletion type (Table 45–10). Therapy in all instances depends on the histologic type and clinical stage. Staging to determine the extent of disease involves the presence or absence of systemic symptoms such as fever, night sweats, weight loss; blood tests including leukocyte, renal, and liver function studies, erythrocyte sedimentation rate, serum copper, and fibrinogen; radiologic examination including lymphangiography and CT scan; biopsy; laparotomy; and splenectomy.

After a complete workup, the patient is staged according to the modified Ann Arbor Staging System: stage I, involvement of a single lymph node region; stage II, 2 or more lymph node regions on the same side of the diaphragm; stage IIIa, lymph node regions on both sides of the diaphragm and abdominal disease limited to the upper abdomen; stage IIIb, lymph node regions on both sides of the diaphragm and abdominal disease with or without disease in the upper abdomen; stage IV, diffuse or disseminated involvement of one or more extralymphatic organs or tissues, with or without associated lymph node enlargement.

Treatment consists of radiotherapy for localized disease, with the addition of multiagent chemotherapy for disseminated disease, using MOPP (mechlorethamine, vincristine [Oncovin], procarbazine, prednisone).

Approximately 75% of all patients with Hodgkin's disease are cured by appropriate therapy. However, because of the long-term survival that ensues, second neoplasms may appear years later. These include acute granulocytic leukemia (7%) and non-Hodgkin lymphoma (15%). There is also male and female infertility secondary to chemotherapy, as well as hypothyroidism and bone marrow depression.

NEOPLASMS OF THE MONONUCLEAR PHAGOCYTE SYSTEM

Neoplasms of the mononuclear phagocyte system include acute and chronic monocytic leukemia and the various types of malignant histiocytosis. The latter are a confusing group, because so many different histiocytic processes are usually included. Further confusion has resulted from the inclusion of a histiocytic lymphoma category in the Rappaport classification. Current evidence indicates that true histiocytic neoplasms are rare. To call them "histiocytic lymphomas" is a misnomer, since "lymphoma" by definition means a neoplasm of lymphocytes. Nevertheless, there are true malignant neoplasms of histiocytes, which have distinctive morphologic, cytochemical, ultrastructural, and immunophenotypic features. If tumor masses or infiltrates of cytologically malignant histiocytes are present, a diagnosis of true histiocytic lymphoma may be made. However, these proliferations must be distinguished from reactive macrophage infiltrates, benign histiocytes seen in the lipid storage diseases, granulomatous diseases, and metastatic carcinoma cells that may be phagocytic.

HISTIOCYTIC MEDULLARY RETICULOSIS

This is a rare disorder seen primarily in males in their 30s. Clinically, there is wasting, severe hemolytic anemia, fever, weakness, and short-duration weight loss. Peripheral lymphadenopathy, spleno-

megaly, and hepatomegaly are common, as are nodules and papules of the skin. The hemolytic anemia is apparently due to erythrophagocytosis by the malignant histiocytes, and there is also thrombocytopenia, apparently from splenic sequestration. Leukopenia is common, and, rarely, there is a leukemic phase. Median survival is approximately 6 months, although complete remission has occurred with combination chemotherapy. Central nervous system relapse is common. Three types of histiocytes are seen; in lymph node sinuses, splenic red pulp, and the marrow. These include immunoblastlike cells, pleomorphic histiocytes showing erythrophagocytosis, and normal-appearing histiocytes with quite prominent erythrophagocytosis. Lymph nodes frequently show complete filling of the medullary and subcapsular sinuses with neoplastic histiocytes. The cells typically are α-naphthyl acetate esterase-positive and stain by immunoperoxidase techniques with α_1-antichymotrypsin and α_1-antitrypsin.

The differential diagnosis includes other malignant histiocytoses and the virus-associated hemophagocytic syndrome.

OTHER MALIGNANT HISTIOCYTOSES

Very few patients have true histiocytic neoplasms; however, the clinical disease is very similar to lymphocytic lymphomas. Most patients are males with an average age of onset of 50–60 years, although younger patients have been described. Splenomegaly, peripheral lymphadenopathy, and skin lesions are common, the skin lesions being multiple, rapidly growing, bluish-red nodules. There may be a mild anemia, but laboratory work is generally normal and the bone marrow is only rarely involved. Information about prognosis and therapy is of little use because of the rareness of the disease and the inconsistently applied diagnostic criteria.

Lymph nodes show extensive accumulations of neoplastic histiocytes with abundant eosinophilic cytoplasm and atypical nuclei. Sinusoidal involvement is the usual prominent pattern of growth. In some cases the pattern makes it difficult to distinguish from metastatic carcinoma. Prominent vascular proliferation is common. Individually the cells are indistinguishable from the atypical histiocytes in histiocytic medullary reticulosis. Phagocytic activity is not always a prominent feature, and cytochemical and ultrastructural studies may be necessary to indicate that the neoplastic cells are histiocytes. The cells may be PAS-positive and show nonspecific esterase activity. Muramidase activity may be detected by immunocytochemistry, but this is frequently not helpful. Some of the cells are labeled by α_1-antichymotrypsin, but ultrastructural examination is frequently required for diagnosis of the more primitive neoplasms.

ACUTE MYELOMONOCYTIC LEUKEMIA

Acute myelomonocytic leukemia accounts for about 20–30% of the acute myeloid leukemias in the USA. Males and females are affected equally, with an average age of onset of 55 years. The disease is quite rare in children. Patients present with bone marrow failure and anemia, thrombocytopenia, hemorrhage, and infection. Some complain of bone and joint pain. Up to 50% will have hepatosplenomegaly and adenopathy. Leukocyte counts tend to be in the range of 55,000/μL, with a high proportion of blast cells. The response to multiagent chemotherapy is generally poor, with a median duration of complete response of 10 months.

The bone marrow is generally heavily infiltrated with immature granulocytes and monocytes. Monocyte progenitors, myeloblasts, and promyelocytes are all present, and Auer rods may be seen.

The neoplastic cells are Sudan black-positive and PAS-positive. The monocyte progenitor cells stain for α-naphthyl acetate (or butyrate) esterase, and the granulocyte precursors are chloroacetate esterase-positive. Examination by electron microscopy shows the distinctive filaments and nuclei of monocytic and granulocytic cells.

ACUTE MONOCYTIC LEUKEMIA

A. Clinical Features: Acute monocytic leukemia is very rare in the USA and affects males and females equally. It affects 2 age groups: those younger than 10 years and those older than 40 years (mean, 58 years). The clinical features are generally similar to those of acute granulocytic leukemia, including bone marrow failure with anemia, thrombocytopenia, bleeding, and infection. Hepatosplenomegaly and lymphadenopathy are present in approximately half of all patients. The leukocyte count is high (above 100,000/dL in about 50% of patients). Monoblasts are frequent, and the cells show various degrees of staining for esterase, Sudan black, and PAS. Rearrangements of chromosome 11 have been reported.

B. Pathology: The bone marrow is diffusely and homogeneously involved. The neoplastic cells show the nuclear folding and abundant cytoplasm of monocytes. Some are large blasts with weak or negative cytochemical staining, and others are Sudan black-, PAS-, and esterase-positive promonocytes. Granulocytic components usually make up less than 10% of the cells.

C. Immunologic Features: Acute myelomonocytic leukemia and acute monocytic leukemia have been characterized with monoclonal antibodies. Both cell types generally stain with monoclonal antibodies that recognize myeloid and monocyte differentiation antigens. These include CD14, CD13, CD33, and CD11b.

D. Differential Diagnosis: This includes acute and chronic myelomonocytic leukemias.

E. Therapy: The response to combination chemotherapy is similar to that of acute granulocytic leukemia, with complete remission in approximately 40–60% of patients for less than 1 year. Central nervous system relapse is common.

INTERRELATION OF GRANULOCYTIC & LYMPHOCYTIC LEUKEMIAS

After approximately 3 years, patients with chronic myelogenous leukemia frequently develop an acute phase of the disease called blast crisis. Because the blast cells may show a lineage different from myeloid cells, immunophenotyping of these cells is important for therapeutic decisions. The blast cells may express antigens and enzymes characteristic of B lymphoblasts, T lymphoblasts, erythroblasts, myeloblasts, or megakaryoblasts. The cells of approximately one-third of patients with blast crisis have the phenotype of B immunoblasts (TdT+, CD10 [CALLA]+, Ia+, CD20+, cytoplasmic IgM+, with rearrangements of immunoglobulin heavy and light chain genes). Rarely do the blasts have the phenotype of T lymphoblasts (TdT+, CD5+, CD3+, CD2+). Patients with lymphoid blast crisis may respond to vincristine and prednisone chemotherapy, whereas patients with myeloid blast do less well with this combination. Myeloid blast cells tend to be positive for CD13, CD33, and CD11b. All of the blast cells, no matter what the differentiation, retain the Philadelphia chromosome.

NATURAL KILLER (NK) CELL/ LARGE GRANULAR LYMPHOCYTE (LGL) LEUKEMIA (T-Gamma Lymphoproliferative Disease)

A subset of T lymphocytes, the so-called T-gamma lymphocytes, are characterized by an Fc receptor for IgG and with large cytoplasmic granules. They are also called large granular lymphocytes (LGLs). These cells seem to be largely responsible for NK activity. In a smaller number of patients with leukemia, the phenotype and morphology of the leukemic cells indicate that they are proliferations of large granular lymphocytes. Patients are generally elderly males, and the LGLs infiltrate bone marrow and spleen and are present in peripheral blood. The patients typically have chronic neutropenia. The cells may express the phenotype of cytotoxic/suppressor T cells or NK cells, or both. Some investigators consider this to be a nonneoplastic lymphoproliferation, whereas others believe it is a type of T-CLL.

Recently, clonal chromosomal abnormalities have been observed, indicating that the condition is a true neoplasm. The phenotype and reduced NK activity suggest that the LGLs are immature. The cells usually are acid phosphatase-positive and β-glucoronidase-positive, and express CD3, CD2, CD8, and the NK-associated antigen CD57. They are generally sheep erythrocyte rosette-positive. Trisomy 14 (47xy, +14) and trisomy 8 (47xy, +8) have been reported, and there is clonal rearrangement of the gene for the β-chain of the T cell receptor.

The rather indolent course of this leukemia suggests that it may be an early stage of disease similar to B-CLL, which slowly evolves to a more aggressive disease.

Although most of the patients have a chronically progressive disease, others may have a more aggressive course, with a lymphoma of LGLs. In these patients the disease progresses rapidly, and high-dose chemotherapy is needed. In addition, some patients with T-ALL may have cells with characteristics of NK cells.

Not only do the cells from patients with LGL leukemia demonstrate in vitro NK activity, but they also show antibody-dependent cell-mediated cytotoxicity (ADCC). They also suppress T cell proliferation and immunoglobulin synthesis in vitro, but most produce erythroid colony-forming units and burst-forming units. Most of the patients with chronic disease do not require cytotoxic chemotherapy, but they must be treated with antibiotic therapy because of repeated bacterial infections related to their neutropenia.

BENIGN CONDITIONS MIMICKING OR ASSOCIATED WITH NEOPLASMS OF THE IMMUNE SYSTEM

There are several benign proliferations of cells of the immune system that may be confused with lymphomas or leukemias or, in some cases, may evolve into true neoplasms. Many of these conditions are associated with aberrant immune responses. Immunophenotyping may help to distinguish reactive from neoplastic processes by virtue of identifying monoclonality with or without gene rearrangement confirmation. These conditions include the following:

(1) **Benign follicular hyperplasia:** This may be so severe as to mimic FCC lymphomas and the follicular hyperplasia seen in the AIDS-related complex (ARC). It may occur in certain infections, rheumatoid arthritis, drug reactions, and, rarely, immunodeficiencies, but frequently there is no apparent underlying primary disease. The cells have a B cell phenotype but are polyclonal.

(2) **Angiofollicular hyperplasia:** Follicular centers are enlarged, but there is also an increase in interfollicular plasmacytoid cells. These cells have a polyclonal B cell phenotype but express CD4 as well. Large asymptomatic mediastinal masses may be present. Patients have anemia, polyclonal hypergammaglobulinemia, thrombocytopenia, and marrow plasmacytosis. Some may progress to malignant lymphoma or Kaposi's sarcoma.

(3) **Sjögren's syndrome (see Chapter 31):** This is characterized by inflammation of the salivary glands (sialadenitis) with proliferations of lymphocytes, plasmacytoid cells, and immunoblasts. There is an increased risk of developing IBS-B and plasmacytoid lymphocytic lymphomas.

(4) **Hashimoto's thyroiditis (see Chapter 32):** The thyroid contains lymphoid follicles with hyperplastic follicular centers. The frequency of lymphomas is 1% or less, but most of those that do arise in the thyroid (FCC lymphomas) are in elderly female patients with Hashimoto's thyroiditis.

(5) **Systemic lupus erythematosus (see Chapter 31):** This disease usually affects young women with cervical or generalized lymphadenopathy who have follicular hyperplasia and interfollicular expansion of plasma cells and immunoblasts. These patients only rarely develop IBS-B.

(6) **Immunoblastic reactions in infectious mononucleosis, vaccinations, and herpes zoster:** Following stimulation of the immune system by certain infections or vaccinations, lymph nodes may enlarge and show clusters of small and transformed lymphocytes (immunoblasts) in the interfollicular areas, with focal necrosis and occasional Reed-Sternberg-like cells. Atypical lymphocytes are seen in the peripheral blood. The resemblance to IBS-B and Hodgkin's disease may create diagnostic problems. However, the cells are phenotypically polyclonal.

(7) **Drug reactions:** Drugs, particularly phenytoin (Dilantin), may produce a follicular hyperplasia and lymphadenopathy with areas of focal necrosis. Lymph nodes contain eosinophils, and the pathology may suggest Hodgkin's disease. Rarely do lymphomas develop in these patients.

(8) **Abnormal immune reactions, including immunoblastic lymphadenopathy (IBL) (angioimmunoblastic lymphadenopathy):** IBL is a diffuse involvement of lymph nodes characterized by the presence of plasmacytoid immunoblasts and plasma cells, branching small vessels with PAS-positive walls, and general hypocellularity due to an overall decrease in the number of lymphocytes. Deposits of granular pale acidophilic interstitial material separate these cells. Phenotypically, the B cells and plasma cells are polyclonal and T cells appear to be benign.

However, T cell receptor β-chain gene rearrangements have been reported in cases of angio-immunoblastic lymphadenopathy, suggesting clonal T cell proliferations. However, some patients also show T cell receptor γ-chain and immunoglobulin heavy-chain gene rearrangements. Approximately 10–20% of patients with this condition develop IBS-B, and others develop T cell neoplasms.

(9) Gluten-sensitive enteropathy (see Chapter 35): These patients with malabsorption show small bowel atrophy with increased numbers of lymphocytes and plasma cells. The incidence of malignant lymphoma (IBS-B) is increased but the onset is insidious. Most patients have IBS-B with monoclonal cytoplasmic IgM.

(10) X-linked lymphoproliferative syndrome (Duncan's syndrome) (see Chapter 19): Lymph nodes and the spleen show heavy immunoblastic infiltrates, separating and replacing the lymphoid follicles and associated with a marked plasmacytosis and decreased T cell numbers. The liver and bone marrow may be involved. This syndrome is rare; it usually affects males between 5 months and 23 years of age. Most die of infectious mononucleosis, aplastic anemia, or hypogammaglobulinemia, but some develop malignant lymphomas. The latter are usually monoclonal B cell lymphomas, although the initial B cell immunoblastic proliferation is polyclonal. Even if progression to IBS-B has not occurred, the immunoblastic proliferation may be confused with this lymphoma.

(11) Immunosuppressed patients: These include organ transplant patients (see Chapters 44 and 57) and AIDS patients with B cell lymphomas (see Chapter 52). The risk of lymphoma in patients receiving transplants following or during immunosuppression is approximately 40 times that of the normal population. The lymphoproliferative disorder may occur in the transplanted organ, particularly the heart, or in other organs. Multiple allotransplants increase the risk even more. Lymphomas that arise are almost always B cell in origin; however, they may not express surface immunoglobulin, or when surface and cytoplasmic immunoglobulin is expressed it may be monoclonal or polyclonal. Heavy- and light-chain gene rearrangements have been reported, even when the immunoglobulin phenotype is polyclonal. A role for EBV in the etiology has been proposed, but the constant antigenic stimulation of the graft in conjunction with the suppressed immune response has suggested that the neoplastic clones of B cells arise by somatic mutation from rapidly proliferating reactive B lymphocytes.

AIDS. Since the early 1980s, it has been clear that patients with AIDS and ARC have a high incidence of lymphomas, almost all of which are B cell lymphomas. Most, if not all, individuals with asymptomatic HIV infection will eventually progress to ARC and then to AIDS. Because there are an estimated 1–1.5 million individuals in the USA who are currently infected but asymptomatic and another estimated 250,000 who have ARC, the number of patients with AIDS and AIDS-related lymphoma will continue to increase. Immunophenotyping studies on these lymphomas have demonstrated that most are of B cell origin, with the majority expressing monoclonal surface immunoglobulin staining for κ or λ (κ predominating), and a variety of B cell differentiation antigens. Immunoglobulin gene rearrangements are also identified. Some lymphomas, however, have polyclonal immunoglobulin patterns and others lack surface immunoglobulin. Initially, some of these lymphomas appear as a multiclonal B cell expansion followed by evolution to a monoclonal phenotype. The similarity to the lymphomas arising in immunosuppressed organ transplant patients is striking.

The great majority of the AIDS-related lymphomas are high-grade, IBS-B, or small noncleaved FCC lymphomas, Burkitt or non-Burkitt in type. Discrepancies between reported histologic types and the course and response to therapy in different centers are explained by differences in histologic classification. However, most agree that they are high-grade lymphomas and have distinctive features including a high incidence of central nervous system involvement by the lymphomas, particularly by IBS-B. In addition, almost all patients present with disseminated disease and systemic symptoms at time of diagnosis. An unusual generalized involvement by lymphomas occurs in the myocardium, adrenals, ear lobes, maxillae, popliteal foci, gall-bladder, orbit, and rectum.

The chromosomal abnormalities in the AIDS-related lymphomas are the same as those commonly reported in Burkitt's lymphoma, ie, translocations between chromosomes 8 and 14 and between 8 and 22. The survival time of AIDS patients with lymphomas has been extremely short with or without therapy. Various centers have reported median survivals ranging from 5 to 28 months for patients on therapy. Various high-dose multiagent combinations and radiation therapy have been attempted, generally with poor results. Chemotherapy in conjunction with hematopoietic growth factors and antiretroviral therapy is being explored.

REFERENCES

General

Aisenberg AC: *Malignant Lymphomas. Biology, Natural History and Treatment.* Lea & Febiger, 1991.

Lennert K: *Malignant Lymphomas Other than Hodgkin's Disease. Histology, Cytology, Ultrastructure, Immunology.* Springer-Verlag, 1978.

Lennert K, Collins RD, Lukes RJ: Concordance of the Kiel and Lukes/Collins classifications of non-Hodgkin lymphomas. *Histopathology* 1983;**7**:549.

Lukes RJ, Collins RD: Immunologic characterization of human malignant lymphomas. *Cancer* 1974;**34**:1488.

Lukes RJ, Collins RD: Tumors of the hematopoietic system. In: *Atlas of Tumor Pathology,* Second Series, fascicle 28. US Armed Forces Institute of Pathology, 1992.

Lukes RJ et al: A morphologic and immunologic surface marker study of 299 cases of non-Hodgkin's lymphomas and related leukemias. *Am J Pathol* 1978;**90**:461.

National Cancer Institute Sponsored Study of Classifications of Non-Hodgkin's Lymphomas: *Cancer* 1982; **49**:2112.

Immunologic Features, Immunophenotyping, Therapy

Bray RA, Landay AL. Identification and functional characterization of mononuclear cells by flow cytometry. *Arch Pathol Lab Med* 1989;**113**:579.

Braylan RC, Benson NA: Cell surface markers and cell cycle analysis of lymphomas. *Cytometry* (Suppl) 1988;**3**:73.

Colombat P et al: The role of autologous bone marrow transplantation in 46 adult patients with non-Hodgkin's lymphoma. *J Clin Oncol* 1990;**8**:630.

Coon JS, Weinstein RS: Diagnostic flow cytometry. In: *Techniques in Diagnostic Pathology Series.* United States and Canadian Academy of Pathology. Williams & Wilkins, 1991.

Greaves NF et al: Lineage promiscuity in hemopoietic differentiation and leukemia. *Blood* 1986;**67**:1.

Knowles DN II: Lymphoid cell markers: Their distribution and usefulness in the immunophenotypic analysis of lymphoid neoplasms. *Am J Surg Pathol* 1985; **9(Suppl)**:85.

LeBien TW, McCormack RT: The common acute lymphoblastic leukemia antigen (CD10): Emancipation from a functional enigma. *Blood* 1989;**73**:625.

Lukes RJ et al: Immunologic approach to non-Hodgkin lymphomas and related leukemias. Analysis of the results of multiparameter studies of 425 cases. *Semin Hematol* 1978;**15**:322.

Parker JW: Flow cytometry in the diagnosis of lymphomas. *Cytometry* (Suppl) 1988;**3**:38.

Parker JW: Immunological basis for the redefinition of malignant lymphomas. *Am J Clin Pathol* 1979; **72(Suppl)**:679.

Peterson FB et al: Autologous marrow transplantation for malignant lymphomas: A report of 101 cases from Seattle. *J Clin Oncol* 1990;**8**:638.

Roholl PJM et al: Immunologic marker analysis of normal and malignant histiocytes. *Am J Clin Pathol* 1988;**89**:187.

Schuurman HJ et al: Immunophenotyping of non-Hodgkin's lymphoma: Correlation with relapse-free survival. *Am J Pathol* 1988;**131**:102.

Turner RR et al: Flow cytometric measurements of proliferation-associated nuclear antigen p105 and DNA content in non-Hodgkin's lymphomas. *Arch Pathol Lab Med* 1989;**153**:907.

DNA Content & Cell Proliferation

Bauer KD et al: Prognostic implications of ploidy and proliferative activity in diffuse large cell lymphomas. *Cancer Res* 1986;**46**:3173.

Shackney SE et al: The biology of tumor growth in the non-Hodgkin's lymphomas. A dual parameter flow cytometry study of 220 cases. *J Clin Invest* 1984; **3**:1201.

Wain SL, Braylan C, Borowitz MJ: Correlation of monoclonal antibody phenotyping and cellular DNA content in non-Hodgkin's lymphoma. *Cancer* 1987;**60**:2403.

Weiss LM et al: Proliferative rates of non-Hodgkin's lymphomas as assessed by Ki-67 antibody. *Hum Pathol* 1987;**18**:1155.

Cytomolecular Genetics

Berliner N et al: Detection of clonal excess in lymphoproliferative disease by kappa/lambda analysis: Correlation with immunoglobulin gene DNA rearrangement. *Blood* 1986;**67**:80.

Cossman J et al: Molecular genetics in the diagnosis of lymphoma. *Arch Pathol Lab Med* 1988;**112**:117.

Korsmeyer SJ: Antigen receptor genes as molecular markers of lymphoid neoplasms. *Clin Invest* 1987;**79**:1291.

Korsmeyer SJ: Immunoglobulin and T cell receptor genes reveal the clonality, lineage, and translocations of lymphoid neoplasms. In: *Important Advances in Oncology,* V DeVita (editor). Lippincott, 1987.

Kristoffersson U et al: Prognostic implication of cytogenetic findings in 106 patients with non-Hodgkin lymphoma. *Cancer Genet Cytogenet* 1987;**25**:55.

Lebeau M, Rowley J: Recurring chromosomal abnormalities in leukemia and lymphoma. *Cancer Surv* 1984;**3**:372.

Nowell PC, Croce CM: Chromosomes, genes and cancer. *Am J Pathol* 1986;**125**:8.

Nowell PC et al: The most common chromosome change in 86 chronic B cell or T cell tumors: A 14q32 translocation. *Cancer Genet Cytogenet* 1986;**19**:219.

Rowley JD: Chromosome studies in the non-Hodgkin's lymphomas: The role of the 14:18 translocation. *J Clin Oncol* 1988;**6**:919.

Sklar J, Weiss LM: Application of antigen receptor gene rearrangement to the diagnosis and characterization of lymphoid neoplasms. *Annu Rev Med* 1988;**39**:315.

Waldmann TA: The arrangement of immunoglobulin and T cell receptor gene in human lymphoproliferative disorders. *Adv Immunol* 1987;**40**:247/

B Cell Neoplasms

Bartl R et al: Histologic classification and staging of multiple myeloma: A retrospective and prospective study of 674 cases. *Am J Clin Pathol* 1987;**87**:342.

Browman GP, Neame PB, Soamboonsrup P: The contribution of cytochemistry and immunophenotyping to the reproducibility of the FAB classification of acute leukemia. *Blood* 1986;**68**:900.

Dutcher TF, Fahey JL: The histopathology of the macroglobulinemia of Waldenstrom. *J Natl Cancer Inst* 1959;**22**:887.

Horning SJ, Rosenberg SA: The natural history of initially untreated low-grade non-Hodgkin's lymphomas. *N Engl J Med* 1984;**311**:1471.

Kubagawa H et al: Studies on the clonal origin of multiple myeloma. Use of individually specific (idiotype) antibodies to trace the oncogenic event to its earliest point of expression in B cell differentiation. *J Exp Med* 1979;**150**:792.

Nadler LM et al: B cell origin of non-T cell acute lymphoblastic leukemia. A model for discrete stages of neoplastic and normal pre-B cell differentiation. *J Clin Invest* 1984;**74**:332.

Rai R et al: Clinical staging of chronic lymphocytic leukemia. *Blood* 1975;**46**:219.

Schwartz RS, Beldotti L: Malignant lymphomas following allogenic disease: Transition from an immunological to a neoplastic disorder. *Science* 1965;**149**:1511.

York JC et al: Changes in the appearance of hematopoietic and lymphoid neoplasms: Clinical, pathologic and biologic implications. *Hum Pathol* 1984;**15**:11.

T Cell Neoplasms

Bertness V et al: T cell receptor gene rearrangements as clinical markers of human T cell lymphomas. *N Engl J Med* 1985;**313**;534.

Borowitz MJ et al: The phenotypic diversity of peripheral T cell lymphomas: A Southeastern Cancer Study Group experience. *Hum Pathol* 1986;**17**:567.

Chan WC et al: Heterogeneity of large granular lymphocyte proliferations: Delineation of two major subtypes. *Blood* 1986;**68**:1142.

Greer JP et al: Peripheral T cell lymphoma: A clinicopathologic study of 42 cases. *J Clin Oncol* 1984; **2**:788.

Horning SJ et al: Clinical and phenotypic diversity of T cell lymphomas. *Blood* 1986;**67**:1578.

Knowles DN, Pelicci PG, Dalla-Favera R: T cell receptor beta chain gene rearrangements: Genetic markers of T cell lineage and clonality. *Hum Pathol* 1986;**17**:546.

Lutzner M et al: Cutaneous T cell lymphomas: The Sezary syndrome, mycosis fungoides, and related disorders. *Ann Intern Med* 1979;**83**:534.

Nasu K et al: Immunopathology of cutaneous T cell lymphomas. *Am J Pathol* 1985;**119**:436.

Sausville EA et al: Histologic assessment of lymph nodes in mycosis fungoides/Sezary syndrome (cutaneous T cell lymphoma). Clinical correlations and prognostic import of a new classification system. *Hum Pathol* 1985;**16**:1098.

Waldmann TA et al: Rearrangements of genes for the antigen receptor on T cells as markers of lineage and clonality in human lymphoid neoplasms. *N Engl J Med* 1985;**313**:776.

Watanabe S: Pathology of peripheral T cell lymphomas and leukemias. *Hematol Oncol* 1986;**4**:45.

Weiss LM et al: Clonal rearrangements of T cell receptor genes in mycosis fungoides and dermatopathic lymphadenopathy. *N Engl J Med* 1985;**313**:539.

Hodgkin's Disease

Drexler HG et al: Is the Hodgkin cell a T- or B-lymphocyte? Recent evidence from geno- and immunophenotypic analysis and in vitro cell lines. *Hematol Oncol* 1989;**7**:95.

Forni M et al: B and T lymphocytes in Hodgkin's disease: An immunohistochemical study utilizing heterologous and monoclonal antibodies. *Cancer* 1985; **55**:728.

Lukes RJ, Butler JJ: The pathology and nomenclature of Hodgkin's disease. *Cancer Res* 1966;**26**:1063.

Lukes RJ et al: Report of the nomenclature committee. *Cancer Res* 1966;**26(Part 1)**:1311.

Mononuclear Phagocyte Neoplasms

Roholl PMJ et al: Immunologic marker analysis of normal and malignant histiocytes. *Am J Clin Pathol* 1988;**89**:187.

Conditions Mimicking Neoplasms or Associated with a High Incidence of Neoplasms of the Immune System

Butler JJ: Nonneoplastic lesions of lymph nodes of man to be differentiated from lymphomas. *Natl Cancer Inst Monogr* 1969;**32**:233.

Childs CC, Parham DM, Berard CW: Infectious mononucleosis. The spectrum of morphologic changes simulating lymphoma in lymph nodes and tonsils. *Am J Surg Pathol* 1987;**11**:122.

Cleary ML, Warnke R, Sklar J: Monoclonality of lymphoproliferative lesions in cardiac transplant recipients: Clonal analysis based on Ig-gene rearrangements. *N Engl J Med* 1984;**310**:477.

Dorfman RF, Warnke R: Lymphadenopathy simulating the malignant lymphomas. *Hum Pathol* 1974;**5**:519.

Hartsock, RJ: Reactive lesions in lymph nodes. Chap 9, p 196, in: *The Reticuloendothelial System.* Rebuck JW, Berard CW, Abell MR (editors). Williams & Wilkins 1975. Monograph 16.

Levine AM: AIDS-associated malignant lymphoma. *Med Clin North Am* 1992;**76**:253.

Lukes RJ, Tindle BH: Immunoblastic lymphadenopathy: A prelymphomatous state of immunoblastic sarcoma. *Recent Results Cancer Res* 1978;**64**:241.

Purtilo DT: X-linked lymphoproliferative syndrome: an immunodeficiency disorder with acquired agammaglobulinemia, fatal infectious mononucleosis, or malignant lymphoma. *Arch Pathol Lab Med* 1981; **105**:119.

Symmers WS: Drug-induced lymphoma-like lymphadenopathies and their relation to lymphomas. Pages 696–701 in: *Systemic Pathology.* Vol 2. Churchill Livingstone, 1978.

46

Mechanisms of Immunity to Infection

John Mills, MD, & David J. Drutz, MD

The environment in which we live is populated by microorganisms, many of which are capable of causing disease. The immune system probably evolved primarily as a defense against infection by these omnipresent pathogenic microorganisms. However, nonimmunologic defenses against infectious disease (Table 46–1) are at least as important as immunologic defenses, especially in preventing early stages of infection. Collectively, these immunologic and nonimmunologic defense mechanisms are responsible for maintaining our internal milieu free of microorganisms. Host defense mechanisms maintain the sterility of distal portions of the "external" portions of the host despite continuous exposure to contamination. The best example of this is the respiratory tract, in which the tracheobronchial tree distal to the carina is normally sterile.

As our understanding of the immune system has improved, the boundary between specific and nonspecific immune resistance to infection has blurred. For example, natural killer (NK) cells and macrophages function in nonspecific immune defense mechanisms, but they may be activated by lymphokines produced as a result of the specific interaction between immune lymphocytes and antigens. These cells may also become specific effectors through cooperation with antibody.

Host defenses against infection—whether specific or nonspecific—are also characterized by considerable redundancy. This may explain why profound defects in one sector of host defenses ordinarily result in only a minimal increase in the overall susceptibility to infection.

NONIMMUNOLOGIC DEFENSES AGAINST INFECTION

Host Defenses at Body Surfaces

For an invading pathogen to produce infection, it must first slip through an impressive barrier of surface defenses that operate wherever intact body tissues interface with the environment. These barriers—the skin and mucosal epithelial surfaces—are largely nonspecific and nonimmunologic, but they constitute a vital component of host defense.

Many pathogens initiate infection by attaching to mucosal epithelial cells. All epithelial cells are covered with a mucus layer, which serves in part to prevent microorganisms from attaching to the cell surface. Coordinated movement of the underlying cilia sweeps organisms entrapped in the mucus layer out of the body. This process may be assisted by coordinated movements of these organs, such as coughing or peristalsis. Intestinal epithelial cells have a short (30-hour) half-life, which also limits the efficiency of infection. If the invading microorganism happens to attach to a desquamating epithelial cell, infection will not occur. Exposure of epithelial cells to many microorganisms triggers a coordinated response in the cell, which may augment host resistance to infection.

Many substances coating body surfaces serve as local disinfectants and antimicrobial substances. The skin has a high content of fatty acids, which are inhibitory to bacteria and fungi. The stomach secretes hydrochloric acid with a pH between 1 and 2, which is sufficient to kill most gastrointestinal pathogens. Factors that reduce gastric acidity, such as treatment with antacids or H_2 blockers, can increase the susceptibility of the host to enteric pathogens. A number of specific bactericidal or fungicidal proteins are formed on body surfaces. For example, the enzyme lysozyme, which is present in tears and many other mucosal secretions, is bactericidal for many gram-positive bacteria. Most of the bacteria susceptible to lysozyme are classified as nonpathogens, but it may be that they are nonpathogenic because of the large amounts of lysozyme in secretions. Many other mucosal proteins with specific activity against microorganisms, eg, lactoferrin, have been described. Lactoferrin is an iron-binding protein that maintains the concentration of free iron necessary for bacterial replication below levels at which most bacteria grow.

Most animal and human surfaces that are exposed

Table 46–1. Nonimmunologic host defense mechanisms.

Surface defenses
  Mucus
  Coughing/peristalsis
  Epithelial-cell turnover
  Local disinfectants (gastric acid, skin lipids)
  Normal microbial flora
Inflammatory reaction
  Cells
    Phagocytic cells
      PMN
      Monocyte-macrophages
    NK cells
  Complement (alternative pathway)
  Prostaglandins and leukotrienes
  Cytokines (interferons, IL-1, etc)

to the environment are colonized by nonpathogenic (or weakly pathogenic) bacteria and fungi collectively known as the normal flora. Sites populated by the normal flora include the mouth, skin, and gastrointestinal tract (Table 46–2). Anaerobic bacteria are important components of the normal flora at all sites. The density of the normal flora also varies greatly depending on the location; for example, the gastrointestinal tract at the stomach and proximal small bowel is virtually sterile, whereas the contents of the distal colon may contain 10^{11} bacteria/g of contents.

The normal flora clearly serves a protective role. For example, elimination of the anaerobic component of the gastrointestinal normal flora by antimicrobial therapy has been shown to increase the susceptibility of patients to infection by enteric pathogens such as *Shigella* and *Salmonella.* However, the extent to which the normal flora participates in host defense and the mechanisms by which it prevents colonization or infection by pathogens are incompletely defined. Some mechanisms that have been identified

Table 46–2. The normal flora.

Site	Representative Organisms
Oral mucosa	Viridans streptococci Anaerobic streptococci
Vagina	Anaerobic streptococci *Lactobacillus*
Dental plaque	*Fusobacterium* (anaerobes) *Veillonella* (anaerobes) Actinomycetes (anaerobes) Spirochetes (anaerobes)
Colonic mucosa	*Bacteroides* (anaerobes) *Fusobacterium* (anaerobes) *Escherichia coli* (anaerobes) *Clostridium* (anaerobes) *Lactobacillus* Anaerobic streptococci and staphylococci
Skin	*Propionibacterium* (anaerobes) *Staphylococcus epidermidis* *Corynebacterium* *Pityrosporum, Malassezia*

include stimulation of antibodies and T cells cross-reactive with pathogenic microorganisms, competition for nutrients, competition for receptor sites on epithelial cells, and secretion of substances toxic to pathogens (eg, secretion of bactericidal short-chain fatty acids by intestinal anaerobes).

Inflammation

Immunoglobulins and phagocytic cells play a major role in host defenses at external surfaces; they are also critical to host defenses within the body.

Cells whose major function is phagocytosis of foreign materials and killing of microorganisms are frequently referred to as "professional phagocytes," to differentiate them from other cells, including epithelial cells, that have some capacity to ingest foreign material (Table 46–3). These cells include neutrophils, basophils, eosinophils, and cells of the monocyte-macrophages series, including blood monocytes and tissue macrophages such as Kupffer's cells and alveolar macrophages. Professional phagocytes also have specialized surface receptors (eg, for the Fc portion of IgG and IgA, complement, and the products of inflammation) that are essential to their function, and they contain proteins in granules that will kill eukaryotic and prokaryotic cells. NK cells are lymphoid cells that have surface Fc receptors, but they are nonphagocytic and do not contain microbicidal systems such as lysosomes. They primarily mediate lysis of virus-infected cells (see below and Chapter 48).

Invasion of a host by a pathogen that is able to evade the surface defenses described above usually results in an inflammatory response. The components of this response include phagocytic cells, soluble factors (eg, complement, arachidonic acid metabolites), and the response of local host tissues and organs (eg, the vascular tree; see Chapters 10 and 11). In viral infections, NK cells and interferons (see Chapters 9 and 11) are probably important in early nonspecific defense mechanisms. Invasion by microorganisms produces changes in the host that attract phagocytic cells (especially PMN); in addition, some substances produced by pathogens (eg, the N-formyl peptides produced by bacteria) are chemotactic (attractive for phagocytic cells) in themselves. The PMN, which are usually the first cells at the site of infection, attack the invading pathogen and simultaneously produce

Table 46–3. Phagocytic cells.

Neutrophilic leukocytes
Eosinophilic leukocytes
Basophilic leukocytes
Blood monocytes
Tissue macrophages
Kupffer's cells of the liver
Alveolar macrophages
Astroglial cells

chemoattractants to call in additional phagocytic cells, both PMN and monocyte-macrophages. PMN products also produce important changes in host tissues (eg, vasodilatation). Monocyte-macrophages and other cells produce cytokines such as interleukin-1 (IL-1), tumor necrosis factor (TNF), and interferons. These cause fever and further augment the inflammatory reaction by attracting additional cells, augmenting the activity of these cells, and inducing vasodilatation (see Chapter 9).

Fever

Elevation of body temperature (fever) in response to infection is nearly universal in humans and other animals; this response has been highly conserved during evolution. It is therefore reasonable to conclude that fever is an important host defense mechanism. However, this contention has been difficult to prove. The main problem in proving the role of fever in antimicrobial defense in homoiothermic animals has been in dissociating the effects of the endogenous pyrogens (IL-1, TNF) that produce fever from the complex effects of fever per se. Fever has a salutory effect on the course of infection, whereas hypothermia has deleterious effects. Although these data would argue for not reducing fever in patients with infections (eg, through tepid sponging or antipyretic drugs such as aspirin), high fever itself may be deleterious. In addition, the role of fever as a host defense mechanism is probably adjunctive rather than central, and it becomes insignificant if effective antimicrobial chemotherapy is being administered.

IMMUNOLOGIC DEFENSES AGAINST INFECTION

Immunologic defenses are, by definition, those host defense mechanisms which have specificity to-

ward the invading pathogen and which are augmented on second and subsequent exposures. The specificity of the host response to invading microorganisms is determined primarily by immunoglobulins and T lymphocytes. However, the response frequently requires recruitment of otherwise nonspecific components such as complement and phagocytic cells.

Antibody-Mediated Host Defenses

Antibodies serve a variety of important host defense functions, both alone and in conjunction with nonspecific effectors (Table 46–4) (see Chapter 6). Functions of antibodies include neutralization of the biologic activity of microbial toxins (the mechanism by which tetanus and diphtheria toxoid vaccines protect against disease), inhibition of enzyme activity (eg, the neuraminidase of influenza virus), blocking of the adherence of microorganisms to mucosal surfaces, and inhibition of the growth of some prokaryotes such as *Mycoplasma*. Viruses may be neutralized in the presence of antibody alone, but many enveloped viruses are neutralized more efficiently if complement is also present. Although in vitro lysis of virus-infected cells by specific antibody and complement has been documented, the overall role of this phenomenon in host defense is unclear. Opsonization—preparing material for ingestion by phagocytic cells—also may occur with antibody alone, although the combination of antibody and complement usually increases the efficiency of ingestion. Killing of gram-negative bacteria by IgM antibody has an absolute requirement for complement.

T Lymphocyte-Mediated Host Defenses

Although T lymphocytes play a central and critical role in the generation of the immune response to invading microorganisms (see also Chapter 2), their role is predominantly one of recruiting, facilitating,

Table 46–4. Principal antibody-mediated host defense.

Immunologic Function	Pathogens Affected[1]	Principal Antibody Classes Involved	Nonspecific Cofactors Required
Opsonization	V, B, F	IgG, IgM	Phagocytic cells and complement (in some cases)
Neutralization	V	IgG, IgM, IgA	Complement (in some cases)
Inhibition of binding	B, F(?)	IgA	None
Cytolysis	V,[2] B, P	IgG, IgM	Complement
Toxin neutralization	B	IgG	None
Enzyme inhibition	V, B(?)	IgG	None
ADCC	V, F(?), ?P(?)	IgG, IgA	None
Growth inhibition	*Mycoplasma* B[3]	IgG, IgA IgA	None Lactoferrin

[1]V, viruses; B, bacteria; F, fungi; P, parasites.
[2]Lysis of virus-infected cells.
[3]IgA against bacterial nonbinding proteins synergistically inhibits growth with lactoferrin.

and augmenting other effectors, especially macrophages, rather than of directly attacking the pathogens themselves. Viruses are the major exception to this generalization, as the T lymphocyte-mediated attack on virus-infected cells constitutes a major host defense against established viral infection. The specific T cell response to virus-infected cells is mediated by CD8 cytotoxic T lymphocytes (CTLs); in addition, for some viral infections (eg, by herpes simplex virus) NK cells and macrophages are important in recovery from infection. Secretion of lymphokines, especially gamma interferon, by immune lymphocytes is responsible for augmented NK and CTL activity. Lymphokines (especially gamma interferon) also activate macrophages, which constitute a major host defense against many bacterial, fungal, and parasitic infections. Interferons produced by virus-infected cells that are not a part of the immune system (eg, alpha interferon from fibroblasts) have a direct antiviral effect, but they also augment NK cell and macrophage function.

In vitro testing has shown that T cells may play a direct role in defense against prokaryotic and eukaryotic pathogens by a number of mechanisms. Sensitized T lymphocytes have been shown to lyse certain bacteria, fungi, and parasites both directly and in the presence of antibody (antibody-dependent cell-mediated cytotoxicity). Macrophages infected with some intracellular bacterial pathogens are recognized and lysed by specific T cell clones (both CD4 and CD8 types). However, the in vivo significance of these mechanisms has generally not been validated. In some experimental bacterial infections T cells have been shown to have a direct protective effect, perhaps by secreting poorly characterized bactericidal proteins or lymphokines.

Complement

Complement acts by inactivating microorganisms and by facilitating phagocytosis (opsonization); in both roles it is often assisted by antibody (Table 46–4) (see Chapter 10). In addition, complement breakdown products induce vasodilation and are chemoattractants. The alternative complement pathway alone can be stimulated to kill some gram-negative bacteria and inactivate some viruses in the absence of antibodies. Specific antibody, however, is required for activation of the classic complement pathway, which plays an important role in host defenses to bacterial and other infections (Table 46–4). Early in infection, prior to synthesis of specific antibodies, the ability of the alternative complement pathway to nonspecifically opsonize or kill certain bacteria may be critical to recovery from infections.

Phagocytic Cells

Phagocytic cells fulfill a number of important functions in host defense (Table 46–5) (see Chapter 11). They subserve nonspecific roles such as phago-

Table 46–5. Functions of phagocytic cells thought to be important in host defenses.

Chemotaxis
Phagocytosis
  Nonfacilitated
  Facilitated (opsonization)
Killing
  Intracellular
    Oxygen-dependent
    Oxygen-independent
  Extracellular
    Nonfacilitated
    Antibody-facilitated (ADCC)
Secretion
  Monokines (IL-1, TNF, etc)
  Enzymes (proteases, etc)
  Inflammatory mediators (kinins, prostaglandins, etc)
  Growth factors

cytosis and secretion of monokines and enzymes, but these functions are often augmented by lymphokines secreted as the result of a specific immune response, as described above. Many organisms have extracellular products (eg, the polysaccharide capsule on pneumococci) that inhibit phagocytosis. Once ingested by phagocytic cells, the microorganisms are attacked by a variety of microbicidal systems (Table 46–5). Recent work has identified an array of microbicidal proteins in phagocytic cells (Table 46–6). Organisms that can survive and replicate within the professional phagocyte are termed "facultative intracellular pathogens."

In addition, Fc-bearing phagocytic cells and NK cells may have immunologic specificity imposed upon them by antibody: the so-called ADCC reaction (Table 46–4). When coated with specific IgG antibody, virus-infected cells and perhaps fungi and other eukaryotic pathogens become susceptible to killing by these NK cells and macrophages (and perhaps by PMN in some cases). The immunologic specificity of this reaction is wholly imparted by the antibody. The importance of the ADCC mechanism has been demonstrated conclusively in some experimental viral infections (eg, adult and neonatal murine herpes simplex virus infection), but it is thought to play some role in many other infections.

IMMUNOPATHOLOGY OF INFECTION

Disease may result directly from injury induced by a pathogen, for example, the paralysis and death caused by secretion of tetanus toxin by *Clostridium*

Table 46–6. Microbicidal proteins of phagocytic cells

Bactericidal permeability-increasing protein
Defensins
Serprocidins

tetani. However, in other cases the host response to the pathogen may contribute to the resulting disease and, in a few instances, may be solely responsible for the resulting clinical findings. In addition, the host immune response may facilitate or augment infection in some cases, such as the antibody-mediated enhancement of dengue virus and human immunodeficiency virus (HIV) infection of Fc-bearing cells such as macrophages. Lastly, some pathogens, particularly viruses, may injure the immune system itself, producing transient or even longstanding immunosuppression. Infection with HIV is the most important example of this type of host-parasite interaction (see Chapter 52).

Nonspecific host immune responses to invading pathogens, ie, the inflammatory response or some component of it, may be injurious in many cases. Release of inflammatory mediators causes pain and swelling, and the enzymes secreted by PMN and macrophages may produce permanent tissue damage. In most instances the beneficial effects of the local inflammatory response far outweigh any deleterious ones. However, for the patient suffering from the discomfort of a large staphylococcal abscess, this may be a difficult point to make!

Endotoxin-mediated host injury, which clinically results in the sepsis syndrome or septic shock, is usually consequent to severe infection by gram-negative bacteria such as meningococci. In this instance, much of the resulting disease is attributable to the host response to the endotoxin, not to direct injury by the endotoxin itself. The most important host response to endotoxin is probably direct stimulation of IL-1 and TNF synthesis by macrophages, which results from binding of endotoxin to specific receptors on the macrophage surface. TNF is quite probably the principal mediator of the lethal action of endotoxin, since pretreatment of animals with antibodies to TNF reduces the mortality from experimental endotoxic shock. Some of the effects of TNF itself may also be indirect, mediated through other products of inflammation such as arachidonic acid metabolites or kinins.

There are many examples of host injury secondary to the humoral immune response to a pathogen. The most important examples occur in immune-complex disease (see Chapter 27). Poststreptococcal glomerulonephritis results from formation of complexes between streptococcal antigens and host IgG antibody, which are deposited in the kidney, attracting complement and inflammatory cells. Chronic antigen-antibody complex disease may occur in hepatitis B virus infection, with a clinical syndrome of polyarteritis nodosa. Infection by *Mycoplasma pneumoniae* induces antibody to the I blood group antigen on erythrocytes, even though the I antigen is not found on the organisms. In some patients who develop high titers of this antibody, hemolytic anemia may develop.

Clear examples of host injury secondary to the cellular immune response are more difficult to identify. It is likely that some of the clinical features of tuberculosis are attributable to delayed hypersensitivity to the proteins of *M tuberculosis,* but as the organism itself produces injury, this has been difficult to prove. Liver cell damage by hepatitis B virus is probably due wholly or partly to the CTL response to viral antigens, but direct proof of this point is also lacking.

REFERENCES

Elsbach P, Weiss J: The bactericidal/permeability-increasing (BPI) protein, a potent element in host-defense against gram-negative bacteria and lipopolysaccharide. *Immunobiology* 1993;**187:**417.

Gabay JE, Almeida RP: Antibiotic peptides and serine protease homologs in human polymorphonuclear leukocytes: Defensins and azurocidin. *Curr Opin Immunol* 1993;**5:**97.

Galanos C, Freudenberg MA: Mechanisms of endotoxic shock and endotoxin hypersensitivity. *Immunobiology* 1993;**187:**246.

Kluger MJ: Fever revisited. *Pediatrics* 1992;**90:**846.

Mims CA: *The Pathogenesis of Infectious Diseases,* 3rd ed. Academic Press, 1986.

Notkins A, Oldstone MBA (editors): *Concepts in Viral Pathogenesis.* Springer Verlag, 1984.

Roth JA (editor): *Virulence Mechanisms of Bacterial Pathogens.* Am Soc Microbiol, 1988.

Smith H: The influence of the host on microbes that cause disease (The Leeuwenhoek Lecture, 1991). *Proc R Soc London Ser B* 1991;**246:**97.

Southern P, Oldstone MB: Medical consequences of persistent viral infection. *N Engl J Med* 1986;**314:**359.

Sprunt K, Leidy G: The use of bacterial interference to prevent infection. *Can J Microbiol* 1988;**34:**332.

Styrt B, Sugarman B: Antipyresis and fever. *Arch Intern Med* 1990;**150:**1589.

Tramont EC: General or nonspecific host defense mechanisms. Chapter 4 in: *Principles and Practice of Infectious Diseases,* 3rd ed. Mandell GL, Douglas RG Jr, Bennett JE (Editors). Wiley, 1990.

Ulevitch RJ: Recognition of bacterial endotoxins by receptor-dependent mechanisms. *Adv Immunol* 1993;**53:**267.

Urbaschek B (editor). Perspectives on bacterial pathogenesis and host defense: Proceedings of a Symposium. *Rev Infect Dis* 1987;**9:**S431.

Wick MJ et al: Molecular cross talk between epithelial cells and pathogenic microorganisms. *Cell* 1991;**67:**651.

Bacterial Diseases

47

John L. Ryan, PhD, MD

Immunity to bacterial infections is mediated by both cellular and humoral mechanisms. Bacteria express many different surface antigens and secrete a variety of virulence factors (eg, toxins) that may trigger immune responses. Since the topic of bacterial immunity is vast, attention in this chapter will be focused on 3 principal types of immunity to bacteria, with examples for which pathogenesis and host responses are well characterized.

(1) The first is immunity to **toxigenic bacterial infections.** Bacterial exotoxins and endotoxins are important in the pathogenesis of specific diseases. Exotoxins are the sole virulence factor in certain toxigenic bacterial infections, and immunity directed against these toxins can completely prevent disease.

(2) The second is immunity to **encapsulated bacteria.** These organisms evade phagocytosis by coating themselves with innocuous polysaccharide. Encapsulated bacteria may be gram-positive or gram-negative, and vaccines containing purified capsular antigens generate protective immunity.

(3) The third is immunity to **intracellular bacteria.** These bacteria avoid the host immune response because they grow inside cells, particularly phagocytes. The same evasive mechanism is utilized by many fungal and parasitic pathogens. Cellular immunity mediated by macrophages that are activated by specific lymphocytes and their products is the critical mode of host defense against this group of bacteria.

SERODIAGNOSIS

Serodiagnosis of bacterial diseases is of value only in specific circumstances. IgG antibody is long-lived, and its presence, although indicative of exposure to antigenic stimulation from previous infection or immunization, gives little or no information on current bacterial infection. IgM antibody is usually produced within days to a few weeks after exposure to antigen, and thus its presence suggests recent exposure in

most cases. As with viral diseases, serial determinations of antibody levels with rising titers are of greater diagnostic value, but because of the time intervals required, they are usually of little clinical value.

In general, culture of specific pathogens is required to confirm the diagnosis of a bacterial disease. Serologic tests may aid in diagnosis when diseases are caused by bacteria that are difficult to grow. *Brucella* is one such species. These organisms are difficult to culture from patients' specimens, and there is no useful delayed hypersensitivity skin test. Even though many mycobacteria are also difficult to grow, antibody titers are not helpful in diagnosis. Thus, in contrast to viral and fungal pathogens, the serologic tests in bacterial infections remain primarily a tool for epidemiologic studies rather than for clinical diagnosis in individual cases. Nevertheless, most bacteria induce specific antibody responses, which, in most cases, can be easily measured in serum. As discussed below, these antibody responses are often critical in determining the host response to an infecting agent.

EXOTOXINS & ENDOTOXINS

Exotoxins are noxious proteins that are secreted by many bacteria. These toxins are often heat-labile and thus can be heat-inactivated for use as vaccines to prevent toxigenic bacterial disease. Many bacteria produce more than one protein exotoxin, making vaccine development more difficult. Endotoxins are somatic lipopolysaccharide-protein complexes. These complex antigens are located in the outer membrane of all gram-negative bacteria. Toxicologic activity is associated with the lipid A component of the endotoxin, whereas the serologic determinants are polysaccharides. Antibody directed against specific polysaccharides can be protective both by enhancing phagocytosis directly and by fixing complement for lysis. Unfortunately, from an immune standpoint, there are usually antigenic differences in the polysaccharide components of endotoxins among strains of bacteria. Thus, in general, infection with one strain does not generate protective immunity to reinfection with a different strain of the same species. IgM and IgG antibodies directed against the lipid A component of lipopolysaccharide have different capacities to neutralize the infectivity of gram-negative bacteria. It appears that IgM is a more potent neutralizing antibody than IgG. This is particularly true for cross-reacting antibody directed against core polysaccharide or lipid A determinants of gram-negative bacteria. Passive administration of human or murine IgM directed against core determinants of endotoxin has been attempted for treatment of gram-negative sepsis. These attempts have not been efficacious except in selected subgroups of patients.

TOXIGENIC BACTERIAL DISEASES

In this section, 2 groups of toxigenic diseases will be considered. In the first group, an exotoxin is the sole virulence determinant, and vaccines directed at the exotoxin can generate effective immunity. In the second group, toxins are major virulence factors, but other pathogenic factors exist, making specific immune responses less effective in disease prevention (Fig 47–1). Antibody to toxins can neutralize the toxin by several mechanisms, including enhancing clearance by macrophages or blocking binding sites on toxin for its cellular receptors.

Clostridium Species

Clostridia are obligate anaerobic, sporeforming gram-positive rods, which cause a variety of clinical diseases. *Clostridium tetani* is the cause of tetanus. Disease occurs when spores are introduced into wounds from contaminated soil or foreign bodies. After these spores germinate, a potent neurotoxin called tetanospasmin is produced. Tetanospasmin binds to specific glycolipids in nerve cells in the peripheral nervous system and ascends to the spinal cord from nerves in the periphery. The toxin blocks normal postsynaptic inhibition of spinal reflexes, leading to generalized muscular spasms, or "tetany." A vaccine prepared from the inactivated toxin, termed "toxoid," prevents disease by generating antibodies that neutralize the toxin. It is recommended that all children be immunized with tetanus toxoid soon after birth (see Chapter 55). Subsequent boosts of immunity to toxoid are required every 10 years during adult life to maintain a protective level of antibody. There does not appear to be significant antigenic variation in tetanus toxins, since the single vaccine is protective.

Clostridium botulinum is another exotoxin-producing species for which immunity requires neutralizing antibodies to the toxin (antitoxin). *C botulinum* causes botulism, which is primarily a food-borne disease, occurring when spores or toxin are ingested from contaminated food. The botulinum toxin acts by inhibiting the release of acetylcholine neurotransmitter at the neuromuscular junctions. This produces diplopia, dysphagia, and, in severe cases, respiratory arrest. Botulism is treated with antitoxin, which is equine antiserum directed against the 3 most com-

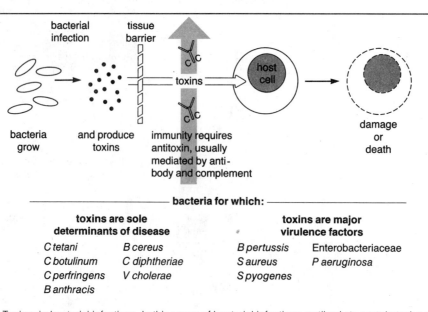

toxins are sole determinants of disease		toxins are major virulence factors	
C tetani	B cereus	B pertussis	Enterobacteriaceae
C botulinum	C diphtheriae	S aureus	P aeruginosa
C perfringens	V cholerae	S pyogenes	
B anthracis			

Figure 47–1. Toxigenic bacterial infections. In this group of bacterial infections, antibody to protein toxins and complement play a protective role in enhancing survival.

mon toxin serotypes: A, B, and E. A pentavalent toxoid (A, B, C, D, E) is distributed by the Centers for Disease Control and Prevention (CDC). This toxoid is prepared from formalin-treated toxins, which are adsorbed to aluminum phosphate to enhance immunogenicity. Natural immunity does not occur, because immunogenic doses of these toxins are lethal.

Several other *Clostridium* strains cause pyogenic infections that are mediated, in part, by cytopathic exotoxins. The most common are soft tissue infections caused by *Clostridium perfringens,* which releases a potent lecithinase called α toxin. This toxin has been associated with massive intravascular hemolysis in uncontrolled infection. *C perfringens* also secretes several other toxins, including an enterotoxin that is an important cause of food poisoning. Therapy with antitoxins has not been useful in treating diseases caused by *C perfringens,* because the organism secretes such a wide variety of toxins.

Bacillus Species

Bacillus species are facultative anaerobic gram-positive rods that can form spores. They are similar to clostridia, except for their facultative anaerobic metabolism. One of the first pathogenic bacteria to be studied was *Bacillus anthracis,* the only nonmotile species in the genus. The disease anthrax is caused by human contact with animal products contaminated by *B anthracis.* Animals are infected by ingestion of the bacteria or spores in the environment. Pathogenicity depends on toxin production, and the disease can be prevented by vaccination against attenuated bacteria. Pasteur was the first to show that vaccination could prevent anthrax in animals. The anthrax exotoxin is complex, consisting of at least 3 components: protective antigen, edema factor, and lethal factor. The protective antigen, which is not toxic alone, induces immunity and is the major component of current vaccines. *B anthracis* has also been shown to have a polysaccharide capsule, which may contribute to the virulence of this organism.

Bacillus cereus, the other toxigenic *Bacillus* species, is a common cause of food poisoning. Several toxins, including a pyogenic toxin and enterotoxins, are produced. Little is known about protective immunity to these bacteria.

Corynebacterium diphtheriae

Corynebacteria are facultative anaerobic gram-positive rods that do not form spores. The most important species is *Corynebacteria diphtheriae,* the cause of diphtheria. This organism colonizes the mucuous membranes of the posterior pharynx and elaborates a potent exotoxin. The toxin kills cells by covalently linking adenosine diphosphoribose to elongation factor 2, which is required for cellular protein biosynthesis. Immunity to diphtheria depends on the presence of antibody to the toxin. Diphtheria toxoid, a formalin-inactivated toxin preparation, is cur-

rently used worldwide to vaccinate infants against diphtheria. Immunity to diphtheria is assessed by using the Schick test. In this test, small amounts of toxin and toxoid are injected intradermally at different sites. If no response is observed at either site after 48 hours, the patient is immune to the toxin (has circulating antitoxin) and is not hypersensitive to the toxoid. If there is necrosis at the toxin site and response at the toxoid site, the patient does not have protective antibody. An immediate reaction at both sites indicates allergy to the proteins. A delayed reaction at one or both sites indicates cellular immunity to the proteins. The Schick test has been very useful in assessing immunity to *C diphtheriae.* It is no longer used very often and has been replaced with antibody titers. Nevertheless, it has provided insight into the importance of maintaining adequate circulating antibody to toxin to ameliorate or prevent clinical infection.

Vibrio cholerae

The vibrios are curved, gram-negative bacilli with polar flagellae. Infection with *Vibrio cholerae,* the agent of cholera, occurs after ingestion of contaminated water. Organisms multiply in the gut and release an enterotoxin, which binds to epithelial cells and triggers massive secretion of fluid and electrolytes. Severe diarrhea may occur within hours after infection, and the fluid loss is often life-threatening, particularly in infants and young children. Cholera is unique among the toxigenic diseases in that antibody to the toxin does not fully prevent disease. Infection with *V cholerae* induces systemic and mucosal antibody. Mucosal IgA, which prevents attachment of the bacteria in the gut, may be the most important form of immunity. Cholera vaccines induce short-term protection and elicit only IgM and IgG responses unless administered orally. Neither IgM nor IgG functions well in the intestinal lumen. Further research is needed to develop cholera vaccines that confer lifelong immunity.

Bordetella pertussis

Pertussis (whooping cough) is caused by mucosal infection with *Bordetella pertussis,* a small, gram-negative coccobacillary organism that replicates in bronchial mucosa. Infection is characterized by paroxysmal coughing, which can result in significant morbidity in young children. *B pertussis* contains several antigens that may elicit immune responses, but the critical factors in immunity to this organism are not fully understood. Killed whole bacteria are currently used as a vaccine, but acellular vaccines are under active development. Pertussis vaccine is given in combination with diphtheria toxoid and tetanus toxoid (DPT) to infants at 2, 4, and 6 months of age, with boosters usually given 1 year later and again before the children begin to attend school. Immunity to pertussis is relatively short-lived, lasting only 3 years after completion of primary immunization or boosting. Antibody that prevents attachment of the bacteria to respiratory epithelium appears to be the first line of defense, with antitoxin providing further protection against a protein exotoxin produced by the bacteria.

The presence of *B pertussis* in the DPT combination vaccine may enhance the antibody response to both protein toxoids (DT). The lipopolysaccharide in the outer membrane of *B pertussis* is a potent immune adjuvant. Thus, it is advantageous as well as convenient to use the combined vaccine.

Staphylococcus aureus

Staphylococci are facultative anaerobic, nonmotile gram-positive cocci that are most often seen as clusters in gram-stained specimens. *Staphylococcus aureus* is probably the single most prevalent pathogen in skin and soft tissue infections. Its virulence has been studied intensively, but the mechanism remains obscure. The primary line of defense against staphylococci is the polymorphonuclear leukocyte, which phagocytoses and kills the bacteria. *S aureus* produces a vast number of virulence factors, including toxins, which may contribute to its pathogenicity. Production of coagulase, a factor that can bind and activate fibrinogen, defines the species *S aureus*. At least 4 separate hemolysins are also produced. A nonhemolytic leukocidin is cytotoxic for granulocytes. In addition, *S aureus* secretes several enterotoxins, an exfoliative toxin associated with epidermal necrolysis, and an exotoxin associated with the toxic shock syndrome.

The immune response to *S aureus* infections is inadequate in that previous infection does not protect the host from reinfection. The few strains of *S aureus* that have significant capsules do generate protective antibody, but these strains are not commonly pathogenic. Most staphylococci contain small amounts of capsular polysaccharides that do not generate protective antibody. However, conjugation of these polysaccharides to protein carriers may elicit protective antibody. Similarly, antibodies to the toxic shock exotoxin and to the exfoliative exotoxins seem to prevent the specific clinical syndromes caused by these toxins. Pyogenic *S aureus* infections occur, however, despite the presence of multiple antibodies against cellular components in the host. Only the number and functional capacity of granulocytes are critically important in the defense against *S aureus*.

Another *Staphylococcus* strain associated with human disease is *Staphylococcus epidermidis*. This strain produces few toxins and is associated primarily with bacteremias in patients with plastic catheters or other foreign objects in the bloodstream. *S epidermidis,* as the name implies, is one of the most common bacteria of the skin flora. It adheres to catheters or other materials by means of an extracellular polysaccharide slime, which inhibits the ability of granulocytes to function properly. Protective immunity to this organism does not appear to develop, since repeated infections may occur in susceptible hosts.

Streptococcus Species

Streptococci are a diverse group of catalase-negative, facultatively anaerobic gram-positive cocci, which cause a variety of toxigenic and pyogenic infections in humans. *Streptococcus pyogenes* is the most important bacterial cause of pharyngitis. Late sequelae, such as rheumatic fever and glomerulonephritis, may follow infection with certain strains of this species.

Most streptococcal infections do not confer immunity unless the syndrome is mediated by toxins, such as the streptococcal pyogenic exotoxins associated with scarlet fever. The antigenic composition of streptococci is complex, with approximately 18 group-specific carbohydrate antigens lettered A–R. These antigens are useful for classifying streptococci, but they do not elicit protective immunity. Group A streptococci contain another set of type-specific M antigens, known as M proteins (more than 80 types exist). These proteins are antiphagocytic factors and enhance the virulence of group A streptococci. The M proteins do generate protective IgG antibody, but since there are many serotypes of M protein, reinfection with another strain is common.

Streptococci of groups A, B, C, F, and G produce many extracellular products that may elicit protective immunity. Streptolysins O and S are cytopathic proteins that inhibit phagocytosis and killing by leukocytes. A variety of proteinases exist, including streptokinase and other degradative enzymes such as hyaluronidase and deoxyribonuclease, which enhance the pathogenicity of the organism. Antibodies may be produced to all of these factors during infection. The widely used Streptozyme test is a hemagglutination procedure that detects a variety of antibodies against streptococcal enzymes.

Group D streptococci have recently been reclassified as enterococci and are antigenically distinct from other streptococci in that they do not possess a group-specific carbohydrate antigen, but they do have a group-specific glycerol teichoic acid antigen.

Most of the streptococci that normally colonize the human oropharynx do not possess group-specific antigens and are classified in the viridans group. Many individual strains may be defined by biochemical tests, but none of these streptococci are prominent toxin producers. They are active in causing periodontal diseases and are the most common causes of infective endocarditis. Little is known about protective immunity to this diverse group of organisms.

Gram-Negative Rods

Gram-negative rods produce a variety of toxins and are responsible for many infectious diseases. The family Enterobacteriaceae is composed of 5 major genera: *Escherichia, Klebsiella, Proteus, Yersinia,* and *Erwinia.* These are all glucose-fermenting, nonsporeforming bacilli. All members of the family Enterobacteriaceae, but particularly *Escherichia* and *Salmonella,* have undergone extensive immunologic analyses. They are serotyped on the basis of O antigens (polysaccharides associated with the lipopolysaccharide component of the outer membrane), K antigens (polysaccharide capsular components), and H antigens (proteins associated with flagella).

Some of these organisms are partially responsible for contributing to the immune pathogenesis of the spondyloarthropathies. The well-known association of the class MHC I molecule HLA-B27 and ankylosing spondylitis, as well the association of the disease with preceding enteric infection, has stimulated a search for molecular mimicry, ie, identity between epitopes on a bacterium and one in the human host. The immune response to *Klebsiella pneumoniae* elicits antibody that can bind to HLA-B27 on the surface of synovial lining cells. Similar molecular mimicry has been shown for *Shigella flexneri,* which produces an arthritogenic epitope that is shared by HLA-B27 antigen. Thus, the immune response to certain members of the Enterobacteriaceae may result in autoimmune disease in selected hosts.

Each member of the family Enterobacteriaceae contains an endotoxin. This endotoxin is a lipopolysaccharide-protein complex in the outer membrane and contains the O-specific serologic group. The biologically active components of the endotoxin are the lipid A and certain lipoproteins associated with the lipopolysaccharide.

Enterotoxins are also produced by many members of the Enterobacteriaceae, particularly *Escherichia coli.* *E coli* has at least 2 enterotoxins, an immunogenic heat-labile toxin and a nonimmunogenic heat-stable toxin. More typical exotoxins are also related to certain strains of *E coli, Shigella,* and *Yersinia.*

Immunity to the Enterobacteriaceae is achieved early in life after colonization of the gut with *E coli.* Antibodies against K and O antigens are generated and are protective against autologous serotypes. Prior to the development of antibody, the neonate is susceptible to systemic and particularly to central nervous system infection by *E coli.* In adult life, these bacteria cause opportunistic as well as enteric diseases. Attempts to transfer passive immunity with antiserum to *E coli* have proved effective in both animal and some human studies. Antibodies directed against the endotoxin component may be able to help prevent the morbidity and mortality associated with sepsis in certain patient groups.

Pseudomonas aeruginosa is the most clinically important nonfermenting gram-negative rod and has been the subject of extensive immunologic analysis. It characteristically produces exotoxin A, a cytolytic

factor with a similar mechanism of action to diphtheria toxin. Antibodies directed against exotoxin A as well as the lipopolysaccharide appear to be important in immunity to infection with *P aeruginosa.* Different serotyping schemes have been used to define *P aeruginosa* for epidemiologic purposes. Multivalent vaccines containing several serotypes to protect immunocompromised patients from invasive *Pseudomonas* infection are under investigation. *Pseudomonas* is a virulent opportunistic pathogen that commonly invades immunocompromised patients. The role of antibody to endotoxin in ameliorating human disease has been shown in animals by using homologous and heterologous antisera to protect them against lethal *P aeruginosa* infections.

ENCAPSULATED BACTERIA

Bacteria that express capsular polysaccharide present a unique problem for the immune system. Capsular polysaccharide inhibits phagocytosis by both macrophages and polymorphonuclear leukocytes. Effective phagocytosis requires functional leukocyte receptors for the Fc region of immunoglobulin and C3b or C3bi (Fig 47–2). Opsonization of encapsulated bacteria with antibody and complement is necessary for phagocytes to efficiently ingest and kill these pathogens. The charge and hydrophilicity of unopsonized encapsulated bacteria inhibit phagocytosis by interfering with attachment of leukocytes and bacteria. Immaturity of humoral immunity in the very young and decline of humoral immunity in the elderly probably account for the susceptibility of individuals at these stages of life to invasive disease by encapsulated bacteria.

Bacterial vaccines hold great promise for enhancing immunity against encapsulated bacteria. Since polysaccharides are relatively poor immunogens, complexes of protein with polysaccharides may represent more effective vaccine candidates. Coupling of weak antigens with other types of adjuvants may also improve the efficacy of vaccines.

Streptococcus pneumoniae

Streptococcus pneumoniae strains, commonly called pneumococci, differ from other streptococci in that they contain complex polysaccharide capsules that determine the major virulence determinant in the species. Pneumococci are respiratory pathogens that colonize upper airways and cause bronchitis or pneumonia after aspiration of respiratory secretions. The capsule inhibits alveolar macrophage phagocytosis and allows the pneumococcus to multiply in the lung. Patients with abnormal mucocillary reflexes or decreased alveolar macrophage function are more susceptible to infection. Patients with decreased sys-

A

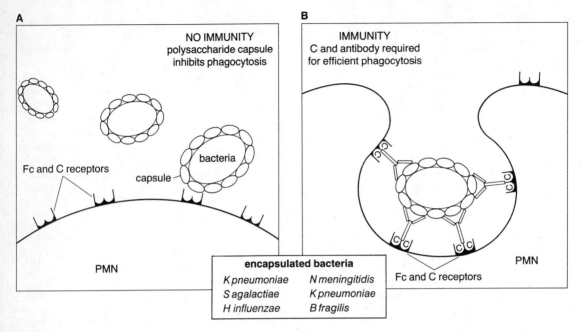

NO IMMUNITY
polysaccharide capsule
inhibits phagocytosis

Fc and C receptors

capsule

bacteria

PMN

B

IMMUNITY
C and antibody required
for efficient phagocytosis

Fc and C receptors

PMN

encapsulated bacteria	
K pneumoniae	N meningitidis
S agalactiae	K pneumoniae
H influenzae	B fragilis

Figure 47–2. Encapsulated bacteria. Polysaccharide capsules allow bacterial multiplication by avoiding receptor-mediated phagocytosis. If specific antibody to the capsule is present, both antibody and complement serve as opsonins to enhance the uptake of bacteria by host phagocytes.

temic clearance of bacteria are susceptible to disseminated disease.

Type-specific antibody is elicited and is protective, but there are more than 80 serotypes of pneumococci. Thus, reinfection with a different serotype is common in susceptible persons. The polysaccharide capsule is sometimes cross-reactive with the capsular polysaccharides of different genera, including *Haemophilus* and *Klebsiella*. A vaccine containing capsular polysaccharide from the 23 most prevalent or virulent serotypes is available for adult patients at high risk for pneumococcal disease. Conjugated protein-polysaccharide vaccines are under development to prevent disease in infants.

Streptococcus agalactiae (Group B)

The group B streptococci are a leading cause of neonatal meningitis. Most disease occurs because of colonization of the infant by members of the vaginal flora during parturition. Group B organisms contain 4 major capsular serotypes. Sialic acid, one of the carbohydrate components of group B streptococcal capsular polysaccharide, can block complement activation. This prevents a key nonspecific defense mechanism in infants who are without adequate antibody levels. Type-specific antibodies are protective for group B streptococcal disease. Both passive immunization with IgG antibody to capsular polysac-

charides and active immunization with polysaccharides to prevent group B streptococcal disease in the neonatal period are under investigation.

Haemophilus influenzae

Of the several species of *Haemophilus* that are known, *Haemophilus influenzae* is the most prevalent pathogen. Several distinct capsular serotypes have been defined, but type b *H influenzae* is responsible for most clinical disease. *H influenzae* is a respiratory pathogen that colonizes the oropharynx and causes bronchitis, pneumonia, or disseminated infection when local or systemic host defense factors are compromised. The type b capsule is a polyribitol phosphate. The susceptibility of a given host to infection is directly related to serum levels of bactericidal antibody. Maternal IgG is lost within a few months after birth, and natural antibody is acquired by 3–4 years of age. The development of natural antibody may be related to colonization and subsequent immunization with nonpathogenic members of the family Enterobacteriaceae that contain cross-reactive capsular polysaccharides. *H influenzae* type b capsular polysaccharide (PRP) is a weak immunogen, and vaccines have not been effective in children younger than 2 years. Recently, conjugate vaccines with diphtheria toxin and outer membrane proteins linked to PRP have proven effective in immunizing children between 6 months and 2 years of age. There are few bacterial diseases in which the protective role of antibody has been so clearly demonstrated as in *H influenzae* type b disease.

Neisseria Species

These are gram-negative cocci containing high levels of cytochrome *c* oxidase. The 2 pathogenic species are *Neisseria gonorrhoeae* (gonococcus) and *Neisseria meningitidis* (meningococcus). There is no definite role of anticapsular antibody in immunity to gonococci. Repeated infections with gonococci are quite common. Mucosal antibody directed against surface proteins appears to have some protective value, and the complement system is particularly important in the maintenance of bactericidal activity. The meningococcus normally inhabits the pharynx without producing disease. This provides a reservoir for outbreaks and produces some immunity in the host. The critical antigenic components of the meningococcus are capsular polysaccharides, and 9 distinct serotypes can elicit group-specific protective antibody. IgM antibody appears to be more protective than does IgG, perhaps because of its more potent complement-fixing activity. Patients deficient in the terminal complement components C6, C7, C8 or properdin are susceptible to recurrent neisserial infections. Vaccines are available to both group A and group C *N meningitidis*. Group B capsular polysaccharides are cross-reactive with *E coli* capsular polysaccharides (K1 antigens), and no vaccine is available against this strain. The importance of antibody in protection against meningococcal disease is underscored by the peak incidence of disease, which occurs at about 1 year of age, when maternal antibody has waned and acquired antibody has not yet been produced.

Klebsiella pneumoniae

Klebsiella species are members of the family Enterobacteriaceae that are characterized by polysaccharide capsules with more than 70 serotypes. Although they are predominantly intestinal organisms that cause opportunistic infections, they are also associated with primary pneumonias. This is probably related to the ability of these bacteria to avoid phagocytosis in the absence of antibody. The capsular polysaccharides found in *Klebsiella* are related to those in *Streptococcus* and *Haemophilus*. The role of specific anticapsular antibodies in *Klebsiella* has not been elucidated. Immunity appears to be multifactorial, with disease most commonly occurring in debilitated patients with depressed host defenses.

Bacteroides fragilis

Bacteroides fragilis and closely related species are obligate anaerobic nonsporeforming gram-negative rods, which colonize the intestinal tract and are often associated with intra-abdominal abscess formation.

Unless the mucous membrane barrier of the gastrointestinal or respiratory tract is damaged, *B fragilis* is a member of the harmless normal flora. In the presence of tissue necrosis or trauma, *B fragilis* may be released into a relatively low-oxygen environment, allowing growth and elaboration of several enzymes that potentiate tissue damage. *B fragilis* also contains a capsular polysaccharide that is a key virulence factor in animal models of infection. The capsule mediates resistance to phagocytosis, and capsular antibody enhances the phagocytic killing of these bacteria.

INTRACELLULAR BACTERIAL PATHOGENS

Many bacteria have developed the ability to avoid host defense systems by invading cells so that serum antibody and complement cannot harm them and granulocytes cannot recognize them (Fig 47–3). These bacteria induce T cell-mediated immunity in the same fashion as fungi, parasites, and viruses. Serum antibody and complement are not markers of resistance for these bacteria. The presence of sensitized T lymphocytes and activated macrophages is the key factor in immunity. Microbial antigens are expressed on the surface of macrophages after the antigens are processed, in conjunction with products of the major histocompatibility complex. In this configuration, macrophages interact with T lymphocytes to produce macrophage-activating factors such as gamma interferon. This complex series of events is required for the expression of effective immunity to intracellular pathogens.

Salmonella Species

Salmonella species are members of the family Enterobacteriaceae and cause a significant proportion of enteric disease. Three major species (*Salmonella typhi, Salmonella choleraesuis,* and *Salmonella enteritidis*) exist. Based on serologic reactions, there are more than 1700 types of *S enteritidis*. Most invasive disease, such as typhoid fever, is caused by *S typhi*, and it is of great interest that this is the only species of *Salmonella* with a surface capsular antigen. This capsule, therefore, is a key virulence factor for *S typhi*. Antibody against the capsule is not protective, and many typhoid carriers have circulating antibody. This reflects the ability of salmonellae to reside within cells of the reticuloendothelial system. Salmonellae usually enter the body by ingestion and cause enterocolitis if they are present in sufficient numbers to survive the acidic environment of the stomach. If they invade mucosal tissues, they can cause disseminated disease. Immunity to *Salmonella* involves activation of macrophages by sensitized T lymphocytes through lymphokine secretion. Circulating antibodies

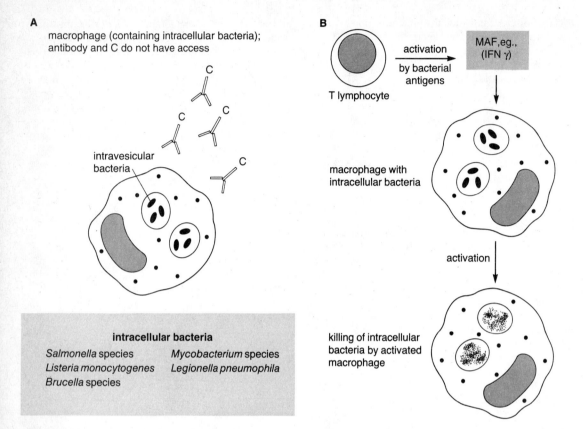

A

macrophage (containing intracellular bacteria);
antibody and C do not have access

intravesicular
bacteria

intracellular bacteria

Salmonella species   Mycobacterium species
Listeria monocytogenes   Legionella pneumophila
Brucella species

B

T lymphocyte

activation
by bacterial
antigens

MAF, eg.,
(IFN γ)

macrophage with
intracellular bacteria

activation

killing of intracellular
bacteria by activated
macrophage

Figure 47–3. Intracellular bacterial pathogens. Antibody and complement have no access to intracellular pathogens. Lymphokines mediate macrophage activation, which allows the killing of these bacteria by both oxidative and nonoxidative mechanisms.

do not penetrate the cell to eradicate intracellular bacteria. Thus circulating antibody represents a marker of infection, but not of immunity.

Other Intracellular Bacterial Pathogens

Bacterial strains other than *Salmonella* that are intracellular pathogens include *Legionella, Listeria,* and *Brucella. Legionella pneumophila* and related strains are obligate intracellular parasites of macrophages. These bacteria exhibit optimal growth only within cells. Antibodies to serogroup-specific antigens are produced and are useful for diagnostic or epidemiologic studies, but they have not proved to be protective. Antigen-specific T lymphocyte activation with release of gamma interferon and other macrophage-activating factors enhances immunity to *Legionella.*

Listeria monocytogenes is a gram-positive rod similar to *Corynebacterium;* it causes meningeal infections or sepsis in adults and a variety of infections in neonates. Although antibody may play some role in preventing invasion, it is clear that the macrophage is the primary mode of defense against these bacteria. Investigations in animal models have demonstrated

that T lymphocyte function is important in macrophage activation for immunity to *Listeria.*

Brucella species are small coccobacillary gram-negative bacteria that resemble *Haemophilus* in appearance and are spread to humans through contact with animals (zoonosis). Three species are pathogenic for humans and cause systemic disease that may be chronic or subacute. The first is *Brucella abortus* from cattle, the second is *Brucella suis* from pigs, and the third is *Brucella melitensis,* usually from goats and sheep. Diagnosis is often made by serology, but antibody does not confer immunity. Immunity to *Brucella* species is conferred by activated macrophages produced by specifically sensitized T lymphocytes and lymphokines derived from them. The specific antigens that elicit cellular immunity to brucellosis have not been defined.

Mycobacterium Species

The genus *Mycobacterium* comprises a unique group of bacteria characterized by a lipid-rich cell wall that contains N-glycolylneuraminic acid. The major pathogenic strain is *Mycobacterium tuberculosis,* although *Mycobacterium avium* complex (MAC) has emerged as a significant pathogen in patients with acquired immunodeficiency syndrome (AIDS). Tuberculosis has been one of the great infectious scourges of mankind throughout history and remains a major world health problem today. One reason is that despite decades of excellent research into the immune mechanisms relating to tuberculosis, an effective vaccine has not been found. Bacillus Calmette-Guérin (BCG), an attenuated *Mycobacterium bovis* strain, has been used for more than 60 years and is able to confer delayed cutaneous hypersensitivity but no clear-cut cellular immunity. Serum antibody plays no role in immunity to mycobacterial diseases. Sensitized T lymphocytes and activated macrophages are the critical factors in immunity. The components of the cell wall of *M tuberculosis* that may confer immunity have been analyzed in detail. Both proteins and polysaccharides have immunogenic potential, and there are data supporting a substantive role for the polysaccharide components as the key epitopes for cellular immunity. A purified protein derivative is used as an intradermal antigen to measure delayed hypersensitivity to *M tuberculosis*. A positive delayed skin test demonstrates previous exposure to the bacteria and is often correlated with immunity. There is not a one-to-one correlation between a positive skin test and immunity, however, and further definition of the protective antigens in the tubercle bacillus is needed before immunity to *M tuberculosis* can be understood.

The need to develop more effective vaccines against *M tuberculosis* has been accentuated by the recent striking increase in the incidence in AIDS patients of tuberculosis due to bacteria with multiple drug resistance.

Immunity to mycobacteria such as MAC and *Mycobacterium leprae* (the agent of Hansen's disease, ie, leprosy) is also mediated by cellular immunity, with serum components playing an insignificant role. The occurrence of MAC infections in AIDS patients underscores the critical importance of cell-mediated immunity in resistance to mycobacterial infections.

CONCLUSIONS

Immunity to bacterial infections is extremely complex because of the diverse virulence factors used by bacteria to enhance their survival. Primary nonspecific defense against bacterial infections is afforded by granulocytes, which ingest and kill most potential pathogens. Specific immunity is needed for protection against encapsulated or intracellular bacteria. This requires the development either of antibody, which can enhance killing by its opsonic or complement-fixing activity, or of T cell immunity, which can activate the microbicidal activity of macrophages. In many infections, a complex interaction of immune mechanisms is required to achieve protective immunity. Thus, antibody, complement, granulocytes, lymphocytes, and macrophages are all needed to permit the development of protective immunity to many bacterial pathogens.

REFERENCES

General

Braude AI (editor): *Infectious Diseases and Medical Microbiology,* 2nd ed. Saunders, 1986.

Sherris JC (editor): *Medical Microbiology: An Introduction to Infectious Diseases.* Elsevier, 1984.

Specific

Bloom BR et al: Tuberculosis: Commentary on a reemergent killer. *Science* 1992;**257**:1005.

Daniel DM: Antibody and antigen detection for the immunodiagnosis of tuberculosis: Why not? What more is needed? Where do we stand today? *J Infect Dis* 1988;**158**:678.

Densen P et al: Familial properdin deficiency and fatal meningococcemia. *N Engl J Med* 1987;**316**:922.

Dezfulian M, Bitar RA, Bartlett JG: Kinetics study of immunologic response to *Clostridium botulinum.* toxin. *J Clin Microbiol* 1987;**25**:1336.

Fattom A et al: Laboratory and clinical evaluation of conjugate vaccines composed of *Straphyloccus aureus* type 5 and type 8 capsular polysaccharides bound to *Pseudomonas aeruginosa* recombinant exotoxin A. *Infect Immun* 1993;**61**:1023.

Fierer J: *Pseudomonas* and *Flavobacterium,* Chap 33, pp 314–320, in: *Infectious Diseases and Medical Microbiology,* 2nd ed. Braude AI (editor). Saunders, 1986.

Gazapo E et al: Changes in IgM and IgG antibody concentrations in brucellosis over time: Importance for diagnosis and follow-up. *J Infect Dis* 1989;**159**:219.

Greenman RL et al: A controlled clinical trial of E5 murine monoclonal antibody to endotoxin in the treatment of Gram-negative sepsis. *JAMA* 1991;**266**:1097.

Griffiss JM et al: Vaccines against encapsulated bacteria: A global agenda. *Rev Infect Dis* 1987;**9**:176.

Harriman GR et al: The role of C9 in complement-mediated killing of *Neisseria. J Immunol* 1981;**127**:2386.

Johnston RB: Recurrent bacterial infections in children. *N Engl J Med* 1984;**310**:1237.

Kasper DL: The polysaccharide capsule of *Bacteroides fragilis* subspecies *fragilis:* Immunochemical and morphologic definition. *J Infect Dis* 1976;**133**:79.

McCabe WR et al: Immunization with rough mutants of *Salmonella minnesota:* Protective activity of IgM and IgG antibody to the R595 (Re Chemotype) mutant. *J Infect Dis* 1988;**158**:291.

Orskov F, Orskov I: Enterobacteriaceae. Chap 31, pp

292–303, in: *Infectious Diseases and Medical Microbiology*, 2nd ed. Braude AI (editor). Saunders, 1986.

Ryan KJ: *Corynebacteria and Other Non-Spore Forming Microorganisms. An Introduction to Infectious Diseases.* Sherris JC (editor). Elsevier, 1984.

Santosham M et al: The efficacy in Navajo infants of a conjugate vaccine consisting of *Haemophilus influenzae* type b polysaccharide and Neisseria meningitidis outer-membrane protein complex. *N Engl J Med* 1991;**324:**1767.

Schwimmbeck MD, Oldstone MBA: Molecular mimicry between human leucocyte antigens B27 and *Klebsiella. Am J Med* 1988;**85(Suppl 6A):**51.

Ziegler EJ et al: Treatment of Gram-negative bacteremia and septic shock with HA-1A human monoclonal antibody against endotoxin. *N Engl J Med* 1991;**324:**429.

Viral Infections

48

John Mills, MD

The interactions between viruses and the host immune system are not only complex and fascinating but also critical in determining the outcome of infection and strategies for its prevention. Viruses share the qualities of being complex immunogens with other pathogens that replicate in the host. They can stimulate both cellular and humoral immune responses, which then have a major influence on the outcome of infection. However, because viruses parasitize cellular metabolic processes during their own replication, they have a unique capacity to directly alter cell structure and function. This chapter considers some representative viral diseases of humans, selected either because of their clinical relevance or because they illustrate important facets of the interaction between virus infection and host immunity. Viruses that chiefly infect cells of the immune system are considered in Chapter 52.

Viruses are obligate intracellular parasites. Thus, clinical features of infection by a specific virus are determined by which cells are infected and whether the virus itself produces cellular pathology. In addition, for many viruses, the host immune response to viral antigens induces additional injuries, called **immunopathic effects,** which are qualitatively different from viropathic effects. Much of the disease morbidity associated with some viruses is, in fact, secondary to the host response. The outcome of virus infection may be broadly classified into those in which the virus is eliminated (eg, influenza virus and poliovirus) and those in which the virus persists. In the latter instance the virus persists either in latent form, with or without intermittent replication (eg, herpes simplex virus), or as a chronic infection (eg, human immunodeficiency virus). Other infections have late immunologic sequelae (Table 48–1). For some viruses, the host immune response is one determinant of whether the infection becomes latent.

INFLUENZA VIRUS

Major Immunologic Features
- Viral surface proteins show marked antigenic variation, resulting from mutation and recombination.
- In the naive host, CTL are responsible for elimination of virus after infection.
- Serum antibodies to viral surface proteins mediate resistance to pneumonia; mucosal (IgA) antibodies protect against rhinotracheitis.

General Considerations
Influenza is a respiratory infection with systemic manifestations; it is caused by influenza viruses. The disease occurs chiefly in epidemics, predominantly during the winter months. Although all age groups are affected, the severity of the illness is greatest at the extremes of age, and the mortality rate is highest in the elderly and in individuals with underlying chronic cardiorespiratory disease. Recurrent epidemics of influenza contribute significantly to the premature death of patients in these risk groups.

Virology
Influenza virus has an envelope and an antisense RNA genome that is segmented (7–8 pieces) rather than continuous as is found in most viruses. The virus has several important structural proteins (Table 48–2), and, in general, each genome segment specifies one protein.

Three types of influenza virus, A, B, and C, are known; the classification is based on the antigenic characteristics of the ribonucleoprotein and matrix proteins, as well as other features. Influenza A virus is unique in part because it infects both humans and other animals (pigs, horses, fowl, and seals) and because it is the principal cause of pandemic influenza. When a cell is infected by 2 different influenza A viruses, the segmented RNA genomes of the 2 parental virus types mix during replication, so that virions of the progeny may contain RNA and protein from both

Table 48–1. Viral infections with immunologic sequelae.

Acute Viral Infection	Immunologic Sequelae
Measles virus	Encephalitis (early), subacute sclerosing panencephalitis (SSPE) (late)
Rubella virus	Encephalopathy, arthritis
Hepatitis B virus	Polyarteritis nodosa, glomerulo-nephritis
Respiratory syncytial virus	Asthma (unproved association)
Epstien-Barr virus	Guillain-Barré syndrome

parents (so-called "recombinants," even though they are really reassortants). Influenza A virus thereby varies its surface hemagglutinin and neuraminidase molecules by recombining with other strains (including animal strains) as well as by mutation. Like other viruses with an RNA genome, influenza virus has a high rate of mutation, which underlies its rapid antigenic variation. These phenomena result in new epidemic strains (Fig 48–1). Influenza B virus does not have an animal reservoir from which it can select novel hemagglutinin types, and thus the range of antigenic variation observed is narrower than that for influenza A virus. Influenza C virus appears to have only one serotype and differs from types A and B in some other features as well.

The principal targets for influenza virus infection are the ciliated epithelial cells of the upper and lower respiratory tract. Influenza virus infection kills these cells, which regenerate slowly during convalescence. Virus shedding terminates with recovery from infection, and neither chronic nor latent infection occurs.

Clinical Features

Influenza is spread through both aerosols and fomites. The clinical features of influenza are fever, cough, myalgia, headache, and malaise. Mild pharyngeal or conjunctival irritation is common, and gastrointestinal symptoms may occur as well, especially in children. There are no characteristic abnormalities on routine laboratory testing. Influenza may be diagnosed by culture of the virus from nasopharyngeal or pulmonary secretions, by direct detection of viral antigens on desquamated respiratory epithelial cells with labeled monoclonal antibodies, or by demonstration of an antibody response to the virus in convalescent-phase sera.

Table 48–2. Major structural proteins of influenza virus.

Protein	Location	Function
Hemagglutinin	Surface (envelope)	Acts as ligand for cell receptor acetylneuraminic acids
Neuraminidase	Surface (envelope)	Releases progeny virus from cell
Matrix protein	Internal	Stabilizes virus coat
RNA polymerase	Internal	Replicates RNA genome
Nucleoprotein	Internal	Stabilizes RNA within virion

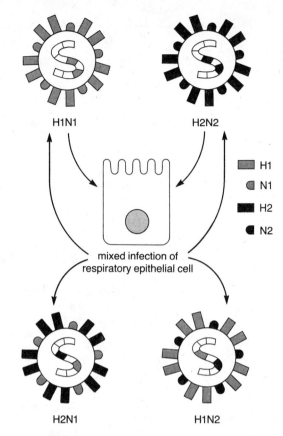

H1N1   H2N2

H1
N1
H2
N2

mixed infection of respiratory epithelial cell

H2N1   H1N2

Figure 48–1. Schematic reproduction of genetic reassortment in influenza viruses. Shown are the major surface proteins and their corresponding gene segments.

Immunologic Pathogenesis

Although influenza virus stimulates a vigorous host immune response, including specific antibodies and cytotoxic T cells, most of the clinical findings are probably due to the cytopathic effects of this virus and to stimulation of alpha interferon production. In animal models of influenza, immunosuppression has a variable effect on the course of the infection, but virus replication is invariably prolonged. Patients with a wide variety of immunodeficiency disorders do not clearly show increased symptoms following influenza virus infection, although virus shedding may be prolonged, particularly in the context of cellular immune deficiency.

Cellular immunity, measured by either skin test reactivity or in vitro lymphocyte activation to antigens, is slightly depressed during acute influenza. The mechanism of this effect is uncertain, although it may be related to production of inhibitors of interleukin-1 (IL-1). This brief period of cellular immunosuppression appears to have no adverse clinical sequelae and does not interfere with the antiviral immune response. In contrast, influenza virus infection suppresses normal pulmonary antibacterial defenses, so that patients recovering from influenza have a greatly increased risk of developing bacterial pneumonia. The mechanism of this effect is unknown, but it may be the disruption of the mucociliary escalator combined with impaired function of pulmonary alveolar macrophages or neutrophils.

Infection with influenza virus stimulates interferon synthesis and also a vigorous cytotoxic T cell (CTL) response, and both contribute to eradicating the virus. Antibody is also produced, but this appears to have only a marginal role in recovery from infection. Nude mice (which lack cellular immunity) cannot control influenza infection, and administration of antibody results in only transient cessation of virus shedding. In contrast, reconstitution with cloned influenza-specific CTL eradicates the infection. Natural killer (NK) cells do not appear to play an important role in resistance to influenza.

Influenza is associated with a number of postinfectious disorders including encephalitis (see Chapter 38), myopericarditis (see Chapter 34), and Goodpasture's syndrome (see Chapters 36 and 43). The pathogenesis of these complications is unknown.

Antibodies directed against hemagglutinin and neuraminidase surface proteins are critical determinants of host resistance to influenza virus. Antibodies to the hemagglutinin prevent the virus from attaching to cells and neutralize infectivity. Alone, they can prevent infection. Antibodies to neuraminidase inhibit the release of virus from cells and its subsequent spread to other cells within the host or to other people. Although antineuraminidase antibodies do not prevent infection, they ameliorate disease. Recent studies with mice have shown clearly that serum antibodies to influenza prevent pulmonary infection but not rhinotracheitis; in contrast, mucosal IgA antibody is primarily responsible for resistance to upper respiratory infection. The limited data available from humans suggest that this is true in humans as well.

Treatment

Amantadine and rimantadine are cyclic amines that arrest influenza A virus replication in vitro and are effective clinically for both prophylaxis and treatment. However, the utility of these drugs is limited by a relatively high incidence of adverse reactions, their narrow antiviral spectrum (influenza A virus only), and the propensity of this virus to become resistant.

Prevention

As mentioned above, serum (IgG) antibody to the major influenza surface proteins, the hemagglutinin and neuraminidase, prevents pulmonary infection, whereas mucosal (IgA) antibody is required to prevent infection of the upper respiratory tract and trachea. The presence of influenza-specific CTL also limits influenza virus infection. Although the protective antibody response is highly serotype-specific,

the CTL response tends to be much broader (so-called heterotypic immunity), in part because it is directed toward viral proteins (eg, the nucleoprotein), which are much more highly conserved among strains than are the hemagglutinin and neuraminidase.

Vaccines against influenza virus were developed within a few years after identification of the virus in 1933. Current vaccines are made from virus inactivated with formalin or β-propiolactone, but the viral antigens are separated from egg proteins to avoid sensitization or reaction to egg proteins. Vaccines are standardized by hemagglutinin concentration, the only viral antigen found in significant amounts in the vaccine. Influenza vaccine is given parenterally and thus stimulates serum IgG antibody but not mucosal IgA antibody or CTL. The strains of influenza A and B viruses used for vaccine production (influenza C virus is not included because of its minor public health importance) are changed annually to reflect the antigenic characteristics of current isolates, on the recommendations of the Centers for Disease Control and Prevention.

When given annually, influenza vaccines induce protection against both severe and mild influenza. Protection against infection per se is usually minimal or nonexistent. Protection is due entirely to the stimulation of antibodies directed against the hemagglutinin protein (see Table 48–2). The efficacy of the vaccine is limited by continuing antigenic variation in influenza A and B viruses, especially the extreme antigenic changes that occur in influenza A virus.

Influenza vaccines are relatively free of serious side effects, although painful local reactions are relatively common. At least one type of influenza virus—the swine influenza virus—has been associated with production of Guillain-Barré syndrome when administered as a vaccine. No other influenza virus type has yet been associated with this complication.

Research on improving influenza vaccines centers on development of live attenuated vaccines, insertion of hemagglutinin and neuraminidase genes into other vectors such as vaccinia virus, and attempts to find protective epitopes on molecules that are not subject to antigenic variation.

RESPIRATORY SYNCYTIAL VIRUS

Major Immunologic Features

- There is moderate antigenic variation of viral surface proteins.
- Immunity is imperfect, resulting in repeated infections throughout life.
- Infection of infants causes bronchospasm, perhaps as a result of IgE antibodies to respiratory syncytial virus.
- The host immune response probably contributes to disease.

General Considerations

Respiratory syncytial virus causes respiratory infections in children and adults. Infections occur in annual epidemics, commonly during the winter or rainy months. The disease causes severe pneumonia and bronchiolitis in infants, whereas upper respiratory infection predominates in adults.

Virology

Respiratory syncytial virus is an enveloped virus with a continuous, negative-stranded RNA genome. On the basis of antigenic and sequence analysis of the virion surface glycoproteins, F and G, two major groups (A and B) have been identified and there are subgroups of both, although the exact number is still uncertain. Most of the observed antigenic variation is in the G protein. The virus infects respiratory epithelium and causes extensive cytopathology, including characteristic syncytia. Recovery from infection is complete, and neither latent nor chronic infection occurs.

Clinical Features

The virus is spread through airborne droplets and by interpersonal contact through fomites. In infants 4–24 months of age, respiratory syncytial virus infection is frequent and is often associated with lower respiratory tract disease. It is the most common cause of bronchiolitis—pneumonia associated with bronchospasm and air trapping (Fig 48–2). The severity of disease is greatest in infants with underlying chronic cardiorespiratory conditions. Infection is diagnosed by recovery of the virus in tissue culture, by identification of viral antigens on desquamated respiratory epithelial cells with monoclonal antibodies, or by documentation of a serum antibody response. Precise virologic diagnosis is important because chemotherapy is available.

Immunologic Pathogenesis

Infection with respiratory syncytial virus stimulates both humoral and cellular immunity. Eradication of established infection is primarily a function of intact CTL, since patients with defective cellular immunity may become persistently infected with the virus. Antibody (against the F and G proteins) appears to partially protect against reinfection and disease, and maternal IgG antibody transferred transplacentally to the fetus confers some protection against

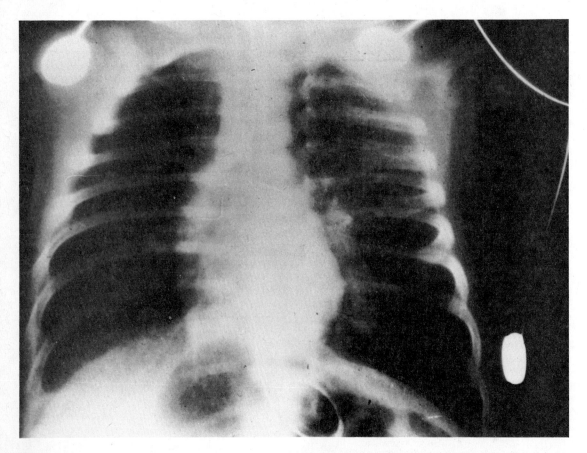

Figure 48–2. Chest x-ray of 1-year-old child with bronchiolitis due to respiratory syncytial virus, showing diffuse hyperinflation and air trapping with a left upper lobe infiltrate.

disease early in life. Passive transfer of antibody to both the F and G proteins, but particularly the former, is protective in experimental respiratory syncytial virus infection and in infants.

The pathogenesis of the wheezing and air trapping associated with respiratory syncytial virus infection in infancy is not fully understood. Allergy to the virus is one possibility, since infection stimulates virus-specific IgE antibody, which can result in mast cell degranulation. The severity of bronchiolitis is directly proportionate to the quantity of mast cell products in respiratory secretions. Some of the histopathologic changes are probably due to the CTL response to respiratory syncytial virus. In experimental animals, administration of CD4- and CD8-expressing respiratory syncytial virus T cell lines worsens pulmonary lesions. In vitro studies have also shown that respiratory syncytial virus infection of lymphocytes and macrophages can directly depress the function of these cells, perhaps restricting the protective antiviral immune response.

Treatment

A nucleotide analog, ribavirin, has been shown to accelerate the recovery of children with respiratory syncytial virus infection, and is licensed for this indication in the USA. The drug is aerosolized and administered by inhalation. Because of its high cost and marginal efficacy, this drug is generally used only for children with underlying chronic cardiorespiratory disease who are at risk for severe morbidity or mortality from respiratory syncytial virus infection.

In experimental animals, passive administration of antibodies to the F and G proteins (particularly the former) accelerates resolution of disease, and preliminary studies in infants are promising. Passive immunotherapy with various respiratory syncytial virus antibodies (high-titer human immune globulin and a humanized mouse anti-F monoclonal) are in progress.

Prevention

Many efforts to produce a vaccine have been made because of the morbidity and mortality rates associated with respiratory syncytial virus infection in infants. An immunogenic, formalin-inactivated whole respiratory syncytial virus vaccine was field-tested in the 1960s. In a placebo-controlled trial, the vaccine recipients had more severe disease after respiratory syncytial virus infection than did those who received the placebo. Recent studies of respiratory syncytial virus infection in animal models have shown that the CTL response to this virus is both critical to recovery from infection and a major determinant of severity of illness. A formalin-inactivated vaccine similar to that used in that clinical trial produced a feeble CTL response in mice and accentuated disease after respiratory syncytial virus challenge. This vaccine also produces a vigorous humoral response to the F and G

proteins, but the antibodies lack potent virus-neutralizing activity. Thus, although the mechanism(s) is still not wholly clear, the paradoxic response to this inactivated respiratory syncytial virus vaccine appears to have been immunologically mediated.

Promising new approaches to the prevention of respiratory syncytial virus infection include passive immunoprophylaxis with antibodies to the F (or F and G) virion surface proteins and an F protein vaccine. Clinical studies using both these approaches are under way.

MEASLES VIRUS

Major Immunologic Features

- There is a single viral serotype; either infection or immunization results in lifelong immunity.
- Acute infection depresses cellular immunity.
- The rash is due to the cellular immune response to virus in the skin.
- "Unbalanced" immune response to inactivated measles vaccine may produce atypical and severe disease after natural infection.

General Considerations

Measles virus causes an important acute exanthem of childhood and a chronic, slowly progressive neurologic disease, subacute sclerosing panencephalitis (SSPE), which may follow decades after an acute infection. The highly infectious virus is spread via respiratory secretions. Acute infection is associated with significant morbidity and mortality rates, especially in individuals in developing countries. An effective live, attenuated vaccine is available; if used widely, it could prevent nearly all cases.

Virology

Measles virus is a paramyxovirus with an envelope and a negative-stranded RNA genome. There is only one serotype, although minor sequence changes may occur in the surface glycoproteins of the virus. The virus has internal proteins, including a ribonucleoprotein and an RNA-dependent RNA polymerase, a matrix protein, and 2 envelope proteins, the fusion protein and a hemagglutinin. Acute infection of cells results in their death, commonly accompanied by syncytial giant cell formation.

Clinical Features

The virus is spread primarily via the airborne route, through the upper respiratory tract. After an incubation period of 9–11 days, during which the virus undergoes subclinical replication at unknown sites, perhaps in the lymphoreticular system, patients develop fever, cough, coryza, and conjunctivitis. Within 1 or 2 days, an erythematous, maculopapular rash develops, which quickly spreads over the entire body. In malnourished children, the disease is severe and enteritis is prominent. The main complications are bacterial superinfections, such as otitis media and pneumonia, and a postviral encephalitis.

Decades after the primary infection, a very small proportion of individuals develop SSPE, a chronic, progressive neurologic disorder due to persistent infection of the central nervous system. SSPE is caused by variants of measles virus with defects in the synthesis of matrix and envelope (fusion and hemagglutinin) genes. As a consequence, extracellular virus is not produced; infected cells do not produce viral antigens on their surface and thus are not removed by immune surveillance. A low-grade, persistent infection results in gradual neurologic injury. SSPE is particularly common in those who acquired measles before the age of 2 years.

In children who are vaccinated with inactivated measles virus vaccine, an "atypical" form of measles can occur, with acute infection, characterized by pleomorphic skin eruptions, including a vesicular rash, and pneumonitis. This condition is thought to be due to an unbalanced immune response to the virus (see below).

The diagnosis of measles can be made clinically in most cases. Lymphopenia is a characteristic laboratory abnormality in acute cases. The diagnosis may be confirmed by recovering the virus from blood or oropharyngeal secretions in tissue culture, by demonstrating viral antigen on leukocytes or respiratory epithelium, or by documenting the development of IgG antibodies to the virus during convalescence. The presence of IgM antibody to measles virus during the illness also confirms the diagnosis.

Immunologic Pathogenesis

Acute infection with measles virus markedly depresses cellular immunity, as measured by delayed hypersensitivity, skin test reactivity, or lymphocyte activation in vitro (see Chapter 13). In some cases, this immunosuppression is associated with reactivation of infections such as tuberculosis. Some suppression of antibody responses also occurs. The mechanism of the immunosuppression is unclear but is probably related to a direct effect of the virus on B and T lymphocytes. The postviral encephalitis that rarely complicates measles is probably due to the host immune response to viral antigens, perhaps cross-reacting with neural antigens.

Control of measles virus replication is a function of cellular immunity, and patients with defects in cellular immunity often develop progressive, fatal infections. In contrast, the virus is quickly eradicated in patients with intact cellular immunity. Immunodeficient patients usually fail to develop a rash, suggesting its dependence on T cell immunity.

Resistance to measles virus infection is primarily due to humoral immunity, specifically antibodies to the viral envelope proteins. Evidence for this is that resistance to measles virus may be conferred by passive administration of human IgG containing antibodies to the virus. Protective antibodies elicited by infection persist for life. Antibodies that develop in response to immunization may not persist as long, particularly if the vaccine was administered before 1–2 years of age.

The first measles vaccines were made from inactivated virus. Natural infection following such vaccination often resulted in severe disease, but with very atypical clinical features such as pneumonitis and vesicular skin rash. These early vaccines stimulated antibody to the viral hemagglutinin, but not to the fusion protein—in contrast to live virus vaccines or natural infection, in which a vigorous antibody response occurs to both proteins. This "unbalanced" immune response may be responsible for the atypical disease. Because the inactivated vaccine has not been used for decades, cases of atypical measles should now be rare.

Prevention

Resistance to disease following measles virus infection is predominantly a function of serum antibody, which results from natural infection, infection with attenuated vaccine strains of measles virus, or passive immunization. Passive administration of pooled human IgG (immune serum globulin [ISG] or intravenous immunoglobulins [IVIG]) is not a long-term control measure but is useful for postexposure prophylaxis of nonimmune subjects. It will prevent measles even if given up to 1 week after exposure.

Current measles vaccines are live, attenuated viruses given parenterally. They are extremely effective and prevent disease in more than 95% of those immunized. However, because measles virus is extremely infectious and highly communicable, herd immunity is negligible and epidemics can still occur even if more than 95% of the population has protective antibodies (ie, less than 5% of the population is susceptible). Thus, control of the disease requires high compliance with immunization guidelines. All children should be immunized unless they have a congenital or acquired defect in cellular immunity contraindicating live virus vaccination (see Chapter 55). Current cases of measles in the USA are largely attributable to immigration of unvaccinated individuals or poor vaccination of the indigenous population, although some recent cases have occurred in vaccinated individuals with subprotective antibody titers.

HEPATITIS B VIRUS

Major Immunologic Features

- There is a single viral serotype, with 8 major subtypes.
- Liver damage is secondary to antiviral cellular immune response.

- Acute and chronic immune complex disease may occur.
- Infection and immunization usually result in long-lasting, complete resistance to infection.
- Perinatal transmission can be prevented by passive antibody administration followed by active immunization.

General Considerations

Hepatitis B virus (HBV) is a major cause of acute and chronic hepatitis as well as hepatic carcinoma. The virus causes either acute, self-limited infection or a chronic infection that persists for the life of the host. Chronic carriers may remain infectious for life and are the major reservoir for the virus. It is estimated that there are more than 200 million chronic hepatitis B carriers worldwide.

Virology

HBV is a nonenveloped DNA virus with a unique structure and mode of replication. It is related to several other animal hepatitis viruses, which collectively are known as hepadnaviruses. They contain double-stranded DNA with a nicked or single-stranded region, and they replicate via an RNA intermediate. Virion genomic DNA is synthesized from the RNA intermediate, by a virion-encoded RNA-dependent DNA polymerase, which is structurally closely related to the reverse transcriptases of retroviruses, which are enveloped viruses with an RNA genome. The major proteins of HBV are the surface antigen (HBsAg) and core antigen (HBcAg). Although over 8 subtypes of the virus are recognized, this distinction is rarely of clinical importance. Following infection, the virus replicates primarily in hepatocytes, with production of large amounts of excess surface antigen, HBsAg, which then circulates in the blood. Acute infection may resolve, with complete elimination of the virus, or may be followed by chronic persistent infection in which viral cDNA persists and replicates either as an episome or integrated into the host genome. Persistent infection is associated with a high risk of hepatic carcinoma.

A defective RNA virus, hepatitis delta virus (HDV), can replicate only in HBV-infected cells, and thus causes infection only in patients with HBV infection. The delta virus genome codes for only one protein, delta antigen, and following replication, genomes of the progeny are packaged in HBsAg. HDV may be cotransmitted with HBV or may superinfect patients with chronic HBV infection.

Clinical Features

HBV is transmitted almost exclusively by sexual contact; parenteral inoculation of blood or blood products through transfusion, parenteral drug abuse, tattooing, or acupuncture; and from infected mothers to their infants during birth (perinatal transmission). The incubation period varies from 3–4 weeks to nearly 6 months; however, it is generally 1–2 months. The majority of infections are asymptomatic, although laboratory testing reveals "chemical" hepatitis with elevated transaminase levels and the presence of HBV infection (see below). Some 10–20% of infected patients will have symptomatic hepatitis, and about 1% of those will develop fatal fulminant hepatitis. A proportion of patients who recover from acute infection will then go on to chronic infection, which, in turn, may be asymptomatic or associated with chronic hepatitis. Chronic infection is a major risk factor for the development of hepatoma; the incubation period may be up to 40 years.

Age and ethnicity are major variables in determining the outcome of HBV infection. Infection of the neonate during birth is rarely associated with acute hepatitis, but more than half of those children will become lifelong carriers of HBV. In contrast, although hepatitis occurs in 10–20% of HBV infections acquired in adult life, chronic carriage occurs in fewer than 5% of cases. Asians appear to be at higher risk than whites for developing chronic carriage.

HDV is transmitted primarily by intravenous drug use, although some infections have been transmitted by sexual contact, particularly between homosexual men. HDV coinfection with HBV usually results in more severe disease than HBV infection alone; in some instances, the course of the disease is bimodal. HDV superinfection of patients chronically infected with HBV often results in marked worsening of the chronic hepatitis.

HBV infection was initially recognized and now is most frequently diagnosed by detection of the excess HBsAg present in serum during both acute and chronic infection. This antigen can be detected by a variety of standard immunologic tests; all are highly sensitive and specific. More than 95% of patients with acute and chronic infection will have antigen detected by these techniques. Screening of blood donors for HBsAg, as well as exclusion of paid donors, has dramatically reduced the incidence of HBV infection among recipients of blood and blood products.

Another useful test for the diagnosis of acute HBV infection is detection of the IgM antibody to core antigen (IgM anti-HBcAG), which, unlike HBsAg, is present only in patients with acute HBV infection. This test is useful for differentiating acute and chronic HBV infection and non-A, non-B hepatitis (Table 48–3). The antibody response to HBsAg tends to be delayed for several months following infection and hence is seldom used for diagnosis. However, the presence of either anti-HBsAg or anti-HBcAg indicates past infection. Fig 48–3 shows the time course of HBV serologic markers and the resulting host immune response in relation to infection.

Immunologic Pathogenesis

Hepatic damage following HBV infection is attributable primarily to the cellular immune response to

Table 48–3. Use of HBV markers for the diagnosis of hepatitis.

Markers Present in Serum			Diagnosis
HBsAg	IgM Anti-HBcAg	Anti-HBsAg	
+	+	−	Acute HBV infection.
−	+	−	Acute HBV infection (after HBsAg has disappeared).
+	−	±	Chronic HBV infection.
−	−	+[1]	Past HBV infection or HBV vaccination. Indicates immunity,.

[1]IgG-class anti-HBcAg also present if infection has occurred (not present following immunization).

the virus. HBV infection of hepatocytes by itself is noninjurious, and the clinical and laboratory findings of hepatitis do not appear unless CTL directed against the virus are generated. Thus, infection in patients with reduced cellular immunity (eg, neonates) tends to be asymptomatic. However, resolution of the acute infection and elimination of the virus also depend upon the same cellular immune response; hence, immunodeficient patients also have a much higher incidence of chronic persistent infection.

HBV infection is associated with overproduction (occasionally massive) of HBsAg. In some patients with acute HBV infection, simultaneous synthesis of anti-HBsAg results in immune-complex disease, manifested by fever, skin rashes, arthralgia, and arthritis. Glomerulonephritis is rare. These findings wane as HBsAg antibody levels increase and HBsAg levels fall, resulting from control of the infection by the cellular immune response. A small proportion of

patients with chronic HBV infection develop polyarteritis, which is probably also due to HBsAg immune complexes.

Treatment

Chronic HBV infection is associated with considerable morbidity and mortality, and given the large number (> 200 million) of chronic carriers known globally, there is an obvious need for chemotherapy. Alpha interferon has been licensed for treatment of chronic HBV infection in many countries, and with one or more courses of treatment about 50% of patients temporarily clear HBsAg and up to 25% appear to be cured. Interferon is probably not primarily an antiviral agent but instead acts by increasing the expression of class I HLA antigens on the surface of the hepatocytes, which facilitates their recognition by cytotoxic T lymphocytes. Several nucleoside analogues (including ganciclovir and penciclovir) have

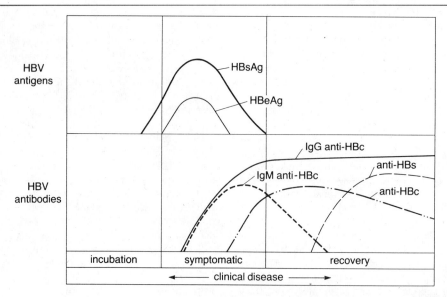

Figure 48–3. Schematic diagram showing temporal pattern of viral markers, illness, and antibody response in acute HBV infection.

shown anti-HBV activity in early clinical trials and may be useful adjuncts to alpha interferon therapy in the future.

Prevention

Cytotoxic T lymphocytes are critical to recovery from HBV infection and elimination of the virus. In contrast, resistance to HBV infection is mediated effectively by antibody to HBsAg alone. Administration of antibody to HBsAg prevents infection, and eliciting anti-HBsAg by immunization with inactivated or recombinant HBsAg confers resistance as well.

Preventive measures for HBV infection employ either pooled human immune serum globulin with high titers of antibody to HBsAg (hepatitis B immune globulin [HBIG]) or HBV vaccine. The latter consists of HBsAg, either purified from the plasma of chronic carriers or prepared by recombinant DNA techniques. Both types of vaccines are extremely safe and induce protective antibodies in more than 95% of individuals immunized.

Control measures may be implemented either in anticipation of infection or after infection has already occurred; the latter is known as "postexposure prophylaxis." Postexposure prophylaxis is indicated when a susceptible individual has been exposed to someone with active infection (ie, a patient with HBsAg in the blood), for example through sexual contact or a needle-stick injury. It is also administered postpartum to infants born to mothers with HBV infection. Passive immunity is achieved immediately by administration of HBIG. Then active immunity is stimulated by administration of HBV vaccine. Postexposure prophylaxis is highly effective, particularly if it is initiated within a few days of the exposure.

Preexposure immunization against HBV infection was formerly recommended only for individuals at high risk of HBV infection—for example, health care workers and intravenous drug users. However, there is now a reasonable consensus that universal hepatitis B immunization has a favorable cost-benefit ratio and should be instituted in most countries, including the USA. HBIG has no role in preexposure prophylaxis.

HEPATITIS A VIRUS

Hepatitis A virus (HAV) is closely related to other picornaviruses (small, nonenveloped RNA viruses) such as poliovirus. However, HAV has a different cell receptor and tissue tropism from other picornaviruses, and there are important although subtle differences in the replicative cycles. There is only a single strain. HAV is transmitted primarily by the fecal-oral route. Following ingestion, the virus travels via the bloodstream to the liver, the exclusive site of virus replication. Replication in the liver results in a brief period of viremia (5–10 days) and shedding of virus in the stools for 1–2 weeks. The infection resolves completely in all cases, except for rare instances of fatal infection. In contrast to HBV, chronic or latent infection does not occur. Resolution of infection is dependent on intact cellular immunity, since patients with cellular immunodeficiency may experience prolonged virus shedding and disease, similar to the case with other enteroviruses (see the section below on poliovirus).

The incubation period of HAV infection averages 30 days and ranges from 10 to 50 days. Most infections, especially those in children, are asymptomatic, although evidence of "chemical" hepatitis is usually found on laboratory testing. Liver cell injury is thought to be due primarily to the host cellular immune response, as in HBV infection. The mortality rate during acute infection is about 0.1% overall, but it is lower in children and increases with increasing age.

HAV infection generates a vigorous antibody response, which protects against reinfection and serves as the basis for diagnosis. Detection of the transient anti-HAV IgM response is the single most useful test for acute infection, whereas detection of the long-lasting anti-HAV IgG response is the best marker for past infection and resistance to subsequent infection. Infection may also be documented by demonstrating the development of IgG antibody response by comparing acute- and convalescent-phase serum specimens. However, this approach is cumbersome and may yield false-negative results, especially if the acute-phase serum specimen was obtained too long after the initial antibody response; thus, it is little used today. Unlike HBV, there is no serologic test for HAV antigen.

Resistance to HAV infection is mediated solely by serum antibody to the virus. This has been demonstrated by studies showing passive transfer of protection by immune globulin that contains antibody to HAV. Protection from HAV infection can be achieved with pooled human ISG given every 3–6 months. The intramuscular preparation is usually used, although intravenous immune globulin is also effective. Protection from illness may also be achieved by administration of ISG within 1 week following exposure to HAV. An inactivated HAV vaccine is now licensed in many countries; it is entirely safe and provides long-lasting protective antibodies. At present it is recommended primarily for residents of developed countries who are traveling to developing countries and who otherwise would have received immune globulin for protection. In the future, it may become part of the recommended panel of vaccines for universal immunization.

RABIES VIRUS

Rabies virus infection is enzootic in many wild animal species, including foxes, skunks, and bats. It can infect many domestic animals (dogs are the most commonly infected), although infection of domestic animals is unusual in developed countries because of the widespread application of control measures. When rabies virus infects humans, generally as the result of an animal bite, the resulting disease is virtually 100% fatal. Hence, preventive measures are of the utmost importance.

Rabies virus is an enveloped RNA virus that is related to several other animal viruses. Although only one serotype is detectable by the usual clinical criteria, studies with monoclonal antibodies have identified strains with differing geographic and host ranges. Following a bite wound, the virus replicates in muscles and nerves, extends centripetally along peripheral nerves over a period of days to months or even years, finally reaching the spinal cord and central nervous system. At this stage the hyperexcitability and hydrophobia characteristic of rabies occur. There are no effective antiviral drugs, and even with maximum supportive care, virtually every affected individual dies.

Because of the tremendous epidemiologic and public health implications of a case of rabies, the clinical diagnosis of rabies must be supported by laboratory data. Viral antigens can be detected by immunofluorescence with specific antisera or monoclonal antibodies in the brains of animals and humans and in corneal epithelial cells of humans. This technique is more sensitive than the histopathologic demonstration of Negri bodies. A diagnosis can also be made by demonstrating a rise in antibody titer following infection, although this is less useful clinically.

Animal data support a role for the host immune response in the pathogenesis of rabies. Although immunosuppression of animals prior to infection shortens the latency period and increases the mortality rate, immunosuppression after infection may delay mortality, even though brain virus titers are increased. In immunosuppressed animals with high brain virus titers, administration of rabies hyperimmune serum markedly worsens disease, further supporting the role of the immune system in production of illness.

Antibody to the virus surface glycoprotein (G protein) is protective. Individuals with serum antibody elicited by immunization are resistant to infection, and protection from disease can be achieved even after infection by administration of hyperimmune animal or human antibodies. These antibodies are effective only if given shortly after infection, and their efficacy is increased by local administration around the site of the bite wound, suggesting that they act by local neutralization of the virus.

The first rabies vaccines were prepared by Pasteur, who used virus that had been adapted to growth in rabbit neural tissue and then inactivated by heating and drying. Currently, many rabies vaccines are available; however, the only one used widely in developed countries is inactivated virus grown in human fibroblasts. This vaccine is highly immunogenic, protective if given either before or immediately after infection, and relatively free of serious side effects. Although animal-derived vaccines from rabbit or monkey brain or embryonated egg are effective in preventing rabies and are still available in many developing countries, the nervous-tissue antigens present in these products may cause allergic encephalitis in vaccine recipients. A vaccinia virus recombinant expressing the rabies virus G protein will infect animals if given orally (food bait laced with vaccine) and has proven effective in control of rabies in wildlife. G-protein vaccines made by recombinant DNA technology may be available for humans in the near future.

POLIOVIRUS

Poliovirus is the cause of poliomyelitis, an acute encephalomyelitis that results in asymmetric paralysis with muscle atrophy. Although cases of paralysis almost certainly due to poliovirus have been recognized for thousands of years, the 20th century has seen a marked increase in the incidence of the disease and a change from endemic to epidemic spread. Development of poliovirus vaccine in the middle of the twentieth century and its widespread application in developed countries have resulted in the virtual elimination of the disease in vaccinated populations.

Poliovirus is a member of the picornavirus family, which consists of small, nonenveloped positive-stranded RNA viruses and includes other enteroviruses (echovirus, coxsackie-virus etc), rhinoviruses, and HAV. Although closely related by structure, mode of replication, and RNA sequence homology, these viruses exhibit tremendous antigenic diversity, and there is little or no serologic relatedness or cross-resistance among them. Poliovirus has 3 non-cross-reactive serotypes, serotypes 1, 2, and 3. Infection generates a vigorous cellular and humoral immune response to the coat proteins of the virus.

Patients infected with poliovirus and the other enteroviruses shed large amounts of virus in the feces, often for periods of weeks or months. Infection is transmitted when a susceptible individual ingests food or water contaminated by infected feces. The virus replicates in the intestinal tract, and viremia occurs; this is followed by seeding of the spinal cord and central nervous system. Although most patients (> 99%) recover without sequelae, the remainder suffer some degree of motor nerve dysfunction, which varies from minimal weakness of an extremity to severe paralysis of all major muscle groups. Partial or complete recovery may occur after the acute illness.

Resolution of infection and elimination of the virus appear to require intact cellular immune mechanisms, since patients with defective cellular immunity continue to shed poliovirus as well as other enteroviruses for months or years after infection. However, antibodies play some role in recovery from infection, since patients with isolated hypogammaglobulinemia have persistent enterovirus infections. Resistance to disease is mediated by serum neutralizing antibody to virion surface antigens. Administration of pooled human ISG containing antibodies to poliovirus will prevent the disease, even if given a few days after exposure. In addition, inactivated vaccines that stimulate humoral but not cellular immunity are also highly protective. Intestinal infection can still occur in the presence of serum antibodies; however, viremia with seeding of the central nervous system does not occur. Intestinal mucosal IgA (coproantibody) antibody to poliovirus is stimulated by natural infection and immunization with live attenuated (Sabin-type) vaccine and will prevent infection.

The first poliovirus vaccine consisted of tissue-culture-grown suspensions of poliovirus types 1–3, which were inactivated with formalin. Although in-activated (Salk) vaccine is highly effective for preventing paralytic poliomyelitis, it has several disadvantages. It requires parenteral injection (hence, there is an increased cost for needles and syringes); booster doses are required to maintain immunity; and it does not displace wild-type poliovirus circulating in the community. Live, attenuated (Sabin) vaccine can be given orally; it does not routinely require booster doses; and when immunization is widespread in a community, the vaccine virus displaces the wild-type virus in the environment, thus reducing the risk of paralytic disease among the unimmunized. However, live poliovirus may rarely revert to virulence, producing paralytic disease in vaccinees or their contacts.

Both inactivated and live attenuated poliovirus vaccines are manufactured and used today, although either one or the other is usually selected by national vaccination programs. For example, the live attenuated virus is used in the USA; inactivated virus is used in Scandinavia. Although the choice between live and inactivated virus vaccine is often the subject of heated debate, either type of vaccine will virtually eliminate paralytic poliomyelitis if used widely. Active investigation is under way to improve both the live attenuated and inactivated vaccines.

REFERENCES

General

McChesney MB, Oldstone MBA: Virus-induced immunosuppression: Infections with measles virus and human immunodeficiency virus. *Adv Immunol* 1989; **45**:335.

Quinnan GV Jr: Immunology of viral infections. Chapter 5 in: *Textbook of Human Virology.* Belshe RB (editor). PSG Publishing Co, 1984.

Tyler KL, Fields BN: Pathogenesis of viral infections. Chapter 10 in: *Virology,* 2nd ed. Fields BN et al (editors). Raven Press, 1990.

Whitton JL, Oldstone MBA: Virus-induced immune response interactions: Principles of immunity and immunopathology. Chap 15 in: *Virology,* 2nd ed. Fields BN et al (editors), Raven Press, 1990.

Influenza Virus

Ada GL, Jones PD: The immune response to influenza infection. *Curr Top Microbiol Immunol* 1986;**128**:1.

Air GM, Laver WG, Webster RG: Antigenic variation in influenza viruses. *Contrib Microbiol Immunol* 1987; **8**:20.

Askonas BA, Taylor PM, Esquivel F: Cytotoxic T cells in influenza infection. *Ann NY Acad Sci* 1988; **532**:230.

Bender BS, Small PA: Influenza: Pathogenesis and host defense. *Semin Respir Infect* 1992;**7**:38.

Klenk HD, Rott, R: The molecular biology of influenza virus pathogenicity. *Adv Virus Res* 1988;**34**:247.

Murphy BR, Webster RG: Orthomyxoviruses. Chapter 40 in: *Virology,* 2nd ed. Fields BN et al (editors). Raven Press, 1990.

Respiratory Syncytial Virus

Conners M et al: Pulmonary histopathology induced by respiratory syncytial virus (RSV) challenge of formalin-inactivated RSV-immunized BALB/c mice is abrogated by depletion of CD4+ T cells. *J Virol* 1992; **66**:7444.

Groothuis JR et al: The RSVIG Study Group. Use of intravenous gamma globulin to passively immunize high-risk children against respiratory syncytial virus: Safety and pharmacokinetics. *Antimicrob Agents Chemother* 1991;**35**:1469.

Graham BS et al: Role of T lymphocyte subsets in the pathogenesis of primary infection and rechallenge with respiratory syncytial virus in mice. *J Clin Invest* 1991;**88**:1026.

Josephs S et al: Parainfluenza 3 virus and other common respiratory pathogens in children with human immunodeficiency virus infection. *Pediatr Infect Dis J* 1988;**7**:207.

Kakuk TJ et al: A human respiratory syncytial virus (RSV) primate model of enhance pulmonary pathology induced with a formalin-inactivated RSV vaccine but not a recombinant FG subunit vaccine. *J Infect Dis* 1993;**167**:553.

McIntosh K, Chanock RM: Respiratory syncytial viruses. Chapter 38 in: *Virology,* 2nd ed. Fields BN et al (editors). Raven Press, 1990.

Tristram DA et al: Immunogenicity and safety of respiratory syncytial virus subunit vaccine in seropositive children 18–36 months old. *J Infect Dis* 1993;**167:**191.

Measles Virus

Johnson ERT, Griffin DE, Moench TR: Pathogenesis of measles immunodeficiency and encephalomyelitis: Parallels to AIDS. *Microb Pathog* 1988;**4:**169.

Norrby E, Oxman MN: Measles. Chapter 37 in: *Virology,* 2nd ed. Fields BN et al (editors). Raven Press, 1990.

ter Meulen V: Autoimmune reactions against myelin basic protein induced by corona and measles viruses. *Ann NY Acad Sci* 1988;**540:**202.

Hepatitis B Virus

Chisari FV: Hepatitis B virus biology and pathogenesis. *Mol Genet Med* 1992;**2:**67.

Ferrari C et al: Immune pathogenesis of hepatitis B. *Arch Virol Suppl* 1992;**4:**11.

Gowans EJ, Bonino F: Hepatitis delta virus pathogenicity. *Prog Clin Biol Res* 1993;**382:**125.

Hepatitis A Virus

Coulepsis AG, Anderson BN, Gust ID: Hepatitis A. *Adv Virus Res* 1987;**32:**129.

Rabies Virus

Baer GM: Rabies virus. In: *Virology.* Fields BN et al (editors). Raven Press, 1990.

King AA, Turner GS: Rabies: A review. *J Comp Pathol* 1993;**108:**1.

Poliovirus

Kinnunen L, Poyry T, Hovi T: Genetic diversity and rapid evolution of poliovirus in human hosts. *Curr Top Microbiol Immunol* 1992;**176:**49.

Minor PD: Attenuation and reversion of the Sabin vaccine strains of poliovirus. *Dev Biol Stand* 1993;**78:**17.

Fungal Diseases

49

David J. Drutz, MD

Infectious disease caused by fungi are called **mycoses.** Fungi, like mammalian cells, are eukaryotes; ie, they possess a true nucleus containing several chromosomes, bounded by a nuclear membrane. In contrast, bacteria are prokaryotes, with a single linear chromosome and no true nucleus. The principal sterol of the mammalian cell membrane is cholesterol; that of fungi is ergosterol. Ergosterol is the target of amphotericin B and the antifungal azoles and triazoles. Fungal cell walls have no counterpart in mammalian cells, and they differ from those of bacteria by lacking peptidoglycans, teichoic acids, and lipopolysaccharides (endotoxin). In their place are the external and antigenic **peptidomannans** embedded in matrices of **α-** and **β-glucans**; structural rigidity is provided by sheets, disks, or fibrils of **chitin** (poly β-1,4-N-acetylglucosamine). Recent RNA typing studies and electron-microscopic analysis have suggested that *Pneumocystis carinii* might be more appropriately classified as a fungus rather than a protozoon. The reclassification is unsettled. Although chitin and β-glucans are components of the *P carinii* cyst wall, the organism does not contain ergosterol or the characteristic protein elongation factor 3 found in fungi. Moreover, antifungal drugs have no effect on *P carinii,* whereas antiprotozoal drugs do.

Although there are thousands of fungi in nature, relatively few are pathogenic for normal humans. Table 49–1 lists common mycoses according to the usual sites of infection. Superficial mycoses usually occur on the body external to common immunologic influences. Cutaneous mycoses produced delayed hypersensitivity responses to the local presence of keratinolytic fungi. Subcutaneous and systemic mycoses represent successful challenges to major immunologic host defense mechanisms. Some systemic mycoses (eg, blastomycosis, coccidioidomycosis, histoplasmosis, and paracoccidiodomycosis) are due to primary pathogens, theoretically capable of infecting anyone present in an endemic area. Others (eg, candidiasis, cryptococcosis, aspergillosis, and muc-

ormycosis [zygomycosis]) are due to opportunistic pathogens, which seldom cause life-threatening tissue invasion in the absence of impaired host defenses. Except for *Malassezia* and *Pityrosporum* spp, *Candida albicans, C tropicalis,* and *C glabrata,* most fungi reach the body from the external environment. Most primary invasive mycoses are acquired by the inhalation of specialized forms (conidia and spores) that are progeny of filamentous soil forms of the fungi. Once inhaled, some fungi reproduce in the body in the original filamentous (mycelial, hyphal) form. Others adopt specialized forms (yeasts, spherules, and endospores) more suitable for host survival and tissue invasion. The latter fungi are referred to as **dimorphic fungi.** Table 49–1 indicates the forms assumed by common fungi when invading host tissues. A major attribute of all opportunistic filamentous fungi is the tendency to invade blood vessels (**angioinvasion**), with resultant tissue infarction (Table 49–2).

Immunity to the mycoses is principally cellular, involving neutrophils, macrophages, lymphocytes, and probably natural killer (NK) cells. With the possible exception of the dermatophytes and *Rhizopus arrhizus,* the principal etiologic agent of mucormycosis (zygomycosis), fungi are not susceptible to direct killing by antibody and complement. Patients with neutropenia or defective neutrophil function appear predisposed to hematogenously disseminated infection with yeastlike fungi (eg, *Candida* spp, *Trichosporon beigelii*), or with filamentous fungi (eg, *aspergillus,* agents causing mucormycosis, and *Fusarium* spp). Patients with defective cell-mediated immunity (CMI) (eg, acquired immunodeficiency syndrome [AIDS] sufferers) are predisposed to mucosal candidiasis or hematogenously disseminated cryptococcosis, histoplasmosis and coccidioidomycosis (Table 49–3). Allergy to fungi is discussed in Chapters 24–28.

Salient features of the superficial, cutaneous, and subcutaneous mycoses may be found in Tables 49–1

Table 49–1. Common mycoses according to usual sites of disease production.

Site and Disease	Etiologic Agents	Origin	Invasive Form	Pathophysiologic Basis	Principal Clinical Features
Superficial mycoses Pityriasis (tinea) versicolor	*Malassezia* and *Pityrosporum* spp.	Hair follicle (yeasts)	Yeasts and/or mycelia	Decreased epithelial turnover allows normal flora to produce disease.	Flat, branny skin lesions; variously pigmented or nonpigmented.
Pityrosporum folliculitis	*Malassezia* and *Pityrosporum* spp	Hair follicle (yeasts)	Yeasts	Obstructed hair follicles are damaged by follicular flora.	Acneiform folliculitis.
Tinea nigra	*Phaeoannelomyces werneckii*	Soil (mycelia)	Mycelia	Hyperhidrosis permits infection from environment.	Brown-black nonscaly macules (especially on palms).
White piedra	*Trichosporon beigelii*	Soil, skin (mycelia)	Mycelia and yeasts	Poor personal hygiene permits infection from environment or by normal flora.	Soft whitish nodules on hair shaft.
Black piedra	*Piedraia hortai*	Soil (mycelia)	Mycelia	Poor personal hygiene permits infection from environment.	Hard gritty black nodules on hair shaft.
Cutaneous mycoses Dermatophytosis	*Epidermophyton, Trichophyton,* and *Microsporum* spp	Soil and animal fur (mycelia)	Mycelia	Etiologic agents are keratinolytic; infection is potentiated by warmth, moisture, and occlusion; cutaneous inflammation is due to delayed-hyper-sensitivity reaction.	Tinea pedis (scaly, vesicular, ulcerative), tinea cruris (dry, red, scalloped, expanding), tinea corporis (ringworm), tinea barbae (suppuration, beard), tinea capitis (scalp; resembles seborrhea), tinea unguium (nails).
Subcutaneous mycoses Chromoblastomycosis	*Cladosporium, Fonsecaea, Philaophora,* and *Rhinocladiella* spp	Soil (mycelia)	Mycelia and sclerotic bodies	Traumatic implantation.	Papules, warty tumors, plaques, cauliflowerlike growths.
Mycetoma	*Acremonium, Exophiala, Leptosphaeria, Madurella, Microsporum, Neotestudina,* and *Pseudallescheria* spp	Soil (mycelia)	Mycelia and grains	Traumatic implantation.	Swelling, draining fistulae, pus, and grains.
Sporotrichosis	*Sporothrix schenckii*	Vegetation (mycelia)	Yeasts	Traumatic implantation.	Subcutaneous nodules along lymphatics.
Systemic invasive mycoses Primary pathogens Blastomycosis	*Blastomyces dermatitidis*	Soil (mycelia)	Yeasts	Inhalation of conidia.	Pulmonary, spreading to skin, bones, male reproductive tract.
Coccidioidomycosis	*Coccidioides immitis*	Soil (mycelia)	Spherules and endospores	Inhalation of arthroconidia.	Pulmonary, spreading to skin, bones, joints, meninges.

(continued)

Table 49–1. Common mycoses according to usual sites of disease production (*continued*).

Site and Disease	Etiologic Agents	Origin	Invasive Form	Pathophysiologic Basis	Principal Clinical Features
Histoplasmosis	*Histoplasma capsulatum*	Soil (mycelia)	Yeasts	Inhalation of microconidia.	Pulmonary, spreading to reticuloendothelial system, mucous membranes, adrenals.
Paracoccidioidomycosis	*Paracoccidioides brasiliensis*	Soil (mycelia)	Yeasts	Inhalation of conidia.	Pulmonary, spreading to reticuloendothelial system, skin, mucous membranes, adrenals.
Opportunistic pathogens Candidiasis	Principally *Candida albicans,* *C tropicalis,* and *T glabrata*	Mucosal surfaces (yeasts, pseudomycelia)	Yeasts, pseudomycelia, mycelia	Local extension; bloodstream invasion from colonization sites (mucosal disruption).	Mucosal site, spreading to eyes, skin, kidneys, myocardium, other sites.
Cryptococcosis	*Cryptococcus neoformans*	Soil (yeast, possibly mycelia)	Yeasts	Inhalation of desiccated yeasts or basidiospores.	Pulmonary, spreading to meninges, brain, bone, skin.
Aspergillosis	*Aspergillus fumigatus, A flavus,* and *A niger,* principally	Soil (mycelia)	Mycelia	Inhalation of conidia.	Invasive pulmonary or sinus disease, leading to hematogenous dissemination.
Mucormycosis (zygomycosis)	*Rhizopus, Absidia, Cunninghamelia, Mortierella,* and *Saksenaea* spp	Soil (mycelia)	Mycelia	Inhalation of spores.	Invasive sinus or pulmonary disease, leading to hematogeneous dissemination.
Pneumocystosis	*Pneumocystis carinii*	Unknown	Cysts and trophozoites	Inhalation of infective particles or arousal from latency.	Progressive interstitial lung disease with or without cysts, pneumothorax.
Phaeohyphomycosis	Approximately 40 genera of pigmented fungi (eg, *Alternaria, Bipolaris, Cladosporium, Exserohilum, phialophora, Wangiella*)	Soil (mycelia)	Mycelia	Inhalation or implantation of common environmental fungi (pigmented; dematiaceous).	Invasive sinus or pulmonary disease, leading to hematogenous dissemination.
Hyalohyphomycosis	Diverse nonpigmented fungi (eg, *Fusarium, Paecilomyces, Pseudaliescheria, Scopulariopsis*)	Soil (mycelia)	Mycelia	Inhalation or implantation of common environmental fungi (nonpigmented)	Invasive sinus or pulmonary disease, leading to hematogenous dissemination.

Table 49–2. Pathologic features of subcutaneous and systemic mycoses.

Mycosis	Predominant Location of Fungi	Suppuration	Granulomas	Caseation	Fibrosis	Calcification	Other
Subcutaneous Chromomycosis	Extracellular (sclerotic bodies)	Dominant	Dominant	Rare	Dominant	Rare	PH[1]; transdermal elimination.
Mycetoma	Extracellular (grains)	Dominant	Dominant	Rare	Dominant	Rare	Grain color varies by etiologic agent; grains surrounded by amorphous material reflecting immune complex deposition (Hoeppli-Splendore phenomenon).
Sporotrichosis	Intracellular and extracellular (yeasts)	Dominant	Dominant	Occasional	Occasional	Rare	Asteroid bodies with Hoeppli-Splendore phenomenon.
Systemic Primary pathogens Blastomycosis[2]	Extracellular (yeasts)	Dominant	Dominant	Rare	Occasional	Occasional	PH.
Coccidioidomycosis[2]	Extracellular (spherules)	Dominant (endospores)	Dominant (spherules)	Rare	Occasional	Occasional	PH.
Histoplasmosis	Intracellular (yeasts)	Rare	Dominant	Occasional	Dominant	Dominant	Proliferative endarteritis (lungs).
Paracoccidioidomycosis[2]	Extracellular (yeasts)	Dominant	Dominant	Rare	Dominant	Occasional	PH.
Opportunistic pathogens Cryptococcosis[2]	Extracellular (yeasts)	Rare	Dominant	Rare	Rare	Rare	Extensive accumulation of extracellular capsular material may produce local anatomic distortions.
Candidiasis[3]	Intracellular (yeasts), extracellular (pseudomycelia, mycelia)	Dominant	Rare	Rare	Rare	Rare	Granuloma formation common only with CMCC.
Aspergillosis[3]	Extracellular (mycelia)	Dominant	Rare	Rare	Rare	Rare	Angioinvasion and infarction.
Mucormycosis (zygomycosis)[3]	Extracellular (mycelia)	Dominant	Rare	Rare	Rare	Rare	Angioinvasion and infarction.
Pneumocystosis	Extracellular (trophozoites, cysts)	Rare	Rare	None	Occasional	Rare	Foamy intra-alveolar infiltrate and alveolar epithelial damage.

[1]PH, Pseudoepitheliomatous hyperplasia of skin and mucosal lesions.
[2]Severely depressed CMI is often associated with poor granuloma formation and increased suppuration with increased numbers of microorganisms (blastomycosis, coccidioidomycosis, paracoccidioidomycosis) or with gelatinous masses of encapsulated fungi (cryptococcosis).
[3]Severe neutropenia is often associated with loss of suppurative tissue response.

Table 49–3. Effect of common immunologic abnormalities on disease course of common mycoses.

Mycosis	Reduction in PMN[1]	Reduction in CMI[2]	Other
Superficial			
Pityriasis (tinea) versicolor	None	None	Lipid hyperalimentation therapy is associated with *Malassezia* and *Pityrosporum* fungemia and pulmonary vasculitis, especially in infants
Pityrosporum folliculitis	None	None	Treatment with corticosteroids predisposes to folliculitis
Tinea nigra	None	None	
White piedra	Hematogenous dissemination of *T beigelii* [4]	None	
Black piedra	None	None	
Cutaneous			
Dermatophytosis	None	Increased severity and chronicity of *T rubrum* infection	
Subcutaneous			
Chromomycosis	None	None	
Mycetoma	None	None	
Sporotrichosis	None	Increase in severity and likelihood of dissemination	
Systemic, invasive			
Primary pathogens			
Blastomycosis	None	Increase in severity and likelihood of dissemination	Frequency of meningitis is increased in patients with AIDS
Coccidioidomycosis	None	Definite increase in severitry and dissemination	Possible increase in severity and dissemination in second and third trimesters of pregnancy
Histoplasmosis	None	Definite increase in severity and dissemination	
Paracoccidioidomycosis	None	Probable increase in severity or likelihood of dissemination	
Opportunistic pathogens			
Candidiasis	Hematogenous dissemination	Increased severity of mucosal disease	
Cryptococcosis	None	Definite increase in severity and dissemination	
Aspergillosis	Invasive paranasal sinus and respiratory infection, and hematogenous dissemination	Probable increase in severity	
Mucormycosis (zygomycosis)	Invasive paranasal sinus and respiratory infection, and hematogenous dissemination	Possible increase in severity	Diabetic ketoacidosis predisposes to invasive paranasal sinus infection
Pneumocystosis	None	Drastic increase in incidence and severity in AIDS	
Phaeohyphomycosis	Invasive paranasal sinus infection and hematogenous dissemination	None	
Hyalohyphomycoses	Invasive paranasal sinus infection and hematogenous dissemination	None	

[1] < 500 PMN/dL.
[2] Principally AIDS. Histoplasmosis, coccidioidomycosis, and cryptococcosis also occur with increased severity and/or extent of dissemination in patients with other causes of depressed CMI (eg, immunosuppression for organ transplantation).
[3] *Malassezia* and *Pityrosporum* are lipophilic fungi. Lipid hyperalimentation therapy allows them to gain access to the bloodstream. Patients with *Malassezia* and *Pityrosporum* fungemia do not have tinea versicolor or folliculitis.
[4] Patients with *T beigelii* sepsis do not necessarily have white piedra.

to 49–4. The major systemic invasive mycoses found in the Western hemisphere are described below.

SYSTEMIC INVASIVE MYCOSES: PRIMARY PATHOGENS

BLASTOMYCOSIS

Major Immunologic Features
- Yeasts are large and singly-budding and commonly exceed the size of phagocytes.
- Islands of suppuration (microabscesses) amid granulomas are produced.
- Both neutrophils and CMI may play important and concomitant roles in host defense.
- It may be more severe in patients with defective CMI, including those with AIDS.

General Considerations
Blastomycosis is an inhalation-acquired mycosis that can produce primary pulmonary infection or hematogenously disseminated disease involving predominantly skin, bones, and the male genitourinary tract. *Blastomyces dermatitidis,* the cause of this disease, is a spherical multinucleated yeast with thick walls and single broad-based buds. The mycelial form of *B dermatitidis* is a soil organism found on river banks predominantly in the south-central USA and around the Great Lakes. A closely related fungus occurs in Africa. Infection occurs by inhalation of fungal microconidia in endemic areas (eg, by hunters, trappers, campers, or boaters). Hunters and their dogs have been simultaneously infected. There are sporadic and occasionally common-source outbreaks. Areas where the disease is endemic are defined by the occurrence of cases and by seroconversions. There is no reliable skin test to gauge population exposures. No convincing sex or age prevalence is apparent in common-source outbreaks. Men are more susceptible than women to progressive pulmonary or hematogenous disease. There is no known genetic predisposition.

Pathology
See Table 49–2.

Clinical Features
A. Signs and Symptoms: Primary exposure may be asymptomatic, or it may produce an influenzalike syndrome. Pneumonia, pleuritis, pulmonary cavitation, and mediastinal adenopathy may occur. Hematogenous dissemination may occur in the presence or absence of apparent pulmonary disease. Favored sites of metastic infection include skin (pap-

ules, pustules, or verrucous granulomas that heal centrally and extend peripherally); bone (lytic lesions, especially vertebrae and long bones, with or without draining sinuses); and prostate, testis, and epididymis. Central nervous system infection occurs in about 5% of cases, but this increases to 40% in patients with AIDS. Gastrointestinal tract involvement almost never occurs.

B. Laboratory Findings: These include leukocytosis, abnormal chest x-ray, and evidence of specific organ dysfunction at metastatic loci. Diagnosis is established by finding large budding yeasts on smears or histologic sections and by recovering the fungus in culture.

C. Immunologic Diagnosis: See Table 49–4. With the possible exception of antibody directed against the A antigen, immunologic tests lack either sensitivity or specificity.

D. Differential Diagnosis: This includes diverse granulomatous infectious diseases (eg, other mycoses and tuberculosis), sarcoidosis, and pulmonary cancer.

E. Treatment: Itraconazole is highly effective and has fewer side effect than ketoconazole when used to treat chronic, indolent forms of blastomycosis. For patients with meningitis or acute life-threatening infections, intravenous amphotericin B is preferable.

F. Prevention: No vaccine is available.

G. Complications and Prognosis: Untreated extrapulmonary blastomycosis carries a 20–90% mortality rate, depending on the individual series. The mortality rate with therapy is less than 10%. Most relapses occur within 1 year of treatment, but they have been documented after as long as 9 years.

COCCIDIOIDOMYCOSIS

Major Immunologic Features
- Inhaled arthroconidia have an antiphagocytic surface.
- Spherules exceed the size of phagocytes and have an antiphagocytic surface.
- Endospores are released in packets that exceed the size of phagocytes.
- Mixed granulomas and suppuration occur.
- Primary infections may be signaled by erythema nodosum or erythema multiforme.
- Negative skin test (coccidioidin, spherulin) and high complement fixation antibody titer suggest hematogenous dissemination.
- Disease is much more severe with defective CMI (including AIDS).
- Infection confers solid immunity.

General Considerations
Coccidioidomycosis is an inhalation-acquired mycosis that can produce primary pulmonary infection,

Table 49–4. Immunologic diagnosis of subcutaneous and systemic mycoses.

Mycosis	Serologic Tests[1]		Delayed Hypersensitivity Skin Test[1,2]	Comments[1,3]
	Antibody	Antigen		
Subcutaneous Chromoblasto-mycosis	None	None	None	Chromoblastomycosis is diagnosed by its characteristic clinical appearance (warty plaques, nodules, and cauliflowerlike excrescences), together with the demonstration of characteristic pigmented sclerotic bodies in histologic sections. Specific etiologic diagnoses must be established by culture.
Mycetoma	None	None	None	Mycetoma is diagnosed by its characteristic clinical picture (sinuses discharging pus and grains). Specific etiologic diagnosis rests upon microscopic examination of grains and cultures of grains and biopsy material.
Sporotrichosis	EIA, TA, LPA (sensitive/specific) CF, ID (less sensitive)	None	Investigational only	Serologic tests are generally valuable only in extracutaneous and disseminated infection. A slide latex agglutination titer of ≥ 1:8 is presumptive evidence of disseminated or systemic infection.
Systemic Primary pathogens Blastomycosis	ID, CF (blastomycin as antigen); ID, CF EIA (A antigen)	None	Blastomycin (mycelial phase), BASWS (investigational only)	The blastomycin skin test and serologic tests lack sensitivity and specificity; there is major cross-reactivity with histoplasmosis. Tests for antibody to A antigen are more specific (especially ID and EIA).
Coccidioidomy-cosis	IgM (TP, IDTP, LPA); IgG (CF, IDCF) (coccidioidin as antigen)	Experimental only	Coccidioidin (mycelial phase), spherulin (spherule phase)	IgM tests are positive early and transiently; IgG tests are positive later and more persistently. A CF antibody titer in blood > 1:16 suggests hematogenous dissemination, especially if skin tests are negative. A positive CF titer in the cerebrospinal fluid is virtually diagnostic of meningitis.
Histoplasmosis	CF (whole yeast cells as antigen); CF (histoplasmin as antigen); ID (histoplasmin as antigen); LPA (histoplasmin as antigen)	Experimental only: RIA useful for antigen detection in urine serum CSF (see text); not available commercially	Histoplasmin (mycelial phase), histolyn CYL (yeast phase)	A positive histoplasmin skin test can artificially elevate CF antibody titers and produce a positive ID test ("m" band). Histolyn CYL is less likely to do this. An ID antibody "h" band suggests active infection. An LPA antibody titer ≥ 1:32 suggests active infection. A CF antibody titer ≥ 1:32 or a four-fold titer rise suggests active infection.
Paracoccidioido-mycosis	ID, CIE (simple, more specific) CF, EIA (sensitive; less specific)	None	Various "paracoccidioidins" (mycelial phase), investigational only	Elevated precipitin titers (transient) precede elevated CF titers (more persistent). The number and duration of precipitin bands are directly proportional to disease activity. The CF titer is directly proportional to the severity of illness. The skin test is commonly negative with active disease.

(continued)

Table 49–4. Immunologic diagnosis of subcutaneous and systemic mycoses (*continued*).

Mycosis	Serologic Tests[1]		Delayed Hypersensitivity Skin Test[1,2]	Comments[1,3]
	Antibody	Antigen		
Opportunistic pathogens Cryptococcosis	IFA, EIA, TA	Capsular polysaccharide (LPA, EIA)	"Cryptococcin" (investigational only)	Cryptococcal skin tests and tests for antibody lack sensitivity and specificity. The LPA for cryptococcal antigen is highly sensitive and specific. Rare (low-titer) cross-reactivity with *T beigelii*. A positive cerebrospinal fluid test is diagnostic of cryptococcal meningitis.
Candidiasis	Multiple, diverse serologic tests (precipitins, agglutinins most common; CIE, IHA, IFA, RIAID, LPA	Mannan (LPA, EIA, RIA, coagglutination), enolase 48-k Da cytoplasmic protein (LIA, EIA, DIA), undefined heat-labile glycoprotein antigen (LPA), D-arabinitol, D-mannose (GLC)	Oidiomycin	Skin tests lack diagnostic value (healthy persons are positive). Antibody tests lack sensitivity and specificity, especially in immunosuppressed patients. Mannan antigen tests are positive in low titer, generally too late in the course of illness to be useful diagnostically. Heat-labile antigen lacks sensitivity and specificity in immunocompromised patients. Tests for mannose and arabinitol are not of proven diagnostic efficacy.
Aspergillosis	Multiple, diverse serologic tests (precipitins most common)	Galactomannan (RIA, EIA)	"Aspergillin"	More than 90% of patients with ABPA have positive *Aspergillus* skin tests and precipitin titer elevation. More than 90% of patients with aspergilloma have precipitin titer elevation. Serologic tests for antibody lack sensitivity and are without value in patients with invasive aspergillosis. Galactomannan antigen detection (experimental) is not of proven efficacy in diagnosis.
Mucormycosis (zygomycosis)	EIA, ID	None	None	Serologic tests for zygomycosis have been unsuccessful owing to poor antibody response to the antigens that have been tested. The disease moves with such rapidity that death may occur before characteristic antibody uses can be documented.

[1]Abbreviations: BASWS, an alkali-soluble, water-soluble blastomycosis skin test preparation; BF, bentonite flocculation; CIE, counterimmunoelectrophoresis; CF, complement fixation; DIA, dot immunoassay; EIA, enzyme immunoassay; ID, immunodiffusion; IDCF, immunodiffusion with the CF antigen; IDTP, immunodiffusion with the TP antigen; IFA, indirect immunofluorescence assay; IHA, indirect hemagglutination; GLC, gas-liquid chromatography; LIA, liposomal immunoassay; LPA, latex particle agglutination; PHA, passive hemagglutination; RIA, radioimmunoassay; TA, tube agglutination; TP, tube precipitin; YCA, whole yeast cell agglutination.

[2]Skin tests are predominantly of epidemiologic importance, defining loci of endemnicity. A positive skin test indicates only that infection has occurred in the past. Some skin tests (especially histoplasmin) can influence serologic test results.

[3]In vitro correlates of CMI (eg, lymphocyte blastogenesis and migration inhibition) have been studied extensively, but are insufficiently standardized for routine diagnostic use.

progressive pulmonary disease, or hematogenously disseminated disease involving predominantly skin, subcutaneous tissues, bones, joints, and meninges. It is caused by *Coccidiodes immitis,* a fungus characterized uniquely by large spherules that rupture to release hundreds of endospores which mature, in turn, to more spherules. The mycelial form of *C immitis* is a soil organism found in semidesert areas of the USA (eg, California, Arizona, and Texas), contiguous areas of Mexico, and scattered areas of Central and South America. Infection occurs by inhalation of arthroconidia in endemic areas (eg, by tourists, travelers, farmers, archeologists, or construction engineers).

Sporadic and, occasionally, common-source outbreaks occur (eg, dust storm in central California). Endemic areas are defined by skin test (coccidioidin, spherulin) reactivity. Susceptibility to hematogenous dissemination is greatest at the extremes of age. It is also positively correlated with male sex, race (blacks and Filipinos are the commonest victims), deficient CMI, and hormonal status (it occurs more often in the second and third trimesters of pregnancy than in the first). The growth of *C. immitis* is stimulated by estrogen. There is a suspected HLA-related susceptibility to infection (HLA-A9).

Pathology

See Table 49–2.

Clinical Features

A. Signs and Symptoms: Primary exposure may be asymptomatic (60%) or associated with an influenzalike syndrome. In some patients (especially white women) there may be transient arthralgias, erythema nodosum, or erythema multiforme (also known as valley fever, and desert rheumatism). Similar immunologic phenomena have been observed with histoplasmosis and blastomycosis. Pneumonia, pleuritis, and pulmonary cavitation may occur; cavitary lung disease may be chronic or progressive. Hematogenous dissemination usually occurs in the absence of apparent pulmonary disease. Among the usual manifestations of metastatic infection are skin lesions including nodules, ulcers, sinus tracts from deeper loci, and verrucous granulomas. Also involved are bones, joints, tendon sheaths, and meninges. Meningitis may be the sole apparent locus of metastasis. The gastrointestinal tract is rarely involved.

In patients with AIDS, disease is more acute and more severe. Manifestations of fungemia, including hematogenous (miliary) pneumonia, acute respiratory distress syndrome (ARDS), cellulitis, and papulopustular skin lesions in a hematogenous pattern, may dominate. Meningitis is commonly present.

B. Laboratory Findings: These include leukocytosis, eosinophilia (including cerebrospinal fluid), abnormal chest x-ray, and evidence of specific organ dysfunction at metastatic loci. Diagnosis is established by demonstrating endosporulating spherules on smears and histologic sections and by recovering the fungus in cultures.

C. Immunologic Diagnoses: See Table 49–4. Immunologic tests are useful in diagnosis and prognosis. Negative delayed-hypersensitivity skin tests and an elevated (or rising) complement fixation (CF) titer suggest hematogenous dissemination. An elevated CF titer in the cerebrospinal fluid is virtually diagnostic of coccidioidal meningitis, which is often culture-negative. Coccidioidin (and presumably spherulin) skin testing in a patient with active erythema nodosum may produce a violent, necrotic skin test reaction.

D. Differential Diagnosis: This includes diverse granulomatous infectious diseases (eg, mycoses, tuberculosis), sarcoidosis, and cancers.

E. Treatment: Amphotericin B is the drug of choice in immunocompromised patients acutely ill with hematogenous dissemination; it must be given intrathecally for meningitis. Ketoconazole, itraconazole, and fluconazole are ameliorative and may be useful for long-term maintenance therapy of nonmeningeal disease. Fluoconazole is often effective in suppressing chronic coccidioidal meningitis.

F. Prevention: A spherule vaccine has failed to demonstrate effective protection.

G. Complications and Prognosis: Most patients recover spontaneously from primary infection. Erythema nodosum and erythema multiforme are considered particularly good prognostic signs. Some 2–4% of primary infections go on to progressive cavitary lung disease (poorly responsive to antifungal drugs; extirpative surgery may be required) or hematogenously disseminated disease. Meningitis is fatal without therapy. AIDS-associated infections require life-long suppressive therapy to prevent relapse.

HISTOPLASMOSIS

Major Immunologic Features

- It is a reticuloendothelial system disease in which tiny yeasts reside in macrophages.
- Granulomas with or without caseation are present.
- Cavitary lung disease may have a partial immunologic basis (subintimal arterial proliferation; pulmonary infarction).
- Progressive ocular histoplasmosis syndrome (POHS) is probably immunologic in origin.
- The disease is more severe in patients with defective CMI (including AIDS).
- Prominent calcification and fibrosis occur during healing.
- Immunity to reinfection occasionally wanes.

General Considerations

Histoplasmosis is an inhalation-acquired mycosis that can produce primary pulmonary infection, progressive pulmonary disease, or hematogenously disseminated disease involving predominantly the reticuloendothelial system, mucosal surfaces, and adrenal glands. It is caused by *Histoplasma capsulatum,* a tiny intracellular yeast. *H capsulatum* is a soil saprobe (mycelial form) that is found worldwide. In the USA it is particularly common in river valleys of the southeastern and central states. It grows particularly well in soil fertilized by bird droppings and bat guano, especially in caves. Infection occurs by inhalation of microconidia in areas where the infection is endemic, eg, by farmers, cave explorers, tourists, or construction workers. Sporadic and, occasionally, common-source outbreaks occur (eg, during construction in Indianapolis). A positive delayed-hypersensitivity skin test is extremely common in endemic areas. Hematogenous dissemination is especially common at the extremes of age. Progressive pulmonary disease, strongly resembling tuberculosis, is especially common in white men with chronic obstructive pulmonary disease. There is no known genetic predisposition.

Pathology
See Table 49–2.

Clinical Features
A. Signs and Symptoms: Primary exposure may be asymptomatic or associated with a flulike syndrome. Pneumonia, pleuritis, pulmonary cavitation,and mediastinal adenopathy may occur. Except in infants, hematogenous dissemination usually occurs in the absence of apparent pulmonary disease. Favored sites of metastatic infection include the reticuloendothelial system (hepatosplenomegaly; lymphadenopathy; bone marrow involvement with anemia, leukopenia, and thrombocytopenia); mucous membranes (oronasopharyngeal ulcerations); gastrointestinal tract (malabsorption); and adrenals (adrenal insufficiency). An intense fibrotic response during healing may lead to fibrous mediastinitis. Calcification is common at healed loci ("buckshot" granulomas of the lungs; splenic calcifications). The progressive ocular histoplasmosis syndrome (POHS) may represent an immunologic response to fungi that otherwise are found without symptoms at the posterior pole of the eye. In patients with AIDS, disease is more acute and may be fulminating, resembling bacterial septicemic shock. Manifestations include hematogenous (miliary) pneumonia, ARDS, DIC, hematogenously distributed papulopustules, and meningitis.

B. Laboratory Findings: These include leukocytosis or leukopenia, thrombocytopenia, and anemia. There is evidence of specific organ dysfunction at metastatic loci. Diagnosis is established by the presence of intracellular yeasts on smears (eg, buffy coat smears in AIDS patients); histologic specimens (eg, mucosal biopsies); or cultures of sputum, blood, bone marrow, and liver biopsy material.

C. Immunologic Diagnoses: See Table 49–4. Serologic tests may be useful in assessing disease activity and, less frequently, in establishing the diagnosis. A positive histoplasmin skin test may spuriously elevate antibody titers detected serologically. The detection of polysaccharide antigen in urine, blood, or CSF may be especially helpful in diagnosis and in assessing the response to therapy. Unfortunately, this test is not available commercially.

D. Differential Diagnosis: This includes diverse granulomatous infectious diseases (eg, mycoses, tuberculosis, leishmaniasis, and toxoplasmosis), sarcoidosis, Whipple's disease and other causes of malabsorption, and lymphohematogenous cancer. *Penicillium marneffei,* a filamentous fungus with a yeastlike intracellular form, is an emerging pathogen in AIDS patients in Southeast Asia. The disease, and the fungus, bear a superficial resemblance to histoplasmosis and its causative fungus.

E. Treatment: Amphotericin B is the drug of choice in immunocompromised patients acutely ill with hematogenous dissemination. Itraconazole is highly effective for nonmeningeal, non-life-threatening forms of the disease and has a superior side effect profile to that of ketoconazole. AIDS-associated infections require lifelong suppressive therapy to prevent relapse.

F. Prevention: No vaccine is available.

G. Complications and Prognosis: Most primary infections resolve spontaneously. Progressive cavitary pulmonary disease is difficult to treat and may contribute to death from underlying pulmonary insufficiency. Hematogenous dissemination is generally fatal in the absence of therapy. Relapses are common in those with severe underlying immunodeficiency. Adrenal insufficiency may occur years after the original disease is quiescent.

PARACOCCIDIOIDOMYCOSIS

Major Immunologic Features
- Large, multiply budding yeasts may exceed the size of phagocytes.
- Mixed granulomas and suppuration occur.
- It may be more severe with defective CMI.

General Considerations
Paracoccidioidomycosis is an inhalation-acquired mycosis that can produce primary pulmonary infection or hematogenously disseminated disease involving predominantly the skin, mucous membranes, reticuloendothelial system, and adrenals. It is caused by *Paracoccidioides brasiliensis,* a large, spherical, uninucleate yeast with highly characteristic multiple buds attached by narrow necks. The mycelial form of *P brasiliensis* is a soil saprobe that has only rarely been recovered from the environment in the area where it is endemic in tropical and subtropical forests of Latin America, particularly Brazil, Venezuela, and Colombia. Paracoccidioidomycosis is the most common systemic mycosis in South America. Infection occurs by inhalation of conidia and is most common among agricultural workers. The disease is sporadic. Skin test surveys suggest that men and women are equally susceptible. However, men are 12–48 times as likely to experience hematogenous dissemination as women, perhaps because physiologic concentrations of estrogen can prevent the conversion of conidia to invasive yeasts. In Brazilians, HLA-B40 antigen is more common in patients than controls; in Colombians, HLA-A9 and -B13 are more common.

Pathology

See Table 49–2.

Clinical Features

A. Signs and Symptoms: Primary exposure may be asymptomatic, or pneumonia, pleuritis, pulmonary cavitation, and mediastinal adenopathy may occur. Hematogenously disseminated disease occurs in 2 main forms, juvenile and adult. In the juvenile pattern (3–5% of cases), the primary pulmonary infection disseminates rapidly, with predominant reticuloendothelial system involvement. In the adult form (90% of cases), fungi, presumably aroused from latency, give rise to progressive localized lung disease, skin lesions, mucocutaneous lesions, reticuloendothelial system infection, and adrenal involvement. Oropharyngeal mucosal invasion is characteristic, with ulcerating lesions that involve most of the oral adventitia. Lesions are so painful that eating is difficult; tooth loss is common. Involvement of the gastrointestinal tract may lead to malabsorption; adrenal involvement can produce adrenal insufficiency.

B. Laboratory Findings: These include leukocytosis and evidence of specific organ dysfunction at metastatic loci. Diagnosis is established by demonstrating multiple-budding yeasts on smears or histologic sections and by recovering the fungi in culture.

C. Immunologic Diagnosis: See Table 49–4. Serologic tests are of use in monitoring the course of established disease.

D. Differential Diagnosis: This includes diverse granulomatous infectious diseases (eg, mycoses, tuberculosis, leishmaniasis, yaws, and syphilis), sarcoidosis, and cancer.

E. Treatment: Both ketoconazole and itraconazole are useful for the treatment of paracoccidioidomycosis. Itraconazole has become the drug of choice because of its improved side effect profile and shorter required duration of therapy.

F. Prevention: No vaccine is available.

G. Complications and Prognosis: Disseminated paracoccidioidomycosis is generally fatal in the absence of therapy. Disease that was originally acquired asymptomatically may present as disseminated infection years after the infected individual has emigrated from the area where the infection is endemic.

SYSTEMIC INVASIVE MYCOSES: OPPORTUNISTIC PATHOGENS

CANDIDIASIS

Major Immunologic Features

- The source of the infection is usually the normal host flora.
- Intact mucosal barriers represent the major nonspecific host defense mechanism.
- Phagocytes ingest yeasts but attack pseudomycelia and mycelia by extracellular apposition.
- Neutropenia predisposes to hematogenous dissemination.
- Defective CMI predisposes to invasive mucosal disease.
- Thrush, esophagitis, and vaginitis are major presenting features of AIDS.
- Chronic mucocutaneous candidiasis is a specific syndrome in patients with defective immunoregulation.

General Considerations

Candidiasis is a general term for diseases produced by *Candida* species and encompasses colonization, superficial infection (eg, thrush, vaginitis, cystitis, and intertrigo), deep local invasion (eg, esophagitis), and hematogenous dissemination (eg, to the eyes, skin, kidneys, and brain). The species that most commonly cause candidiasis are *C albicans* (yeasts, pseudomycelia, and mycelia), *C tropicalis* (yeasts and pseudomycelia), and *Torulopsis glabrata* (yeasts only). *Candida* species are found in nature, but human infection usually arises from normal flora. *C albicans, C tropicalis,* and *T glabrata* are commonly found on mucous membranes (eg, vagina, and gastrointestinal tract) but rarely on the skin. Vaginal colonization is increased by diabetes mellitus, pregnancy, and the use of oral contraceptive agents. Carriage at all sites is increased by antibiotics. Hematogenous dissemination occurs most commonly in a setting of neutropenia or gastrointestinal mucosal disruption after repeated abdominal surgery. Neonates may be colonized or infected by passage through a colonized birth canal; premature infants in intensive care units are at particularly high risk of life-threatening *Candida* sepsis. Vaginal colonization occurs after menarche. Disseminated infection occurs in both sexes and at all ages as a function of immunologic impairment. Chronic mucocutaneous candidiasis (CMCC) shows a familial tendency in about 20% of cases. In about 50% of cases there is associated endocrinopathy (eg, hypoparathyroidism, hypoadrenalism, hypothyroidism, or diabetes mellitus). The cause of this association is not known.

Pathology

See Table 49–2.

Clinical Features

A. Signs and Symptoms: Mucosal candidiasis is characterized by thrush, laryngitis, esophagitis, gastritis (especially in patients with drug-induced hypochlorhydria), vaginitis, cystitis, and intestinal candidiasis (the assumed source of hematogenous dissemination in most neutropenic patients). Vulvovaginitis is probably the most common overall manifestation of *Candida* infection. CMCC is manifested by persistent infection of skin, scalp, nails, and mucous membranes and is often accompanied by chronic dermatophyte infections. Associated findings include alopecia, depigmentation, cheilosis, blepharitis, keraconjunctivitis, corneal ulcers, and cutaneous horn formation. Hematogenously disseminated candidiasis can be either acute or chronic. The acute syndrome is characterized by involvement of the eyes (chorioretinitis), muscles (myalgias), skin (macronodular skin lesions), and kidneys (parenchymal destruction, papillary necrosis, and bezoar formation). Hematogenous (miliary) pulmonary infection is common, but *Candida* aspiration pneumonia is rare. Other manifestations include myocardial abscesses, meningitis, cerebral abscesses, and arthritis. Chronic disseminated candidiasis occurs most commonly in patients recovering from neutropenia who remain febrile despite broad-spectrum antibacterial therapy. Imaging studies reveal abscesses in the liver, spleen, lungs, and kidneys. The former designation of this syndrome as "hepatosplenic" candidiasis is not adequately descriptive and should be dropped.

B. Laboratory Findings: These include leukopenia or leukocytosis and evidence of specific organ dysfunction at metastatic loci. Diagnosis is established by direct histologic demonstration of fungal tissue invasion and/or recovery of fungi in culture from normally sterile areas. Candidemia should be regarded as indicative of invasive infection in all but the most exceptional circumstances. Candiduria indicates cystitis more frequently than it indicates progressive renal infection.

C. Immunologic Diagnosis: See Table 49–4. Serologic tests are not helpful in neutropenic patients.

D. Differential Diagnosis: This includes diverse septicemic syndromes (eg, *Staphylococcus aureus* and *Pseudomonas aeruginosa* infections) and diverse opportunistic infectious diseases of neutropenic patients, including mycoses.

E. Treatment: Topical imidizoles are used for thrush and vaginitis, ketoconazole or fluconazole for vaginitis or progressive mucocutaneous infection, amphotericin B for deep local invasive infection or hematogenous dissemination, and amphotericin B plus flucytosine (depending on renal function) for disseminated infections that involve the eyes or central nervous system. Fluconazole may be useful for prolonged follow-up therapy of acute or chronic disseminated candidiasis, but amphotericin B is the only therapy with proven efficacy for invasive infection. Candiduria can usually be cured by removal of a urinary catheter plus a short course of amphotericin B or flucytosine.

F. Prevention: Prophylactic administration of nystatin or ketoconazole to immunocompromised patients has not been clearly shown to prevent *Candida* infections. Prophylactic ketoconazole may actually predispose to infection by *C tropicalis, T glabrata,* or *Aspergillus* spp, which are not susceptible to ketoconazole. Similarly, prophylactic fluconazole may predispose to infections with *C krusei* or *T glabrata.*

G. Complications and Prognosis: CMCC can be ameliorated but not cured by chronic ketoconazole therapy. *Candida* endocarditis is essentially incurable without valve replacement. Empirical amphotericin B therapy in febrile neutropenic patients has led to an improved prognosis for recovery in these patients, who are otherwise extremely difficult to diagnose and often die untreated. Reversal of neutropenia is the most important single predictor of recovery from infection.

CRYPTOCOCCOSIS

Major Immunologic Features

- Unencapsulated environmental yeasts acquire a capsule in the lungs.
- Encapsulated yeasts evade phagocytosis.
- Free capsular polysaccharide triggers suppressor cells, down-regulating host defenses.
- Disease is much more common and severe in patients with defective CMI, particularly AIDS sufferers.
- Detection of free capsular polysaccharide is extremely helpful in diagnosis.

General Considerations

Cryptococcosis is an inhalation-acquired mycosis that is initiated by symptomatic or asymptomatic pulmonary infection. It most commonly presents with meningitis. Less common sites of hematogenous dissemination include skin, bones, eyes, and prostate. It is caused by *Cryptococcus neoformans,* an encapsulated yeast with 4 serotypes (A, B, C, and D) based on antigenic differences in the capsular polysaccharide. Virulence is linked to encapsulation and the capacity to synthesize melanin. Cryptococci are ubiquitous, and the disease occurs worldwide. Serotypes A and D are most commonly found in avian habitats (eg, in pigeon dung); serotypes B and C may be associated with eucalyptus trees. Serotype A causes most disease worldwide; serotype D is common only in Europe. Disease caused by serotypes B and C is found predominantly in subtropical areas (including Southern California). Serotypes A and D are the most common causes of cryptococcal infection in immuno-compromised patients and are overwhelmingly the most common serotypes recovered from patients with AIDS. Studies with poorly standardized "crypto-coccin" skin tests suggest that asymptomatic infection may be common. Immunosuppression (including AIDS) causes the disease to emerge from apparent latency. Some 6–13% of AIDS patients will develop a *C neoformans* infection. Cryptococcosis is more common in males, even excluding the current AIDS population. Infection is rare in children. The disease is sporadic. There is no known genetic predisposition.

Pathology
See Table 49–2.

Clinical Features
A. Signs and Symptoms: Cryptococcal infection commonly presents as isolated meningitis. Disease of the lungs is generally not apparent, even though this is the site of fungal entry. However, in patients who do present with pulmonary infection, meningeal involvement may be inapparent or absent. The most common manifestations of pulmonary cryptococcosis are solitary or multiple infiltrates or nodules. Cryptococcal meningitis is commonly a subtle or subacute process characterized by headache, impaired mentation, optic neuritis or papilledema, cranial nerve palsies, and seizures. Hydrocephalus may lead to progressive mental deterioration. In patients with AIDS, meningeal involvement may also be subtle, despite disproportionately huge numbers of fungi in the cerebrospinal fluid. In addition, manifestations of widespread hematogenous dissemination may also be present. (eg, diffuse skin lesions, miliary pulmonary infiltrates, ARDS) and may lead rapidly to death. Other sites of hematogenous dissemination include the skin (particularly prominent in AIDS patients), bones, prostate, kidneys, and liver.

B. Laboratory Findings: Meningitis is usually low-grade, with lymphocytosis and low sugar levels in cerebrospinal fluid. The diagnosis is usually established by cryptococcal antigen detection, India ink stains, and positive cultures of the cerebrospinal fluid. Organisms may also be cultured from blood, skin lesions, urine, and prostatic secretions.

C. Immunologic Diagnosis: See Table 49–4. Demonstration of cryptococcal antigen in cerebrospinal fluid or blood is extremely helpful in establishing the diagnosis. In AIDS patients, antigen titers are extremely high.

D. Differential Diagnosis: The differential diagnosis of pulmonary cryptococcosis includes diverse infections and cancers. Cryptococcal meningitis may be confused with diverse chronic hypoglycorrhachic syndromes, including tuberculosis or

coccidioidomycosis. Symptoms may be erroneously attributed to a primary psychiatric disorder. In AIDS patients the differential diagnosis includes the gamut of opportunistic infections commonly encountered in this disorder.

E. Treatment Because of its rapidity of action, amphotericin B, with or without flucytosine, should be used to initiate therapy. Fluconazole may be substituted once the infection has stabilized. AIDS-associated infection requires lifelong suppressive therapy to prevent relapse.

F. Prevention: The value of prophylactic triazole treatment is under investigation. No vaccine is available.

G. Complications and Prognosis: Patients with any alteration in mental status at the time of presentation are more likely to die then those with normal mentation. The likelihood of cure is inversely proportional to the severity of underlying immunosuppression. Although the cryptococcal antigen test is very helpful in establishing a diagnosis, the decrease in antigen titer may not be proportionate to the extent of clinical therapeutic response. Thus, disappearance of antigen from cerebrospinal fluid may not be a realistic therapeutic goal.

ASPERGILLOSIS

Major Immunologic Features
- Infection is caused by inhalation of conidia (common environmental contaminants).
- Conidia are ingested and killed by alveolar macrophages.
- Phagocytes attack mycelia by extracellular apposition.
- Neutropenia or neutrophil dysfunction predisposes to respiratory tract invasion, angioinvasion, and hematogenous dissemination.
- Balls of fungi may colonize previously damaged respiratory tissues (aspergilloma).
- Allergy may develop to inhaled conidia or to fungi colonizing the bronchial tree (atopic asthma, extrinsic allergic alveolitis, allergic bronchopulmonary aspergillosis).

General Considerations
Aspergillosis is a poorly descriptive term, which includes disease processes characterized by colonization, allergy, or tissue invasion. In addition, *Aspergillus* spp produce mycotoxins. Aflatoxin (*A flavus*) is linked epidemiologically to hepatocellular carcinoma; gliotoxin (*A fumigatus*) is toxic to macrophages and cytotoxic T cells. The focus of this section is on invasive aspergillosis. Allergic bronchopulmonary aspergillosis (ABPA) is discussed elsewhere (see Chapter 28). *Aspergillus* spp are among the most common environmental saprophytic fungi. Only a few thermotolerant species are pathogenic for

humans, most notably *A fumigatus, A flavus,* and *A niger. Aspergillus* infections occur worldwide. Outbreaks of invasive aspergillosis have followed exposure to conidia released by hospital construction, contaminated air-conditioning ducts and filters, and fireproofing materials above false ceilings. Invasive infection occurs in both sexes at all ages, as a function of immunologic impairment. There is no known genetic predisposition.

Pathology
See Table 49–2.

Clinical Features
A. Signs and Symptoms: Invasive pulmonary aspergillosis occurs characteristically in immunosuppressed, neutropenic patients. Widespread bronchial ulceration, parenchymal invasion, and angioinvasion lead to patchy necrotizing pneumonia, thrombosis, and infarction. Widespread metastatic infection may occur. Infarcted lung tissue may contain necrotic sequestrae that resemble aspergillomas. A similar process may take place in the paranasal sinuses, resulting in a clinical picture identical to that of rhinocerebral mucormycosis (see below). An indolent, semi-invasive pulmonary infection occasionally occurs in immunocompetent patients with underlying chronic obstructive pulmonary disease.

B. Laboratory Findings: These include neutropenia, abnormal chest or sinus x-rays, and evidence of specific organ dysfunction at metastatic loci. Diagnosis depends on histologic demonstration of tissue invasion by an exclusively mycelial fungus. Cultivation of *Aspergillus* spp from respiratory secretions may reflect only transient colonization; blood cultures are virtually never positive.

C. Immunologic Diagnosis: See Table 49–4. Serologic tests for antibody are not useful in diagnosis for invasive aspergillosis; antigen tests are promising, but still experimental. Delayed-hypersensitivity skin tests and precipitin titers may be quite helpful in diagnosis of ABPA.

D. Differential Diagnosis: This includes diverse opportunistic pulmonary infections (bacterial and fungal), pulmonary infarction, diverse septicemic syndromes, and rhinocerebral mucormycosis.

E. Treatment: Amphotericin B is the only drug of proven therapeutic value. It must be used early and aggressively if the patient is to survive. Itraconazole may be useful for long-term follow-up therapy or in patients whose disease is not acutely life-threatening.

F. Prevention: Hospital rooms with enclosed filtered ventilation systems provide some degree of protection from environmental fungi.

G. Complications and Prognosis: Invasive aspergillosis is commonly fatal. An aggressive approach to diagnosis and treatment is essential. Surgical debulking of infected, infarcted tissues may be of particular value. Empirical amphotericin B therapy in febrile neutropenic patients who are not responding to broad-spectrum antibacterial agents is commonly used in an attempt to prevent this and other opportunistic mycoses. Reversal of neutropenia is the single most important predictor of recovery from this infection.

MUCORMYCOSIS (ZYGOMYCOSIS)

Major Immunologic Features
- Infection is caused by inhalation of spores.
- Spores are ingested and prevented from germinating by alveolar macrophages.
- Phagocytes attack mycelia by extracellular apposition.
- Acidotic states predispose to invasive paranasal sinus infection.
- Neutropenia predisposes to paranasal sinus, pulmonary, and disseminated infection.

General Considerations
Mucormycosis is a suppurative opportunistic mycosis that produces predominantly paranasal sinus (rhinocerebral) disease in patients with acidosis and rhinocerebral, pulmonary, or disseminated disease in patients with neutropenia. The most common etiologic agent is *Rhizopus arrhizus;* others include *Absidia, Cunninghamella, Mortierella,* and *Saksenaea* spp. These are all common environmental contaminants. Colonization and infection are uncommon in healthy persons; mucormycosis is less common than invasive aspergillosis in immunocompromised patients. Infection occurs sporadically; clusters of infection occurs sporadically; clusters of infection are rare. Wound infections may occur, and CNS infection may complicate intravenous drug abuse. Invasive infection occurs in both sexes and at all ages as a function of acidosis or immunosuppression. There is no known genetic predisposition.

Pathology
See Table 49–2.

Clinical Features
A. Signs and Symptoms: These are virtually identical to those of invasive aspergillosis. Rhinocerebral mucormycosis accounts for about 50% of all cases of mucormycosis; more than 75% of cases occur in patients with acidosis, especially diabetic ketoacidosis. However, increasing numbers of cases are being seen in association with neutropenia and immunosuppression. Early clinical features include nasal stuffiness, bloody nasal discharge, facial swelling, and facial and orbital pain. Later manifestations include orbital cellulitis, proptosis, endophthalmitis, orbital apex syndrome, cranial nerve palsies, and cerebral extension.

B. Laboratory Findings: These include acidosis (principally diabetic ketoacidosis), neutropenia, abnormal paranasal sinus or chest x-rays, and evidence of specific organ dysfunction at sites of local extension (central nervous system) or metastatic loci. Diagnosis depends on histologic demonstration of tissue invasion by an exclusively mycelial fungus. Cultures are positive in fewer than 20% of patients, and even positive cultures may represent the presence of fungal contaminants.

C. Immunologic Diagnosis: See Table 49–4. There are no useful tests available.

D. Differential Diagnosis: This includes diverse opportunistic paranasal sinus infections (aspergillosis, phaeohyphomycosis, hyalohyphomycosis) and diverse opportunistic pulmonary bacterial and fungal infections.

E. Treatment: Amphotericin B is the only drug of proven value. Aggressive surgical debridement is required for paranasal sinusitis or rhinocerebral mucormycosis.

F. Prevention: No effective preventive measures are known.

G. Complications and Prognosis: Rhinocerebral mucormycosis advances at an extremely rapid rate; an aggressive approach to diagnosis and treatment is essential. Survival is more likely in the setting of diabetic ketoacidosis than that of neutropenia.

PNEUMOCYTOSIS

The cause of pneumocytosis (*Pneumocystis carinii*) is tentatively classified as a fungus. However, there is considerable evidence that the microorganism is a protozoan.

Major Immunologic Features

- Infection is apparent only in patients with impaired CMI or in infants with severe protein-calorie malnutrition (marasmus).
- It is the most common index diagnosis for AIDS.
- Disease is predominantly alveolar and interstitial; extrapulmonary spread is distinctly rare.

General Considerations

Pneumocystis carinii pneumonia (PCP) is an apparently inhalation-acquired disease, but the environmental form of the pathogen has never been identified. PCP occurs predominantly in patients with impaired CMI and is classically the defining opportunistic infection for AIDS. *P carinii* is a unicellular eukaryote with a proposed life cycle consisting of trophozoites and cysts. It can be maintained transiently in cell culture but has never been cultivated independently in cell-free media. Seroepidemiologic studies indicate that over more than two-thirds of normal children have acquired antibody to *P carinii* by 3–4 years of age. Clinical attributes of the presumed in-

fecting event are unknown, and autopsy studies have failed to provide evidence of residual pulmonary microorganisms in persons who have died of unrelated causes. The occurrence of PCP in immunocompromised adults could represent either new infection or arousal of inapparent disease from latency. When PCP occurs in infants with AIDS or marasmus, it is assumed to represent primary infection. Common-source outbreaks of PCP have occurred, suggesting that infection may be spread by aerosol. Most cases, however, appear to be sporadic. Diverse animal species harbor *P carinii,* as evidenced by spontaneous occurrence of PCP in response to immunosuppression. There is no evidence of spread from animals to humans; there are antigenic differences among human and animal strains. Prevalence is directly related to the occurrence of marasmus or impaired CMI. Neutropenia is not a risk factor. There is no independent age or sex-related susceptibility. Approximately 75% of AIDS patients will experience at least one episode of *P. carinii* pneumonia if no prophylaxis is given. There is no known genetic predisposition.

Pathology

See Table 49–2.

Clinical Features

A. Signs and Symptoms: These include fever, cough, and shortness of breath, especially in patients with prolonged fatigue and weight loss.

B. Laboratory Findings: These include CD4 T cell counts of generally less than 200/μL; elevated nonspecific serum lactic dehydrogenase level; and diffuse alveolointerstitial infiltrates on chest x-ray, sometimes with cystic changes or pneumotoceles. Hypoxemia and alveolar-to-arterial O_2 tension differences are common, especially in response to exercise. Gallium lung scanning is sensitive, but not specific. Diagnosis is established by visualizing characteristic organisms, in expectorated sputum, induced sputum, bronchoalveolar lavage specimens, or lung biopsy specimens obtained transbronchially or by open thoracotomy.

C. Immunologic Diagnosis: See Table 49–4. There are several experimental techniques for detecting an antibody response to *P carinii* or free *P carinii* antigen. However, these are not of current clinical value. An immunofluorescent antibody test utilizing a monoclonal antibody specific for *P carinii* has enhanced recognition of the organism (over that by Giemsa and fast silver stains) in clinical specimens.

D. Differential Diagnosis: This includes the gamut of diseases caused by the opportunistic pulmonary pathogens in patients with AIDS or profoundly depressed CMI. Among these are tuberculosis, histoplasmosis, cryptococcosis, toxoplasmosis, cytomegalovirus infection, bacterial pneumonia, lymphomas, and Kaposi's sarcoma.

E. Treatment: Trimethoprim-sulfamethoxazole (TMP-SMZ) and intravenous pentamidine isethionate are both effective for the treatment of *P carinii*. However, TMP-SMZ is associated with fewer and less severe side effects, particularly in patients without AIDS. Other drugs shown to be effective include dapsone, TMP-dapsone, pyrimethamine-sulfadoxine, trimetrexate, clindamycin-primaquine, and eflornithine. Corticosteroids are useful in the prevention and treatment of *P carinii*-induced ARDS.

F. Prevention: *P carinii* prophylaxis is central to the clinical management of AIDS patients. A regimen of TMP-SMZ given 3 days per week is highly effective. Aerosolized pentamidine administered once weekly is also effective. No vaccine is available.

G. Complications and Prognosis: Aggressive use of prophylaxis in AIDS patients is decreasing the frequency of PCP as an index diagnosis. Aerosolized pentamidine may delay or change the presentation of PCP to less easily recognized forms (eg, apical cystic disease and hematogenously disseminated disease, both of which are extremely rare at present). Pneumothorax is a late but important complication of PCP.

REFERENCES

GENERAL

Anaissie E et al: Focus on fungal infections: An update on diagnosis and treatment. *Clin Infect Dis* 1992;**14**:S-1.

Armstrong D: Treatment of opportunistic fungal infections. *Clin Infect Dis* 1993;**16**:1.

Beck-Sagué CM et al: Secular trends in the epidemiology of nosocomial fungal infections in the United States, 1980–1990. *J Infect Dis* 1993;**167**:1247.

Chandler FW, Watts, JC: *Pathologic Diagnosis of Fungal Infections.* ASCP Press, 1987.

Cox GM, Perfect JR: Fungal infections. *Curr Opin Infect Dis* 1993;**6**:422.

Cox RA: *Immunology of the Fungal Diseases.* CRC Press, 1989.

Gradon JD et al: Emergence of unusual opportunistic pathogens in AIDS: A review. *Clin Infect Dis* 1992;**15**:134.

Kwon-Chung KJ, and Bennett JE: *Medical Mycology.* Lea & Febiger, 1992.

Kaufman L, Reiss E: Serodiagnosis of fungal diseases. Chap 78, 506, in: *Manual of Clinical Laboratory Immunology,* 4th ed. Chapter 78. American Society for Microbiology, 1992.

SUPERFICIAL MYCOSES

Pityrosporum & Malassezia

Danker WM et al: *Malassezia* fungemia in neonates and adults: Complication of hyperalimentation. *Rev Infect Dis* 1987;**9**:743.

Marcon MJ, Powell DA: Human infections due to *Malassezia* spp. *Clin Microbiol Rev* 1992;**5**:101.

White Pledra; *Trichosporon beigelii*

Anaissie E et al: Azole therapy for trichosporonosis: Clinical evaluation of eight patients, experimental therapy for murine infection, and review. *Clin Infect Dis* 1992;**15**:781.

Steinman HK, Papenfort RB: White piedra—A case report and review of the literature. *Clin Exp Dermatol* 1984;**9**:591.

Walsh TJ: Trichosporonosis. *Infect Dis Clin N Am* 1989;**3**:43.

SUBCUTANEOUS MYCOSES

Dermatophytosis

Feingold DS: What the infectious disease subspecialist should know about dermatophytes. Page 154 in: *Current Clinical Topics in Infectious Diseases.* Vol 8. Remington JS, Swartz MN (editors). McGraw-Hill, 1987.

Wright DC et al: Generalized chronic dermatophytosis in patients with human immunodeficiency virus type I infection and CD4 depletion. *Arch Dermatol* 1991;**127**:265.

Chromomycosis

Fader RC, McGinnis MR: Infections caused by dematiaceous fungi: Chromoblastomycosis and phaeohyphomycosis. *Infect Dis Clin N Am* 1988;**2**:925.

Mycetoma

McGinnis MR, Fader R: Mycetoma: A contemporary concept. *Infect Dis Clin N Am* 1988p;**2**:939.

Sporotrichosis

Penn CC et al: *Sporothrix schenckii* meningitis in a patient with AIDS. *Clin Infect Dis* 1992;**15**:741.

Winn RE: Sporotrichosis. *Infect Dis Clin N Am* 1988;**2**:899.

SYSTEMIC INVASIVE MYCOSES

Blastomycosis

Al-Doory Y, DiSalvo AF: *Blastomycosis.* Plenum, 1992.

Bradsher RW: Clinical considerations in blastomycosis. *Infect Dis Clin Pract* 1992;**1**:97.

Pappas PG et al: Blastomycosis in patients with the acquired immunodeficiency syndrome. *Ann Intern Med* 1992;**116**:847.

Coccidioidomycosis

Ampel NM et al: Coccidioidomycosis during human immunodeficiency virus infection: Results of a prospective study in a coccidioidal endemic area. *Am J Med* 1993;**94**:235.

Einstein HE, Johnson RH: Coccidioidomycosis: New aspects of epidemiology and therapy. *Clin Infect Dis* 1993;**16**:349.

Galgiani JN: Coccidioidomycosis. *Infect Dis Clin Pract* 1992;**1:**357.

Histoplasmosis

Alsip SG, Dismukes WE: Approach to the patient with suspected histoplasmosis. Page 254 in: *Current Clinical Topics in Infectious Disease.* Vol 7. Remington JS, Swartz MN (editors). McGraw-Hill, 1986.

Graybill JR: Histoplasmosis and AIDS. *J Infect Dis* 1988;**158:**623.

Wheat LJ et al: Effect of successful treatment with amphotericin B on *Histoplasma capsulatum* variety *capsulatum* polysaccharide antigen levels in patients with AIDS and histoplasmosis. *Am J Med* 1992; **92:**153.

Penicillium marneffei

Supparatpinyo K et al: *Penicillium marneffei* infection in patients infected with human immunodeficiency virus. *Clin Infect Dis* 1992;**14:**871.

Paracoccidioidomycosis

Brummer E et al: Paracoccidioidomycosis: An update. *Clin Microbiol Rev* 1993;**6:**89.

Candidiasis

Crislip MA, Edwards JE Jr: Candidiasis. *Infect Dis Clin N Am* 1989;**3:**103.

Walsh TJ et al: Detection of circulating *Candida* enolase by immunoassay in patients with cancer and invasive candidiasis. *N Engl J Med* 1991;**324:**1026.

Cryptococcosis

Perfect JR: Cryptococcosis. *Infect Dis Clin N Am.* 1989; **3:**77.

Powderly WG: Treatment of cryptococcal meningitis. *Infect Dis Clin Pract* 1992;**1:**164.

White M et al: Cryptococcal meningitis: Outcome in patients with AIDS and patients with neoplastic disease. *J Infect Dis* 1992;**165:**960.

Aspergillosis

Denning DW, Stevens DA: Antifungal and surgical treatment of invasive aspergillosis: Review of 2,121 published cases. *Rev Infect Dis* 1990;**12:**1147.

Minamoto GY et al: Invasive aspergillosis in patients with AIDS. *Clin Infect Dis* 1992;**14:**66.

Tang CM, Cohen J: Invasive aspergillosis: Diagnosis, treatment, and prevention. *Infect Dis Clin Pract* 1992;**1:**217.

Mucormycosis (Zygomycosis)

Paparello SF et al: Hospital-acquired wound mucormycosis. *Clin Infect Dis* 1992;**14:**350.

Rinaldi MG: Zygomycosis. *Infect Dis Clin N Am* 1989; **3:**19.

Pneumocystosis

Edman JC et al: Ribosomal RNA sequence shows *Pneumocystis carinii* to be a member of the fungi. *Nature* 1988;**334:**519.

Huges WT: *Pneumocystis carinii* infection: An update. *Medicine* 1992;**71:**175.

Raviglione MC: Extrapulmonary pneumocystosis: The first 50 cases. *Rev Infect Dis* 1990;**12:**1127.

Smulian AG et al: Geographic variation in the humoral response to *Pneumocystis carinii*. *J Infect Dis* 1993; **167:**1243.

Phaeohyphomycosis & Hyalohyphomycosis

McGinnis MR, Hilger AE: Infections caused by black fungi. *Arch Dermatol* 1987;**123:**1300.

50

Parasitic Diseases

James McKerrow, MD, PhD, & Donald Heyneman, PhD

Parasitic diseases such as malaria, schistosomiasis, and leishmaniasis are among the most important health problems in developing countries. Not only is an understanding of the immunology of parasitic disease essential to control these diseases by immunization, but also the study of the host response to parasites continues to lead to important discoveries about the immune response itself. For example, the response to schistosome (blood fluke) eggs by infected mice represents one of the best experimental models for studying the formation and regulation of granulomatous inflammation. Immature schistosomes (schistosomula) and eggs have also provided an in vitro experimental model for elucidating the function of the eosinophil. New models of regulation of cytokine production and the role of cytokines in the immune response have come from studies of leishmaniasis, a protozoan parasite infection.

Immune responses to the complex antigenic structures of parasites have diverse manifestations and do not always lead to complete protective immunity. Unfortunately, as is often the case with infectious diseases, the immune response to parasites can even produce more serious disease than the parasite itself. Examples are the hepatic granulomas of schistosomiasis, antigen-antibody complex glomerulonephritis in quartan malaria, and antibody-mediated anaphylactic shock from a ruptured hydatid cyst or from too-rapid killing of filarial microfilariae.

Some of the most fascinating and perplexing aspects of parasitic disease are the variety of mechanisms by which the parasite evades the immune response (Fig 50–1). A parasite can "hide" within a host's own cells, as in leishmaniasis, produce successive waves of progeny with different surface antigens, as in African trypanosomiasis, or disguise itself as "self" with host antigens, as in schistosomiasis. Nonspecific immunosuppression, due to a variety of stimuli, is characteristic of a number of parasitic infections. The ability of parasites to adapt to the host environment is the essence of successful parasitism,

and it increases immeasurably the difficulty of developing immunization procedures against parasitic infection.

IMMUNE RESPONSE TO PROTOZOA

Protozoa are important agents of worldwide disease. Falciparum malaria, for example, is still considered one of the most lethal diseases in humans despite massive efforts at eradication and control. These parasites also offer unlimited immunologic challenges, the immune responses induced being as diverse as the protozoa themselves. In developing countries, especially in Africa, malaria and trypanosomiasis take enormous tolls of life and are significant barriers to economic development. Amebiasis, giardiasis, and toxoplasmosis are widespread even in highly developed countries. The use of immunosuppressive drugs to treat cancer and to prevent rejection of transplanted organs has resulted in activation of otherwise subclinical infections with protozoa such as *Toxoplasma* or induced an overwhelming systemic infection with the nematode *Strongyloides stercoralis*. Finally, the global epidemic of AIDS has led to exacerbation of preexisting parasitic infections as well as complicated multiple infections by protozoa such as *Cryptosporidium, Toxoplasma,* and Microsporidium.

MALARIA

Major Immunologic Features
- Complex partial humoral and cellular immunity occurs with multiple exposure.
- Nonimmune individuals in areas where malaria is

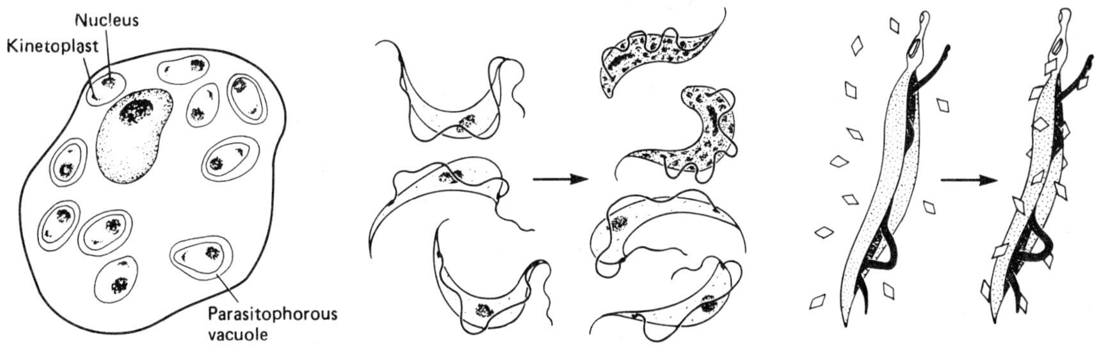

A Living within a host cell (*Leishmania* living in macrophage within a parasitophorous vacuole)

B Rapidly changing surface antigens (trypanosomes)

C "Camouflaging" surface with host antigens

Figure 50–1. Some of the devious ways in which parasites evade the host immune response.

endemic have significantly higher mortality rates from cerebral malaria.

- Species-specific protective IgG antibody is produced against merozoites after multiple infections.
- Genetic variability in immune response to specific antigens has hindered vaccine development.

General Considerations

Human malaria is caused by species of *Plasmodium*. It is transmitted by female anopheline mosquitoes that ingest the sexual forms of the parasite in blood meals. The infective sporozoites develop in the mosquito and are injected into the definitive (human) host during insect bites. In the human, the parasites first develop in an exoerythrocytic form, multiplying within hepatic cells without inducing an inflammatory reaction. The progeny, or merozoites, invade host erythrocytes to begin the erythrocytic cycle and initiate the earliest phase of clinical malaria. The gametocyte is the sexual stage taken up by the mosquito.

Destruction of erythrocytes occurs on a 48-hour cycle with *Plasmodium vivax* and *Plasmodium ovale* and every 72 hours with *Plasmodium malariae*. The characteristic chills-fever-sweat malarial syndrome follows this cyclic pattern, being induced by synchronous rupture of infected erythrocytes by the mature asexual forms (schizonts), releasing merozoites that quickly invade new erythrocytes. The syndrome associated with *Plasmodium falciparum*, although classically thought to occur on a 48-hour cycle, is, in fact, frequently not synchronous. In contrast to the exoerythrocytic stage, the erythrocytic merozoites induce an array of humoral responses in the host, as demonstrated by complement fixation, precipitation, agglutination, and fluorescent-antibody reactions.

In *P vivax* and *P ovale* infections, relapse after a period of dormancy may result from periodic release of merozoites from the liver (hypnozoites), owing to

the lack of an immune response to the intracellular parasites. When the erythrocytic cellular and humoral protection is deficient (from concurrent infection, age, trauma, or other debilitating factors), the reappearing blood-stage forms induce a new round of clinical malaria until the erythrocytic cycle is again controlled by antibody and T cell host responses. This is a true relapse, as opposed to a recrudescence of erythrocytic infection. Relapses can occur for up to 5 years with some strains of *P vivax* and possibly 2–3 years for *P ovale*. *P malariae* appears to recur only as a recrudescent erythrocytic infection, sometimes appearing 30 or more years after the primary infection. *P falciparum* may have a short-term recrudescence but does not develop a true relapse from liver-developed merozoites.

Blackwater fever, formerly a common and rapidly fatal form of falciparum malaria among colonists in Africa, has declined in frequency with reduction in quinine therapy. It is associated with repeated falciparum infection, inadequate quinine therapy, and possibly genetic factors more frequently found in whites. The resulting rapid, massive hemolysis of both infected and uninfected erythrocytes is thought to result from autoantibodies from previous infections that react with autoantigens (perhaps an erythrocyte-parasite-quinine combination) derived from a new infection with the same falciparum strain. With increased use of quinine to prevent or treat chloroquine-resistant falciparum malaria, blackwater fever may again increase in frequency in coming years.

Quartan malaria, caused by *P malariae* has been associated with a serious complement-dependent immune complex glomerulonephritis and nephrosis in African children, resulting in edema and severe kidney damage unless the disease is arrested early. After resolution of the edema, persistent symptomless proteinuria or slowly deteriorating renal function is common. Stable remissions with corticosteroid therapy occur when proteinuria is restricted to only a few classes of protein and histologic changes are minimal. However, patients with poorly controlled generalized proteinuria are probably not benefited by antimalarial or immunosuppressive therapy. Chronic *P malariae* infection probably triggers autoimmunity, perpetuating the immune complex glomerulonephritis, but the antigen involved is not yet identified.

Innate, nonacquired immunity to malaria is well demonstrated. Africans, African Americans, and African descendants elsewhere lacking Duffy blood group antigen Fy(a–b–) are immune to *P vivax*, since this genetic factor appears to be necessary for successful merozoite penetration of the human erythrocyte by this plasmodial species. Intracellular growth of the malaria parasites is also affected by the molecular structure of hemoglobin. Sickle cell (SS) hemoglobin inhibits growth of *P falciparum*. The sickle cell gene is widespread in areas of Africa where falciparum malaria is hyperendemic. Although the prevalence of infection appears unaffected by the sickling trait, *severe* infections in individuals with hemoglobin A/S (sickle cell trait) are very much reduced compared with those in homozygous individuals without the sickling trait. Similarly, *P falciparum* growth is retarded in erythrocytes with the fetal hemoglobin (F)—hence the selective advantage of β-thalassemia heterocygotes, in whom postnatal hemoglobin F declines at a lower than normal rate. Other red cell abnormalities such as glucose-6-phosphate dehydrogenase deficiency appear to be protective of the erythrocyte and thereby reduce the severity of plasmodial infection.

Immunity to *P falciparum* malaria is species- and strain-specific. If immune individuals migrate to other, geographically distinct areas of endemicity, they may acquire new disease. Both acquired and innate specific or nonspecific resistances to malaria are influenced by a number of genetic traits that reflect strong selective pressure in areas with specific mosquito-human-*Plasmodium* combinations. A very gradual long-term resistance to hyperendemic falciparum malaria is acquired in African populations. The resistance develops years after the onset of disease among nearly all children over 3 months of age. Initial passive protection is present owing to transplacental maternal IgG. Nonetheless, there are estimates of a million malaria deaths a year in Africa, chiefly among children under 5 years of age. Even after surviving a childhood infection, a large proportion of adults remain susceptible to infection and show periodic parasitemia, while their serum contains antiplasmodial antibodies, some with demonstrated protective action. Susceptibility to a low-level chronic infection provides the population with a protective **premunition** (prevention of subsequent infection). It is believed that in areas of Africa, where malaria is hyperendemic, nearly all residents harbor throughout their lives a continuous series of falciparum infections of low to moderate pathogenicity. Antibodies are produced that inhibit the entry of merozoites into erythrocytes. All immunoglobulin classes are elevated in the serum of malaria patients, but IgG levels appear to correlate best with the degree of malaria protection (or control of acute manifestations).

In addition to the variables of parasite genetics and vector biology, it is clear that there is significant variability within human populations in the ability to mount an immune response to the malaria parasite. This has somewhat dampened the optimism for early development of a subunit vaccine against malaria, because preliminary clinical trials of the first vaccine candidate were disappointing, raising fears that subunit vaccines would be poorly immunogenic in many individuals of a target population. Genetic variability in induction of immune response by a vaccine is by no means a new observation. Even in a very effective recombinant vaccine such as that against hepatitis B, one finds a bell-shaped curve of response, with some individuals failing to produce sufficient levels of antibodies in the standard vaccination protocol. The situation in malaria is even more heterogeneous and is seen in inbred strains of mice as well as in outbred human populations. In mice, the variability in immune response is linked to variability in the major histocompatibility complex (MHC). However, is it apparent that immune response to malaria in humans is probably also regulated by genes outside the MHC region that have yet to be fully defined.

The failure to induce protective antibodies in vaccinated individuals led research investigators to focus on the role of cell-mediated immunity and especially T cell-derived cytokines, already known to be important in control of other parasitic diseases. The following striking observation indicates that our understanding of the immune response to malaria is still murky. In areas where there is a high proportion of both malaria and HIV, no significant effect of HIV infection on the course of malaria or, for that matter, of malaria on the course of HIV infection has been noted, even though specific individuals with low T cell counts and malaria infections were studied. This suggests that humoral immunity may indeed be important in control of malaria or that other types of T cells, for example γδ T cells, generate cytokines that can control malaria but may not be affected in HIV infection.

TOXOPLASMOSIS

Major Immunologic Features
- Specific antibody is present.
- There is a nonspecific increase in serum immunoglobulins.
- Natural acquired immunity is widespread; cell-mediated immunity is probably the major mechanism.

■ Disseminated toxoplasmosis is a frequent complication in HIV-infected individuals with low T cell counts.

General Considerations

Toxoplasma infection in humans is generally asymptomatic; it has been estimated that as much as 40% of the adult population worldwide is infected, as well as all species of mammals that have been tested for the presence of this ubiquitous parasite. Clinical disease, which develops in only a small fraction of those infected, ranges from benign lymphadenopathy to an acute and often fatal infection of the central nervous system. The developing fetus and the aged or otherwise immunologically compromised host are most vulnerable to the pathologic expression of massive infection and resulting encystation in the eye or brain. Damage to the fetus is greatest during the first trimester, when the central nervous system is being organized, and nearly all such instances end in fetal death. Infection of the mother during the second trimester may produce hydrocephaly, blindness, or various less degrees of neurologic damage in the fetus. Most cases of fetal infection occur during the third trimester, resulting in chorioretinitis or other ophthalmic damage, reduced learning capacity or other expressions of central nervous system deficit, or asymptomatic latent infection that may become clinically apparent years later. Women exposed *before* pregnancy—as indicated by a positive indirect immunofluorescent or Sabin-Feldman dye test—are thought to be unable to transmit the infection in utero.

In most cases, the diagnosis of toxoplasmosis is made by serology. Positive tests for IgM and IgG appear approximately 5 days and approximately 1–2 weeks, respectively, after infection. Because an IgG reaction may persist for months to years, IgM is diagnostically more useful, since a single high titer is indicative of acute infection. For confirmation, 2 specimens are generally drawn at a 3-week interval and tested simultaneously. A serial rise in titer is a reliable indication of recent infection.

In ocular toxoplasmosis, no rise in titer is observed, but a negative serologic test can be used to rule out chorioretinitis. The IgM serologic test can also be used during pregnancy and on cord blood, but serologic positivity may be suppressed by immunosuppressive therapy or AIDS.

Many potential sources of infection have been suggested, including tissue cysts in raw or partially cooked pork or mutton and oocysts passed in feces of infected cats (the true final hosts). However, these sources seem insufficient to account for such large numbers of infections. The major reservoirs of infection are therefore unknown. *Toxoplasma* infection usually occurs through the gastrointestinal tract, and the protozoa can apparently penetrate and proliferate (as rapidly multiplying tachyzoites) in virtually every cell in the body. They ultimately produce cysts filled with minute slow-growing infective bodies (bradyzoites) that remain viable for long periods. Following successful cellular and humoral immune responses only encysted parasites can survive.

The tachyzoites of *Toxoplasma* and the promastigotes of *Leishmania* (discussed below) are 2 examples of parasite protozoa that replicate inside human macrophages. These protozoa are, of course, not the only infectious agents that can replicate inside a cell of the human immune system. HIV is the best-known example, but in many ways the adaptation of protozoan parasites, which are themselves eukaryotes, is even more remarkable. *Toxoplasma* invades a cell in a process that is independent of normal phagocytosis. The tachyzoite attaches to the cell membrane and induces changes in membrane topology as well as secretion from the specialized parasite structures called rhoptries. The parasite enters the cell through a moving membrane junction and forms a parasitophilus vacuole in the cytoplasm. This vacuole is a specialized structure that is probably the result of rhoptry secretions and which contains no recognizable host membrane proteins. The "parasite nature" of the vacuole prevents it from becoming acidified or fusing with host cell lysosomes. Before invasion, parasites become coated with extracellular matrix protein such as laminin, which, by interacting with host cell integrins (cell surface receptors), inhibit phagocytosis and the oxidative burst of macrophages that could result in parasite killing.

The ability of macrophages to kill intracellular parasites is greatly increased if the parasites are first exposed to antibody. In that case, the antibody-coated *Toxoplasma* cell is recognized by the Fc receptors of the macrophage. This triggers normal phagocytosis and the formation of reactive oxygen and nitrogen intermediates that ultimately kill the parasite.

An intact immune system is necessary for protection against *Toxoplasma*; thus, immunosuppression to control transplant rejection or malignancies, or infection with HIV, may result in active toxoplasmosis. This phenomenon may result either from the elimination of sensitized lymphocytes previously limiting an apparent infection or from inability of the immunosuppressed host to mount an adequate protective response to new infection.

LEISHMANIASIS

Leishmania is a genus of obligate intracellular parasites that infect macrophages of the skin and viscera to produce disease in both animals and humans. Sandflies, the principal vectors, introduce the parasites into the host while taking blood meals. In leishmaniasis, a range of host responses interact with a number of parasite leishmanial species and strains to produce a panoply of pathologic and immunologic responses. Leishmaniasis teaches 2 important lessons: (1) how different species or strains of the same parasite can produce drastically different diseases in a given host and (2) how genetic differences in the host can also lead to vastly different immune responses to infection by the same parasite.

1. CUTANEOUS LEISHMANIASIS

Major Immunologic Features
- Cell-mediated immunity is a critical factor.
- There is little or no specific serum antibody.

General Considerations
Old World cutaneous leishmaniasis, or tropical sore, is caused by several species of *Leishmania: Leishmania tropica, Leishmania major,* and *Leishmania aethiopica*. These agents induce an immune response characterized by nonprotective antibody but strong cell-mediated immunity. In cutaneous leishmaniasis, it is chiefly the patient's immune response to the infection that determines the form taken by the clinical disease; however, the strain of parasite may also determine part of the host response. If the patient mounts an adequate but not excessive cell-mediated immune response to the parasite, healing of the ulcerative lesions and specific protection result. However, if cell-mediated immunity to the parasite is inadequate or suppressed, the result may be diffuse cutaneous disease, in which there is little chance of spontaneous cure. In the Old World, this condition is due chiefly to *L aethiopica* in East Africa. A similar form, caused by *L mexicana* subsp *pifanoi*, occurs in Venezuela, again in specifically anergic patients. On the other hand, an excessive cell-mediated immune response produces lupoid or recidiva leishmaniasis, caused by *L tropica*, in which nonulcerated lymphoid nodules form at the edge of the primary lesion; these lesions persist indefinitely, although parasites are not easily demonstrated. Recidiva leishmaniasis may occur from 2 to 10 years after the initial lesion. Thus, a spectrum of host responses to cutaneous leishmaniasis exists, ranging from multiple disseminated parasite-filled ulcers or nodules (anergic response) to single, spontaneously cured immunizing sores to recidiva hyperactive host responses with few or no parasites (allergic response).

Cutaneous leishmaniasis of the New World is caused by a number of leishmanial pathogens now divided into 2 species complexes: *Leishmania mexicana* (subdivided into 4 or more subspecies) and *Leishmania braziliensis* (subdivided into 4 or more subspecies). The parasite subspecies (considered distinct species by many specialists) are distinguished on the basis of growth characteristics in the vector and in culture, isoenzyme electrophoresis patterns, kinetoplast DNA analysis, lectin-binding specifities, excreted factor serotyping, and monoclonal antibody probes. Geographic factors, hosts, and the character of the disease produced in humans are also important.

The most significant clinical distinction in the *L mexicana* complex is the high frequency of ear cartilage lesions (chiclero ulcer) and rare diffuse cutaneous leishmaniasis. In the *L braziliensis* complex, metastatic lesions develop, usually within 5 years of healing of the initial ulcer, which itself may be large, persistent, and disfiguring. Nasal cartilage and other nasopharyngeal tissues are attacked and destroyed by the subsequent massive ulceration (espundia), which may erode away much of the face and cause death by septic bronchopneumonia, asphyxiation, or starvation. This manifestation of American leishmaniasis is frequently nonresponsive to treatment. Parasites are abundant in the early stages of espundia but subsequently are rare, where was persistent infiltration of giant cells, plasma cells, and lymphocytes is characteristic. Delayed and perhaps immediate hypersensitivity and circulating antibody levels are higher in espundia than in cases of the primary lesion alone. The mucocutaneous form is thought to be an allergic or abnormal immunologic manisfestation of infection with the type subspecies *L braziliensis* subsp *braziliensis*.

A skin test (Montenegro test) is rapidly positive with cutaneous leishmaniasis, particularly the New World forms. Assays for lymphocyte proliferation or production of cytokines such as gamma interferon are also positive. Dermal response to kala-azar is slower, becoming positive only after cure of the visceral infection. Serodiagnosis of cutaneous leishmaniasis is still unsatisfactory because of low serum antibody levels and, in Latin America, because of cross-reactions with Chagas' disease antibodies. An exciting advance in field analysis of species (*L mexicana* versus *L braziliensis* complexes) is the application of nonradioactive species-specific DNA probes. By using the polymerase chain reaction (PCR), the *Leishmania* species infecting a patient can be determined from a small amount of parasite material in a cutaneous lesion.

The different clinical courses produced by infection with *Leishmania* species constitute a paradigm for the immune response to intracellular parasites. *Leishmania* parasites enter cells by a different pathway from that used by *Toxoplasma* organisms discussed above. *Leishmania* promastigotes enter passively through phagocytosis into macrophages. One of the unusual features of this infection is the predilection of the organisms for infection of the macrophage, a cell that is itself key to the host immune response. *Leishmania* parasites have adapted to replication in an unusual environment, the phagolysosomal vacuoles. Nevertheless, in cases of spontaneous cure of cutaneous leishmaniasis, parasite killing does occur. Recent studies in a mouse model of infection have begun to shed light on this interplay between host and intracellular parasite. First, a single dominant genetic locus, called *Bcg*, appears to govern whether mice are resistant to infection by both *Leishmania* and mycobacteria. This locus includes a gene that codes for a membrane channel protein which may be key in the transport of precursors of nitric oxide or oxygen radicals used by the macrophage for parasite killing. It is noteworthy that lessons from studying the immune response to intracellular parasites can cross-fertilize research on host response to mycobacteria and other fungal or bacterial infections in which macrophages play a key role. T cell products are also key to a successful host response to *Leishmania*. Gamma interferon is critical to parasite killing. In *L major* infections of mice, 2 CD4 T cell subtypes have been identified. In genetically resistant mice, the TH1 subtype predominates. This is a T cell population that produces interferon γ in its cytokine repertoire. In contrast, genetically susceptible mice have a predominant TH2 T cell subtype response with no production of gamma interferon but, rather, production of cytokines such as IL-5, IL-4, and IL-10. Although the existence of distinct T cell subtypes in human infections is more controversial, the mouse studies point out how a particular cytokine profile is key to activating infected macrophages to successfully kill the intracellular parasites. This work has had practical application, in that administration of recombinant gamma interferon enhances the response to chemotherapy in patients with visceral leishmaniasis.

2. VISCERAL LEISHMANIASIS

Major Immunologic Features
- Delayed hypersensitivity occurs only after spontaneous recovery or chemotherapy.
- Nonspecific immunoglobulin levels are increased.
- It causes polyclonal B cell hypergammaglobulinemia.
- Parasites in cells throughout the body produce systemic disease, characterized by leukopenia and splenomegaly and release of cachectin (TNFα).

General Considerations
The immune response to visceral leishmaniasis (kala-azar)—caused by various subspecies of *Leishmania donovani* (considered separate species by some authors)—is significantly different from that of cutaneous leishmaniasis, although the parasites are distinguishable only by enzyme analysis with zymodemes or other forms of molecular characterization. Massive polyclonal hypergammaglobulinemia with little or no evidence of cell-mediated immunity is the rule in visceral leishmaniasis. There is no quantitative relationship between the elevated serum immunoglobulin levels and antiparasite antibodies, which are, moreover, not species-specific. The immunoglobulin level diminishes rapidly when treatment be-

gins. Delayed cutaneous hypersensitivity to parasite antigens becomes demonstrable only after spontaneous recovery or treatment, which suggests that cell-mediated mechanisms play a role in the resolution of the infectious process. Under certain circumstances, post-kala-azar dermal "leishmanoid" occurs. Nodules containing many parasites form papules as a result of incomplete or defective cell-mediated immunity or a persistent allergic reaction to parasite antigens. Many cases of severe disseminated infection in HIV-infected individuals have now been reported in Mediterranean countries. This underscores the importance of cell-mediated immunity in controlling disease.

AFRICAN TRYPANOSOMIASIS

Major Immunologic Features
- There is a succession of parasite populations in the bloodstream, each with a different antigenic coating.

General Considerations
Trypanosoma brucei subsp *gambiense*, also called *T gambiense,* is the agent of chronic Gambian or West African sleeping sickness. *Trypanosoma brucei* subsp *rhodesiense*, also called *T rhodesiense*, is the agent of acute Rhodesian or East African sleeping sickness. Both cause human disease, and the Rhodesian form is the one most responsible for denying vast areas of Africa to human occupation, chiefly in the flybelt regions where the tsetse fly vectors are found. Tsetse-borne trypanosomes (*Trypanosoma brucei* subsp *brucei* as well as several other species) infect domestic animals with similar or even greater virulence. The impact of this dual threat—one to humans and the other to domestic animals, especially cattle—has had an enormous effect on human history in Africa. The great herd of wild herbivores, once abundant everywhere, have survived in this region because of their natural tolerance to heavy infections. The trypanosomes multiply extracellularly in successive waves in the human and animal bloodstream but produce very little disease in spite of their numbers. Only when the parasites enter the central nervous system does the ravaging disease sleeping sickness develop. It is this pathologic phase of an otherwise harmless chronic or recurrent infection to which humans and domestic animals succumb and which most native antelope and other herbivores resist.

Greatly increased levels of immunoglobulins, especially of the IgM class, are regularly present in infected humans and animals. The increased immunoglobulin levels, which do not correlate positively with protection, may result from B cell stimulants produced by the trypanosomes themselves or by the increased IgG production by helper T cells, which act nonspecifically to increase immunoglobulin levels. A large proportion of the immunoglobulin in infected hosts is nonspecific.

Although trypanosomes are continually exposed to the host immune system in the bloodstream, they evade the host defenses. The first hint of how this is accomplished was noted in 1910, when the periodicity of fever in patients with trypanosomiasis was correlated with a sharp rise and fall in the number of trypanosomes found in the blood. More recently, it was discovered that when individual organisms are cloned in culture, each clone displays a unique antigenic surface protein. When organisms first enter the host (Fig 50–2), the host immune system generates antibodies against the predominate surface antigen (variable surface glycoprotein [VSG]). Antibodies can kill over 90% of the original infecting trypanosome population. The reason why not all of the trypanosomes are killed is that some have switched on a different VSG antigen not recognized by the initial immune response. This switch occurs spontaneously and can be detected in immune-deficient mice. It is therefore not dependent on the host immune response. The switch is very rapid, so that by 5 days into an infection, parasites with more than one antigen type can be detected. By 6 days, as few as 15% of the trypanosomes may still have the initial surface VSG. This switching from one VSG to another explains the waves of parasitemia and periodicity of the fever characteristic of trypanosomiasis. The potential VSG repertoire is not known, although parasites derived from a single parent trypanosome have been found with more than 100 distinct VSGs.

What is the mechanism by which the trypanosome can so quickly switch its surface coat? Recombinant DNA techniques have been used to unravel part of the mystery. One copy of the VSG gene is located on a specific trypanosome (Fig 50–3). If that VSG is to be expressed, a copy of the gene is made and translocated to another chromosome close to the telomere. In this new location, and only in the new location, it is transcribed into messenger RNA to which a 35-nucleotide sequence is added. This small 35-nucleotide sequence has been transcribed from yet another site, where many of these small sequences are found closely linked to each other. Most trypanosome proteins have this small sequence at the beginning of their messenger RNA. Therefore, it is assumed that it is necessary for expression of the messenger RNA. However, some of the VSGs come from genes that are already near the telomere and therefore do not translocate before expression. Although the mechanism of "gene jumping" and subsequent expression has been elucidated, the exact mechanism by which one VSG is switched to another is still unclear. Understanding of this switching mechanism might provide a means of interrupting the ability of trypanosomes to change their antigenic disguises.

Serodiagnosis of trypanosomiasis is possible by using indirect immunofluorescence, enzyme-linked immunosorbent assay (ELISA), indirect hemagglutination, direct agglutination, gel precipitation for IgM titration, and gel precipitation with trypanosomal antigen. However, none of these methods are yet suitable for field studies or surveys in Africa.

Specific antibodies to trypanosomes can either lyse the parasites or clump them. Clumping allows for more efficient removal of the parasites by the reticuloendothelial system. It is controversial whether hu-

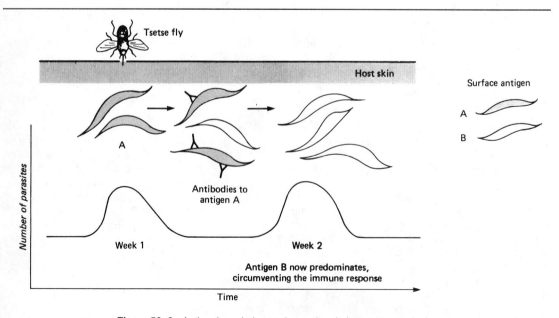

Figure 50–2. Antigenic variation and parasitemia in trypanosomiasis.

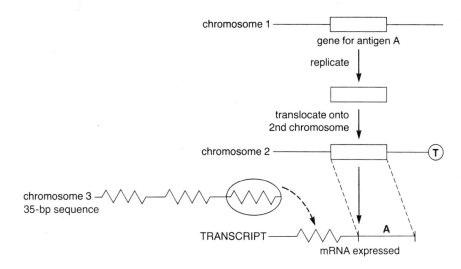

Figure 50–3. Molecular mechanism of antigenic diversity in trypanosomiasis.

mans or domestic animals living in areas where the infection is endemic develop resistance to infection, although epidemiologic observations suggest that resistance does arise. The fact that there are healthy human carriers of *T rhodesiense*—which usually produces a fatal infection—implies that some protective mechanism must exist.

Suppression of immune responses to other, unrelated antigens may be observed during trypanosomal infections. It is not known whether the suppression results from exhaustion of B cells, the presence of suppressor T cells, a lack of helper T cells, or the availability of fewer T cells to interact with new antigens.

The multiplicity of antigenic variants observed during field studies in bovines makes vaccination an unlikely solution to trypanosomiasis unless common antigens can be found.

IMMUNE RESPONSE TO HELMINTHS

Multicellular parasites, by reason of their size, more complex tissue and organ structure, and varied and active metabolism, include very complex host responses. Further complicating the picture is the fact that several forms of the parasite may be present in the host, each eliciting a unique immune response.

The primary antigens of helminths may often be metabolic by-products, enzymes, or other secretory products. For example, the eggs of *Schistosoma mansoni* have been shown to secrete unique antigens that induce granuloma formation; the various stages of developing nematodes have stage-specific antigens, often molting fluids, to which the host responds in various ways; and the granules in the stichocytes, special cells located in the "neck" of *Trichuris trichiura* elicit specific antibody.

Trematodes, cestodes, and nematodes probably all share common antigens. The two most frequent responses to helminths—eosinophilia and reaginic antibody (IgE)—are both T cell-dependent. Moreover, certain helminths have been shown to potentiate the immune response to other antigens, perhaps by common metabolic by-products acting as nonspecific adjuvants.

TREMATODES

Trematodes are important pathogens of humans and domestic animals. Fascioliasis debilitates and kills domestic animals in large numbers and renders the livers unfit for human consumption. Schistosomiasis is a major disease of humans. The lung flukes of the genus *Paragonimus* cause central nervous system complications in humans if they encyst in the brain. In the lungs, considerable mechanical damage results. *Clonorchis sinensis*, the fish-borne Chinese liver fluke, causes much morbidity both in the Orient and among recent emigrants from areas, where the infection is endemic, producing infection that may last the lifetime of the host.

1. SCHISTOSOMIASIS

Major Immunologic Features
- Response to invading worms is both humoral (IgE, IgM, IgG) and cellular (eosinophils, lymphocytes, macrophages).
- A serum sickness-like acute disease (Katayama fever) may develop.
- Chronic disease occurs owing to granulomatous reaction to eggs with subsequent fibrosis.
- Developing larvae and adult worms evade immune response by camouflaging their surface with host antigens.

Schistosomiasis in humans is caused by *Schistosoma mansoni*, *Schistosoma japonicum*, *Schistosoma haematobium*, and *Schistosoma mekongi*. The advent of new high dams in many areas of the world, especially Africa, has increased the prevalence of schistosomiasis, because the additional irrigation made possible by the dams has vastly enlarged the habitat of the freshwater snails that serve as intermediate hosts to the worms. The life cycle of this parasite depends on skin penetration of the definitive host by infective larvae produced in large numbers in the snail. Because attempts to reduce snail populations have largely failed, infection has become rampant in these areas. *S mansoni*, now widespread in Africa and the Middle East, has also spread extensively in South America. *S haematobium* is found in all watered areas of Africa and the Arabian peninsula. *S japonicum* is found in the Yangtze River watershed in China, where it has been subjected to a vast control effort but is still common in Szechwan province and may be returning to the main river valley. It is also common in the central Philippines. A purely animal-infecting (zoophilic) form is found in Taiwan. *S mekongi*, a newly described species similar to *S japonicum*, causes human disease in Thailand, Laos, and Cambodia, with a scattering of cases in Malaysia, recently described as being due to *S malaysiensis*. There is also a focus of *S japonicum* in Sulawesi (Celebes) that may prove to be a distinct species.

In brief, the life cycle of the schistosomes that infect humans is as follows. Infected humans and animals excrete eggs that hatch in water, releasing miracidia; these actively penetrate snails, in which several generations of multiplying larvae (sporocysts) develop. These in turn produce great numbers of fork-tailed cercariae, the stage infective for humans, which leave the host snail at a rate of 300–3000 per day. The cercariae penetrate the skin of the definitive host, leaving the tail outside, and enter the bloodstream as minute motile immature schistosomula, which migrate in 3–8 days to the lungs and eventually to the liver. Further development and adult worm pairing take place about 5 weeks after skin penetration. The paired mature schistosomes then migrate against the venous flow into the mesenteric or vesical venules, where the female deposits eggs. The embryo (miracidium) within the egg secretes proteases, which may facilitate passage through the blood vessel and adjacent tissue into the lumen of the intestine (or bladder in the case of *S haematobium*). Alternatively, some investigators have suggested that the granuloma produced by the host around the egg "chaperones" it through the wall of the intestine. Egg movement is also probably aided by peristalsis of the intestine or contractions of the bladder.

Unfortunately, not all the eggs reach the lumen of the intestine or bladder. Some become trapped in the submucosa, and others do not leave the bloodstream but instead are carried with the venous flow to the liver portals or by collateral circulation to other organs of the body. Because of their size, eggs reaching the liver become trapped in the portal venules and do not enter the sinusoids. When eggs are trapped in the liver, the wall of the intestine, or the bladder, they elicit a granulomatous inflammation that is the hallmark of the chronic stage of schistosomiasis. An early infiltrate of neutrophils and lymphocytes may be seen around eggs, but distinctive granulomas containing a core of macrophages and eosinophils, surrounded by a cuff of lymphocytes, appear shortly thereafter. The early stages of inflammation may be seen by 6 weeks, but granulomas reach their maximal cellularity within 9–12 weeks. Later, an increasing number of fibroblasts or lipocytes (Ito cells) can be seen in association with the granulomas, and the cellular lesion becomes slowly replaced by collagen. In the liver, older lesions become periportal scars. Since numerous eggs are deposited, a circumferential periportal fibrosis called Symmer's clay pipestem fibrosis develops; this is particularly well demarcated in *S mansoni* infection. This fibrosis blocks normal blood flow from the portal venous system to the sinusoids, resulting in portal hypertension and its complications.

The factors that initiate granuloma formation are soluble proteins secreted through pores in the eggshell by the embryonic micracidium. These soluble egg products, some of which have been purified, are used in one serodiagnostic test for schistosomiasis. As might be expected from the complex group of cells that form the granuloma, the mechanisms of granuloma formation, modulation, and subsequent fibrosis are complex. Pleiotropic cytokines are involved, as well as factors from the egg itself that may be both chemotactic and mitogenic for fibroblasts. The importance of cellular immunity in granuloma formation has been underscored by the observation that both the granulomatous reaction to schistosome eggs and subsequent periportal fibrosis are absent or significantly diminished in thymus-deficient ("nude") mice and in mice with severe combined immunodeficiency (*scid* mice). *scid* mice have no functional T and B cells, and in the absence of a granulomatous response, schistosome eggs produce a frequently fatal acute hepatotoxic effect. Therefore, one conclusion made from these observations in *scid* mice was that the granulomatous reaction to the eggs protects the host from diffusible egg products which can directly damage liver cells. On the other hand, an unexpected observation was than an intact cellular immune response was necessary for egg production by schistosome females and passage of eggs through the intestinal wall. Injection of supernatant from cultures of T cell clones led to reconstitution of the host granulomatous response as well as egg production and transmission. This suggested that specific T cell-derived cytokines were required as key elements in the host-parasite interplay. These observations confirm that the host-parasite relationship is an extremely intricate, complicated, and highly evolved phenomenon in which elements of the host immune response are sometimes subverted by the parasite for its own replication and transmission.

Although the immune response to schistosome eggs is the central immunopathologic mechanism in chronic schistosomiasis, it is not the only immune response of importance in schistosome infection. In some previously infected individuals, invading cercariae may elicit a dermatitis with features of both immediate and delayed hypersensitivity. This is similar to the "swimmers' itch" produced by nonhuman schistosomes that enter the skin of previously sensitized individuals. Some schistosomes species may produce any acute form of schistosomiasis (Katayama fever) characterized by fever, eosinophilia, lymphadenopathy, diarrhea, splenomegaly, and urticaria. This appears to be an anaphylactic (IgE) or serum sickness (IgG) reaction. In fact, cases of glomerulonephritis secondary to schistosome antigen-antibody complexes have been reported.

An important unresolved question is whether protective immunity to schistosomiasis develops in humans after infection. Studies in Kenya and Gambia have shown that schistosome-infected individuals in an area of endemicity who had been treated with anti-schistosome drugs showed an age-dependent resistance to reinfection. Children were much more easily reinfected than were adults, suggesting that true human immunity can be acquired with age. Identification of "resistant" groups of children may help to identify important parasite antigens. Augmentation of the response to these antigens would be one rational approach to vaccine development.

The question of immunity to reinfection has been studied intensively by using animal models. Two models in particular have been used. In the first of these, called the **concomitant immunity model**, mice are infected with 20–30 normal *S mansoni* cercariae 6 weeks prior to challenge. In the second, called the **attenuated vaccine model**, mice are immunized with 400–500 cercariae attenuated by 20–50 kilorads of gamma radiation 2 weeks before challenge. The mechanisms by which the host eliminates

the challenge infection may be different in each of these 2 models. Studies with the concomitant immunity model in mice or in rats, a naturally nonpermissive host, emphasized the importance of specific antiparasite IgG and eosinophils. In fact, these models help to elucidate many of the cellular functions of eosinophils. Eosinophilia is a common denominator in helminth parasite infections, and histologic examination of parasites and host tissue invariably confirms the presence of numerous eosinophils around dead or dying organisms. On the other hand, studies with attenuated vaccine model pointed to macrophages as the principal effector cells in elimination of the challenge infection. Whether one or both of these mechanisms is key in the human immune response to schistosome infection remains an active area of research and debate.

By comparing normal with various immune-deficient mouse strains, the cellular and antibody requirements of vaccine immunity have been investigated. Vaccinated mice with T lymphocyte deficiencies, as well as mice immunosuppressed from birth, have a sharply diminished resistance to challenge infection. On the other hand, mice deficient in complement, mast cells, natural killer (NK) lymphocytes, and IgE show no difference in resistance compared with normal controls. In a theme common to many parasitic infections, CD4 T cells secreting gamma interferon and macrophages appear key to killing of larvae in vaccinated mice.

The exact site of killing schistosomula in vaccinated mice remains controversial. Most studies indicate that killing occurs in the lungs. However, some evidence also exists for immune killing in the skin.

Immunodiagnosis of schistosome infection in the absence of egg excretion by the host can be accomplished in various ways, both humoral and cellular. Stage-specific humoral responses can be used to produce circumoval precipitation; schistosomule growth inhibition or death; and complement fixation, hemagglutination, and various precipitation reactions. None of these reactions can be positively correlated with protection. Immediate and delayed cutaneous hypersensitivity develop in most individuals during the course of the disease, although the specificity of these reactions is often suspect, owing to antigens that cross-react with those of other worms. However, the purification of novel antigenic fractions and sensitive ELISA or radioimmunoassays may improve the specificity of tests based on these responses.

CESTODES

There are 2 types of immune response to cestodes. One is directed against the intestinal lumen-dwelling adult tapeworms such as *Diphyllobothrium latum* and *Taenia saginata*, which have restricted, nonhumoral immunogenic contact. The response is chiefly cell-mediated, is induced primarily by the scolex, affects growth and strobilation of challenge worms, and varies considerably with the host species. The other is directed against migratory tissue-encysting larval tapeworms such as *Hymenolepis nana* (in its intravillous larval phase), *Echinococcus granulosus* (hydatid cysts), and *Taenia solium* (cysticercosis), which have intimate and continuous tissue contact and induce a strong parenteral host response detectable as serum antibody and strongly protective against reinfection. Serodiagnostic tests are available only for the larval tissue cestode parasites, and humoral responses that protect the challenged host have only recently been described for this form of cestode parasitism. ELISA for serodiagnosis of cysticercosis—with some cross-reactivity—has been developed.

1. ECHINOCOCCOSIS

Major Immunologic Features

- IgE levels are elevated.
- Anaphylaxis may occur after rupture of hydatid cysts and release of cyst fluids.
- The Casoni skin test is of questionable use.
- Diagnostic antibody is present.

General Considerations

The most serious human cestode infection is that caused by *Echinococcus*. These tiny tapeworms do not produce pathologic lesions in the definitive host, the dog, but severe complications occur when their eggs are ingested by humans and other animals. The larval form of the tapeworm hatches from the egg in the intestine of the intermediate host, eg, humans, and then claws its way through the intestinal mucosa and is transported through the lymphatic and blood vessels to sites in which it grows to enormous proportions, although it is enclosed by a heavy cyst wall laid down by both the host and the parasite. In humans, *Echinococcus* normally forms fluid-filled cysts in the liver, but these can also occur in the lungs, brain, kidneys, and other parts of the body. Hydatid cysts are highly immunogenic and result in production of higher titers of IgE and other immunoglobulins. If a cyst is ruptured, anaphylactic response to the cyst fluid can cause death. Little or no immune protection is elicited by this highly immunogenic cestode, because the hydatid cysts remain alive for years and, in animals, can be shown to increase in number as the host ages. Humans are usually a dead-end host, for the cysts must be eaten by a canid to become sexually mature. There is some evidence that complement-mediated lysis of protoscoleces (the numerous future scoleces in hydatid fluid or "hydatid sand") might be protective in the infected human or other intermediate host.

The Casoni skin test indicates past or present echinococcosis. It consists of intradermal injection of hy-datid cyst fluid, resulting in both immediate and delayed hypersensitivity. The specificity of this test is in doubt because of cross-reactions with other helminths. Heating the cyst fluid slightly increases the specificity of the test. Serodiagnosis can be made by hemagglutination, complement fixation, and flocculation tests, ELISA, and radioimmunoassay, with serum from the patient and specially fractionated antigenic components made from cyst fluid. These tests are not species-specific.

NEMATODES

Nematodes are the most common, varied, and widely distributed helminths that infect humans. As with other parasites, immunogenicity is a reflection of the degree and duratin of parasite contact with the host tissues. Even with the intestinal lumen dwellers such as *Ascaris*, there is a migratory larval phase in which such contact is made—in most cases, in the pulmonary capillaries and alveolar spaces. The hookworms of humans (*Ancylostoma duodenale* and *Necator americanus*) also migrate, except that the infective larvae enter via the skin or buccal mucosa rather than as hatchlings in the small bowel. *Strongyloides stercoralis*, the small intestinal roundworm of humans, undergoes a similar hookwormlike migration (as well as a stage of internal autoinfection or reinvasion via the mucosa of the large intestine).

The immature stages are particularly immunogenic, probably because of their high production of antigens from secretory glands and of enzymes or other products from these metabolically active stages. Commercially prepared vaccines are available only for nematodes, and all are living larval worms, irradiated to arrest their development but not their immunogenicity. These are the cattle and sheep lungworms *Dictyocaulus viviparus* and *Dictyocaulus filaria* and the dog hookworm *Ancylostoma caninum*. Another important group of human parasites are the filariae (chiefly *Wuchereria bancrofti, Brugia malayi, Loa loa, Onchocerca volvulus*, and the related guinea worm, *Dracunculus medinensis*). Diagnosis of these infections is often difficult, in part because of the presence of common antigens that preclude highly specific immunologic tests. Hypersensitivity reactions may occur after drug treatment (such as with diethylcarbamizine for *Onchocerca*), when large numbers of dead or dying microfilariae produce severe skin reactions and edema or dangerous reactions in the eye or (with *Loa*) when dead adult worms induce central nervous system reactions.

1. TRICHINOSIS

Major Immunologic Features
- Skin tests for immediate and delayed hypersensitivity are positive.
- Diagnostic antibody is present.

General Considerations

Trichinosis is acquired by ingestion of the infective larvae of *Trichinella spiralis* in uncooked or partially cooked meat. Pork is the primary source of infection in humans. The larvae are released from their cysts in the meat during digestion and rapidly develop into adults in the mucosa of the host small intestine. After copulation in the lumen, the males die and the females return to the intestinal mucosa, where for about 5–6 weeks each female produces 1000–1500 larvae, which migrate through the lymphatic system to the bloodstream. These larvae travel in the blood to all parts of the body and develop in voluntary muscles, especially in the diaphragm, tongue, masticatory and intercostal muscles, larynx, and eyes. Within the sarcolemma of striated muscle fibers, the larvae coil up into cysts whose outer walls are rapidly laid down by histiocytes. Larvae may remain viable and infective for as long as 24 years, even though the cysts calcify. The encysted larvae apparently do not elicit immune protection. The migrating larvae and adult forms of the parasite excrete antigens that appear to be responsible for induction of the strong protection from subsequent challenge infections. An important expression of host resistance is active expulsion of developing or adult worms from the gut of a parasitized host—the so-called self-cure phenomenon. This occurs when a new infection initiates a host response, resulting in elimination of the old one—the opposite of concomitant immunity.

The expulsion of *T spiralis* in humans appears to follow the mechanism proposed by Ogilvie and coworkers for the rodent hookworm, *Nippostrongylus brasiliensis*. A two-step mechanism is proposed: antibody-induced metabolic damage that blocks feeding by the worms followed by worm expulsion induced by activated lymphocytes. Both antibodies and cells are probably required for full expression of intestinal resistance, and the effect is synergistic rather than additive. As in the case of leishmaniasis, discussed above, TH1 subtype CD4 lymphocytes may be key in cellular immunity via their production of gamma interferon.

Trichinella infection sometimes presents characteristic clinical symptoms, such as edema of the eyelids and face, but often presents less specific clinical signs such as eosinophilia, which can also be suggestive of several other parasitic infections. Specific immunodiagnostic tests may thus be of great importance. The bentonite flocculation test for human trichinosis is of value because of its high degree of specificity. A skin test (Bachman intradermal test) produces both immediate and delayed responses.

In humans, infection with *Trichinella* initially elicits IgM antibody followed by an IgG response. IgA antibody has been reported, which is not surprising, because the female worms are in the intestinal mucosa, although the locally produced protective gut antibodies probably are IgG rather than IgA or IgM. This antibody reaction against the feeding worms is complement-independent and, as noted, precedes the rapid expulsion of the antibody-damaged worms by T lymphocytes.

Although *Trichinella* is extremely immunogenic in its hosts, it can also exert an immunosuppressive action. Certain viral infections are more severe during infection with this parasite, and skin grafts show delayed rejection. On the other hand, cellular immunity to BCG seems to be potentiated when *T spiralis* is present, and *T spiralis*-infected mice are less susceptible to *Listeria* infections.

2. ASCARIASIS

Major Immunologic Features
- Specific antibody is detectable.
- IgE levels are elevated.

General Considerations

Ascaris, the giant roundworm in humans, is a lumen-dwelling parasite as an adult and causes little inconvenience to the host except in the heaviest infections, although even single adult worms may produce mechanical damage by entering the bile or pancreatic ducts and penetration through an amebiasis intestinal lesion may result in peritonitis. Ingestion of eggs is followed by their hatching and then by penetration of the mucosa by the larvae which eventually reach the lung via the bloodstream. In a previously infected host, hypersensitivity reactions in the lung as a result of high levels of IgE can cause serious pneumonitis. Acute hypersensitivity to *Ascaris* antigens often develops in laboratory workers and makes it virtually impossible for them to continue working with the nematode.

Cases of sudden death in Nigeria have been ascribed to *Ascaris*-induced anaphylactic shock syndrome, heretofore rarely diagnosed or recognized. Death probably resulted from the release of a mast cell degranulator by the worms, since degranulated mast cells were found throughout the body tissues in these children, or from a reagin-*Ascaris* allergen interaction at the mast cell surface. Allergy to ascariasis may underlie many of the symptoms of *Ascaris* infection, including abdominal pain.

3. FILARID NEMATODES

Major Immunologic Features

- Induction of host immune response to adults or microfilariae leads to disease.

General Considerations

Filarid nematodes are introduced into the human host by insect vectors. Nematoses of the genus *Brugia* or *Wuchereria* are spread by a mosquito vector, whereas *Onchocerca volvulus* is transmitted by blackflies. Although the stages of each life cycle are similar, the type of disease produced varies considerably. A common theme is that morbidity is due primarily to the host immune response to the parasite rather than any toxic product of the parasite itself.

O volvulus is the causative agent of onchocerciasis, or African river blindness. This is the major cause of blindness in areas of West Africa and Central America where the infection is endemic. Infectious larvae that are deposited by a blackfly bite migrate in the subcutaneous tissue and develop into adults in approximately 1 year. The adults elicit an unusual fibrogenic host response, resulting in a subcutaneous collagenous nodule in which the worm lives. The female produces large numbers of microfilariae, which migrate out of the nodule and are distributed widely in subcutaneous tissue. This dispersal of microfilariae increases the likelihood that they will be picked up again by the insect vector to continue the life cycle. Humans react to migrating microfilariae by production of both circulating antibody and cellular immunity. An intense delayed hypersensitivity-like reaction to dead or dying microfilariae can lead to a disseminated skin reaction or a more serious eye disease. Microfilariae can enter all chambers of the eye and elicit a keratitis or retinitis, which, over a period of years, can lead to total blindness.

Parasites of the genera *Brugia* and *Wuchereria*, in contrast, produce lymphatic filariasis. In this case, the damaging response is due to adult worms residing in lymphatics, most commonly in the groin. Over time, the lymphatic lumen may be compromised by scarring, leading to blockage of lymph drainage from the lower extremities and production of a disfiguring condition called "elephantiasis" that characterizes severe chronic disease.

REFERENCES

General

Ash C: Macrophages at the centre of infection. *Parasitol Today* 1991;**7**:2.

Cox FEG, Liew EY: T-cell subsets and cytokines in parasitic infections. *Parasitol Today* 1992; **8**:371.

Desowitz RS: *Ova and Parasites. Medical Parasitology for the Laboratory Technologist.* Harper & Row, 1980.

Ellner JJ, Mahmoud AF: Phagocytes and worms: David and Goliath revisited. *Rev Infect Dis* 1982;**4**:698.

Finkelman FD, Urban, JF Jr: Cytokines: Making the right choice. *Parasitol Today* 1992;**8**:311.

Kagan IG, Maddison SE: Immunology of parasites: General aspects. Pages 315–325 in: *Immunology of Human Infection*, Part 2, *Viruses and Parasites: Immunodiagnosis and Prevention of Infectious Diseases.* Nahmias AJ, O'Reilly RH (editors). Plenum, 1982.

Kay AB et al: Leukocytes activation initiated by IgE-dependent mechanisms in relation to helminthic parasitic disease and clinical models of asthma. *Int Arch Allergy Appl Immunol* 1985;**77**:69.

Klei TR: Experimental immunologic studies on lymphatic filariasis. Pages 31–42 in: *Molecular & Immunological Aspects of Parasitism.* Wang CC (editor). American Association for the Advancement of Science, 1991.

Mitchell GF et al: Examination of strategies for vaccination against parasitic infection or disease using mouse models. Pages 323–328 in: *Contemporary Topics in Immunobiology.* Vol 12. Marchalonis JJ (editor). Plenum, 1984.

Scott P: IL-12: Initiation cytokine for cell-mediated immunity. *Science* 1993;**260**:496.

Soulsby EJL (editor): *Immune Responses in Parasitic Infections: Immunology, Immunopathology, and Immunoprophylaxis.* Vol 1: *Nematodes.* Vol 2: *Trematodes and Cestodes.* Vol 3: *Protozoa.* Vol 4: *Protozoa, Arthropods, and Invertebrates.* CRC Press, 1987.

Wakelin D: Immunity to parasites. In: *How Animals Control Parasitic Infection.* Arnold, 1984.

Wakelin D: Genetic control of immunity to helminth infections. *Parasitol Today* 1985;**1**:17.

Serodiagnostic Tests

Centers for Disease Control: *Reference and Disease Surveillance.* Center for Infectious Diseases, CDC, 1985.

Sun, T: *Pathology and Clinical Features of Parasitic Diseases.* Masson Monograph in Diagnostic Pathology. Vol 5. Masson, 1982.

Leishmaniasis

Reiner SL et al: T_H1 and T_H2 cell antigen receptors in experimental leishmaniasis. *Science* 1993;**259**:1457.

Scott P, Sher A: A spectrum in the susceptibility of leishmanial strains to intracellular killing by murine macrophages. *J Immunol* 1986;**136**:1461.

Malaria

Butcher GA: HIV and malaria: A lesson in immunology? *Parasitol Today* 1992;**8**:307.

Greenwood B, Marsh K, Snow R: Why do some African

children develop severe malaria? *Parasitol Today* 1991;**7**:277.

Jensen JB et al: Induction of crisis forms in cultured *Plasmodium falciparum* with human immune serum from Sudan. *Science* 1982;**216**:1230.

Riley EM, Olerup O, Troye-Blomberg M: The immune recognition of malaria antigens. *Parasitol Today* 1991;**7**:5.

Sinigaglia F, Pink JRL: A way round the 'real difficulties' of malaria sporozoite vaccine development? *Parasitol Today* 1990;**6**:277.

WHO Scientific Working Group on the Immunology of Malaria: Development of malaria vaccines: Memorandum from a USAID/WHO meeting. *Bull WHO* 1983;**61**:81.

Zavala F et al: Rationale for development of a synthetic vaccine against *Plasmodium falciparum* malaria. *Science* 1985;**228**:1436.

Schistosomiasis

Butterworth AE et al: Studies on the mechanism of immunity in human schistosomiasis. *Immunol Rev* 1982;**61**:5.

Capron A et al: Mechanisms of immunity to schistosomes and their regulation. *Immunol Rev* 1982;**61**:41.

Cheever AW: Schistosomiasis: Infection versus disease and hypersensitivity versus immunity. *Am J Pathol* 1993; **142**:699.

Damian RT et al: *Schistosoma mansoni*; Parasitology and immunology of baboons vaccinated with irradiated cryopreserved schistosomula. *Int J Parasitol* 1985;**15**:333.

Hagan P, Wilkins HA: Concomitant immunity in schistosomiasis. *Parasitol Today* 1993;**9**:3.

McLaren DJ: The role of eosinophils in tropical disease. *Semin Hematol* 1982;**19**:100.

Mitchell GF et al: Analysis of infection characteristics and antiparasite immune responses in resistant compared with susceptible hosts. *Immunol Rev* 1982; **61**:137.

Nogueira-Machado JA et al: *Schistosoma mansoni*: Cell-mediated immunity evaluated by antigen-induced leukocyte adherence inhibition assay. *Immunol Lett* 1985;**9**:39.

Phillips SM, Lammie PJ: Immunopathology of granuloma formation and fibrosis in schistosomiasis. *Parasitol Today* 1986;**2**:296.

Stadecker MJ, Colley DG: The immunobiology of the schistosome egg granuloma. *Parasitol Today* 1992; **8**:218.

Von Lichtenberg F: Conference on contend issues of immunity to schistosomes. *Am J Trop Med Hyg* 1985; **34**:78.

Warren KS: Immunology. In: *Schistosomiasis: Epidemiology, Treatment, Control*. Jordan P, Webbe G (editors). Pitman, 1982.

Trypanosomiasis

Donelson JE, Turner MJ: How the trypanosome changes its coat. *Sci Am* (Feb) 1985;**252**:44.

Esser KL, Schornblecher MJ: Expression of two variant surface glycoproteins on individual African trypanosomes during antigen switching. *Science* 1985; **229**:290.

Parsons M et al: Antigenic variation in Africana trypanosomes: DNA rearrangements program immune evasion. *Immunol Today* 1984;**5**:43.

51

Spirochetal Diseases

Charles S. Pavia, PhD, & David J. Drutz, MD

Spirochetes are a highly specialized group of motile gram-negative bacteria, with a slender and tightly helically coiled structure. They range from 0.1 to 0.5 μm in width and from 10 to 50 μm in length. One of the unique features of spirochetes is their motility by rapidly drifting rotation, often associated with a flexing or undulating movement along the helical path. These bacteria belong to the order Spirochaetales, which includes 2 families: Spirochaetaceae and Leptospiraceae. Important members of these groups include *Treponema, Borrelia,* and *Leptospira.*

Spirochetal infections leading to such diseases as syphilis and the other treponematoses, Lyme disease, relapsing fever borreliosis, and leptospirosis are important worldwide health problems. A better understanding of the immunobiology of the disease-causing spirochetes has become crucial in efforts to develop effective vaccines, because there has been no significant modification in excessive sexual activity, personal hygiene practices, or vector control. Further knowledge of immune responses to spirochetes is essential for their eventual control by immunization, and studies of the host-spirochete relationship have led to important new insights into the immune system itself. Serologic techniques have now become indispensable diagnostic tools for detection of many of the spirochetal diseases, especially syphilis and Lyme disease (Fig 51–1). The response of small laboratory animals to *Treponema pallidum* infection is an excellent experimental model for studying the development of resistance to syphilitic reinfection and the relative roles of humoral versus and immunity in protection against syphilis. Unfortunately, the immune response to spirochetal infections, as in other infections, may paradoxically cause immunologically induced disease in the host, such as aortitis, immune-complex glomerulonephritis, the gummatous lesions of syphilis, and the neuropathies and arthritis of Lyme disease.

SYPHILIS

Major Immunologic Features

- Both nonspecific, anticardiolipin, and specific antitreponemal antibodies are detectable following primary infection.
- Cell-mediated immunity becomes activated during or after the late secondary stage.
- Immunosuppression occurs during various phases of the disease.
- A complex state of partial immunity develops late following an untreated primary infection.

General Considerations

T pallidum is the spirochetal bacterium responsible for the sexually transmitted disease syphilis, which can have severe pathologic consequences if untreated and for which there is no vaccine. The organism is noncultivable, highly motile, and infectious, and it replicates extracellularly in vivo.

With the institution of antibiotic therapy in the mid-1940s, the incidence of syphilis fell sharply from a high of 72 cases per 100,000 in 1943 to about 4 per 100,000 in 1956. For the past several years, however, the Centers for Disease Control and Prevention have periodically reported significant increases in primary and secondary syphilis cases, which can be attributed, in part, to changing lifestyles, sexual practices, and other factors such as an unusually high prevalence and resistance to antibiotics in patients with acquired immunodeficiency syndrome (AIDS). The estimated annual rate per 100,000 increased nationwide from 10.9 cases in 1986 to 13.3 cases in 1987 and 17.3 cases in 1991. This represents the largest rise in more than 10 years. Syphilis continues to rank annually as the third or fourth most frequently reported communicable disease in the USA.

The course of syphilis in humans is marked by several interesting phenomena. Without treatment the disease will usually progress through several well-defined stages. This is unlike most other infectious

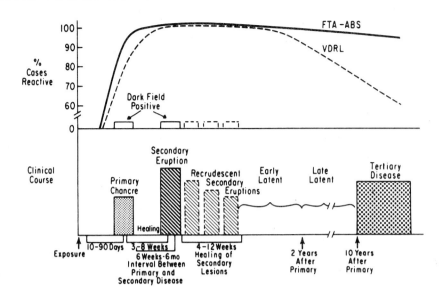

Figure 51–1. The course of untreated syphilis. (Reproduced, with permission, from Joklik WK et al (editors). *Zinsser Microbiology,* 20th ed. Appleton-Century-Crofts, 1992.)

diseases, which are ultimately eliminated by the host's immune system or, in severe cases, result in death. The relatively slow generation time of treponemes, which is estimated at 30–33 hours, contributes to this unique course. During the first 2 stages (primary and secondary syphilis) there is almost unimpeded rapid growth of *T pallidum,* leading to an early infectious spirochetemic phase of disease. The third stage (tertiary syphilis) occurs much later, following a prolonged latency period. Alterations in this stage are due primarily to tissue-damaging immune responses elicited by small numbers of previously deposited or disseminated spirochetes.

Syphilis activates both humoral and cell-mediated immunity, but this protection is only partial. The relative importance of each type of immune response is not fully known. Protective immunity against reexposure is incomplete, especially during early stages, when it develops relatively slowly. Evidence for the participation of humoral immunity in syphilis is as follows:

(1) A variety of nonspecific "reaginic" or Wassermann cardiolipin and specific antibodies are routinely present in the sera of patients with syphilis.

(2) *T pallidum*-immobilizing antibodies (TPIA) are regularly present in the sera of syphilitic patients.

(3) The frequency with which TPIA are found increases as syphilis progresses to latent and tertiary infection.

(4) Partial immunity can be conferred in experimentally infected laboratory animals by passive transfer of serum from syphilis-immune donors. This protection is apparent when treponemes are injected intradermally into these animal hosts. Chancres may

be either prevented or delayed, and dissemination of treponemes from the primary focus of infection may be reduced by passive immunization.

Interestingly, humans who have been experimentally infected with *T pallidum* also develop increased local resistance to rechallenge at a cutaneous site. This local resistance is referred to as **chancre immunity**. Chancre immunity persists if primary infection remains untreated and syphilis progresses to a latent stage. Although chancre immunity is indicative of heightened local resistance, it does not prevent the systemic spread of *T pallidum* from the site of initial challenge. Chancre immunity may be attributable to antibody, because both the immunity and reaginic antibodies wane after treatment of primary syphilis. The time required depends on the titer of antibody and the severity of the illness. For several reasons, it is not likely that the antibodies are completely protective:

(1) Treponemes from the initial infection persist systemically during latent syphilis, even though there is resistance to a second challenge. This suggests that the organism has found sanctuary in some sort of privileged residence, where it resists or is unaffected by host defenses.

(2) Some antibodies are nonspecific and are found in other diseases such as systemic lupus erythematosus. They might even be directed against host rather than treponemal antigens.

(3) By preventing the attachment of treponemes to cells in tissue culture, antibodies might, in fact, aid the organism in escaping host defense mechanisms.

(4) Circulating immune complexes are formed during infection with *T pallidum.* They are demonstrable in sera of both rabbits and patients with syphilis.

They may be composed of cardiolipin-anticardiolipin as well as of treponemal antigen-antitreponemal antibody. They may act to depress the synthesis of IgG against independent antigens, such as sheep erythrocytes. It is conceivable that circulating immune complexes prevent the host from synthesizing treponemicidal antibody during primary syphilis or from synthesizing antitreponemal antibody that might act in concert with cell-mediated immunity against *T pallidum.*

(5) The patterns of antibody production change during the course of untreated syphilis. Patients with secondary syphilis have antitreponemal antibody as well as anticardiolipin antibody. These antibodies are of both IgG and IgM classes. As the disease enters latency, antitreponemal IgM antibody production ceases and patients are left with antitreponemal IgG and anticardiolipin IgM and IgG. The clinical significance of this sequence of events is uncertain.

Recent investigations in animal models have increasingly implicated cell-mediated immunity as a critical element in host response to *T pallidum.* Evidence for the participation of cell-mediated immunity in syphilis is as follows:

(1) Passive transfer of syphilis immune serum is only partially protective and does not follow classic models of humoral immunity.

(2) Syphilis progresses through the primary and secondary stages despite the presence of antibodies that immobilize the infecting organism.

(3) Delayed hypersensitivity to treponemal antigens is absent in primary and early secondary syphilis but develops late in secondary infection and is regularly present in latent and tertiary syphilis.

(4) Granulomatous lesions characterize tertiary syphilis.

(5) Immunization with killed microorganisms is usually unsuccessful, whereas immunization with live attenuated organisms has produced immunity.

(6) In vitro lymphocyte reactivity to treponemal and nontreponemal antigens and T lymphocyte counts are suppressed during primary and secondary syphilis.

(7) Infecting rabbits with *T pallidum* stimulates acquired cellular resistance to *Listeria;* this reaction is mediated by T lymphocytes.

(8) Both T and B cells are effective in conferring antisyphilis immunity when transferred from nonimmune recipients to normal challenged recipients.

It is puzzling why so much time is required for patients to develop humoral and cellular immunity to syphilis. One theory holds that the mucoid envelope of *T pallidum* renders it highly resistant to phagocytosis; only after the treponemes have remained in the host for some time is the mucoid coat broken down sufficiently for phagocytosis to occur. (Treponemal mucopolysaccharides also suppress lymphocyte blastogenic response to concanavalin A.) As a result, treponemal proliferation outstrips the rate of anti-

genic processing for stimulation of humoral and cellular immune mechanisms; a condition of "antigen overload" then occurs, with production of secondary immunosuppression. An alternative explanation is that sensitization with treponemal antigen leads primarily to generation of antibodies that then block antigenic sites, thereby inhibiting an appropriate cell-mediated immune response.

The proposed immunologic mechanisms are highly speculative.

Clinical Features

The severe late manifestations or complications of syphilis occur in the blood vessels and perivascular areas. However, sexual contact is the common mode of transmission, with inoculation on the mucous membranes of genital organs.

The first clinically apparent manifestation of syphilis (primary syphilis) is an indurated, circumscribed, relatively avascular and painless ulcer (chancre) at the site of treponemal inoculation. Spirochetemia with secondary metastatic distribution of microorganisms occurs within a few days after onset of local infection, but clinically apparent secondary lesions may not be observed for 2–4 weeks. The chancre lasts 10–14 days before healing spontaneously.

The presence of metastatic infection (secondary syphilis) is manifested by highly infectious mucocutaneous lesions of extraordinarily diverse description as well as headache, low-grade fever, diffuse lymphadenopathy, and a variety of more sporadic phenomena. The lesions of secondary syphilis ordinarily go on to apparent spontaneous resolution in the absence of treatment. However, until solid immunity develops—a matter of about 4 years—25% of untreated syphilitic patients may be susceptible to repeated episodes of spirochetemia and metastatic infection.

Following the resolution of secondary syphilis, the disease enters a period of latency, with only abnormal serologic tests to indicate the presence of infection. During this time, persistent or progressive focal infection is presumably taking place, but the precise site remains unknown in the absence of specific symptoms and signs. One site of potential latency, the central nervous system, can be evaluated by examining the cerebrospinal fluid, in which pleocytosis, elevated protein levels, and a positive serologic test for syphilis are indicative of asymptomatic neurosyphilis.

Only about 15% of patients with untreated latent syphilis go on to develop symptomatic tertiary syphilis. Serious or fatal tertiary syphilis in adults is virtually limited to disease of the aorta (aortitis with aneurysm formation and secondary aortic valve insufficiency), the central nervous system (tabes dorsalis, general paresis), the eyes (interstitial keratitis), or the ears (nerve deafness). Less frequently, the disease becomes apparent as localized single or multiple

Table 51–1. Serologic tests for syphilis.[1]

Antigen	Antigen Source	Tests[2]	Percent Reactivity During		
			Primary Stage	Secondary Stage	Tertiary Stage
Nontreponemal	Extracts of tissue (cardiolipin-lecithin-cholesterol	Complement fixation (Wassermann, Kolmer) Flocculation (VDRL, Hinton, Kann)	78	90	77
Treponemal	*T pallidum* Reiter strain *T pallidum*	RPCF TPI FTA-ABS MHA-TP	61 56 85 85	85 94 99 98	72 92 96 95

[1] Reproduced, with permission, from Joklik WK et al (editors). *Zinsser Microbiology.* 20th ed. Appleton-Century-Crofts, 1992.
[2] FTA-ABS, Fluorescent treponemal antibody-absorption; MHA-TP, microhemagglutination assay for *T pallidum;* RPCF, Reiter protein complement fixation; TPI, *T pallidum* immobilization.

granulomas known as "gummas." These lesions are typically found in skin, bones, liver, testes, or larynx. The histopathologic features of the gumma resemble those of earlier symphilitic lesions, except that the vasculitis is associated with increased tissue necrosis and often frank caseation.

Immunologic Diagnosis

In its primary and secondary stages, syphilis is best diagnosed by dark-field microscopic examination of material from suspected lesions. Diagnostic serologic changes do not begin to occur until 14–21 days following acquisition of infection. Serologic tests provide important confirmatory evidence for secondary syphilis but are the only means of diagnosing latent infection (Fig 51–1; Table 51–1). Many forms of tertiary syphilis can be suspected on clinical grounds, but serologic tests are important in confirming the diagnosis. Spirochetes are notoriously difficult to demonstrate in the late stages of syphilis.

Two main categories of serologic tests for syphilis (STS) are available: tests for reaginic antibody and tests for treponemal antibody.

A. Tests for Reaginic Antibody: This is an unfortunate and confusing designation; there is no relationship between this antibody and IgE reaginic antibody. Patients with syphilis develop an antibody response to a tissue-derived substance (from beef heart) that is thought to be a component of mitochondrial membranes and is called cardiolipin. Antibody to cardiolipin antigen is known as Wassermann, or reaginic, antibody. Numerous variations (and names) are associated with tests for this antigen. The simplest and most practical of these are the VDRL test (Venereal Disease Research Laboratory of the US Public Health Service), which involves a slide microflocculation technique and can provide qualitative and quantitative data, and the rapid plasma reagin (RPR) circle card test. Positive tests are considered to be diagnostic of syphilis when there is a high or increasing titer or when the medical history is compatible with primary or secondary syphilis. The tests may also be of prognostic aid in monitoring the response

to therapy, because the antibody titer will revert to negative within 1 year of treatment for seropositive primary syphilis or within 2 years of that for secondary syphilis. Because cardiolipin antigen is found in the mitochondrial membranes of many mammalian tissues as well as in diverse microorganisms, it is not surprising that antibody to this antigen should appear during other diseases. A positive VDRL test may be encountered, for example, in patients with infectious mononucleosis, leprosy, hepatitis, and systemic lupus erythematosus. Although the VDRL test lacks specificity for syphilis, its great sensitivity makes it extremely useful.

B. Tests for Treponemal Antibody: The first test used for detecting specific antitreponemal antibody was the *T pallidum* immobilization (TPI) test. Although highly reliable, it proved to be too cumbersome for routine use. A major test development was the fluorescent *T pallidum* antibody (FTA) test. If virulent *T pallidum* from an infected rabbit testicle is placed on a slide and overlaid with serum from a patient with antibody to treponemes, an antigen-antibody reaction will occur. The bound antibody can then be detected by means of a fluoresceinated antihuman immunoglobulin antibody. The specificity of the test for *T pallidum* is enhanced by first absorbing the serum with nonpathogenic treponemal strains. This modification is referred to as the FTA-ABS test. (If specific anti-IgM antibody to human gamma globulin is used, the acuteness of the infection or the occurrence of congenital syphilis can be assessed. However, this test is sometimes falsely positive or negative in babies born of mothers with syphilis.)

The FTA-ABS test is reactive in approximately 80% of patients with primary syphilis (versus 50% for the VDRL test). Both tests are positive in virtually 100% of patients with secondary syphilis. Whereas the VDRL test shows a tendency to decline in titer after successful treatment, the FTA-ABS test may remain positive for years. It is especially useful in confirming or ruling out a diagnosis of syphilis in patients with suspected biologic false-positive reactions to the VDRL test. However, even the FTA-ABS test may be susceptible to false-positive reactions, especially in the presence of lupus erythematosus.

The microhemagglutination-*T pallidum* (MHA-TP) test, a simple passive hemagglutination test, is a satisfactory substitute for the FTA-ABS test. Its principal advantages are economy of technician time and money. Its results correlate closely with those of the FTA-ABS test, except during primary and early secondary syphilis, when both the VDRL and FTA-ABS are more likely to show reactivity. The VDRL test is the only one that can be used with reliability in the evaluation of cerebrospinal fluid.

The interpretation of serologic data from patients with syphilis may be extremely complex in some cases. For example, a prozone phenomenon may be encountered in secondary syphilis; serofastness may characterize late syphilis; and the VDRL test may be negative in up to one-third of patients with late latent syphilis.

Differential Diagnosis

Syphilis produces sufficiently diverse clinical manifestations that a textbook of general internal medicine should be consulted for a discussion of the differential diagnosis.

Prevention

If used properly, condoms can be an effective barrier against the sexual transmission of syphilis. Early treatment with antibiotics is the only way known to prevent the later ravages of syphilis.

Treatment

Penicillin is the drug of choice for syphilis in all its stages. Because the lesions of tertiary syphilis may be irreversible, it is crucial to identify and treat the disease before tertiary lesions begin. AIDS patients with syphilis must be treated more intensively with penicillin. This reinforces the notion that curing syphilis depends on interactions between an intact immune system and the treponemicidal effects of antibiotics.

Complications & Prognosis

The most frequent complication of treatment is the **Jarisch-Herxheimer reaction,** which occurs in up to half of patients with early syphilis and is manifested by fever, headache, myalgias, and exacerbation of cutaneous lesions. The intensity of a Jarisch-Herxheimer reaction reflects the intensity of local inflammation prior to treatment and is thought to result from the release of antigenic material from dying microorganisms. The reaction is of short duration (2–4 hours) and is generally not harmful, although shock and death have been attributed to this reaction in tertiary forms of the disease. (The Jarisch-Herxheimer reaction has also been described in the treatment of louse-borne borreliosis, brucellosis, and typhoid fever.)

Other immunologic complications of syphilis include paroxysmal cold hemoglobinuria and nephrotic syndrome.

It is estimated that one in 13 patients who receive no treatment for syphilis will develop cardiovascular disease, one in 25 will become crippled or incapacitated, one in 44 will develop irreversible damage to the central nervous system, and one in 200 will become blind.

NONVENEREAL TREPONEMATOSES

The causes of yaws (*T pallidum* subsp *pertenue*), pinta (*Treponema carateum*), and bejel (*T pallidum* subsp *endemicum*) are human pathogens responsible for this group of contagious diseases, which are endemic among rural populations in tropical and subtropical countries. Unlike syphilis, these diseases are transmitted not by sexual activity but primarily by direct contact, mostly among children living under poor hygienic conditions. These 3 treponemal species are morphologically and antigenically similar to *T pallidum,* yet give rise to slightly different disease manifestations. Pinta causes skin lesions only; yaws causes skin and bone lesions; and bejel (so-called endemic syphilis) affects the mucous membranes, skin, and bones. They do resemble venereal syphilis by virtue of the self-limiting primary and secondary lesions, a latency period with clinically dormant disease, and late lesions that are frequently highly destructive. The serologic responses for all 3 diseases are indistinguishable from one another and from that of venereal syphilis, and there is the same degree of slow development of protective immunity associated with prolonged, untreated infection.

LYME DISEASE

Major Immunologic Features
- Multisystem spirochetal disease involves inflammation of skin, joints, and nervous system.
- Specific antibody is diagnostic following infection.
- Cell-mediated immunity is activated during or shortly after the early stage of disease.

General Considerations

In the mid-1970s a geographic clustering of an unusual rheumatoid arthritis-like condition involving mostly children and young adults occurred in northeastern Connecticut. This condition proved to be a newly discovered disease, named Lyme disease after the town of its origin. The arthritis is characterized by intermittent attacks of asymmetric pain and swelling primarily in the large joints (especially the knees) over a period of a few years. Epidemiologic and clinical research showed that the onset of symptoms was preceded by an insect bite and unique skin rash probably identical to that of an illness following a tick bite, first described in Europe at the turn of the century. The beneficial effects of penicillin or tetracycline in early cases suggested a microbial origin for what was initially called Lyme arthritis.

Lyme disease is now the most common tick-transmitted illness in the USA and it has been reported in at least 43 states. However, it occurs primarily in 3 geographic regions: the coastal areas of the Northeast from Maine to Maryland, the Midwest in Wisconsin and Minnesota, and the far West in parts of California and Oregon. These geographic areas parallel the location of the primary tick vector of Lyme disease in the USA—*Ixodes scapularis* (formerly *dammini*) in the East and Midwest and *Ixodes pacificus* in the far West. Lyme disease has been reported in many other countries, especially in western Europe, corresponding to the distribution of *Ixodes ricinus* ticks. The greatest concentration of cases is in the northeastern USA, particularly in New York state, where the disease is endemic on Long Island and just north of New York City in neighboring Westchester County.

In the early 1980s spirochetal organisms were isolated and cultured from the midguts of *Ixodes* ticks taken from Shelter Island, NY (an endemic focus), and shortly thereafter they were cultured from the skin rash site, blood, and cerebrospinal fluid of patients with Lyme disease. This newly discovered spirochete, called *Borrelia burgdorferi,* is microaerophilic, resembles other spirochetes morphologically, and is slightly larger than the treponemes. Unlike the pathogenic treponemes, *B burgdorferi* can be readily cultivated in vitro in a highly fortified growth media.

As with syphilis, protection against *B burgdorferi* may develop slowly and it is unclear whether resistance to reinfection occurs. Experimental animal studies have shown that immune sera can transfer protection to normal recipients challenged with *B brugdorferi*. Monoclonal antibodies to borrelial outer surface proteins are also protective and have thus become the major target antigens for a vaccine.

Clinical Features

Lyme disease is an illness having protean manifestations with symptoms that include (1) an erythematous expanding red annular rash with central clearing; (2) fever, headache, stiff neck, nausea, and vomiting; (3) neurologic complications such as facial nerve (Bell's) palsy and meningitis; and (4) arthritis in about 50% of untreated patients. These symptoms occur most frequently from May to November, when ticks are active and numerous and people are engaged in many outdoor activities. The most characteristic feature of early Lyme disease is a skin rash, often referred to as erythema migrans (EM), which appears shortly (3–32 days) after a bite from an infected tick. The lesion typically expands almost uniformly from the center of the bite and is usually flat or slightly indurated with central clearing and reddening at the periphery. It is noteworthy, however, that many

Lyme disease victims do not recall being bitten by a tick or do not develop classic EM. On the other hand, at various intervals after the initial rash, some patients develop similar but smaller multiple secondary annular skin lesions that last for several weeks to months. Biopsy of these skin lesions reveals a lymphocytic and plasma-cytic infiltrate. Various flulike symptoms such as malaise, fever, headache, stiff neck, and arthralgias are often associated with EM. The late manifestations of Lyme disease may include migratory and polyarticular arthritis, neurologic and cardiac involvement with cranial nerve palsies and radiculopathy, myocarditis, and arrhythmias. Lyme arthritis typically involves a knee or other large joint. It may enter a chronic phase, leading to destruction of bone and joints if left untreated. Interestingly, Lyme arthritis is less common in Europe than in the USA but neurologic complications are more prevalent in Europe. Unique strain variations expressing antigenic subtypes between European and North American isolates of *B burgdorferi* probably explain these dissimilarities.

In most cases, humoral and cell-mediated immune responses are activated during borrelial infection. Antibody, mostly of the IgM class, can be detected shortly after the appearance of EM; thereafter, there is a gradual increase in overall titer and a switch to predominant IgG antibody response for the duration of an untreated infection. Most notably, very high levels of antibody have been found in serum and joint fluid taken from patients with moderate to severe arthritis. Although the presence of such high antibody titers against *B burgdorferi* may reduce the spirochete load somewhat, they appear not to ameliorate the disease process completely and, indeed, may actually contribute to some of the pathologic changes. These serologic responses form the basis of laboratory tests to aid in the diagnosis of Lyme borreliosis. On the basis of lymphoctye transformation assays, peripheral blood T cells from Lyme disease patients respond to borrelial antigens primarily after early infection and following successful treatment. Also, addition of antigens to synovial cells in vitro from infected patients triggers the production of interleukin-1, which could account for many of the harmful inflammatory reactions associated with this disease. Human mononuclear and polymorphonuclear phagocytes can both ingest and presumably destroy *Borrelia*. Thus, borrelial antigen-stimulated T cells or their products may activate macrophages, limiting dissemination and resulting in enhanced phagocytic activity and the eventual clearance of spirochetes from the primary lesion.

Immunologic Diagnosis

Successful isolation and culture of *B burgdorferi* from skin lesions, blood, and joint and cerebrospinal fluid in suspected cases of Lyme disease is rare, although procedures based on the polymerase chain reactions (PCR) are now being developed (as they are for other difficult-to-culture microorganisms) for sensitive detection of *B burgdorferi* in certain patient specimens. Antibody responses important in diagnosis typically begin to occur 3–5 weeks after the onset of EM, but they can be obliterated by early antibiotic therapy. Serologic tests provide important confirmatory evidence for all stages of Lyme disease and may be the only way of diagnosing atypical cases. There is some evidence that a small percentage of untreated patients with Lyme disease produce few or no detectable antibodies throughout the course of infection. The most commonly used serologic tests are the enzyme-linked immunosorbent assay (ELISA) and indirect fluorescent-antibody assay (IFA). Because of its sensitivity, adaptability to automation, and ease of quantitation, the ELISA is probably the preferred method. Standard indirect IFA and newer quantitative solid-phase IFAs are available. Although not standardized, commercial Western immunoblot test kits are now being offered for further confirmation of a serologic response to specific borrelial antigens. Most of these tests are designed to detect total serum antibody to *Borrelia* without differentiating between IgG or IgM antibodies. Some have been developed for specifically detecting IgM where this class of antibody usually shows preferentially elevated levels early in primary infection or relapse and in sera of newborn infants following transplacentally acquired infections. For all these assays, false-positive reactions are relatively rare but can occur if a patient has syphilis, infectious mononucleosis, systemic lupus erythematosus, or rheumatoid arthritis. Serum from Lyme disease patients is sometimes reactive in specific treponemal antibody tests but is consistently negative for the nontreponemal (VDRL) tests. In the absence of the hallmark skin rash or with an unclear clinical presentation, laboratory serologic testing assumes a vital role in establishing or confirming the diagnosis.

Differential Diagnosis

Like syphilis, Lyme disease produces such a diverse number of clinical symptoms that a textbook of general internal medicine should be consulted for a detailed account of differential diagnosis. Patients with Lyme disease are usually distinguished by their characteristic skin lesions and diagnostic serologic changes. Distinctions must be made from syphilis, rheumatoid arthritis, and chronic fatigue syndrome, which produce similar symptoms.

Prevention

Avoiding *Borrelia*-infected ticks or tick-infested areas will guarantee protection against Lyme disease. For those living in areas where the infection is endemic, a few simple precautions will help minimize possible exposure. These include wearing clothing that fully protects the body and using repellents that contain DEET (diethyltoluamide). If a tick does attach to the skin, careful removal with tweezers shortly after it attaches followed by application of alcohol or another suitable disinfectant will make borrelial transmission unlikely.

There is considerable attention to the development of a vaccine for Lyme disease. A canine vaccine consisting of whole inactivated organisms (Bacterin) has existed for a few years, whereas those being developed for humans consist of recombinant outer surface proteins of *B burgdorferi*. One such vaccine is now undergoing phase I and phase II clinical trials, and other prototypes for both humans and dogs are in the early developmental or testing stages.

Treatment & Prognosis

Early disease is adequately treated with a 2–3 week course of penicillin or tetracycline. Later complications such as arthritis and the neuropathies may require more intense and prolonged antibiotic therapy. There are, however, some concerns regarding the universal efficacy of treatment. Despite the use of very aggressive and repeated antibiotic therapy, there are reports of some patients with persisting Lyme disease-like symptoms, indicating that irreversible damage may have occurred in a manner analogous to late-stage syphilis. It is unclear whether this phenomenon is due at least in part to persistence of pathogenic *Borrelia*, possibly because of antibiotic resistance.

RELAPSING-FEVER BORRELIOSIS

Relapsing fever is an acute febrile disease of worldwide distribution and is caused by arthropod-borne spirochetes belonging to the genus *Borrelia*. Two major forms of this illness are louse-borne relapsing fever (for which humans are the reservoir and the body louse, *Pediculus humanus,* is the vector) and tick-borne relapsing fever (for which rodents and other small animals are the major reservoirs and ticks of the genus *Ornithodorus* are the vectors). *B recurrentis* causes louse-borne relapsing fever and is transmitted from human to human following the ingestion of infected human blood by the louse and release of newly acquired organisms onto the skin or mucous membranes of a new host. The disease is endemic in parts of central and east Africa and South America. The causative organisms of tick-borne relapsing fever are numerous and include *B hermsii, B turicatae,* and *B parkeri* in North America; *B hispanica* in Spain; *B duttonii* in east Africa; and *B persica* in Asia. Ticks become infectious by biting and sucking blood from a spirochetemic animal. The infection is transmitted to humans or animals when saliva is released by a feeding tick through bites or penetration of intact skin.

After an individual has been exposed to an infected

louse or tick, *Borrelia* organisms penetrate the skin and enter the bloodstream and lymphatic system. After a 1–3 week incubation period, spirochetes replicate in the blood and there is an acute onset of shaking chills, fever, headache, and fatigue. Concentrations of *Borrelia* can reach as high as 10^8 spirochetes/mL of blood, and these are clearly visible after staining blood smears with Giemsa or Wright's stain. During febrile disease, *Borrelia* organisms are present in the patient's blood but disappear prior to afebrile episodes and subsequently return to the bloodstream during the next febrile period. Jaundice can develop in some severely ill patients as a result of intrahepatic obstruction of bile flow and hepatocellular inflammation; if left untreated, patients can die from damage to the liver, spleen, or brain. The majority of untreated patients, however, recover spontaneously. They produce borrelial antibodies that have agglutinating, complement-fixing, borreliacidal, and immobilizing capabilities and that render patients immune to reinfection with the same *Borrelia* serotype. Serologic tests designed to measure these antibodies are of limited diagnostic value because of antigenic variation among strains and the coexistence of mixed populations of *Borrelia* within a given host during the course of a single infection. Diagnosis in the majority of cases requires demonstration of spirochetemia in febrile patients.

LEPTOSPIROSIS

Leptospirosis is an acute, febrile disease caused by various serotypes of *Leptospira*. Often referred to as Weil's disease, infection with *Leptospira interrogans* causes diseases that are extremely varied in their clinical presentations and that are also found in a variety of wild and domestic animals. Transmission to humans occurs primarily after contact with contaminated urine from leptospiruric animals. In the USA, dogs are the major reservoir for exposure of humans to this disease. After entering the body through the mucosal surface or breaks in the skin, leptospiral bacteria cause an acute illness characterized by fever, chills, myalgias, severe headaches, conjunctival suffuseness, and gastrointestinal problems. Most human infections are mild and anicteric, although in a small proportion of victims, severe icteric disease can occur and be fatal, primarily owing to renal failure and damage to small blood vessels. After infection of the kidneys, leptospiras are excreted in the urine. Liver dysfunction with hepatocellular damage and jaundice is common. Antibiotic treatment is curative if begun during early disease, but its value thereafter is questionable.

Diagnosis of leptospirosis depends upon either seroconversion or the demonstration of spirochetes in clinical specimens. The macroscopic slide agglutination test, which uses formalized antigen, offers safe and rapid antibody screening. Measurement of antibody for a specific serotype, however, is performed with the very sensitive microscopic agglutination test involving live organisms. This method provides the most specific reaction with the highest titer and fewer cross-reactions. Agglutinating IgM-class-specific antibodies are produced during early infection and persist in high titers for many months. Protective and agglutinating antibodies often persist in sera of convalescent patients and may be associated with resistance to future infections.

REFERENCES

General

Barbour AG: Laboratory aspects of Lyme borreliosis. *Clin Microbiol Rev* 1988:**1**:399.

Benach JL, Bosler EM (editors): Lyme disease and related disorders. *Ann NY Acad Sci* 1988:**539**:1.

Fitzgerald TJ: Pathogenesis and immunology of *Treponema pallidum Annu Rev Microbiol* 1981;**35**:29.

Schell RF, Musher DM (editors): *Pathogenesis and Immunology of Treponemal Infections.* Marcel Dekker, 1983.

Syphilis

Baseman JB et al: Virulence determinants among the spirochetes. Page 203 in: *Microbiology—1979.* Schlessinger D (editor). American Society for Microbiology, 1979.

Baughn RE, Tung KS, Musher DM: Detection of circulating immune complexes in the sera of rabbits with experimental syphilis: Possible role in immunoregulation. *Infect Immun* 1980;**29**:575.

Bryceson AD: Clinical pathology of the Jarisch-Herxheimer reaction. *J Infect Dis* 1976:**133**:696.

Hanff PA et al: Humoral immune response in human syphilis to polypeptides of *Treponema pallidum. J Immunol* 1982:**129**;1287.

Lukehart SA et al: Invasion of the central nervous system by *Treponema pallidum:* Implications for diagnosis and treatment. *Ann Intern Med* 1988:**109**:855.

Pavia CS, Niederbuhl CJ: Acquired resistance and expression of a protective humoral immune response in guinea pigs infected with *Treponema pallidum* Nichols. *Infect Immun* 1985:**50**:66.

Pavia CS, Niederbuhl CJ: Adoptive transfer of antisyphilis immunity with lymphocytes from *Treponema pallidum*-infected guinea pigs. *J Immunol* 1985;**135**:2829.

Pavia CS, Folds JD, Baseman JB: Cell-mediated immunity during syphilis: A review. *Br J Vener Dis* 1978;**54**:144.

Schell RF, Chan JK, Le Frock JL: Endemic syphilis: Passive transfer of resistance with serum and cells in hamsters. *J Infect Dis* 1979;**140:**378.

Lyme Disease

Barbour AG, Heiland RA, Howe TR: Heterogeneity of major proteins of Lyme disease borreliae: A molecular analysis of North American and European isolates. *J Infect Dis* 1985:**152:**478.

Barbour AG, Tessier SL, Hayes SF: Variation in a major surface protein of Lyme disease spirochetes. *Infect Immun* 1984:**45:**94.

Benach JL et al: Interactions of phagocytes with the Lyme disease spirochete: Role of the Fc receptor. *J Infect Dis* 1984:**150:**497.

Burgdorfer W et al: Lyme disease: A tick-borne spirochetosis? *Science* 1982:**216:**1317.

Craft JE, Grodzicki RL, Steere AC: Antibody response in Lyme disease: Evaluation of diagnostic tests. *J Infect Dis* 1984:**149:**789.

Dattwyler RJ et al: Seronegative Lyme disease: Dissociation of specific T- and B-lymphocyte responses to *Borrelia burgdorferi. N Engl J Med* 1988;**319:**1441.

Magnarelli LA, Anderson JF, Johnson RC: Cross-reactivity in serological tests for Lyme disease and other spirochetal infections. *J Infect Dis* 1987:**156:**183.

Schwartz I et al: Diagnosis of early Lyme disease by polymerase chain reaction amplication and culture of skin biopsies from erythema migrans lesions. *J Clin Microbiol* 1992;**30:**3082.

Steere AC: Lyme disease. *N Engl J Med* 1989;**321:**586.

Steere AC et al: The spirochetal etiology of Lyme disease. *N Engl J Med* 1983;**308:**733.

Leptospirosis

Adler B, Faine S: The antibodies involved in the human immune response to leptospiral infection. *J Med Microbiol* 1978;**11:**387.

Alexander AD: Serological diagnosis of leptospirosis. Chap 69, pp 435–439, in: *Manual of Clinical Laboratory Immunology,* 3rd ed. Rose NR, Friedman H, Fahey JL (editors). American Society for Microbiology, 1986.

Relapsing Fever Borreliosis

Meier JT, Simon MI, Barbour AG: Antigenic variation is associated with DNA rearrangements in a relapsing fever *Borrelia. Cell* 1985;**41:**403.

Southern PM, Sanford JP: Relapsing fever: A clinical and microbiological review. *Medicine* 1969;**48:**129.

Virus Infections of the Immune System

52

Suzanne Crowe, MBBS, FRACP, & John Mills, MD

Although measles virus infection has been recognized for decades as a cause of immunosuppression, Epstein-Barr virus (EBV) was the first pathogen shown to cause immune dysfunction as a result of directly infecting cells of the immune system. Since then, other viruses, especially herpesviruses and retroviruses, have been identified that can infect cells of the immune system and produce immune suppression, immune stimulation, or both. The discovery of the human immunodeficiency virus (HIV), which primarily infects immune cells, has provided additional impetus for understanding the mechanisms by which virus infection results in immune dysfunction.

HUMAN IMMUNODEFICIENCY VIRUS

Major Immunologic Features

- CD4 cells of the immune system, including T lymphocytes, monocyte-macrophages, follicular dendritic cells, and Langerhans' cells, are infected.
- Infection causes progressive global defects of humoral and cell-mediated immunity.
- CD4 (helper/inducer) T lymphocytes are depleted.
- There is polyclonal activation of B lymphocytes with increased immunoglobulin production.
- Disease progresses despite vigorous humoral and cell-mediated responses to the virus.

General Considerations

The acquired immune deficiency syndrome (AIDS) was first recognized in 1981. The identification of HIV as the causative agent of AIDS in 1983–1984 was rapidly followed by characterization of this virus and the target cells that it infects and by elucidation of the multiple consequences of infection. Epidemiologic studies have identified the major populations at risk of acquiring infection and the routes by which the virus can be transmitted. The clinical illnesses associated with HIV infection have been classified, and therapeutic strategies to treat or suppress them

have been designed. By 1985, diagnostic kits had been developed for the detection of antibody to HIV, potentially therapeutic compounds were being screened for in vitro activity against this virus, and clinical trials for safety and efficacy of these potential drugs had begun. In 1987, only 6 years after the initial recognition of the AIDS epidemic and 3 years after identification of the etiologic agent, zidovudine (2′-azido-3′-deoxythymidine [AZT]), the first antiretroviral agent, was licensed by the US Food and Drug Administration for treatment of HIV infection.

Infection with HIV results in an acquired defect in immune function, especially involving cell-mediated immunity. Infected individuals may be asymptomatic or have progressive disease associated with recurrent opportunistic infections, certain cancers, severe weight loss, and central nervous system degeneration.

The recognition of the viral etiology of AIDS has stimulated immunologists to investigate the pathogenesis of the disease. Rational development of effective antiretroviral compounds can be aided by knowledge of the mechanisms by which HIV can damage the immune system. Although research on HIV has probably provided us with more pathogenetic information than we have on any other virus, the genesis of the characteristic and profound immune dysfunction caused by HIV still remains incompletely understood.

Etiology

A. Virology: HIV is a member of the retrovirus family, a group of enveloped viruses possessing the enzyme reverse transcriptase. This enzyme allows the virus to synthesize a DNA copy of its RNA genome. HIV was previously termed "human T lymphotrophic virus type III (HTLV-III)," "lymphadenopathy-associated virus (LAV)," and "AIDS-related virus (ARV)." However, molecular characterization of these retroviruses demonstrated their relatedness, and they are regarded as variants of the same virus. HIV has been subclassified within the lentivirus family, a group of transforming retroviruses with a long latency period from infection to the onset of clinical features and similar morphologic features and nucleotide sequence homology. Other members of the lentivirus family include visna and caprine arthritis-encephalitis viruses, which cause chronic, progressive neurodegenerative disease in sheep and goats, respectively. The clinical picture of lentivirus infection in sheep and goats is similar to that resulting from HIV infection in humans and is characterized by a slow and progressive disorder of the immune system and the brain. HIV is also closely related to simian immunodeficiency virus (SIV), which causes an AIDS-like illness in macaque monkeys. There are 2 subtypes of HIV: HIV-1 is most prevalent in central Africa, USA, Europe, and Australia, and HIV-2 is found in west Africa, parts of Europe, and less commonly elsewhere. At the molecular level, HIV-2 more closely resembles SIV, supporting data which suggest that HIV originated from primate lentiviruses. When compared with HIV-1, HIV-2 has a longer clinical latency period from the time of infection to the development of symptoms and has a lower rate of vertical transmission (Table 52–1; Fig 52–1).

B. Genomic Organization: HIV consists of an inner core, containing an RNA genome, surrounded by a lipid envelope. The HIV genome (Fig 52–2) contains the standard retroviral structural genes, *env*, *gag*, and *pol*, encoding the viral envelope proteins, viral core protein, and viral enzymes (reverse transcriptase, integrase, and protease), respectively. The virus possesses at least 6 other genes, a feature that makes it unique among retroviruses. Many of these gene products are made as precursor proteins, which require cleavage by viral proteases or cellular enzymes later in the replicative cycle. Within the DNA provirus, the viral genes are flanked by long terminal repeats (LTR) at both 5' and 3' ends. The LTR contains enhancer and promoter elements, which are necessary for transcription. HIV is initially transcribed into a full-length mRNA, which is translated into the structural Gag and Pol proteins. Production of singly and multiply spliced mRNA is necessary for the synthesis of the envelope proteins and accessory proteins, respectively.

The first of the additional gene products to be recognized was the transactivating protein Tat, a positive-feedback regulator of HIV replication, which can accelerate viral protein production by several thousandfold. Tat-binding protein, a cellular protein, attaches to Tat and thereby can modify its function. Current data suggest that Tat can act via TAR (transactivating response) structures within the LTR at both the DNA and RNA levels. *rev* encodes proteins that regulate viral mRNA expression. The Rev protein permits unspliced mRNA to leave the nucleus and thus inhibits transcription of the regulatory genes while enhancing expression of the viral structural genes. Rev protein binds to the REV-responsive element (RRE), an RNA structure found in all mRNA species that are unspliced. The product of the virion infectivity gene, *vif*, increases viral infectivity and may be responsible for the efficient cell-to-cell transmission observed with HIV. The function of the *nef* gene is still being evaluated. Its product appears to act predominantly to inhibit viral replication. Two further genes have been described: the *vpr* (viral protein R) gene, whose function is not yet known, and the *vpu* (viral protein U) gene whose protein product is thought to influence release of infectious virus (Figure 52–2).

C. Pathogenesis of Infection: HIV infection affect predominantly the immune system and the brain. The dominant immunologic feature of HIV infection is progressive depletion of the CD4 (helper/inducer) subset of T lymphocytes, thereby reversing the normal CD4:CD8 ratio and inexorably worsening immunodeficiency. The depletion of CD4 lymphocytes is predominantly due to the tropism of HIV for these and other CD4-bearing cells because the CD4 cell surface molecule functions as a receptor for the virus. The CD4 lymphocyte is necessary for the proper functioning of the immune system. It interacts with antigen-presenting cells, B cells, cytotoxic T cells, and natural killer (NK) cells (see Chapter 8) Thus, it is easy to see that infection and depletion of this cell population could induce profound immunodeficiency. Early in situ hybridization studies suggested that only very few (about 1 in 10,000) CD4 lymphocytes contain replicating HIV. More recently, studies of peripheral blood lymphocytes have demonstrated that up to 1 in 10 of these cells are infected with HIV, particularly in persons with advanced disease. Although the data are limited, the number of infected cells in tissues appears to be larger than that in peripheral blood.

The finding that the CD4 molecule is present on cells other than helper/inducer T lymphocytes was accompanied by evidence that HIV could infect other cell populations which expressed this molecule on their surface. Other cells susceptible to HIV infection include monocyte-macrophages, microglial cells, Langerhans cells, follicular dendritic cells, immortal-

Table 52–1. Classification of retroviruses.

Oncoviruses	Lentiviruses	Spumiviruses
Avian retroviruses	Visna/maedi virus	Human foamy virus
Bovine leukemia virus	Caprine arthritis encephalitis virus	Simian foamy virus
Murine retroviruses	Equine infectious anemia virus	
Feline leukemia virus	HIV-1 and HIV-2	
HTLV-I and HTLV-II	Simian immuno-deficiency virus	

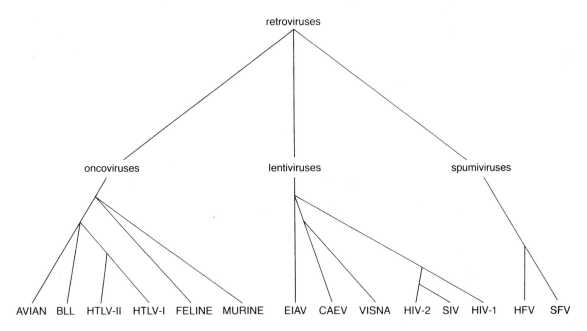

Figure 52–1. Schematic evolutionary relationships among retroviruses.

ized B cells, retinal cells, and colonic mucosal cells. Dendritic cells in the blood can transmit HIV infection to T lymphocytes. It is controversial as to whether or not these dendritic cells are susceptible to HIV infection. While HIV infection of macrophages and T lymphocytes has been clearly demonstrated in vivo, there is no conclusive evidence that blood dendritic cells, Langerhans cells, stem cells or B lymphocytes are infected in vivo (Table 52–2). Monocyte-macrophages are thought to provide a major reservoir for HIV in vivo and may contribute to the pathogenesis of the immune deficiency by functioning abnormally. For example, HIV-infected monocyte-macrophages secrete an inhibitor of interleukin-1 (IL-1), a cytokine of major importance in T cell proliferative responses (see Chapter 9). Although the pathogenesis of immune dysfunction associated with HIV infec-

tion is incompletely understood, it is likely that the process occurs through collective dysfunction of both antigen-presenting cells, such as macrophages, and T lymphocytes, especially the CD4 subset.

During the course of HIV infection there is a progressive depletion of CD4-bearing T lymphocytes. The loss of these cells may occur as a result of a number of possible mechanisms. These include the death of uninfected CD4 T cells as a result of cell fusion with HIV-infected cells, the development of pores in the cell membrane of the infected lymphocyte as HIV buds from the cell surface, the accumulation of unintegrated viral DNA within the cell cytoplasm, and the killing of both uninfected CD4 T cells (innocent bystanders) which have found free HIV envelope glycoprotein gp120 and HIV-infected cells expressing gp120 by gp120-specific clones of cytotoxic lympho-

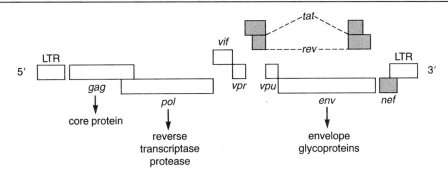

Figure 52–2. Genomic organization of HIV. The 9.6-kb genome of HIV consists of both structural and regulatory sequences (see text for details). HIV has a far more complex genome than that of many other retroviruses.

Table 52–2. Cells infected by HIV.

CD4 T lymphocytes
Monocyte-macrophages
Follicular dendritic cells
Langerhans' cells
Microglial cells
Immortalized B cells
Retinal cells
Colonic mucosal cells
Endothelial cells in brain

cytes. Recently, apoptosis, or programmed cell death, has been implicated in the depletion of CD4 T lymphocytes. HIV enters the cell through a specific interaction between the V1 region of the CD4 molecule on the cell surface and a specific region within the HIV envelope glycoprotein. Whether HIV is able to infect macrophages or lymphocytes (cell tropism) is determined largely by the amino acid sequence of the HIV envelope. The binding of the gp120 to CD4 results in exposure of the transmembrane protein, gp41, facilitating virus-cell fusion and viral entry. Certain cells (eg, fibroblast cell lines and brain-derived glial cells) that do not bear the CD4 molecule may also be infected by HIV. These cells possess other molecules that may act as receptors for HIV, including galactosyl ceramide on brain-derived cells, Fc and complement receptors, and possibly members of the leukocyte adhesion molecule family. HIV replication within monocyte-macrophages occurs at a leisurely pace compared with that within lymphocytes, with little cytopathology, supporting their role as a viral reservoir in vivo. Resting T lymphocytes can also be infected with HIV, but the virus replication cycle is blocked at the reverse transcription step. If the cell is activated within a few days, infectious virus is produced; otherwise, the infection is aborted. Thus resting or nonactivated lymphocytes provide and additional reservoir of HIV in infected persons. The factors that trigger latently infected cells to produce virus are not completely known. A number of intracellular and viral factors can influence the production of HIV. These include cellular transcription factors such as the DNA-binding protein nuclear factor kappa B (NF-κB), as well as cytokines including tumor necrosis factor alpha and (TNFα), and the colony-stimulating factors GM-CSF and M-CSF, which have been found to augment HIV replication. A number of viruses (herpes simplex virus, cytomegalovirus, adenovirus, human T lymphotropic virus type I, Epstein-Barr virus, and hepatitis B virus) stimulate HIV replication in vitro, but these findings have not been substantiated clinically. In addition, HIV regulatory genes themselves can influence viral production.

Early in infection, when the individual is asymptomatic, macrophage-tropic strains of HIV are isolated predominantly from peripheral blood. At this stage, the virus generally does not produce the char-

acteristic cytopathology of multinucleated giant cells or syncytia in cell culture and is described as non-syncytium-inducing (NSI). A change in viral phenotype from NSI to syncytium-inducing (SI) occurs at approximately the same time as decline in CD4 numbers and the onset of HIV-related clinical disease. The tropism of the viral strains also broadens to include T lymphocytes and other cell populations as disease progresses. Another major feature of HIV infection is involvement of the central nervous system. The clinical findings range from minor memory defects to personality changes to progressive, fatal dementia. The mechanism of brain damage is obscure. As there is no evidence to support direct neuronal infection with HIV, it is more likely that soluble factors such as quinolinic acid or TNFα secreted by infected cells that transport the virus to the brain may alter the function of neurons and contribute to the dementia. In infected brain tissue, HIV has been detected in multinucleated giant cells composed predominantly of monocyte-macrophages, and in microglia, suggesting a major pathogenetic role for these cells. An alternative hypothesis is that HIV may competitively inhibit neuroleukin from binding to neurons. This neurotrophic factor shares homology with a conserved region of the HIV envelope glycoprotein, gp120.

Epidemiology

By mid-1993, there were approximately 250,000 reported cases of AIDS in the USA. The disease is recognized as a global health problem, with cases of AIDS being reported in virtually all countries. In the USA, Europe, and Australia, transmission of HIV has been documented to occur via sexual contact, administration of infected blood or blood products, artificial insemination with infected semen, exposure to blood-containing needles or syringes, and transmission from an infected mother to her fetus or to the infant during or after birth. Homosexual activity accounts for the majority of sexually transmitted cases in these countries. Male-to-female transmission is more commonly reported than female-to-male transmission; whether this is secondary to epidemiologic factors (a larger number of infected males) or to greater efficacy of transmission is not known. HIV has been detected in up to 30% of seminal and vaginal fluid specimens from HIV-infected persons. Transmission from mother to offspring occurs by transplacental passage of the virus at the time of delivery or, less commonly, through breast feeding, with estimates for the incidence of transmission of HIV from an infected mother to her child varying from 15 to 30%. The diagnosis of HIV in a neonate can be difficult (see the section on neonatal diagnosis). Following the introduction of programs to exclude blood donors who are members of high-risk groups and the serologic testing of donated blood, the risk of acquiring HIV from infected blood or blood products has been virtually eliminated. Thus, the groups presently at highest risk are homosexual and bisexual men, injecting drug users who share needles or syringes, sexual partners of people in high-risk groups, and children born to infected mothers (Table 52–3). Health care workers are at risk of HIV infection, but this risk is considered to be very low (approximately 1:250 HIV positive needle stick exposures results in infection) Epidemiologic data do not support transmission of HIV by casual contact, insects, or sharing of utensils (tableware, toothbrushes, etc). There are no data to suggest aerosolized transmission of the virus. HIV can be detected in less than 10% of saliva samples from HIV-infected persons, at extremely low titer (less than one infectious particle per ml). Similarly, urine, feces, sweat, tears and amniotic fluid are considered unlikely to transmit HIV because of their extremely low viral titers.

In central and western Africa, cases of AIDS are equally distributed among men and women, and heterosexual transmission (especially from infected female prostitutes to their clients) is thought to account for the majority of cases. In Africa, risk factors associated with HIV infection in heterosexuals include large numbers of sexual partners, prostitution, sex with prostitutes, a history of sexually transmitted disease such a as gonorrhea or syphilis, and genital ulceration of any cause. Although both bowel mucosa and cervical epithelium can be infected with HIV, the chance of infection is markedly increased if abrasions or ulceration are present. Other risk factors include multiple use of needles or syringes in health clinics and ritualistic practices in which unsterilized instruments are used; these include scarification, tattooing, and ear-piercing.

Exposure to HIV does not always result in infection. However, one exposure may be sufficient to cause infection, depending on inoculum size, route of entry, and, perhaps, host factors. The dose to infect 50% of exposed individuals (ID_{50}) is not known for humans, but it is presumed to be low (less than 10–100 virions). Both cell-free and cell-associated viruses are infectious. About 50% of HIV-infected individuals will contract AIDS over an 8–10 year period from the time of infection. The latency period (from time of infection to onset of disease) may vary according to viral inoculum and possibly virulence of the strain, route of entry, and age of the patient.

Clinical Features

A. Acute HIV mononucleosis: Following infection with HIV, an individual may remain asymptomatic or develop an acute illness that resembles infectious mononucleosis. This syndrome usually occurs within 2–6 weeks after infection, with reported periods ranging from 5 days to 3 months. The predominant symptoms are fever, headache, sore throat, malaise, and rash. Clinical findings include pharyngitis (which may be exudative and may be accompanied by mucosal ulceration); generalized lymphadenopathy; a macular or urticarial rash on the face, trunk, and limbs; and hepatosplenomegaly (Table 52–4). During the acute illness, antibodies to HIV are generally undetectable. Although the illness is often severely incapacitating, requiring bed rest or even hospitalization, some individuals experience only mild symptoms and do not seek medical attention.

Acute infection with HIV has also been associated with neurologic disease, including meningitis, encephalitis, cranial nerve palsies, myopathy, and peripheral neuropathy. These findings are usually accompanied by features of the acute HIV mononucleosis syndrome.

B. AIDS-related complex (ARC): This poorly defined condition basically encompasses patients chronically infected with HIV but not with acute mononucleosis who have clinical findings short of those fulfilling the Centers for Disease Control and Prevention (CDC) criteria for AIDS. The condition is regarded as evidence of progressive immune dysfunction. Constitutional symptoms and signs include persistent fever, night sweats, weight loss, unexplained chronic diarrhea, eczema, psoriasis, seborrheic dermatitis, generalized lymphadenopathy, herpes zoster, oral candidiasis, and oral hairy leukoplakia. The last 3 conditions are regarded as poor prognostic indicators and herald progression to AIDS. HIV-related thrombocytopenia (defined as a platelet count of $< 50,000/\mu L$ without other known causes) is found in less than 10% of individuals and usually does not result in a bleeding diathesis.

C. AIDS: The criteria for diagnosis of AIDS have been defined by the CDC and comprise certain opportunistic infections and cancers, HIV-related encephalopathy, HIV-induced wasting syndrome, and a broader range of AIDS-indicative diseases in individuals who have laboratory evidence of HIV infection.

Table 52–3. Individuals at risk of HIV infection.

High risk
Homosexual and bisexual men
Injecting drug users who share needles or syringes
Sexual partners of people in high-risk groups
Children born to infected mothers
Low risk
Health care workers, including nurses, doctors, dentists, and laboratory staff

Table 52–4. Clinical features of acute HIV infection.

Fever and sweats
Myalgia and arthralgia
Malaise and lethargy
Lymphadenopathy and splenomegaly
Pharyngitis
Anorexia, nausea, and vomiting
Headaches and photophobia
Macular rash

Recently, the CDC has altered the definition to include adults and adolescents with diagnosed HIV infection who have a CD4 lymphocyte count of less than 200 cells/μL of blood or a CD4 T lymphocyte level of less than 14% regardless of clinical symptoms. In addition, pulmonary tuberculosis, recurrent bacterial pneumonia, and invasive cervical cancer have been added to the list of AIDS-defining conditions.

The most common opportunistic infections encountered are *Pneumocystis carinii* pneumonitis; disseminated cryptococcosis; toxoplasmosis; mycobacterial disease (both *Mycobacterium avium* complex infection and tuberculosis); chronic, ulcerative, recurrent herpes simplex virus infection; disseminated cytomegalovirus infection; and histoplasmosis (Table 52–5). Patients with AIDS also have a higher incidence of *Salmonella* bacteremia, staphylococcal infections, and pneumococcal pneumonia. Children with AIDS may develop opportunistic infections such as *P carinii* pneumonia, but they have a higher incidence of lymphocytic interstitial pneumonitis and recurrent bacterial infections than adults do.

The most common cancer diagnosed in AIDS patients is Kaposi's sarcoma, a neoplasm or neoplasm-like disease involving endothelia and mesenchymal stroma. Once common, this tumor is now less frequently seen as a presenting illness. The reason for this is obscure. Late in the course of immune dysfunction, high-grade B cell lymphomas are encountered; these are generally resistant to therapy.

Laboratory Diagnosis
A. Serology:
1. Seroconversion—During the early phase of the primary illness, antibodies to HIV are not detected in the serum; they generally appear 2–8 weeks after the onset of illness. IgM antibodies, detected by immunofluorescence, generally precede IgG antibody detection by Western immunoblot. During seroconversion, antibodies directed against the various viral proteins do not develop simultaneously. Those directed against HIV p24 (core) and gp41 (transmembrane) proteins can be detected before those directed at the *pol* gene products on Western blot. There may be a "window" period during which time the screening enzyme-linked immunosorbent assay (ELISA) is negative but antibodies can be demonstrated by Western blot. HIV antigenemia (predominantly HIV p24, measured by enzyme im-

munoassay) usually precedes seroconversion. Following the appearance of antibodies (specifically anti-HIV p24), HIV p24 antigen levels decline. They may later reappear, coincident with a loss of anti-HIV p24 antibody (Fig 52–3). Whereas about 70% of AIDS patients have detectable HIV antigen in their sera, the HIV antigen test is positive in fewer than 20% of asymptomatic individuals. The complexing of p24 antigen with specific antibody is largely responsible for the fluctuation of antigen titer during the course of disease. Newer methods to detect p24 antigen by ELISA involve an acid dissociation technique to remove the antigen from antibody. African patients rarely have detectable HIV antigenemia, perhaps owing to higher antibody levels. Persistence of HIV antigen following the acute infection in an asymptomatic carrier is probably associated with a more rapid progression to symptomatic disease. By using sensitive methods of detection (eg, polymerase chain reaction), HIV can be identified in the peripheral blood mononuclear cells and plasma of virtually all infected persons, regardless of the stage of disease. During acute HIV infection, virus titers of up to 5000 infectious particles/mL have been reported. Lower titers of HIV are usually present in blood following HIV seroconversion, remaining low during the asymptomatic phase of infection. As disease progresses and immune function declines, there is an increase in viral load.

2. Screening for HIV—ELISA is the basic screening test currently used to detect antibodies to HIV. Purified whole virus is disrupted, and viral proteins are then immobilized on plastic beads or multiwell trays. Test serum containing antibodies to HIV will bind to these viral proteins. An enzyme-linked

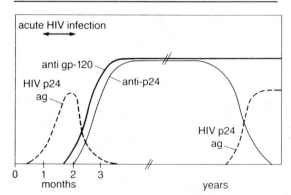

Figure 52–3. Common pattern of serologic response following HIV infection. p24 antigen (p24 ag) may be first detected during the acute HIV mononucleosis phase of infection. The initial antibody to appear in the serum is usually that directed against the HIV envelope glycoprotein gp120 (anti-gp120), and its level remains elevated throughout the course of the disease. Antibody directed against the core protein (anti-p24) appears in the serum coincident with the decline in p24 antigen levels.

Table 52–5. Common opportunistic infections encountered in AIDS patients.

Pneumocystis carinii pneumonia
Toxoplasmosis
Mycobacterium avium complex disease
Disseminated *Mycobacterium tuberculosis* infection
Persistent, ulcerative herpes simplex virus infection
Disseminated cytomegalovirus infection

anti-human antibody added to the reaction will bind to the complex and be detected calorimetrically. The ELISA is both highly sensitive (> 99%) and highly specific (> 99% in high-risk populations). The genomic diversity between HIV-1 and HIV-2 is greatest within the envelope region. As there is significant homology between the *gag* and *pol* gene products of the subtypes of HIV, HIV-2 can usually be detected by HIV-1 ELISAs. However, the sensitivity of HIV-1 ELISA for HIV-2 is unacceptably low, and blood banks should now routinely screen for both HIV-1 and HIV-2 proteins to ensure detection.

3. Confirmatory Tests–A repeatedly reactive ELISA should be confirmed by either a Western blot or, less commonly, a radioimmune precipitation assay, immunofluorescence assay, or ELISA with recombinant antigens. Because of its high sensitivity, a negative ELISA does not usually warrant confirmatory testing. The Western blot detects specific antibodies directed against the various HIV proteins. Purified viral proteins are run on a polyacrylamide gel, transferred to a nitrocellulose membrane, and then reacted with the test serum. Antibodies to HIV present in the serum will bind to the specific viral protein (Fig 52–4).

B. Neonatal Diagnosis: Neonates with HIV infection pose a difficult serodiagnostic problem because maternal IgG antibody crosses the placenta. Thus, the infant will passively acquire anti-HIV antibody, which may persist for up to 15 months. The predictive value of specific IgM antibodies in the diagnosis of neonatal and perinatal infection awaits clarification. Culture of the virus from peripheral blood or tissue or demonstration of HIV antigen is therefore necessary to be confident of the diagnosis of HIV infection in asymptomatic infants born to HIV-infected mothers. The PCR, which amplifies HIV genome present in cells or serum, provides a useful adjunct to diagnosis.

Immunologic Findings

A. CD4 Lymphocyte Depletion: The immunologic hallmark of AIDS is a defect in cell-mediated immunity, characteristically associated with a decrease in the number and function of the CD4 T lymphocytes. CD4 T lymphocytes are functionally separated into the TH1 subset, which produces gamma interferon and IL-2, and the TH2 subset, which produces IL-4, IL-6, and IL-10. In advanced HIV infection, the TH1 subset is markedly decreased in number.

There is a spectrum of CD4 cell numbers in all clinical stages of HIV infection: Occasional asymptomatic individuals have very low counts, whereas rarely the values are normal in individuals with AIDS. Individuals who present with Kaposi's sarcoma frequently have higher CD4 cell counts than those who initially present with AIDS-defining opportunistic infections. This suggests that patients who

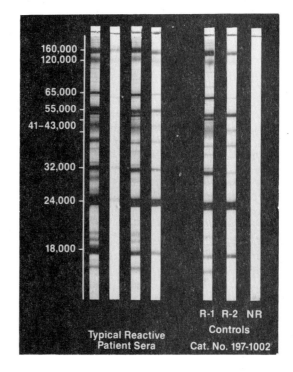

Figure 52–4. Western blot analysis. Reactive sera typically contain demonstrable antibodies to envelope proteins gp160, gp120, and gp41, as well as to core proteins p55 and p24 and to reverse transcriptase p32. Detection of antibody to p24 alone is insufficient to meet the diagnostic criteria for a positive Western blot and may be due to a nonspecific reaction. Alternatively, a reactive band at 24,000 may represent an early serologic response during seroconversion. (Photograph courtesy of Bio-Rad Laboratories, Richmond, Calif.)

present with opportunistic infections have more severe immunologic dysfunction than those with Kaposi's sarcoma. CD4 cell levels are of prognostic value: The risk of progression to AIDS in a given time interval increases as the CD4 count declines. The CD4 number can also provide a guide to the risk of development of individual opportunistic infections and malignancies (Fig 52–5). Not unexpectedly, certain infections with organisms of high virulence (eg, *Mycobacterium tuberculosis*) are manifest when the CD4 count is well preserved, whereas others with organisms of lower virulence (eg *Mycobacterium avium* complex) tend to occur only when the CD4 number is much smaller. In general the CD4 lymphocyte number is less than 200 cells/μL of blood at the time of AIDS diagnosis, and with the routine use of prophylaxis for common opportunistic infections and antiretroviral drugs, the CD4 number is in fact commonly smaller than 100/μL at the onset of the first AIDS-defining illness.

The CD4:CD8 ratio invariably becomes inverted

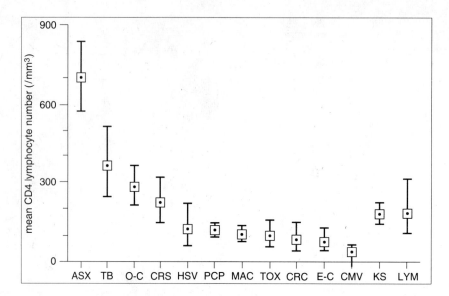

Figure 52–5. The mean CD4 lymphocyte numbers and approximate 95% confidence intervals for individuals with asymptomatic HIV infection, oral candidiasis, or AIDS-defining opportunistic infections or malignancies. Assessments were performed between 2 months preceding or 1 month following diagnosis of the illness, with 55% being determined at the time of diagnosis. A total of 307 events in 222 patients were examined. ASX, asymptomatic infection; TB, disseminated tuberculosis; O-C, oral candidiasis; CRS, cryptosporidium; HSV, recurrent mucocutaneous herpes simplex virus; PCP, *P carinii* pneumonia; MAC, disseminated *M avium* complex; TOX, *T gondii* encephalitis; CRC, cryptococcal meningitis; EC, esophageal candidiasis; CMV, cytomegalovirus retinitis; KS, Kaposi's sarcoma; LYM, lymphoma. (Reproduced, with permission, from Crowe SM et al: Predictive value of CD4 lymphocyte numbers for the development of opportunistic infections and malignancies in HIV-infected persons. *J Acquired Immune Defic Syndr* 1991;**4:**770.)

primarily as a consequence of CD4 lymphocyte depletion. However, a variety of other conditions, including infection with EBV, hepatitis B virus, and cytomegalovirus (CMV), can cause inversion of the CD4:CD8 ratio, primarily owing to an increase in the CD8 subset. Thus, this ratio is of no diagnostic value.

B. Abnormal Delayed-Type Hypersensitivity Responses: Delayed-type hypersensitivity responses are usually normal in the early phase of HIV infection and decreased or absent in patients with advanced disease.

C. T Cell Proliferative Responses: The normal in vitro proliferative responses of CD4 T lymphocytes to soluble antigens (such as tetanus toxoid) and mitogens (such as concanavalin A, phytohemagglutinin, or pokeweed mitogen) are impaired in HIV-infected individuals, especially AIDS patients. This abnormality may be due to a selective loss of a subset of CD4 lymphocytes, to defective antigen presentation by monocyte-macrophages, or to direct viral suppression of CD4 lymphocyte function. Current evidence favors a functional defect of this cell population rather than an abnormality of antigen-presenting cells. Responses to mitogens tend to vary and are less severely impaired than responses to antigen. Antigen responses but not mitogen responses strictly require the interaction of the CD4 molecule on the surface of the lymphocyte with the class II MHC molecule. The HIV envelope glycoprotein (gp120) binds to the CD4 molecule, and its presence could interfere with the interaction with the class II MHC molecule, thus explaining why mitogen responses are less impaired than antigen responses.

D. Cytotoxic Lymphocyte Responses: Cells infected with HIV provide a target for lysis by the various types of cytotoxic cells, including MHC-restricted cytotoxic lymphocytes, MHC-nonrestricted NK cells, and lymphokine-activated cells. Cytotoxic T lymphocyte (CD8 or CD4) responses and NK cell activity are present but quantitatively defective in cells from HIV-infected individuals with late stages of infection. Although the number of NK cells is relatively normal when compared with that in uninfected controls and binding of these cells to their target is unimpaired, their cytotoxic capacity is moderately diminished. Recent in vitro studies suggest that reduced NK activity may be restored by IL-12. Cytotoxic CD8 cells kills infected cells of the same class I MHC type that express HIV proteins (envelope, core, and some regulatory proteins). In addition to this cytotoxic role, CD8 lymphocytes can suppress HIV replication in CD4 lymphocytes.

E. B Cell Responses:
(1) Polyclonal B cell activation resulting in hyper-

gammaglobulinemia is commonly found in HIV-infected individuals, resulting predominantly in increases in serum IgG1, IgG3, and IgM levels. This spontaneous secretion of immunoglobulin by B cells is not always present, and in HIV-infected infants panhypogammaglobulinemia may occur.

(2) Autoantibodies directed against erythrocytes, platelets, lymphocytes, neutrophils, nuclear proteins, myelin and spermatozoa have been found in patients infected with HIV. In some instances these have been associated with disease (eg, HIV-associated thrombocytopenia and peripheral neuropathy).

(3) Antibody capable of neutralizing HIV in vitro is present in low titer in the sera of infected individuals. However, there is no evidence that this antibody has a protective role. Neutralizing antibody is directed against envelope and core proteins.

(4) The enhancement of in vitro HIV infection by antibodies has been reported, although the in vivo significance of this phenomenon is uncertain. Antibody-enhanced viral uptake is mediated by Fc and complement receptors.

(5) B cell proliferative responses to T cell-independent specific B cell mitogens (such as formalinized *Staphylococcus aureus* Cowan 1 strain) are impaired.

(6) Despite depression of helper T cell function and abnormalities of humoral immunity, HIV-infected individuals at early stages of infection can often mount appropriate antibody responses to commonly used vaccines. However, a decrease in response to hepatitis B vaccine, pneumococcal vaccine, and influenza vaccine is generally found as HIV disease progresses.

F. Monocyte-Macrophage Responses: The HIV-infected monocyte-macrophage is probably the major reservoir for HIV in vivo. There are conflicting data about the degree of monocyte-macrophage dysfunction and the specific functions that are altered as a result of HIV infection. Current evidence suggests that phagocytosis and killing of organisms, antigen presentation, and chemotaxis are moderately impaired. Infected macrophages produce an inhibitor of IL-1 termed contra-IL-1, which may contribute to the impairment of T cell proliferative responses observed in HIV-infected individuals (Table 52–6).

G. Other Immunologic Responses: Other ab-

normal immunologic parameters include decreased lymphokine production (in particular, IL-2 and gamma interferon), decreased expression of IL-2 receptors, and an increase in the level of circulating immune complexes. Elevated serum levels of β_2-microglobulin and neopterin are of some prognostic importance in predicting progression to AIDS.

H. Hematologic Findings: Subjects with acute HIV mononucleosis generally have leukopenia with an atypical lymphocytosis. Transient thrombocytopenia occurs in some patients. With disease progression, the total leukocyte count falls, with an associated lymphopenia, reflecting depletion of CD4 lymphocytes. The hemoglobin and hematocrit decrease as a result of anemia due to chronic disease, the presence of an opportunistic infection, or related to therapy. Mild thrombocytopenia is common.

Differential Diagnosis

Acute HIV mononucleosis must be distinguished from infectious mononucleosis caused by EBV, CMV infection, and less commonly, rubella, secondary syphilis, hepatitis B, human herpesvirus type 6 infection, and toxoplasmosis (Table 52–7). Once there is evidence of immunodeficiency, it should be ascertained that this is an acquired rather than a congenital defect and that there is no other underlying explanation for the clinical and immunologic manifestations, such as hematologic cancer or tissue transplantation. However, any individual with laboratory-confirmed HIV infection and a definitively diagnosed disease that meets the CDC criteria for AIDS is considered to have AIDS, regardless of the presence of other potential causes of immune deficiency.

Treatment

A. Life Cycle of HIV: The initial phase of the replicative cycle of HIV involves binding of specific epitopes of the CD4 molecule on the surface of the target cell to defined regions of gp120. Following this, HIV enters the cell and is uncoated. Viral RNA is then used as a template by reverse transcriptase to make a minus-strand DNA copy, thus forming an RNA-DNA hybrid. Soon thereafter, the RNA strand is degraded by the ribonuclease H activity of reverse transcriptase. A positive DNA strand is synthesized, and the linear double-stranded DNA molecule changes conformation to become circular. Some of this DNA migrates to the nucleus and subsequently

Table 52–6. Potential role of macrophages in the pathogenesis of AIDS.

Act as target for HIV
Provide reservoir for HIV
Contribute to immune deficiency through abnormal function
Defective phagocytosis
Defective chemotaxis
Defective antigen presentation
Abnormal cytokine production
Contribute to T cell depletion through a cell fusion process[1]

[1]Shown in vitro only.

Table 52–7. Differential diagnosis of acute HIV infection.

EBV infectious mononucleosis
CMV infection
Rubella
Secondary syphilis
Hepatitis B
Toxoplasmosis
Human herpesvirus type 6.

becomes integrated into the cellular DNA to form the HIV provirus, through the action of the viral integrase. Further replication of HIV depends on changes within the cell that are only partly understood. Cellular transcription factors that bind to HIV LTR are dependent on the activation of the lymphocyte; differentiation of monocytes into macrophages is associated with increased replication of HIV; cytokines can influence HIV replication through the above mechanisms as well as by their independent activities. The replication cycle continues with the translation of viral genomic RNA and viral proteins from unspliced, singly spliced, and multiply spliced mRNA species. These proteins undergo posttranslational protein cleavage and glycosylation. Within the cytoplasm the final stage of assembly of viral proteins occurs and is followed by the budding of the mature virion through the cell membrane, with simultaneous acquisition of envelope (Fig 52–6).

B. Antiretroviral Therapy: The complicated machinery used by HIV in its replicative cycle has provided many specific target sites for potential intervention (Table 52–8). Because reverse transcriptase is not normally present in human cells, selective inhibitors of this enzyme have been a major focus of drug development. Zidovudine (AZT) is a thymidine

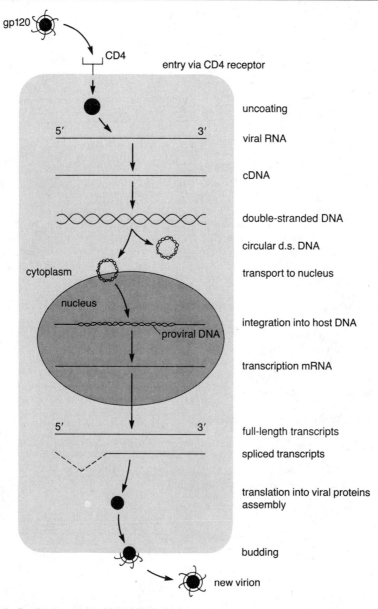

Figure 52–6. Replicative cycle of HIV. Lifelong infection is a consequence of the viral replicative cycle.

Table 52–8. Targets for antiretroviral therapy.

Target	Therapy
HIV binding and cell entry	Soluble recombinant CD4, dextran sulfate, castanospermine, heparin
Reverse transcription	Zidovudine, Foscarnet, Didanosine, Zalcitabine, Second-site RT inhibitors (eg, TIBO, nevirapine)
Regulatory proteins	Tat inhibitors
HIV translation and protein assembly	Ribavirin, protease inhibitors
Budding from cell	Interferons

analogue that requires phosphorylation by host nucleoside kinases to the triphosphate derivative within the infected cell for it to be active. Once phosphorylated, the drug inhibits the virus-encoded reverse transcriptase enzyme, since it has about 100 times the affinity for this enzyme as it does for the host DNA polymerase. Zidovudine further prevents HIV replication by becoming incorporated into the transcribed DNA strand and thus preventing further HIV DNA synthesis. In clinical trials, individuals with symptomatic HIV infection treated with zidovudine have had lower mortality rates and less frequent opportunistic infections than those receiving placebo. In asymptomatic HIV-infected persons with a preserved CD4 count, studies to assess the use of zidovudine therapy have provided conflicting data. Many clinicians advocate initiation of antiviral therapy (usually with zidovudine) when the CD4 lymphocyte number falls below 500/μL. During zidovudine therapy, CD4 lymphocytes initially increase in number but usually return to baseline levels within 6 months of the start of therapy. Zidovudine resistance develops over a similar period, but the precise clinical significance for this observation remains uncertain. Resistance is due to the development of mutations within the reverse transcriptase gene (codons 67, 70, 215, and 219; mutations in other amino acid positions have also been reported).

Dideoxyinosine (ddI, didanosine) and dideoxycytidine (ddC, zalcitabine) are related nucleoside analogues with the same mechanism of action as zidovudine; they are licensed for the treatment of HIV-infected persons who are intolerant to or failing idovudine therapy. Whereas the toxicity of zidovudine is predominantly hematologic (anemia and neutropenia), didanosine and zalcitabine may cause a peripheral neuropathy and pancreatitis. In vitro resistance to didanosine and zalcitabine has been reported but at a lower incidence than that to zidovudine. Other reverse transcriptase inhibitors, such as the pyrophosphate analogue foscarnet, do not require cellular phosphorylation for activity and act directly on the enzyme. Second-site reverse transcriptase inhibitors (TIBO compounds, nevirapine, L-639,697) are currently being evaluated in clinical trials. The rapid emergence of resistance in early clinical trials has led to the development of protocols in which these drugs are used in combination with other antiretroviral therapies. Agents acting at other sites in the replicative cycle (including protease inhibitors and inhibitors of Tat protein) are in clinical trials.

C. Immunorestorative Therapy: Attempts to restore the defective immune system have to date generally been ineffective. The alleged immune stimulator inosine pranobex (Isoprinosine) has been associated with only transitory immunologic benefit; bone marrow and peripheral blood lymphocyte transplantation is not regarded as useful, because the transplanted cells also become infected with HIV. The augmentation of general immune or cytotoxic responses by IL-2 and IL-12 is currently being investigated. Inhibitors of cytokines (such as pentoxifylline, a TNFα inhibitor) may provide additional immune and antiviral benefit. It is possible that combination therapy with an immunomodulatory agent together with one or more antiretroviral agents will be more effective than either alone. In certain patients with Kaposi's sarcoma, administration of high-dose alpha interferon has been beneficial. Interferon inducers such as the mismatched doubled-stranded RNA compound Ampligen are effective in vitro in inhibiting HIV replication. Early clinical trials with this drug suggested temporary clinical improvement with restoration of immune responses, but these studies have not been confirmed. GM-CSF has been used in clinical trials for treating cytopenias occurring in AIDS patients, whether they are due to drugs, opportunistic infections, or HIV itself. However, this compound may in fact increase viral replication within monocyte-macrophages unless used in combination with an antiretroviral agent.

Passive immunotherapy to enhance HIV-specific humoral immunity is being evaluated in a number of clinical trials. Approaches include the use of humanized monoclonal antibodies directed against either the CD4-gp120-binding site of the viral envelope or the immunodominant V3 loop of HIV gp 120. Another approach to boost or augment the immune response to HIV involves using a therapeutic vaccine administered to persons already infected with HIV. Jonas Salk, the polio vaccine pioneer, has developed a vaccine made from inactivated HIV (without the envelope); studies to date suggest that it is safe and that it can boost delayed hypersensitivity responses to vaccine antigens. A number of other candidate vaccines are in clinical trial. The immunogens include envelope proteins made in insect and mammalian cell systems, as well as a novel approaches such as HIV core protein produced in such a way that the HIV p24 is presented to the immune system as a viruslike particle. It is anticipated that these vaccines will stimulate both cell-mediated and humoral immune responses, resulting in greater clinical benefit than that provided by immunogens which induce only neutralizing antibodies to HIV.

Prevention

A. Vaccines: The development of an effective vaccine has been hampered by the genomic diversity of HIV (Table 52–9). Strains of HIV vary in their nucleic acid sequence by up to 20% as a result of high-frequency point mutations that occur during the replication of the virus. This variation is most evident in the envelope region of HIV. Of interest, certain regions are conserved between different isolates (for example, the region of gp120 that interacts with CD4), and other regions of the envelope are highly variable. Unfortunately, the major antigenic epitopes (and therefore, predictably, the major protective epitopes) are in the regions associated with the highest degree of strain-to-strain variation. This includes the immunodominant third variable loop (V3) within gp120. The V3 loop contains the GPGRA amino acid sequence, which is regarded as the principal neutralizing domain. This genomic diversity is one of the many major obstacles hampering vaccine development, as an effective vaccine should provide protection against all strains of HIV. Another impediment to vaccine development is the fact that HIV is spread from cell to cell via a fusion process as well as by cell-free virus.

Prophylactic vaccines (for HIV-negative persons) containing attenuated virus or inactivated whole virus would meet with ethical concerns because of difficulty in guaranteeing their safety. Recombinant HIV envelope glycoproteins expressed in a cell culture system (eg, mammalian cells, bacteria, or yeasts) and HIV genes inserted into an attenuated vector (eg, vaccinia virus) are currently undergoing trials in chimpanzees. Neutralizing antibodies have been produced to these viral proteins in vaccinated animals. Some of these vaccines have resulted in various degrees of success in providing protection against subsequent challenge with strains of HIV. Because chimpanzees are not an ideal animal model for human HIV infection and because of the shortage of supply of these animals, trial vaccination of humans is now under way. Other strategies in vaccine development include production of anti-idiotype vaccines and construction of synthetic peptides. The recognition of the importance of mucosal immunity, the possible ad-

vantages of live vectors such as vaccinia virus or canarypox virus, and the ability of various adjuvants to provide differing immunologic responses are influencing the design of future vaccines.

B. Education: The major thrust of strategies to prevent HIV infection lies in education of individuals about practicing safer sex, in which the transmission of bodily fluids (specifically semen, vaginal secretions, and blood) is prevented, and not sharing needles or syringes.

CYTOMEGALOVIRUS

Major Immunologic Features

- CD8 lymphocyte numbers increase and CD4 lymphocyte numbers transiently decrease.
- Cell-mediated immunity is depressed.

General Considerations

Cytomegalovirus (CMV) is a member of the herpesvirus family, a group that includes the human pathogens EBV, herpes simplex virus types 1 and 2, varicella-zoster virus, and human herpesvirus type 6, as well as many animal pathogens. Similar to other herpesviruses, CMV is associated with persistent, latent, and recurrent infection, the last being due to reactivation of latent virus.

The prevalence of infection within a community varies with socioeconomic status, being as low as 40% in upper strata and approaching 100% in lower groups.

Clinical Features

Infection with CMV can result in a variety of clinical syndromes, depending partially on the immune state of the infected individual (Table 52–10). In healthy subjects, infection is usually subclinical, occasionally causing an infectious mononucleosis-like syndrome resembling that due to EBV or primary HIV infections (however, pharyngitis is unusual). There is a tendency to develop allergic skin rashes to antibiotics, similar to that observed during acute EBV infection. If infection is acquired in utero, following primary maternal infection, the infant may be born with cytomegalic inclusion disease (CID), with features of hepatosplenomegaly, microcephaly, chorioretinitis, thrombocytopenia, and jaundice. Although only about 5–10% of infants with prenatal infection

---

Table 52–9. Obstacles to development of HIV vaccine.

Genomic diversity of HIV strains
Progression of infection despite vigorous immune response
Transmission of HIV in vivo by cell fusion as well as by cell-free virus
Lack of a good animal model
Potential enhancement of HIV replication by neutralizing antibody

---

Table 52–10. Clinical manifestations of CMV infection.

Prenatal infection
  Cytomegalic inclusion disease
Immunocompetent host
  Subclinical infection
  CMV mononucleosis
Immunocompromised host
  Disseminated CMV: retinitis, esophagitis, colitis, pneumonitis, other sites

are born with CID, another 2–5% develop abnormalities such as deafness, spasticity, intellectual retardation, and dental defects within the first 2 years of life. Asymptomatic perinatal infection may be acquired as a result of exposure to CMV in the birth canal or through breast-feeding.

Immunocompromised patients, such as those with AIDS or those being treated with immunosuppressive drugs, are prone to disseminated CMV infection. In this instance, the infection involves predominantly the retinas, gastrointestinal tract (especially the colon, esophagus, and liver), and lungs. Such individuals often have progressive disease, despite high levels of serum-neutralizing antibody. Organ transplant recipients develop generalized and occasionally fatal CMV disease more commonly following primary than reactivated infection.

Immunologic Findings

A. CMV Serology: IgM antibodies are produced following initial infection and generally persist for 3–4 months. IgG antibodies appear at the same time, peak about 2 or 3 months after infection, and persist for many years and often for life. However, complement-fixing IgG antibody levels may fluctuate and even disappear within a few years of infection. Reactivation of infection generally fails to produce an IgM response.

B. Cellular Immunity: Primary infection is followed by activation of both MHC-restricted cytotoxic CD8 T lymphocytes, whose function is to specifically destroy CMV-infected cells, and MHC-nonrestricted NK cells. Both the humoral and cellular responses that occur following infection develop relatively slowly. The cell-mediated response, specifically directed against CMV intermediate-early (IE) antigens, is the most important aspect of host defense. However, CMV infection results in a general impairment of cellular immunity, characterized by impaired blastogenic responses to nonspecific mitogens and specific CMV antigens, diminished cytotoxic ability, and elevation of the CD8 lymphocyte subset with a moderate but transient decrease in the number of CD4 lymphocytes. Recently is has been shown that infection with CMV causes selective interference with class I MHC presentation of the major IE antigen, thus hampering the recognition of infected cells by IE-specific cytotoxic T lymphocytes. Thus, there is a delicately balanced relationship between the CMV-mediated immune dysfunction and the ability of the host to control the virologic response. This balance is in part temporal: Initially, viral replication and cell-mediated immunopathology occur unhindered, with the immune function being restored during convalescence. Furthermore, the underlying immune status of the infected individual is of major prognostic importance.

In the immunocompetent individual, specific defects in the cell-mediated immune response are re-stored within a few months following infection. However, seropositive individuals may intermittently excrete CMV for many years or perhaps for life, owing to low-grade chronic infection or reactivation of latent infection.

The immune response following primary CMV infection in transplant recipients is usually severely impaired; there is usually marked depression of cytotoxic T cell and NK cell responses, diminished antibody-dependent cell-mediated cytotoxicity, depressed proliferative responses to CMV and nonspecific antigens and mitogens, and decrease or loss of delayed hypersensitivity reactions. Although an IgM and IgG antibody response is usually detected, occasionally there may be failure to mount an antibody response following primary infection in these patients. Transplant recipients who were previously seropositive for CMV invariably undergo reactivation of latent virus following transplantation. Patients with AIDS who develop reactivation of latent CMV infection do not mount an IgM response.

The immaturity of the immune response in infants with congenital or perinatal infection results in chronic excretion of CMV in nasopharyngeal secretions and urine. Blastogenic responses of lymphocytes in response to CMV is impaired in these chronically infected children. This defect, the major feature of cell-mediated dysfunction in these children, is eventually restored coincident with cessation of viral excretion.

Treatment

There are 2 antiviral agents effective against CMV: foscarnet and ganciclovir. Treatment with these agents is limited to immunocompromised individuals. Both of these drugs are administered by the intravenous route: there is currently no effective oral therapy. Combination therapy with ganciclovir plus high-dose intravenous immunoglobulin has been successful in treating interstitial pneumonitis due to CMV following allogeneic bone marrow transplantation.

EPSTEIN-BARR VIRUS

Major Immunologic Features

- B lymphocytes are target cells.
- There is atypical T cell lymphocytosis.
- Heterophil antibodies are produced.
- There is in vitro transformation of B lymphocytes.

General Considerations

EBV is a member of the herpesvirus family and, as such, shares certain features with the other members, including the ability to establish persistent and latent infection. EBV can transform B lymphocytes and has clinically relevant oncogenic potential. Primary infection, which may be subclinical, results in a life-long carrier state.

Pathogenesis

The virus initially replicates within the pharyngeal epithelium, with subsequent infection of B lymphocytes in subjacent lymphoid tissue. Circulating lymphocytes are responsible for generalized infection. Following the acute infection, EBV remains latent within the B lymphocyte population; these cells most probably provide a lifelong reservoir of the virus. Intermittent seeding of the pharyngeal epithelia, with low-level replication within these cells, allows potential transmission of infection to susceptible members of the community.

The incubation period varies from 3 to 7 weeks; most commonly adolescents and young adults develop symptomatic infection.

Shedding of EBV from salivary tissue continues for a number of months postinfection. Recently, EBV has been found in both semen and cervical epithelium: it is now known whether sexual transmission occurs. Transmission of EBV by blood transfusion and bone marrow transplantation has been rarely described.

Clinical Features

In 1964, Epstein, Achong, and Barr described the presence of viral particles in cultured fibroblasts from tissue from a patient with Burkitt's lymphoma. Since then, this DNS virus has been causally associated with acute infectious mononucleosis, nasopharyngeal carcinoma, lymphomas in immunocompromised individuals, X-linked lymphoproliferative syndrome (Duncan's syndrome), and 2 HIV-related conditions, oral hairy leukoplakia and lymphocytic interstitial pneumonitis (Table 52–11). EBV has been proposed as the cause of the chronic fatigue syndrome. At this time there is substantial evidence against this causal association.

Infectious mononucleosis is the most common illness caused by EBV. This disease occurs most frequently in young adults. Typical features include fever; sore throat, often with exudate; generalized lymphadenopathy; and splenomegaly. Chemical hepatitis is present in most patients, and a few develop frank jaundice. About 10% of patients develop a macular rash; therapy with amoxicillin or ampicillin frequently produces an eruption. Rare complications of infectious mononucleosis include hemolytic anemia, aplastic anemia, encephalitis, Guillain-Barré syndrome, myocarditis, nephritis, and hepatic failure.

Laboratory Diagnosis of Infectious Mononucleosis

Usually a mild leukopenia precedes the development of a leukocytosis (and absolute lymphocytosis) during the second to third week of illness. From 50 to 70% of the lymphocytes are atypical. IgM heterophil antibodies, which agglutinate sheep erythrocytes, are present. These antibodies must be distinguished from Forssman's antibodies present in patients with serum sickness, which also agglutinate sheep erythrocytes. Differentiation of the various heterophil antibodies is based on absorption techniques, with guinea pig kidney and bovine erythrocytes. EBV-associated heterophil antibodies are found in the sera of more than 90% of individuals with infectious mononucleosis. They persist for 3–6 months.

The pattern of antibody response to EBV initially reflects the synthesis of viral antigens involved in cell lysis, notably the early antigen (EA), viral capsid antigen (VCA), and EBV-induced membrane antigen (MA). VCA and MA are classified as late antigens, since their expression is suppressed in the presence of inhibitors of DNA synthesis. The appearance of antibody directed against the EBV nuclear antigen (EBNA) usually occurs weeks to months after infection. EBNA is present in all cells containing the viral genome, whether latently or productively infected (Fig 52–7).

Immunologic Features of EBV Infection

The host immune response plays a critical role in restricting the primary infection. The importance of the immune system can be observed following infection of individuals with normal versus depressed immune function. Subjects with severe cellular immunodeficiency, such as renal transplant recipients, may develop fulminant mononucleosis or monoclonal B cell malignancy. The X-linked lymphoproliferative syndrome occurs in males who have an inherited immune defect that predisposes them to a severe, often fatal form of infectious mononucleosis. Uncontrolled EBV replication within the pharyngeal epithelia may be central to the development of EBV-associated nasopharyngeal carcinomas and lymphomas. By comparison, individuals with intact immune function can control the proliferative potential of EBV-infected lymphocytes and regulate replication within pharyngeal epithelia, thus preventing the emergence of lymphoproliferative disorders and cancer.

EBV infects B lymphocytes through binding to the CD21 molecule on the cell surface. CD21 is expressed on a variety of cells besides mature B lym-

Table 52–11. Diseases associated with EBV.

Infectious mononucleosis
Burkitt's lymphoma
Nasopharyngeal carcinoma
Lymphomas in immunocompromised host
X-linked lymphoproliferative syndrome
Oral hairy leukoplakia[1]
Lymphocytic interstitial pneumonitis[1]

[1]In HIV-infected individuals.

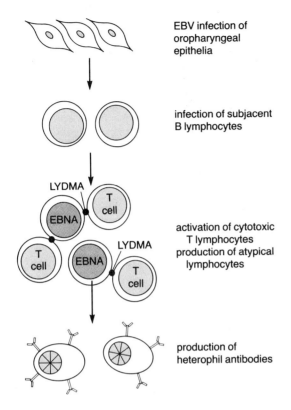

EBV infection of
oropharyngeal
epithelia

infection of subjacent
B lymphocytes

activation of cytotoxic
T lymphocytes
production of atypical
lymphocytes

production of
heterophil antibodies

Figure 52–7. Pathogenesis of infectious mononucleosis. Following infection of oropharyngeal epithelia, EBV infection spreads to the subjacent B lymphocytes. Activation of cytotoxic T lymphocytes by EBV antigens results in the appearance of atypical lymphocytes in the peripheral blood.

phocytes, including follicular dendritic cells, and pharyngeal and cervical epithelia. CD21 is a receptor for the C3d component of complement as well as for EBV. Following infection, large numbers of atypical lymphocytes appear within the circulation which are not, in fact, virus-infected B cells but result from polyclonal activation of cytotoxic/suppressor (CD8) cells (Fig 52–8). These activated T cells, which are not MHC-restricted or EBV-specific, are responsible for preventing the unchecked expansion of EBV-transformed B lymphocytes. In addition, EBV-specific, MHC-restricted cytotoxic T cells are produced. Of interest, these cells appear to specifically recognize virus-infected B lymphocytes expressing **lymphocyte-determined membrane antigen (LYDMA),** without requiring MHC restriction. The true specificity of cytotoxic T cell responses in infectious mononucleosis remains to be completely elucidated. The mechanism for viral persistence may involved inhibition of the normal replicative cycle of EBV within B cells prior to the expression of LYDMA, the target antigen for cytotoxic T cells.

Differential Diagnosis of Infectious Mononucleosis

Streptococcal pharyngitis and, less commonly, diphtheria may resemble infectious mononucleosis. In individuals who present with jaundice, hepatitis A, B, C, E, and delta should be considered. The hematologic changes in infectious mononucleosis, together with serology, generally clarify the issue. In persons at risk of HIV infection a negative heterophil antibody test should alert the clinician to the possibility of acute HIV infection. Other causes of mononucleosislike illness are discussed under the HIV section in this chapter.

Treatment

Therapy for infectious mononucleosis is symptomatic. Although EBV is sensitive to acyclovir in vitro, the drug is of no clinical benefit. However, oral hairy leukoplakia (an HIV-associated EBV infection) responds clinically and virologically to acyclovir.

HUMAN T CELL LEUKEMIA VIRUS TYPES I AND II (HTLV-I AND HTLV-II)

The field of human retrovirology is relatively young: The first human retrovirus was isolated from the T lymphocytes of 2 black men with aggressive T cell cancers in the USA in 1980. This virus, now called HTLV-I, has since been causatively linked with adult T cell leukemia and an incurable progressive neuromyelopathy called tropical spastic paraparesis. HTLV-II has been associated with unusual T cell malignancies in humans.

Molecular studies have shown that leukemic cells from patients with adult T cell leukemia contain provirus, that is, a DNA copy of virion genomic RNA integrated into the host cell genome. Although a variety of cells will support the replication of HTLV-I, T lymphocytes are the preferential target cells for this virus. HTLV-I-infected cells express high levels of IL-2 receptors; however, these cells do not produce IL-2, and IL-2 mRNA is absent.

On morphology, HTLV-I is a type C retrovirus of the oncovirus subfamily (Table 52–1). This virus can transform normal T lymphocytes, allowing these cells to become immortalized. This can occur even though this retrovirus does not possess an *onc* gene. It is not clear by what mechanism HTLV-I transforms cells; integration of the provirus in proximity to the c-*myc* gene (a cellular *onc* gene) may result in subsequent expression of this gene.

Endemic HTLV-I infection exists in parts of the Caribbean region, Japan, and Africa. Worldwide, up to 20 million persons are estimated to be infected with HTLV-I. The modes of transmission of HTLV-I are virtually identical to those for HIV: via infected blood, through sexual contact, and from mother to

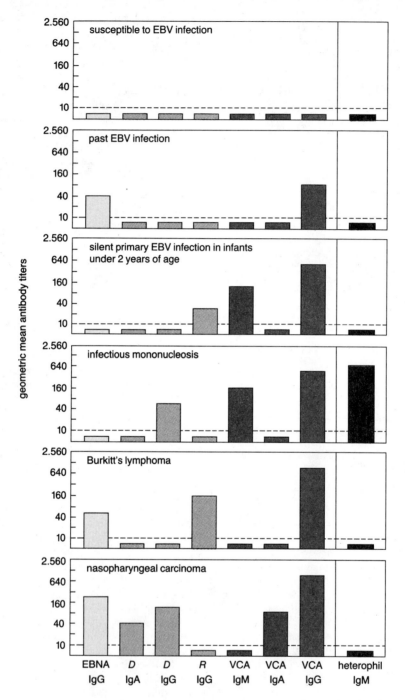

Figure 52–8. Serologic response to EBV infection. Typical antibody patterns are observed in different clinical conditions caused by EBV. Abbreviations: D, diffuse; R; restricted.

child. There is no direct evidence for transplacental transmission of HTLV-I; however, transmission to the infant commonly occurs via the mother's milk, analogous to transmission of bovine leukemia virus.

There is a high rate of infection with HTLV-II in certain populations, including injecting drug users. Screening of blood bank donations in the US for HTLV-I/II began in 1988. Seroprevalence ranged from 0 to 0.1%. Since HTLV-I is difficult to distinguish serologically from HTLV-II, assays that detect both together have been developed. A number of assays are available for the detection of HTLV-I/II, including enzyme immunoassays, particle agglutination assays, Western blot, immunoprecipitation, and PCR. Standardization of these assays is not currently at the same level of development for HIV.

HUMAN HERPESVIRUS TYPE 6 (HHV-6)

The T lymphotropic HHV-6, initially described in 1986, is the most recent addition to the human herpesvirus family. Although this virus replicates primarily in T cells, the virus was initially called "human B lymphotropic virus (HBLV)" because it was isolated from B cells of 6 individuals with lymphoproliferative disorders. HHV-6 also infects fibroblasts, monocyte-macrophages, and glial cells. Molecular studies indicate that HBLV and HHV-6 are different strains of the same human herpesvirus. Cells infected with HHV-6 develop nuclear and cytoplasmic inclusions, with electron-microscopic features typical of other herpesviruses. Infection in infancy occurs as maternal antibody levels decline. Infection may be subclinical or may result in the development of fever and rash (exanthema subitum or roseola infantum). Infection of older persons causes an illness similar to infectious mononucleosis. There is a high seroprevalence of antibody in healthy children and adults (up to 80%). It is postulated that reactivation of latent infection can occur in immunocompromised individuals.

REFERENCES

Human Immunodeficiency Virus

Connolly KJ, Hammer S: Minireview. Antiretroviral therapy: Reverse transcription inhibition. *Antimicrob Agents Chemother* 1992;**36:**245.

Crowe SM, et al: Predictive value of CD4 lymphocyte numbers for the development of opportunistic infections and malignancies in HIV-infected persons. *Acquired Immune Defic Syndr* 1991;**4:**770.

Cullen BR: Mechanism of action of regulatory proteins encoded by complex retroviruses. *Microbiol Rev* 1992;**56:**375.

Haynes BF: Scientific and social issues of human immunodeficiency virus vaccine development. *Science* 1993;**260:**1279.

Levy JA: Pathogenesis of human immunodeficiency virus infection. *Microbiol Rev* 1993;**57:**183.

Salk J, et al: A strategy for prophylactic vaccination against HIV. *Science* 1993;**260:**1270.

Cytomegalovirus

Gilbert MJ, et al: Selective interference with class I major histocompatibility complex presentation of the major intermediate-early protein following infection with human cytomegalovirus. *J Virol* 1993;**67:**3461.

Koszinowski UH, Reddehase MJ, Del VM: Principles of cytomegalovirus antigen presentation in vitro and in vivo. *Semin Immunol* 1992;**4:**71.

Onorato IM et al: Epidemiology of cytomegalovirus infections: Recommendations for prevention and control. *Rev Infec Dis* 1985;**7:**479.

Stagno S et al: Congenital and perinatal cytomegalovirus infections: Clinical characteristics and pathogenic factors. Pages 65–85 In: *CMV: Pathogenesis and Prevention of Human Infection. Birth Defects: Original Article Series.* Vol 20, no. 1. Plotkin SA et al (editors). March of Dimes Birth Defects Foundation, 1984.

Epstein-Barr Virus

Strauss SE: Epstein-Barr virus infections: Biology, pathogenesis and management. *Ann Intern Med* 1993; **118:**45.

Human T Lymphotropic Virus Type I

Hollsberg P, Hafler DA: Pathogenesis of diseases induced by human lymphotropic virus type I infection. *N Engl J Med* 1993;**328:**1173.

Yodoi J, Uchiyama T: Diseases associated with HTLV-I: Virus, IL-2 receptor dysregulation and redox regulation. *Immunol Today* 1992;**13:**405.

Human Herpesvirus Type 6

Caserta MT, Hall CB: Human herpesvirus-6. *Annu Rev Med* 1993;**44:**377.

Niederman JC, et al: Clinical and serological features of human herpesvirus-6 infection in three adults. *Lancet* 1988;**2:**817.

Oren I, Sobel JD: Human herpes virus type 6: Review. *Clin Infect Dis* 1992;**14:**741.

53

Opportunistic Infections in the Immunocompromised Host

Lowell S. Young, MD

"Immunocompromised host" is a term that refers to a patient who either has an underlying immunologic defect which predisposes to infection or is being treated with medication or therapy (eg, radiation) which impairs host resistance to infection. Mechanisms responsible for immunodeficiency are discussed in Chapter 18. Typical examples of patients with compromised host defenses are those who have a hematologic cancer, those who are being treated with pharmacologic doses of corticosteroids, and those who have had organ transplants and are receiving immunosuppressants. The immunosuppression that accompanies many forms of treatment has created a large and growing population of patients who must be considered immunocompromised (see Chapter 58).

The term "opportunistic" relates to the ability of organisms of relatively low virulence to cause disease in the setting of altered immunity. Most of these microorganisms are part of the human normal gastrointestinal or skin flora or are usually harmless components of the environment. More virulent organisms such as staphylococci or pneumococci (see Chapter 47), which cause infection even in normal hosts, can cause even more serious clinical syndromes of infection in the setting of impaired host resistance.

HOST DEFECTS
PREDISPOSING TO INFECTION

Mechanical barriers to microorganisms play an important role in limiting the access of potentially invasive organisms to the host. These are nonspecific barriers and represent a first line of defense. Beyond these barriers are the components of host defense, which are summarized in Table 53–1. Specific immunity is the functional effect of antibodies or cell-mediated immune responses. Mobile (eg, neutrophils) or fixed (eg, Kupffer's cells) phagocytes function more efficiently after antibody binding to microorganisms,

a process known as opsonization. Table 53–1 summarizes the important host defenses and shows that certain forms of therapy, usually drugs or radiation, may result in defects that mimic those present in disease states.

Table 53–1 also suggests typical infecting pathogens that may complicate disease states. These associations are by no means absolute, but they summarize patterns that have been repeatedly observed in such patients. For instance, mycobacterial, pneumocystic, and cryptococcal infections are those against which the bulwark of host defense is considered to be the cell-mediated immune system. These opportunistic infections do not occur in the typical patient with acute myelocytic leukemia, a disease characterized by a defect in the absolute number of circulating neutrophils. Patients with leukemia are more typically prone to infections caused by aerobic gram-negative bacteria and staphylococci (so-called pyogenic bacteria). Thus, gram-negative bacillary infections are less common in patients with acquired immunodeficiency syndrome (AIDS) or Hodgkin's disease than in those with leukemia, but the associations are not absolute. Noteworthy is that medical treatment, such as immunosuppressive therapy, can blur these associations. Radiation that results in pancytopenia can cause functional defects or a reduction in the number of circulating neutrophils and thus predisposes to acute bacterial infection. Deficiencies in specific antibodies are common in chronic lymphatic leukemia and multiple myeloma. Impaired synthesis to antibodies results in less efficient opsonization and impaired clearance of microorganisms.

APPROACH TO THE
IMMUNOCOMPROMISED PATIENT

Although an underlying disease may suggest an association with an opportunistic pathogen, the converse is also true. Detection of *Pneumocystis carinii*

Table 53–1. Impaired host defenses, therapy mimicking disease states, and infectious complications.

Host Defense Element	Disease State	Therapy Mimicking Disease State	Infectious Complications
Polymorphonuclear neutro-phil	Acute myelocytic leukemia	Cyclophosphamide, cytarabine	Staphylococci, gram-negative bacteria, *Aspergillus* spp. *Candida* spp
Monocyte-macrophage, lymphocyte	Hodgkin's disease, AIDS	Corticosteroids, cyclosporin, Antithymocyte globulin	Mycobacteria, *Nocardia* spp, *Pneumocystis* spp, *Candida* spp
Circulating antibody	Multiple myeloma, chronic lymphatic leukemia	Corticosteroids, antimetabolites	Pneumococci, other encapsulated bacteria

in lung sections or pulmonary secretions suggests a disorder such as lymphoma or AIDS. What these introductory concepts have emphasized is there are, indeed, 3 approaches to patients with opportunistic infection in the setting of compromised host defenses. One is the immunologic approach; this involves considering the nature of the defect that predisposes to infection. The second is the syndrome-oriented approach; this involves considering the presentation of a cluster of signs and symptoms (eg, meningitis, diarrhea, or pneumonia) and hence inferring the most likely causative organisms in the process known as differential diagnosis. Finally, there is the organism-oriented approach; this involves considering the likely sites of infection and the type of immunologic defect when a specific pathogen is isolated from body fluids such as blood. The clinician should integrate these 3 approaches in diagnosing and treating the patient with suspected opportunistic infection.

DISEASE ASSOCIATIONS

Table 53–1 suggests specific host defects that are associated with opportunistic infection. There are additional patterns derived from clinical experience. These are discussed below.

Leukemia and Lymphoma

These diseases (see Chapter 45) often represent the more dramatic examples of compromised host defense. Patients with acute leukemia, by virtue of their functional neutropenia, are at risk of developing precipitous, overwhelming opportunistic bacterial and fungal infection. The same is true of recipients of bone marrow transplants who are treated with immunosuppressants. As soon as neutrophil function is reconstituted (circulating cells $\geq$ 500/mL), serious infections may abate.

Splenectomy

It has long been recognized that the spleen serves an important function, both as a site of antibody synthesis and as a reservoir of phagocytic cells capable of filtering out organisms that are circulating in the

bloodstream. Splenectomized patients are particularly prone to infections caused by *Streptococcus pneumoniae, Haemophilus influenzae,* meningococci, and staphylococci.

Sickle Cell Anemia

This disorder has been associated with pneumococcal sepsis, meningitis, and *Salmonella* osteomyelitis.

Diabetes Mellitus

Diabetes (see Chapter 32) has been clinically associated with increased susceptibility to infection, but the specific mechanisms are multifactorial. At high blood glucose concentrations (high osmolarity) and during ketoacidosis, phagocytic and bactericidal activity is reduced. A leukocyte chemotactic defect has been reported at elevated blood glucose levels.

Chronic Renal Failure

Decreased movement of neutrophils rather than impaired killing has been reported to occur in this condition.

Alcoholism & Hepatic Cirrhosis

In liver disease, the role of the liver as filter for microorganisms may be impaired and organisms can "bypass" this filter. Antibody responses are normal, but leukocyte mobilization may be impaired. Alcohol has a direct inhibitory effect on leukocyte proliferation.

Rheumatic Diseases

Complement deficiencies have been reported to occur in systemic lupus erythematosus (see Chapter 31). Circulating immune complexes present in hypersensitivity states per se have been postulated to impair particle clearance in vivo. Some rheumatoid disorders are associated with neutropenia and lymphopenia.

Hypocomplementemia

This has also been postulated to be a factor in increased susceptibility to infection (see Chapter 23). Low complement levels (particularly of the terminal lytic components) have been associated with meningococcal disease.

Infections

In certain immunodeficiency disorders, amplification of infections may be related to factors elaborated by the organisms themselves. Such factors are the production of toxins or the ability to secrete factors that enhance intracellular survival even within host tissues.

APPROPRIATE DIAGNOSIS

A high index of suspicion for unusual pathogens and an appreciation of the causes of a specific clinical syndrome form the cornerstone of the clinical approach to the immunocompromised patient. It is important that appropriate cultures of all body fluids or sites suspected of being infected are taken prior to the initiation of treatment. Proper diagnosis may involve invasive studies, such as lumbar puncture and lung biopsy, and noninvasive imaging, such as magnetic resonance imaging or radionuclide scans. Table 53–2 is a summary of the clinical syndromes and the organisms that should be suspected in specific settings.

A useful clinical approach is to work backward from the clinical presentation to the organisms that have been associated with infections in the specific body sites and in patients with specific immunologic defects. For instance, central nervous system infection in patients with impaired cellular immunity is

most likely to be due to listerias or cryptococci. In patients with leukemia or neutropenia, infection that spreads by vascular routes and is caused by pseudomonads or staphylococci is relatively more common.

DIAGNOSTIC TESTS

Although treatment will clearly have to be initiated in the acute stages of any opportunistic infection, immunologic screening tests may be of some use in determining the nature of the underlying defect when an unusual infection appears (see Chapters 12, 13, and 17). As mentioned above, patients with known defects in immune function are prone to the types of infections summarized in Table 53–1.

Conversely, the question may arise at the bedside about the potential underlying defect in a patient with an unusual infection. The tests that are summarized in Table 53–3 may not be available in some medical centers. Some, such as quantitation of total antibody classes, total and differential leukocyte counts, and lymphocyte subsets, may be used as initial screening procedures to ascertain immunologic defects. More sophisticated tests are necessary in certain circumstances to elucidate the exact mechanism of the defect in host defense. This is particularly true in the phagocyte disorders, in which a variety of specific enzymatic defects exist. Screening for some of the neutrophil disorders is possible by using the Nitro

Table 53–2 Infectious syndromes and differential diagnoses.

Syndrome	Potential Causative Agent			
	Bacteria	**Fungi**	**Viruses**	**Parasites**
Fever, suspected septicemia, skin lesions	*Staphylococcus aureus*, gram-negative bacilli, *Nocardia* spp	*Candida* spp, *Aspergillus* spp, *Cryptococcus* spp, *Trichosporon* spp, zygomycetes	Herpes simplex virus	(May be significant in tropics)
Central nervous system infection	*Listeria* spp, *Nocardia* spp, *Staphylococcus aureus*, *Pseudomonas aeruginosa*, *Mycobacterium tuberculosis*	Cryptococcus spp, *Aspergillus* spp, zygomycetes, *Candida* spp	Varicella-zoster virus, herpes simplex virus, human immunodeficiency virus	*Strongyloides* spp
Pulmonary infection	Gram-positive bacteria (pneumococci, staphylococci, nocardias, mycobacteria); gram-negative bacteria (enteric bacilli, legionellas, pseudomonads)	*Aspergillus* spp, *Coccidioides* spp, *Histoplasma* spp, *Petriellidium* spp, *Cryptococcus* spp, *Candida* spp, *Pneumocystis* spp	Cytomegalovirus, adenovirus, herpes simplex virus, varicella-zoster virus	*Toxoplasma* spp, *Stronglyoides* spp
Oroesophageal ulceration or inflammation	Anaerobic bacteria, streptococci, gram-negative bacilli (especially pseudomonads)	*Candida* spp, *Aspergillus* spp, zygomycetes, *Histoplasma* spp	Herpes simplex virus, cytomegalovirus	
Diarrhea	*Clostridium difficile, Salmonella* spp, *Shigella* spp, *Campylobacter* spp		Rotavirus, enteroviruses, Norwalk virus	*Giardia* spp, *Cryptosporidium* spp, *Entameba histolytica*

Table 53–3. Immunologic screening tests.[1]

Immune System Component	Tests
Antibody response	Quantitative levels of IgG, IgM, IgA; Isohemagglutinin titers; rubella titer. diphtheria-tetanus titer; response to *Haemophilus influenzae* type B or other nonattenuated or live vaccines.
Complement level	Total hemolytic complement; C3, C4, C5, factor B.
Phagocyte function	Leukocyte and differential cell count; Nitro Blue Tetrozolium (NBT) test; other tests for oxidative burst of phagocytosis.
Cell-mediated immunity	PMN chemotaxis; skin tests (*Candida albicans*, purified protein derivative, diphtheria-tetanus, mumps); total T cells and T cell subsets; mitogen responses.

[1]See Chapters 12. 13. and 17.

Blue Tetrazolium dye test or other measures of oxidative killing.

TREATMENT

The specifics of treatments of opportunistic infection are clearly beyond the scope of this chapter. Currently, a wide variety of broad-spectrum antibacterial agents are available, and this is the area in which the greatest progress has been made. Treatment of fulminating bacterial infections with broad-spectrum antibiotics has resulted in a significant decrease in mortality and morbidity rates, particularly from infections due to gram-negative bacteria, in the past 20 years. Persistence of infection is often associated with persistence of the immunologic defect, but other factors, such as a foreign body (eg, an in-dwelling vascular catheter), must be considered. The treatment of parasitic, fungal, and viral infections has been more frustrating because there are fewer effective antimicrobial drugs for these organisms.

REVERSAL OF UNDERLYING IMMUNOLOGIC DEFECTS

Although antibiotics have definitely prolonged life and reduced morbidity, the ultimate ability to control and prevent such infections rests on the ability to correct the immunologic impairment. When the defect that predisposes to infection is caused by essential drug therapy, the clinical dilemma is obvious. Sometimes, reducing immunosuppression will have a major role in the control of an opportunistic infection. With some congenital neutrophil disorders, a variety of investigational therapies have been tried, eg, gamma interferon for chronic granulomatosis disease (see Chapter 22).

Realistically, neutrophil replacement has not been a practical approach, simply because of the enormous requirements for adequate quantities of leukocytes for transfusion. New approaches for stimulating the neutrophil pool, such as the use of colony-stimulating factors, may ultimately prove useful. Immunoglobulin for replacement therapy in hypogammaglobulinemia has long been available, but more recent advances in the technology allow the delivery of large quantities of more specific antibodies that have been modified for intravenous infusion (see Chapter 19).

In the future, monoclonal antibodies may make it possible to deliver even larger amounts of specific antibodies for prophylaxis and treatment. Treatment of disorders of cell-mediated immunity has not yet responded to attempts at cell replacement (see Chapters 20–22). Theoretically, immune modulators such as interleukins or interferons could help reconstitute these important components of the immune system (See Chapters 54 and 59). More controversial approaches include plasma exchange for removal of immune complexes, toxins, and other factors.

PROPHYLAXIS

Since organisms that cause significant infection in the immunocompromised host are often part of the normal flora or are abundant in the environment, attempts to suppress these potentially infectious agents have met with variable success. Isolation of the patient is controversial and expensive, but it may limit exposure of selected patients to some important disease-causing microorganisms (eg, *Legionella pneumophila* or *Aspergillus* spp.) Organisms that part are part of the normal flora are clearly more difficult to suppress or eliminate. Prophylactic antimicrobial drugs have a limited role, but they have been successful against *Pneumocystis* infection and gram-negative bacteremia in immunocompromised cancer patients. Prophylaxis of infection may be achieved by immunization or passive administration of antibodies.

REFERENCES

Anaissie E: Opportunistic mycoses in the immunocompromised host: Experience at a cancer center and review. *Clin Infect Dis* 1992;**14(suppl 1):**S43.

EORTC International Antimicrobial Therapy Cooperative Group: Ceftazidime combined with a short or long course of amikacin for empirical therapy of gram-negative bacteremia in cancer patients with granulocytopenia. *N Engl J Med* 1987;**317:**1692.

Lieschke GJ, Burgess AW: Granulocyte colony-stimulating factor and granulocyte-macrophage colony-stimulating factor. *N Engl J Med* 1992;**327:**28, 99.

Pizzo PA: Drug therapy: Management of fever in patients with cancer and treatment-induced neutropenia. *N Engl J Med* 1993;**328:**1323.

Ross SC, Densen P: Complement deficiency states and infection: Epidemiology, pathogenesis and consequences of neisserial and other infections in an immune deficiency. *Medicine* 1984;**63:**243.

Rubin RH, Young LS: *Clinical Approach to Infection in the Compromised Host*, 3rd ed. Plenum Press, 1993.

Section IV.
Immunologic Therapy

Immunologic Therapy

54

Abba I. Terr, MD

Immunologic therapy in its broadest sense encompasses the treatment and prevention of a large number and variety of immunologic and nonimmunologic diseases. Historically, therapeutic immunology began in 1796, well before the dawn of scientific and clinical immunology, when William Jenner showed that an ancient viral scourge, smallpox, could be successfully prevented by immunization. Jenner was an English physician who accomplished this feat alone, using only his astute clinical observations. As a result smallpox was completely eradicated as a human disease after the last case was reported in 1977. Ironically, only 3 years later a new and lethal viral disease, acquired immune deficiency syndrome (AIDS), appeared and rapidly became a major worldwide public health problem. The causative virus, human immunodeficiency virus (HIV), infects the CD4 T cell, which is the central focus of the immune response itself. As the subject of widespread research by thousands of immunologists and other scientists, AIDS has generated an enormous expansion of our knowledge of human immunology; however, it has thus far eluded all attempts at successful treatment or prevention by immunization.

The chapters to follow in Section IV discuss major categories of therapy for immunologic diseases and the treatment of these and other diseases by manipulation, alteration, and exploitation of the immune response. Some of these treatment modalities, such as immunization against infections and toxins, allergy desensitization, and certain drugs, arose from empirical clinical observations. Others, such as the use of genetically engineered interleukins, are products of fundamental laboratory investigations. Both well-established and promising new therapies will be discussed. These chapters will address pharmacologic properties and mechanisms. Clinical indications

or details of drug administration are included in the previous sections where specific diseases are discussed.

This chapter is an overview of those that follow. To best understand the mechanisms and clinical indications for the many forms of treatment, the immune system can be divided functionally into two categories: the **immune response** and the **inflammatory response.** Therapy directed at the immune response can be either **antigen-specific** or **antigen-nonspecific.** Some diseases require that the immune response be stimulated, whereas others require suppression. The therapeutic armamentarium to accomplish these diverse goals now includes chemically defined drugs obtained from natural sources such as fungal products, synthetic chemicals, specific antibodies, and many of the actual cellular and chemical components of the immune system itself. Genetically engineered cloning techniques make available adequate quantities of virtually any cytokine, adhesion molecule, cell membrane molecule, or receptor in remarkably short time after their discovery. Some mention will be made in this section of therapies that are currently theoretical or in the process of animal experimentation or clinical trials.

Increasingly, antibodies are being used as drugs because of their ability to target a particular structure within the body with great specificity. Monoclonal antibody technology has largely supplanted the traditional use of serum gamma globulin from animals immunized with the relevant antigen. Although this greatly increases specificity and eliminates the problem of allergic reactions to irrelevant serum proteins, the monoclonal antibody is itself antigenic and may in time become ineffective by neutralization or by an allergic reaction to it. In some cases in which target cell death is the therapeutic goal, the monoclonal antibody has been coupled to a potent toxin such as ricin, diphtheria toxin, or *Pseudomonas* exotoxin A.

MODULATION OF THE IMMUNE RESPONSE

ANTIGEN-SPECIFIC THERAPY

Immune Stimulation

A. Active Immunization: Prophylaxis against the future occurrence of an **infectious** or **toxic disease** is possible by means of active immunization. In this case, natural host immune response to a primary microbial infection is stimulated by immunization with an antigenically active killed or attenuated microorganism, an antigenically cross-reactive but nonpathogenic living organism, an antigenically active product or constituent of the organism, or a modified form of a microbial toxin that is antigenic but nontoxic. The resulting immune response can be transient or lifelong, depending on a number of factors related to the immunizing antigen (often referred to as a vaccine), the host, and the mode of administration of the antigen. The response can generate effector T cells, antibodies, or both. Furthermore, the antibodies produced can include any one or more of the immunoglobulin classes and subclasses (isotypes). The type of immune response determines efficacy in prophylaxis. Chapter 55 details immunization procedures and effectiveness for all of the currently available vaccines.

Immunization to ameliorate **allergic disease** has been clinically successful for many years, but the precise mechanism of the effect is still unknown. The various immunologic changes that ensue from injecting allergen into patients with IgE-mediated diseases are addressed in detail in Chapter 56. These changes include (eventually) both suppression of IgE antibodies and production of IgG antibodies. This shifting of the profile of isotypes of the allergen-specific antibody is presumed to occur because the route of allergen exposure has changed from mucosal absorption to subcutaneous injection. Other explanations may apply, but this one suggests that antigen processing is important in successful allergy desensitization. In mice there are two subpopulations of helper T cells, TH1 and TH2, which have different cytokine profiles for their activation and which signal B cells for antibody production of differing isotypes. Limited evidence to date suggests that there are similar subpopulations of human helper T cells. In theory, therefore, administration of appropriate cytokines with or without antigen could be used to tailor a desired immune response pathway for treatment of allergic and other diseases.

Adjuvants are chemicals added to the immunizing antigen to enhance the host immune response by increasing the availability of the antigen to the antigen-presenting cell (APC), prolonging the persistence of antigen in tissues, or stimulating the APC directly. Examples of adjuvants, discussed in more detail in Chapter 55, are alum (used to insolubilize the antigen), water-in-oil emulsions, muramyl dipeptide, and liposomes.

B. Passive Immunization: The transfer of the active product of the immune response (antibody or effector T cell) from an immune individual to a nonimmune recipient is called passive immunization. The protection afforded in this way is immediate but transient, since no ongoing immune response or memory is involved. The immune donor of the passive antibody can be human or animal. The latter is preferable for producing antibodies to particularly dangerous immunogens, but the resultant antibody is foreign and therefore itself antigenic to the human recipient. The therapeutic benefit of passive immunization is thus limited by immune elimination, neutralization or possible allergic reaction by the recipient's own immune response to the administered antibody.

Passive antibody protection is standard therapy for patients with any of the antibody deficiency diseases with or without concomitant cellular immunodeficiency. These conditions are described in Chapters 19 and 21. The treatment usually is given in the form of the gamma globulin fraction of normal human plasma pooled from many donors, yielding a product with a broad range of antibodies. These are almost exclusively IgG antibodies, because ethanol fractionation used in its preparation excludes other immunoglobulin classes. For specific protection of anyone (ie, normal or immunocompromised) with an anticipated exposure to certain infections or toxins, hightiter preparations of the specific antibody are available from hyperimmunized individuals or animals.

Antigen-specific passive cellular immunization by transfer of effector lymphocytes has been demonstrated repeatedly in animal experiments, but to date it has had no role in human treatment. Cellular immunodeficiency diseases are treated instead by adoptive immunity (discussed below).

C. Adoptive Immunity: Transplantation of immunocompetent cells from normal donors is the method used to achieve immune function in children with congenital cellular immunodeficiency. Since the recipient lacks the ability to mount an immune response, rejection of the transplanted cells does not occur, but a graft-versus-host reaction is still possible, so histocompatible donors are preferred. The usual source is the bone marrow from which the cells are transfused intraperitoneally or intravenously. Long-term immunologic restoration in children with severe combined immunodeficiency has been achieved in a number of cases. When histocompatible bone marrow is not available, fetal liver or thymus has been used, but to date results have been less satisfactory than with bone marrow.

Rare cases of immunodeficiency arise from congenital deficiency of an enzyme in the purine metabolic pathway, eg, adenosine deaminase or nucleoside phosphorylase. In some cases of adenosine deaminase deficiency, immune competence has been restored by the administration of the enzyme and recently by somatic gene therapy, in which the gene encoding the enzyme is inserted into the genome of bone marrow stem cells by using a viral vector.

Treatment of specific immunodeficiency diseases is covered in Chapters 18–22.

Immune Suppression

A. Active Suppression: A variety of strategies, both tested and theoretical, are designed to actively suppress antigen-specific immune responses. A unique form of highly effective antigen-specific therapy is available for prevention of erythroblastosis fetalis. In this case anti-Rh antibodies are administered to Rh-negative mothers during or promptly after their delivery of an Rh-positive offspring. Although the mechanism is not thoroughly understood, the administered antibody suppresses the ability of the mother to make her own Rh antibody to fetal Rh-positive red cells that enter her circulation during the pregnancy.

In theory, both allergic diseases and disorders caused by autoantibodies to known self-antigens could be cured if a state of specific acquired immunologic tolerance (**anergy**) to the relevant allergen or autoantigen could be permanently induced. As discussed in Chapter 56, the currently used procedure of allergen injection therapy for IgE-mediated atopy or anaphylaxis does create a state of partial immunological tolerance in some patients, so a fully successful application of this therapeutic principle may be possible in the future. Specific therapy for allergy requires a form of allergen administration that avoids systemic reactions, and therapeutic trials involving genetically engineered peptide epitopes are currently under way. In patients with autoimmune diseases the challenge is to identify the autoantigen, which in most of these diseases is unknown. Recently, prevention and reversal of experimental allergic encephalomyelitis in mice, the animal model of human multiple sclerosis, were reported as a result of injections of peptide fragments of myelin basic protein. In theory the peptide epitope can bind to the T cell receptor-major histocompatibility complex (TCR-MHC) molecular structure with the same immunologic specificity as does the complete autoantigen but without activating the T cell.

A possible approach to antigen-specific immune suppression is the elimination of the T cells or B cells bearing the specific TCR or B cell surface immunoglobulin, respectively, by using an appropriate monoclonal antibody. This is possible only when the antigenic epitope is known, so that the corresponding TCR or immunoglobulin idiotypic specificity can be recognized. This approach has had limited success in certain animal models of autoimmune disease and in treatment of a human B cell lymphoma.

Another theoretical means of achieving antigen-specific immune suppression would be to prevent the MHC molecule expressed on the surface of the T cell from undergoing its requisite association with the antigen in question. This could be accomplished with anti-MHC monoclonal antibodies. Since the number of possible MHC molecules is much more limited than the number of possible antigenic sites, and since presentation of a specific antigen or even a single antigenic epitope may occur in association with more than one MHC molecule, this approach may lack sufficient specificity to avoid eliminating desirable immune responses as well.

Another form of treatment that appears to operate through a "partially specific" mechanism is intravenous normal pooled immunoglobulin (IGIV). Ironically, administration of large amounts of IGIV not only corrects antibody deficiency by passively supplying antibodies from pooled normal plasma but also seems to suppress antibody production when given to patients with certain autoimmune diseases, notably acute idiopathic thrombocytopenic purpura and Kawasaki disease. Although the mechanism of this effect is unknown, current speculation centers on immunomodulation by blocking of Fc receptors for IgG.

B. Passive Suppression: Plasmapheresis consists of repeated removal of blood with replacement of the cells and exchange of patient's plasma for normal plasma, thereby removing circulating antibodies along with other plasma proteins. The procedure does not suppress specific antibody production, but it does selectively, albeit transiently, remove antibodies of the IgM isotype and circulating immune complexes. This makes it a reasonable short-term therapy for certain diseases caused by pathogenic IgM antibodies or antigen-antibody complexes.

ANTIGEN-NONSPECIFIC THERAPY

Immune Stimulation

Techniques for generalized stimulation or up-regulation of the immune response are currently being pursued in clinical trials. This general approach to treatment is also called **immune system modulation** or **biologic response modification.** It is of particular interest in cancer therapy as a means of enhancing the patient's own immunity to the cancer cells. Unfortunately, there are only a few available means to achieve this result, and they are of limited efficacy and often highly toxic, so application of immune stimulation to other conditions with impaired immunity must await development of newer drugs. The current state of knowledge and application is described in Chapter 59.

Adjuvants (see above) have been used alone without exogenous antigen in an effort to enhance an endogenous immune response to putative (ie, unknown) tumor cell antigens. To date this experimental form of treatment has been unsuccessful, but future efforts with other adjuvants or modes of administration may prove fruitful.

Certain **cytokines** cloned by genetic engineering technology are potential nonspecific immune stimulators (or inhibitors), because they act as secondary signals in the presence of the antigenic epitope to activate lymphocytes, as discussed in Chapter 9. In fact, clinical trials of various cytokines have been under way in recent years, especially in experimental cancer therapy.

Monoclonal antibodies to various antigenic sites on molecules and cells involved in the immune response can potentially be used in treatment to exploit the ability of the antibody to (1) sterically block a ligand molecule or its receptor to prevent a particular activation or binding step, (2) eliminate the target molecule or lyse the target cell, or (3) stimulate a receptor by acting as a surrogate for the ligand.

The **T cell receptor-CD3 complex** itself is, of course, the principal site where the immune response is driven, so therapy that sends activation signals to this complex could be nonspecifically immunostimulating, and in fact experiments with an anti-CD3 antibody in mice have yielded antitumor effects. It has been shown in vitro that antigen-mediated activation of T cells is stimulated by monoclonal antibodies to certain **T cell membrane molecules** such as CD5 and CD28, even though the normal function of these molecules is currently unknown. It remains to be shown whether these antibodies act similarly when administered in vivo and may therefore be of use in treating disease. Monoclonal antibodies to **interleukin receptors** on lymphocytes have the potential for stimulating the receptor by mimicking the action of the interleukin, thereby stimulating the target cell and enhancing the immune response.

Another approach to achieving nonspecific immune stimulation involves the therapeutic use of lymphocytes. In one strategy, natural killer **(NK)** cells are activated by in vitro incubation with interleukin-2 **(IL-2)** to enhance their tumoricidal function. These cells, called lymphokine-activated killer **(LAK)** cells have been used for cancer therapy with promising results, although their use has been complicated by IL-2 systemic toxicity. The use of lymphocytes isolated directly from the patient's own tumor and then incubated with IL-2, called tumor-infiltrating lymphocytes **(TIL)**, is another strategy that provides greater tumor cell antigen specificity. These are discussed further in Chapter 59.

Immune Suppression

A variety of immunomodulating techniques are also being used to suppress undesirable immune responses. As the role of the various **cytokines** in immunoregulation becomes clearly delineated, strategies for using cloned cytokines, their receptors, or antibodies to cytokines or their receptors are being developed and tried in animal models of various immunologic diseases to down-regulate aberrant or pathologically exuberant immune responses. This approach is particularly appealing as therapy for autoimmune diseases or to suppress graft rejection.

As discussed above, administration of antibodies to lymphocyte membrane molecules can either stimulate or suppress immunity. Originally, the antibodies were produced in animals by injecting purified human cell preparations, but currently monoclonal antibodies to various T lymphocyte cell surface molecules are being used or undergoing clinical trials. Antibodies to **CD4** are immunosuppressive in animals, and results of limited human trials suggest that they hold promise in treatment of autoimmune disease. There is some evidence that this form of therapy may induce acquired immunologic tolerance as well. Monoclonal antibodies to lymphocytes have also been tried with some success in preventing graft rejection and to a lesser extent in treating graft-versus-host reactions.

One way to focus the immunosuppressant effect of anti-lymphocyte antibodies is to target only cells engaged in an active immune response. For example, activated T cells up-regulate their expression of the IL-2 receptor **(IL-2R)** on the cell surface, so anti-IL-2R antibodies have been considered for immunosuppression in graft rejections. Further discussion can be found in Chapter 58.

Certain drugs and ionizing radiation have the ability to destroy cells during cell division. For years the use of **cytotoxic drugs** has been the primary approach to nonspecific immunosuppression, because expansion of nonspecific lymphocyte population by cell division is an essential element in the active immune response. Since all dividing cells are similarly affected, toxicity of this form of treatment reflects the loss of dividing cells in other tissues, as well as the suppression of desirable (eg, antimicrobial) along with the undesirable (eg, autoantibody) immune responses. The types of cytotoxic drugs used for nonspecific immunosuppression and their individual modes of action are discussed thoroughly in Chapter 58. They are used therapeutically with various degrees of success in many diseases characterized by autoimmune phenomena. During the course of treatment of these diseases, the effect of the cytotoxic drugs on autoantibody production is variable and does not necessarily correlate with clinical improvement in disease activity.

A major breakthrough in nonspecific immunosuppression was the discovery of **cyclosporin,** a drug that selectively blocks T cell activation, thereby inhibiting immune responses and immunoregulation. Recently, 2 more drugs, FK506 and rapamycin, with similar properties but fewer side effects, have become available and promise to replace cyclosporin.

Corticosteroids are commonly thought of as immunosuppressant, because they are effective therapy for so many human diseases with pathologically overactive immune responses to known or unknown antigens. In fact, their benefit to patients with these disorders is largely anti-inflammatory, although some of their properties result in modest inhibition of the immune response too. The profound loss of lymphocytes from the peripheral blood circulation that occurs rapidly with pharmacologic doses of glucocorticoids represents primarily a shift of these cells into tissues. However, inhibition of IL-1 production from monocytes down-regulates T lymphocyte synthesis and secretion of IL-2 and T cell mitosis. Clinically, patients on prolonged steroid therapy may have reduced levels of total serum IgG, although there is little evidence for impaired antibody production when this occurs.

MODULATION OF THE INFLAMMATORY RESPONSE

The inflammatory phase of the immune response is one of the effector mechanisms by which the immune response protects the host from infection. The same immune-mediated inflammation, on the other hand, is responsible for the deleterious effects of the allergic diseases, some autoimmune diseases, graft rejection, and the graft-versus-host response. Therefore, drugs that reduce or inhibit the inflammatory response are necessary in the treatment of many immunologic diseases. In general, anti-inflammatory therapy is independent of the cause of the inflammation, and therefore these drugs are also useful for tissue inflammation induced by physical injury or toxic insults. Some anti-inflammatory drugs such as the corticosteroids, however, have limited immunosuppressive activity as well.

The various types of inflammatory responses are addressed in Chapter 11 as effector consequences of the immune response in vivo. Different immune response pathways lead to different specific pathologic and clinical forms of inflammation. For example, IgE antibody-mediated inflammation is characterized by vasodilation, stimulation of visceral organ smooth muscle contraction, and an eosinophilic infiltrate, whereas effector T cell inflammation generates tissue infiltration by lymphocytes and monocytes with granuloma formation. Some drugs inhibit only one of these inflammatory pathways, whereas others have a more global anti-inflammatory effect. Most of the inflammation-inhibiting treatments used today have acquired their clinical status empirically, and their precise modes of action are incompletely understood.

The anti-inflammatory mechanisms of steroid (glucocorticoid) and nonsteroid (aspirin and nonsteroidal anti-inflammatory drugs [NSAID]) chemicals share in common the ability to inhibit metabolites of arachidonic acid from inflammatory cell membranes, particularly the prostaglandins. As described in Chapter 60, they do so in quite different ways, however. The NSAID inhibit amino acid transport across the cell membrane, whereas the glucocorticoids prevent synthesis of arachidonic acid metabolites by stimulating the cell to synthesize and release lipomodulin, which in turn inhibits phospholipase A_2. Both classes of drugs have other therapeutic actions, side effects, and toxicities, but if the specific property that inhibited cellular inflammation can be pinpointed, there is the possibility in the future of designing a molecule with limited activity, eg, at the level of the arachidonic acid oxygenation products.

Drugs with a more restricted anti-inflammatory effect are available for treatment of IgE-mediated allergic disorders. Cromolyn (disodium cromoglycate) and nedocromil act on the mast cell to prevent mediator release, although the mechanism is unknown. The numerous antihistaminic drugs specifically inhibit histamine H_1 receptors on target cells. Unfortunately, histamine is only one of a number of mast cell-derived mediators in allergy (see Chapters 10 and 11), but there are as yet no clinically useful receptor antagonists for any of the other mediators. Other drugs used in allergy, such as sympathomimetic and anticholinergic drugs and theophylline are indirectly anti-inflammatory, because they favorably modulate the function of target tissues involved in the allergic inflammatory process.

REFERENCES

Allison AC, Byars NE: Adjuvant formulations and their mode of action. *Semin Immunol* 1990;**2**:369.

Chatenoud L, Bach J-F: Monoclonal antibodies to CD3 as immunosuppressants. *Semin Immunol* 1990;**2**:437.

Cournoyer D, Caskey CT: Gene therapy of the immune system. *Annu Rev Immunol* 1993;**11**:297.

Gefter M (editor): T cell epitope-based immunotherapy. *Semin Immunol* 1991;**3**:193–255 (entire issue).

Greenberger PA (editor): Immunotherapy of IgE-mediated disorders. *Immunol Allergy Clin North Am* 1992;**12**:1. [Entire issue.]

Oettgen HF: Human cancer immunology II. *Immunol Allergy Clin North Am* 1991;**11**:1. [Entire issue.]

Schreiber SL, Crabtree GR: The mechanism of action of cyclosporin A and FK506. *Immunol Today* 1992; **13**:136.

Waldmann H: Manipulation of T-cell responses with monoclonal antibodies. *Annu Rev Immunol* 1989; **7**:407.

Waldmann T: Immune receptors: Targets for therapy of lekemia/lymphoma, autoimmune diseases, and for prevention of allograft rejection. *Annu Rev Immunol* 1992;**10**:675.

Wofsky D, Carteron NL: CD4 antibody therapy in systemic lupus erythematosus. *Semin Immunol* 1990; **2**:419.

Immunization

55

Moses Grossman, MD

The goal of immunization in any one individual is the prevention of disease. The goal of immunization of population groups is the eradication of disease. Immunization has accounted for some spectacular advances in health around the world. Childhood immunizations have been accepted as part of routine health care; in the USA, the federal government has financed the purchase of vaccines for the public sector and all states have passed legislation requiring proof of immunization as a condition for school entry. As a result, poliomyelitis, diphtheria, and tetanus have all but disappeared in developed nations; measles, rubella, and pertussis have become rare. Smallpox has been eradicated, and the World Health Organization has made poliomyelitis the next target for eradication.

HISTORICAL OVERVIEW

It has been recognized for centuries that individuals who recover from certain diseases are protected from recurrences. The moderately successful but hazardous introduction of small quantities of fluid from the pustules of smallpox into the skin of uninfected persons (variolation) was an effort to imitate this natural phenomenon. Jenner's introduction of vaccination with cowpox virus (1796) to protect against smallpox was the first documented use of a live, attenuated viral vaccine and the beginning of modern immunization. Koch demonstrated the specific bacterial cause of anthrax in 1876, and the causes of several common illnesses were rapidly identified thereafter. Attempts to develop immunizing agents followed (Table 55–1).

TYPES OF IMMUNIZATION

Immunization may be **active,** in which administration of an antigen (usually a modified infectious agent or toxin) results in active production of immunity, or **passive,** in which administration of antibody-containing serum or sensitized cells provides passive protection for the recipient.

ACTIVE IMMUNIZATION

Active immunization results in the production of antibodies directed against the infecting agent or its toxic products; it may also initiate cellular responses mediated by lymphocytes and macrophages. The most important protective antibodies include those that inactivate soluble toxic protein products of bacteria (antitoxins), facilitate phagocytosis and intracellular digestion of bacteria (opsonins), interact with the components of serum complement to damage the bacterial membrane and hence cause bacteriolysis (lysins), or prevent the proliferation of infectious virus (neutralizing antibodies). Newly appreciated are the antibodies that interact with components of the bacterial surface to prevent adhesion to mucosal surfaces (antiadhesins). Some antibodies may not be protective and, by "blocking" the reaction of protective antibodies with the pathogen, may actually depress the body's defenses.

Antigens react with antibodies in the bloodstream and extracellular fluid and at mucosal surfaces. Antibodies cannot readily reach intracellular sites of infection, where viral replication occurs. However, they are effective against many viral diseases in 2 ways: (1) by interacting with the virus before initial intracellular penetration occurs and (2) by preventing locally replicating virus from disseminating from the

Table 55–1. Historical milestones in immunization.

Variolation	1721
Vaccination	1795
Rabies vaccine	1885
Diphtheria toxoid	1925
Tetanus toxoid	1925
Pertussis vaccine	1925
Viral culture in chick embryo	1931
Yellow fever vaccine	1937
Influenza vaccine	1943
Viral tissue culture	1949
Poliovaccine, inactivated (Salk)	1954
Poliovaccine, live, attenuated (Sabin)	1956
Measles vaccine	1960
Tetanus immune globulin (human)	1962
Rubella vaccine	1966
Mumps vaccine	1967
Hepatitis B vaccine	1975
Smallpox eradicated	1980
First recombinant vaccine (hepatitis B)	1986
Conjugate polysaccharide vaccine for *H influenzae* B	1988

site of entry to an important target organ, as in the spread of poliovirus from the gastrointestinal tract to the central nervous system or of rabies virus from a puncture wound to peripheral neural tissue. Lymphocytes acting alone and antibody interacting with lymphoid or monocytic effector K cells may also recognize surface changes in virus-infected cells and destroy these infected "foreign" cells.

Types of Vaccines

The agent used for active immunization is loosely termed "antigen" or "vaccine." It may consist of live, attenuated viruses (measles virus) or bacteria (bacillus Calmette-Guérin [BCG]) or killed microorganisms *(Vibrio cholerae)*. It may also be an inactivated bacterial product (tetanus toxoid) or a specific single component of bacteria (polysaccharide of *Neisseria meningitidis*). Such a polysaccharide component may be conjugated to a protein in order to produce immunogenicity at an earlier age (conjugated *Haemophilus influenzae*). It may be a recombinant DNA segment (hepatitis B virus), in which case it would be expressed in another living cell (yeasts, *Escherichia coli*). In each case, it usually contains—in addition to the desired antigen—other ingredients including other antigens, suspending fluids that may be complex and may contain protein ingredients of their own (tissue culture, egg yolk), preservatives, and adjuvants for enhanced immunogenicity (aluminum, protein conjugate). Undesirable reactions may occur not only to the antigen itself but also to these added components.

Active immunization with living organisms is generally superior to immunization with killed vaccines in inducing a long-lived immune response. A single dose of a live, attenuated virus vaccine often suffices for reliable immunization. Multiple immunizations are recommended for poliovirus in case intercurrent enteroviral infection or interference among 3 simulta-

neously administered virus types in the trivalent vaccine prevents completely successful primary immunization. The persistence of immunity to many viral infections may be explained by repeated natural reexposure to new cases in the community, the unusually large antigenic stimulus provided by infection with a living agent, or other mechanisms such as the persistence of latent virus.

All immunizing materials—live organisms in particular—must be properly stored to retain effectiveness. Serious failures of smallpox and measles immunization have resulted from inadequate refrigeration prior to use. Agents presently licensed for active immunization are listed in Table 55–2.

Factors in Immunization

Primary active immunization develops more slowly than the incubation period of most infections and must therefore be induced prior to exposure to the etiologic agent. By contrast, "booster" reimmunization in a previously immune individual provides a rapid secondary (anamnestic) increase in immunity.

Previous infection can also substantially alter the response to an inactivated vaccine. For example, volunteers who have recovered from cholera or who live in a cholera-endemic area respond to parenteral immunization with an increase in anticholera secretory IgA, which is not seen in immunized control subjects.

The route of immunization may be an important determinant of successful vaccination, particularly if nonreplicating immunogens are used. Thus, immunization intranasally or by aerosol, which stimulates mucosal immunity, often appears to be more successful than parenteral injection against viral or bacterial respiratory challenges.

The route of administration recommended by the manufacturer and approved by the FDA should be used. Vaccines containing adjuvants such as aluminum hydroxide should always be given deep into the muscle and not subcutaneously. The ideal intramuscular injection site is the anterolateral portion of the upper thigh.

The timing of primary immunization, the interval between doses, and the timing of booster injections are based on both theoretic considerations and vaccine trials. The resulting recommendations should be followed closely. Many factors are involved. For instance, the age at which measles immunization is administered in the USA was changed from 12 to 15 months because the persistent maternal antibody, although present in small amounts only, was shown to interfere with active antibody formation by the child. Ironically, now that most mothers have induced immunity rather than naturally acquired measles antibody, their lower antibody titer may require that childhood immunization be changed back to 12 months of age.

Because of the clonal nature of immunity, it is possible—and, in fact, routine practice—to give many

Table 55–2. Materials available for active immunization.[1]

Disease	Product (Source)	Type of Agent	Route of Administration	Primary Immunization	Duration of Effect	Comments
Cholera	Cholera vaccine	Killed bacteria	SC, IM, ID	2 doses 1 week or more apart.	6 months[2]	50% protective; International Certificate may be required for travel.
Diphtheria	DTP, DT (adsorbed for child under age 7; Td (adsorbed) for all others.	Toxoid	IM	3 doses 4 weeks or more apart, with an additional dose 1 year later for a child under age 7. (Can be given at same time as polio vaccine if doses at least 8 weeks apart.) A fifth dose before entering school is recommended if the fourth dose was given before the fourth birthday.	10 years[3]	Regular booster injections are recommended every 10 years. After the seventh birthday use the adult-type tetanus-diphtheria toxoid (Td). This product has a lower antigenic content and is less likely to produce reactions in older individuals.
Hameophilus influenzae influenza	Polysaccharide capsule conjugated with protein	Polysaccharide protein conjugate	IM	2 or 3 doses and a booster depending on type of vaccine used.	1 1/2–3 1/2 years	As of 1992, 3 vaccines are available, conjugated to different proteins. Immunization to be started at 2 mo of age. The vaccine can be given at the same time as DPT. A combined product is expected to be available in the future.
Hepatitis B	Hepatitis B vaccine (human carriers). (Recombin·nt DNA, produced in yeast cells. Human carrier-derived vaccine is no longer being manufactured in the USA but is still available commercially.)	Recombinant antigen or formalin-treated purified antigen	IM	2 doses 1 month apart, followed by a booster given 6 months later. *Do not freeze vaccine;* this causes aggregation and loss of potency. The simultaneous administration of hepatitis B immune globulin (HBIG) in a separate syringe at a separate site does not appear to impair the effectiveness of the vaccine.	Variable, about 5 years	A stable, adjuvant-supplemented vaccine from highly purified formalin-activated HBsAg harvested from human carriers or recombinant antigen expressed in yeast cells. Recommended for all individuals at high risk of exposure to HBV infection, including health care personnel such as surgeons, anesthesiologists, autopsy staff, phlebotomists, operating room and dialysis nurses, medical technologists, dentists, and other staff exposed to patients with a high rate of HBV carriage; for patients undergoing chronic hemodialysis or repeatedly receiving plasma or clotting factor concentrates for clotting disorders; in the first week of life for newborn children of carrier mothers; for sexual and household contacts of HBV carriers (families accepting children from countries with high endemic rates of HBV infection should have the child screened and should be vaccinated if the child is HBsAg-positive); for male homosexuals, intravenous drug abusers, and prison populations with problems of homosexuality and drug use; for clients and staff of institutions for the mentally retarded, and classroom contacts of aggressively behaving deinstitutionalized mentally retarded HBV carriers; for heterosexually active persons with multi-

(continued)

Table 55–2. Materials available for active immunization[1] (continued).

Disease	Product (Source)	Type of Agent	Route of Administration	Primary Immunization	Duration of Effect	Comments
Hepatitis B (cont'd.)						ple partners; for travelers to areas endemic for more than 6 months (begin series at least 6 months prior to departure), especially if sexual contacts are anticipated in these areas; and for morticians. Anti-HBs titers in individuals repeatedly exposed to the risk of HBV infection should be checked at intervals of 2–3 years as well as at the time of definite exposure to blood or saliva suspected of being HBsAg-positive, if not measured within the previous year. A single booster dose should be given if a nonprotective level of anti-HBs is found. There is no evidence that the vaccine can transmit acquired immunodeficiency syndrome (AIDS). Very recently this vaccine has been recommended for the routine immunization of all children starting at birth.
Influenza	Influenza virus vaccine. Monovalent or bivalent (chick embryo). Composition of the vaccine is varied depending upon epidemiologic circumstances.	Killed whole or split virus types A and B	IM	1 dose. (Two doses 4 weeks or more apart are recommended in individuals who have not previously received the current antigenic components or been otherwise exposed to the current strain of virus. Two doses of the split virus products should be used in persons 12 years or age or under because of fewer side effects.)	1 year	Give immunization by November. Recommended annually for individuals with chronic cardiovascular or pulmonary disease, for residents of nursing homes and other chronic care facilities, for medical personnel who may spread infection to high-risk patients, and for healthy individuals over 65 years of age, as well as for patients with chronic metabolic disorders, renal dysfunction, anemia, immunosuppression, or asthma. Patients receiving chemotherapy for malignant disease are likely to respond better if immunized between courses of treatment.
Measles[4]	Measles virus vaccine, live (chick embryo)	Live virus	SC	2 doses, one at 15 months, the other at 6–12 years of age.	Permanent	Usually given as MMR (with mumps and rubella). Two doses are required as proof of immunity for school or college entry and for health care workers. May prevent natural disease if given less than 48 hours after exposure.
Meningococcus	Meningococcal polysaccharide vaccine (combination vaccine against groups A, C, Y, and W135).	Polysaccharide	SC	1 dose. Since primary antibody response requires at least 5 days, antibiotic prophylaxis with rifampin (600 mg or 10 mg/kg every 12 h for 4 doses) should be given to household contacts.	?Permanent in older children and adults; transient in children < 2 years.	Recommended in epidemic situations, for use by the military to prevent outbreaks in recruits, for patients with anatomic or functional asplenia, for individuals with a congenital deficiency of terminal components of the complement cascade, and possibly as an adjunct to antibiotic prophylaxis in preventing secondary cases in family contacts. Not reliably effective in infants, who re-

Meningococcus (cont'd.)						quire booster injections if antibody is to last for a year (especially antibody to group C). Revaccination may be indicated for individuals at high risk of infection, particularly if first immunized before age 4. The need to reimmunize adults and older children is unknown.
Mumps[4]	Mumps virus vaccine, live (chick embryo)	Live virus	SC	2 doses	Permanent	Usually given as MMR (with measles and rubella).
Pertussis	DTP.	Killed bacteria. Also an "acellular" vaccine containing 2 or more antigens but not the whole cell.	IM	As for DTP.	Up to 5 years[3]	Not generally recommended after the seventh birthday. Contraindications to beginning or continuing pertussis immunization include a history of seizures or the development of seizures before the 4-dose primary series is completed. Immunization of these children should be deferred until it can be determined whether an evolving neurologic illness is present. For infants who have received fewer than 3 doses of DTP, the decision to pursue immunization should be made before 1 year of age; children with seizures have a higher risk of adverse outcome from pertussis itself and are at increased risk of exposure as they grow older and contact other children. If the neurologic condition is stable and seizures are well controlled, the benefits of immunization outweigh the hazards, although the parents should be warned of an 8-fold increased risk of postimmunization convulsions if febrile convulsions have occurred previously. Definitive contraindications to further administration of DTP include hypersensitivity to the vaccine, an evolving neurologic disorder, or history of a severe reaction. The latter usually occurs within 48 hours of vaccination and is characterized by collapse in a shocklike state, persistent uncontrolled screaming for 3 hours or more, a temperature of 40.5 °C (105 °F) or higher, convulsions or a severely altered state of consciousness, general or local neurologic signs, or a systemic allergic reaction. An acellular pertussis vaccine producing fewer local reactions, in use in Japan for 10 years, has now been licensed in the USA but only for children over 15 months of age.
Plague	Plague vaccine.	Killed bacteria	IM	3 doses 4 weeks or more apart.	6 months[3]	Recommended only for occupational exposure and not for residents of endemic area in the southwest USA.

(continued)

Table 55–2. Materials available for active immunization[1] (continued).

Disease	Product (Source)	Type of Agent	Route of Administration	Primary Immunization	Duration of Effect	Comments
Pneumococcus	Pneumococcal polysaccharide vaccine, polyvalent.	Polysaccharide	SC, IM	0.5 mL, if possible before splenectomy or before instituting chemotherapy.	Uncertain—probably at least 5 years in adults, but erratic in children under age 5	Recommended for patients with cardiorespiratory disease or other chronic illness, for patients with sickle cell disease, for patients with functional, congenital, or postsurgical asplenia, and for patients with nephrotic syndrome or with cerebrospinal fluid leakage. Also suggested for immunosuppressed or alcoholic patients and for patients aged 65 or older. Only the 23 most common serotypes are incorporated in the vaccine. Children up to age 2, splenectomized children, and some chronically ill patients respond unreliably. *Caution:* Because of a marked increase in adverse reactions following revaccination, booster doses should generally *not* be given, even to recipients of the earlier less comprehensive and less immunogenic vaccine. However, a booster is warranted after 3–5 years for high-risk children and is recommended after 3–4 months off chemotherapy for children first immunized while receiving it. Can be given at the same time as influenza or DTP vaccines.
Poliomyelitis	Poliovirus vaccine, live, oral, trivalent (monkey kidney, human diploid).	Live virus types I, II, III	Oral	2 doses 6–8 weeks or more apart, followed by a third dose 8–12 months later. (Can be given at the same time as primary DTP immunization.) A fourth dose before entering school is recommended if the third dose was given before age 4.	Permanent	Recommended for adults only if at increased risk by travel to epidemic or highly endemic areas or occupational contact. Individuals who have completed a primary series may take a single booster dose if the risk of exposure is high.
	Poliomyelitis vaccine, inactivated.	Killed virus types I, II, III	IM	3 doses 4–8 weeks apart, followed by a fourth dose 6–12 months later. A fifth dose before entering school is recommended if the fourth dose was given before age 4. A single booster dose should be given every 5 years until age 18, after which the need is uncertain.	5 years[3]	Killed virus vaccines are preferred for immunologically deficient patients and their household contacts. Adults who have not previously received oral polio vaccine and who are at risk because of travel or, minimally, from immunization of their children should receive the inactivated vaccine. A new "enhanced" inactivated vaccine contains more antigenic material and is more immunogenic.

Rabies	Rabies vaccine (human diploid).	Killed virus	IM or preexposure only) ID	2 years[3] if titer < 1:16	Preexposure immunization only for occupational or avocational risk or residence in hyperendemic area.
			Preexposure: 2 doses 1 week apart, followed by a third dose 2–3 weeks later.		For animal bite, consider antitetanus and other antibacterial measures as well. *Caution:* Several reports document unexpectedly poor response to intradermal immunization. If the intradermal route is used, rabies antibody must be measured 2–3 weeks after the third dose of vaccine. If the antibody titer is < 1:16, an additional dose should be given and the antibody level retested 2–3 weeks later. If the antibody response of an individual who has received intradermal vaccine within the past 12 months is unknown, the level should be checked; if more than 12 months have elapsed, a booster should given and the titer tested 2–3 weeks later. If a rabies exposure takes place following preexposure immunization by the intradermal route and there is no documentation of an adequate antibody level, a full course of HRIG and IM rabies vaccine should be given. Serologic testing does not appear to be necessary if preexposure prophylaxis was given by the IM route.
			Postexposure: Always give rabies immune globulin as well. If not previously immunized, give a total of 5 doses, on days 0, 3, 7, 14, and 28 (WHO recommends a sixth dose 90 days after the first dose). If the vaccinee is immunocompromised (or if only DEV is available), a serum specimen should be collected on day 28 or 2–3 weeks after the last dose and tested for rabies antibody[5] If the antibody level is insufficient, a booster should be given and the titer remeasured 2–3 weeks later. *If previously immunized* with diploid vaccine, do not give serum therapy. Give 2 booster doses, one immediately and one 3 days later. *Note:* Unexplained immediate-type (anaplylactic) hypersensitivity reactions have occurred during primary rabies immunization with vaccine from different manufacturers. Immunization of such individuals should be discontinued unless there is actual exposure to rabies virus or inapparent or unavoidable rabies contact is truly likely to occur. In the later situations, the serologic		

(continued)

Table 55–2. Materials available for active immunization[1] (*continued*).

Disease	Product (Source)	Type of Agent	Route of Administration	Primary Immunization	Duration of Effect	Comments
Rabies (cont'd.)				response to rabies should be checked and booster doses omitted if protective titers have already been attained; vaccination should be continued only under careful supervision. Rabies vaccine, Adsorbed (RVA Michigan Department of Public Health), a newly licensed vaccine, can be used for both preexposure and postexposure prophylaxis. There is limited experience with and limited availability of this vaccine, but it appears to have a far decreased incidence of hypersensitivity reactions.		
Rubella[4]	Rubella virus vaccine, live (human diploid).	Live virus	SC	2 doses	Permanent	Give after 15 months of age. Second dose at 6–11 years of age. Usually given as MMR (with measles and mumps) for children. Because a history of rubella is unreliable and because the vaccine is innocuous in immune recipients, unimmunized women of childbearing age should be vaccinated without serologic testing. Vaccination should be avoided during pregnancy on theoretic grounds unless there is a risk of exposure due to an outbreak; however, there is no evidence of vaccine-induced fetal damage in over 200 recipients. Vaccination is contraindicated for those receiving systemic corticosteroids for more than 2 weeks; for leukemic or immunosuppressed patients for at least 3 months after chemotherapy has been discontinued; for recipients of immune globulin treatment other than anti-Rh therapy within the following 2 weeks or prior 3 months; and for individuals with allergy to neomycin but not to eggs or penicillin. If a female is immunized posparturm and has received blood products or Rh immune globulin,

Rubella (cont'd.)						serologic testing should be done 6–8 weeks later to confirm successful immunization. Viremia can occur if antibody has fallen to low levels; the frequency and thus the clinical importance of this phenomenon are unknown.
Smallpox	Smallpox vaccine (calf lymph, chick embryo). Available from CDC[7].	Live vaccinia virus	ID	1 dose.	3 years	Smallpox has been eradicated, and smallpox vaccine is no longer available to civilian populations.
Tetanus	DTP, DT (adsorbed) for children under age 7; Td, T (adsorbed) for all others.	Toxoid	IM	3 doses 4 weeks or more apart.	10 years[3,5]	Recipients aged 7 or above should be given a third dose 6–12 months after second. (See Table 56–4 regarding use of hyperimmune globulin.)
Tuberculosis	BCG vaccine.	Live attenuated Mycobacterium bovis	ID, SC	1 dose.	?Permanent[6]	Recommended in USA only for PPD-negative contacts of ineffectively treated or persistently untreated cases and for other unusually high risk groups.
Typhoid	Typhoid vaccine.	Killed bacteria	SC	2 doses 4 weeks or more apart, or 3 doses 1 week apart (less desirable).	3 years[3]	70% protective. Recommended only for exposure from travel, epidemic, or household carrier and not, for example because of floods.
		Live attenuated bacteria	Oral	4 doses on alternate days	5 years	Oral vaccine has similar effectiveness.
Yellow fever	Yellow fever vaccine (chick embryo).	Live virus	SC	1 dose	10 years[2]	Certificate may be required for travel. Recommended for residence or travel to endemic areas of Africa and South America. Avoid administration to an immunologically incompetent host or an individual on long-term (> 2 weeks) corticosteroid therapy.

[1]Dosages for the specific product, including variations for age, are best obtained from the manufacturer's package insert. Immunizations should be given by the route suggested for the product.

[2]Revaccination interval required by international regulations.

[3]A single dose is a sufficient booster at any time after the effective duration of primary immunization has passed.

[4]Combination vaccines available.

[5]For contaminated or severe wounds, give booster if more than 5 years have elapsed since full immunization or last booster. A single booster any time after primary immunization is effective.

[6]Test for PPD conversion 2 months later, and reimmunize if there is no conversion.

[7]Drug Immunologic and Vaccine Service, Center for Infectious Diseases, Telephone: (404) 329–3311 (main switchboard, day) or (404) 329–3644 (nights and weekends).

different antigens simultaneously. Some antigens are premixed (measles, mumps, rubella [MMR] and diphtheria, tetanus, pertussis [DPT], whereas others may be given on the same day at different sites (DTP and *H influenzae*). However, live virus vaccines that are not given on the same day should be given at least 1 month apart.

Splenectomy may markedly impair the primary antibody response to thymus-independent antigens such as bacterial polysaccharides, although many splenectomized patients respond normally to polysaccharide antigens because of priming by natural exposure prior to splenectomy.

Technique of Immunization

When administering vaccines intended for subcutaneous or intramuscular deposition, it is essential to pull back on the syringe before depressing the plunger to make certain that the product will not be injected intravenously, resulting in lessened immunizing effect and increased untoward reactions. It is particularly important to use a sufficiently long needle (usually >1 in) for intramuscular delivery of adjuvant-containing (eg, alum [aluminum phosphate]-adsorbed) vaccines; subcutaneous inoculation of adjuvants may result in tissue necrosis.

Recent studies of injection techniques suggest that the anterolateral thigh or deltoid site is preferable to the buttocks. Even with the usual precautions, use of the latter site occasionally leads to sciatic nerve damage, and in adults most injections meant for intramuscular delivery are instead delivered into fat.

The intradermal route of immunization is under intensive study as a means of obtaining an earlier or greater immune response with the same amount of antigen or of inducing a satisfactory immune response with a smaller quantity of expensive immunogens such as the hepatitis B and rabies vaccines.

Adverse Reactions & the Risk:Benefit Ratio

All vaccines approved and licensed in the USA have been shown to be safe and effective. However, each of them has also been shown to cause adverse reactions. Sometimes these are minimal in occurrence rate and severity, as in tetanus toxoid. Historically, some immunizing agents produced adverse reactions that were so severe they would be unacceptable today; variolation and the original rabies vaccine made from spinal cord material are 2 examples. Smallpox vaccination with vaccinia virus carried a very acceptable risk at a time when smallpox posed an imminent and serious threat. However, as the risk of smallpox declined to the point at which the disease was eradicated, the risk:benefit ratio of the vaccine has increased and is now infinite. At present, the most controversial vaccine in routine use is the whole-cell pertussis vaccine. It is only about 70% effective for protection, causes very frequent minor

reaction, and occasionally results in serious neurologic reactions. However, it is still used because the risk:benefit ratio is acceptably low. Japan, the United Kingdom, and Sweden have experienced a significant rise in the fatality rate from pertussis since the use of the vaccine was discontinued. An acellular pertussis vaccine is expected to replace the whole-cell vaccine in the future.

Unique Hazards of Live Vaccines

Because of their potential for infection of the fetus, live vaccines should *not* be given to a pregnant woman unless there is a high immediate risk (eg, a poliomyelitis epidemic). A pregnant woman traveling in an area where yellow fever is endemic *should* be immunized because the risk of infection exceeds the small theoretic hazard to fetus and mother. If yellow fever vaccination is being performed solely to comply with a legal requirement for international travel, however, the woman should seek a waiver with a letter from her physician. Live vaccines, furthermore, can cause serious or even fatal illness in an immunologically incompetent host. They generally should not be given to patients receiving corticosteroids, alkylating drugs, radiation, or other immunosuppressive agents or to individuals with known or suspected congenital or acquired defects in cell-mediated immunity (eg, severe combined immunodeficiency disease, leukemias, lymphomas, Hodgkin's disease, and acquired immunodeficiency syndrome [AIDS]). Patients with pure hypogammaglobulinemia but no defect in cell-mediated immunity usually tolerate viral infections and vaccines well but have a 10,000-fold excess of paralytic complications over the usual one case per million recipients, in part because of the frequent reversion of attenuated poliovirus strains to virulence in the intestinal tract. Since live poliovirus is shed by recipients, it should not be given to household contacts of these patients either.

Even in immunocompetent hosts, live vaccines may result in mild or, rarely, severe disease.

The early measles vaccines caused high fever and rash in a significant proportion of recipients. Subacute sclerosing panencephalitis, a rare complication of natural infection, has occurred following administration of live, attenuated measles vaccine (see Chapter 38), but the rate of about one case per million is one-tenth to one-fifth the rate following natural measles, and the number of cases of measles encephalitis has fallen 100-fold since the introduction of the vaccine. The mild, recurrent arthralgia or arthritis that can follow rubella immunization may represent the consequences of a secondary rather than a primary infection in an individual who has low levels of antibodies not detected by all assays and who has in vitro evidence of cell-mediated immunity.

Because passage through the human intestinal tract occasionally results in reversion of oral attenuated poliovirus vaccine (particularly type III) to neurovirulence, paralytic illness has occurred in recipients or, rarely, their nonimmune contacts, especially adults. The success of live polio vaccines in preventing widespread natural infection has resulted in the paradox that the vaccine itself now accounts for a large fraction of the few cases of paralytic poliomyelitis seen each year in the USA. Killed (Salk) vaccine also appears to be effective in abolishing polio, and the major advantages of live (Sabin) vaccine, which sustain its use despite the small risk of paralysis (5 cases per million doses in nonimmune recipients), are its ease of administration and more durable immune response.

Live vaccines may contain undetected and undesirable contaminants. Epidemic hepatitis resulted in the past from vaccinia and yellow fever vaccines containing human serum. More recently, millions of people received SV40, a simian papovavirus contained in live or inactivated poliovirus vaccine prepared in monkey kidney tissue culture. Although a virus closely related to SV40 has been isolated from the brains of patients with progressive multifocal leukoencephalopathy, a lethal degenerative disease, there is no known history of polio immunization in these cases. An increased incidence of cancer in children of mothers who received inactivated polio vaccine during pregnancy was suggested in 2 studies but not in a 20-year follow-up of a large number of childhood recipients. SV40 can now be detected and excluded from human viral vaccines, but other undetected viruses might be transmitted by vaccines grown in nonhuman cell lines. Yellow fever vaccine has been reported to be probably contaminated with avian leukosis virus. Bacteriophages and probably bacterial endotoxins have also been shown to contaminate live virus vaccines, although without known hazard thus far.

Live viral vaccines probably do not interfere with tuberculin skin testing, although they depress some measurements of lymphocyte function.

Unlike live vaccines, inactivated vaccines may safely be given to immunocompromised hosts. They may not, however, dependably elicit an adequately protective immune response.

The risk:benefit ratio of live measles vaccine is sufficiently low to recommend its use in patients with human immunodeficiency virus (HIV) infection—even immunocompromised patients.

Other Adverse Effects

Allergic reactions may occur on exposure to egg protein (in measles, mumps, influenza, and yellow fever vaccines) or antibiotics or preservatives (eg, neomycin or mercurials) in viral vaccines. Patients with known IgE-mediated sensitivity to a vaccine component (eg, egg albumin in yellow fever vaccine grown in eggs) should not receive the vaccine unless successfully desensitized (in cases when immunization is essential). Occasionally, the product of a dif-

ferent manufacturer does not contain the offending allergen. Improvements in antigenicity and better purification procedures in vaccine production decrease the amount and number of foreign substances injected and result in fewer side effects.

Reporting Adverse Effects & Legal Liability

Lawsuits arising from adverse reaction to vaccines have led to steep increases in the cost of vaccines in recent years. Because of the high costs of litigation and liability insurance, the threat to development and production of new vaccines prompted the passage of the National Childhood Vaccine Injury Act of 1986. This Act provides for compensation of those injured by adverse reactions and at the same time mandates that certain adverse effects be reported and that physicians use vaccine information pamphlets prepared by the Centers for Disease Control and Prevention (CDC) which provide information on benefits and risks of vaccines. These pamphlets are mandatory when government-purchased vaccine is used and can be obtained by called (800) PIK-VIPS. Physicians and clinics purchasing their own vaccines may prepare their own information pamphlets.

The reportable events are listed in Table 55–3. The information in this table is currently undergoing some modifications, particularly in the area of interval after immunization. Reports are to be made to the Vaccine Adverse Event Reporting System, 1–800–822–7267. Preventable adverse effects can be minimized by reading vaccine labels, storing vaccines carefully, using the correct method of administration at the proper site, and being aware of contraindications, particularly by identifying immunocompromised hosts.

PASSIVE IMMUNIZATION

Immunization may be accomplished passively by administering either performed immunoreactive serum or cells.

Antibody, either as whole serum or as fractionated, concentrated immune (gamma) globulin that is predominantly IgG, may be obtained from human or animal donors who have recovered from an infectious disease or have been immunized. These antibodies may provide immediate protection to an antibody-deficient individual. Passive immunization is thus useful for individuals who cannot form antibodies or for the nonimmunocompromised host who might develop disease before active immunization could stimulate antibody production, which usually requires at least 7–10 days.

Additionally, passive immunization is useful when no active immunization is available, when passive immunization is used in conjunction with vaccine administration (eg, in rabies vaccination), in the man-

Table 55–3. Reportable events following vaccination.[1]

Vaccine/Toxoid	Event	Interval from Vaccination
DTP.P, DTP/Polio combined	Anaphylaxis or anaphylactic shock Encephalopathy (or encephalitis)[2] Shock-collapse or hypotonic hyporesponsive collapse[2] Residual seizure disorder[2] Any acute complication or sequela (including death) of above events Events (such as convulsions) described in manufacturer's package insert as contraindications to additional doses of vaccine[3]	Immediate 7 days 7 days Variable[2] No limit See package insert
Measles, mumps, and rubella; Td, tetanus toxoid	Anaphylaxis or anaphylatic shock. Encephalopathy (or encephalitis)[2] Residual seizure disorder[2] Any acute complication or sequela (including death) of above events. Events described in manufacturer's package insert as contraindications to additional doses of vaccine[3]	Immediate 15 days for measles, mumps, and rubella vaccines; 7 days for DT, Td, and T toxoids Variable[2] No limit See package insert
Oral polio vaccine	Paralytic poliomyelitis in a nonimmunodeficient recipient in an immunodeficient recipient in a vaccine-associated community case Any acute complication or sequela (including death) of above events Events described in manufacturer's package insert as contraindications to additional doses of vaccine[3]	 30 days 6 months No limit No limit See package insert
Inactivated polio vaccine	Anaphylaxis or anaphylactic shock Any acute complication or sequela (including death) of above event Events described in manufacturer's package insert as contraindications to additional doses of vaccine[3]	Immediate No limit See package insert

[1]The schedule of reportable events is currently undergoing some revisions, and changes are expected in the near future.
[2]Aids to interpretation: Shock-collapse or hypotonic-hyporesponsive collapse may be evidenced by signs or symptoms such as decrease in or loss of muscle tone, paralysis (partial or complete), hemiplegia, hemiparesis, loss of color or turning pale, white, or blue, unresponsiveness to environmental stimuli, depression of or loss of consciousness, prolonged sleeping with difficulty arousing, or cardiovascular or respiratory arrest. Residual seizure disorder may be considered to have occurred if no other seizure or convulsion unaccompanied by fever or accompanied by a fever of less than 102°F occurred before the first seizure or convulsion after the administration of the vaccine involved. AND, if in the case of measles, mumps, or rubella-containing vaccines, the first seizure or convulsion occurred within 15 days after vaccination OR in the case of any other vaccine, the first seizure or convulsion occurred within 3 days after vaccination. AND, if 2 or more seizures or convulsions unaccompanied by fever or accompanied by a fever of less than 102°F occurred within 1 year after vaccination. The terms "seizure" and "convulsion" include grand mal, petit mal, absence, myoclonic, tonic-clonic, and focal motor seizures and signs. "Encephalopathy" means any significant acquired abnormality of, injury to, or impairment of function of the brain. Among the frequent manifestations of encephalopathy are focal and diffuse neurologic signs, increased intracranial pressure, or changes lasting at least 6 hours in the level of consciousness, with or without convulsions. The neurologic signs and symptoms of encephalopathy may be temporary with complete recovery, or they may result in various degrees of permanent impairment. Signs and symptoms such as high-pitched and unusual screaming, persistent unconsolable crying, and bulging fontanel are compatible with an encephalopathy but, in and of themselves, are not conclusive evidence of encephalopathy. Encephalopathy usually can be documented by slow wave activity on an electroencephalogram.
[3]The health care provider must refer to the Contraindication section of the manufacturer's package insert for each vaccine.

agement of specific effects of certain toxins and venoms, and, finally, as an immunosuppressant.

Antibody may be obtained from humans or animals, but animal sera give rise to an immune response that leads to rapid clearance of the protective molecules from the circulation of the recipient and the risk of allergic reactions, particularly serum sickness or anaphylaxis (see below). Thus, to obtain a similar protective effect, much more animal antiserum must be injected compared with human antiserum (eg, 3000 units of equine tetanus antitoxin versus 300 units of human tetanus immune globulin).

Human Immune Globulin

This preparation is derived from alcohol fractionation of pooled plasma. The antibody content of immune globulin is almost all of the IgG isotype and reflects the infection and immunization experience of the donor pool. Three types of preparations are available: standard immune gamma globulin for intramuscular use (IGIM), standard immune globulin adapted for intravenous use (IGIV), and special immune globulins with a known high content of antibody against a particular antigen; the last may be available for intravenous or intramuscular use.

Immune globulin should be given only when its efficacy has been established. Although its side effects are minimal, the administration is painful and rare anaphylactoid reactions have been described. It is not useful for the immunologically normal child or adult with frequent viral infections. There is no evidence that HIV infections can be transmitted by the administration of immune globulin. *Caution:* The intramuscular form should *never* be given intravenously; very serious systemic reactions may result from the presence of high-molecular-weight aggregated immunoglobulins.

IGIV is derived from the same pool of adult donors and also consists almost solely of IgG antibodies. The immune globulin has been adapted to intravenous use by eliminating high-molecular-weight complexes that may activate complement in the recipient. The advantages of the intravenous route are the ability to administer large doses of immune globulin, the more rapid onset of action, and the avoidance of intramuscular injections, which are painful and may be contraindicated because of a tendency to bleed. IGIV is particularly valuable as replacement therapy for antibody deficiency disorders and for the management of idiopathic thrombocytopenic purpura. The cost, however, is approximately 5 times the cost of IGIM. Approximately 2.5% of patients receiving IGIV will experience side effects of fever or vasoactive phenomena (usually vasodilatation), but these reactions can usually be prevented by slow administration of the material.

Special Preparations of Human Immune Globulin

Many preparations with a high titer of a specific antibody are available. These are prepared either by hyperimmunizing adult donors or by selecting lots of plasma tested for a high specific antibody content. Most of these are available in the intramuscular form; a few are currently being made available for intravenous use (Table 55–4).

Animal Sera & Antitoxins

These preparations are used only when human globulin is not available, because they carry a much higher risk of anaphylactic reactions. They are usually prepared from hyperimmunized horses or rabbits.

No antiserum of animal origin should be given without carefully inquiring about prior exposure or allergic response to any product of the specific animal source. Whenever a foreign antiserum is admin-

istered, a syringe containing aqueous epinephrine, 1:1000, should be available. If allergy is suspected by history or shown by skin testing and no alternative to serum therapy is possible, desensitization may be attempted as outlined in Chapter 56.

The various materials available for passive immunization, of both human and animal origin, are detailed in Table 55–4.

Passive Immunization in Noninfectious Diseases

A. Prevention of Rh Isoimmunization: Rh-negative women are at hazard of developing anti-Rh antibodies when Rh-positive erythrocytes enter their circulation. This occurs regularly during pregnancy with an Rh-positive fetus, whether the pregnancy ends in a term or preterm delivery or in abortion. It may also occur with other events listed below. The development of anti-Rh antibodies threatens all subsequent Rh-positive fetuses with erythroblastosis. This can be prevented by administration of Rh immune globulin to the mother.

Rh-negative females who have not already developed anti-Rh antibodies should receive 300 μg of Rh immune globulin within 72 hours after obstetric delivery, abortion, accidental transfusion with Rh-positive blood, chorionic villus biopsy, and, probably, amniocentesis, especially if the needle passes through the placenta. This passive immunization suppresses the mother's normal immune response to any Rh-positive fetal cells that may enter her circulation, thus avoiding erythroblastosis fetalis in future Rh-positive fetuses; it may protect in a nonspecific manner as well, analogous to the "blocking" effect of high-dose IgG in ameliorating autoimmune diseases such as idiopathic thrombocytopenic purpura. Even if more than 72 hours has elapsed after the exposures listed above, Rh immune globulin should be administered, since it will be effective in at least some cases. Three of 6 subjects were protected from the immunogenic effect of 1 mL of intravenous Rh-positive erythrocytes by 100 μg of anti-Rh globulin given 13 days later. Some workers have also suggested the administration of anti-Rh globulin to Rh-negative newborn female offspring of Rh-positive mothers to prevent possible sensitization from maternal-fetal transfusion.

A significant number of Rh isoimmunizations occur during pregnancy rather than at the time of delivery. This can be almost completely prevented by administration of anti-Rh globulin at 28 weeks of gestation. The American College of Obstetricians and Gynecologists recommends routine administration of 300 μg of Rh immune globulin at 28 weeks of gestation and again at delivery as soon as it is determined that the infant is Rh-positive. Prior to 28 weeks of gestation, any condition associated with fetomaternal hemorrhage (abortion, amniocentesis, ruptured ectopic pregnancy) should be treated with

Table 55–4. Materials available for passive immunization. (All are of human origin unless otherwise stated.)

Disease	Product	Dosage	Comments
Black widow spider bite	Antivenin widow spider, equine.	1 vial IM or IV.	A second dose may be given if symptoms do not subside in 3 hours.
Botulism	ABE polyvalent antitoxin, equine.	1 vial IV and 1 vial IM; repeat after 2–4 hours if symptoms worsen, and after 12–24 hours.	Available from CDC.[1] A 20% incidence of serum reactions. Only type E antitoxin has been shown to affect outcome of illness. Prophylaxis is not routinely recommended but may be given to asymptomatic exposed persons.
Cytomegalovirus	CMV immune globulin		CMV immune globulin may be used intravenously for prophylaxis or for treatment (with an antiviral agent) of CMV infections in the immunocompromised host.
Diphtheria	Diphtheria antitoxin, equine.	20,000–120,000 units IM depending on severity and duration of illness.	Active immunization and perhaps erythromycin prophylaxis, rather than antitoxin prophylaxis, should be given to nonimmune contacts of active cases. Contacts should be observed for signs of illness so that antitoxin may be administered if needed.
Hepatitis A	Immune globulin.	0.02 mL/μg IM as soon as possible after exposure up to 2 weeks. A protective effect lasts about 2 months.	Modifies but does not prevent infection. Recommended for sexual and household contacts of infected persons including diapered children and their staff contacts in a child care center if one case occurs among them or if cases are recognized in the households with more than 2 children. (If cases occur in more than 3 homes, consider prophylaxis for all households with diapered children attending the center.) In centers without diapered children, prophylaxis is recommended only for classroom contacts of an index case. Prophylaxis is also suggested for coworkers of an infected food handler (but not generally for patrons) and for persons exposed to a common source *if* cases have not yet begun to occur. Prophylaxis is not recommended for personal contacts at offices, schools, hospitals, or institutions for custodial care *except* in an outbreak centered in these areas.
		For continuous risk of exposure, a dose of 0.05 mL/kg is recommended every 5 months.	Personnel of mental institutions, facilities for retarded children, and prisons appear to be at chronic risk of acquiring hepatitis A, as are those who work with nonhuman primates. Also recommended for travelers who will remain in endemic areas for more than 2 months.
Hepatitis B	Hepatitis B immune globulin (HBIG).	0.06 mL/kg IM up to a maximum of 5 mL as soon as possible after exposure, preferably within 24 hours, but up to 14 days for sexual exposure. HBV vaccination begun within 7 days of exposure is recommended in preference to a second HBIG injection 25–30 days after the first.	Administer to nonimmune individuals as postexposure prophylaxis following sexual contact with HBsAg-positive individuals (one dose of HBIG appears to be as effective as 2 doses for sexual exposure). For percutaneous or mucosal exposure to known HBsAg-positive or high-risk material, prophylactic strategy depends upon testing the source and upon the vaccination history of the exposed person (see Table 55–2). Of no value for persons

(continued)

Table 55–4. Materials available for passive immunization. (All are of human origin unless otherwise stated.) (*continued*)

Disease	Product	Dosage	Comments
Hepatitis B (cont'd)			already demonstrating anti-HBsAg antibody. Administration of various live virus vaccines should be delayed for at least 2 months after this concentrated immune globulin has been given. Pregnant women should be screened before delivery or as soon as possible thereafter, and newborn infants of all carriers should be given HBIG, 0.5 mL, within 12 hours of birth. Immunization with HBV vaccine should be started within the first week of life (see Table 55–2). High-risk mothers include women of Asian, Pacific island, or Alaskan Eskimo descent, whether immigrant or US-born; women born in Haiti or sub-Saharan Africa; and women with a history of acute or chronic liver disease work or treatment in a hemodialysis unit, work or residence in an institution for the mentally retarded, repeated blood transfusion, frequent occupational exposure to blood in a medicodental setting, rejection as a blood donor, household exposure to an HBV carrier or a hemodialysis patient, multiple episode of sexually transmitted disease, or percutaneous use of illicit drugs. HBIG has no effect upon non-A, non-B hepatitis.
Hypogamma-globulinemia	Immune globulin.	0.6 mL/kg IM every 3–4 weeks.	Give double dose at onset of therapy. Immune globulin is of no value in the prevention of frequent respiratory infections in the absence of demonstrable hypogammaglobulinemia.
	Immune globulin IV.	100–150 mg/kg IV about once a month, depending on maintenance of serum IgG levels.	Ordinary immune globulin cannot safely be given intravenously because of complement-activating aggregates. It is difficult to administer sufficient IM globulin to maintain normal IgG levels in immunodeficient children or to passively protect acutely infected individuals who lack a specific antibody. This material contains a very small amount of IgA and can cause an allergic reaction in a sensitive IgA-deficient recipient. The IgE in some preparations may cause some reactions; although one product causes symptoms, particularly if confirmed by skin testing, another preparation may not.
Measles	Immune globulin.	0.25 mL/kg IM as soon as possible after exposure. This dose may be ineffective in immunoincompetent patients, who should receive 20–30 mL.	Live measles vaccine will usually prevent natural infection if given within 48 hours following exposure. If immune globulin is administered, delay immunization with live virus for 3 months. Do not vaccinate infants under age 15 months.
Rabies	Rabies immune globulin.[2]	20 IU/kg, 50% of which is infiltrated locally at the wound site if anatomically feasible, and the remainder given IM. (See also rabies vaccine in Table 55–2.) If the equine produce is used, the dose is 40 IU/kg.	Give as soon as possible after exposure. Recommended for all bite or scratch exposures to carnivores, especially bat, skunk, fox, coyote, or raccoon, despite animal's apparent health, if the brain cannot be immedi-

(*continued*)

Table 55–4. Materials available for passive immunization. (All are of human origin unless otherwise stated.) (*continued*)

Disease	Product	Dosage	Comments
Rabies (cont'd.)			ately examined and found rabies-free. Give also even for abrasion exposure to known or suspected rabid animals as well as for bite (skin penetration by teeth) of escaped dogs and cats whose health cannot be determined. Not recommended for individuals with demonstrated antibody response from preexposure prophylaxis.
Rh isoimmuniza-tion (erythro-blastosis fetalis)	Rh_o (D) immune globulin.	1 dose IM within 12 hours of abortion, amniocentesis or chorionic villus bi-opsy, obstetric delivery of an Rh-posi-tive infant, or transfusion of Rh-positive blood in an Rh_o (D)–nega-tive female.	For nonimmune females only. May be effective at much greater postexpos-ure interval. Give even if more than 72 hours have elapsed. One vial contains 300 µg of antibody and can reliably in-hibit the immune response to a fetomaternal bleed of 7.5–8 mL as es-timated by the Betke-Kleihauer smear technique. Some groups also recom-mend administration of 100 µg of anti-body at 28 and 34 weeks of pregnancy to prevent prepartum isoimmunization. Transient seroposi-tivity for anti-HAV and anti-HBV anti-bodies may follow the administration of large doses.
Snakebite	Antivenin coral snake, equine. Antivenin rattle-snake, copperhead, and moccasin, equine.	At least 3–5 vials IV.	Dose should be sufficient to reverse symptoms of envenomation. Consider antitetanus measures as well.
Tetanus	Tetanus immune globulin.[3]	Prophylaxis: 250–500 units IM. Ther-apy: 3000–5000 units IM.	Give in separate syringe at separate site from simultaneously administered toxoid. Recommended only for major contaminated wounds in individuals who have had fewer than 2 doses of toxoid at any time in the past (fewer than 3 doses if wound is more than 24 hours old). (See tetanus toxoid in Table 55–2.) There is some evidence that 250 units given intrathecally to mildly affected patients prevents pro-gression to severe disease and death, but intrathecal therapy is not effective in severe cases with generalized re-peated spasms.
Vaccinia	Vaccinia immune globulin. (Available from CDC.[1])	Prophylaxis: 0.3 mL/kg IM. Therapy: 0.6 mL/kg IM. VIG may be repeated as necessary for treatment and at in-tervals of 1 week for prophylaxis.	Give at a different site if used to pre-vent dissemination in a patient with skin disease who must undergo vacci-nation. May be useful in treatment of vaccinia of the eye, eczema vaccinatum, generalized vaccinia, and vaccinia necrosum and in the preven-tion of such complications in exposed patients with skin disorders such as eczema or impetigo. Also recom-mended to prevent fetal vaccinia when a pregnant woman must be vac-cinated. VIG should rarely be needed, since smallpox vaccination is now lim-ited to military personnel and at-risk laboratory workers.
Varicella	Varicella-zoster immune globulin (VZIG).[4]	1 vial/10 kg or fraction thereof, up to a maximum of 5 vials, given IM within 96 hours of exposure.	It should be administered to nonim-mune leukemic, lymphomatous, or im-munosuppressed children, children receiving prednisone at ≥2 mg/kg/d for any reason, or other immunoincompet-

(*continued*)

Table 55–4. Materials available for passive immunization. (All are of human origin unless otherwise stated.) (*continued*)

Disease	Product	Dosage	Comments
Varicella (cont'd.)			ent children <15 years of age who have had household, hospital (same room containing ≤4 beds or adjacent beds in large ward), or playmate (>1 hour play indoors) contact with a known case of varicella-zoster. Should also be given to exposed bone marrow transplant patients regardless of immune history of donor, to exposed infants born before 28 weeks of gestation, and to neonates whose mothers have developed varicella <5 days before or 48 hours after delivery or who are exposed postnatally and whose mothers have uncertain or negative histories of varicella. VZIG should be considered for adults—especially pregnant women and immunocompromised patients—having close contact with a case of varicella-zoster as defined above for children and whose history suggests susceptibility. A negative history for varicella is extremely unreliable (only about 8% of adults who believe they are nonimmune become infected after household exposure) and should if possible be checked by a serologic test such as the fluorescent-antibody test against membrane antigen, because of the high cost of VZIG (an adult dose costs approximately $400). Protective antibody levels can be attained using immune globulin IV in a dose of 6 mL/kg if VZIG is unavailable.

[1]Available from the Centers for Disease Control and Prevention. Telephone: (404) 329–3311 (main switchboard, day) or (404) 329–3644 (night).
[2]Antirabies serum, equine, may be available but is much less desirable.
[3]Bovine and equine antitoxins may be available but are not recommended. They are used at 10 times the dose of tetanus immune globulin.
[4]Contact the regional blood center of the American Red Cross.
Note: Passive immunotherapy or immunoprophylaxis should always be administered as soon as possible after exposure to the offending agent. Immune antisera and globulin are always given intramuscularly unless otherwise noted. Always question carefully and test for hypersensitivity before administering animal sera.

Rh immune globulin (a 50-µg "minidose" is used before 12 weeks and a standard 300-µg dose is used thereafter). A larger dose is necessary when a significant fetomaternal hemorrhage (more than 25 µg/mL of incompatible cells) has taken place.

B. Serum Therapy of Poisonous Bites: The toxicity of the bite of the black widow spider, the coral snake, and crotalid snakes (rattlesnakes and other pit vipers) may be lessened by the administration of commercially available antivenins. These are of equine origin, so the risk of serum sickness is high and the possibility of anaphylaxis must always be considered.

Antisera for scorpion stings and rarer poisonous bites, especially of species foreign to North America, may also be available.

Information on the use and availability of antivenins is often available from Poison Control Centers, particularly those in cities having large zoos, such as New York and San Diego. A Snakebite Trauma Center has been established at Jacobi Hospital in New York ([212] 430–8183). In addition, an antivenin index listing the availability of all such products is maintained by the Poison Control Center in Tucson, Arizona ([602] 626–6016 or 626–6000).

C. Kawasaki Syndrome: This severe disease, a form of generalized vasculitis, produces coronary artery aneurysms that may result in myocardial infarction in a significant number of cases. There is a large and convincing body of evidence that IGIV given during the acute phase of the disease substantially improves the outcome. The dose and duration that have been successful in clinical trials are 400 mg daily for 5 days given as early as possible during the acute phase. A single 2-g/kg dose of IVIG administered over 10 hours is equally efficacious.

D. Thrombocytopenic Purpura: In this disease, IGIV is given because it presumably prolongs platelet survival by blocking Fc receptors for IgG on macrophages that ingest antibody-coated platelets.

Hazards of Passive Immunization

Illness may arise from a single injection of foreign serum but more commonly occurs in patients who have previously been injected with proteins from the same or a related species. Reactions range in severity from serum sickness arising days to weeks following treatment to acute anaphylaxis with hives, dyspnea, cardiovascular collapse, and even death (see Chapter 26). Typical manifestations of serum sickness include adenopathy, urticaria, arthritis, and fever (see Chapter 27). Demyelinating encephalopathy has been reported.

Rarely, the administration of human immune globulin is attended by similar allergic reactions, particularly in patients with selective IgA deficiency (see Chapter 19). Viral hepatitis may be transmitted by whole human plasma or serum but not by the purified gamma globulin fraction.

The administration of intact lymphocytes to promote cell-mediated immunity is hazardous if the recipient is immunologically depressed. The engrafted donor cells may "reject" the recipient by the graft-versus-host reaction, producing rash, pancytopenia, fever, diarrhea, hepatosplenomegaly, and death (see Chapter 57).

COMBINED PASSIVE-ACTIVE IMMUNIZATION

Passive and active immunization are often undertaken simultaneously to provide both immediate, transient protection and slowly developing, durable protection against rabies or tetanus. The immune response to the active agent may or may not be impaired by the passively administered antibodies if the injections are given at separate sites. Tetanus toxoid plus tetanus immune globulin may give a response superior to that generated by the toxoid alone, but after antiserum has been given for rabies, the course of immunization is usually extended to ensure an adequate response.

Parenterally administered live virus vaccines such as measles or rubella virus should not be given until at least 6 (and preferably 12) weeks after the administration of immune globulin.

CLINICAL INDICATIONS FOR IMMUNIZATION

Immunizing procedures are among the most effective and economical measures available for preservation and protection of health. The decision to immunize a specific person against a specific pathogen is a complex judgment based upon an assessment of the risk of infection, the consequences of natural unmodified illness, the availability of a safe and effective immunogen, and the duration of its effect.

HERD IMMUNITY

The organisms that cause diphtheria and tetanus are ubiquitous, and the vaccines have few side effects and are highly effective, but only the immunized individual is protected. Thus, immunization must be universal. By contrast, a nonimmune individual who resides in a community that has been well immunized against poliovirus and who does not travel has little opportunity to encounter wild (virulent) virus. Here the immunity of the "herd" protects the unimmunized person since the intestinal tracts of recipients of oral polio vaccine fail to become colonized by or transmit wild virus. If, however, a substantial portion of the community is not immune, introduced wild virus can circulate and cause disease among the nonimmune group. Thus, focal outbreaks of poliomyelitis have occurred in religious communities objecting to immunization.

ANTIGENIC SHIFT & ANTIGENIC VARIATION

Each immunologically distinct viral subtype requires a specific antigenic stimulus for effective protection. Immunization against adenovirus infection has not benefitted civilian populations subject to many differing types of adenovirus, in contrast to the demonstrated value of vaccine directed against a few epidemic adenovirus types in military recruits. Similarly, immunity to type A influenza virus is transient because of major mutations in surface chemistry of the virus every few years (antigenic shifts). These changes render previously developed vaccines obsolete and may not permit sufficient production, distribution, and utilization of new antigen in time to prevent epidemic spread of the altered strain. Antigenic variation may also be an important impediment to immunization against HIV infection.

SPECIFIC DISEASES

Pertussis

Several acellular vaccines used in Japan for the past 8 years are saline suspensions of 2 or more antigens: formalin-treated lymphocyte proliferative factor (pertussis toxin) and filamentous hemagglutinin. The degree of protection afforded by acellular vaccine appears to be about the same (70%) as that for the whole-cell product, and minor reactions (fever, pain) are less frequent. Acellular pertussis vaccine (in combination with diphtheria and tetanus toxoids [DT] has now been licensed for children older than 15 months. Licensing for younger children awaits the completion of studies currently in progress.

Poliomyelitis

Two forms of polio vaccine are available. The live, attenuated oral (Sabin) vaccine, used in the USA and many parts of the world, is cheap, effective, and easily administered. Infection causing paralysis occurs in only one per 7 million immunodeficient recipients or members of their households. The killed virus vaccine (Salk) is also effective, particularly in the new "enhanced" form. It requires injection and gives a shorter duration of immunity but is free of the danger of producing paralysis in the recipient or household members. Immunodeficient individuals should receive the killed vaccine. Adults who have never been immunized are protected by herd immunity in developed countries and should therefore be immunized with the killed (Salk) vaccine prior to travel to areas endemic for polio.

Hepatitis B

Vaccine for hepatitis B, both plasma-derived and recombinant, has been available for some 10 years and is used for special populations—health care workers, infants of surface antigen- positive mothers. A new 1992 recommendation is for universal immunization against hepatitis B in infancy.

Rabies

Previously available rabies vaccines did, if only rarely, give rise to severe reactions. The risk of exposure is low, and preexposure immunization is thus reserved for travelers to hyperendemic areas and for persons with occupational or avocational hazard. Human diploid vaccine may change this risk:benefit assessment. Approximately 30,000 courses of antirabies treatment are given annually in the USA, and perhaps only 20% of these are necessary when the recommended treatment guidelines are carefully followed.

Cholera

Cholera immunization offers only temporary and incomplete protection. It is of little use to travelers and should be given only when the risk of exposure is high or in fulfillment of local regulations.

AGE AT IMMUNIZATION

The natural history of a disease determines the age at which immunization is best undertaken. Pertussis, polio, and diphtheria often infect infants; immunization against these diseases is therefore begun shortly after birth. Serious consequences of pertussis are uncommon beyond early childhood, and pertussis vaccination is not usually recommended after 6 years of age. Since the major hazard of rubella is the congenital rubella syndrome, and since nearly half of congenital rubella cases occur with the first pregnancy, it is very important to immunize as many females as possible prior to puberty. In this way the theoretic hazard of vaccinating a pregnant female and endangering the fetus is avoided, although inadvertently immunized fetuses have thus far not been reported to be damaged by their exposure to the attenuated virus.

The efficacy of immunization may also be age-related. Failure may occur because of the presence of interfering antibodies or an undeveloped responsiveness of the immune system. Infants cannot be reliably protected with live measles, mumps, or rubella vaccines until maternally derived antibody has disappeared. Because a proportion of children immunized as late as 1 year of age fail to develop antibody after measles vaccination, the age recommended for measles vaccine administration has been changed to 15 months (see above), and some workers have made the same suggestion for rubella vaccine administration. Most of the children without antibody, however, may actually have been protected, based on the lack of an IgM response to reimmunization and in vitro evidence of cell-mediated immunity. Furthermore, delay in immunization is attended by a decrease in the number of children actually immunized, which approximates the improved rate of seroconversion. Individuals who were vaccinated at an earlier age in accordance with recommendations in effect at that time should be revaccinated. Infants frequently develop severe infections with *H influenzae* type b, pneumococci, or meningococci, but injecting them with purified capsular polysaccharide has failed to reliably yield a good antibody response, despite the excellent activity of the same antigen in older children and adults. This issue has now been addressed by the development of several conjugated *H influenzae* vaccines (polysaccharide conjugated to protein). A similar effort is under way for *N meningitidis* and *Streptococcus pneumoniae* polysaccharide vaccines.

Recommendations for Childhood Immunization

Despite the extraordinary impact of immunization in the developed world, WHO estimates that of every

1000 children born today, 5 are crippled by poliomyelitis, 10 die of neonatal tetanus, 20 die of pertussis, and 30 die of measles and its complications. A rational program of immunization against infectious diseases begins in childhood, when many of the most damaging and preventable infections normally appear. Table 55–5 summarizes the current guidelines for immunization in childhood recommended by the Immunization Practices Advisory Committee (ACIP). The need for childhood immunization has increased because unimmunized individuals in a partially immune population will be less exposed to such childhood diseases as measles and mumps and will therefore develop them later than they otherwise would. When these illnesses do occur in adolescence or adulthood, they are often diagnostically bewildering to the physician unprepared for such illnesses in this age group. Epidemic measles has recently been occurring in college students.

The physician should provide the patient with a clear and up-to-date record of all immunizations, which is useful in future medical encounters and in fulfilling school registration and other institutional requirements. Physicians can improve immunization rates by developing recall systems to identify children who are due for immunizations and by using the occasion of a visit for intercurrent illness to investigate and augment a patient's immune status. It is *not* necessary to restart an interrupted series of vaccinations or to add extra doses. If the vaccine history is unknown and there are no obvious contraindications, the child or adult should be fully immunized appropriately for his or her age. Reimmunization poses no significant risk.

For developing nations in which much preventable serious infection occurs in the first few years of life, WHO recommends an accelerated immunization program: at birth, oral poliovirus and BCG; at ages 6, 10, and 14 weeks, oral poliovirus and DTP; at age 9 months, measles (to be repeated in the second year of life if given before age 9 months).

Immunization of Adults & the Elderly

Childhood immunization programs have significantly decreased the incidence of preventable infections in developed countries. However, optimal immunization of adult populations has not yet been achieved. Much disease preventable by immunization continues to exist. Table 55–6 lists the most important immunizations for the adult and elderly population.

SIMULTANEOUS IMMUNIZATION WITH MULTIPLE ANTIGENS

The simultaneous inoculation of the nonliving antigens of diphtheria, tetanus, and pertussis (DTP) elicits a response equal to that seen with their separate injection. Similarly, the single injection of a mixture of live, attenuated measles, rubella, and mumps viruses elicits good responses to each component of the mixture. However, between 2 and 14 days following the administration of one live virus vaccine, there is a period of suboptimal response to a subsequently injected live virus vaccine. Live vaccines that are not given simultaneously should be given at least 4 weeks apart if time permits. The administration of cholera and yellow fever vaccines within 1–3 weeks

Table 55– 5 Recommended schedule of vaccinations for all children.[1]

Vaccine	At birth[2]	1–2 months	2 months	4 months	6 months	12 months	15 months	6–18 months	4–6 years[3]
DTP			X	X	X		X[4]		X
Polio			X	X			X[4]		X
MMR							X[5]		X[6]
HbCV[7]									
Option 1			X	X	X		X		
Option 2			X	X		X			
HBv									
Option 1	X	X[8]						X[8]	
Option 2		X[8]		X[8]				X[8]	

[1]Polio, live oral polio vaccine drops (OPV) or killed (inactivated) polio vaccine shots (IPV); HbCV, *H influenzae* type b conjugate vaccine; HBv, hepatitis B vaccine.
[2]Before hospital discharge.
[3]Before beginning school.
[4]Many experts recommend these vaccines at 18 months.
[5]In some areas this dose of MMR vaccine may be administered at 12 months.
[6]Many experts recommend this dose of MMR vaccine be administered at entry into middle school or junior high school
[7]HbCV is administered in either a 4-dose schedule (1) or a 3-dose schedule (2), depending on the type of vaccine used.
[8]HBv can be administered at the same time as DTP and/or HbCV.

Table 55–6. Vaccines and toxoids[1] recommended for adults, by age groups, in the USA

Age group (years)	Vaccine/toxoid					
	Td[2]	Measles	Mumps	Rubella	Influenza	Pneumococcal Polysaccharide
18–24	X	X	X	X		
25–64	X	X[3]	X[3]	X		
≥65	X				X	X

[1]Refer also to sections in text on specific vaccines or toxoids for indications, contraindications, precautions, dosages, side effects, adverse reactions, and special considerations.
[2]Td, Tetanus and diphtheria toxoids, adsorbed (for adult use), which is a combined preparation containing <2 flocculation units of diphtheria toxoid.
[3]Indicated for persons born after 1956.

of each other decreases the antibody response to both agents. Therefore, these immunizations also should be given at the same time or at least 4 weeks apart.

The recent addition of conjugated *H influenzae* vaccine and recombinant hepatitis B vaccine to childhood immunizations has created a serious problem with multiple needle sticks necessary at each well-baby visit. Further combinations of vaccines (such as DPT and *H influenzae* or DPT and hepatitis B) are essential, and many of them are in the process of development.

IMMUNIZATION FOR FOREIGN TRAVEL

National health authorities may require an International Certificate of Vaccination against cholera or yellow fever from travelers, usually depending upon the presence of these diseases in countries on their itinerary. Cholera vaccination may be given by any licensed physician; because it is not very effective, it is not generally recommended except when required. The certificate must be completed in all details and then validated with an officially approved stamp. Yellow fever vaccination may be administered and the certificate validated only at an officially designated center, which may be located by contacting the state or local health department. In addition to these legal requirements, all adults are advised to be adequately immunized against measles, tetanus, and diphtheria and to undergo additional immunizations (against poliomyelitis, typhoid, hepatitis A, and meningococcal meningitis) if they are visiting areas where the frequency of illness in the population or the level of sanitation increases the risk of infection. Travelers should be immunized against plague if contact with wild rodents or rabbits in an endemic rural area is anticipated and to hepatitis B if sexual contacts are anticipated in Southeast Asia or sub-Saharan Africa. A formalin-inactivated vaccine against Japanese B encephalitis, not licensed in the USA, is available in several Asian countries where the infection is endemic; long-term travelers to areas with a significant risk of infection (China, India, Japan, Korea, Nepal, and Thailand) should ask at their embassies how vaccine may be obtained.

Travelers to malaria-endemic areas should be specifically advised to use mosquito repellents, malaria chemoprophylaxis, and acute therapy of presumptive infections.

No special immunizations are generally recommended for persons traveling from the USA to Western Europe, Canada, Australia, or Japan. Detailed suggestions of the USPHS are given country by country in its *Health Information for International Travel Supplement* (see References).

VACCINES FOR SPECIAL POPULATIONS

The greatest application of vaccines is in routine immunization of children and adults in large population groups. However, some vaccines are used only for population groups at greater hazard of disease by virtue of geography, occupation, or special exposure. The armed forces use an oral adenovirus vaccine containing types 4 and 7, as well as a polyvalent meningococcal vaccine, for all recruits.

Veterinarians and animal handlers usually receive preexposure rabies vaccination, whereas postexposure rabies immunization is appropriate for the general public. Hepatitis B vaccine is recommended for those with increased occupation, household, or lifestyle risks.

VACCINES CURRENTLY IN DEVELOPMENT

Many vaccines are currently in various stages of development. New ones produced by recombinant DNA technology can be anticipated. The first of these to be licensed and marketed is hepatitis B recombinant vaccine; many others are in various stages of design and production. Synthetic analogs of antigen and possibly anti-idiotype antibodies may be developed in the future.

Varicella vaccine (live attenuated varicella-zoster virus) is almost ready for licensing and marketing. An effective vaccine against hepatitis A has been developed. Its application remains to be determined. Vaccines against cytomegalovirus, herpes simplex virus, gonococci, *Plasmodium, Pseudomonas aeruginosa,* respiratory syncytial virus, rotavirus, *Shigella,* and many other pathogens are undergoing active development in the laboratory and in clinical trials. An effort is under way to conjugate the polysaccharide capsule of pneumococci to protein in a manner analogous to what has been accomplished with *H influenzae.*

Special immunoglobulin pools high in specific antibodies are being developed. The use of monoclonal antibodies in clinical practice is discussed in Chapter 59.

HIV INFECTION

Active efforts are under way to develop a recombinant DNA vaccine utilizing HIV viral components. Candidate vaccines have been targeted both for prevention of HIV infection in uninfected individuals and for boosting the immune response of those already infected. Many obstacles stand in the way of the effort, among them the frequent antigenic shift of this virus (see Chapter 48). The current recommendation for HIV-infected individuals is that they receive all the normal childhood immunizations (Table 55–4), with the exception that polio immunization be restricted to the inactivated form (Salk). This is principally to protect other members of the household who may be seriously immunocompromised. Live measles vaccine is recommended, despite the theoretic hazard, because of the severe form of measles infection that occurs in HIV-infected children. Vaccines against influenza and *S pneumoniae* should also be administered to the appropriate individuals in this group.

REFERENCES

American Academy of Pediatrics: *Report of Committee on Infectious Diseases.* American Academy of Pediatrics, 1991.

Brunell P: Chickenpox—examining our options. *N Engl J Med.* 1991;**325**:1577.

Centers for Disease Control: Update on adult immunization. *MMWR* 1991;**40**(no. RR-12):1.

Centers for Disease Control: *Immunization—Survey of Recent Research.* HHS Publication no. (CDC) 91–8391, 1992.

Centers for Disease Control: Prevention and control of influenza. *MWWR.* 1992;**41** (no. RR-9):1.

Centers for Disease Control and Prevention: *Health Information for International Travel,* 1993. HHS Publication no. (CDC) 93–8280. [Revised annually.]

Glode M et al: Safety and immunogenicity of acellular pertussis vaccine combined with diphtheria and tetanus toxoids—17- to 24-month-old children. *Pediatr Infect Dis* 1992;**11**:530.

Granoff DM et al: Differences in the Immunogenicity of three *Haemophilus influenzae* type B conjugate vaccines in infants. *J Pediatr* 1992;**121**:187.

Kaplan LJ et al: *Severe measles in immunocompromised patients. JAMA* 1992;**267**:1237.

National Vaccine Advisory Committee: The measles epidemic: The problems, barriers and recommendations. *JAMA* 1991;**266**:1547.

Schlenker TL: Measles herd immunity. The association of attack rates with immunization rates in preschool children. *JAMA* 1992;**267**:823.

Stienhoff MC (editor): Use of vaccines in the prevention of childhood pneumonia in developing countries. *Rev Infect Dis* 1991;**13(Suppl)**:S528.

Stiehm ER: New developments: Recent progress in the use of intravenous immunoglobin. *Curr Probl Clin Pediatr* 1992;**22**:335.

Weber DJ, Rutala WA: Prevention of mumps, measles and rubella among hospital personnel. *J Pediatr* 1991; **199**:322.

Werzberger A et al: Controlled trial of formalin inactivated hepatitis A vaccine in healthy children. *N Engl J Med* 1992;**327**:453.

West DJ, Margolis HS: Prevention of hepatitis B virus infection. *Pediatr Infect Dis J* 1992;**11**:866.

Allergy Desensitization

56

Abba I. Terr, MD

Allergy **desensitization** is a form of treatment in which allergens are injected into the patient for the purpose of reducing or eliminating the allergic response. It is also called allergen immunotherapy, hyposensitization, or allergy injection therapy. The term "desensitization" will be used here to avoid confusion with the use of the term "immunotherapy" elsewhere in this book to describe other forms of therapeutic manipulation of the immune system. It is most often used in IgE antibody-mediated diseases, but it has been used in other forms of allergy as well. Ideally, the treatment goal is complete abolition of the sensitivity, but in practice the result is usually a significant diminution in symptoms. It is an adjunct to allergen avoidance and symptomatic drug therapy, not the primary mode of treatment or a substitute for avoidance of allergens. Nevertheless, it is usually effective in situations where allergen avoidance is not possible.

Noon published the first report of desensitization for hay fever in England in 1911. Since then it has been extensively used in allergy practice to treat hay fever and allergic asthma. Since 1949 a sufficient number of controlled clinical trials have been completed to clearly establish its effectiveness in allergic rhinitis and Hymenoptera venom anaphylaxis. So far there have been too few definitive studies of its use in asthma to draw firm conclusions, but results to date support efficacy. Short-term desensitization has been accomplished in some cases of penicillin and insulin allergy. Successful oral desensitization has been reported for some drug-induced cutaneous eruptions, but these findings are uncontrolled. Desensitization is often attempted in *Rhus* contact dermatitis (poison ivy or poison oak), but as yet it has not been shown to be effective in this disease.

The mechanism of desensitization is still uncertain, but it is immunologically specific to the injected allergens. A variety of specific immunologic responses are induced during desensitization treatment. Promising improvements in the procedure are currently under study.

METHODS

The general procedure for desensitization in allergic rhinitis used today is similar to the method used originally by Noon. Sterile allergen extracts are administered subcutaneously in increasing doses once or twice a week until a dose is reached that produces a transient small local area of inflammation at the injection site. This dose is then given as a maintenance dose once every 2–4 weeks. Originally the course of treatment was preseasonal for a single-season pollen allergy, beginning 3–6 months before the expected onset of the season and terminating at the onset of the season. Because most patients with allergic rhinitis have allergies to different pollens at different times of the year as well as year-round dust or mold allergy, perennial (year-round) injection therapy is the most common schedule used by allergists today. The injections include a mixture of all relevant inhalant allergens, and after the maximum tolerated dose of the mixture is reached, the maintenance injections are continued for several years.

The injections are given subcutaneously. Oral, sublingual, inhaled, and local nasal routes of desensitization have been tried, but none has been shown to be effective in preventing diseases caused by IgE antibodies.

Extracts used in immunotherapy are the same as those used for testing (see Chapter 25). In most cases they are crude or partially purified aqueous extracts of the common inhalant allergens. Some are now standardized for content of the major allergen to ensure uniformity among different batches of extracts. Purified isolated major allergens, such as ragweed Amb a I, formerly called antigen E, have been used in clinical studies and may be effective in treatment of certain patients with restricted sensitivity to that allergen. Many allergic patients, however, have multiple sensitivities and therefore require the multiple allergens present in crude allergen extracts.

Injection Technique

Details of the proper technique for administering therapeutic allergen injections to patients with atopic or anaphylactic disease are important for the success and safety of the treatment. Because of possible risk of systemic reactions, facilities must be available to treat such reactions. Potentially fatal reactions usually begin within 30 minutes after the injection. Treatment should be withheld on a day when the patient is experiencing acute asthma or a fever. Small local swelling with itching at the injection site is acceptable. Excessive local swelling or any systemic reaction requires a reduction in dose. The dose should also be reduced if there has been a lapse in treatment.

Duration of Treatment

There are insufficient data to set guidelines for the overall length of desensitization in atopy. The variability in the natural course of disease, the vagaries of environmental exposure for the many different indoor (dust, molds, animals) and outdoor (pollens, molds) allergens, and the effect of nonallergic factors (weather, pollution, infections, stress) make definitive controlled long-term studies technically difficult. The immunologic changes induced by desensitization (see below), either singly or in combination, do not correlate sufficiently with symptomatic relief to justify in vitro immunologic monitoring to assess the optimal duration of therapy. Clinically, there is a progressive reduction of symptoms of pollen allergy for the first 3 or 4 years of preseasonal ragweed injections, after which the therapeutic effect levels off. There are no data yet on recurrence of symptoms after the injections are stopped. Some allergists recommend that treatment be discontinued after 2 or 3 successive symptomless years.

Desensitization for Hymenoptera venom anaphylaxis has been shown to be highly effective in reducing the risk of reactions from spontaneous stings throughout the period of active treatment at the maintenance dosage. Studies are now being conducted to assess the effects of discontinuing treatment, but until results are available, patients with life-threatening reactions should continue venom desensitization indefinitely.

Clinical Results

The results of the first controlled clinical trial of desensitization were published in 1949. Since then, results from dozens of placebo-controlled double-blind studies have shown clearly that desensitization is effective in seasonal and perennial allergic rhinitis when sufficient allergen is given to induce an immunologic response. The effect is immunologically specific. Fig 56–1 shows the results of one such study on

patients with seasonal ragweed hay fever. On average, symptoms are considerably reduced, especially at the peak of the pollen season. Similar efficacy has been shown for other pollens and for molds, house dust, dust mites, and cat allergen.

Controlled trials on patients with allergic asthma are more difficult to perform because the disease is exacerbated by so many nonallergic factors such as respiratory infections, atmospheric irritants, and emotions. Nevertheless, one study showed that desensitization treatment of asthma caused by allergy to cats reduced the bronchoprovocation response to cat allergen inhalation.

Hymenoptera insect venom anaphylaxis responds exceedingly well to desensitization: 95% of treated patients are protected from reactions to deliberate or unintentional stings, whereas about 50% of untreated or placebo-treated controls continue to experience systemic reactions to insect stings. Venom desensitization also appears to be effective in patients who respond to insect stings with urticaria or with consistently large local swellings at the sting site, but these conditions are not considered serious enough to warrant the treatment.

Desensitization has not been evaluated as a treatment for atopic dermatitis because exacerbations of the skin lesions usually do not correlate with inhalant allergen exposure. Food allergen injection therapy has not yet been definitively evaluated for efficacy against any of the clinical manifestations of food allergy, including anaphylaxis.

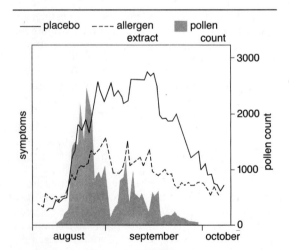

Figure 56–1. Desensitization therapy in patients with allergic rhinitis. Results of a placebo-controlled double-blind trial of ragweed allergen injections on the allergic symptoms of patients with ragweed hay fever during the ragweed pollinating season. (Modified and reproduced, with permission, from Norman PS, Winkenwerder WL, Lichtenstein LM: Trials of alum-precipitated pollen extracts in the treatment of hay fever. *J Allergy Clin Immunol* 1972;**50:**31.)

IMMUNOLOGIC EFFECTS

Several different immunologic effects are induced in allergic patients by desensitization therapy.

Hyposensitization

The term "desensitization" implies that the treatment eliminates the preexisting allergen-specific IgE antibody, converts the wheal-and-erythema skin test to negative, prevents the target organ response to the allergen by provocative-dose testing, and cures the disease. In practice, true desensitization is rare, being achieved in only about 5% of patients on an adequate course of therapy. Most treated atopic patients are hyposensitized. That is, immunologic and clinical measures of the specific IgE-mediated allergy are significantly lessened but not eliminated, even after many years of the injection treatment. The level of circulating IgE antibody falls below pretreatment levels only after many months of treatment (Fig 56–2). It is important to note that IgE antibody production is enhanced transiently during the first few months of low-dose allergen injections, and some patients experience a corresponding temporary worsening of symptoms during that time.

Immunization

An allergen-specific IgG antibody is induced by treatment (Fig 56–2). The antibody is often called "blocking antibody," because it inhibits the effect of IgE antibody in the passive-transfer (Prausnitz-Küstner) skin test and in the passive-transfer in vitro histamine release assay. Blocking antibodies of the IgA isotype may also be detected in the serum of treated patients, but blocking activity in secretions does not occur to a significant extent. Recent studies suggest that blocking antibody of the IgG4 subclass may correlate better with clinical improvement than that of other IgG subclasses. The presence of blocking antibody in serum is sustained as long as the maintenance injections are continued; the level then drops off gradually after treatment is stopped.

Regulation of IgE Antibody Production

There is limited evidence from a few studies that desensitization therapy alters regulatory factors in the production of allergen-specific IgE antibody. Some in vitro experiments indicate that treatment generates specific T cells with suppressor activity on IgE antibody production. One study detected the induction of auto-anti-idiotypic antibodies.

Combination Effects

It is likely that the beneficial effect of desensitization treatment in allergic diseases may derive from an optimal combination of some or all of the immunologic changes described above—and perhaps others—since no single effect, such as the quantity of blocking

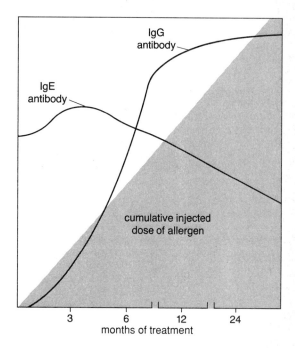

Figure 56–2. Immunologic changes during prolonged desensitization therapy for IgE-mediated diseases. The level of circulating IgE antibody is initially increased and later decreases below pretreatment levels. IgG antibody appears rapidly after the start of treatment, and its level is sustained while treatment continues.

antibody, correlates well with clinical improvement. Regardless of the precise mechanism, desensitization is specific for the allergens injected, is dose-related, and requires repeated and prolonged parenteral administration.

ADVERSE EFFECTS

The possible adverse effects of desensitization are both immediate and long-term. The immediate hazard is a systemic anaphylactic reaction. The risk is greatest both during the early weeks or months of treatment while the dose is being increased before a significant level of blocking antibody has been achieved and again when the dose is at or near the maintenance level. Systemic reactions are unpredictable and may occur after years of uneventful injections. They are more likely to happen during the patient's pollen and allergy season than during the off-season. Fever and physical exercise increase blood flow, causing more rapid absorption of the injected allergen and hence enhancing the risk of reaction.

The prevalence of systemic reactions is unknown. Recent studies show that on average, between one and 5 deaths occur per year in the USA from allergy injection treatment or skin testing, some because of dosage errors. About half of these occur in patients with active asthma.

Other immediate adverse effects are the same as for any subcutaneous injection, such as vasovagal reactions, infections, or injury from injecting the needle into the wrong tissue.

There appear to be no late or long-term ill effects from immunotherapy. With the use of aqueous allergen extracts, there is no evidence that repeated injections induce de novo allergic sensitization to components to which the patient was not previously sensitive. There are no proven instances in which allergen desensitization produces systemic immune-complex disease or other late sequelae.

INDICATIONS

Atopy

Desensitization has been used for almost 80 years to treat allergic rhinitis, and today it is widely accepted as beneficial. It is indicated for patients who are allergic to unavoidable inhalant allergens such as pollens and fungi and whose symptomatic periods of illness are severe, prolonged, and not well controlled by antihistamines or other symptomatic medications. House dust and dust mite desensitization is used in conjunction with a program of dust and mite elimination, since the latter is rarely completely effective. Allergists are currently divided in their opinion about injections of animal dander extracts for treatment of allergy to pets in the home or for occupational animal allergy. Opponents point out the paucity of controlled studies, presumed excessive risk of systemic reactions, and concern about unknown long-term effects of immunization with animal protein. Although there are insufficient controlled clinical trials for firm recommendations, the indications for desensitization of allergic asthma parallel those for allergic rhinitis. Desensitization is not indicated for treatment of atopic dermatitis or allergic gastroenteropathy. Patients with atopic dermatitis may receive injections for concomitant allergic rhinitis or asthma if indicated, but starting doses should be low and the buildup in dosage should be slow, because injected allergens may cause a flare of the dermatitis. Desensitization is not indicated for food allergy.

Anaphylaxis

Desensitization is indicated for any patient with a history of systemic anaphylaxis from a Hymenoptera insect sting who has a positive skin test to one or more Hymenoptera venoms. Many authorities exclude from treatment those patients whose reaction to the sting was limited to urticaria, regardless of the skin test results, because such patients generally do not have an excessive risk of systemic anaphylaxis on future stings. There is no indication for desensitization treatment of localized swelling from an insect sting, no matter how large the swelling, since these responses also do not predict future anaphylaxis. The injected allergens for treatment of anaphylaxis should include all of the venoms that give a positive skin test, since identification of the stinging insect under field conditions of a spontaneous sting is usually unreliable.

Desensitization for anaphylaxis in response to drugs has been successful for selected cases of penicillin and insulin allergy. In those instances, injection of increasing doses at intervals of approximately 30 minutes achieves a clinical state of desensitization permitting therapeutic use of the drug on a regular basis. If the drug is withdrawn, the patient may again become allergic.

Urticaria

Desensitization has never been known to be effective therapy for urticaria, and it is not indicated for this condition.

Immune-Complex Allergies

Desensitization is not necessary for treatment of cutaneous Arthus reactions or for serum sickness. These are self-limited reactions, which subside when the allergen has been eliminated.

Allergic Contact Dermatitis

Oral and subcutaneous desensitization with extracts of *Rhus* oil has been used for many years, but there is no evidence for its effectiveness in prevention of *Rhus* allergic dermatitis (from poison ivy and poison oak), and therefore it is not indicated for these conditions.

Hypersensitivity Pneumonitis

Desensitization is not indicated for this disease.

MONITORING DESENSITIZATION

Desensitization of respiratory atopic disease is a treatment that continues for years. Indications for starting this long-term process are usually clear, but selection of allergens, dosages and frequency of injections, and duration of therapy must be individualized. The beneficial and adverse responses are difficult to predict in advance. It is therefore important to establish a long-term goal and a program for monitoring treatment at the outset.

Changes in serum levels of specific IgE antibody and induced IgG blocking antibody correlate poorly with clinical improvement, so these are not useful monitors of progress in individual cases. Some allergists repeat skin testing at regular intervals, but clinical improvement can occur without change in skin test reactivity. The principal reason for retesting is to diagnose new sensitivities when symptoms worsen or appear at new seasons.

At present, assessing desensitization for effectiveness requires monitoring of symptoms and physical signs of illness, as well as performing objective tests such as pulmonary functions when applicable. It is reasonable to discontinue the injections after 2 or 3 successive disease-free years.

DESENSITIZATION WITH MODIFIED ALLERGENS

There has been a continuing effort to improve the effectiveness of specific injection therapy and to reduce the risk of reactions and the number of injections through the use of adjuvants and by chemical alteration, modification, and polymerization of the allergen.

Adjuvants

Incomplete Freund's adjuvant—an emulsion of aqueous antigen in mineral oil—enhances the immune response by providing an insoluble lipid depot in the subcutaneous tissue from which droplets of allergen are gradually released, thereby simulating repeated injections of allergen over time. It has been used in research to generate large quantities of antibodies in animals. In the early 1960s this method of "one-shot" desensitization given preseasonally underwent extensive clinical trials. The treatment was probably similar in effectiveness to conventional multi-injection desensitization, but mineral oil persists indefinitely in tissues and causes long-lasting nodules, cysts, and sterile abscesses that might require surgical removal. This form of therapy was abandoned because of concern about potential carcinogenicity.

Adsorption of allergens onto alum produces an in-soluble antigen that is more efficiently phagocytosed by macrophages. Alum-adsorbed allergens have had limited acceptance in practice for many years. The hoped-for advantages over aqueous allergens—fewer injections and improved efficacy—have not been achieved.

Allergoids

Formalin treatment of toxic antigens such as tetanus toxin yields a toxoid, a molecule without toxicity that retains antigenicity, thereby permitting complete and safe active immunity. The same principle has been exploited with allergens for desensitization, but to date attempts to modify allergens with formalin, propylene glycol, urea, and other chemicals to eliminate or reduce allergenicity and risk of systemic reactions while preserving immunogenicity to the native allergen have been unsuccessful.

Polymerized Allergens

The most promising method to date for improving desensitization is the technique of polymerizing protein allergens with glutaraldehyde. Covalently linked allergen monomers provide a molecule with low allergenicity in proportion to the degree of polymerization. Theoretically, monomeric and polymeric molecules are equally effective in bridging IgE antibodies for (undesired) allergy-producing mediator release, whereas the polymer, when phagocytosed and processed by the antigen-presenting macrophage, presents more antigenic epitopes per molecule for the (desired) protective immune response. Although not yet released for clinical practice, several different polymerized inhalant allergens have been confirmed by therapeutic trials to have the theoretic advantages of this form of desensitization.

REFERENCES

American Academy of Allergy and Immunology Executive Committee: Personnel and equipment to treat systemic reactions caused by immunotherapy with allergenic extracts. (Position statement.) *J Allergy Clin Immunol* 1986;**77:**271.

Castracane JM, Rocklin RE: Detection of human auto-anti-idiotypic antibodies (Ab2). *Int Arch Allergy Appl Immunol* 1988;**86:**295.

Grammer LC, Shaughnessy MA, Patterson R: Modified forms of allergen immunotherapy. *J Allergy Clin Immunol* 1985;**76:**397.

Johnstone DE, Dutton A: The value of hyposensitization therapy for bronchial asthma in children: A 14-year study. *Pediatrics* 1968;**47:**793.

Lichtenstein LM, Norman PS, Winkenwerder WL: Clinical and in vitro studies on the role of immunotherapy in ragweed hay fever. *Am J Med* 1968;**44:**514.

Lowell FC, Franklin W: A double-blind study of the effectiveness and specificity of injection therapy in ragweed and hay fever. *N Engl J Med* 1965;**273:**675.

Noon L: Prophylactic inoculation against hay fever. *Lancet* 1911;**1:**1572.

Norman PS: Immunotherapy for nasal allergy. *J Allergy Clin Immunol* 1988;**81:**992.

Norman PS: An overview of immunotherapy: Implications for the future. *J Allergy Clin Immunol* 1980;**65:**87.

Ohman JL: Allergen immunotherapy in asthma: Evidence for efficacy. *J Allergy Clin Immunol* 1989;**84:**133.

Rocklin RE: Clinical and immunologic aspects of allergen-specific immunotherapy in patients with seasonal allergic rhinitis and/or allergic asthma. *J Allergy Clin Immunol* 1983;**73:**323.

Sherman WB, Connell JT: Changes in skin-sensitizing antibody titer (SSAT) following two to four years of injection (aqueous) therapy. *J Allergy Clin Immunol* 1966;**37:**123.

Marvin R. Garovoy, MD, Peter Stock, MD, Ginny Bumgardner, MD, PhD,
Fraser Keith, MD, & Charles Linker, MD

Transplantation of organs is becoming increasingly successful. What was once an experimental and life-saving emergency procedure is being transformed into a life-enhancing and technologically advanced form of therapy.

The first successful renal transplant was performed in 1954. Subsequently, advances in histocompatibility testing and immunosuppressive drug therapy made renal transplantation a clinical reality in the 1960s. Improved skills and handling of immunosuppressive drugs (prednisone and azathioprine) resulted in a decline in infectious complications and marked reduction in mortality rates. The 1970s witnessed the beneficial effects of blood transfusions and antilymphocyte globulin (ALG) as graft-enhancing treatments. The 1980s may be characterized as the era of cyclosporin and the advent of monoclonal antibody therapy—immunosuppressive agents that have greatly improved the success rate of kidney transplants and have also made possible heart, liver, lung, and pancreas engraftment with better results than before. Transplant outcome has become so promising that it is now being offered early in the care of many patients with chronic and debilitating diseases.

KIDNEY TRANSPLANTATION

Patients with end-stage renal disease can be considered for renal transplantation. Absolute contraindications are conditions that would interfere with the safe administration of anesthesia or immunosuppressive therapy. These include debilitating cardiopulmonary disease, cancer, and untreated peptic ulcer disease or infection. Preoperative immunologic evaluation includes ABO blood grouping, histocompatibility testing (determination of the patient's and potential donor's human leukocyte antigens [HLA antigens] and the degree of haplotype matching) (see Chapter 16), state of presensitization to HLA antigens,

and viral serology (hepatitis B and C viruses, human immunodeficiency virus [HIV], cytomegalovirus [CMV], and Epstein-Barr virus). Medical evaluation to rule out contraindications to transplantation frequently includes voiding cystourethrography, dental and pulmonary evaluations, and assessment of cardiac status.

ABO TESTING

ABO testing is performed on all recipients and potential donors. The ABO system is present not only on erythrocytes but also on the vascular endothelium of the graft. The danger of transplanting across the ABO barrier is the production of very rapid graft rejection owing to preformed isohemagglutinins that injure the vascular endothelium and elicit a coagulation reaction in situ. The same rules that apply to blood transfusion compatibility also apply to renal transplantation: For a type O recipient the donor should be type O; for a type A recipient the donor may be type A or O; for a type B recipient the donor may be type B or O; and for a type AB recipient the donor may be type A, B, or O. It is possible to overcome the ABO barrier by plasmapheresis to lower the natural titer of anti-A or anti-B antibodies and by administration of cyclophosphamide to prevent new antibody formation, but graft survival has been disappointing.

Living Related Donor Transplantation

All recipients and their potential donors should have complete testing for HLA-A, -B, -C, -DR, and -DQ antigens (see Chapter 16). On the basis of family typings, it is usually possible to determine the genotype or haplotype (chromosome) assignment for each identified antigen. The value of haplotype matching (zero, one, or 2) was established clinically: a sibling matched for 2 haplotypes and a parent or sibling matched for one haplotype achieve 90% graft survival at 1 year. Because of improved immunosuppression, zero-haplotype-matched family members can now also achieve 90% graft survival at 1 year.

Presensitization

Prior exposure to transplantation antigens can lead to sensitization manifested by the development of cytotoxic antibodies against HLA antigens. Patients who have antibodies to HLA antigens may have a poorer graft outcome. Moreover, patients who are sensitized and receive second and subsequent transplants are more likely to reject these grafts than are those who receive a primary graft. This likelihood is especially increased in patients who rapidly rejected their first graft (in < 3 months). Whether repeated rejection is caused by specific sensitization to transplantation antigens or reflects a high immune reactivity of the recipient is under investigation.

Cross-Matching

The cross-match test is used to determine the presence of any performed antibodies (presensitization) to donor HLA antigens. A cross-match typically is performed by using the patient's most recent serum and donor lymphocytes (either peripheral blood mononuclear cells or isolated T or B lymphocytes) (see Chapter 16). Positive cross-matches are a contraindication to transplantation, since they are associated with very early and uncontrollable rejection episodes, leading to irreversible graft loss.

Cadaveric Transplantation

In circumstances when the recipient has no family members as potential donors, the opportunity exists to receive a kidney from a recently deceased individual (cadaveric transplantation). Recipients referred for this type of treatment undergo comparable immunologic evaluation of ABO grouping, HLA typing, and antibody screening and are then placed on a waiting list. The most likely causes of formation of anti-HLA antibodies include pregnancy and previously rejected grafts. To monitor the extent of anti-HLA antibodies produced, serum from each recipient is collected monthly and tested in a manner known as screening. The patient's serum is cross-matched against a panel of lymphocytes obtained from many individuals. The number of individuals whose cells are killed is often expressed as a percentage of the panel (eg, 10% panel-reactive antibody). By this procedure, it is possible to determine the extent of presensitization, ie, how often the patient is likely to have a positive cross-match, assuming that the transplant organ is taken from the same genetic pool of donors as the lymphocyte panel. In addition, knowing the HLA antigens on the lymphocyte panel cells that have been lysed makes it possible to analyze the specificities of the antibodies present in the serum and responsible for the positive reactions.

Donor Selection

When a potential cadaveric donor's organs are harvested, a section of spleen, some lymph nodes, and some peripheral blood are collected. The donor ABO blood group and HLA antigens are determined from these samples. The waiting list of recipients can then be cross-matched against the donor tissues, using the patient's current serum and the recipient's highest-reacting serum within the past 2 years to exclude the possibility of a positive cross-match. Recipients who are ABO-compatible and cross-match-negative become available for further consideration. Often, there may be a second round of cross-match testing among this smaller pool of recipients, in which additional past sera are chosen to be certain of no hidden presensitization. From among the ABO-compatible, cross-match-negative recipients, the best-matched recipients may then be selected. In programs in which a large enough choice of recipients is not available to find a perfectly matched recipient, additional criteria such as length of time on the waiting list, urgency of medical condition, and whether this is a first or second transplant are considered in recipient selection.

Donor Evaluation & Procedures

Candidacy for living related donation is determined by evaluating the potential donors for heart disease, renal dysfunction, diabetes, infection, and malignancy. A preoperative angiogram guides selection of the right or left kidney for living related donation. Factors that influence the choice of kidney are operating safety for the donor, vascular and internal anatomy, and occasionally differential creatinine clearance by renal scan. The living-donor nephrectomy procedure includes a flank incision through which the kidney and vascular pedicle are removed. The ureter is removed with all periureteral soft tissue in order to preserve the ureteral blood supply and prevent distal ureteral avascular necrosis.

Family studies conducted to evaluate a potential family donor include a complete medical evaluation. There is no long-term change in survival or life-style of individuals who have undergone uninephrectomy for donation. Because of increased success rates of related-donor transplantation, owing to improved immunosuppression and preoperative conditioning, it is now possible to consider living donors who share 2, one, or no haplotypes with the recipient. With the increasing demand for kidneys, many centers are now performing transplants from living unrelated donors. Recent results indicate that a 90% 1-year survival rate can be achieved. Evaluation of donor motivation and psychologic factors is necessary.

Cadaveric donors can be considered when determined to be neurologically dead from a variety of causes, including spontaneous intracerebral hemorrhage and head trauma. Cadaveric donors must be free from metastasizing tumors, kidney dysfunction, or active infection (particularly with hepatitis viruses or HIV). There are evolving criteria for selecting organs for transplantation from donors who are positive for hepatitis C antibody. Hemodynamic stabilization with volume expansion and the conservative use of vasopressors and desmopressin acetate maintain optimal organ function. Organ recovery from cadaveric donors includes removal of both kidneys with renal arteries and veins frequently left en bloc with the donor aorta and vena cava. Both ureters are removed, including all periureteral soft tissue, in order to include the ureteral blood supply and prevent distal ureteral avascular necrosis. Samples of spleen and lymph nodes are also removed for donor tissue typing and cross-matching against potential recipients.

Once removed, the kidney is flushed with preservation fluid to remove all donor blood. Cadaveric kidneys can be stored by either of 2 methods. Cold storage involves storing in ice to maintain subphysiologic temperatures. Alternatively, the aorta or renal arteries are cannulated, and a cold mixed-electrolyte solution is instilled by continuous cold pulsatile perfusion. Cadaver renal transplantation within the first 48 hours after donor nephrectomy is preferred.

Blood Transfusion

In the past, recipient preconditioning with blood transfusion has led to improved graft survival. Mechanisms for the transfusion effect include elimination of immunologic responders who will demonstrate cytotoxic antibodies contraindicating transplantation, development of specific and nonspecific suppressor T cells, and generation of blocking or anti-idiotypic antibodies. With improved immunosuppressive protocols, the benefits of pretransplant transfusions have been more difficult to demonstrate. Furthermore, many centers now believe that the infectious risks associated with blood transfusions outweigh the potential benefits.

Transplant Surgery

The operative procedure for the recipient includes an incision over the iliac fossa through which the graft is placed in the retroperitoneal position against the psoas muscle (Fig 57–1). A renal artery anastomosis to either the internal or external iliac artery and renal vein anastomosis to the external iliac vein are standard. Ureteroneocystotomy involving anastomosis of the ureter to bladder mucosa through an anterior cystotomy incision is a usual approach. The ureter is often passed through a short submucosal tunnel in the bladder wall to prevent vesicoureteral reflux.

Postoperatively, hemodynamic stability is achieved with central venous pressure monitoring and careful fluid and diuretic management. Careful monitoring of urine output, electrolytes, blood urea nitrogen, and serum creatinine to evaluate renal function is mandatory. All cadaveric kidneys have some degree of acute tubular necrosis, ranging from very mild to

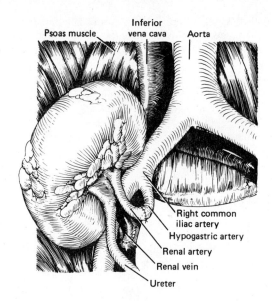

Figure 57–1. Technique of renal transplantation. (Reproduced, with permission, from Way LW (editor): *Current Surgical Diagnosis & Treatment,* 9th ed. Appleton & Lange, 1991.)

very severe. Dialysis is required in approximately 20% of cadaveric renal transplant recipients during the early period of severe acute tubular necrosis (usually 5–10 days). Acute tubular necrosis is rare in patients receiving related-donor transplants since donor nephrectomy and recipient transplant are performed sequentially, minimizing cold-storage time.

Postoperative Immunosuppression

Postoperative immunosuppression is the most variable aspect of recipient care. Standard immunosuppression to prevent rejection includes corticosteroids, and additional immunosuppression is chosen depending on the type of allograft and tissue match (see Chapters 58 and 60). The use of cyclosporin (5–15 mg/kg/d) has clearly improved long-term allograft success in recipients of cadaveric and some related-donor transplants. Cyclosporin is definitely nephrotoxic, and monitoring of drug dosages and drug levels (100–400 μg/mL) is required.

Azathoprine, an antimetabolite that interferes with new DNA formation in proliferating cells, is frequently used (1–2 mg/kg/d) in combination with prednisone and cyclosporin. Azathoprine is potentially hepatotoxic, whereas cyclophosphamide is a nonhepatotoxic alternative. Antilymphocyte globulin (ALG; 10–20 mg/kg) and antithymocyte globulin (ATG; 10–20 mg/kg) heterologous sera prepared in animals immunized with human lymphocytes or thymocytes, respectively, are potent immunosuppressive reagents and act through antilymphocytic properties. These heterologous animal proteins can be made in horses, sheep, goats, or rabbits. Monoclonal antibodies (OKT 3, OKT 4) against specific T cell subsets are also in clinical use. Lymphoplasmapheresis occasionally is used to remove recipient lymphocytes and immunoglobulin while immunosuppressive drugs are concurrently administered. Local graft irradiation has been used but has not provided reliable immunosuppression. A number of newer immunosuppressive agents with different mechanisms of action are in clinical trials (FK-506, RS-61443 [mycophenolate mofetil], 15-deoxysporgualin).

Rejection

Classic signs and symptoms of acute rejection include swelling and tenderness over the allograft and decrease in renal function. Systemic manifestations such as temperature elevation, malaise, poor appetite, and generalized myalgia can be seen. Decrease in renal function is diagnosed by a decrease in urine volume, increasing blood urea nitrogen and creatinine levels, poorly controlled hypertension, fluid retention, and radiographically by ultrasonography (blurring of corticomedullary junctions, increased resistive index, prominent pyramids) and by radionuclide renal scans showing decreased uptake and excretion of the tracer. In the presence of a decline in renal

function, however, the differential diagnosis includes prerenal azotemia and obstruction, acute tubular necrosis, pyelonephritis, and other drug-induced toxicity. In addition, recurrence of the primary renal disease and de novo glomerulonephritis can be late causes of decreased renal function. Renal biopsy is frequently performed to histologically diagnose the cause of graft dysfunction.

Mechanisms of Rejection

A. Acute: Evidence suggests that at least 2 pathways of antigen presentation may be operative. The "direct path" of antigen presentation suggests that blood-borne antigen-presenting cells ("passenger cells") in grafts provide the primary stimulus. These are dendritic cells and monocytes expressing allogeneic class I and II HLA molecules. The "indirect path" of antigen presentation suggests that host antigen-presenting cells can present shed allogeneic class I and II HLA antigens found on donor parenchymal cells. Both donor and host type antigen-presenting cells provide second signals, interleukin-1 (IL-1), and IL-6, which aid in triggering lymphocyte activation (Fig 57–2). IL-1 not only is involved in the activation of helper/inducer CD4 T cells but probably also is

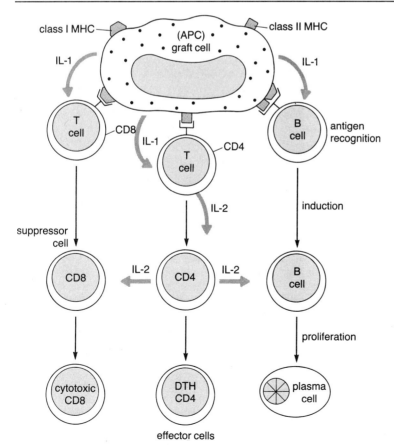

Figure 57–2. Generation of allograft rejection response (primary).

important for the activation of unprimed cytotoxic CD8 T cells and B lymphocytes. The activation of helper/inducer T cells by alloantigen is pivotal to the development of cell immune responses against the graft. Once activated, these cells release IL-2, which is an essential cofactor in the activation of both CD8 T cells and B cells. As a consequence of exposure to antigen plus the interleukins, there is clonal proliferation and maturation of alloantigen-reactive cells. This leads to the development of effector T cells, which migrate from lymphoid tissue via the blood to all tissues, including the graft, where they mediate damage at antigen-containing sites, and antibody, which is released into the blood or locally within the graft, where it has access to these antigens.

The precise mechanism by which T cells destroy the graft is still under study. Effector T cells that can destroy graft tissue develop from both CD8 and CD4 subclasses (Fig 57–3). The results are similar except that CD8 T cells recognize HLA-A and HLA-B antigen-bearing cells, whereas CD4 T cells recognize HLA-DR antigen-bearing cells. Both CD4 and CD8 subclasses of effector cells probably can directly destroy graft cells by classic cytotoxic T cell mechanisms. However, another important consequence of T cell activation is their release of other lymphokines, especially gamma interferon (IFN γ), which can produce 2 important effects. First, IFN γ induces increased expression of HLA-A, -B, and -DR on graft tissue, which potentially makes the graft more vulnerable to effector mechanisms. Second, it activates monocytes to mediate a destructive delayed hypersensitivity response against the graft.

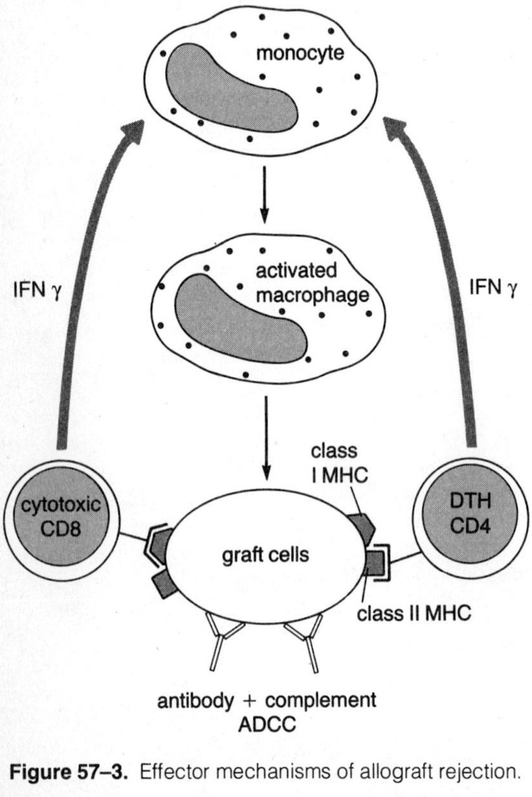

Hence, T cells can directly cause target cell injury or activate macrophages into nonspecific destruction. Lymphokines in addition to IL-2 and IFN γ are released from activated T cells; they include IL-4 and IL-5, which play a role in directing B cell production of antibody. Antibody-mediated damage may then take place directly through complement activation or by recruitment of antibody-dependent cell-mediated cytotoxic (ADCC) effector cells (Fig 57–3). Most of the cells that arrive in the graft early after transplantation are lymphocytes, which migrate out of the capillary and venous beds, but after 4–7 days a remarkably heterogeneous collection of cell types appears. Those of the lymphocytic series predominate over the monocyte/macrophage and include also a few polymorphonuclear neutrophils. Although a variety of cell types are present, there is some evidence that early rejection of solid-tissue allografts is associated with T lymphocytes having direct cytotoxic activity against donor target cells. A significant number of B lymphocytes, null cells, and monocytes also appear in the early infiltrate, and although cytotoxic T cell activity is easily demonstrated at first, later stages of rejection may involve a non-T killer cell. In all phases, the presence of antibodies and ADCC effector cells makes this mechanism an additional possibility. Macrophages appear to play an effector and suppressor role, whereas some B lymphocytes become activated and begin immunoglobulin synthesis in situ. When the host has been primed to donor antigens before transplantation, an accelerated process, often marked by antibody-mediated vasculitis, may result.

Recent applications of anti-T cell monoclonal antibodies in staining biopsies and in vivo as therapy add considerable support to the key role of T lymphocytes in most cases of rejection. When immunofluorescence or immunoperoxidase techniques are used with renal graft biopsies, 50–90% of the infiltrating cells generally express CD3 and CD6, with variable proportions of CD4 and CD8 cells. Although the peripheral blood often shows an increased proportion of CD4 cells in association with acute rejection episodes, many investigators relate rejection in the kidney to a preponderance of CD8 cells. More precisely, there is a preponderance of CD8 cells in the blood and perivascular areas in the grafts of patients experiencing irreversible rejection (ratio of CD4 to CD8 cells < 1.0). When peripheral blood CD4:CD8 ratios are higher, perivascular ratios are also higher, and rejection usually is reversible with therapy. High-dose corticosteroids, given either intravenously (methylprednisolone, 1 g/d for 3 days) or orally (prednisone, 5–10 mg/kg/d for 5 days) are often used to treat acute

Figure 57–3. Effector mechanisms of allograft rejection.

rejection. Corticosteroids function through several pathways. They reduce the capacity of antigen-presenting cells to express class II antigens and to release IL-1. They also inhibit the alloactivation of T cells and consequently the release of IL-2. Their effect on migration and function of effector cells, as well as their capacity to release IFN γ, may explain their efficacy in reversing acute rejection. In this regard, they are known to produce lymphocytopenia, especially of CD4 T cells, by delaying transit of the lymphocytes through marrow and lymphoid tissues.

If there is no response or only a partial response to corticosteroids, ALG or ATG may be given (10–20 mg/kg/d for 5–14 days). ALG lyses lymphocytes, especially T cells, making it an excellent agent for treatment of acute rejection. ALG, however, is associated with anaphylaxis, serum sickness, and fever. Biologic effects also vary, since there is no effective measure for standardization.

More commonly, monoclonal antibodies (OKT 3 antibodies) are used to treat rejection refractory to steroids. A mouse IgG2, a monoclonal antibody to the T cell surface molecule CD3, is used for the treatment of rejection. Not only is it effective for the treatment of initial bouts of rejection, but rejection episodes that are resistant to high-dose steroids usually respond to OKT 3 therapy (5 mg/d intravenously for 10 days). OKT 3 initially causes an acute T lymphocyte depletion as the antibody-coated T lymphocytes are opsonized by the reticuloendothelial system. After 48 hours of therapy, there is a slow return of T lymphocytes to the circulation; however, the T cell receptor-CD3 complex is modulated (cleared) from the cell surface. Without a sufficient number of CD3 molecules present, T cell activation is impaired. One side effect of therapy with this foreign protein may be the production of antimouse antibodies in a small percentage of patients; this can limit the effectiveness of a subsequent course of therapy, and prolonged or high-dose OKT 3 therapy has been associated with an increased incidence of lymphoproliferative disease. In the future, monoclonal antibodies against lymphokine receptors and adhesion molecules as well as soluble cytokine receptors may be found useful.

B. Hyperacute: Preformed anti-ABO isohemagglutinins or anti-class I HLA antibodies, when present in sufficient quantity, will bind to the vascular endothelium and trigger a cascade of immunologic events. Initially, fixation of complement components and complement activation ensues, followed by activation of the clotting pathway. This series of events, if severe enough, can result in microthrombi within glomerular capillary loops and arterioles, leading to severe ischemia and necrosis of the graft. At present, there are no effective means of treating this lesion once it begins. Emphasis is therefore placed on prevention by careful assessment of ABO blood type and donor-specific sensitization to

HLA antigens by cross-match testing prior to transplantation.

C. Chronic: Chronic rejection, which can occur months to years after transplantation, is characterized by a narrowing of the vascular arterial lumen owing to growth of endothelial cells that line the vascular bed. The actual control mechanisms for this response are unknown but may include immunologic injury signals, monocyte release of IL-1, and platelet and endothelial cell release of platelet-derived growth factor. Initially, the proliferating endothelial cell lesion is reversible, but once it progresses to fibrotic changes within the blood vessel wall itself, it is unresponsive to current modes of immunosuppression and progresses to graft ischemia, extensive interstitial fibrosis, and ultimate loss of renal function. Since there is no specific therapy for this form of rejection, emphasis is again placed on minimizing chronic immunologic stimuli by seeking the greatest possible degree of histocompatibility between recipients and donors.

Outcome

Survival of patients after renal transplantation is not significantly different from that of patients undergoing dialysis. In most series, patient survival at 2 years is 90–95%. Graft survival, defined as allograft function adequate to maintain life without dialytic treatment, is 85% at 2 years in cadaveric renal allograft recipients treated with corticosteroids and either cyclosporin or ALG/OKT 3. Related-donor transplants have greater than 90% success at 2 years.

Surviving renal allografts have normal function, with mean creatinine levels of less than 2 mg/dL in most series. A functioning allograft therefore affords the recipient an optimal chance for normalization of health and is associated with minimal morbidity and mortality rates.

LIVER TRANSPLANTATION

Extensive experimental work in the field of liver transplantation has been performed since the early 1950s. Early investigators, using a variety of animal models, demonstrated that liver transplantation was feasible. The use of large-animal models indicated potential problem areas such as control of the splanchnic circulation during cross-clamping (the predecessor of the venovenous bypass) and rejection in grafts progressing to liver failure in animals untreated with immunosuppressive agents. The first human liver transplant was performed in 1963. Although this and the next several transplants were all unsuccessful, liver transplantation later became a successful procedure because of improved surgical techniques, intraoperative management, and methods of immunosuppression. In 1992, more than 3500 liver transplants were performed in the USA, and over 100 liver transplant centers exist throughout the world at this time.

Although liver grafts were initially thought to be immunologically privileged from results of experimental liver transplantation in animals, rejection is commonly encountered in human liver transplantation. In certain strains of pigs and rats, liver grafts between the same donor and recipient combination have prolonged survival even though allogeneic kidney allografts are rejected within a short time. In addition, animals tolerate subsequent skin grafts from the same donor for prolonged periods but promptly reject third-party skin grafts. These effects are specific to only limited strains. There is, however, evidence that liver transplant rejection occurs by substantially different mechanisms from kidney transplant rejection. As a consequence of these different mechanisms and the difference of expression of major histocompatibility complex (MHC) antigens on the surface of liver cells and bile duct cells, the rejection response of the liver is distinctly different from that of other whole organs.

Indications

The indication for liver transplantation is the certainty that an individual's disease process is likely to progress to death within 2 years or that the compromise in life-style is so severe as to merit the risk of transplant. Although some diseases are known to be fatal in the long term, it is only recently that the use of longitudinal studies in primary biliary cirrhosis and sclerosing cholangitis has elucidated specific factors that can predict for short-term survival. Liver transplantation is usually not indicated until the life expectancy of the individual is expected to be less than 2 years. Hepatic dysfunction may be manifested by alterations in either synthetic or regulatory ability.

Signs and symptoms of progressive liver deficiency include malaise, weight loss, encephalopathy, ascites, coagulopathy, hypoalbuminemia, hyperbilirubinemia, and renal insufficiency. Complications of cholestatic disease include intractable pruritus, metabolic bone disease, recurrent biliary sepsis, and xanthomatous neuropathy. In addition, progressive complications of portal hypertension (gastroesophageal bleeding, ascites) in the context of liver deficiency require intervention. With the development of transjugular intrahepatic portasystemic shunts (TIPS), variceal bleeding and refractory ascites can often be managed effectively until a donor organ becomes available. At present, many potential liver transplant recipients (particularly children) die before a suitable organ becomes available. The most common indication for liver transplant in the adult population to date has been non-A, non-B hepatitis virus postnecrotic cirrhosis or chronic active hepatitis. Other diagnoses for which liver transplantation has been performed include primary biliary cirrhosis, sclerosing cholangitis, hepatitis B cirrhosis, hepatitis C cirrhosis, alco-

holic cirrhosis, fulminant hepatic failure, hemochromatosis, Wilson's disease, Budd-Chiari syndrome, hepatitis C, and inborn errors of metabolism. Some patients with hepatocellular tumors or cholangiocarcinomas have received transplants, and a few patients have survived long term (3–5 years), but in the vast majority of patients the tumor has recurred with fatal consequences. Similarly, patients with antigen-positive chronic active hepatitis B frequently have recurrent hepatitis B antigenemia following transplantation. A large number of these patients have developed recurrent hepatitis and cirrhosis, although the rapidity of progression of chronic active hepatitis leading to cirrhosis and liver failure has been questioned. Techniques to decrease hepatitis B antigenemia, such as the use of hepatitis B hyperimmune globulin, may prove useful. Although liver transplantation in patients with alcohol-related liver failure was initially quite controversial, this indication has become more widely accepted because of the increasing evidence that these patients have results comparable to those of patients with other causes of liver failure. Most transplant centers require that these patients remain abstinent from alcohol for 6–12 months and that they can comply with posttransplant treatment regimens.

The most common diagnosis for which liver transplantation is performed in infants and children is extrahepatic biliary atresia. This disease occurs in between 1:8,000 and 1:12,000 live births in the USA. Children commonly undergo the Kasai procedure, which has long-term effectiveness in one-third to one-half of all patients. For patients with failed hepaticojejunostomy, liver transplantation is the only viable solution. Other indications for liver transplants in children are inborn errors of metabolism such as α_1-antitrypsin deficiency, tyrosinemia, and Wilson's disease. As outcome has improved, liver replacement has been used to treat liver-based inborn errors of metabolism that result in extrahepatic organ system failure. For example, one patient with homozygous familial hypercholesterolemia has received a heart-liver transplant, and several patients with α_1-antitrypsin deficiency and renal involvement have received combination liver-kidney transplants.

Contraindications to liver transplantation vary from center to center. General guidelines are to exclude potential recipients whose disease conditions are associated with poor prognosis (HIV seropositivity, hepatitis B surface and/or E antigen seropositivity, extrahepatic malignancy, or evidence of metastatic disease). Further contraindications include behavioral and social issues that may predict a poor outcome because of noncompliance. Examples are active substance abuse and the recipient's inability to meet with the rigors of postoperative management (compliance and medication protocol) and/or postoperative follow-up. Finally, medical contraindications to liver transplantation include advanced cardiopulmonary disease, anatomic considerations that preclude surgical reconstruction, and active infection (especially with fungal pathogens).

Procedure

Orthotopic liver transplantation is the most commonly used method to date. This involves the removal of the host liver and replacement with the transplanted liver in the orthotopic position. Heterotopic transplantation is less frequently performed, as the clinical results have been less successful than with orthotopic transplantation. In heterotopic transplantation, the native liver is left in place and the transplanted liver is placed at an ectopic site. After removal from the donor, the donor liver is flushed with heparinized UW solution and then preserved in preservation solution and stored in the cold. The recently developed UW solution enables the liver to be preserved for more than 24 hours in some cases. This has greatly expanded the ability to transport organs long distances and to use back-up recipients if the first recipient proves unacceptable for transplantation. However, to minimize the risk of intrahepatic biliary strictures associated with prolonged hepatic preservation time, an attempt is made to transplant within 12 hours after harvest. The recipient hepatectomy is technically the most difficult phase of the transplant operation because of frequent portal hypertension, previous surgery, and coagulopathy. Often there is excessive bleeding due to numerous adhesions at the operative site. The liver is mobilized al-

though not removed until the donor organ is brought into the operative field and examined. The anhepatic phase is the time of greatest physiologic stress, because at this point the liver is removed and clamping of the portal vein and vena cava results in decreased venous return to the heart. This may in part be overcome by the use of venovenous bypass, which serves to bypass the splanchnic circulation and the infrahepatic vena caval circulation. The anhepatic phase lasts from the time when the host liver is removed until the vascular clamps are released, reperfusing the new liver. The revascularization phase requires attention to hemostasis. Revascularization involves supply to the liver via either the portal vein or the hepatic artery, or both, depending on the individual's anatomy and stability on venovenous bypass. The specific type of arterial revascularization depends on the blood supply to the donor organ. Complex revascularization may be required if multiple arteries are supplying the donor liver. The bile duct is reconstructed by using a choledochocholedochostomy, preferably when the recipient common duct is of good quality, or a choledochojejunostomy if the recipient duct is poor quality (eg, in biliary atresia) or of marked unequal size compared with the donor's common bile duct (Fig 57–4). Improvements in surgical technique, new technologic advances such as the venovenous bypass, the availability of UW solution, and the ability to control coagulation have decreased operative mortality rates and expanded the preservation time.

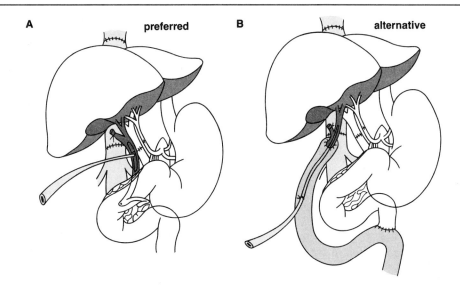

Figure 57–4. Liver transplantation. The preferred method **(A)** and the alternative technique **(B)** are shown. The donor suprahepatic vena cava, infrahepatic vena cava, portal vein, and hepatic artery are anastomosed end to end to the corresponding recipient vessels. When the recipient common duct is intact and the size matches the donor common duct, a choledochocholedochostomy **(A)** is performed. When the recipient duct is not intact (eg, biliary atresia or sclerosing cholangitis), a choledochojejunostomy **(B)** is used.

Outcome

Early graft failure, also known as primary non-function, may be a devastating complication if the patient does not receive a second transplant. Primary nonfunction is really a spectrum of diseases that range from no graft function (and certain death without retransplantation) to a liver whose function is mildly impaired at the outset but regains function within the first few days or weeks after transplantation. Factors related to primary nonfunction include the nature of the donor injury, the donor retrieval operation, the preservation solution, the length of preservation, host immunologic factors, the transplant operation, and host cardiovascular factors. Infectious complications after transplantation are frequent. Survival after infection relates to the type of offending organisms. Bacterial infections from pulmonary, bladder, and vascular sites usually respond to antibiotics, but fungal or viral infections may be associated with higher mortality and morbidity rates. Rejection is common after liver transplantation and may be seen in 75% of patients when defined by histologic means alone (see below). Rejection can be readily diagnosed (see below) by frequent percutaneous biopsies and is easily and successfully treated when diagnosed early. Late failure is due to chronic rejection or recurrence of the original disease. A particularly virulent type of rejection that is associated with damage to bile ducts and disappearance of bile ducts may be associated with early graft loss. The survival rate at 1 year following liver transplantation ranges between 70 and 90% and is about 60% at 5 years.

Cross-matching & Immunosuppression

Decisions regarding the suitability of the donor organ for liver transplantation are currently based on ABO blood matching and organ size. HLA antigen typing is not used to match donors and recipients, although an inverse relationship between matching and survival has been reported. Many liver transplants are performed in children, so the donor liver must be of an appropriate size to fit into the child's abdominal cavity. Recently the use of livers that are made surgically smaller has drastically changed the approach to transplant in small recipients. The use of partial grafts from live donors is an extension of the work with pared-down organs from cadavers. Cross-matches are not routinely performed preoperatively but usually postoperatively. There are only a few reports of hyperacute rejection when the liver recipient has preformed antibodies against the donor. The apparent resistance of the liver to hyperacute rejection is interesting, but its cause is unknown. It has been suggested that perhaps the liver is not sensitive to preformed antibodies or that the liver mass itself results in dilution of the antibody titer to a level that is not harmful. There have been reports of combination liver and kidney transplants in recipient-donor combinations with a positive cross-match that becomes

negative upon completion of the liver transplant. There has been no demonstration of increased antibody fixation to the graft. However, loss of cytotoxic antibodies could be due to the formation of soluble immune complexes. Alternatively, it may be that the blood loss associated with the liver transplant operation may dilute the antibody titers.

Rejection is readily diagnosed by percutaneous biopsy, and consensus is accumulating regarding the histologic features of acute rejection. Nonetheless, other causes of hepatic malfunction must be considered. Biliary obstruction, vascular thrombosis, viral hepatitis, drug toxicity, and recurrence of the underlying disease must all be excluded. Signs and symptoms of rejection include fever, abdominal pain, ascites, hepatomegaly, and decreased appetite, all of which are nonspecific. Laboratory abnormalities do not predict for rejection but include elevation of serum bilirubin, alkaline phosphatase, and transaminases. The histopathologic features that suggest rejection include a mixed cellular portal infiltrate with bile duct epithelial damage and central vein or portal vein endothelial damage. Treatment of rejection includes the use of methylprednisolone, antilymphoblast globulin, or monoclonal antibody OKT 3; more recently, FK-506 has been used to treat refractory rejection. The use of these drugs depends on an assessment of the severity of the rejection process.

Cyclosporin has had a major impact on the results after liver transplantation. Prior to the cyclosporin era, the 1-year patient survival was in the range of 30–40%. This changed markedly after 1979 with the introduction of cyclosporin. Current protocols at most centers call for cyclosporin and prednisone with or without azathioprine as prophylaxis against rejection. A few centers use antilymphocyte preparations in addition as rejection prophylaxis. Bile salts are necessary for the gastrointestinal absorption of cyclosporin, and if bile output is poor, inadequate absorption may necessitate intravenous administration of the drug. Although hepatotoxicity has been reported with cyclosporin, it is rare, and elevated postoperative liver function tests usually have another cause. The use of cyclosporin may be limited by its nephrotoxicity, which is compounded in patients with recent hepatorenal syndrome. The bone marrow suppression seen with azathioprine may be more pronounced in hypersplenic cirrhotic patients. New immunosuppressive agents in clinical trials include FK-506, RS-61443 (mycophenolate mofetil), and 15-deoxysporgualin. Advances in the field of immunosuppression are eagerly awaited to avoid the complications of the currently used immunosuppressive agents.

PANCREAS TRANSPLANTATION

Unlike liver transplantation, which often is life-saving, pancreas transplantation can be considered only life-enhancing at present. The rationale for the use of pancreas transplantation is that replacement of the ability to metabolize glucose normally will prevent the secondary sequelae of diabetes: nephropathy, neuropathy, and retinopathy. Pancreas transplantation can be performed with the whole organ, a segmental graft, or dispersed islets of Langerhans. The purpose of all three techniques is to provide biologically responsive insulin-producing tissue. Most uremic diabetic patients improve considerably with a kidney transplantation, but other long-term complications of diabetes, ie, retinopathy, angiopathy, and neuropathy, do not improve. The autoimmune pathogenesis of type I insulin-dependent diabetes mellitus is evidenced by mononuclear cell infiltrate, which is seen surrounding the islets of Langerhans, and by the presence of circulatory autoantibodies directed against islet cytoplasm and cell surface antigen, which can be found in the sera of some type I diabetics (see Chapter 32). There is also a strong association of insulin-dependent diabetes mellitus with other organ-specific autoimmune endocrinopathies, and there is an association with certain HLA types of HLA-DR3 and -DR4 and -DQµ3.2 alleles. The histologic finding that the infiltrating lymphocytes are of the cytotoxic/suppressor T cell (CD8) phenotype resembles that seen in other autoimmune diseases and in allograft rejection. Therefore, distinguishing recurrent autoimmune disease from rejection in transplanted pancreatic tissue may prove difficult. More than 1500 pancreas transplants have been performed throughout the world. It may be expected that higher graft survival would be associated with transplants between HLA-identical siblings and with pancreases from donors who previously had given a kidney to the recipient. However, insulitis has occurred in a number of living-related transplants between identical twins and in a number of failed transplants from related donors. These findings have decreased the enthusiasm for the use of well-matched grafts from relatives.

Indications

Ideally, pancreas transplantation should be performed before the patient has developed any of the secondary complications of diabetes. However, not all diabetic patients suffer from secondary complications, and in fact only about 40% of individuals with type I diabetes will develop uremia. It has been difficult to balance the risk of long-term immunosuppression against the risks of developing systemic complications of diabetes. Therefore, pancreas transplantation to date has been performed on patients who were uremic and required a simultaneous renal transplant. However, a few centers now perform pancreas transplants in patients who have neither uremia nor kidney transplantation but have other progressive secondary complications that outweigh the risk of long-term immunosuppression. Changes in renal glo-

merular basement membrane thickness before other evidence of renal malfunction may be an indication for the progression of the diabetic process.

Procedure

For the whole-organ or segmental pancreas graft, the pancreas is removed from the donor and preserved in cold storage so that it can be transported from a distant retrieval site to the facility where transplantation will take place. Preservation time in UW solution has exceeded 20 hours. Pancreas transplantation can either be done simultaneously with implantation of the kidney or sequentially in a post-kidney transplant patient with stable renal function. Simultaneous implantation of the kidney allows the use of kidney function and kidney biopsy as a marker for rejection. Various surgical techniques are used for implantation of the pancreas graft. The grafts are implanted either as a whole organ with a small button of donor duodenum or as a distal segment of the pancreas.

Outcome

The major complications following pancreas transplantation are infection, vascular thrombosis, preservation injury, rejection, and pancreatitis. Overall graft function and patient survival rates have improved steadily since the first clinical pancreas transplant was performed in 1966. The present overall pancreas graft survival at 1 year in patients who have received a simultaneous kidney transplant is over 80%. In the past, the pancreas graft survival for isolated pancreas transplants was often less than 50%. The poorer outcome of isolated pancreas transplants has been attributed to the lack of good markers for rejection in the absence of a simultaneously rejecting kidney. However, the graft survival of isolated pancreas transplants has improved dramatically over the last 2 years. This improved survival has been attributed to stricter matching criteria and better techniques for monitoring rejection.

Cross-matching & Immunosuppression

Pancreas transplant donors and recipients are typed and matched for ABO and HLA antigens, and a transplant is not performed in the face of a positive cross-match. The exact role of tissue typing has not been clearly defined, largely owing to small numbers of patients. In patients who have received simultaneous pancreas-kidney transplant, both organs are not uniformly rejected, but rejection of their kidney graft can frequently be used to predict ongoing rejection of the pancreas. Nonetheless, in some instances the pancreas has failed (presumably owing to rejection) while the kidney graft continues to function. The benefits of HLA-DR matching in isolated cadaveric pancreas transplantation have clearly been demonstrated.

Rejection of the vascularized pancreatic allograft is recognized by a loss of control over blood glucose levels. This, however, is unfortunately a relatively insensitive and late finding. Disappearance of insulin from the circulation usually parallels the plasma glucose levels and consequently cannot be used as an early indicator of rejection. Corticosteroids used for immunosuppression also tend to cause diabetogenic effects. Serum amylase levels have not been useful previously in diagnosis of rejection. However, in transplants drained into the urinary system, low levels of urinary amylase are suggestive of graft failure. This finding usually precedes changes in blood glucose levels by 24 or 48 hours, therefore allowing time for institution of antirejection therapy.

The current practice at some centers is to perform a biopsy of the graft when there is a question of rejection, even when diagnosis is not assured. The presence of vasculitis is the only certain histologic evidence for rejection because parenchymal fibrosis and inflammatory-cell infiltrate may be secondary to foreign body reaction, particularly in grafts with polymer-injected ducts or grafts associated with recurrent disease. Successful immunosuppression for pancreas transplantation appears to be more difficult than for kidney or liver transplantation. Rejection is usually treated with intravenous bolus corticosteroids, an increase in the oral prednisone dose, or a temporary course of OKT 3.

Islet Cell Transplantation

A successful placement of isolated islets between nonidentical donor-recipient pairs has been a goal for some time. Initially it was hoped that unmodified islet transplants might display the prolonged survival of other endocrine tissue. However, survival of isolated islet allografts is shorter than survival of allografts of skin, kidney, or heart regardless of placement site. Syngeneic grafts implanted in the liver, under the kidney capsule, produce insulin and are able to reverse hyperglycemia, virally induced diabetes, diabetes induced by beta cell toxins, and spontaneous diabetes in BB rats and NOD mice. Since autografts cannot be used in most clinical situations, the major experimental thrust has been to perfect allograft islet transplantation.

Islet cells are obtained from either adult or fetal pancreas. The fetal pancreas contains less connective tissue, so that the relative yield of viable islets is greater but still not sufficient to render a recipient normoglycemic. The basic method for retrieving islets is via mechanical separation followed by enzymatic digestion, usually with collagenase. Secondary steps of separation are required to remove as much nonislet tissue as possible; this usually necessitates manual removal of islet tissue. The purer the islet cell separation, the longer the graft survives. Nonetheless, islets themselves contain dendritic cells and other cells capable of stimulating an immune response. A number of investigators have tried different means of reducing immunogenicity of islet tissue, such as

treatment with anti-class II monoclonal antibody or irradiation. Culturing of pure islets in an oxygen-rich atmosphere has been successful in decreasing tissue immunogenicity. An alterative method that has been successful in rats and mice involves encapsulation of individual islets within a semipermeable biologic membrane across which immunocompetent cells cannot pass. All of these experiments have been performed in animal models, with prolonged reversal of the diabetic state when modified islet allografts were used. Although islet transplantation has been slow to develop as a therapy for type I diabetes, recent success of allotransplanted islets from a single cadaveric donor has been reported. In these cases, unpurified islets from a single pancreas were transplanted into the portal vein of the uremic recipient simultaneously with a kidney from the same donor. Two recipients have remained normal for over 6 months. The further clinical application of this work remains to be realized.

HEART TRANSPLANTATION

In 1983 the International Society of Heart and Lung Transplantation (ISHLT) began to maintain a registry of patients undergoing all forms of thoracic organ transplantation. The 1992 report listed almost 22,000 patients who had undergone cardiac transplantation since the registry was begun. Annually, about 2700 patients throughout the world undergo transplants in more than 200 centers, most of which are in the USA.

The indication for cardiac transplantation is the presence of end-stage cardiac disease that is not amenable to conventional medical-surgical treatment. In adults, the main indications are coronary artery disease and idiopathic dilated cardiomyopathy. Among children, the main indications are congenital heart disease that cannot be successfully treated or palliated by conventional means and cardiomyopathy. All age groups have been transplanted successfully, and operative techniques have been developed to deal with even the most complex congenital cardiac venous and arterial anatomic malformations. The current operative mortality is less than 10% for most patients. Even patients requiring intravenous pharmacologic or mechanical circulatory support (intra-aortic balloon pump, ventricular assist device, total artificial heart) can undergo cardiac transplantation with outcomes that are not significantly different from those in less critically ill patients. Elevated pulmonary vascular resistance, congenital heart disease, and repeat transplantation are the most important operative risk factors. The only absolute contraindications are irreversible pulmonary vascular disease, uncontrollable infection or cancer, and the presence of a separate life-threatening disease. Relative contraindications include advanced generalized organ dysfunction (CNS, hepatic, renal) as a consequence of poor cardiac function, a recent pulmonary infarct, or a separate disease process that would significantly affect or be affected by immunosuppression (cholelithiasis, peptic ulcer disease, diverticulosis, peripheral vascular disease, etc). Patients with a history of medical noncompliance or who are at increased risk of noncompliance because of drug and/or alcohol addiction or psychiatric conditions are not good candidates for any form of organ transplantation.

Cardiac donors are heart-beating brain-dead cadavers with good cardiac function and no significant history or risk factors for cardiac disease. Donors and recipients are matched in terms of ABO blood group compatibility and approximate size. Recipients are screened pretransplant for HLA antibodies, and an elevated panel-reactive antibody (> 15%) or a highly specific antibody specificity is an indication for prospective donor-recipient cross-matching. The extreme shortage of cardiac donors in recent years has led to considerable relaxation of the criteria for donor suitability. Currently, advanced donor age is no longer a contraindication provided cardiac function is satisfactory and any coronary disease is either mild or else amenable to conventional coronary artery bypass or angioplasty. Clinical outcomes following cardiac transplantation from donors older than 50 years are only marginally inferior to those seen with younger donors. Ventricular hypertrophy, requirement for moderate inotropic support, and short periods of severe hypotension or cardiac arrest are no longer exclusionary provided Echocardiographic and visual assessment of cardiac function are adequate.

Heart procurement occurs at the donor's hospital, usually remote from the recipient and almost always in conjunction with multiorgan retrieval. The coronary circulation is flushed with a cold electrolyte solution at the time of procurement. The heart is then excised and stored under hypothermic conditions until it is implanted in the recipient. The maximal safe duration of ex vivo preservation with current techniques is about 6 hours, and most groups try to limit preservation times to less than 4 hours. With high-speed civilian jet travel this limits the maximal radius for cardiac procurement to within 2000 miles from the transplant center. It also limits the time available for HLA matching or cross-matching. Methods to extend the tolerable limits of cardiac ischemia are currently the subject of a lot of laboratory and clinical research.

There are 2 operative techniques for cardiac transplantation. Both require cardiopulmonary bypass. In the heterotopic or piggy-back technique, the recipient's heart remains in its usual location and the donor heart is connected in a parallel configuration, which results in the donor heart being positioned in the right pleural space. In the orthotopic technique the recipient's ventricles are completely excised and the donor heart is positioned in its normal mediastinal

location. The heterotopic technique is technically more difficult, offers few advantages over the orthotopic technique, and is infrequently performed at present. There is commonly a transient period of systolic and diastolic biventricular dysfunction accompanied by bradycardia in the first few days posttransplantation. In most cases this responds to pharmacologic treatment, and in the absence of rejection in the late posttransplant period, resting hemodynamics are remarkably normal.

Maintenance immunosuppression is usually initiated with cyclosporin, azathioprine, and corticosteroids. Doses of the individual drugs are then continuously monitored and adjusted to produce the desired level of immunosuppression with minimum toxicity or side effects. Many patients have been successfully weaned from chronic corticosteroids. Early trials with FK-506 in cardiac transplantation indicate that this drug may be as effective as cyclosporin. Induction of immunosuppression therapy with anti-lymphocyte sera or monoclonal anti-T cell antibodies is also practiced by many groups.

Hyperacute rejection has been observed only rarely in cardiac transplantation and then usually only on the basis of postmortem examination. There is no effective treatment other than retransplantation, which is rarely possible under the circumstances. Prospective donor-recipient cross-matching of recipients with high levels of HLA antibodies reduces but does not entirely eliminate this problem. Acute rejection occurs frequently, the incidence diminishing with time over the first 6–12 months posttransplant and then remaining at a low but stable level thereafter. There are few symptoms and signs associated with early rejection and no noninvasive diagnostic studies that are completely reliable. The diagnosis of acute allograft rejection therefore rests on the basis of the histologic findings on endomyocardial biopsies, which must be performed at intervals throughout the remainder of the posttransplant period. Diagnosis of allograft rejection is made on the basis of endomyocardial biopsy performed through a transvenous catheter placed in the right jugular vein. A mononuclear cell infiltrate is the characteristic hallmark of rejection. Lymphocytes, lymphoblasts, and monocytes are the predominant cell types in acute rejection. Evidence of tissue damage is found in necrosis of myocardial fibers and edema, which further impairs perfusion and function. Electrocardiographic changes of decreased voltage, sometimes associated with arrhythmias and signs of congestive heart failure, can also be demonstrated during rejection episodes. Treatment of rejection includes the use of ALG and increased levels of corticosteroids. Chronic rejection is the major cause of late deaths (> 1 year posttransplant) among cardiac transplant recipients. It manifests as a diffuse obliterative coronary vasculopathy, which results in myocardial infarction and cardiac arrhythmias. The angiographic incidence of any coronary disease at 4 years posttransplant may be as high as 40%. To date there has been no specific treatment that has been shown to either prevent or halt the progression of the disease. Interestingly, the disease is seen almost exclusively in recipients who develop HLA antibodies in the posttransplant period, suggesting that humoral mechanisms may be playing an important role.

Acute allograft rejection is treated with short-term augmented corticosteroids (normal allograft function and moderate rejection) or cytolytic therapy, anti-lymphocyte sera, or OKT 3 (abnormal allograft function, corticosteroid-resistant rejection, or severe rejection, respectively). Most rejection episodes resolve without long-term hemodynamic or functional sequelae. Selected recipients with particularly frequent episodes of rejection may benefit from total lymphoid irradiation.

Currently, the average patient and graft survivals in the ISHLT registry are 78.3, 66.8, and 52.5% at 1, 5, and 10 years, respectively. At 2 years after transplantation 85% of recipients are in New York Heart Association functional class I and 13% are in class II; up to 60% have been able to return to work or school full-time.

COMBINED HEART-LUNG & LUNG TRANSPLANTATION

Before 1980, more than 35 attempts at pulmonary transplantation including 3 combined heart lung-transplants were performed in humans. The median survival for the entire group was less than 2 weeks. One patient survived for 10 months, but the function of the graft in this case was poor. The excellent early results with cyclosporin-based immunosuppression protocols in both animal and human cardiac transplantation in the early 1980s encouraged investigators at Stanford University to reattempt combined heart-lung transplantation first in primates and shortly thereafter in humans. In these early experiments, healing of the supracarinal tracheal anastomosis was almost always successful, which had not been the case in the previous experience with isolated lung transplantation, in which bronchial anastomotic complications (eg, dehiscence or stenosis) were the major cause of death among patients who survived beyond the first week. Thus, combined heart-lung transplantation was initially thought to be the safest operative procedure for all patients with end-stage cardiopulmonary or pulmonary disease and isolated lung transplantation was relegated to the laboratory. Then in a series of well-designed canine experiments, investigators at the University of Toronto defined the adverse effects of high-dose perioperative corticosteroid therapy, the neutral effect of cyclosporin therapy, and the beneficial effect of omental wrap-

ping on bronchial anastomotic healing. They also performed the first successful human single-lung transplant in 1983 in a patient with pulmonary fibrosis and rekindled worldwide interest in single-lung transplantation. In the past decade, single-lung transplantation has emerged as the preferred procedure for most types of end-stage pulmonary disease. Patients with pulmonary sepsis (eg, those with cystic fibrosis) require bilateral lung replacement and now undergo either combined heart-lung transplantation or simultaneous bilateral single-lung transplantation.

The ISHLT also maintains a registry for patients undergoing combined heart-lung and lung transplantation. In 1992 there were 1212 patients in the registry who had undergone combined heart-lung transplantation, 716 patients who had undergone single-lung transplantation, and 289 patients who had undergone bilateral lung replacement. As in cardiac transplantation, the major limiting factor affecting further transplantation remains the limited donor organ availability.

The indication for combined heart-lung or lung transplantation is still the presence of an end-stage disease for which there are no alternative treatments that can restore satisfactory survival or function. Major clinical categories include (1) pulmonary vascular disease, either primary pulmonary hypertension or Eisenmenger's syndrome secondary to congenital heart disease; (2) restrictive lung disease including idiopathic pulmonary fibrosis; (3) obstructive lung disease such as emphysema secondary to α_1-anti-trypsin deficiency; and finally (4) diseases such as bronchiectasis and cystic fibrosis, which produce a mixed restrictive and obstructive picture. All age groups have undergone transplantation successfully, and the indications for single-lung transplantation have been extended to include patients with Eisenmenger's syndrome and correctable intracardiac shunts (atrial septal defects, ventricular septal defects, patent ductus arteriosus). Current operative mortalities for single-lung, bilateral-lung and combined heart-lung transplantation are 12.6, 13.6, and 21% respectively.

Absolute contraindications for single- or bilateral-lung transplantation include concomitant cardiac failure, particularly severe right ventricular dysfunction; uncontrollable infection or cancer; and the presence of a separate life-threatening disease. Preoperative low-dose steroids, prior intrathoracic surgery, and tracheostomy are relative contraindications. A few ventilator-dependent patients have undergone transplantation successfully, but the presence of severe cachexia or multiorgan failure has invariably proven fatal.

Lung donors are heart-beating brain-dead cadavers with good pulmonary function, no evidence of pulmonary sepsis, and a negative history or risk factors for pulmonary disease. Obviously, combined heart-lung donors must also satisfy the requirements for cardiac donation. Donors and recipients are matched in terms of approximate size including thoracic dimensions and ABO compatability. If pretransplant screening of the recipient for HLA antibodies was positive, a preoperative cross-match is also performed. For purposes of single-lung transplantation, unilateral lung disease in the donor is not necessarily a contraindication provided function of the contralateral lung is satisfactory.

Combined heart-lung or lung procurement occurs at the donor's hospital almost always as part of a multiple-organ retrieval. If necessary the heart and lungs can be separated and used in 3 recipients. Both the pulmonary artery and coronary circulation are flushed with hypothermic electrolyte solutions at the time of procurement. Lungs preserved in this way can be safely maintained for up to 10 hours, which markedly extends the safe procurement radius over that available for cardiac transplantation, providing additional time for sequential bilateral lung transplantation and HLA typing or cross-matching if they are required.

Immunosuppression following lung transplantation is carried out with cyclosporin, azathioprine, and corticosteroids, with dosages adjusted for maximal immunosuppressive efficacy and minimal toxicity. Some groups withhold routine corticosteroid therapy for 2–3 weeks following transplantation to allow for tracheal/bronchial anastomotic healing. Others believe that with modification of the bronchial anastomotic technique, routine postoperative corticosteroid administration is not detrimental and that by avoiding early acute rejection episodes the ultimate clinical result is better. The optimal early immunosuppression protocol is unknown at present.

Acute rejection in the early postoperative period must be differentiated from the effects of organ preservation, interruption of lymphatic drainage, and infection. This is often a difficult distinction. The initial attempts to diagnose pulmonary rejection by bronchoscopic and pulmonary function tests have evolved from the early animal experiments, and now characteristic histologic findings for both acute and chronic rejection have been described on the basis of endobronchial biopsy results. Acute pulmonary rejection occurs frequently, and asynchronous rejection of the heart and lungs in recipients of combined heart-lung transplantation has been observed. Chronic pulmonary rejection evidenced as obliterative bronchiolitis occurs with equal frequency in recipients of combined heart-lung transplantation and isolated lung transplantation. At least 30% of the operative survivors ultimately develop symptoms and signs of obliterative bronchiolitis, and in most it follows a progressively downhill and ultimately fatal course. In some patients obliterative bronchiolitis may be associated with repetitive pulmonary infections with CMV or *Pseudomonas* species. Augmentation of immunosuppression has halted the progression of disease in others.

Acute pulmonary rejection is treated with short-term augmented corticosteroids or cytolytic therapy (ALG or OKT 3), and most rejection episodes resolve without long-term sequelae. Pulmonary infections remain an important long-term source of morbidity and mortality. Currently, the average patient survivals in the ISHLT registry are 59% and 42% for combined heart-lung transplantation at 1 and 5 years, respectively; 69 and 62.5% for single-lung transplantation at 1 and 2 years, respectively; and 62 and 51% for bilateral lung transplantation at 1 and 2 years, respectively.

James Hardy at the University of Mississippi attempted the world's first human heart transplant in 1964. This occurred prior to the acceptance of the concept of a heart-beating brain-dead human organ donor, and consequently a chimpanzee donor was used. Although the operation was described as technically successful, there was a substantial size difference and the recipient died within a few hours as a result of inadequate cardiac output. The next 2 attempts were performed on separate continents in December 1967. The second recorded attempt was performed between 2 adults, the donor having first suffered a cardiac arrest before the heart was resuscitated and transplanted by Christiaan Barnard in Cape Town, South Africa. The recipient survived for 18 days. The third attempt was carried out a few days after the Cape Town transplant by Adrian Kantrowitz at Columbia University in New York. The donor in this instance was an anencephalic infant and the recipient was a child with severe congenital heart disease. This attempt was unsuccessful as well. However, the interest of the cardiovascular community was captured, and during the following year over 100 heart transplants were performed in more than 20 centers worldwide. The 1-year survival for this group of patients was only 20%, a reflection of inappropriate recipient and donor selection as well as inadequate perioperative care, particularly immunosuppression. Faced with these dismal results, most groups abandoned clinical cardiac transplantation. However, the few groups who persisted with both laboratory and clinical programs throughout the 1970s were able to solve many of the problems, and their patient survival rates improved considerably. Undoubtedly the next most significant step was the development of cyclosporin-based immunosuppression protocols in the early 1980s, which resulted in markedly reduced early mortality from acute rejection and infection. Subsequently there was an exponential growth worldwide both in the number of centers and in the number of patients undergoing cardiac transplantation until 1988, when further increase was limited by the donor supply.

BONE MARROW TRANSPLANTATION

Modern clinical bone marrow transplantation began in 1968, when a small number of patients with severe combined immunodeficiency disease (SCID), Wiskott-Aldrich syndrome, or advanced leukemia received infusions of marrow from HLA-identical siblings. Previous observations in animals had shown that matching the donor and recipient at the MHC loci reduced the incidence of graft-versus-host (GVH) disease and improved survival rates. Many patients have now survived for more than 2 decades after bone marrow transplantation for a variety of malignant and nonmalignant hematologic diseases. Laboratory and clinical advances in such areas as histocompatibility typing, prevention of GVH disease, improved supportive care, and reduction of the risk of relapse have made bone marrow transplantation a realistic and successful form of treatment for several previously uniformly fatal diseases (Tables 57–1 and 57–2).

Until recently, most donors for bone marrow transplantation have been either identical twins (syngeneic) or genotypically HLA-identical individuals (allogeneic). However, only 30% of patients can be expected to have an HLA-identical donor, and efforts to use marrow from partially matched family members or phenotypically matched unrelated donors are beginning to be successful. For diseases not involving the marrow, autologous transplantation allows the use of high-dose chemoradiotherapy and avoids the risk of GVH disease. Provocative studies with monoclonal antibodies to leukemic and other malignant cells or with in vitro chemotherapy treatment have given credence to the idea that such marrow "purging" techniques could greatly extend the benefit of autologous transplantation to patients assumed to have indiscernible neoplastic cells remaining in the marrow.

Table 57–1. Diseases treatable by bone marrow transplantation.

Allogeneic/Syngeneic	Autologous
Aplastic anemia	Leukemia
Leukemia	AML
AML	ALL
ALL	Multiple myeloma
CML	Non-Hodgkin lymphoma
Myelodysplasia	Hodgkin disease
Multiple myeloma	Solid tumors
Non-Hodgkin lymphoma	Breast
Hodgkin disease	Lung
Immunodeficiencies	Ovarian
Common variable	Testicular
SCID	Neuroblastoma
Wiskott-Aldrich syndrome	
Agranulocytosis	
Osteopetrosis/genetic diseases	

Table 57–2. Genetic diseases treatable by bone marrow transplantation.

SCID
Wiskott-Aldrich syndrome
Fanconi's anemia
Kostmann's syndrome
Chronic granulomatous disease
Osteopetrosis
Ataxia-telangiectasia
Diamond-Blackfan syndrome
Mucocutaneous candidiasis
Chédiak-Higashi syndrome
Cartilage-hair hypoplasia
Mucopolysaccharidosis
Gaucher's disease
Thalassemia major
Sickle cell anemia

Indications & Results

A. SCID: Bone marrow transplantation is the treatment of choice for children with congenital SCID and its variants. For HLA-matched transplants, no immunosuppressive conditioning is necessary. Partially matched recipients require conditioning, usually with cyclophosphamide and busulfan. The removal of T cells from donor marrow by lectin agglutination or monoclonal antibody and complement lysis enables parents of haploidentical children with these disorders to serve as donors.

B. Aplastic Anemia: Severe aplastic anemia has a mortality rate of 90% when treated with supportive care. Allogeneic bone marrow transplantation increases survival to 60% overall and to 80% in patients younger than 30 years. Furthermore, if patients are able to avoid pretransplantation transfusions—and hence presensitization—the overall actuarial survival at 10 years increases to 80–90%. Unlike the case for leukemia, rejection of the donor marrow in patients with aplastic anemia has been a major cause of failure (15–30% versus 1% for leukemia); this is probably due to the underlying autoimmune nature of the aplasia in some patients, to presensitization by transfusions, and to the lack of radiotherapy in the stand and conditioning regimen. New immunosuppressive regimens appear to be beneficial in reducing graft rejection without causing excessive toxicity. These approaches include the addition of either ATG or total lymphoid irradiation to high-dose cyclophosphamide.

For patients without marrow donors or for those over age 55, the treatment of choice is immunosuppressive therapy with ATG (possibly combined with cyclosporin). This therapy produces responses and 5-year survival in 60% of patients. However, long-term survivors may develop myelodysplasia, reflecting underlying bone marrow injury.

C. Acute Myelogenous Leukemia (AML): AML is now a curable malignancy, in both children and adults. With improvements in supportive care, adults up to age 60 should now be approached with curative intent. Once an initial complete remission has been achieved with intensive chemotherapy, several potentially curative options are available. Nonablative intensive chemotherapy offers a 30–40% chance of long-term survival.

For patients with histocompatible siblings, allogeneic bone marrow transplantation in first remission offers a 60% long-term cure rate. However, this comes at the expense of a 20–25% treatment-related mortality rate in the first 6 months. The improved disease control (15–20% relapse rate compared with 55–65% for chemotherapy) is due both to the high-dose ablative chemoradiotherapy and to an alloimmune function of the marrow graft, "graft-versus-leukemia" (GVL) effect.

For patients without suitable donors or in older patients, autologous bone marrow transplantation offers the advantage of improved disease control from ablative therapy. However, in the absence of GVL, the relapse rate would be expected to be higher than in allogeneic bone marrow transplantation. Autologous bone marrow transplantation is a far less morbid procedure, with treatment-related mortality less than 5%. Preliminary results of autologous bone marrow transplantation report relapse rates of 20–40% and long-term survival in 40–70% of cases.

D. Chronic Myelogenous Leukemia (CML): For patients with chronic myelogenous leukemia (CML) there had been no hope for cure and no improvement in survival over the past 50 years. Data now clearly show that allogeneic bone marrow transplantation will provide a 60–80% relapse-free survival in patients with CML in chronic phase. More favorable results are produced when the transplant is performed within 1 year of diagnosis and when patients are younger than 30 years. Results in patients with more advanced CML are inferior. For patients without suitable sibling donors, a search for a matched correlated donor should be performed through the National Marrow Donor Program (NMDP).

E. Acute Lymphoblastic Leukemia (ALL): ALL is now a curable malignancy in both children and adults. Conventional nonablative chemotherapy is curative in 60–90% of children and 30–60% of adults, depending on a number of factors. Allogeneic bone marrow transplantation is usually reserved for patients in second remission or in those with high-risk cytogenetics that predict a poor outcome with conventional therapy. Allogeneic bone marrow transplantation offers a 30–50% cure rate in second remission. Autologous bone marrow transplantation is not as successful as in AML but remains on option for patients without donors.

Procedure

Unlike other organ transplants, bone marrow aspirated from the iliac crests of a donor is entirely regenerated in 8 weeks. Since the amount harvested is less than 20% of the total, the donor is not harmed immunologically or hematologically. Multiple aspirations of 5 mL each, yielding a total of 10 mL/kg of the recipient's body weight (600–1200 mL), are obtained in a single procedure under general or epidural anesthesia. The marrow is drawn through heparinized needles and placed into heparinized, buffered culture medium. This mixture is then gently filtered through fine stainless steel mesh screens to produce a single-cell suspension. Nucleated-cell counts are checked to ensure the adequacy of the withdrawn marrow. If the donor and recipient are ABO-compatible, 2×10^8 to 6×10^8 nucleated marrow cells/kg of the recipient's weight are infused intravenously together with erythrocytes (erythrocyte volume of 20–30%). If the donor and recipient are not ABO-compatible, the erythrocytes must be removed from the donor's marrow in vitro.

Except in patients with SCID, destruction of the recipient's immune system is necessary to prevent rejection and to allow transplantation of an entirely new hematopoietic system, including new immunocompetent cells. This is usually accomplished by giving cyclophophamide, 50–60 mg/kg for 4 or 2 days (the higher dose for patients not receiving total-body irradiation). The dose of total-body irradiation is 1000–1400 cGy, which is usually administered in fractions over 3–5 days rather than in a single dose, to avoid toxicity to the lungs and eyes. This combination of chemotherapy and radiotherapy provides a potent immunoablative and antineoplastic function for most cancer patients.

Following preparative chemoradiotherapy and infusion of the marrow, patients are extremely vulnerable to infections. The early and aggressive use of broad-spectrum antibiotics and amphotericin B is critical. The role of trimethoprim-sulfamethoxazole in preventing *Pneumocystis carinii* pneumonia is clearly established. Ganciclovir is effective in reducing the risk of CMV infections and pneumonitis. Platelet transfusions, on the other hand, are given to keep the platelet count above 15,000/μL to prevent serious spontaneous hemorrhage. All blood products must be irradiated to prevent GVH disease due to viable lymphocytes in transfused cellular components or plasma.

Engraftment is heralded by a rising leukocyte count and the appearance of circulating mature neutrophils 2–4 weeks after transplantation. In general, all hematopoietic and immune cells of the recipient are replaced by donor cells, although there are rare examples of mixed "chimerism," most often in children who receive transplants for immunodeficiency diseases. As peripheral counts improve, antibiotics can be discontinued and transfusions become unnecessary. Patients can be discharged when they can be observed closely as outpatients for at least the first 100 days after transplantation.

Posttransplantation Complications

The major obstacles to successful bone marrow transplantation are GVH disease, infections, interstitial pneumonia, venoocclusive liver disease, and relapse of the underlying disease. GVH disease and infections are responsible for 10–30% of morbidity and mortality in the first 100 days following transplantation.

Graft-versus-Host (GVH) Disease

The presence of immunocompetent donor cells in an immunocompromised host is a prerequisite for GVH disease. In patients who are HLA-identical with their donors, the occurrence of GVH disease is attributed to "minor," presently undetectable differences in histocompatibility.

The clinical syndrome of acute GVH disease in humans consists of skin rash, severe diarrhea, and jaundice. Pathophysiologically, immunocompetent CD8 T cells can be found in biopsy specimens of the skin, intestine, and liver. These tissues appear to be especially at risk because they are rich in surface DR antigens. The skin rash of acute GVH disease usually begins at the time of engraftment, 10–28 days after transplantation. It is a fine, diffuse, erythematous, macular rash often beginning on the palms, soles, or head and spreading to involve the entire trunk and sometimes the extremities. In severe GVH disease, the rash can become desquamative—the clinical equivalent of an extensive second-degree burn. Watery diarrhea is associated with malabsorption, cramps, and gastrointestinal bleeding when severe. Hyperbilirubinemia is due to GVH disease-induced inflammation of small bile ducts and is usually accompanied by an elevated serum alkaline phosphatase level. Elevations of alanine aminotransferase and aspartate aminotransferase are mild to moderate. A staging and grading system for GVH disease developed at the University of Washington has become standard (Table 57–3).

Successful prevention of acute GVH disease began with the use of methotrexate after transplantation. Initial studies found that approximately 50% of patients treated with methotrexate alone developed acute GVH disease within 10–70 days after grafting and that up to half of these died. More modern immunosuppressive therapy with both methotrexate and cyclosporin has reduced the risk of acute GVH disease to 20–40, with only 5–10% of cases being severe (grade III–IV). Cyclosporin is continued for the first 6 months after transplantation. Infusions of ATG, prednisone, and monoclonal antibodies have been used with limited success to treat established acute GVH disease. T cell depletion of donor marrow is highly successful in reducing GVH disease. Unfortunately, studies of patients receiving T cell-depleted marrow have shown an increased risk of rejection, higher relapse rate of leukemia, and increased risk of

Table 57–3. Clinical staging of GVH disease by organ system.

Stage	Skin	Liver	Gastrointestinal Tract
+	Maculopapular rash < 25% body surface	Serum bilirubin 2–3 mg/dL	> 500 mL diarrhea/d
+ +	Maculopapular rash 25–50% body surface	Serum bilirubin 3–6 mg/dL	> 1000 mL diarrhea/d
+ + +	Generalized erythroderma	Serum bilirubin 6–15 mg/dL	> 1500 mL diarrhea/d
+ + + +	Generalized erythroderma with bullous formation and desquamation	Serum bilirubin > 15 mg/dL	Severe abdominal pain with or without ileus

fungal infections. These findings support the concept that donor T cells have an active GVL effect. Efforts to fine-tune T cell depletion (by elective or incomplete depletion) are under way.

Chronic GVH disease affects 25–45% of patients surviving longer than 180 days. It occurs more frequently in older patients and in those with preceding acute GVH disease. Clinically, it most closely resembles the spectrum of rheumatic or autoimmune disorders, and its main clinical effect is to produce severe immunodeficiency, leading to recurrent and life-threatening infections, much like those seen in the congenital and acquired immunodeficiency syndromes. Treatment with prednisone, alone or in combination with azathioprine, can effectively reverse many of the manifestations of chronic GVH disease in 50–75% of affected patients.

Venoocclusive Disease of the Liver

High doses of chemoradiotherapy, such as that used to condition patients prior to marrow transplantation, can cause a fibrous obliteration of small hepatic venules, known as venoocclusive disease of the liver. About 20% of patients undergoing bone marrow transplantation develop venoocclusive disease, manifested clinically as hepatomegaly, ascites, hepatocellular necrosis, and encephalopathy within 8–20 days after transplantation. The disease resolves in 60% of patients but is fatal in 5–20%. There is no effective treatment.

The most important risk factor is the presence of hepatitis before transplantation, which, by serology and natural history, is usually non-A, non-B viral hepatitis associated with transfusions. Patients with transaminasemia before bone marrow transplantation are 3–4 times more likely to develop venoocclusive disease than are those with normal serum liver enzymes. Venoocclusive disease must be distinguished from GVH disease of the liver and from viral and fungal infections.

Infections

Infectious complications following bone marrow transplantation are from the profound lack of granulocytes and lymphocytes following ablation by the pretransplant conditioning regimen. Since full recovery of these 2 major elements of the immune system occurs separately following transplantation, it is not surprising that the risk of infection can be separated into 3 distinct phases (Table 57–4).

The first, and most dangerous, phase is the 2–4-week period prior to engraftment, when no circulating leukocytes are present. During this time, patients are at risk for both bacterial and fungal infections, which can advance extremely rapidly and cause death. Clinical experience and trials over the past 15 years have led to the aggressive, empirical use of broad-spectrum antibiotics (both antibacterial and antifungal). The recent increase in infections due to resistant species of staphylococci, especially *Staphylococcus epidermidis* responsive only to vancomycin, is most probably due to the use of tunneled, central intravenous catheters in these patients. As a result, vancomycin is empirically added to the antibiotic regimen when fever persists.

Two to 4 weeks after transplantation, the marrow begins to export granulocytes successfully to the blood; when the absolute neutrophil count reaches 500/μL and is rising, the greatest threat of bacterial infection is past. The second phase of potential infectious complications is due to the paucity and immaturity of the lymphocytes, and the greatest risk is due to fungal and viral agents during the second and third posttransplant months. An especially prominent and potent pathogen is *Aspergillus fumigatus,* which can cause vascular invasion in the lungs and brain. Although these infections can be treated with amphotericin B, they are difficult to eradicate and may be fatal. The most prominent viral pathogen is CMV. Ganciclovir prophylaxis has had a major impact on this problem. CMV pneumonitis, formerly uniformly fatal, can now be effectively treated with ganciclovir plus intravenous immunoglobulin.

The third phase of infectious complications occurs after the third month and lasts until the maturation of the lymphocytic arm of the immune system. This parallels the neonatal period and takes 6–18 months. During this time, there is an abnormal ratio of CD4 to CD8 T cells, T cells respond poorly to antigens, and immunoglobulin production is abnormal. This leads to a risk of infection by encapsulated bacteria such as pneumococci because of a lack of opsonic immunoglobulins. The higher risk of viral infection diminishes as T cell function gradually improves. Patients must remain relatively isolated until the immune system has fully recovered. Patients with chronic GVH disease may never recover full function of the immune system. However, the majority of surviving patients do recover full immunity and lead lives free from infection, requiring no antibiotics or other supplements. Unlike patients with solid-organ transplants, they do not need to take immunosuppressive medications to ensure engraftment, since the immune and hematopoietic systems are replaced. Once tolerance is achieved (by about 6 months after transplantation), all medications can gradually be discontinued, and patients are able to live completely normal lives.

BONE TRANSPLANTATION

Bone is more commonly transplanted than any other tissue. In general, bone-grafting operations are performed to promote healing of nonunited fractures, to restore structural integrity of the skeleton, and to facilitate cosmetic repair. Human skull defects larger than 2–3 cm are closed by neurosurgeons to protect the brain and restore bone integrity. Plastic surgeons, oral surgeons, and periodontists use fresh autografts and freeze-dried allografts in oral and maxillofacial surgery. Various bone grafts are used to promote stability of the spine and to correct spinal deformity. Autografts and allografts are used to repair the appendicular skeleton (arms and legs). When autograft sources are insufficient, allogeneic bone may be used but only in combination with an autograft, which provides a greater degree of early repair. Bone is procured for implantation by aseptic removal or by removal and subsequent sterilization by ethylene oxide or γ irradiation. Except for a fresh autograft, all other bone tissues are used after freezing because of the re-

Table 57–4. Sequence of infections after bone marrow transplant.

Phase	Infection
I Up to engraftment	Gram-positive cocci/central lines Gram-negative bacteria *Candida* *Aspergillus*

II
After initial engraftment
	Fungal
	  Aspergillus
	  Candida esophagitis
	Viral
	  CMV
	  Adenovirus
	  EBV
	  Respiratory syncytial virus, enterovirus, parainfluenza, papovaviruses

III Late	Sinopulmonary (sicca syndrome, IgA deficiency) *Streptococcus pneumoniae/ Haemophilus influenzae* Varicella-zoster virus

duction in immunogenicity achieved by this storage technique.

Posttransplantation Course

Following grafting, one of 3 courses can occur: (1) the bone graft may become viable, acquiring the mechanical, cosmetic, and biologic characteristics of adjacent bone; (2) it may partially or completely resorb without satisfactory new-bone formation, leaving disfigurement or instability; or (3) it may become sequestrated, encapsulated, and treated by the host as a foreign body. The most likely graft to achieve optimal function in humans is the fresh autograft. However, allogeneic implants are becoming more widely used.

A bone graft transferred to a recipient undergoes several adaptive phases before ultimate incorporation into the skeletal system. Osteogenesis from surviving cells of the graft itself is characteristic only of fresh autografts. By contrast, cells from an allograft usually elicit antibody production and cell-mediated immunity and start to decay. These alloimplants slowly revascularize by invasion of capillary sprouts from the host bed during the process of resorption of the old matrix. Finally, in both autografts and allografts, osteoinduction occurs by the process of recruitment of mesenchyme-type cells into cartilage and bone under the influence of a diffusible bone morphogenetic protein derived from the bone matrix. Bone morphogenetic protein is a recently discovered glycoprotein of MW 17,500. The target cell for its activity is an undifferentiated, perivascular mesenchymal cell whose protein synthesis is reprogrammed in favor of new-bone formation.

Temporally, healing of bone grafts follows a well-known pattern. For the initial 2 weeks, an inflammatory response occurs, associated with infiltration of the graft by vascular buds and the presence of fibrous granulation tissue, osteoclast activity, and osteocyte autolysis. There occurs a "creeping substitution" of graft bone, manifested as differentiation of mesenchymal cells into osteoblasts that deposit osteoid over devitalized trabeculae. Dead trabeculae are later remodeled internally. Thus, through appositional new-bone formation, the graft is strengthened. In contrast to cancellous bone, cortical bone grafts undergo a somewhat longer period of resorption and slower appositional phases of new-bone formation. This results in only half strength being acquired during the first 6 months and full strength 1–2 years after grafting.

Immunologic Rejection

Since bone is a composite of cells, collagen, ground substance, and inorganic minerals, all but the minerals are potentially immunogenic. Cell surface transplantation antigens associated with the MHC are the most potent immunogens within osteochondral allografts and are found on cells of osteogenic, chondrogenic, fibrous, neuronal, fatty, hematopoietic, and mesenchymal origin. Cell-rich marrow contributes significantly to immunogenicity.

Fresh allogeneic bone can sensitize the host and cause the production of circulating antibodies. Nevertheless, cellular immunity is thought to be more important than humoral antibodies in causing rejection of allogeneic bone transplants. Cartilage seems to resist destruction by antibody and cellular resorptive mechanisms, but if an immune response by the recipient develops, this protection is only relative and a low-grade, slow, immunologically mediated inflammatory response ensures, characterized by an increase in synovial fluid, leukocyte counts, antibody response, and pannus reactions.

Rejection of allogeneic bone (cortical or cancellous) elicits a response that delays healing at the site of osteosynthesis and blocks revascularization, resorption, and appositional new-bone formation. Clear-cut rejection or failure of the graft occurs in only about 10% of bone grafts.

Immunosuppression

Temporary systemic immunosuppression has been used, since MHC antigens are present in bone for only 2–3 months after transplantation. Drugs that have successfully allowed bone union include azathioprine, corticosteroids, cyclosporin, and cyclophosphamide. Because of side effects and the low rate of graft failure, these agents are no longer routinely used in human musculoskeletal transplantation. A promising new technique to diminish the antigenicity of grafts is the use of a temporary biodegradable cement that coats the donor bone and hides the bone cell antigens until these cells have died and their MHC antigens have deteriorated.

Clinical Recovery

Early ambulation and mild exercise stimulate blood flow and osteogenesis within the graft. External splinting helps to stabilize the graft. Education of the patients in proper posture, weight-bearing, turning, and exercise has been helpful in allowing sufficient time for healing.

FUTURE OF TRANSPLANTATION

The current shortage of hearts, livers, and lungs is a major impediment to offering this therapy to the growing number of eligible recipients. Stimulated by this urgent need, research into the use of xenogeneic organs (from species other than humans) is proceeding. In addition to the usual rejection problems, a more severe form of hyperacute rejection must be overcome before this approach can become a clinical reality.

Closer to implementation, however, are transplants of specific types of celss that can be used to replace missing genes or enzymes. One can imagine trans-planting hepatic parenchymal cells for thier synthesis of clotting factors, proteins, and even hematopoietic stem cells.

REFERENCES

Kidney Transplantation

Cho YW, Terasaki PI: Chap 29, p 277 in: *Long Term Survival in Clinical Transplants.* Terasaki P (editor). UCLA Tissue Typing Laboratory, 1988.

Halloran PF, Broski AP, Batiuk TD, Madrenas J: The molecular immunology of acute rejection: An overview. *Transplant Immunol* 1993;**1**:3.

Mizel SB: The interleukins. *FASEB J* 1989;**3**:2379.

Strom TB, Kelley VE: Toward more selective therapies to block undesired immune responses. *Kidney Int* 1989;**35**:1026.

Warvariv V, Garovoy MR: Transplantation immunology. Page 752 in: *Textbook of Internal Medicine.* Kelley WN (editor). Lippincott, 1989.

Liver Transplantation

Jenkins RL et al: Liver transplantation. *Surg Clin North Am* 1985;**65**:103.

Lake JR (editor): Advances in liver transplantation. *Gastroenterol Clin North Am* 1993;**22**:213.

Shaw BW et al: Transplantation of the liver. In: *Surgical Treatment of Digestive Disease.* Moody FG, Carey LC (editors). Yearbook, 1986.

Starzl TE, Demetris AJ, Von Thiel D: Liver transplantation. *N Engl J Med* 1989;**329**:1014, 1092.

Pancreas & Islet Cell Transplantation

International Symposium on Complications of Diabetes: Current status of prevention and treatment. *Transplant Proc* (In press).

Starzl TE et al: Pancreaticoduodenal transplantation in humans. *Surg Gynecol Obstet* 1984;**159**:265.

Sutherland DER, Kendall DM: Pancreas transplantation: Registry report and a commentary. *West J Med* 1985;**143**;845.

Sutherland DER, Moundry-Munns KE: Pancreas transplants in blacks and whites. *Transplant Proc* 1989;**21**:3968.

Sutherland DER et al: One institution's experience with pancreas transplantation. *West J Med* 1985;**143**:838.

Transplantation of pancreatic islet cells. (Progress Symposium.) *World J Surg* 1984;**8**:135.

Heart & Lung Transplantation

Barnard CN: The operation. A human cardiac transplant: An interim report of a successful operation performed at Groote Schuur Hospital, Cape Town. *S Afr Med J* 1967;**41**:1271.

Cooper JD: The evolution of techniques and indications for lung transplantation. *Ann Surg* 1990;**212**:249.

Egan TM, Kaiser LR, Cooper JD: Lung transplantation. *Curr Probl Surg* 1989;**10**:673.

Hardy JD et al: Heart transplantation in man: Develop-mental studies and report of a case. *JAMA* 1964; **188**:1132.

Hardy JD et al: Lung homotransplantation in man. *JAMA* 1963;**186**:1065.

ISHLT: A working formulation for the standardization in the diagnosis of heart and lung rejection. *J Heart Transplant* 1990;**9**:587.

Kaye MP: The Registry of the International Society for Heart and Lung Transplantation *J Heart Lung Transplant* 1992;**4**:599.

Reitz BA et al: Heart and lung transplantation. Autotransplantation and allotransplantation in primates with extended survival. J Thorac Cardiovasc Surg 1980;**80**:360.

Reitz BA et al: Orthotopic heart and combined heart and lung transplantation with cyclosporin-A immune suppression. *Transplant Proc* 1981;**1**:393.

Reitz BA et al: Heart-lung transplantation. Successful therapy for patients with pulmonary vascular disease. *N Engl J Med* 1982;**306**:557.

Reitz BA et al: Clinical heart-lung transplantation. *Transplant Proc* 1983;**1**:1256.

The Toronto Lung Transplant Group: Unilateral lung transplantation for pulmonary fibrosis. *N Engl J Med* 1986;**314**:1140.

Veith FJ, Koerner SK: Lung transplantation 1977. *World J Surg* 1977;**1**:177.

Bone Marrow Transplantation

Biggs JC et al: Treatment of chronic myeloid leukemia with allogeneic bone marrow transplantation after preparation with BuCy2. *Blood* 1992;**80**:1352.

Blaise D et al: Allogeneic bone marrow transplantation for acute myeloid leukemia in first remission: A randomized trial of busulfan-cytoxan vs. cytoxan-total body irradiation as preparative regimen: a report from the Groupe D'etudes de la Greffe de Moelle Osseuse. *Blood* 1992;**79**:2578.

Bortin MM et al: Changing trends in allogeneic bone marrow transplantation for leukemia in the 1980's. 1992;**268**:607.

Bosly A et al: Bone marrow transplantation—prolonged survival after relapse in aggressive lymphoma patients treated with the LNH-84 regimen. *J Clin Oncol* 1992;**10**:1615.

Carey PJ: Autologous bone marrow transplantation for high-grade lymphoid malignancy using melphalan/irradiation conditioning without marrow purging or prior preservation. *Blood* 1991;**77**:1593.

Chao NJ et al: Allogeneic bone marrow transplantation for high-risk acute lymphoblastic leukemia during first complete remission. *Blood* 1991;**78**:1923.

Chopra R et al: The place of high-dose BEAM therapy and autologous bone marrow transplantation in poor-risk Hodgkin's disease: A single center eight year study of 155 patients. *Blood* 1993;**81:**1137.

Copelan EA et al: Treatment for acute myelocytic leukemia with allogeneic bone marrow transplantation following preparation with BuCy2. *Blood* 1991;**78:**838.

Gluckman E et al: Bone marrow transplantation for severe aplastic anemia: influence of conditioning and graft vs. host disease prophylaxis regimens on outcome. *Blood* 1992;**79:**269.

Gribben JG et al: Immunologic purging of marrow assessed by PCR before autologous bone marrow transplantation for B-cell lymphoma. *N Engl J Med* 1991;**325:**1525.

Horowitz MM: Chemotherapy compared with bone marrow transplantation for adults with acute lymphoblastic leukemia in first remission. *Ann Inter Med* 1991;**115:**13.

Jagannath S et al: Low-risk intensive therapy for multiple myeloma with combined autologous bone marrow and blood stem cell support. *Blood* 1992;**80:**1666.

Linker CA et al: Autologous bone marrow transplantation for acute myeloid leukemia using busulfan plus etoposide as a preparative regimen. *Blood* 1993; **81:**311.

McGlave P et al. Unrelated donor marrow transplantation therapy for chronic myelogenous leukemia: initial experience of the National Marrow Donor Program. *Blood* 1993;**81:**543.

Bone Transplantation

Prolo DJ, Rodrigo JJ: Contemporary bone graft physiology and surgery. *Clin Orthop* 1985;**200:**322.

Immunosuppressive Therapy

58

Alan Winkelstein, MD

The growth of clinical immunology has uncovered increasing numbers of diseases that are due to aberrant immune responses. This has resulted in a search for drugs capable of inhibiting these unwanted responses. Particularly, the technical ability to successfully transplant many organs created a strong impetus for the development of safe and effective immunosuppressive regimens. Over the past 2 decades, considerable progress has been made in identifying a group of compounds capable of achieving *nonspecific* inhibition of immune response. The eventual goal in this area is to develop *specific* immunosuppression or tolerance directed only at the immune response to selected antigens. This currently remains an elusive goal.

CORTICOSTEROIDS

The glucocorticoid steroid hormones are widely and effectively used to suppress manifestations of numerous inflammatory and immune reactions. The pharmacology and anti-inflammatory effects of corticosteroids are discussed in Chapter 60. Although a clear-cut distinction between the immunosuppressive and anti-inflammatory actions of these drugs is not always possible, this section will emphasize glucocorticoid effects on the cells involved in the immune response.

Clinical research studies have often been confused by a failure to recognize that lymphocytes from different animal species vary in their susceptibility to steroid-induced lysis. In mice, rats, and rabbits, these hormones cause extensive lymphoid destruction. By contrast, normal lymphocytes from guinea pigs, monkeys, and humans are highly resistant to steroid-induced lysis. Not all human lymphocytes are resistant to steroid-induced lympholysis; these drugs will effectively kill acute lymphoblastic leukemic cells and are moderately cytolytic for neoplastic B cells in chronic lymphocytic leukemia and non-Hodgkin lymphomas.

The anti-inflammatory and immunosuppressive activities of corticosteroids can be grouped conveniently into 3 general categories: the effect of these drugs on leukocyte circulation, their ability to alter specific cellular functions, and other miscellaneous anti-inflammatory activities.

Effects on Cellular Traffic

One of the most important effects of corticosteroids is to alter transiently the number of circulating leukocytes. This is illustrated in Fig 58–1, which depicts the quantitative changes in each cell type following a single intravenous injection of a glucocorticoid. There is a prompt increase in the number of neutrophils and a concomitant decrease in the total number of lymphocytes, monocytes, eosinophils, and basophils. Maximum changes are observed 4–6 hours after injection, and all counts have returned to baseline-values within 24 hours.

The neutrophilia resulting from steroid administration appears to be due to at least 2 distinct activities: release of mature neutrophils from marrow reserves and reduced neutrophil egress from intravascular spaces into inflammatory exudates. As a result, the half-life of circulating neutrophils is increased.

In contrast to the neutrophilia, steroids cause a striking reduction in the number of circulating lymphocytes. This effect results from the sequestration of recirculating lymphoid cells into lymphoid tissues, including the bone marrow. The total numbers of circulating T cells are markedly decreased, B cell numbers are only modestly reduced, and numbers of null cells are unchanged. Among the T cell subsets, numbers of CD4 cells are reduced to a greater extent than are numbers of CD8 cells.

One of the important steroid-induced changes is a pronounced monocytopenia. Monocyte counts frequently decline to less than 50 cells/μL, and the re-

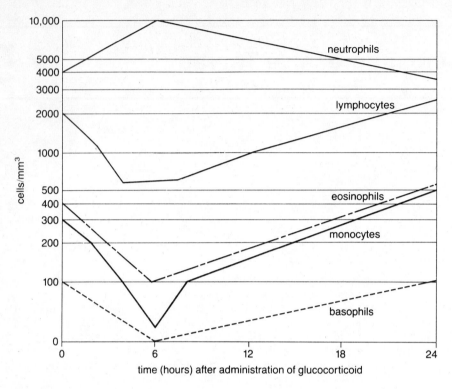

Figure 58–1. Glucocorticoids, whether given as a single dose or repetitively on alternate days, cause a decrease in lymphocyte, monocyte, basophil, and eosinophil counts and a rise in neutrophils within 4–6 hours, with a return to baseline within 24 hours. (Reproduced, with permission, from Claman HN: Glucocorticosteroids. I. Anti-inflammatory mechanisms. *Hosp Pract* 1983;**18**:123.)

duced availability of these cells has been postulated to be of prime importance in mediating steroid-induced anti-inflammatory activities. Eosinophil and basophil numbers are also reduced in the circulation because of redistribution.

Functional Change

In addition to affecting the distribution of leukocytes, corticosteroids alter important functional activities of both lymphocytes and monocytes. Neutrophilic activities such as chemotaxis and lysosomal enzymes are not significantly impaired, but the release of nonlysosomal proteolytic enzymes such as collagenase and plasminogen activator is decreased by steroids.

T lymphocyte activities are considerably altered by corticosteroids. In vitro lymphoproliferative responses are inhibited, in part from an impairment in the synthesis and secretion of interleukin-2 (IL-2), which is essential for the clonal expansion of activated lymphocytes (Fig 58–2). The decreased availability of IL-2 is most probably an indirect result of suppressed IL-1 production by monocytes. IL-2 receptor expression is not impaired. Steroids do not

alter the release of 2 other lymphokines, gamma interferon and migration inhibitory factor (MIF).

Corticosteroids can block the progression of phytohemagglutinin (PHA)-stimulated lymphocytes through the mitotic cycle (see below). They inhibit the entry of cells into the G_1 phase and arrest the progression of activated lymphocytes from the G_1 to the S phase.

Corticosteroids have less effect on B lymphocytes. Patients receiving moderate doses of prednisone are able to respond normally to test antigens. On the other hand, high-dose corticosteroid therapy modestly reduces the serum concentrations of IgG and IgA but not IgM. These changes may be observed as early as 2–3 weeks after initiation of the course of steroids and are reversible. In one study using cultured spleen cells from patients with idiopathic thrombocytopenic purpura, steroids inhibited the ability of B lymphocytes to synthesize IgG in vitro. Steroid therapy does not alter the activities of either natural killer (NK) cells or effectors of antibody-dependent cell-mediated cytotoxicity (ADCC).

Parelleling their profound effects on the number of circulating monocytes, corticosteroids induce strik-

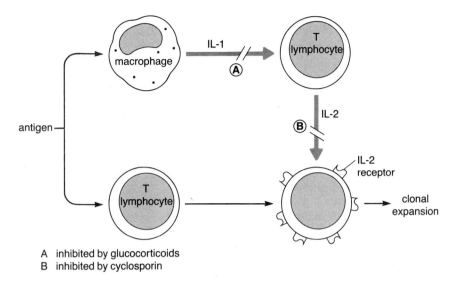

Figure 58–2. Antigen stimulation in vivo induces monocytes to release the cytokine IL-1. This soluble mediator has numerous effects including inducing helper T cells to synthesize IL-2. Antigen stimulation also induces responsive T cells to express receptors for IL-2. When IL-2 combines with IL-2 receptor (IL-2R)-bearing lymphocytes, these cells undergo clonal expansion. Corticosteroids act primarily to inhibit IL-1 synthesis and release. Cyclosporin suppresses the release of IL-2 and inhibits IL-2R expression. The letters A and B indicate inhibition by glucocorticoids and cyclosporin, respectively.

ing impairment in the functions of monocyte-macrophages in vitro. They suppress the bactericidal activities of these phagocytic cells, thereby lowering resistance to infection. Steroids also interfere with the antigen-presenting function of these cells. Other effects include impaired directed migration in response to chemotactic factors, decreased response to MIF, blocking of the differentiation of monocytes to macrophages, and suppression of the capacity of monocytes to express Fc and complement receptors, which may contribute to impaired phagocytic activities.

Steroids suppress the ability of reticuloendothelial cells to phagocytose antibody-coated cells, probably by decreasing the binding of immune complexes to Fc and C3b surface membrane receptors. This impaired binding may account for their beneficial effects in diseases such as idiopathic thrombocytopenic purpura and autoimmune hemolytic anemia.

Delayed-hypersensitivity skin tests to recall antigens are inhibited by prolonged treatment with corticosteroids. In general, these hormones must be administered for 10–14 days before skin test reactivity is impaired.

Clinical Use

Pharmacologic quantities of corticosteroids can effectively inhibit a spectrum of clinical manifestations associated with immune-mediated diseases. In numerous circumstances, these effects can be lifesaving. The beneficial effects result from a combina-

tion of two separate activities, immunosuppressive and nonspecific anti-inflammatory properties. The relative contributions of each cannot be accurately quantified; either can produce the desired therapeutic goal, suppression of the underlying clinical disease. In general, statements to the effect that corticosteroids have "broad immunosuppressive activities" usually refer to this inhibition of disease-associated features, not to the effect of the drug on specific immune responses.

In clinical trials, corticosteroids, as a single therapeutic agent, do not appear to be potent immune inhibitors. By contrast, in combination with other immunosuppressants they have considerable activity as an adjunctive agent. Thus drug combinations containing steroids are extremely useful both in suppressing transplant rejection reactions and in inhibiting manifestations of autoimmune diseases.

Steroid therapy appears to exert differential effects on acute and chronic manifestations of immune-associated diseases. These agents are primarily active in suppressing acute inflammatory reactions and in inhibiting the short-term consequences of aberrant immune responses. However, in many disorders, they do not alter the ultimate course of the underlying disease or reduce the concentrations of pathogenic autoantibodies. For example, these hormones are potent inhibitors of acute articular inflammatory reactions in patients with rheumatoid arthritis. By contrast, they do not decrease the incidence of chronic complications such as deforming arthritis. Likewise, steroids can suppress the carditis associated with acute rheumatic fever but do not change the frequency of chronic valvular disease. They inhibit the accelerated cell destruction resulting from autoantibody formation in autoimmune hemolytic anemia or idiopathic thrombocytopenic purpura. However, these effects often occur without reductions in the concentrations of pathogenic autoantibodies, and when the steroid dose is reduced, the cellular destructive processes often recur.

Clinical protocols for corticosteroid administration in immunologic diseases vary with the disease; they are discussed in the relevant chapters. There are 3 general patterns to steroid therapy protocols, depending on the circumstances. The first is often used if these drugs are to be administered for extended periods. It entails the use of the smallest amount needed to partially suppress disease manifestations. An example of this is the treatment of rheumatoid arthritis with 7.5–10 mg of prednisone daily. The second approach uses larger doses in an attempt to rapidly and completely suppress manifestations of an immunologically mediated disease. Prednisone at 1–2 mg/kg is given daily, in one or divided doses. This type of therapy is often used in disorders such as autoimmune hemolytic anemia, idiopathic thrombocytopenic purpura, and various types of immune-induced glomerulonephritis. The third pattern is the pulse administration of very large doses of an intravenous corticosteroid preparation (eg, methylprednisolone at 10–30 mg/kg). These ultralarge doses are generally reserved for unusually severe or potentially life-threatening illnesses. They have also been used successfully in reversing acute allograft rejection reactions. Most studies suggest that the immunologic effects of these massive-dose steroid protocols do not differ significantly from those resulting from more conventional doses. Although the therapeutic superiority of these regimens has not been proven in controlled trials, numerous reports imply effectiveness.

Prolonged therapy with corticosteroids is not innocuous; these drugs have numerous and potentially serious side effects (see Chapter 60). It is important to be aware of these side effects so that high-dose prolonged therapy does not cause greater morbidity than the underlying disease.

CYTOTOXIC DRUGS

Cytotoxic drugs are a group of chemicals with the pharmacologic property of killing cells capable of self-replication. Immunologically competent lymphocytes make up such a susceptible cell population. These drugs were originally introduced into clinical medicine for anticancer therapy; however, the initial studies revealed that many also possessed immunosuppressive activities. Thus, their use was extended

to treatment of diseases caused by aberrant immune responses and to inhibition of transplant rejection reactions. There are 4 cytotoxic drugs currently in clinical use for immunosuppression: cyclophosphamide, azathioprine, methotrexate, and chlorambucil.

Although the antigen-specific cells responsible for the unwanted immune response are potentially susceptible to cytotoxic immunosuppression, it must be recognized that the immunosuppressive activities of these drugs are not limited to a single lymphocyte subset. To various degrees, they can affect all immunologically competent cells, so that therapy leads to a generalized suppression of the immune defense system. As a result, treated patients are more susceptible to both opportunistic infections and certain neoplastic diseases.

Cytotoxic drugs are not selectively toxic for lymphocytes. They can kill nonlymphoid proliferating cells, including hematopoietic precursors, gastrointestinal mucosal cells, and germ cells in the gonads. Thus, predictable side effects of all these drugs include pancytopenia, gastrointestinal toxicities, and reduced fertility.

The lymphocytotoxic activities of different cytotoxic drugs can be related to their toxicities for cells in specific phases of the mitotic cycle (Fig 58–3). There are 4 phases in mitosis: G_1 (the pre-DNA syn-

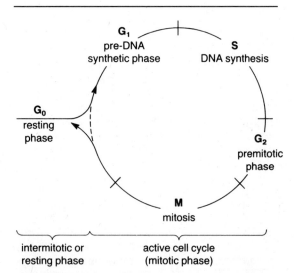

Figure 58–3. Mitotic cycles. Drugs that are selectively toxic for cells in a discrete phase of their cycle are designated phase-specific agents: most exert their toxicity for cells in the S phase. Examples include azathioprine and methotrexate. Cycle-specific agents, such as cyclophosphamide and chlorambucil, are toxic for both intermitotic and proliferating cells but show greater toxicity for those in active cycle. Cycle-nonspecific agents show equal toxicity for all cells regardless of the mitotic activity. Radiation is considered a cycle-nonspecific therapeutic modality.

thetic phase), S (the DNA synthetic phase), G_2 (the premitotic phase), and M (the actual mitosis). Cells in a prolonged intermitotic period are considered to be in a G_0 phase. One group of drugs, which includes azathioprine and methotrexate, are termed "phase-specific." These drugs are cytolytic to cells as they enter a selective phase of the mitotic cycle. For example, both azathioprine and methotrexate are cytolytic for cells only when they are in the S (DNA synthetic) phase.

Cyclophosphamide and chlorambucil are classified as "cycle-specific." They are toxic for cells at all stages of the mitotic cycle, including intermitotic (G_0) lymphocytes. However, they show differential cytolytic activities; they are more toxic for actively cycling than for resting (G_0) cells. The third group, the "cycle-nonspecific" compounds, are equally cytotoxic for proliferating and intermitotic cells.

Based on animal experiments, certain principles have been formulated concerning the immunosuppressive activities of cytotoxic drugs. By extension, these principles form the basis for the use of the drugs in clinical situations. They are summarized as follows:

(1) A primary immune response is more readily inhibited than is a secondary or anamnestic reaction. Drugs that are effective in suppressing an immune response in an unsensitized animal usually show only minimal inhibitory activity in a sensitized animal. The same effect is observed in patients. For example, the primary immune response elicited by a renal transplant is readily impaired by a combination of azathioprine and corticosteroids. However, if the recipient has been presensitized to donor histocompatibility antigens, this immunosuppressive regimen is relatively ineffective in inhibiting rejection reactions.

(2) The stages of an immune response differ markedly in their susceptibility to immunosuppressants. The cellular events associated with an antigenic challenge can be subdivided into 2 phases, designated the induction phase and the established or effector phase (Fig 58–4). The former is the interval between exposure to antigen (sensitization) and the production of sensitized T cells or mature plasma cells; it is characterized by the rapid proliferative expansion of antigen-sensitive precursors. Thereafter, the reaction is considered to have entered an established phase. Most cytotoxic drugs are effective if the period of drug administration coincides with the induction phase; once the reaction has entered the established

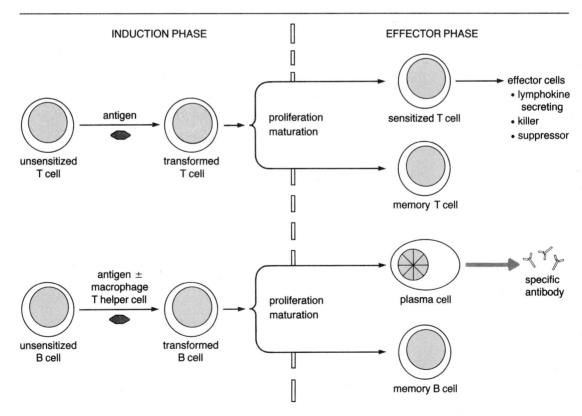

Figure 58–4. Development of an immune response. The period from antigenic challenge through the proliferative expansion of transformed lymphocytes is considered the induction phase. The period following cellular expansion is defined as the established (effector) phase.

phase, they are considerably less active. Furthermore, memory lymphocytes are unresponsive to immunosuppressive drugs.

(3) The effectiveness of an immunosuppressive drug in a primary response is highly dependent on the timing of its administration relative to the initial antigenic challenge. On the basis of their effective interval, immunosuppressive agents are divided into 3 groups:

Group I: This group includes modes of therapy that exert their maximum immunosuppressive activity when administered just before the antigen and are considerably less effective if used after the immunologic challenge. Included in this group are corticosteroids, irradiation, and the cycle-nonspecific cytotoxin, nitrogen mustard.

Group II: This group includes drugs that show immunosuppressive properties only if administered in the period immediately following the antigenic challenge. They do not impair responses if used prior to the antigen. This group includes the phase-specific drugs such as azathioprine and methotrexate.

Group III: This group includes drugs that show inhibitory activity if administered either before or after antigenic stimulation, although these compounds show greater suppressive activities if used after the immune challenge. Pharmacologically, they are cycle-specific drugs; cyclophosphamide is the principal immunosuppressant in this group. The differential effects on immunity are illustrated in Fig 58–5, which shows the response to sheep erythrocytes in mice treated with an immunosuppressant either 24 hours before or 24 hours after antigenic challenge.

(4) Immunosuppressive drugs can exert differential toxicities for T and B lymphocytes. Cyclophosphamide causes a proportionately greater reduction in the number of B cells than of T cells; this correlates with its greater suppressive effects on antibody responses than on cell-mediated reactions. In clinical usage, cyclophosphamide is considered more effective in suppressing diseases of aberrant humoral immunity, such as idiopathic thrombocytopenic purpura, than in inhibiting transplant rejection reactions. By contrast, azathioprine appears more potent as an inhibitor of T cell-mediated responses.

(5) In certain circumstances, a paradoxic effect may be elicited by immunosuppressive treatment, namely, augmentation of a specific response. This effect was originally noted with irradiation, which, when administered several days before an antigenic challenge, led to a greater than normal antibody response. Similar effects were then observed with 6-mercaptopurine when used before antigen challenge. With selected treatment protocols, cyclophosphamide can simultaneously suppress humoral responses and augment delayed hypersensitivity reactions to the same antigen. The heightened cellular reactions have been attributed, in part, to its toxicity for suppressor T lymphocytes.

(6) The ability to inhibit manifestations of an immune response may result from pharmacologic activities other than immunosuppression. The expression of many immune responses involves the participation of both immunologically competent cells and nonspecific effector cells such as neutrophils and monocytes. The numbers or functions of these effector cells can be altered by immunosuppressive drugs, an effect that can modify or obliterate the expression of a particular response. Therefore, apparent immuno-

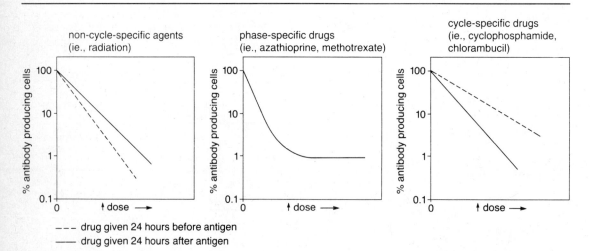

--- drug given 24 hours before antigen
—— drug given 24 hours after antigen

Figure 58–5. Schematic representation of the effects of different classes of immunosuppressants on the numbers of antibody-producing cells. (Reproduced, with permission, from Winkelstein A: Immune suppression resulting from various cytotoxic agents. Pages 296–316 in: *Clinics in Immunology and Allergy.* Vol 4: *Immune Suppression and Modulation,* Mitchell MS. Fahey JL [editors]. Saunders, 1984.)

Table 58–1. Some immunologic disorders in which cytotoxic drugs are effective or probably effective.

Rheumatoid arthritis
Systemic lupus erythematosus
Systemic vasculitis
Wegener's granulomatosis
Polymyositis
Membranous glomerulonephritis
Chronic active hepatitis
Primary biliary cirrhosis
Inflammatory bowel disease
Autoimmune hemolytic anemia
Immune thrombocytopenia
Circulating anticoagulants
Multiple sclerosis
Myasthenia gravis

suppression can result from the anti-inflammatory properties of a specific agent. As an example, corticosteroids are potent suppressors of IgE-mediated allergic asthma and T cell-mediated allergic contact dermatitis. They inhibit inflammation in these diseases without affecting the underlying immune responses.

Clinical Use

These drugs are used to treat many autoimmune disorders. Table 58–1 is a partial list of diseases in which cytotoxic drugs have been reported to be effective.

Despite their usage in these diseases for more than a decade, it is still difficult to ascertain their true effectiveness because there have been only a few controlled clinical trials. Controlled trials are necessary because many autoimmune diseases show unpredictable courses, with both spontaneous remissions and exacerbations. Nevertheless, cytotoxins have been widely accepted as potentially useful therapy for severe immune-related disorders.

Cytotoxic drugs have been used extensively in the treatment of rheumatic diseases. Table 58–2 compares the activities of each of the commonly used cytotoxic immunosuppressants in these diseases.

Individual Cytotoxic Drugs

A. Azathioprine: This compound is a phase-specific drug. It is a nitroimidazole derivative of the purine antagonist 6-mercaptopurine and is rapidly converted in vivo to the parent compound (6-mercaptopurine). Although there are conflicting data, most investigators believe that the addition of the imidazole side chain probably enhances its immunosuppressive potency and increases the therapeutic:toxic ratio.

Biochemically, both azathioprine and 6-mercaptopurine act by competitive enzyme inhibition to block synthesis of inosinic acid, the precursor of the purine compounds adenylic acid and guanylic acid. Therefore, the major effect is to impair DNA synthesis; this results in a decreased rate of cell replication and explains the phase-specific action of the drug. A second and less important activity in impairment of RNA synthesis.

Azathioprine appears to preferentially inhibit T cell responses compared with those resulting from activation of B lymphocytes. Nevertheless, both cell-mediated and humoral responses can be suppressed. In addition, azathioprine appears to effectively reduce the numbers of circulating NK and killer cells. The latter are responsible for ADCC reactions.

Before the development of cyclosporin (see below), combinations of azathioprine and corticosteroids were standard therapy for inhibition of transplant rejection reactions. These 2 agents still maintain an important role in this area. Azathioprine is now frequently used in transplant patients who have developed toxic effects of cyclosporin or in maintaining immunosuppression after discontinuing cyclosporin. In addition, azathioprine is used to treat a spectrum of autoimmune disorders (Table 58–3). There is extensive experience with patients who have severe rheumatoid arthritis, for whom this drug is classified as a "disease-remitting" agent. Beneficial effects have also been reported in patients with other connective tissue diseases, autoimmune blood dyscrasias, and immunologically mediated neurologic diseases. This phase-specific drug may also permit the use of re-

Table 58–2. Clinical efficacy of cytotoxic drugs in rheumatic disorders.[1]

Disease	Efficacy of[2]:			
	Azathioprine	Chlorambucil	Cyclophosphamide	Methotrexate
Rheumatoid arthritis	+	+	+	+
Rheumatoid vasculitis	0	+	+	0
Systemic lupus erythematosus	+	+	+	0
Polyarteritis nodosa	+	0	+	0
Polymyositis	+	0	0	+
Psoriatic arthritis	0	0	0	+
Wegener's granulomatosis	+	+	+	0
Reiter's syndrome	0	0	0	+

[1]Adapted from Nashel DJ: Mechanisms of action and clinical applications of cytotoxic drugs in rheumatic disorders. *Med Clin N Am* 1985;**69:**817.
[2]Symbols: ++, substantial evidence of effectiveness; +, benefit suggested by some studies; 0, not studied or benefit negligible.

Table 58–3. Properties and uses of azathioprine.

Trade name	Imuran
Administration	Orally, 1.25–2.5 mg/kg/d
Mechanism of action	S phase toxin (phase-specific agent) Inhibits de novo purine synthesis
Major indications	Transplant rejection reactions Chronic graft-versus-host reaction Rheumatoid arthritis ? Systemic lupus erythematosus ? Vasculitis ? Other connective tissue diseases Inflammatory bowel disease Chronic active hepatitis/primary biliary cirrhosis ? Myasthenia gravis ? Multiple sclerosis
Toxicities	Bone marrow depression Gastrointestinal irritation Hepatotoxicity (rare) Infections Cancers

Table 58–4. Properties and uses of cyclophosphamide.

Trade Name	Cytoxan
Administration	Orally 1–3 mg/kg/d Intravenously 10–20 mg/kg/every 1–3 months
Mechanism of action	Cycle-specific agent Binds and cross-links DNA strands A affects B cells more than T cells; suppressor T cells more than helper T cells
Major indications	Rheumatoid arthritis and vasculitis Systemic lupus erythematosus Wegener's granulomatosis Systemic vasculitis Autoimmune blood dyscrasias Immune-mediated glomerulo-nephritis
Toxicities	Bone marrow depression Gastrointestinal reactions Sterility (may be permanent) Alopecia Hemorrhagic cystitis Opportunistic infections Neoplasms (lymphoma, bladder carcinoma, acute myelogenous leukemia) Goodpasture's syndrome

duced amounts of corticosteroids in the treatment of primary biliary cirrhosis, chronic active hepatitis, and inflammatory bowel disease. Azathioprine is administered orally, and the maximum beneficial effects generally require continuous therapy for several weeks.

The primary lymphocytotoxic effects of azathioprine are directed against actively replicating cells. Short therapeutic courses do not reduce the numbers of T or B cells in the peripheral blood, but they do decrease the number of large lymphocytes. These cells are believed to be activated lymphocytes that have entered an active proliferative cycle following exposure to appropriate antigens. Immunoglobulin levels and titers of specific antibodies are not appreciably reduced by azathioprine. The numbers of circulating neutrophils and monocytes are reduced in a dose-dependent fashion because of the drug's cytotoxicity for hematopoietic precursors.

B. Cyclophosphamide: Both experimentally and clinically, this cycle-specific drug is a potent lymphocytotoxic immunosuppressant with a comparatively high therapeutic:toxic ratio (Table 58–4). Following pulse administration, there is a dose-dependent reduction in the numbers of both B and T lymphocytes. Cyclophosphamide has diverse effects on immune responses in experimental animals. Depending on such factors as the type of antigen, the dose of the drug, and the timing of the drug relative to antigenic challenge, the targeted immune response may be either inhibited or augmented. Cyclophosphamide is an alkylating agent that appears to cause more pronounced suppression of humoral antibody responses than of responses attributed to cellular reactions. This is illustrated by models in which there is pronounced inhibition of both IgG and IgM antibody responses without significant changes in T cell responses.

The effects of this drug on cell-mediated immune responses are extremely variable. It can prolong the survival of allogeneic skin grafts if administered after grafting. However, if used before grafting, it can be a potent immune enhancer. In part, this augmentation has been attributed to a greater toxicity for suppressor T cells than helper T lymphocytes.

Cyclophosphamide can be administered either orally or intravenously. Recent clinical trials suggest that pulse intravenous therapy, particularly when used with corticosteroids, may be more effective in treating immune-mediated diseases than is daily low-dose oral therapy. The parent drug is inactive until it undergoes hepatic transformation to 4-hydroxy-cyclophosphamide. This compound is further metabolized to form phosphoramide mustard and other alkylators. These can be found in the circulation for only a few hours after administration. Metabolism is not appreciably altered by either hepatic or renal insufficiency.

The cytotoxic effects of cyclophosphamide are primarily due to its ability to bind and cross-link DNA chains. However, it may also react and alter the function of other intracellular macromolecules. The DNA-alkylating activity may result in the immediate death of the target cell, or the cell may incur a lethal injury that is expressed during a subsequent mitotic division. In the latter circumstance, the injured cell may function normally in the intermitotic (G_0) phase of its cycle. Conversely, if DNA repair can be effected, the cell will survive and function normally (Fig 58–6). DNA alkylation is a prime mechanism

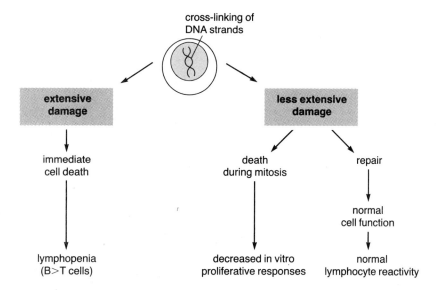

Figure 58–6. The effect of cyclophosphamide on lymphocytes appears to be primarily due to cross-linking DNA strands. This can result in lympholysis and decreased in vitro proliferative response. In cells that are not extensively damaged, repair can occur and the lymphocyte regains its full proliferative capacity. Because of the slow recovery of B cells, the effect is more pronounced than that on T cells.

serving to impair the in vitro proliferative responses of residual lymphocytes.

In animal studies, cyclophosphamide causes a depletion of both T and B lymphocytes; its selectivity for B cells appears to result from their delayed recovery. Clinical studies suggest that the effects on different subsets depend on the dose of the drug; comparatively low doses primarily deplete B cells and CD8 lymphocytes, whereas higher doses results in similar reductions in the total numbers of CD4 and CD8 lymphocytes. Patients with rheumatoid arthritis treated with long-term oral cyclophosphamide have reduced serum immunoglobulin levels. Therapy is also associated with a decrease in the titers of many autoantibodies.

Cyclophosphamide has been used successfully in the treatment of disorders believed to result from aberrant immunity. Beneficial effects have been documented in Wegener's granulomatosis, other forms of vasculitis, severe rheumatoid arthritis, the nephritis associated with systemic lupus erythematosus (SLE), autoimmune blood dyscrasias such as idiopathic thrombocytopenic purpura, autoimmune hemolytic anemia, pure erythrocyte aplasia, Goodpasture's syndrome, and immune forms of glomerulonephritis.

Despite a comparatively high therapeutic:toxic ratio, cyclophosphamide therapy is associated with serious and potentially lethal adverse reactions. In general, the dose-limiting toxicity is suppression of hematopoiesis. Some studies suggest that this drug has less effect on the bone marrow than do other alkylating agents, and it may have a lower incidence of inducing thrombocytopenia. Other side effects include infertility and gastrointestinal symptoms such as abdominal pain, nausea, and vomiting. Teratogenesis is also a well-recognized complication.

In addition, this alkylating agent induces certain toxic manifestations not observed with other immunosuppressants; these include both hemorrhagic cystitis and alopecia. Cystitis has been reported in 9–17% of rheumatic patients chronically treated with this drug. The delayed toxicities include an increased risk of opportunistic infections and a higher than expected occurrence of cancers, specifically non-Hodgkin lymphoma, bladder cancer, acute non-lymphoblastic leukemia, and skin cancers. The incidence of malignancies appears to increase with both the total dose administered and the number of years of treatment. The overall risk for malignancies is difficult to estimate, but 2 long-term studies (7 and 11 years of follow-up) report that the incidence of neoplastic diseases was 24–25% in the group receiving this alkylating drug compared with 7–13% in the control group. Bladder cancer develops in approximately 10% of patients treated for prolonged intervals with oral cyclophosphamide.

C. Methotrexate: This drug is a specific inhibitor of dihydrofolate reductase, an enzyme required for the conversion of folic acid to its active form, tetrahydrofolate (Fig 58–7). The latter compound serves as a donor of one-carbon fragments for the in vivo synthesis of thymidine. Thus, methotrexate is a potent inhibitor of DNA synthesis and is classified as a phase-specific agent.

Methotrexate was one of the earliest anticancer drugs. Shortly after its introduction into clinical med-

Figure 58–7. The folic acid cycle. Methotrexate (MTX) binds to and inhibits the enzyme dihydrofolate reductase (DHFR), thereby preventing the regeneration of tetrahydrofolate (FH_4) from dihydrofolate (FH_2). Leucovorin factor can directly antagonize the effects of methotrexate by providing a source of reduced folate. dUMP, 2-deoxyuridylate; dTMP, thymidylate; TS, thymidine synthase. *One-carbon transfer from $N^{5,10}$ methylene FH_4 to dUMP; **one-carbon transfer for serine to FH_4. (Reproduced, with permission, from Winkelstein A: Immune suppression resulting from various cytotoxic agents. Pages 296–316 in: *Clinics in Immunology and Allergy.* Vol 4: *Immune Suppression and Modulation.* Mitchell MS, Fahey JL [editors]. Saunders, 1984.)

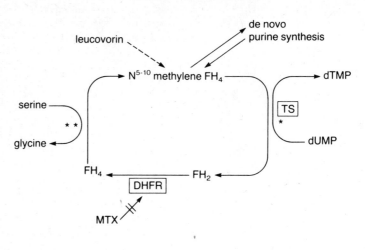

icine, it was found to be effective in the treatment of psoriasis. However, the initial trials had to be terminated because of a high risk of hepatic fibrosis. Subsequently, investigators found that lower doses were equally effective in controlling psoriatic manifestations and could be administered for extended periods without inducing hepatic injury. Psoriatic patients with coexisting arthritis reported concomitant improvement in their joint disease. This led to an evaluation of methotrexate in patients with rheumatoid arthritis, and these studies showed that approximately two-thirds of the patients with severe rheumatoid arthritis achieved either partial or complete remissions. Other studies found that methotrexate effectively suppressed manifestations of polymyositis and Reiter's syndrome. It is also of considerable use in preventing graft-versus-host (GVH) reactions in patients undergoing allogeneic marrow transplants (Table 58–5). Recent preliminary studies suggest that it may also be useful in treating steroid-dependent bronchial asthma.

Although animal studies indicate that methotrexate is a potent inhibitor of both humoral and cellular responses with a high therapeutic:toxic ratio, the mechanisms by which it exerts its beneficial effects in rheumatic diseases are not well understood. It is unlikely that the small doses used to treat immunologically mediated diseases would significantly inhibit immune responses.

A typical treatment regimen for rheumatic diseases consists of administering 2.5 mg of this drug every 12 hours for 3 doses; this course is repeated weekly. The major toxicity of methotrexate is hepatic fibrosis, which appears to be dose-related. Liver disease is rarely a problem until the total dose exceeds 1.5 g. Of particular note, hepatic fibrosis can occur with maintenance of normal liver function tests.

Other toxic manifestations include hypersensitiv-

ity pneumonitis, mucositis, and megaloblastic anemia. With the exception of pneumonitis, these complications are rarely major problems at the doses used to treat rheumatic diseases.

D. Chlorambucil: Chlorambucil is an alkylating drug that has cytotoxic properties similar to those of cyclosphosphamide. Most comparative studies suggest that it is less toxic than cyclophosphamide but not as potent an immunosuppressant.

Chlorambucil has been used extensively in Europe to treat immunologically mediated disease, and most reports suggest that it effectively controls these disorders. These include rheumatoid arthritis, SLE, and Wegener's granulomatosis. It is the drug of choice

Table 58–5. Properties and uses of methotrexate.

Administration	Orally 2.5–5.0 mg every 12 hours × 3 weekly
Mechanisms of action	S phase toxin (phase-specific) Competitively inhibits dihydrofolate reductase, thereby restricting synthesis of tetrahydrofolate. This is required for one-carbon transfer reactions involved in thymidine synthesis.
Major indications	Rheumatoid arthritis Psoriasis and psoriatic arthritis Polymyosititis/dermatomyositis Reiter's syndrome Prophylaxis for graft-versus-host reaction in bone marrow transplants
Toxicities	Gastrointestinal (stomatitis, diarrhea, mucositis) Bone marrow (megaloblastic anemia) Hepatic fibrosis Pneumonitis Decreased fertility

for the treatment of idiopathic cold-agglutinin hemolytic anemia and essential cryoglobulinemia.

Chlorambucil has advantages over cyclophosphamide. It does not cause alopecia or hemorrhagic cystitis and is less irritating to the gastrointestinal tract. Like cyclophosphamide, it will cause marrow suppression and will interfere with gonadal function. It is also a fetal toxin. It increases the risk of both opportunistic infections and certain cancers.

Combinations of Cytotoxic Drugs

Recent clinical studies have attempted to enhance suppression of the manifestations of immunologically related diseases while minimizing toxicities by using combinations of 2 or more cytotoxic drugs. Multidrug therapies, which are derived in part from cancer chemotherapeutic protocols, are based on the concept that lower doses of 2 or more drugs will have an additive or even a synergistic effect on effector lymphocytes. At the same time, the reduced quantities of each agent will result in a decreased incidence of side effects, particularly those that are dose-related. Combinations tested in small series include azathioprine/methotrexate and cyclophosphamide/azathioprine; the initial trials are encouraging, but larger controlled series are required before the ultimate therapeutic role of these combinations is determined.

CYCLOSPORIN

Cyclosporin is a novel immunosuppressant with activities distinct from those of all other compounds. It is able to alter selectively the immunoregulatory activities of helper T cells without affecting suppressor T cells, B lymphocytes, granulocytes, or macrophages. Furthermore, it acts by impairing cellular functions without killing target lymphocytes. Because of its potency, it has become the standard drug for inhibition of allogeneic transplant rejection reactions. Recently, trials with cyclosporin have been initiated for the treatment of several other diseases that are presumed to be immunologically mediated.

Pharmacologically, cyclosporin is a unique cyclic undecapeptide derived from fermentation of certain soil fungi (Fig 58–8). It is not water soluble, but it can be administered either orally or intramuscularly in a lipid vehicle. Immunologically, its effects are highly selective. It specifically inhibits the activities of helper T cells while sparing suppressor T cells. Thus, it selectively blocks the immune responses, including allograft rejection, that are dependent on helper T lymphocytes.

Cyclosporin acts as an immunosuppressant by blocking an early phase of a developing immune response. The principal targets of this drug are CD4 (helper T) lymphocytes. It acts by preventing the transduction of the mitogenic signal resulting from receptor ligation to the nucleus at a stage after the rise in intracellular calcium levels. As a result, there is an inhibition of the synthesis of mRNA for transcription of IL-2 and other cytokines. IL-2 synthesis and secretion (Fig 58–2) are required for the generation and proliferation of cytotoxic T cells responsible for allograft rejection and for activating B cells responsible for T cell-dependent humoral responses (see Chapter 9). By contrast, this fungal metabolite is ineffective in inhibiting the lytic activity of preformed cytotoxic T cells. Cyclosporin may also function as an immune

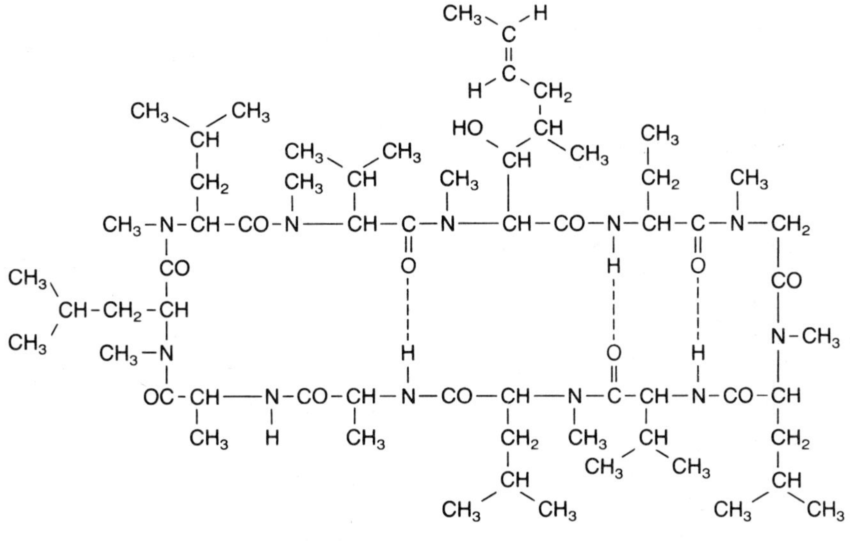

Figure 58–8. Chemical structure of cyclosporin. (Reproduced, with permission, from Cohen DJ et al: Cyclosporine: A new immunosuppressive agent for organ transplantation. *Ann Intern Med* 1984;**101:**667.)

inhibitor by impairing the ability of activated helper T cells to respond to IL-2, perhaps by limiting receptor expression.

Recent studies have shown that cyclosporin inhibits a spectrum of other cellular functions. An intracellular cyclosporin-binding protein, cyclophilin, has been identified, purified, and characterized. This protein is present in nearly all mammalian cells. It is a peptide-prolyl *cis-trans* isomerase (PPIase), an enzyme that catalyzes protein folding. Drug-protein interaction is believed to have a crucial role in impairing the signal transduction required for lymphocyte activation and is also thought to be responsible for the toxic manifestations resulting from cyclosporin therapy. Of potential importance, cyclosporin can modify genes controlling multidrug resistance to cancer-chemotherapeutic agents. Multidrug resistance is commonly associated with the overexpression of the transmembrane transport protein, P glycoprotein, which is responsible for the drug accumulation deficit seen in drug-resistant cancers. Derivatives of cyclosporin have been examined for their immunosuppressive properties; to date none have proven as effective as the parent compound. However, some may be able to block the multidrug resistance gene.

The effectiveness of this immunosuppressant may be increased by the simultaneous administration of moderate doses of corticosteroids. The 2 drugs appear to act synergistically. Cyclosporin directly inhibits IL-2 production, whereas steroids indirectly suppress the synthesis of IL-2 by blocking monocyte-macrophage release of IL-1 (Fig 58–2).

Clinically, cyclosporin has become the principal drug used to inhibit allograft rejection reactions (Table 58–6). Its development is one of the major reasons for the increase in successful transplant surgery with all types of organs, including kidney, heart, heart-lung, liver, and pancreas transplants.

Cyclosporin is also an effective means of preventing GVH reactions in major histocompatibility complex (MHC)-matched allogeneic bone marrow transplants. The drug, however, is comparatively ineffective as treatment for established GVH reactions.

Cyclosporin has a low therapeutic:toxic ratio. Blood levels of the drug should be monitored because of its unpredictable pharmacokinetics. Cyclosporin absorption from the small intestines is normally incomplete and is further reduced by intestinal dysfunction. The drug is metabolized by the liver and excreted in the bile. Blood levels are significantly altered by abnormal liver function, by drugs that induce or inhibit hepatic metabolism, and by low bile flow.

Unlike cytotoxic drugs, cyclosporin is not toxic to bone marrow stem cells and therefore does not cause cytopenias. Renal failure and hypertension are its major toxicities. It causes an increase in renovascular resistance. In its early stages, this is generally reversible; however, longer-term therapy can lead to persistent ischemia, irreversible interstitial fibrosis, and tubular atrophy. The hypertension is probably the result of both renal ischemia and sodium retention.

Cyclosporin treatment has additional side effects. These include gingival hyperplasia, hirsutism, and coarsening of facial features. Reversible hepatotoxicity resulting in elevation of the serum bilirubin and transaminase levels is another common side effect. Neurologic side effects include tremors, paresthesias, and occasionally convulsions. It can increase both serum cholesterol and uric acid levels. It is also a potential diabetogenic agent because it inhibits insulin release from pancreatic islet cells and may increase peripheral insulin resistance. In patients receiving bone marrow transplantation, cyclosporin may cause potentially fatal capillary leak syndromes or hemolytic-uremic syndrome.

Like other immunosuppressants, cyclosporin appears to cause susceptibility to opportunistic infections and certain malignancies. The most frequently encountered neoplasms in organ transplant recipients treated with this immunosuppressant are skin cancers and non-Hodgkin lymphoma. A disproportionally high percentage of the skin cancers are Kaposi's sarcoma. The prevalence of lymphomas in this group has been estimated to be 25–30 times that of an age- and sex-matched control population. This risk does not significantly differ from that observed with other immunosuppressive regimens; however, it appears that lymphomas in the cyclosporin-treated patients have a shorter latent phase.

Table 58–6. Properties and uses of cyclosporin.

Administration	Orally, intravenously Variable dosage, 5–20 mg/kg/d
Mechanisms of action	Effects primarily limited to helper T cells; not cytotoxic Inhibits production of IL-2 ? Reduces expression of IL-2 receptors
Major indications	Inhibition of transplant rejection reactions
Toxicities	Nephrotoxicity Hypertension Hepatotoxicity ? Epstein-Barr virus-induced lymphomas Hirsutism, gingival hyperplasia Neurotoxicity Hemolytic-uremic syndrome

FK-506

This compound, a macrolide antibiotic, has been shown to be an extremely potent immunosuppressant. Comparatively, it is as much as 100 times more potent than cyclosporin in suppressing transplantation rejection reactions and appears to have therapeutic use in certain immune-mediated diseases. FK-506 has significantly fewer side effects than cyclosporin. It has been successful in some trials as the primary therapy for transplantation of liver, heart-lung, intestine, kidney, and other organs. Preliminary results suggest that FK-506 may permit procedures that were previously considered either impractical or impossible.

Although biochemically unrelated to cyclosporin, FK-506 acts by similar mechanisms. Both agents exert their immunosuppressive activities by predominantly affecting the functions of helper T cells. One of the major consequences is the marked inhibition of IL-2 synthesis and secretion. Neither drug is lympholytic or toxic for bone marrow progenitors. Furthermore, FK-506, like cyclosporin, does not inhibit target cell killing by preformed cytotoxic lymphocytes. Recent biochemical studies suggest that the mechanisms of action depend on the binding of both drugs to specific (but different) cytosolic receptors. In both cases, however, one of the major effects of the drug-receptor interaction is to interfere with the function of the enzyme PPIase, which facilitates protein folding.

Current evidence suggests that FK-506 has a better therapeutic index than cyclosporin. Like cyclosporin, it is moderately diabetogenic, since it inhibits the release of insulin from islet cells and possibly increases insulin resistance. Both drugs are neurotoxic. FK-506 appears to cause significantly less hypertension than cyclosporin and is significantly less nephrotoxic.

Other side effects commonly seen with cyclosporin, such as gingival hyperplasia, hirsutism, and coarsening of facial features, are rare with FK-506. Finally, FK-506 does not appear to cause the metabolic disturbances such as hyperuricemia and hypercholesterolemia noted with cyclosporin. Long-term complications appear to include increased incidence of both opportunistic infections and neoplasms associated with chronic immunosuppression.

PLASMAPHERESIS

Diseases due to circulating autoantibodies or toxic antigen-antibody complexes could theoretically benefit from selective removal of the autoantibodies or immune complexes from the plasma. Plasma exchange (plasmapheresis) became clinically feasible with the development of automated cell separators capable of fractionating blood rapidly into its component parts. The procedure has been used experimentally to treat patients with a variety of immunologically related diseases, but there have been insufficient controlled therapeutic trials to ascertain its true effectiveness.

The technique used for plasma exchange is comparatively simple. Blood is removed, the plasma is separated by either centrifugation or membrane filtration and discarded, and the erythrocytes are reinfused into the patient. Fluid volume is maintained by administering either an albumin solution or fresh-frozen plasma. In most treatment protocols, approximately 50% of the patient's plasma is removed with each exchange procedure.

The ability of plasma exchange to remove a specific group of antibodies is dependent on their immunoglobin class. IgG molecules are distributed in both the intravascular and extracellular spaces, with approximately 40% contained in the vascular system. Thus, a single 50% plasma exchange can, at best, remove only 20% of a specific IgG antibody. By contrast, 85–90% of IgM antibodies are intravascular, so that a single exchange procedure can remove almost half the total quantity of pathogenic IgM antibodies. This accounts for the apparent success of plasma exchange in IgM antibody-related disorders such as idiopathic cold-agglutinin hemolytic anemia, essential cryoglobulinenemia, and the hyperviscosity syndrome associated with Waldenström's macroglobulinemia.

Plasma exchange has been most successful for 2 of the IgG antibody autoimmune diseases, myasthenia gravis and Goodpasture's syndrome. It is noteworthy that both of these diseases are characterized by the presence of highly specific tissue autoantibodies. Plasma exchange has been used, with questionable effectiveness, in intractable rheumatoid arthritis, rheumatoid vasculitis, other forms of vasculitis, lupus nephritis, posttransfusion purpura, bleeding from factor VIII antibodies, and immunologically mediated neurologic diseases such as Guillain-Barré syndrome and multiple sclerosis.

INTRAVENOUS GAMMA GLOBULIN

Replacement therapy with intravenous gamma globulin (IVIG) has become standard treatment for severe humoral immune deficiencies (see Chapter 20). IVIG has also been found to influence the course of several autoimmune diseases, particularly immune thrombocytopenia, by functioning paradoxically as an immunosuppressant or an immunomodulator. It has been highly effective in treating children with the acute forms of idiopathic thrombocytopenic purpura. Although prolonged remissions in adults are rare, IVIG can often increase platelet counts transiently, which can be potentially life-saving in cases of bleeding diatheses resulting from severe thrombocytopenia. Although the mechanism of action in idiopathic thrombocytopenic purpura is not fully known, IVIG appears to act primarily by blocking $Fc\gamma R$ on reticuloendothelial cells, thereby inhibiting the phagocytosis of antibody-coated platelets. In some cases, IVIG may also displace platelet-specific antibodies from the cell surface.

Based on the experience with idiopathic thrombocytopenic purpura, several other immunologically mediated diseases have been treated with IVIG. These include autoimmune hemolytic anemia, autoimmune neutropenia, antibody-mediated pure erythrocyte aplasia, other platelet-destructive diseases, autoantibodies against the blood-clotting factor VIII, myasthenia gravis, and Kawasaki disease. With the exceptions of Kawasaki disease and idiopathic thrombocytopenic purpura, the accumulated experience with these conditions to date is too small to determine the true effectiveness of the drug.

Several other mechanisms have been postulated to explain the immune-modulating activities. IVIG has been reported to nonspecifically augment suppressor T cell activities. It may also inhibit the activities of NK cells and reduce the synthesis of specific immunoglobulins. In addition, it may contain anti-idiotypic antibodies that will serve to inactivate autoantibodies.

ANTILYMPHOCYTE ANTIBODIES

The administration of heterologous antisera against lymphocyte membrane antigens is another mode of achieving nonspecific immunosuppression. Two types of antibody preparations have been used: polyclonal antibodies, which react with multiple membrane determinants, and monoclonal antibodies, which are directed at only a single antigen.

Polyclonal Antibodies

Polyclonal antibodies are generally prepared by immunizing animals with human lymphocytes. If cells from the thymus are used, the preparation is termed **antithymocyte serum (ATS)**; this is often further fractionated to obtain the globulin portion, termed **antithymocyte globulin (ATG)**. Other antibodies are prepared from thoracic duct lymphocytes, splenic cells, or peripheral blood lymphocytes obtained by leukophoresis. These are referred to as either **antilymphocyte serum (ALS)** or **antilymphocyte globulin (ALG)**.

Polyclonal antibodies are effective immunosuppressants in animal studies, where the primary effect is the impairment of cell-mediated responses consistent with their specificities for T lymphocytes. However, the mechanisms responsible for their immunosuppressive activities are not fully understood. They do produce lymphopenia in vivo; this is one postulated mode of action. Clinically, they are used primarily to treat organ graft rejection reactions. More recently, they have been used to treat patients with severe GVH reactions and to promote remissions in some cases of aplastic anemia.

Several major problems are associated with the use of polyclonal antibodies. (1) The preparations are not standardized, and there is no objective measure of in vivo immunosuppressive activity of a particular preparation. Thus, the amount needed to achieve a specific clinical effect cannot be predetermined. (2) These reagents are not selective for T cells. They cross-react with other types of cells, including platelets, which may lead to a destructive thrombocytopenia. (3) Heterologous antibodies are recognized as foreign proteins by the patient's immune system, thereby eliciting a humoral immune response, which may cause serum sickness (see Chapter 27).

MONOCLONAL ANTIBODIES

In organ transplant studies, monoclonal antibodies have assumed increasing clinical importance. In fact, some may be capable of inducing a state of selective immunologic unresponsiveness or tolerance, the ultimate goal of therapeutic immunosuppression. A prominent trend in organ transplantation is to use antibodies with increasing specificity for the lymphocyte subsets directly involved in effecting the reaction. This selectivity preserves the function of other immunologically competent lymphocytes and maintains immune defense mechanisms.

Monoclonal antibodies can be divided into 2 general groups, those directed at specific subsets of T cells and those reactive with antigens selectively present on the lymphocyte subset effecting the targeted immune response. The former includes a group of pan-T cell antibodies; the one most widely used clinically is anti-OKT 3, an antibody that reacts with the CD3 determinant on immunologically competent T cells. This monoclonal antibody has been successfully used to treat steroid-resistant acute transplant rejection reactions and is under study as a possible component of an initial immunosuppressive regime.

Monoclonal antibody therapy is not without significant side effects; the immediate complications include severe fevers and chills, headache, meningismus, hypotension, diarrhea, vomiting, respiratory distress, and anaphylactic shock. Fatal reactions to OKT3 have occasionally been reported. Long-term toxicities include an increased prevalence of opportunistic infections and lymphoproliferative neoplasms. Other pan-lymphocytic antibodies with potential clinical usefulness include CAMPATH-1, a lympholytic antibody against an antigen present on most lymphocytes (CDw52), and antibodies directed at the CD5 and CD6 antigens on immunologically competent T cells.

More recently, antibodies specifically directed against either the CD4 or CD8 antigens have been evaluated as agents capable of inhibiting transplant rejection reactions. The initial trials have led to important observations that provide insight into the mechanisms involved in organ rejection. For example, it has been widely assumed that CD8 cytotoxic cells are the prime effectors of graft rejection. However, in experimental models, monoclonal antibodies directed at CD4 cells appear to be more effective than those specific for the CD8 population. CD4 T lymphocytes have been shown to have multiple functions including cytolytic activities for allogeneic cells expressing class II HLA antigens. This reaction appears to be an important mechanism effecting graft rejection reactions. At present, it has not been established whether these antibodies act by depleting CD4 lymphocytes or by functionally inactivating them.

Preliminary data suggest that anti-CD4 monoclonal antibodies may have immunosuppressive potency equal to or greater than that of cyclosporin. There is also evidence suggesting that antibodies to the CD4 determinant may act synergistically with other immunosuppressants such as cyclosporin and anti-CD8 antibodies to promote graft acceptance. In addition, anti-CD4 antibodies may be able to induce tolerance to the murine monoclonal antibody itself, thereby preventing the host from forming neutralizing antibodies.

The second group of immunosuppressive antibodies are those directed at specific T cell activation antigens. These membrane receptors are not expressed on resting T cells but appear shortly after the cells are induced to respond to an immunologic challenge. The best studied of these inhibitors is the anti-Tac monoclonal antibody, which reacts with the p55 peptide of the IL-2 receptor. The Tac antigen is expressed on the effector T lymphocytes of patients with certain autoimmune diseases and in cells participating in organ allograft rejection reactions. They are also present on neoplastic cells of patients with specific T cell leukemias and lymphomas, such as HTLV I-induced acute T cell leukemia.

Both unmodified anti-Tac antibodies and those conjugated with either toxins or radioisotopes are currently being evaluated for their immune inhibitory properties. Initial results indicate that they are potent inhibitors of transplant rejection reactions and are capable of suppressing manifestations of autoimmune diseases. Because of their specificity for activated T cells, they may be able to induce selective immunosuppression without impairing the subsequent ability of the immune system to respond to other antigens. Other activation antigens, such as the transferrin receptor, may also prove to be useful targets for immunosuppressive monoclonal antibodies.

There is a third group of immunosuppressive monoclonal antibodies, those directed at cell adhesion molecules. These membrane determinants appear to be important in transmitting stimuli from antigen-presenting cells to immunologically competent lymphocytes and in effecting the cytolytic responses of antigen-stimulated lymphocytes. By blocking the active sites on these adhesion molecules, it may be possible to inhibit a spectrum of undesired immune responses.

REFERENCES

General

Bach JF: *The Mode of Action of Immunosuppressive Agents.* North-Holland, 1975.

Ben-Yehuda O, Tomer Y, Shoenfeld, Y: Advances in therapy of autoimmune diseases. *Semin Arthritis Rheum* 1988;**17**:206.

Briggs JD: A critical review of immunosuppressive therapy. *Immunol Letts* 1991;**29**:89.

Elion GB. Immunosuppressive agents. *Transplant Proc* 1977;**9**:975.

Fahey JL et al: Immune interventions in disease. *Ann Intern Med* 1987;**106**:257.

Hazleman B: Incidence of neoplasms in patients with rheumatoid arthritis exposed to different treatment regimens. *Am J Med* 1985;**78(Suppl 1A):** 39.

Heppner GH, Calabressi P: Selective suppression of humoral immunity by antineoplastic drugs. *Annu Rev Pharmacol Toxicol* 1976;**16**:367.

Mitchell MS, Fahey JL (editors): *Immune Suppression and Modulation.* Vol 4 of: *Clinics in immunology and Allergy.* Saunders, 1984.

Penn I: The occurrence of malignant tumors in immunosuppressed states. *Prog Allergy* 1986;**37**:259.

Schein PS, Winokur SH: Immunosuppressive and cytotoxic chemotherapy: Long term complications. *Ann Intern Med* 1975;**82**:84.

Spreafico F, Tagliabue A, Vecchi A: Chemical immunodepressants. Pages 315–345 in: *Immunopharmacology.* Sirois CP, Rola-Pleszczynski M (editors). Elsevier, 1982.

Strom TB: Immunosuppressive agents in renal transplantation. *Kidney Int* 1984;**26**:353.

Tsokos GC: Immunomodulatory treatment in patients with rheumatic diseases: Mechanisms of action. *Semin Arthritis Rheum* 1987;**17**:24.

Yunus MB: Investigational therapy in rheumatoid arthritis: A critical review. *Semin Arthritis Rheum* 1988;**17**:163.

Costicosteroids

Claman HN: Glucocorticosteroids. I. Anti-inflammatory mechanisms. II. The clinical response. *Hosp Pract* 1983;**18**:123, 143.

Cupps TR, Fauci AS: Corticosteroid-mediated immunoregulation in man. *Immunol Rev* 1982;**65**:133.

Meulemann J, Katz P: The immunologic effects, kinetics and use of glucocorticosteroids. *Med Clin N Am* 1985;**69**:805.

Parrillo JE, Fauci AS: Mechanisms of glucocorticoid action on immune processes. *Annu Rev Pharmacol Toxicol* 1979;**19**:179.

Zweiman B et al: Corticosteroid effects on circulating lymphocyte subset levels in normal humans. *J Clin Immunol* 1984;**4**:151.

Cytotoxic Drugs

Ahmed AR, Hombal SM: Cyclophosphamide (cytoxan). *J Am Acad Dermatol* 1984;**11**:1115.

Austin HA et al: Therapy of lupus nephritis. *N Engl J Med* 1986;**314**:614.

Berd D et al: Augmentation of the human immune response by cyclophosphamide. *Cancer Res* 1982; **42**:4862.

Clements PJ, Davis J: Cytotoxic drugs: Their clinical application to the rheumatic diseases. *Semin Arthritis Rheum* 1986;**15**:231.

Cupps TR, Edgar LC, Fauci AS: Suppression of human B lymphocytes function by cyclophosphamide. *J Immunol* 1982;**128**:2453.

Felson DT, Anderson J: Evidence for the superiority of immunosuppressive drugs and prednisone over prednisone alone in lupus nephritis. *N Engl J Med* 1984;**311**:1528.

McCune WJ, Fox D: Intravenous cyclophosphamide therapy of severe SLE. *Rheum Dis Clin N Am* 1989; **15**:455.

Moore MJ: Clinical pharmacokinetic of cyclophosphamide. *Clin Pharmacokinet* 1991;**20**:194.

Nashel DJ: Mechanisms of action and clinical applications of cytotoxic drugs in rheumatic disorders. *Med Clin N Am* 1985;**69**:817,.

Turk JL, Parker D: Effect of cyclophosphamide on immunological control mechanisms. *Immunol Rev* 1982;**65**:99.

Winkelstein A: Effects of cytotoxic immunosuppressants on tuberculin-sensitive lymphocytes in guinea pigs. *J Clin Invest* 1975;**56**:1587.

Winkelstein A: Effects of immunosuppressive drugs on T and B lymphocytes in guinea pigs. *Blood* 1977;**50**:81.

Cyclosporin & FK-506

Bennett WM, Norman DJ: Action and toxicity of cyclosporine. *Annu Rev Med* 1986;**37**:215.

Cohen DJ et al: Cyclosporine: A new immunosuppressive agent for organ transplantation. *Ann Intern Med* 1984;**101**:667.

Foxwell BM, Ruffel B: The mechanisms of action of cyclosporin. *Cardiol Clin* 1990;**8**:107.

Freeman DJ: Pharmacology and pharmacokinetics of cyclosporine. *Clin Biochem* 1991;**24**:9.

Harding MW, Handschumacher RE: Cyclophilin, a primary molecular target for cyclosporine. Structural and functional implications. *Transplantation* 1988; **46(Suppl 2)**:296.

Hohman RJ, Hultsch T: Cyclosporin A: New insights for cell biologists and biochemists. *New Biol* 1990;**2**:663.

Holloran PF, Madrenas J: The mechanism of action of cyclosporin: A perspective for the 90's. *Clin Biochem* 1991;**24**:3.

Kropp KA et al: Cyclosporine versus azathioprine: A review of 200 consecutive cadaver renal transplant recipients. *J Urol* 1989;**142**:28.

Starzl TE et al: Selective topics on FK 506 with special reference to rescue of extrahepatic whole organ grafts, transplantation of "forbidden organs," side effects, mechanisms and practical pharmacokinetics. *Transplant Proc* 1991;**23**:914.

Thomson AW: The immunosuppressive macrolides FK-506 and rapamycin. *Immunol Lett* 1991;**29**:105.

Plasmapheresis

Shumak KH, Rock GA: Therapeutic plasma exchange. *N Engl J Med* 1984;**310**:762.

Intravenous Gamma Globulin

Berkman SA, Lee ML, Gale RP: Clinical uses of intravenous immunoglobulins. *Ann Intern Med* 1990; **112**:278.

Polyclonal & Monoclonal Antibodies

Chatenoud L, Bach JF: Monoclonal antibodies to CD3 as immunosuppressants. *Semin Immunol* 1990;**2**:437.

Cobbold SP: Monoclonal antibody therapy for the induction of transplantation tolerance. *Immunol Lett* 1991; **29**:117.

Cosimi AB: Clinical development of orthoclone OKT3. *Transplant Proc* 1987;**19(Suppl 1)**:7.

Goldstein G: Overview of the development of orthoclone OKT3: Monoclonal antibody for therapeutic use in transplantation. *Transplant Proc* 1987;**19(Suppl 1)**:1.

Hall BM: Therapy with monoclonal antibodies to CD4: Potential not appreciated. *Am J Kidney Dis* 1989; **14(Suppl 2)**:71.

Heyworth MF: Clinical experience with antilymphocyte serum. *Immunol Rev* 1982;**65**:79.

Ortho Multicenter Transplant Study Group: A randomized clinical trial of OKT3 monoclonal antibody for acute rejection of cadaveric renal transplants. *N Engl J Med* 1985;**313**:337.

Steunmuler DR et al: Comparison of OKT3 with ALG for prophylaxis for patients with acute renal failure after cadaveric renal transplantation. *Transplantation* 1991;**52**:67.

Waldmann TA, Goldman CK: The multichain interleukin-2 receptor: A target for immunotherapy of patients receiving allografts. *Am J Kidney Dis* 1989; **14(Suppl 2)**:45.

Wood KJ: Transplantation tolerance. *Curr Opin Immunol* 1991;**3**:710.

Immunomodulators

59

Lawrence R. Hennessey, MD & James R. Baker, Jr, MD

Immunomodulators are biologic response-modifying compounds that affect the immune response in either a positive or negative fashion. Although immunosuppressive drugs and some therapeutic uses of gamma globulin can be included in this definition, they are discussed at length elsewhere (see Chapter 58), as are the biologic functions of many of these agents, especially the cytokines (see Chapter 9). In contrast, the focus of this discussion will be the pharmacologic and therapeutic effects of compounds that regulate or stimulate the immune response. These include a large number of compounds, which can be divided into 3 broad categories: general immunostimulatory agents, mostly of bacterial origin; eukaryotic source substances, eg, cytokines and monoclonal antibodies, which tend to have much more specific effects; and biochemical compounds. An ever-increasing array of potential immunomodulators are being examined for therapeutic benefit in a variety of disorders, including but not limited to malignancies, immunodeficient states such as acquired immunodeficiency syndrome (AIDS), and inflammatory diseases. A number of these have reached clinical trials, and some have demonstrated considerable efficacy.

COMPOUNDS DERIVED FROM BACTERIA

Bacterial compounds were among the first to be recognized as immunostimulators. Complete Freund's adjuvant (CFA), which contains mycobacterial derivatives, has long been used as an adjuvant to boost humoral immune responses in animals. Although CFA is not appropriate for human use, the attenuated mycobacterium bacillus Calmette-Guérin (BCG) has been extensively studied in the treatment of certain malignancies. Injection of BCG into lesions of malignant melanoma has led to remission of the local tumor as well as distant metastases, although long-term survival has not in general been af-

fected. It has also been used successfully in the treatment of bladder carcinoma via irrigation. CFA and BCG have been shown to prevent and even reverse the course of autoimmune diabetes in a murine model of this disease, but there are as yet no defined mechanisms for this effect and no data suggesting benefit in human autoimmune disorders. BCG has been shown to stimulate macrophage, T and B lymphocyte, and NK cell function and to augment interleukin-1 (IL-1) production. Various semipurified mycobacterial extracts, eg, methanol extract residue, muramyl dipeptides, and several heat shock proteins, have been examined and found to perform many of the functions of the whole extract.

Certain mycobacterial heat shock proteins and other bacterial substances, eg, toxins from *Staphylococcus aureus*, demonstrate "superantigen" activity; ie, they are capable of activating large numbers of T lymphocytes in a major histocompatability complex-restricted manner. This is thought to occur as a result of binding to subset-specific conserved areas of the T cell receptor variable region, denoted as V_α or V_β subsets, remote from the antigen-binding site. This polyclonal activation of certain T cell subsets may be responsible for some of the immunomodulatory effects seen following the administration of bacterial compounds. These compounds have been reported to stimulate immune responses to certain neoplasms and may be involved in the pathogenesis of certain vasculitides and autoimmune diseases.

OK432, an extract prepared from culture medium following penicillin treatment of a strain of group A *Streptococcus pyogenes*, has been shown to augment macrophage and natural killer (NK) cell activity and has some demonstrated effect in the treatment of human head and neck, gastrointestinal, and lung tumors. Whole or fractionated preparations of a variety of other microorganisms, including *Corynebacterium parvum, Listeria monocytogenes, Salmonella typhimurium, Brucella abortus, Pseudomonas aeruginosa*, and *Nocardia* spp., also have demonstrated immunomodulatory effects. Lipopolysaccharide from gram-negative bacteria has also been studied as an immunostimulatory compound, but the therapeutic usefulness of this preparation is limited by its toxicity.

COMPOUNDS DERIVED FROM EUKARYOTIC ORGANISMS

As knowledge of mammalian immune physiology progressed, attempts to characterize the immune function of certain organs led to the generation of crude immune tissue extracts with biologic functions. Compounds such as thymic extracts and interferons demonstrated varied immunomodulatory activities, and speculations were made regarding the potential clinical usefulness of some of these agents. However, problems with obtaining adequate quantities of appropriately pure preparations limited the study of their role in the treatment of human disease. The advent of recombinant DNA and hybridoma technologies in the 1970s, however, allowed for the appropriate characterization and production of a large number of immunoactive peptides and monoclonal antibodies. The study of the therapeutic potential of these agents is of great interest at present.

1. THYMIC HORMONES

A number of thymic peptide extracts, including thymosins, thymulin, thymopentin, thymostimulin, and thymic humoral factor, have demonstrated immunostimulatory actions. They have purported clinical benefit in a variety of viral infections, including hepatitis B, zoster, and herpes labialis, as well as in chronic *Trichophyton rubrum* infection. They have also been used with limited success in patients with primary immunodeficiency states such as DiGeorge's syndrome and ataxia-telangiectasia. Increased survival of patients with small cell carcinoma of the lung has been demonstrated after administration of thymosin as an adjunct to chemotherapy. Clinical improvement in patients with rheumatoid arthritis has been reported with thymulin and thymopentin. Although increased CD4:CD8 T cell ratios have been demonstrated in some asymptomatic HIV-infected individuals following treatment with thymic humoral factor, the clinical benefit of these compounds in HIV infection has not been conclusively demonstrated. The overall value of these agents in the treatment of human disease will be clarified as defined preparations of the various extracts become available.

2. CYTOKINES

Cytokines are small (< 80-kDa) proteins or glycoproteins that exhibit a variety of autocrine, paracrine and, in some cases, endocrine effects. They are generally subdivided into interferons, interleukins, colony-stimulating factors, and generalized growth and differentiation factors. As a group they have enormous potential for clinical use as immunomodulators and demonstrate a variety of specific as well as generalized influences on the immune system.

Interferons

Although interferons were first recognized for their effect on viral infection, their clinical usefulness as immunomodulators has been demonstrated in certain neoplastic diseases as well.

Alpha interferon (IFN α), a natural product of macrophages, has demonstrated antitumor activity in a number of neoplastic disorders. More than 90% of patients with hairy cell leukemia will respond to treatment with IFN α, although most will relapse shortly after treatment is discontinued. Long-term therapy, unfortunately, is often complicated by adverse effect such as chronic fatigue, and resistance occasionally develops because of the production of anti-interferon antibodies. IFN α also can induce remission in chronic myelogenous leukemia, especially if begun before the accelerated phase of the disease, and it has demonstrated benefit in multiple myeloma, non-Hodgkin lymphoma, and cutaneous T cell lymphoma. It also reportedly has activity against certain solid tumors, including malignant melanoma, renal cell carcinoma, and bladder and ovarian cancers. It is beneficial in the treatment of AIDS-related Kaposi's sarcoma, with a reported response rate of 25–40%, but toxicity at the high doses required for effective treatment (up to 36 million IU/day) is considerable, requiring dose reduction in up to one-third of patients.

Responses to a variety of viral infections have been demonstrated with IFN α. Intralesional and/or topical application has led to improvement in, and in some cases resolution of, condyloma acuminatum, laryngeal papillomatosis, herpetic keratoconjunctivitis, and rhinovirus infections.

Beta interferon (IFN β), naturally produced by fibroblasts, is not yet commercially available. Although it is somewhat less toxic than IFN α, it appears to be less efficacious as an antineoplastic drug. It may, however, be useful in the treatment of central nervous system gliomas, since it is reported to induce partial responses in 10–20% of patients.

Gamma interferon (IFN γ, immune interferon), a product of lymphocytes, also has been reported to have extensive activity in a variety of tumors and viral infections. Although it is structurally unrelated to IFN α and IFN β, IFN γ appears to have a similar spectrum of antitumor activity. It is being used with some success as an alternative treatment in patients with AIDS-related Kaposi's sarcoma who demonstrate resistance to or intolerance of IFN α. Response to IFN γ by tumors that are resistant to the effects of

IFN α (and vice versa) has been described as well. Unlike IFN α and IFN β, IFN γ may have some applicability in the treatment of collagen vascular disorders and has been shown to be effective in the treatment of lepromatous leprosy. There is evidence to support synergy between IFN α and IFN γ in the treatment of some neoplasms. Subjective improvement and increased resistance to opportunistic infections in a small number of AIDS patients treated with IFN γ has been described, but its effect on overall survival has not been demonstrated. Side effects, shared with the other interferons, include acute malaise with a "flulike" syndrome, chronic fatigue, anorexia, and elevation of hepatic enzymes. In addition, however, IFN γ may cause lipidemia, arthralgias, hypocalcemia, and severe headaches. The most effective future use of this agent is thought to be as an adjuvant in the treatment of lymphoproliferative malignancies.

Interleukins

The interleukins are a diverse group of lymphokines, exhibiting a broad array of actions on the immune system. Many possess demonstrated or potential usefulness as therapeutic immunomodulators.

Interleukin-2 (IL-2) has been used successfully in the treatment of certain malignancies, in particular renal cell carcinoma and malignant melanoma. This is in all likelihood due to activation and proliferation of lymphocyte-activated killer (LAK) cells. Direct systemic administration of IL-2 does, however, lead to significant toxicity, including fever, chills, and edema. Severe gastrointestinal and central nervous system toxicity are also seen in most patients. Adoptive immunotherapy, involving IL-2-mediated activation of LAK cells derived from the patients' peripheral blood leukocytes, followed by readministration, has been used, and although it is less toxic than systemic IL-2 administration, it has not shown consistent efficacy in treating neoplasms.

Recently, IL-2 has been used to produce ex vivo activation of a subset of lymphocytes derived from solid tumors, known as tumor-infiltrating lymphocytes (TIL). TIL reportedly possess 50–100 times more antitumor activity than do LAK cells derived from peripheral blood, presumably because they represent a select population directed primarily against the tumor in question. Studies using this approach to immunotherapy are under way.

IL-4, a lymphokine that is known mainly for promotion of IgE production and mast cell stimulation, also has demonstrable antitumor activity in animal models and may have some potential role in the treatment of human malignancies. Its usefulness may be limited because of the possible promotion of adverse allergic responses.

Tumor necrosis factor (TNF), a cytokine that has demonstrated considerable antitumor activity both in vitro and in vivo, has limited therapeutic potential be-cause of its considerable systemic toxicity. Gene therapy strategies in which genes encoding TNF are introduced into TIL in an attempt to make use of the antitumor activity of this cytokine at the microenvironmental level are, however, being developed. This strategy may also prove useful in the application of IL-4 and other cytokines with antitumor activity as immunomodulators.

IL-10, a cytokine with primarily counterregulatory properties, may be useful in the treatment of autoimmune diseases or other disorders of inflammation. It has marked antiproliferative and anti-inflammatory effects in vitro. However, the clinical usefulness of IL-10 is currently not well defined and may be limited by its stimulatory effects on mast cells and IgE production.

Colony-Stimulating Factors

Three cytokines with colony-stimulating properties have been studied extensively and are now being used routinely or experimentally in humans. They are erythropoeitin, now used routinely to treat anemia in patients with chronic renal disease, granulocyte colony-stimulating factor (G-CSF), and granulocyte-macrophage colony-stimulating factor (GM-CSF). G-CSF hastens recovery from neutropenia in patients with nonmyelogenous malignancies who are receiving chemotherapy. GM-CSF is used to accelerate marrow recovery after autologous bone marrow transplantation. CSFs are also being explored experimentally in the treatment of leukopenia of other causes, including primary neutropenia, myelodysplasia, myeloproliferative disorders, aplastic anemia, AIDS, and the neutropenia associated with Felty's syndrome. CSFs appear to have less potential benefit in the treatment of diseases associated with increased peripheral destruction of leukocytes, such as autoimmune neutropenia or Evan's syndrome.

Growth & Differentiation Factors

Perhaps the best studied growth and differentiation factor is transforming growth factor beta (TGF-β), which has a wide range of effects on the immune response. Its uses in a variety of areas are being explored. It has potential benefit as an accelerator of wound healing and may have applications in this regard in ophthalmology, dermatology, and surgical wound healing. It is also reported to have antiproliferative and anti-inflammatory effects in vitro and may prevent postinflammatory fibrotic changes. It also markedly inhibits the IL-4-stimulated synthesis of IgE and may be clinically useful as an antiallergy drug. Other growth factors, such as epidermal growth factor, platelet-derived growth factor, and fibroblast growth factor, are being studied for potential clinical utility in wound healing and revascularization.

There is evidence to suggest that glomerulonephrosis and glomerulosclerosis may be attributable in part to deleterious effects of TGF-β, in particular the excessive accumulation of extracellular matrix proteins. This cytokine has also been suspected in the pathogenesis of systemic sclerosis. A naturally occurring proteoglycan, decorin, has been shown to bind to and effectively inactivate TGF-β and may have potential clinical utility in diseases associated with excessive TGF-β activity.

3. CYTOKINE ANTAGONISTS

A great deal of interest has recently developed in the potential use of cytokine antagonists as immunomodulatory drugs. This has been due primarily to the identification and characterization of a naturally occurring interleukin-1 receptor antagonist (IL-1RA). IL-1RA is a 152-amino-acid peptide, which shares a great deal of sequence homology with both IL-1β and IL-1γ. It binds to the IL-1 receptor with similar affinity; however, it does not lead to receptor-mediated activation of target cells. IL-1RA has demonstrable anti-inflammatory activity in animal models of a variety of human diseases, many attributed at least in part to excessive production of IL-1. These include septic shock, ischemia-reperfusion injury, inflammatory bowel disease, adult respiratory distress syndrome, polyarteritis nodosa, osteoporosis, and glomerulonephritis. IL-1RA does not appear to induce immunosuppression and must be present in at least 100-fold excess over IL-1 to exert its inhibitory effects, suggesting that high doses may be needed to elicit a clinical response. Clinical trials of IL-1RA in the treatment of rheumatoid arthritis, inflammatory bowel disease, and septic shock are under way.

4. MONOCLONAL ANTIBODIES

A variety of monoclonal antibodies have been developed and proposed as potential immunomodulators, and some have been used experimentally in clinical situations. Pilot studies with murine monoclonal anti-TNF antibodies have demonstrated improvement in acute graft-versus-host disease, improved left-ventricular function in septic shock, and possible improvement in hairy cell leukemia. Benefits appeared to be transient, however, and mortality has not been affected in the limited studies performed so far. Studies in a murine model have suggested a possible role for anti-TNF antibodies in the treatment of autoimmune myocarditis, but animal studies of the efficacy of this agent in the treatment of septic shock are inconclusive.

Antiendotoxin monoclonal antibodies have been used in the treatment of gram-negative sepsis, and decreased blood levels of TNF have been documented following their administration. Data on clinical efficacy, however, are still inconclusive.

Animal studies have demonstrated immunomodulatory effects of monoclonal antibodies directed against other mediators of inflammation including IL-6, the adhesion molecule CD11b/18, and the 55-kDa receptor for TNF. The usefulness of monoclonal antibodies in the treatment of human disease is limited in many instances, however, by the development of antimurine antibodies. Future research in this area, for example the splicing of murine variable-region immunoglobulin genes with human constant-region genes to yield less immunogenic "hybrid" monoclonal antibodies, may render these compounds better suited to clinical use.

BIOCHEMICAL AGENTS

Primarily because of the advent of AIDS, a variety of biochemical agents have been explored as potential immunomodulators. Many of these agents, although promising in in vitro studies, unfortunately have demonstrated little benefit in vivo. Some agents, however, have shown clinical benefit in other applications.

Perhaps the best known biochemical immunomodulator is levamisole, an imidathiazole compound originally studied for its anthelmintic activity. It is immunotrophic; however, its mechanism of action is unknown and it exhibits no direct cytotoxic activity. It has little effect in immunocompetent individuals. It has been shown to reverse postviral anergy associated with measles and influenza and has some benefit in chronic infections, malignancies, and neoplastic diseases. A well-defined role for levamisole as an adjunct in the treatment of colon cancer has been established. In a study of 262 patients with Duke's class C colon cancer, addition of levamisole to 5-fluorouracil led to an increased 5-year survival rate from 37 to 49%. The use of levamisole as an adjunct in the treatment of malignant melanoma and other neoplasms is being explored.

A related imidazole drug, inosine pranobex, has been shown in 2 studies of HIV-infected patients to delay the progression to AIDS. Controversy exists, however, about its optimal dose, toxicity, use in combination with other drugs, and overall benefit. The compound diethyldithiocarbamate also has reported activity in the treatment of HIV infection and some cancers.

Other immunostimulatory drugs, among them polyribosinic agents, anthroguinones, and pyrimidinolones, probably act via their ability to induce the production of interferons. Aziridine derivatives, of which Imexone is perhaps the best studied, have been shown to be effective in a murine model of AIDS. A related compound, Azimexone, appears to stimulate delayed hypersensitivity in animal models. However, it paradoxically inhibits graft-versus-host responses via an unknown mechanism. Aziridine derivatives have so far shown no benefit in the treatment of can-

cer. These and many other agents are being evaluated for potential therapeutic benefit in a variety of other immune disorders.

REFERENCES

General

Chirigos MA: Immunomodulators: Current and future development and application. *Thymus* 1992;**19:**S7.

Hadden JW: Immunopharmacology and immunotoxicology. *Adv Exp Med Biol* 1991;**288:**1.

Hassner A, Adelman DC:Biologic response modifiers in primary immunodeficiency disorders. *Ann Intern Med* 1991;**115:**294.

Perren T, Selby P: Biological therapy. *Br Med J* 1992;**304:**1621.

Cytokines

Balmer CM: Clinical use of biologic response modifiers in cancer treatment: An overview. Part II. Colony stimulating factors and interleukin-2. *Drug Intell Clin Pharm* 1991;**25:**490.

Blackwell S, Crawford J: Colony-stimulating factors: Clinical applications. *Pharmacotherapy* 1992;**12:**21S.

Hom DB, Maisel RH: Angiogenic growth factors: Their effects and potential in soft tissue wound healing. *Ann Otol Rhinol Laryngol* 1992;**101:**349.

Pardell DM et al: Molecular engineering of the antitumor response. *Bone Marrow Transplant* 1992;**9:**182S.

Rees RC: Cytokines as biologic response modifiers. *J Clin Pathol* 1992;**45:**93.

Ruocco V et al: Malignant melanoma: Biotherapeutic strategies for management with interferons. *Clin Dermatol* 1992;**9:**505.

Thompson RC et al: Interleukin-1 receptor antagonist (IL-1ra) as a probe and as a treatment for IL-1 mediated disease. *Int J Immunopharmacol* 1992;**14:**475.

Monoclonal Antibodies

Herve P et al: Phase I–II trial of a monoclonal anti-tumor necrosis factor alpha antibody for the treatment of refractory severe acute graft-versus-host disease. *Blood* 1992;**79:**3362.

Biochemical Compounds

Amery W, Bruynseels J: Levamisole, the story and the lessons. *Int J Pharmacol* 1992;**14:**481.

De Simone C et al: Inosine pranobex in the treatment of HIV infection: A review. *Int J Immunopharmacol* 1991;**13:**19S.

Anti-Inflammatory Drugs

James S. Goodwin, MD

The distinction between immunosuppressive and anti-inflammatory drugs is not always clear, because of the extensive interaction of the biologic mechanisms of these interrelated systems. In this chapter, drugs with anti-inflammatory activity mediated at least in part by suppression of the functions of the nonspecific inflammatory cells, especially monocytes, polymorphonuclear leukocytes, and basophils, will be discussed. They are used to treat acute and chronic inflammatory process and are effective in treating inflammation whether or not the inflammation is initiated immunologically. Drugs that primarily suppress the immune response are discussed in Chapter 58.

CORTICOSTEROIDS

Glucocorticoids are the most powerful drugs currently available for the treatment of inflammatory diseases, but their use is associated with significant toxicity (also see Chapter 58). The discovery of corticosteroids was a major advance in the treatment of inflammatory diseases. Since the first successful use in 1948 of hydrocortisone (Cortisol), the principal glucocorticoid of the adrenal cortex, for suppression of the clinical manifestations of rheumatoid arthritis, numerous compounds with glucocorticoid activity have been synthesized and are presently standard therapy for many immunologic and nonimmunologic inflammatory conditions.

Pharmacology & Physiology

Corticosteroids are 21-carbon steroid hormones derived from the metabolism of cholesterol. Fig 60–1 shows the structures of the commonly used synthetic corticosteroids. The activity of corticosteroids depends on the presence of a hydroxyl group on carbon-11. Two of the most commonly used corticosteroids, cortisone and prednisone, are inactive until converted in vivo to the corresponding 11-hydroxyl compounds, cortisol and prednisone.

The clinical potency of the various synthetic steroids depends on the rate of absorption, the concentration in target tissues, the affinity for steroid receptors, and the rate of metabolism and subsequent clearance. Table 60–1 shows the half-lives and relative potencies of the commonly used glucocorticoid preparations. Most are well absorbed after oral administration. Corticosteroid uptake is not usually affected by intrinsic intestinal diseases, and food intake does not influence absorption. Approximately 90% of endogenous circulating cortisol is bound with high affinity to the plasma protein corticosteroid-binding globulin. Another 5–8% is bound to albumin, which is a high-capacity, low-affinity reservoir for steroids. Most synthetic steroids, with the exception of prednisolone, have a low affinity for corticosteroid-binding globulin and are bound predominantly to albumin. Only the small fraction of circulating corticosteroids that are not protein-bound are free to exert a biologic action, whereas those associated with proteins are protected from metabolic degradation.

Corticosteroids are metabolized in the liver. Hydroxylation of the 4,5 double bond and ketone groups and subsequent conjugation with glucuronide or sulfate groups render steroids inactive and water-soluble. The kidney excretes 95% of the conjugated metabolites, and the remainder are lost in the gut. There are individual differences in the half-lives of synthetic steroids, and patients receiving those with prolonged clearance may be at increased risk for side effects from therapy. Clearance rates of corticosteroids are also affected by other drugs and disease states. Phenytoin, phenobarbital, and rifampin can increase steroid clearance by inducing hepatic-enzyme activity. Estrogen therapy and estrogen-containing oral contraceptives impair the clearance of administered steroids and may decrease the steroid requirement. In patients with liver diseases, the metabolism of corticosteroids is not significantly altered and dose

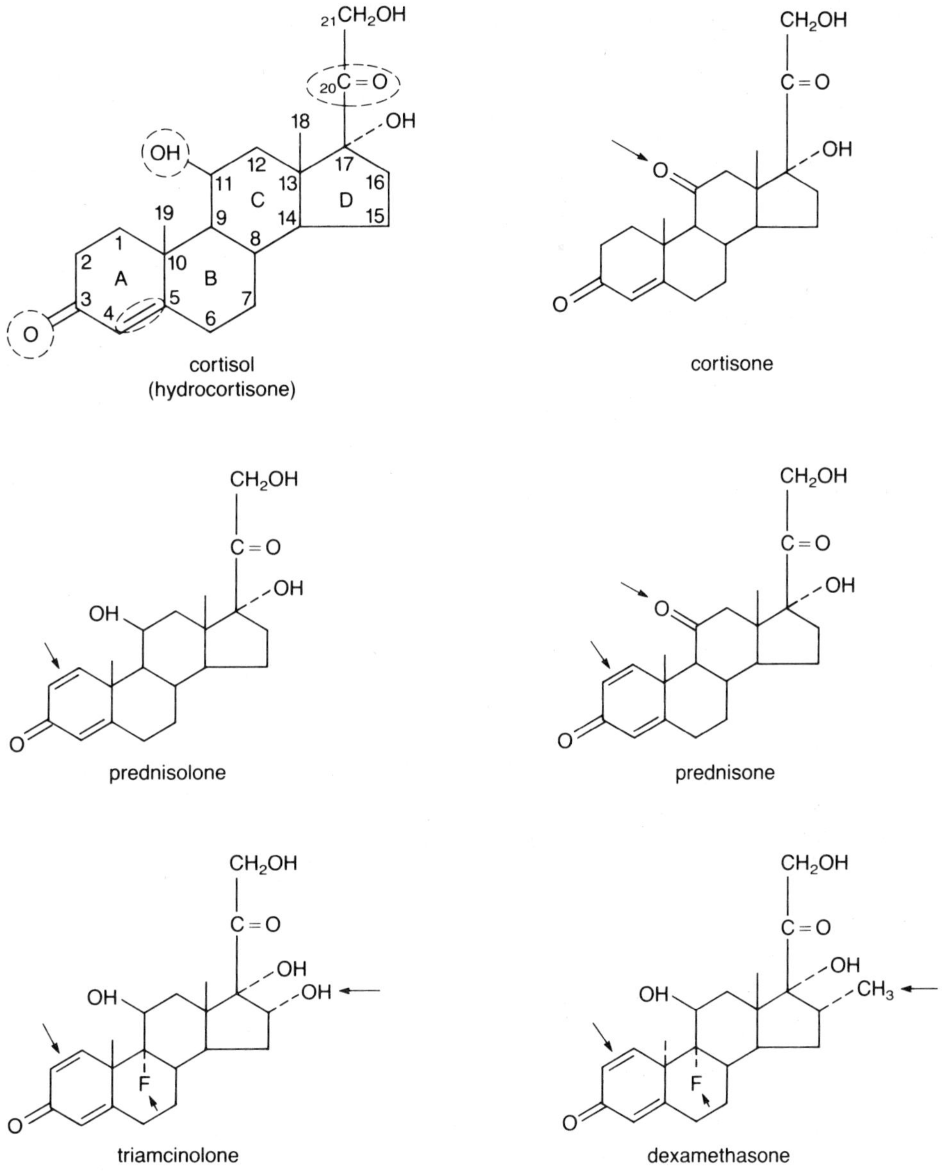

Figure 60–1. Structures of corticosteroid hormones and drugs. The arrows indicate the structural differences between cortisol and each of the other compounds.

adjustments are not necessary. Dose adjustments are also generally not necessary for patients with kidney disease. Corticosteroids can lower plasma salicylate levels by enhancing their renal clearance. Patients on fixed-dose salicylate therapy may develop rapid increases to toxic levels of serum salicylate when glucocorticoids are withdrawn or tapered.

Mechanism of Action

All steroid hormones including vitamin D, corticosteroids, sex hormones, and mineralocorticoid act by binding to high-affinity receptors in the cytoplasm (Fig 60–2). The steroid-receptor complex, in turn, has a high affinity for nuclear interphase chromosomes and thus binds to chromosomal DNA. This triggers DNA transcription, with the formation of messenger RNA, leading to new protein synthesis. The specific genes transcribed and proteins produced after exposure to steroid hormones vary with the different steroid hormones and also with the target cell. Specificity of cell response is manifested in at least 2 ways. (1) The steroid-receptor complex binds to specific

Table 60–1. Half-life relative potency
of commonly used glucocorticoids.

Glucocorticoid	Plasma Half Life (min)	Relative Potency of Glucocorticoid	Mineralocorticoid
Cortisol	80–120	1.0	1.0
Cortisone	80–120	0.8	0.8
Prednisone	200–210	4.0	0.8
Prednisolone	120–300	5.0	0
Triamcinolone	180–240	5.0	0
Dexamethasone	150–270	30–150	0

regulatory sequences, which, in turn, leads to transcription of the particular gene containing that sequence. Presumably the steroid-receptor complex binding vitamin D attaches to regulatory sequences on different genes from those used by the complex binding cortisol. (2) Only a small portion of the genome is capable of induction by steroid hormone because it is contained in an "unraveled" portion of chromatin sensitive to digestion with DNase. This unraveled portion will differ depending on the cell type.

All well-defined physiologic and pharmacologic effects of steroid hormones are thought to be mediated by the process outlined above. However, nonreceptor-mediated effects of steroids, particularly at high doses, may also play an important role in their effects. One implication of this is the delay in appearance of the pharmacologic or physiologic effects after drug administration. Another implication is that glucocorticoid action is indirect; it acts by promoting the synthesis of other compounds.

Cells exposed to glucocorticoids synthesize and re-lease a phospholipase A_2-inhibitory glycoprotein, now termed lipomodulin. The inhibition of phospholipase A_2 leads, in turn, to a reduction in the release of arachidonic acid, thereby slowing production of arachidonic acid metabolites. Lipomodulin appears to be a family of molecules, one of which was recently clones and found to have potent antiinflammatory actions. Thus, the anti-inflammatory actions of glucocorticoids may be related, at least in part, to lipomodulin-induced reduction of arachidonic acid metabolites, the prostaglandins and leukotrienes that are generated by cyclooxygenase and lipoxygenase, respectively. The role of prostaglandins and leukotrienes in mediating various aspects of the inflammatory response is discussed in Chapter 10.

Anti-Inflammatory Effects

Administration of corticosteroids results in a complex series of changes in the actions of cells involved in inflammatory reactions. After a single dose of steroids, there is a net increase in the number of circulat-

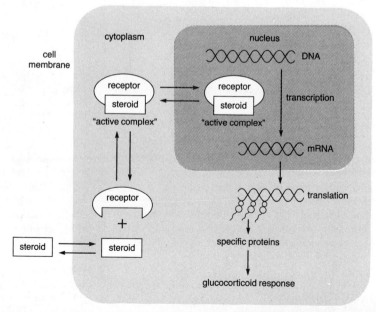

Figure 60–2. Mechanism of action of steroid hormones on a molecular level.

ing neutrophils, accompanied by a decrease in the margination, migration, and accumulation of neutrophils at sites of inflammation, which reduces the signs of acute inflammation and also interferes with the expression of delayed-type hypersensitivity skin reactions.

Corticosteroids also directly suppress the action of cells involved in the inflammatory response, inhibiting phagocytosis by neutrophils and monocytes, the release of degradative enzymes such as collagenase and plasminogen activator by neutrophils and synovial lining cells, and the production of inflammatory lymphokines and monokines such as interleukin-1 and tumor necrosis factor. Other than the clear effects found in vivo and in vitro on migration and accumulation of granulocytes and monocytes, it is difficult to know how the many other effects of corticosteroids on inflammatory cell function contribute to the anti-inflammatory effect, since this information is based largely on in vitro studies of isolated cell populations. It is assumed, however, that the so-called "lysosomal stabilizing" effects and the decreased release of inflammatory mediators and degradative enzymes such as collagenase contribute to the anti-inflammatory clinical effects.

A discussion of related immunosuppressive effects of corticosteroids is in Chapter 58.

Metabolic Effects

Like other hormones, corticosteroids affect many different tissue and organ systems. At physiologic concentrations, their various metabolic effects presumably maintain normal homeostasis, but at the high concentrations used pharmacologically (or from pathologic overproduction), an accentuation of these same metabolic effects leads to target organ dysfunction.

A summary of the metabolic effects of glucocorticoids is given in Table 60–2. In general, steroids promote catabolism. They block glucose uptake by tissues, enhance protein breakdown, and decrease new protein synthesis in muscle, skin, bone, connective tissue, fat, and lymphoid tissue. DNA synthesis and cell proliferation in fibroblasts, lymphocytes, and adipocytes are inhibited. Chronic exposure to supraphysiologic levels of corticosteroids has a type of wasting effect, ie, loss of bone, connective tissue, and muscle and gain in water and fat.

Toxicity

The toxicities of prolonged corticosteroid therapy are numerous and are the major limiting factor in the use of these agents. They are listed in Table 60–3. Susceptibility to side effects varies among patients; the reason for this is unknown. Some patients on prolonged, high-dose therapy appear to tolerate corticosteroids with few adverse effects, whereas others treated with small doses for brief intervals develop devastating side effects such as aseptic necrosis,

Table 60–2. Metabolic effects of glucocorticoids.

Carbohydrate metabolism
Impairs glucose uptake and utilization by peripheral tissues
Increases gluconeogenesis and glycogen deposition in liver

Lipid metabolism
Stimulates lipolysis and increases free fatty acid levels, an effect countered by increased insulin release and gluconeogenesis
Increases fat deposition in truncal and facial areas

Protein metabolism
Inhibits synthesis and enhances breakdown of proteins in many tissues, leading to negative nitrogen balance
Increases plasma free amino acid levels

Nucleic acid metabolism
Stimulates RNA synthesis in liver, inhibits RNA synthesis in other tissues
Inhibits DNA synthesis in most tissues

Fluid and electrolyte metabolism
May enhance sodium retention and potassium loss independent of mineralocorticoid action
Increases glomerular filtration rate

Bone and calcium-metabolism
Decreases intestinal calcium absorption
Decreases renal reabsorption of calcium and phosphate with resulting hypercalciuria
Inhibits osteoblast function

osteoporosis, and vertebral collapse. In part, this differential sensitivity may be related to individual differences in plasma protein binding (with hypoalbuminemic patients at risk) and to variations in metabolism and clearance of synthetic steroids. Sensitivity to glucocorticoids in mice is closely linked to the H-2 histocompatibility region, and there is some evidence of analogous human leukocyte antigen (HLA) linkages in humans.

There are several useful approaches to reducing corticosteroid toxicity. One is through local application, as with topical ointments for dermatitis or administration via inhalers for asthma. Another is the use of so-called steroid-sparing drugs. These are drugs that may not have sufficient activity for use as first-line therapy but may allow a lowering of the dose of corticosteroids required to control disease activity. Drugs touted as steroid-sparing in asthma include those with demonstratable activity in other inflammatory conditions, such as dapsone, chloroquine, methotrexate, and gold. The macrolide antibiotics are "steroid-sparing" by inhibiting metabolism of corticosteroids, resulting in elevated blood levels.

ASPIRIN & OTHER NONSTEROIDAL ANTI-INFLAMMATORY DRUGS (NSAID)

Extracts of the willow tree (Latin, salix) had been used and endorsed by Hippocrates, Pliny, Galen, and other ancient practitioners for the relief of pain and

Table 60–3. Side effects of glucocorticoid therapy.

Very common and should be anticipated in all patients
 Negative calcium balance leading to osteoporosis
 Increased appetite
 Centripetal obesity
 Impaired wound healing
 Increased risk of infection
 Suppression of hypothalamic-pituitary-adrenal axis
 Growth arrest in children

Frequently seen
 Myopathy
 Avascular necrosis
 Hypertension
 Plethora
 Thin, fragile skin/striae/purpura
 Edema secondary to sodium and water retention
 Hyperlipidemia
 Psychiatric symptoms, particularly euphoria or depression
 Diabetes mellitus
 Posterior subcapsular cataracts

Not very common, but important to recognize early
 Glaucoma
 Benign intracranial hypertension
 "Silent" intestinal perforation
 Peptic ulcer disease (often gastric)
 Hypokalemic alkalosis
 Hyperosmolar nonketotic coma
 Gastric hemorrhage

Rare
 Pancreatitis
 Hirsutism
 Panniculitis
 Secondary amenorrhea
 Impotence
 Epidural lipomatosis
 Allergy to synthetic steroids

Table 60–4. NSAID available in the USA.

Drug Name	Approved as Anti-inflammatory	Approved as Analgesic
Diclofenac	X	
Diflunisal	X	
Etodolac	X	X
Fenoprofen	X	X
Flurbiprofen	X	
Ibuprofen	X	X
Indomethacin	X	
Ketoprofen	X	
Meclofenamate	X	X
Mefenamic acid	X	X
Nabumetone	X	X
Naproxen	X	X
Piroxicam	X	
Tolmetin	X	
Tromethamine	X	X

fever. Later, willow bark extract (salicylate) was substituted for the more expensive and frequently unobtainable cinchona bark extract (quinine) in the treatment of pain and fever. Salicylates achieved widespread use by the end of the nineteenth century, when simple and inexpensive ways of synthesizing the drugs were discovered. Today 30 million lb of aspirin are consumed each year in the USA alone. Salicylates can be found in most households. In addition to the many oral formulations, salicylates are present in most skin liniments, plasters, and ointments. The newer nonsteroidal anti-inflammatory drugs (NSAID) are also in widespread use. Hundreds have been synthesized and dozens introduced for clinical use worldwide (Table 60–4). As a class, NSAID are the most frequently prescribed medications for patients older than 65 years. Within the last several years, ibuprofen has become available without a prescription, further contributing to the widespread consumption of NSAID.

Anti-Inflammatory Effects

The anti-inflammatory effects of the different NSAID are very similar in many experimental models, providing indirect support for the concept that they all share a single mechanism of action (discussed below). NSAID prevent the pain, swelling, redness, and loss of function in experimental models of inflammation as diverse as sunburn and carrageenan-induced paw edema in rats. NSAID administration decreases the rate of progressive joint destruction associated with adjuvant-induced arthritis in rats. Clinically, NSAID have been shown to be effective in many acute and chronic inflammatory diseases, such as arthritis, tendinitis, and pericarditis. They are also all analgesics, although only some of them are marketed for pain control.

Mechanism of Action

Since 1971 aspirin and other NSAID at therapeutic levels have been shown to inhibit the production of prostaglandins by inhibiting cyclooxygenase. The relative inhibiting potency in vitro of different NSAID generally parallels their anti-inflammatory potency in vivo. Cyclooxygenase inhibition became the in vitro screening test for new NSAID. However, the simple concept that NSAID are anti-inflammatory because they inhibit cyclooxygenase production of proinflammatory metabolites of arachidonic acid may not be adequate to explain all their clinical effects.

Although prostaglandin E_2 causes vasodilatation and sensitizes pain receptors to agonists such as histamine, other arachidonic acid metabolites have anti-inflammatory or neutral effects. Sodium salicylate, a nonacetylated salicylate, is equally anti-inflammatory as aspirin in vivo but has no demonstrable inhibition of cyclooxygenase activity in vivo or in vitro. Furthermore, aspirin ingested in low doses profoundly inhibits prostaglandin production in blood, kidneys, and vascular endothelium but has no anti-inflammatory effect, and analgesia from aspirin or other NSAID is achieved with considerably lower doses and serum concentrations than is anti-inflammatory activity. There is dose-response relationship of analgesia and prostaglandin inhibition with all

NSAID, but anti-inflammatory effects are seen only at higher doses. Analgesic-antipyretic drugs such as acetaminophen do not inhibit cyclooxygenase and are not anti-inflammatory. Thus, pharmacologic evidence to date links pain and fever, but not inflammation, to in vivo prostaglandin production. The effect of aspirin on prolonging the bleeding time in vivo can be prevented by prior treatment with sodium salicylate or other NSAID.

Other properties of NSAID may better explain their therapeutic anti-inflammatory effects. Inhibition of one or more lipoxygenase enzymes has been described for some NSAID in some in vitro systems. NSAID inhibit cyclic AMP-dependent protein kinase, phospholipase C, amino acid transport across cell membranes, and a variety of other membrane-associated events. The relative potency of various NSAID in inhibiting amino acid transport parallels their anti-inflammatory potency. All NSAID inhibit a variety of neutrophil and monocyte functions, such as aggregation, degranulation, and superoxide anion production.

Some other clinical effects of NSAID could be mediated by prostaglandin E inhibition. NSAID stimulate suppressor T cell activity, possibly explaining the fact that they lower rheumatoid factor levels in patients with rheumatoid arthritis. There may be a therapeutic effect attributable to the inhibition of prostaglandin E stimulation of osteoclast-activating factor production and the excretion of collagenase by monocytes.

Toxicity

The major side effects are listed in Table 60–5. Between 10 and 40% of patients in controlled trials of NSAID will stop using the drug because of upper gastrointestinal symptoms such as pain, nausea, and vomiting. In clinical trials, approximately 1% of patients ingesting any NSAID develop upper gastrointestinal bleeding. It has been estimated that up to 25% of all hospitalizations for peptic ulcer disease are causally associated with NSAID use. The mechanism of gastrointestinal toxicity is thought to involve 3 processes, 2 of which are secondary to cyclooxygenase inhibition: (1) Prostaglandin E is a local feedback inhibitor of hydrochloric acid secretion; (2) prostaglandin E has a cytoprotective effect on gastric mucosa independent of HCl secretion; and (3) all NSAID are organic acids that can directly irritate gastric mucosa.

The major renal complication of NSAID is also related to cyclooxygenase inhibition. In patients with preexisting renal disease or circulatory disease resulting in decreased renal blood flow, NSAID tend to further reduce renal blood flow and glomerular filtration by eliminating prostaglandin-mediated compensatory mechanisms within the kidney. This becomes clinically important in some patients and can lead to total kidney failure, but it is almost always reversible upon cessation of the drug. The prevalence of renal complications from NSAID is difficult to estimate, because it is too rare to be detected in most prospective, controlled clinical trials. In addition, patients most likely to experience renal toxicity because of preexisting renal or heart disease are likely to be excluded from those drug trials. Renal toxicity is very rare in patients whose renal function is normal prior to the start of therapy with NSAID.

COLCHICINE

Colchicine has largely been replaced in the treatment of acute gouty attacks by NSAID, which work quicker, are at least as efficacious, and are less toxic. It is sometimes used as an adjunctive therapy with NSAID in chronic or polyarticular gout and also as a prophylactic agent in low doses (0.6 mg once or twice daily) to prevent attacks.

Recently, prophylactic chronic colchicine ingestion has been found to reduce attacks of familial Mediterranean fever and to prevent the development of amyloidosis in patients with that disease. Colchicine has been reported to slow the progression of cirrhosis in patients with alcoholic liver disease.

The mechanism of action of colchicine is not completely understood. It binds to labile microtubules, so that disruption of neutrophil microtubules leads to decreased chemotaxis, adhesiveness, phagocytosis, and degranulation.

Table 60–5. Side effects of NSAID therapy.

Gastrointestinal
Gastritis
Duodenal ulcer
Gastric ulcer
Renal
Decreased creatinine clearance
Acute renal failure
Interstitial nephritis
Central nervous system
Headache
Confusion, memory loss, personality change, especially in the elderly
Toxicities not shared by all NSAID
Bone marrow failure with phenylbutazone
Rash with meclofenamate

GOLD, D-PENICILLAMINE, & ANTIMALARIALS

Gold, penicillamine, the antimalarial hydroxychloroquine, and perhaps also the various immunosuppressive drugs (see Chapter 58) share a number of properties when used in rheumatoid arthritis and other diseases. (1) They require one to several months before any benefit is noted. (2) They can produce a clinical remission wherein no subjective or objective evidence of continued disease activity remains. (3) They have a narrow therapeutic spectrum. For example, gold has efficacy in rheumatoid arthritis and psoriatic arthritis but not significantly in other chronic inflammatory arthritides such as ankylosing spondylitis or systemic lupus erythematosus. (4) Many of the toxicities of the individual drugs in this class are similar. For example, gold and penicillamine can both cause rash, mouth ulcers, neutropenia, and nephritis. (5) They have little or no activity in experimental animal models of arthritis. (It is ironic that the animal models now used to screen for new treatments for arthritis would not have allowed for the discovery of the most efficacious drugs!) (6)Their mechanism of action is unknown.

In general, gold and penicillamine are considered more efficacious but also more toxic than antimalarial drugs in the treatment of rheumatoid arthritis. Approximately 50% of patients taking gold or penicillamine will have stopped the medication within 5 years of beginning treatment, two-thirds of these because of toxicity and one-third because of lack of efficacy. The major serious side effect of antimalarial drugs is retinal toxicity, which can be prevented by yearly ophthalmologic examinations.

DRUGS THAT SUPPRESS IMMEDIATE-HYPERSENSITIVITY REACTIONS

Cromolyn Sodium

Cromolyn sodium inhibits the release of mediators from mast cells, thereby blocking the tissue response and symptoms of IgE-mediated allergy. The precise mechanism of action of cromolyn sodium is unknown, but there is evidence that it interferes with calcium influx through the cell membrane. It does not interfere with the binding of IgE to mast cells nor with the interaction of antigen with the IgE bound to mast cells. Rather, it suppresses the degranulation reaction normally triggered by the cross-linking of cell surface IgE by antigen.

Cromolyn sodium is effective only prophylactically. It is poorly absorbed after oral administration and is therefore administered by inhaler as a powder, which is effective only when administered topically to mucous membranes. It is available as a micronized powder in a metered-dose inhaler or as a powder for inhalation in a special dispenser for asthma, as a nasal aerosolized solution for allergic rhinitis, as eye drops for allergic conjunctivitis, and as an oral preparation for use in food allergies or for systemic mastocytosis. Nedocromil sodium is chemically unrelated but clinically similar to cromolyn. It was recently released in the USA in a metered-dose inhaler.

The toxicity of cromolyn sodium is low and relates

Table 60–6. Actions of histamine at H_1 receptor sites inhibited by antihistamine.

Increased capillary permeability following histamine or antigen challenge
Smooth muscle constriction, particularly bronchial and gastrointestinal tract
Stimulation of autonomic ganglia
Secretion of exocrine glands

mostly to irritation by the inhaled powdered drug. It has no known utility in other inflammatory diseases.

Antihistamines

There are 2 classes of antihistamines, called H_1 and H_2 blockers, corresponding to the 2 types of histamine receptors found in mammalian tissues. Only H_1 blockers will be considered here because H_2 blockers do not possess noticeable anti-inflammatory activity, although they are sometimes used in allergic diseases. The pharmacologic properties of H_1-blocking antihistamines are listed in Table 60–6.

The major therapeutic role for antihistamines is in the treatment of allergic diseases involving IgE-mediated hypersensitivity reactions. They are effective in reducing nasal and lacrimal secretions in seasonal rhinitis and conjunctivitis (hay fever). They are

Table 60–7. Commonly used antihistamines (H_1 blockers).

Classic	New Generation
Alkylamines Chlorpheniramine Dexchlorpheniramine Brompheniramine Triprolidine	Acrivastine[1,2]
Ethanolamines Diphenhydramine Dimenhydrate Clemastine Cinarrizine[2]	Ketotifen[2] Oxatomide[2]
Ethylenediamines Tripelennamine	
Piperazines Hydroxyzine Meclizine	Cetirizine[1,2,3]
Phenothiazines Promethazine	Mequitazine[1,2,3]
Piperidines Cyproheptadine Azatidine	Loratidine[1,3] Astemizole[1,3] Terfenadine[1] Azelastine[2]
Tricyclics Doxepin Amitriptyline Imipramine Desipramine	

[1]Nonsedative.
[2]Not available in the USA (as of Nov. 1993).
[3]Once-a-day dosage.

also effective in treating urticaria and angioedema, and they reduce pruritus associated with other dermatoses. Another major therapeutic role for antihistamines in the treatment of motion sickness and Meniere's disease.

The principal side effects of antihistamines are sedation, dryness of mucous membranes, and constipation. Recently, several antihistamines have been developed that lack the sedative effect, probably because of their failure to penetrate the blood-brain barrier.

There are a large number of drugs with antihistaminic effects. The chemical classification of these drugs and representative examples are listed in Table 60–7.

Sympathomimetic (Adrenergic) Drugs

These drugs mimic the effects of sympathetic nerve stimulation. They have 2 general mechanisms of action: (1) stimulation of adrenergic receptors and (2) increase in the release of catecholamines from sympathetic nerve endings. Some drugs have both properties.

The sympathetic nervous system is not primarily involved in the pathogenesis of allergic disease, but in certain allergic reactions—particularly anaphylactic shock and acute asthma—the vascular and visceral effects will evoke a secondary sympathomimetic response to maintain homeostasis of function in the affected organs. Sympathomimetic drugs are therefore highly effective in treating many manifestations of IgE-mediated allergy.

The diverse actions of sympathomimetic amines are explained by 2 classes of receptors, α and β, and their subclasses, α_1, α_2, β_1, and β_2 (Table 60–8).

α_1-Adrenergic agonists cause mucosal vasoconstriction and are widely used as nasal decongestants. Examples of such drugs are phenylephrine and phenylpropanolamine. For many years, epinephrine and isoproterenol were the principal sympathomimetic bronchodilators available for treatment of asthma, but their use was limited by the cardiac-stimulating properties of their α and β_1 agonist effects, respectively. A variety of β_2-selective bronchodilators are now available for treatment of asthma. These include metaproterenol, terbutaline, albuterol, pirbuterol, isoetharine, and procaterol. Epinephrine is the drug of choice for anaphylaxis because it has powerful α- and β-stimulating effects necessary to counteract the systemic effects of anaphylaxis.

Methylxanthines

The methylxanthines include caffeine and theophylline. Their principal use is as central nervous system stimulants and as bronchodilators. Theophylline is poorly soluble in water and may be administered as a salt, such as aminophylline or oxytriphylline. Theophylline and its salts are frequently used in treatment of chronic asthma. Side effects include nervousness, insomnia, tachycardia, ventricular arrhythmias, diuresis, anorexia, nausea, vomiting, and abdominal pain. The toxicity of theophylline is related to blood levels, which are easily obtainable in most clinical laboratories.

The mechanism of action is unknown. Methylxanthines inhibit phosphodiesterase, thereby slowing the metabolism of cyclic AMP and increasing cyclic AMP levels. However, phosphodiesterase inhibition requires a much higher theophylline concentration than is clinically effective for bronchodilatation. An-

Table 60–8. Tissue distribution and effects of different adrenergic receptors.

Receptor	Tissue Distribution	Action	Physiologic Effect
α_1	Vascular smooth muscle	Contraction	Vasoconstriction
	Radial muscle of pupil	Contraction	Dilate pupil
	Trigone sphincter muscle	Contraction	Inhibition of urination
	Pilomotor smooth muscle	Contraction	Erect hair
	Liver	Increase gluconeogenesis	Increase blood sugar
α_2	Central nervous system adrenergic receptors	Activation	Diverse
	Platelets	Aggregation	Aggregation
	Presynaptic peripheral adrenergic and cholinergic nerves	Inhibition of transmitter release	Diverse
	Some vascular smooth muscle	Contraction	Vasoconstriction
	Gastrointestinal smooth muscle	Relaxation	Decreased motility
β_1	Heart muscle	Increase cyclic AMP[1]	Increase heart rate, force of contraction, conduction velocity
	Coronary vessel smooth muscle	Contraction	Vasoconstriction
	Fat cells	Increase cyclic AMP	Lipolysis
β_2	Bronchial smooth muscle	Relaxation	Bronchodilation
	Liver	Increase gluconeogenesis	Increased blood sugar
	Kidney	Increase cyclic AMP	Increased renin secretion
	Gastrointestinal smooth muscle	Relaxation	Decreased motility

[1]Activation of all β_1 or β_2 receptors results in increased cyclic AMP. A more distal action is listed, if known.

other potential mechanism is antagonism of adenosine. However, enprophylline, a methylxanthine and bronchodilator, reportedly is not an adenosine antagonist.

REFERENCES

General

Barnes PJ: A new approach to the treatment of asthma. *N Engl J Med* 1989;**321:**1517.

Bray MA, Morley J: *The Pharmacology of Lymphocytes.* Springer-Verlag, 1988.

McCarty DJ, Koopman WJ (editors): *Arthritis and Allied Conditions.* Lea & Febiger, 1993.

Corticosteroids

Behrens TW, Goodwind JS: Glucocorticoids. Pages 604–621 in: *Arthritis and Allied Conditions.* McCarty DJ (editor). Lea & Febiger, 1989.

Davidson F et al: Inhibition of phospholipase A2 by "lipocortins" and calpactins. *J Biol Chem* 1987;**262:**1698.

Duval D, Freyss-Beguin M: Glucocorticoids and prostaglandin synthesis. *Prostaglandins Leukotrienes Essent Fatty Acids* 1992;**45:**85.

Gustavson LE, Benet LZ: Pharmacokinetics of natural and synthetic glucocorticoids. In: *The Adrenal Cortex.* Anderson DC, Winder JSD (editors). Butterworth, 1985.

Lamberts SWJ et al: Cortisol receptor resistance: The variability of its clinical presentation and response to treatment. *J Clin Endicrinol Metab* 1993;**74:**313.

NSAID

Abramson SB, Weissmann G: The mechanism of action of nonsteroidal anti-inflammatory drugs. *Arthritis Rheum* 1989;**32:**1.

Bannwarth B et al: Where are peripheral analgesics acting? *Ann Rheum Dis* 1993;**52:**1.

Brooks PM, Day RO: Nonsteroidal antiinflammatory drugs—Differences and similarities. *N Engl J Med* 1991;**324:**1716.

Goodwin JS, Goodwin JM: Failure to recognize efficacious treatments: A history of salicylate therapy in rheumatoid arthritis. *Perspect Biol Med* 1981;**25:**78.

Vane JR: Inhibition of prostaglandin synthesis as a mechanism of action for aspirin-like drugs. *Nature New Biol* 1971;**231:**232.

Colchicine

Goodwin JS, Goodwin JM: The tomato effect: Rejection of highly efficacious therapies. *JAMA* 1984;**251:**2387.

Putterman C et al: Colchicine intoxication: Clinical pharmacology, risk factors, features and management. *Semin Arthritis Rheum* 1991;**21:**143.

Reibman J et al: Colchicine inhibits inophore-induced formation of leukotriene B4 by human neutrophils: The role of microtubules. *J Immunol* 1986;**136:**1027.

Gold & Other Second-Line Agents for Rheumatoid Arthritis

Berlow BA et al: The effect of dapsone in steroid dependent asthma. *J Allergy Clin Immunol* 1991,**87:**710.

Bunch TW et al: Controlled trial of hydroxychloroquine and D-penicillamine in the treatment of rheumatoid arthritis. *Arthritis Rheum 1984;***27:**267.

Fowler PD et al: Report on chloroquine and dapsone in the treatment of rheumatoid arthritis: A 6-month comparative study. *Ann Rheum Dis* 1984;**43:**200.

Richter JA et al: Analysis of treatment terminations with gold and antimalarial compounds in rheumatoid arthritis. *J Rheumatol* 1980;**7:**153.

Thompson PW, Kirwan JR, Barnes CG: Practical results of treatment with disease-modifying drugs. *Br J Rheumatol* 1985;**24:**167.

Cromolyn Sodium

Kay AB et al: Disodium cromoglycate inhibits activation of human inflammatory cells in vitro. *J Allergy Clin Immunol* 1987;**80:**1.

Antihistamines

Norman PS: Newer antihistaminic agents. *J Allergy Clin Immunol* 1985;**76:**366.

Simons FE, Simons KJ: H_1-receptor antagonists: Clinical pharmacology and use in allergic disease. *Pediatr Clin North Am* 1983;**30:**899.

Sympathomimetics

Fanta CH, Rossing TH, McFadden ER Jr: Treatment of acute asthma: Is combination therapy with sympathomimetics and methylxanthines indicated? *Am J Med* 1986;**80:**5.

Kemp JP: Approaches to asthma management. *Arch Intern Med* 1993;**153:**805.

Skorodin MS: Pharmacotherapy for asthma and chronic obstructive pulmonary disease. *Arch Intern Med* 1993;**153:**814.

Theophylline

Grant JA, Ellis EF: Update on theophylline (Symposium.) *J Allergy Clin Immunol* 1986;**76:**669.

Ward AJ et al: Theophylline—An immunomodulatory role in asthma? *Am Rev Respir Dis* 1993;**147:**518.

Appendices

Glossary of Terms Commonly Used in Immunology

ABO system: A term used to designate the erythrocyte antigens used for blood typing.

Abrin: A potent toxin which is derived from the seeds of the jequirity plant and which agglutinates erythrocytes (a lectin).

Accessory cell: Any nonlymphoid cell that cooperates with lymphocytes in carrying out an immune or inflammatory reaction.

Activated lymphocyte: A lymphocyte in a transient physiologic state characterized by mitotic activity and expression of immunologic functions.

Activated macrophage: A macrophage in a transient physiologic state characterized in part by increased phagocytic, microbicidal, secretory, and antigen-presenting activities.

Activation: Process by which a functionally quiescent cell or protein is induced to express one or more latent biological properties.

Active immunity: Protection acquired by deliberate introduction of an antigen into a responsive host.

Acute-phase response: Transient increase in concentrations of certain liver-derived serum proteins that occurs during some inflammatory reactions.

Adaptive immunity: A series of host defenses characterized by extreme specificity and memory mediated by antibody or T cells.

Addressins: Any surface macromolecule on endothelial cells that serves as an organ-specific ligand for homing receptors on circulating lymphocytes.

Adenosine deaminase: An enzyme that catalyzes the conversion of adenosine to inosine and is deficient in some patients with combined immunodeficiency syndrome.

Adjuvant: Any exogenous substance that, when introduced into a host along with an immunogen, enhances the immune response against that immunogen.

Adoptive transfer: The transfer of immunity by immunocompetent cells from one animal to another.

Adrenergic receptors: Receptors for various adrenergic agents of either the α or the β class that are present on a variety of cells and from which the action of various adrenergic drugs can be predicted.

Affinity chromatography: A technique in which a substance with a selective binding affinity is coupled to an insoluble matrix such as dextran and binds its complementary substances from a mixture in solution or suspension.

Affinity maturation: The tendency for average antibody affinity to be higher in secondary than primary humoral responses against a specific antigen. Also, the processes that give rise to this phenomenon.

Agammaglobulinemia: See **Hypogammaglobulinemia.**

Agglutination: An antigen-antibody reaction in which a solid or particulate antigen forms a lattice with a soluble antibody. In reverse agglutination, the antibody is attached to a solid particle and is agglutinated by insoluble antigen.

Allele: Any of the alternative inheritable forms (sequence variants) of a gene or genetic locus.

Allelic exclusion: The phenomenon in which only one of the 2 copies of a given gene in a diploid cell is phenotypically expressed. Observed in immunoglobulin and T cell receptor genes of lymphocytes but not in most other genes.

Allergens: Antigens that give rise to allergy.

Allergoids: Chemically modified allergens that give rise to antibody of the IgG but not IgE class, thereby reducing allergic symptoms.

Allergy (hypersensitivity): A disease or reaction caused by an immune response to one or more environmental antigens, resulting in tissue inflammation and organ dysfunction.

Allogeneic: Denotes the relationship that exists between genetically dissimilar members of the same species.

Allogeneic effect: A form of general immunopotentiation in which specific stimulation of T cells results in the release of factors active in the immune response.

Allograft (also homograft): A tissue or organ graft between 2 genetically dissimilar members of the same species.

Allotype: Subcategory of immunoglobulin heavy chains based on minor amino acid sequence differences among C_H regions, as a result of allelic variants.

α/β T cells: T lymphocytes that express surface T cell receptors composed of α and β chains.

Alpha-fetoprotein (AFP): An embryonic α-globulin with immunosuppressive properties that is structurally similar to albumin.

Alternative complement pathway (also properdin pathway): The system of activation of the complement pathway through involvement of properdin factor D, properdin factor B, and C3b, finally activating C3 and then progressing as in the classic pathway.

Am marker: The allotypic determinant on the heavy chain of human IgA.

Amboceptor: A term coined by Ehrlich to denote a bacteriolytic substance in serum that acts together with complement ie, antibody.

Anamnesis (also immunologic memory): A heightened responsiveness to the second or subsequent administration of antigen to an immune animal.

Anamnestic: Literally, without loss of memory. Of or concerning the secondary immune response.

Anaphylactoid reaction: Clinical response similar to anaphylaxis but not caused by an IgE mediated allergic reaction.

Anaphylatoxin: A substance produced by complement activation that results in increased vascular permeability through the release of pharmacologically active mediators from mast cells.

Anaphylatoxin inactivator: An α-globulin with a molecular weight of 300,000 that destroys the biologic activity of C3a and C5a.

Anaphylaxis: A reaction of immediate hypersensitivity present in nearly all vertebrates that results from sensitization of tissue-fixed mast cells by cytotropic antibodies following exposure to antigen.

Anergy: A state of diminished or absent cell-mediated immunity, usually defined clinically as the inability to react to multiple common skin test antigens. The same term is also used to describe a state of immunologic nonreactivity involving a specific B or T lymphoid cell or clone.

Angiogenesis factor: Released by macrophages and causes neovascularization of surrounding tissues.

Antibody: Secreted immunoglobulin proteins, particularly those that can bind specifically to a given antigen.

Antibody-dependent cell-mediated cytotoxicity: A form of cytotoxicity in which the effector cell recognizes the target cell by way of immunoglobulins that were preadsorbed to Fc receptors on the effector cell surface.

Antigen: A substance that reacts with antibodies or T cell receptors.

Antigen-binding site: The part of an immunoglobulin that binds antigen.

Antigen-combining site: The chemical moieties on an immunoglobulin or T cell receptor protein that directly contact the target antigen and are required for specific antigen binding.

Antigen presentation: The display of processed antigen as a cell surface complex with MHC protein in a manner that can be recognized by T lymphocytes.

Antigen-presenting cell: Any cell capable of antigen presentation. Unless otherwise stated, the term usually denotes only cells that express class II MHC proteins and so can present antigens to CD4 T cells; these include macrophages, dendritic cells, and activated B lymphocytes.

Antigen processing: The chemical alteration of a protein or other molecule into a form that can associate with MHC proteins and so be recognized by a T cell.

Antigenic competition: The suppression of the immune response to 2 closely related antigens when they are injected simultaneously.

Antigenic determinant. See **Epitope.**

Antigenic modulation: The spatial alteration of the arrangement of antigenic sites present on a cell surface brought about by the presence of bound antibody.

Antigenic shift: Periodic changes over time in the surface antigens of certain viruses. These are caused by genetic mutations.

Antiglobulin test (Coombs test): A technique for detecting cell-bound immunoglobulin. In the direct Coombs tests, erythrocytes taken directly from a sensitized individual are agglutinated by antigammaglobulin antibodies. In the indirect Coombs test, a patient's serum is incubated with test erythrocytes and the sensitized cells are then agglutinated with an anti-immunoglobulin or with Coombs reagent.

Antilymphocyte serum: Antibodies that are directed against lymphocytes and that usually cause immunosuppression.

Antinuclear antibodies (ANA): Antibodies that are directed against nuclear constituents usually in nucleoprotein, and are present in various rheumatoid diseases, particularly systemic lupus erythematosus.

Antiserum: Serum containing antibodies raised against a specific antigen.

Antitoxins: Protective antibodies that inactivate soluble toxic protein products.

Apheresis: Process of removing blood or a blood element from the body.

Apoptosis: A form of programmed cell death, characterized in part by nuclear and cytoplasmic condensation and fragmentation, and by degradation of nuclear DNA. Pronounced "a-po-TO-sis"; the second "p" is silent.

Armed macrophages: Macrophages capable of antigen-specific cytotoxicity as a result of cytophilic antibodies or arming factors from T cells.

Arthus reaction: A focal necrotizing vasculitis due to local deposition of immune complexes.

Association constant (Ka value): The mathematical representation of the affinity of binding between antigen and antibody.

Atopy: A genetically determined state of hypersensitivity to common environmental allergens, mediated by IgE antibodies.

Attenuated: Rendered less virulent.

Autoantibody: Antibody to self antigens.

Autoantigens: Self antigens.

Autocrine: Producing effects on the cell of origin.

Autograft: A tissue graft between genetically identical members of the same species.

Autoimmunity: Immunity to self antigens (autoantigens).

Autoradiography: A technique for detecting radioactive isotopes in which a tissue section containing radioactivity is overlaid with x-ray or photographic film on which the emissions are recorded.

B lymphocyte: Mature lymphoid cells that express surface immunoglobulin proteins.

Bacteriolysin: An antibody or other substance capable of lysing bacteria.

Bacteriolysis: The disintegration of bacteria induced by antibody and complement in the absence of cells.

Band: An immature neutrophil containing a nonsegmented nucleus.

Baseline cellular phagocytosis: Digestion by phagocytic cells and effector mechanisms that have developed for dealing with potential invading pathogens.

BCG (bacillus Calmette-Guérin): A viable attenuated strain of *Mycobacterium bovis* that has been obtained by progressive reduction of virulence and that confers immunity to mycobacterial infection and possibly possesses anti-cancer activity in selected diseases.

Bence Jones proteins: Monoclonal light chains present in the urine of patients with paraproteinemic disorders.

Beta lysin: A highly reactive heat-stable cationic protein that is bactericidal for gram-positive organisms.

Biosynthesis: The production of molecules by viable cells in culture.

Blast: Any cell exhibiting transient nuclear and cytoplasmic enlargement and other morphologic changes prior to undergoing mitotic division.

Blast transformation: The process through which a mitotically inactive cell becomes a blast.

Blocking antibody: See **Blocking factors.**

Blocking factors: Substances that are present in the serum of tumor-bearing animals and are capable of blocking the ability of immune lymphocytes to kill tumor cells.

Bradykinin: A 9-amino-acid peptide that is split by the enzyme kallikrein from serum α_2-globulin precursor and that causes a slow, sustained contraction of the smooth muscles.

Bursa of Fabricius: The hindgut organ located in the cloaca of birds that controls the ontogeny of B lymphocytes.

Bursal equivalent: The hypothetical organ or organs analogous to the bursa of Fabricius in nonavian species.

Bystander activation: Incidental activation, during an immune response, of lymphocytes that do not recognize the immunogen.

C region (constant region): The carboxy-terminal portion of the H or L chain that is identical in immunoglobulin or T cell receptor molecules of a given class and subclass apart from genetic polymorphisms.

C terminus: The carboxy-terminal end of a polypeptide chain.

Cachectin: Tumor necrosis factor α.

Capping: The active translocation and clustering of receptors to one pole of the cell surface, usually caused by binding of a bivalent or polyvalent ligand.

Carcinoembryonic antigen (CEA): An antigen that is present on fetal endodermal tissue and is reexpressed on the surface of neoplastic cells, particularly in carcinoma of the colon.

Cardiolipin: A substance derived from beef heart, probably a component of mitochondrial membranes, that serves as an antigenic substrate for reagin or antitreponemal antibody.

Carrier: An immunogenic substance that, when coupled to a hapten, renders the hapten immunogenic.

Cationic proteins: Antimicrobial substances present within granules of phagocytic cells.

CD (or Cluster of Differentiation): A designation applied, together with a unique identifying number, to a variety of cell surface proteins, most of which are found on one or more hematopoietic cell types, as a standardized system of nomenclature. (See "The CD Classification of Hematopoietic Cell Surface Markers" (p 817).

Cell-mediated immunity: Immunity in which the participation of lymphocytes and macrophages is predominant.

Cell-mediated lymphocytolysis: An in vitro assay for cellular immunity in which a standard mixed-lymphocyte reaction is followed by destruction of target cells that are used to sensitize allogeneic cells during the mixed lymphocyte reaction.

Centimorgan: A unit of physical distance on a chromosome, equivalent to a 1% frequency of recombination between closely linked genes. Also called a map unit.

Central lymphoid organs: see **Primary lymphoid organs.**

CH$_{50}$unit: The quantity or dilution of serum required to lyse 50% of the erythrocytes in a standard hemolytic complement assay.

Charcot-Leyden crystals: Hexagonal dipyramidal extracellular crystals of a lysophospholipase protein derived mainly from eosinophils.

Chase-Sulzberger phenomenon: See **Sulzberger-Chase phenomenon.**

Chemiluminescence: Release of light energy produced by a chemical reaction.

Chemoattraction: Chemotaxis.

Chemokine: Any of a group of chemoattractant cytokines.

Chemokinesis: Reaction by which chemical substances determine rate of cellular movement.

Chemotaxis: Migration of a cell or organism toward increasing concentrations of a chemical substance.

Chromatography: A variety of techniques useful for the separation of proteins.

***cis*-pairing:** Association of two genes on the same chromosome encoding a protein.

Class I MHC protein: Any of the heterodimeric surface glycoproteins encoded by the A, B, or C locus of the major histocompatibility complex, which function mainly in antigen presentation to CD8 (cytotoxic) T lymphocytes.

Class II MHC protein: Any of the heterodimeric surface glycoproteins encoded by the DR, DP, or DQ locus of the major histocompatibility complex, which function mainly in antigen presentation to CD4 (helper) T lymphocytes.

Class III MHC protein: Any of the proteins encoded by a cluster of genes situated between the class I and class II MHC loci but that are functionally and evolutionarily unrelated to the class I and II genes and have no role in antigen presentation.

Class switch: See **Immunoglobulin class switch.**

Classic complement pathway: The sequence of reactions among serum complement proteins that is initiated by binding of C1 protein to a target.

Clonal anergy: Immunologic unresponsiveness of a specific clone of viable lymphocytes.

Clonal deletion: The selective killing of all cells in a particular lymphocyte clone.

Clonal restriction: Any limitation on immune function (such as antigen or MHC specificity) or other characteristics that is shared by all cells in a lymphocyte clone and distinguishes them from other clones.

Clonal selection: The phenomenon in which clonal growth and survival of lymphoid cells having particular characteristics is either favored or inhibited. (See **Negative selection** and **Positive selection**).

Clone: A group of cells all of which are the progeny of a single cell.

Cluster of differentiation: see **CD**

c-Myc: A cellular protein thought to be involved normally in regulating cell proliferation. Abnormal expression of c-Myc contributes to development of certain cancers, including Burkitt's lymphoma.

c-*myc* gene: Member of a candidate set of cancer-related genes or cellular oncogenes.

Cognate: Specifically recognized or bound.

Cohn fraction II: Primarily gamma globulin that is produced as the result of ethanol fractionation of serum according to the Cohn method.

Cold agglutinins: Antibodies that agglutinate bacteria or erythrocytes more efficiently at temperatures below 37 °C than at 37 °C.

Colony-stimulating factor: Any of a diverse group of cytokines that support the growth of specific hematopoietic lineages.

Combinatorial joining: The process in which V-region exons of immunoglobulin or T cell receptor genes are assembled somatically by linking a relatively small number of exon fragments together in a large number of alternative combinations. It is a major source of V-region diversity.

Complement: A system of serum proteins that can be induced to carry out a cascade of enzymatic reactions which may lead to lysis of foreign cells and to formation of certain opsonins and inflammatory mediators.

Complement fixation: A standard serologic assay used for the detection of an antigen-antibody reaction in which complement is fixed as a result of the formation of an immune complex. The subsequent failure of lysis of sensitized erythrocytes by complement that has been fixed indicates the degree of antigen-antibody reaction.

Complementarity: The ability of one gene to substitute for another in producing a specified trait. Alternatively, the relationship between 2 nucleic acid strands in which each can bind to the other through basepairing interactions of the Watson-Crick type.

Complementarity-determining region (CDR): Any of 3 or 4 short regions of extreme sequence variability within the V-region domain of an immunoglobulin or T cell receptor polypeptide, which form the antigen-binding site and are the main determinants of antigen specificity.

Concanavalin A (Con A): A lectin that is derived from the jack bean and stimulates predominantly the T lymphocytes.

Concomitant immunity: The ability of a tumor-bearing animal to reject a test inoculum of its tumor at a site different from the primary site of tumor growth.

Conformational determinant: Any antigenic determinant whose antigenicity is in part dependent on its 3-dimensional structure.

Congenic (originally congenic resistant): Denotes a line of mice identical or nearly identical with other inbred strains except for the substitution at one histocompatibility locus of a foreign allele introduced by appropriate crosses with a second inbred strain.

Contact sensitivity: A type of delayed hypersensitivity reaction in which sensitivity to simple chemical compounds is manifested by skin reactivity.

Copolymer: A polymer of at least 2 different chemical moieties, eg, a polypeptide with 2 different amino acids.

Coproantibody: An antibody present in the lumen of the gastrointestinal tract.

Costimulator: Any stimulus, other than the antigen-MHC complex, that is provided by an antigen-presenting cell and is required for optimal activation of T_H lymphocytes.

Counterimmunoelectrophoresis: See **Electroimmunodiffusion.**

C-reactive protein: An antibacterial serum protein that binds pneumococcal C protein.

CREST phenomenon: A phenomenon that consists of *c*alcinosis, *R*aynaud's phenomenon, *e*sophageal dysmotility, *s*clerodactyly, and *t*elangiectasis and that occurs in patients with progressive systemic sclerosis.

Cross-matching: A laboratory test using cells from a recipient and serum from a donor to detect antibodies directed at recipient's cells.

Cross-reaction: The reaction of an antibody with an antigen other than the one that induced its formation.

Cryoglobulin: A protein that has the property of forming a precipitate or gel in the cold.

Cutaneous basophil hypersensitivity: An immunologically mediated inflammation in the skin with a prominent basophil infiltration occurring about 24 hours after injection of the sensitizing antigen.

Cycle-specific drugs: Cytotoxic or immunosuppressive drugs that kill both mitotic and resting cells.

Cyclooxygenase pathway: Pathway of arachidonate metabolism whereby prostaglandins are produced.

Cytokine: Any of a group of soluble polypeptide mediators that regulate cellular growth or function. (See **Lymphokine** and **Monokine**).

Cytolysin: See **Perforin.**

Cytotoxicity: The ability to kill cells.

Cytotropic antibodies: Antibodies of the IgG and IgE classes that sensitize cells for subsequent anaphylaxis.

D segment: One of a class of short gene fragments that is interposed between the V and J segments during immunoglobulin heavy-chain or T cell receptor gene assembly.

Defensin: Any of a family of small antimicrobial peptides found in neutrophil granules.

Degranulation: The process in which cytoplasmic storage granules fuse with phagosomes or with the cell surface membrane, thereby discharging their contents and disappearing from the cytoplasm.

Delayed-type hypersensitivity (DTH): The pattern of skin test immunoreactivity characterized by local induration and an infiltrate of macrophages and lymphocytes that begin to appear 24 to 48 hours after antigen challenge.

Denature: To eliminate the normal 3-dimensional structure of a macromolecule, usually by heating or chemical treatment.

Dendritic cells: A widely distributed and heterogeneous group of antigen-presenting cells that includes Langerhans cells, interdigitating cells, blood dendritic cells, and others, all of which are developmentally related.

Desensitization: Treatment of allergic disease by repeated injections of allergen extracts. Also called "allergen immunotherapy."

Determinant: Any individual or clustered chemical features on a molecule that determine its antigenic or immunogenic properties.

Determinant groups: Individual chemical structures present on macromolecular antigens that determine antigenic specificity.

Determinant selection: The process by which the immune system selects and attacks a particular subset of antigenic determinants within a complex immunogen.

Dextrans: Polysaccharides composed of a single sugar.

Diapedesis: The outward passage of cells through intact vessel walls.

Diploid: Cell that contains 2 copies of each chromosome; or any organism composed of such cells.

Direct agglutination: The agglutination of erythrocytes, microorganisms, or other substances directly by serum antibody.

Direct immunofluorescence: The detection of antigens by fluorescently labeled antibody.

Disulfide bond: Covalent (S–S) bond between thiol moieties that links 2 cysteine residues located on either the same or different polypeptide chains.

Domain: Any portion of a polypeptide chain that folds to form an independent structural or functional unit.

Double-positive lymphocyte: An immature T cell that expresses both CD4 and CD8. Most thymocytes are double-positive.

Dysgammaglobulinemia: A term not in common use that refers to a selective immunoglobulin deficiency.

E rosette: A formation of a cluster (rosette) of cells consisting of sheep erythrocytes and human T lymphocytes.

EAC rosette: A cluster of erythrocytes sensitized with amboceptor (antibody) and complement around human B lymphocytes.

EAE (experimental allergic encephalomyelitis): An autoimmune disease in which an animal is immunized with homologous or heterologous extracts of whole brain, the basic protein of myelin, or certain polypeptide sequences within the basic protein, emulsified with Freund's complete adjuvant.

ECF-A (eosinophil chemotactic factor of anaphylaxis): An acidic peptide, molecular weight 500, that, when released, causes influx of eosinophils.

Edema: Tissue swelling due to leakage of acellular vascular fluid.

Effector cell: Any cell that actively carries out an immunologic attack. Effector cells of the lymphocyte lineage include helper and cytotoxic T lymphocytes and plasma cells.

Electroimmunodiffusion (counterimmunoelectrophoresis): An immunodiffusion technique in which antigen and antibody are driven toward each other in an electrical field and then precipitate.

Electrophoresis: The separation of molecules in an electrical field.

Endocytosis: Any process whereby external material is taken up into cytoplasmic vesicles in a cell. The 3 major forms of endocytosis are phagocytosis, pinocytosis, and receptor-mediated endocytosis.

Endogenous pyrogen: An outdated term for IL-1, emphasizing its ability to induce fever.

Endotoxins: Lipopolysaccharides that are derived from the cell walls of gram-negative microorganisms and have toxic and pyrogenic effects when injected in vivo.

Enhancement: Improved survival of tumor cells in animals that have been previously immunized to the antigens of a given tumor.

Enterotoxin: A heat-stable toxin produced by bacteria, which produces intestinal disease.

Epithelioid cell: Activated macrophage in a granuloma.

Epitope: The chemical features on a molecule that together form the binding site for a particular immunoglobulin or T cell receptor protein.

Equilibrium dialysis: A technique for measuring the strength or affinity with which antibody binds to antigen.

Equivalence: A ratio of antigen-antibody concentration where maximal precipitation occurs.

Erythema: Redness due to increased local blood flow.

Euglobulin: A class of globulin proteins that are insoluble in water but soluble in salt solutions.

Eukaryote: A cell or organism possessing a true nucleus containing chromosomes bounded by a nuclear membrane.

Exon: Any continuous segment of a gene whose sequence can be found in the mature RNA product of that gene. Most genes are composed of 2 or more exons separated from one another by introns. Most exons contain protein-coding information.

Exotoxins: Diffusible toxins produced by certain gram-positive and gram-negative microorganisms.

F_1 generation: The first generation of offspring after a designated mating.

F_2 generation: The second generation of offspring after a designated mating.

Fab fragment: A monovalent antigen-binding protein fragment that can be prepared from certain immunoglobulin molecules by proteolytic digestion.

F(ab)'$_2$: A divalent antigen-binding protein fragment that can be prepared from certain immunoglobulin molecules by proteolytic digestion.

Fc fragment: A non-antigen-binding protein fragment that can be prepared from certain immunoglobulin molecules by proteolytic digestion, and contains only constant-region sequences.

Fc receptor: Any of a class of cell surface receptors that bind the constant (Fc) portions of antibody molecules and so adsorb these antibodies onto the cell surface. Several types are known, each of which has a unique binding affinity and antibody subclass specificity.

Fetal antigen: A type of tumor-associated antigen that is normally present on embryonic but not adult tissues and that is reexpressed during the neoplastic process.

Fibronectin: A protein that has an important role in the structuring of connective tissue.

Fluorescence: The emission of light of one color while a substance is irradiated with a light of a different color.

Follicular dendritic cell: A supporting cell, found in germinal centers of lymphoid tissues, that is thought to influence memory B cell responses. It is functionally and developmentally distinct from other types of dendritic cells.

Forbidden clone theory: The theory proposed to explain autoimmunity that postulates that lymphocytes capable of self sensitization and effector function are present in tolerant animals, since they were not eliminated during embryogenesis.

Framework region: Any of the regions of relatively low sequence variability that lie between complementarity-determining regions within the V-region domain of an immunoglobulin or T cell receptor polypeptide.

Freund's complete adjuvant: An oil-water emulsion that contains killed mycobacteria and enhances immune responses when mixed in an emulsion with antigen.

Freund's incomplete adjuvant: An emulsion that contains all of the elements of Freund's complete adjuvant with the exception of killed mycobacteria.

G cells: Gastrin-secreting cells in mucosa of the gastric antrum.

Gamma globulins: A group of serum proteins that migrate together with a characteristic mobility on gel electrophoresis and that includes most serum immunoglobulins.

Gammopathy: A paraprotein disorder involving abnormalities of immunoglobulins.

γ/δ T cells: T lymphocytes that express surface T cell receptors composed of γ and δ chains.

Generalized anaphylaxis: A shocklike state that occurs within minutes following an appropriate antigen-antibody reaction resulting from the systemic release of vasoactive amines.

Germinal center: An oligoclonal collection of activated B cells and B cell blasts that develops within a lymphoid follicle during a secondary humoral response. It is the site of memory B cell proliferation and of antibody class switching and affinity maturation.

Graft-versus-host (GVH) reaction: The clinical and pathologic sequelae of the reactions of immunocompetent cells in a graft against the cells of the histoincompatible and immunodeficient recipient.

Granulocyte: Any mature myeloid cell with prominent cytoplasmic granules, including neutrophils, basophils, eosinophils, and mast cells.

Granuloma: A type of cell-mediated immune reaction in which activated macrophages predominate and form dense aggregates around the inciting immunogen.

Granulopoietin: Granulocyte-macrophage colony-stimulating factor.

Granzyme: Any of a family of serine proteases produced by cytotoxic T lymphocytes.

H chain: See **Heavy chain.**

Halogenation: A combination of a halogen molecule with a microbial cell wall that results in microbial damage.

Haplotype: The particular set of alleles found at 2 or more genetic loci on a single chromosome in a given individual. Because these alleles are genetically linked, they are usually inherited together.

Hapten: A substance that is not immunogenic but can react with an antibody of appropriate specificity.

Hassall's corpuscles: Whorls of thymic medullary epithelial cells whose function is unknown.

HBcAg (also core antigen): The 27-nm core of hepatitis B virus, which has been identified in the nuclei of hepatocytes.

HBeAg: Low-molecular-weight component of hepatitis B nucleocapsid indicating infectious state when present in serum.

HBsAg: The coat or envelope of hepatitis B virus.

Heavy chain: In immunoglobulins, one of the 2 polypeptide chains making up the basic 4-chain unit; it contains approximately twice the number of amino acid residues and is twice the molecular weight of the light chain.

Heavy-chain diseases: A heterogeneous group of paraprotein disorders characterized by the presence of monoclonal but incomplete heavy chains without light chains in serum or urine.

Helper factor: Any stimulus that is provided by an activated T<small>H</small> lymphocyte and promotes optimal activation of other T or B lymphocytes.

Helper T cells: Effector T cells whose primary function is to promote the activation and functions of other B and T lymphocytes and of macrophages. Most are CD4 T cells.

Hemagglutination inhibition: A technique for detecting small amounts of antigen in which the agglutination of antigen-coated erythrocytes or other particles by specific antibody is inhibited by homologous antigen.

Hematopoiesis: The production and maturation of blood cells of all types.

Hematopoietic system: All cellular elements of the peripheral blood and the tissues responsible for their production. The term usually excludes secondary lymphoid organs.

Hemolysin: An antibody or other substance capable of lysing erythrocytes.

Heterocytotropic antibody: An antibody that can passively sensitize tissues of species other than those in which the antibody is present.

Heterodimer: A unit composed of two non-identical subunits. For example, each class II MHC protein is a heterodimer of α and β polypeptide chains.

Heterologous antigen: An antigen that serves as the target of a cross-reaction.

High dose (high zone) tolerance: Classic immunologic unresponsiveness produced by repeated injections of large amounts of antigen.

High endothelial venules: Postcapillary venules with specialized, cuboid epithelial cells that mediate specific binding and migration of blood lymphocytes into tissues.

Hinge region: Flexible region in the heavy chains of some immunoglobulin classes that permits movement of the 2 antigen-binding sites with respect to one another.

Histamine: A small organic mediator of inflammation.

Histiocyte: A tissue macrophage.

Histocompatible: The relationship between individuals in which each will tolerate cell or tissue grafts from the other.

Human leukocyte antigen (HLA): Any human class I or class II major histocompatibility complex protein.

Homing receptor: A molecule on the surface of a blood cell that promotes migration of the cell into specific solid tissues.

Homocytotropic antibody: An antibody that attaches to cells of animals of the same species.

Homologous antigen: An antigen that induces an antibody and reacts specifically with it.

Homopolymer: A molecule composed of multiple identical repeating subunits, usually arranged in a chain.

Homozygous typing cells (HTC): Cells derived from an individual who is homozygous at the HLA-D locus used for MLR typing of the D locus in humans.

Horror autotoxicus: A concept introduced by Ehrlich, proposing that an individual is protected against autoimmunity or immunization against self antigens even though these antigens are immunogenic in other animals.

Hot antigen suicide: A technique in which an antigen is labeled with a high-specific-activity radioisotope (^{131}I). It is used either in vivo or in vitro to inhibit specific lymphocyte function by attachment to an antigen-binding lymphocyte, subsequently killing it by radiolysis.

Humoral: Of or pertaining to body fluids, such as the blood or lymph.

Humoral immunity: Immunity or immune responses mediated by soluble factors (especially antibody molecules) in body fluids.

Hybridoma: Any permanent cell line arising from somatic fusion of a transformed cell with an untransformed T or B lymphoid cell and retaining certain properties of the lymphocyte parent, such as secretion of specific antibodies.

Hydrophilic: Having an affinity for water or aqueous solvents.

Hydrophobic: A hydrophobic compound is insoluble in water; a hydrophobic group is pushed to the interior of proteins or membranes, away from water.

Hyperacute rejection: An accelerated form of graft rejection that is associated with circulating antibody in the serum of the recipient and which can react with donor cells.

Hypersensitivity: See **Allergy.**

Hypervariable region: See **Complementarity-determining region.**

Hypogammaglobulinemia (agammaglobulinemia): A deficiency of all major classes of serum immunoglobulins.

Hyposensitization: See **Desensitization.**

Idiotope: Any potentially antigenic epitope formed by the unique antigen-binding region of an immunoglobulin.

Idiotype: The unique antigenic properties of any particular immunoglobulin protein that distinguish it from all others and that results from the potentially antigenic nature of sequences (idiotopes) in its antigen-binding region.

IgA: The predominant immunoglobulin class present in secretions.

IgD: An immunoglobulin class of uncertain function that is present on the surfaces of many B-lymphoid cells but is not secreted.

IgE: The immunoglobulin class that is the predominant mediator of immediate hypersensitivity reactions. Also called **reagin** or **reaginic antibody.**

IgG: The predominant immunoglobulin class produced during secondary immune responses in the blood.

IgM: The predominant immunoglobulin class expressed by virgin B lymphocytes and secreted during primary immune responses.

Immediate hypersensitivity: A pattern of immune reactivity that begins within minutes of antigen exposure and is mediated primarily by mast cells that bear adsorbed IgE antibodies on their surfaces.

Immune adherence: An agglutination reaction between a cell bearing C$\overline{423}$ and an indicator cell, usually a human erythrocyte, which has a receptor for C3b.

Immune complexes: Antigen-antibody complexes.

Immune elimination: The enhanced clearance of an

injected antigen from the circulation as a result of immunity to that antigen brought about by enhanced phagocytosis of the reticuloendothelial system.

Immune exclusion: The normal prevention of entry of antigens across mucosal membranes by secretory IgA.

Immune suppression: A variety of therapeutic maneuvers to depress or eliminate the immune response.

Immune surveillance: A theory that holds that the immune system destroys tumor cells, which are constantly arising during the life of the individual.

Immunization: See **Sensitization.** Natural or artificial induction of an immune response, particularly when it renders the host protected from disease.

Immunobeads: Small plastic spheres coated with antibodies or antigens, which are used to indicate immune reactions by agglutination.

Immunocytoadherence: A technique for identifying immunoglobulin-bearing cells by formation of rosettes consisting of these cells and erythrocytes or other particles containing a homologous antigen.

Immunodominance: The property of certain epitopes within a complex antigen (or certain chemical residues within an epitope) that makes them most critical for immunogenicity or antigenicity.

Immunoelectrophoresis: A technique combining an initial electrophoretic separation of proteins followed by immunodiffusion with resultant precipitation arcs.

Immunofixation electrophoresis: Technique for identification of proteins by electrophoretic separation on a gel followed by precipitation in situ with specific antibodies.

Immunofluorescence: A histo- or cytochemical technique for the detection and localization of antigens in which specific antibody is conjugated with fluorescent compounds, resulting in a sensitive tracer that can be detected by fluorometric measurements.

Immunogen: Any substance that, when introduced into an animal, stimulates an immune response.

Immunogenicity: The property of a substance making it capable of inducing a detectable immune response.

Immunoglobulin (Ig): An extremely diverse group of membrane-bound or soluble antigen-binding proteins, produced only by B lymphoid cells. See **Antibody.**

Immunoglobulin class: A subdivision of immunoglobulin proteins based on major amino acid sequence differences in the C_H region. In humans, there are 5 classes of immunoglobulins, designated IgM, IgG, IgD, IgE, and IgA.

Immunoglobulin class switch: The process by which a B cell expressing immunoglobulins of one class can begin expressing a different class without affecting antigen specificity. The change is irreversible, results from specific deletion of chromosomal DNA, and is passed on to the cell's clonal progeny.

Immunoglobulin domain: The basic 110-amino acid repeating unit of protein structure found in all immunoglobulin proteins.

Immunoglobulin gene superfamily: The large, diverse family of genes whose protein products each include one or more domains that are evolutionarily and structurally related to the 110-amino-acid immunoglobulin domain.

Immunoglobulin subclass: A subdivision within immunoglobulin classes based on moderate amino acid sequence differences in the C_H region. In humans, there are 4 nonallelic subclasses of IgG (designated IgG1, IgG2, IgG3, and IgG4) and 2 of IgA (designated IgA1 and IgA2).

Immunomodulation: A variety of methods for therapeutic manipulation of the immune response.

Immunopathic: Referring to damage to cells, tissues, or organs from immune responses.

Immunopotency: The capacity of a region of an antigen molecule to serve as an antigenic determinant and thereby induce the formation of specific antibody.

Immunoradiometry: A technique of radioimmunoassay that employs radiolabeled antibody rather than antigen.

Immunotherapy: Either hyposensitization in allergic diseases or treatment with immunostimulants or immunosuppressive drugs or biologic products.

Indirect agglutination (also **passive agglutination**): The agglutination of particles or erythrocytes to which antigens have been coupled chemically.

Indirect immunofluorescence (also **double antibody immunofluorescence**): A technique whereby unlabeled antibody is incubated with substrate and then overlaid with fluorescently conjugated anti-immunoglobulin to form a sandwich.

Inflammation: The integrated host response to injury or infection, usually encompassing a neutrophilic or immune response along with any associated defensive phenomena. Primarily neutrophilic reactions are termed acute inflammation; primarily lymphoid and/or macrophage reactions are termed chronic inflammation.

Inflammatory mediator: Any molecule that controls one or more aspects of inflammation.

Innate immunity: Various host defenses present from birth that do not depend on immunologic memory.

Inoculation: The introduction of an antigen or antiserum into an animal to confer immunity.

Integrins: A diverse group of cell membrane proteins that mediate adhesion to other cells and to the extracellular matrix.

Interferon: Any of a group of cytokines that increase the resistance of target cells to viral infection. IFNα and IFNβ are also called type I or leukocyte IFNs; IFNγ is type II or immune IFN.

Interleukin: Any of a diverse family of polypeptide cytokines, most of which act to regulate growth and functions of hematopoietic cells. Most interleukins are evolutionarily and structurally unrelated to one another.

Intron: Any noncoding segment of DNA interposed between 2 exons of a gene. Intron sequences are transcribed into RNA along with the exons but are then removed during RNA processing and so are absent from the mature RNA product.

Invariant chain: A polypeptide that associates with nascent class II MHC molecules in the rough endoplasmic reticulum to prevent binding of endogenous peptides.

Isoagglutinin: An agglutinating antibody capable of agglutinating cells of other individuals of the same species in which it is found.

Isoantibody: An antibody that is capable of reacting with an antigen derived from a member of the same species as that in which it is raised.

Isohemagglutinins: Antibodies to major erythrocyte antigens present in members of a given species and directed against antigenic determinants on erythrocytes from other members of the species.

Isotype: Any of the major groups of immunoglobulin or T cell receptor polypeptides that share a common C region, including the heavy-chain classes and subclasses (μ, γ1, γ2, etc) or the light-chain types (κ and λ).

Isotype switching: See **Immunoglobulin class switching.**

J chain: A glycopeptide chain that is normally found in polymeric immunoglobulins, particularly IgA and IgM.

Jarisch-Herxheimer reaction: A local or occasionally generalized inflammatory reaction that occurs following treatment of syphilis and other intracellular infections; it is presumably caused by the release of large amounts of antigenic material into the circulation.

Jones criteria: Signs and symptoms used to diagnose acute rheumatic fever.

Jones-Mote reaction: See **Cutaneous basophil hypersensitivity.**

K cell: A killer cell responsible for antibody-dependent cell-mediated cytotoxicity.

Kallikrein system: See **Kinin system.**

Kappa (κ) chain: One of the 2 major isotypes of immunoglobulin light chains.

Kinin: A peptide that increases vascular permeability and is formed by the action of esterases on kallikreins, which then act as vasodilators.

Kinin system (also kallikrein system): A humoral amplification system initiated by the activation of coagulation factor XII, eventually leading to the formation of kallikrein, which acts on an α-globulin substrate, kininogen, to form a bradykinin.

Koch phenomenon: A delayed hypersensitivity reaction by tuberculin in the skin of a guinea pig following infection with *Mycobacterium tuberculosis*.

Kupffer's cell: A form of tissue macrophage found within liver sinusoids.

Kveim test: A delayed hypersensitivity test for sarcoidosis in which potent antigenic extracts of sarcoid tissue are injected intradermally and subjected to biopsy 6 weeks later in order to observe the presence of a granuloma, indicating a positive test.

L chain: See **Light chain.**

Lactoferrin: An iron-containing compound that exerts a slight antimicrobial action by binding iron necessary for microbial growth.

Lambda (λ) chain: One of the 2 major isotypes of immunoglobulin light chains.

Langerhans cell: A form of dendritic cell residing within the epidermis.

Late-phase reaction: A pattern of inflammatory events occurring approximately 6–8 hours after antigen exposure in the immediate hypersensitivity response.

Latex fixation test: An agglutination reaction in which latex particles are used to passively adsorb soluble protein and polysaccharide antigens.

LE cell phenomenon: Phagocytic leukocytes that have engulfed DNA, immunoglobulin, and complement and are present as a large homogeneous mass that is extruded from a damaged lymphocyte in systemic lupus erythematosus and other rheumatoid diseases.

Lectin: Any of a diverse group of proteins that have specific carbohydrate-binding activity.

Leukotriene: Any of a group of arachidonic acid metabolites produced through the lipoxygenase pathway.

Ligand: Any molecule that can be bound by, or form a complex with, another.

Light chain: In immunoglobulins, one of the 2 polypeptide chains making up the basic 4-chain unit; it contains approximately half the number of amino acid residues and has half the molecular weight of the heavy chain.

Light-chain type: See **Isotype.**

Lineage infidelity: Expression following neoplastic transformation of molecules on cells that are foreign to the lineage of the cell itself.

Linear determinant: Any antigenic determinant that is entirely specified by the linear amino acid sequence of a protein and is independent of its 3-dimensional structure.

Linkage disequilibrium: The occurrence together of any 2 genetic markers at a frequency higher than would be expected on the basis of independent inheritance.

Lipopolysaccharide: A complex organic compound derived from the cell walls of gram-negative enteric bacteria. Also called endotoxin.

Lipoxygenase pathway: Pathway of enzymatic metabolism of arachidonic acid by which leukotrienes are produced.

Local anaphylaxis: An immediate hypersensitivity reaction that occurs in a specific target organ such as the gastrointestinal tract, nasal mucosa, or skin.

Locus: In genetics, any defined physical location on a chromosome, or the gene that occupies that location. Often used synonymously with the term "gene."

Low dose (low zone) tolerance: A transient and incomplete state of tolerance induced with small subimmunogenic doses of soluble antigen.

Lucio phenomenon (erythema necroticans): A variant of erythema nodosum leprosum in which necrotizing vasculitis produces crops of large polygonal lesions characterized by ulceration and sloughing of large areas of skin.

Lymphocyte: A mononuclear cell 7–12 μm in diameter containing a nucleus with densely packed chromatin and a small rim of cytoplasm.

Lymphocyte-defined (LD) antigens: A series of histocompatibility antigens that are present on the majority of mammalian cells and are detectable primarily by reactivity in the mixed lymphocyte reaction (MLR).

Lymphoid follicle: Nodular cellular aggregate, composed predominantly of B lymphocytes, macrophages, and follicular dendritic cells, found in secondary and tertiary lymphoid organs. See also **Primary follicle** and **Secondary follicle.**

Lymphokine: Any cytokine produced by lymphoid cells.

Lymphokine-activated killer: The cytotoxic cells and activity that can be induced by treating peripheral blood lymphocytes with certain cytokines.

Lymphopoiesis: The growth and maturation of lymphoid cells from uncommitted precursors.

Lymphoreticular: Referring to lymphocyte and monocyte-macrophage system and stromal elements that support its growth.

Lymphotoxin: Tumor necrosis factor β.

Lysosome: Membrane-bounded vesicle containing hydrolytic digestive enzymes, found in the cytoplasm of many cell types.

Lysozyme: An antibacterial enzyme, found in tears, saliva, and other body secretions, that degrades the cell walls of susceptible bacteria.

M cells: Membranous epithelial cells that overlie lymphoid tissues in the small intestine and allow limited passage of intraintestinal antigens.

M protein: Antigenic component of surface of streptococci. Cross-reacts with muscle antigens. See **Myeloma protein.**

Macrophage: Any of the mature phagocytic cells derived from circulating monocytes.

Major basic protein: A toxic protein from the eosinophil membrane that produces tissue damage in allergic and inflammatory diseases.

Major histocompatibility complex: A specific cluster of genes, many of which encode evolutionarily related cell surface proteins involved in antigen presentation, which are among the most important determinants of histocompatibility. See also **class I, class II,** and **class III MHC proteins,** and **human leukocyte antigen.**

Marker: Any surface macromolecule, usually detected using specific antibodies, that provides an indication of the developmental lineage, physiologic status, or other attributes of a cell.

Mast cell: A tissue-resident cell of hematopoietic origin that carries high-affinity Fc receptors for IgE and is the primary effector cell of immediate hypersensitivity reactions.

Membrane attack complex: The multicomponent complex formed from activated complement proteins, which assembles on the surface of a target cell and can cause membrane lysis.

Metabolic burst: Transient rise in oxidative metabolism that occurs in phagocytic cells following phagocytosis.

β$_2$-Microglobulin: A nonpolymorphic glycoprotein that is a component of all class I MHC proteins on cell surfaces and is also found normally in serum.

Mitogen: Any of a variety of lectins or other agents that can stimulate resting cells to undergo mitosis.

Mixed lymphocyte culture (mixed leukocyte culture)
(MLC): An in vitro test for cellular immunity in which lymphocytes or leukocytes from genetically dissimilar individuals are mixed and mutually stimulate DNA synthesis.

Mixed lymphocyte reaction (MLR): See **Mixed lymphocyte culture.**

Molecular mimicry: Immunologic cross-reactivity between determinants on an environmental antigen (such as a virus) and a self antigen, a notion that has been proposed to explain autoimmunity.

Monoclonal antibody: A pure population of immunoglobulin proteins that have identical structure and antigen-specificity. Derived from a single clone of B lymphoid cells, usually either from malignant secretory B cells or from a hybridoma.

Monoclonal gammopathy: Presence in the blood of a monoclonal antibody in detectable amounts, usually observed on serum electrophoresis.

Monoclonal hypergammaglobulinemia: See **Monoclonal gammopathy.**

Monocyte: A mononuclear blood cell that is the precursor of fixed macrophages and other tissue phagocytes.

Monokine: Any cytokine produced by monocytes or macrophages.

Monomer: Any macromolecule composed of a single unit, such as a single polypeptide chain.

Mononuclear phagocyte system: The hematopoietic lineage that includes monocytes and all monocyte-derived phagocytic cells. See **Macrophage.**

Mucosal homing: The ability of immunologically competent cells that arise from mucosal follicles to traffic back to mucosal areas.

Mucosal immune system: The lymphoid tissues associated with the mucosal surfaces of the gastrointestinal, respiratory, and urogenital tracts, which produce a unique immunoglobulin (secretory IgA) and T cell immunity for these mucosal surfaces.

Multiple myeloma: A paraproteinemic disorder consisting typically of the presence of serum paraprotein, anemia, and lytic bone lesions.

Myeloid: Of or related to the bone marrow. Also, a hematopoietic lineage that includes neutrophils, monocytes, basophils, eosinophils, mast cells, megakaryocytes, and their precursors.

Myeloma protein (M protein): Either an intact monoclonal immunoglobulin molecule or a portion of one produced by malignant plasma cells.

Myeloperoxidase: An enzyme that is present within granules of phagocytic cells and catalyzes peroxidation reactions.

N region: Non-germline-encoded nucleotides inserted between gene segments during V/(D)/J joining.

N terminus: The amino-terminal end of a polypeptide chain.

Natural antibody: Any antibody present in the serum in the absence of known prior exposure to the cognate antigen.

Natural killer cell: A lymphoid cell type that is functionally, morphologically, and developmentally distinct from T and B cells and is capable of cellular cytotoxicity without prior immunization.

NBT test: A metabolic assay involving the reduction of

nitro blue tetrazolium dye during activation of the hexose monophosphate shunt in phagocytic cells.

Negative selection: The phenomenon in which particular conditions selectively inhibit growth or survival of cells that have specific characteristics. In T cell ontogeny, the preferential elimination in the thymus of T cells that recognize autoantigens.

Neoantigens: Nonself antigens that arise spontaneously on cell surfaces, usually during neoplasia.

Nephelometry: The measurement of turbidity or cloudiness in a suspension or a solution.

Nephritic factor: Serum immunoglobulin with conglutinin activity that can activate the alternative complement pathway. Often present in serum of patients with membranoproliferative glomerulonephritis.

Neutralization: Biologic inactivation of a toxin, microorganism, or other ligand, occurring as the direct result of antibody binding.

Neutrophil: A marrow-derived phagocyte characterized by a multilobed nucleus and neutrophilic cytoplasmic granules. Also termed a polymorphonuclear leukocyte, PMN, or poly.

Neutrophil microbicidal assay: A test for the ability of neutrophils to kill intracellular bacteria.

Nonresponder: An animal unable to respond to an antigen, usually because of genetic factors.

Northern blot: A technique for detection of specific RNA species within a complex mixture of RNAs after separation by gel electrophoresis.

Nucleoside phosphorylase: An enzyme that catalyzes the conversion of inosine to hypoxanthine and is deficient in some patients with immunodeficiency disorders.

Nude mouse: A hairless mouse that congenitally lacks a thymus and has a marked deficiency of thymus-derived lymphocytes.

Null cell: Any cell, usually of presumed lymphoid origin, that lacks surface markers necessary to assign it to the T or B lineage.

NZB mouse: A genetically inbred strain of mice in which autoimmune disease resembling systemic lupus erythematosus develops spontaneously.

Oligoclonal bands: Immunoglobulins with restricted electrophoretic mobility in agarose gels found in cerebrospinal fluid of patients with multiple sclerosis and some other central nervous system diseases.

Oncofetal antigens: Antigens expressed during normal fetal development that reappear during cancer development, eg, carcinoembryonic antigen.

Oncogene: Any gene of viral or cellular origin that is thought to contribute to malignant transformation of cells when mutated or abnormally expressed. See also **Proto-oncogene.**

Oncogenesis: The process of producing neoplasia or malignancy.

Ontogeny: The process of growth and development of a cell lineage, tissue, or organism during the life of an individual.

Opportunistic infection: The ability of organisms of relatively low virulence to cause disease in the setting of altered immunity.

Opsonin: Any substance capable of enhancing phagocytosis of a particle to which it is bound.

Oral unresponsiveness: The process by which the mucosal immune system normally prevents immune responses to foods and intestinal bacteria while responding to potential pathogens.

Ouchterlony double diffusion: An immunoprecipitation technique in which antigen and antibody are allowed to diffuse toward each other and form immune complexes in agar.

Palindrome: In molecular genetics, any nucleic acid sequence that is identical to its own complementary sequence.

Paracrine: Producing effects on adjacent cells.

Paralysis: The pseudotolerant condition in which an ongoing immune response is masked by the presence of overwhelming amounts of antigen.

Paraproteinemia: A condition occurring in a heterogeneous group of diseases characterized by the presence in serum or urine of a monoclonal immunoglobulin.

Paratope: An antibody-combining site for epitope, the simplest form of an antigenic determinant.

Passive cutaneous anaphylaxis (PCA): An in vivo passive transfer test for recognizing cytotropic antibody responsible for immediate hypersensitivity reactions.

Passive immunity: Protection achieved by introduction of preformed antibody or immune cells into a nonimmune host.

Perforin: A cytotoxic protein produced by cytotoxic T lymphocytes. Also called cytolysin.

Peripheral lymphoid organs: See **Secondary lymphoid organs.**

Peritoneal exudate cells (PEC): Inflammatory cells present in the peritoneum of animals injected with an inflammatory agent.

Peyer's patch: Any of approximately 200 small focal collections of lymphoid tissue normally found in the submucosa of the small intestine.

Phagocyte: Any cell that is capable of, or specialized for, efficient phagocytosis.

Phagocytosis: A form of endocytosis in which particulate material is engulfed by a cell.

Phagolysosome: A phagosome into which lysosomes have fused and emptied their contents.

Phagosome: The membrane-bounded vesicle containing particulate material that has been phagocytosed, prior to fusion with lysosomes.

Phylogeny: The evolutionary history of a group of animals.

Phytohemagglutinin: A lectin derived from the red kidney bean (*Phaseolus vulgaris*) that is predominantly a T lymphocyte mitogen.

Phytomitogen: Any mitogen derived from plants.

Pinocytosis: Non-receptor-mediated endocytosis of soluble materials by imbibing extracellular fluid.

Plaque-forming cells: Antibody-producing cells capable of forming a hemolytic plaque in the presence of complement and antigenic erythrocytes.

Plasma cell: Specialized antibody-secreting cell that is the terminally differentiated effector cell of the B lymphoid lineage.

Plasmin: A fibrinolytic enzyme capable of proteolytically digesting C1.

Plasminogen activator: An enzyme secreted by macrophages that converts a plasma zymogen to active plasmin.

Platelet-activating factor: An organic mediator of inflammation that is released from degranulating platelets.

Pokeweed mitogen: A lectin derived from pokeweed (*Phytolacca americana*) that is a mitogen for T and B lymphocytes.

Polyclonal hypergammaglobulinemia: An increase in γ-globulin of various classes containing different H and L chains.

Polyclonal mitogen: Any mitogen that can act on many different clones of lymphocytes irrespective of their antigen specificities.

Polymer: Any macromolecule composed of multiple identical or nonidentical repeating subunits, which are often arranged as chains.

Polymerase chain reaction: A technique used to replicate specific short regions of DNA exponentially in vitro.

Polymorphonuclear leukocyte: See **Neutrophil.**

Positive selection: The phenomenon in which particular conditions selectively favor growth and survival of cells that have specific characteristics. In T cell ontogeny, the preferential growth, survival, and release from the thymus of T cells that recognize self MHC proteins.

Postcapillary venule: Small, thin-walled blood vessels into which capillaries drain directly; the first and smallest elements of the venous system.

Prausnitz-Küstner reaction: The passive transfer by intradermal injection of serum containing IgE antibodies from an allergic subject to a nonallergic recipient.

Pre-B cell: A B lymphocyte precursor found predominantly in the bone marrow and characterized by the presence of cytoplasmic immunoglobulin heavy chains without surface immunoglobulin expression.

Precipitation: A reaction between soluble antigen and soluble antibody which gives rise to an insoluble precipitate of immune complexes.

Primary follicle: Lymphoid follicles composed predominantly of resting B lymphocytes and lacking a germinal center.

Primary lymphoid organs: Organs that support and are required for B or T lymphopoiesis from undifferentiated precursor cells, ie, the thymus, bone marrow, and fetal liver.

Primed lymphocyte typing (PLT): A variation of the MLR in which cells are primed by allogeneic stimulation and reexposed to fresh stimulator cells. Used to type for HLA-D determinants.

Private antigen: A tumor or histocompatibility antigen restricted either to a specific chemically induced tumor or to the specific product of a given allele.

Pro-B cell: An immature B lymphocyte progenitor that is capable of rearranging its immunoglobulin genes but does not yet express immunoglobulin protein.

Programmed cell death: Cell death that is genetically determined or is carried out by an endogenous cellular suicide mechanism in response to an external stimulus. See also apoptosis.

Proinflammatory: Tending to promote inflammation.

Prokaryote: Any cell that lacks a true nucleus, or organism composed of such cells.

Properdin system: A small group of serum proteins that influence activation of the complement cascade.

Prostaglandin: Any of a class of small organic mediators of inflammation produced through the cyclooxygenase pathway of arachidonic acid metabolism.

Protein tyrosine kinase: Any of a diverse group of enzymes that catalyze phosphorylation of tyrosine residues in other proteins.

Protein tyrosine phosphatases: Any of a diverse group of enzymes that catalyze removal of phosphate from phosphorylated proteins.

Prothymocyte: Any immature thymocyte precursor found in the thymus.

Proto-oncogene: Any oncogene normally found in the mammalian genome.

Prozone phenomenon: Suboptimal precipitation that occurs in the region of antibody excess during immunoprecipitation reactions.

Pruritus: Itching.

Public antigen: Determinant common to several distinct or private antigens.

Pyogenic bacterium: Bacterium belonging to any of several species that induce abundant pus formation.

Pyrogen: Any substance that induces fever.

Pyroglobulins: Monoclonal immunoglobulins that precipitate irreversibly when heated to 56 °C.

Quellung: The swelling of the capsules of pneumococci when the organisms are exposed to pneumococcal antibodies.

Radioallergosorbent test (RAST): A radioimmunoassay capable of detecting IgE antibody directed at specific allergens.

Radioimmunoassay: A variety of immunologic techniques in which a radioactive isotope is used to detect antigens or antibodies in some form of immunoassay.

Radioimmunodiffusion (Rowe's method): A modification of immunodiffusion in which a radioactive antibody is incorporated in order to increase the sensitivity by means of autoradiography.

Radioimmunosorbent test (RIST): A solid-phase radioimmunoassay that can detect approximately 1 ng of IgE.

Ragocytes (RA cells): Polymorphonuclear leukocytes that have ingested characteristic dense IgG aggregates, rheumatoid factor, complement, and fibrin. They are found in the joints of patients with rheumatoid arthritis.

Raji cell test: An assay for immune complexes using the Raji lymphoblastoid cell line.

Reagin: Synonymous with IgE antibody. Also denotes a complement-fixing antibody that reacts in the Wassermann reaction with cardiolipin.

Recombinant: In genetics, a DNA molecule formed by

joining 2 or more DNA molecules of disparate origin; or any organism containing such DNA.

Recombinase: The enzymatic machinery that carries out V/(D)/J rearrangements.

Recombinase signal sequence: The short DNA sequence element, flanking each V, D, or J gene segment, that specifies sites for potential DNA cleavage and rearrangement by recombinase.

Rejection response: An immune response with both humoral and cellular components directed against transplanted tissue.

Respiratory burst: See **Metabolic burst.**

Restriction: In immune function, a genetically determined limitation on the range of immune responsiveness of a cell, clone, or organism that distinguishes it from others of the same type. Antigen restriction is responsiveness to only one or a few antigens; MHC restriction is responsiveness only to antigens complexed with a particular MHC allele.

Restriction enzyme: Any of a group of bacterial endonucleases that cleave DNA at or near specific recognition sequences.

Restriction fragment: DNA fragment produced by cleaving a larger fragment with a restriction enzyme.

Reticuloendothelial system: See **mononuclear phagocyte system.**

Retrovirus: Any of several viruses with RNA genomes, which encode and utilize the enzyme reverse transcriptase.

Reverse transcriptase: Enzyme that catalyzes DNA synthesis by using an RNA template.

Rheumatoid factor (RF): An anti-immunoglobulin antibody directed against denatured IgG present in the serum of patients with rheumatoid arthritis and other rheumatoid diseases.

Ricin: A poisonous substance that derives from the seed of the castor oil plant and agglutinates erythrocytes (a lectin).

Rocket electrophoresis (Laurell technique): An electro-immunodiffusion technique in which antigen is electrophoresed into agar containing specific antibody and precipitates in a tapered rocket-shaped pattern. This technique is used for quantitation of antigens.

Rose-Waaler test: A type of passive hemagglutination test for the detection of rheumatoid factor that employs tanned erythrocytes coated with rabbit 7S IgG antibodies specific for sheep erythrocytes.

S value: Svedberg unit. A standard unit of measurement for the rate of sedimentation of a macromolecule or particle on ultracentrifugation; it is roughly proportionate to density.

Schultz-Dale test: An in vitro assay for immediate hypersensitivity in which smooth muscle is passively sensitized by cytotropic antibody and contracts after the addition of an antigen.

Second set graft rejection: An immunologic rejection of a graft in a host that is immune to antigens contained in that graft.

Secondary follicle: Lymphoid follicle containing a germinal center.

Secondary lymphoid organs: Organs composed predominantly of mature lymphoid and antigen-presenting cells, such as the lymph nodes and tonsils. Organs that contain significant focal collections of lymphoid tissue, such as the spleen, are also included in this category, but the primary lymphoid organs are excluded.

Secretory IgA: The major secreted (11S) form of IgA, comprising a dimer of IgA 4-chain units along with one molecule of J chain and one of secretory component.

Secretory component: A nonimmunoglobulin polypeptide, synthesized by some epithelial cells, that is a component of secretory IgA.

Selectin: Any of a family of cell surface proteins that have lectinlike oligosaccharide-binding activity.

Sensitization: See **Immunization.** Natural or artificial induction of an immune response, particularly when it causes allergy in the host.

Sensitized: Synonymous with immunized.

Sequential determinant: See **Linear determinant.**

Serologically defined (SD) antigens: Antigens that are present on membranes of nearly all mammalian cells and are controlled by genes present in the major histocompatibility complex. They can be easily detected with antibodies.

Serology: Literally, the study of serum. Refers to the study or experimental use of antibodies.

Serum sickness: A pattern of immunologic reactivity in which deleterious effects result from reaction of relatively large amounts of antigen with preformed antibodies, leading to widespread deposition of immune complexes.

Shwartzman reaction: Acute hemorrhagic necrosis and thrombosis that occurs locally following the second of 2 injections of endotoxin.

Single-positive lymphocyte: Any T lymphocyte that expresses surface CD4 or CD8 but not both. Most mature, functional T cells are single-positive.

Single radial diffusion (radioimmunodiffusion): A technique for quantitating antigens by immunodiffusion in which antigen is allowed to diffuse radially into agar containing antibody. The resultant precipitation ring reflects the concentration of the antigen.

Slow virus: A virus that produces disease with a greatly delayed onset and protracted course.

Solid phase radioimmunoassay: A modification of radioimmunoassay in which antibody is adsorbed onto solid particles or tubes.

Somatic hypermutation: The increased rate of mutation that occurs in immunoglobulin V_H regions during memory B cell proliferation.

Southern blot: A technique for detecting specific DNA sequences within a complex mixture of DNA molecules after separation by gel electrophoresis.

Spherulin: A spherule-derived antigen from *Coccidioides immitis* used in delayed hypersensitivity skin testing for coccidioidomycosis.

SS-A: Antibody to RNA found in Sjögren's syndrome and also associated with heart block in infants born to mothers with this antibody.

SS-B: Antibody to RNA found in Sjögren's syndrome and other rheumatic diseases.

Stem cell: Any incompletely differentiated progenitor cell that is capable of mitotic proliferation to produce both stem cells and mature differentiated progeny.

Sulzberger-Chase phenomenon: Abrogation of dermal contact sensitivity to various chemicals produced by prior oral feeding of the specific agent.

Superantigen: Any of a group of bacterial or viral proteins that activate (and may kill) T cells bearing a specific class of V_β chain irrespective of antigen specificity.

Suppressor T cells: A putative, but as yet unproven, subset of T lymphocytes characterized by their ability to suppress immune reactions in an antigen-specific manner.

Surrogate light chain: A polypeptide expressed by immature B cells that can substitute for immunoglobulin light chains in binding to heavy chains but is not involved in antigen recognition.

Switch: See **Immunoglobulin class switch.**

Switch region: The DNA sequences, located between C_H regions, that serve as sites for DNA cleavage and rearrangement in immunoglobulin class switching.

Syngeneic: Denotes the relationship that exists between genetically identical members of the same species.

T antigens: Tumor antigens, probably protein products of the viral genome present only on infected neoplastic cells.

T cell (T lymphocyte): A thymus-derived cell that participates in a variety of cell-mediated immune reactions.

T cell rosette: See **E rosette.**

T lymphocyte: Mature lymphoid cell belonging to the thymus-dependent lineage.

Tail piece: Short C-terminal amino acid sequence in certain secreted immunoglobulin heavy chains, which mediates binding with the J chain.

Tertiary lymphoid organ: Dense, organoid, usually temporary aggregate of lymphoid tissue that may form at sites of intense immunologic reactions.

TH0 lymphocyte: A helper T cell whose spectrum of cytokine production combines features of both TH1 and TH2 lymphocytes.

TH1 lymphocyte: A helper T cell that elaborates cytokines (such as IFNγ) which selectively promote cell-mediated immune responses.

TH2 lymphocyte: A helper T cell that elaborates cytokines (including IL-4, IL-5, IL-6, and IL-10) which selectively promote humoral immune responses.

Theliolymphocytes: Small lymphocytes that are found in contiguity with intestinal epithelial cells and whose function is unknown.

Thymocyte: An immature thymic T lymphoid cell that expresses both CD4 and CD8 and is the predominant cell type in the thymus.

Thymopoietin: One of several peptides elaborated by thymic endothelial cells and proposed to have a role in thymic function.

Thymosin: One of several peptides elaborated by thymic endothelial cells and proposed to have a role in thymic function.

Thymus: A primary lymphoid organ situated in the anterior mediastinum, which is required for and is the site of T lymphopoiesis.

Thymus-dependent antigen: Any immunogen that can efficiently induce humoral (antibody) immune response only when T cells are present.

Thymus-independent antigen: Any immunogen that can efficiently induce a humoral (antibody) immune response in the absence of T cells, usually because it can directly bind and activate B cells.

Tolerance: The state of immunologic unresponsiveness against a potential immunogen.

Toxoids: Antigenic but nontoxic derivatives of toxins.

Transcription: The synthesis of RNA molecules from a DNA template.

Transfer factor: A dialyzable extract of immune lymphocytes that is capable of transferring cell-mediated immunity in humans and possibly in other animal species.

Transgenic: Any organism (usually multicellular) into whose genome a foreign gene has been permanently introduced.

Translation: The process by which genetic information encoded in an RNA template is used to produce a polypeptide chain.

Transplantation antigen: Any antigen whose presence on a cell or tissue can influence the survival or rejection of a graft.

Trophoblast: Cell layer in placenta in contact with uterine lining. Produces various immunosuppressive substances, eg, hormones.

Tryptic peptides: Peptides produced as a result of tryptic digestion of a protein molecule.

Tuftsin: A 4-amino-acid (threonine-lysine-prolinearginine) polypeptide that enhances macrophage functions.

Tumor-specific antigens: Cell surface antigens that are expressed on malignant but not normal cells.

Tumor-specific determinants: Antigens that are found on tumor cells but are also present in different amounts or forms on normal cells.

Ultracentrifugation: A high-speed centrifugation technique that can be used for the analytic identification of proteins of various sedimentation coefficients or as a preparative technique for separating proteins of different shapes and densities.

Ultrafiltration: The filtration of solutions or suspensions through membranes of extremely small graded pore sizes.

Uropods: Long pseudopods extending from lymphocyte cytoplasm covered by cellular plasma membrane.

Urticaria: Hives.

V antigens: Virally induced antigens that are expressed on viruses and virus-infected cells.

V (Variable) region: The N-terminal domain in an immunoglobulin or T cell receptor polypeptide, whose sequence varies widely and determines antigen specificity of the molecule.

V segment: Any of a family of evolutionarily related exon fragments that encode alternative forms of the N-terminal portion of immunoglobulin or T cell receptor variable regions.

V/(D)/J joining: The process of assembling an intact immunoglobulin or T cell receptor gene V/J or V/D/J exon through DNA rearrangement.

Vaccination: Immunization with antigens administered for the prevention of infectious diseases (term originally coined to denote immunization against vaccinia or cowpox virus).

Variolation: Inoculation with a virus of unmodified smallpox (variola).

Viropathic: Damage to host tissues that is produced directly by the presence of pathogenic viral infection.

Viscosity: The physical property of serum that is determined by the size, shape, and deformability of serum molecules. The hydrostatic state, molecular charge, and temperature sensitivity of proteins.

Von Krogh equation: An equation that relates complement to the degree of lysis of erythrocytes coated with anti-red blood cell antibodies under standard conditions. Used to determine hemolytic complement titers in serum.

Wasting disease (also runt disease): A chronic, ultimately fatal illness associated with lymphoid atrophy in mice who are neonatally thymectomized.

Western blot: A technique for detecting specific proteins (usually by using specific antibodies) within a complex mixture of proteins after separation by gel electrophoresis.

Xenogeneic: Denotes the relationship that exists between members of genetically different species.

Xenograft: A tissue or organ graft between members of 2 distinct or different species.

Zone electrophoresis: Electrophoresis performed on paper or cellulose acetate in which proteins are separated almost exclusively on the basis of charge.

Acronyms & Abbreviations Commonly Used in Immunology

2–5A	2′-5′ oligoadenylate.	**BUDR, BUdR**	5-Bromodeoxyuridine.
Ab	Antibody	**C**	Constant region, or complement factor.
ABA	Azobenzenearsenate.	**CAH**	Chronic active hepatitis.
ABPA	Allergic bronchopulmonary aspergillosis.	**CALLA**	Common acute lymphocytic leukemia antigen.
ACTH	Adrenocorticotropic hormone.	**cAMP**	Cyclic adenosine monophosphate.
ADA	Adenosine deaminase.	**CBH**	Cutaneous basophil hypersensitivity.
ADCC	Antibody-dependent cell-mediated cytotoxicity.	**CD**	Cluster of differentiation.
		CDC	Centers for Disease Control
AEF	Allogeneic effect.	**CD3**	Antigenic marker on T cells; complex of signal-transducing proteins associated with T-cell receptor.
AFC	Antibody-forming cells.		
AFP	Alpha-fetoprotein.		
AGN	Acute glomerulonephritis.		
AHA	Autoimmune hemolytic anemia.	**CD4**	Antigenic marker of T cells that recognize antigens bound to class II MHC proteins; most are helper T cells.
AHG	Antihemophilic globulin.		
AIDS	Acquired immunodeficiency syndrome.		
AIHA	Autoimmune hemolytic anemia.	**CD40L**	CD40 ligand: the CD40-binding protein on activated TH cells.
ALG	Antilymphocyte globulin.		
ALL	Acute lymphocytic leukemia.	**CD8**	Antigenic marker of T cells that recognize antigens bound to class I MHC proteins; most are cytotoxic T cells.
ALS	Antilymphocyte serum.		
AMA	Antimitochondrial antibodies.		
AML	Acute myelogenous leukemia.	**cDNA**	Complementary DNA.
AMP	Adenosine monophosphate.	**CDR**	Complementarity-determining region.
ANA	Antinuclear antibody.	**CEA**	Carcinoembryonic antigen.
ANF	Antinuclear factor.	**CF**	Complement fixation.
APC	Antigen-presenting cells.	**CFA**	Colonization factor antigens (also Freund's complete adjuvant).
APSGN	Acute poststreptococcal glomerulonephritis.		
ARC	AIDS-related complex.	**CFU**	Colony-forming unit.
ASO	Antistreptolysin O.	**CFU-C**	Colony-forming unit of cells grown in culture.
ATG	Antithymocyte globulin.		
ATL	Adult T cell leukemia.	**CFU-GEMM**	Colony-forming unit of granulocytes, erythrocytes, monocytes and megakaryocytes.
BAF	B-cell activating factor.		
BAL	Dimercaprol (British anti-Lewisite).	**CFU-GM**	Colony-stimulating factor of granulocytes and macrophages.
BALT	Bronchus-associated lymphoid tissue.		
BCG	Bacillus Calmette-Guérin.	**CFU-S**	Colony-forming unit of cells grown in the spleen.
BCGF-I	B-cell growth factor-I (see IL-4).		
Bcl-2	B cell lymphoma proto-oncogene 2.	**CGD**	Chronic granulomatous disease.
BCSF-I	B cell stimulating factor-I (see IL-4).	**cGMP**	Cyclic guanosine monophosphate.
Bf	Properdin factor B.	**C$_H$**	Constant domain of H chain.
BFP	Biologic false-positive (tests for syphilis).	**CHS**	Chédiak-Higashi syndrome.
BJ	Bence Jones.	**CIg**	Cytoplasmic immunoglobulin.
bp	Base pair(s).	**C$_L$**	Constant domain of L chain.
BPI	Bactericidal permeability-increasing protein.	**CLL**	Chronic lymphocytic leukemia.
BPO	Benzyl penicilloyl.	**cM**	Centimorgan.
BSA	Bovine serum albumin.	**CMCC**	Chronic mucocutaneous candidiasis.
BSF-1	B cell stimulatory factor 1.	**CMI**	Cell-mediated immunity.

CML	Cell-mediated lympholysis, also chronic myelogenous leukemia.
CMPGN	Chronic membranoproliferative glomerulonephritis.
CMV	Cytomegalovirus(es).
C3NeF	C3 nephritic factor.
CNTF	Ciliary neurotropic factor.
Con A	Concanavalin A.
C3PA	C3 proactivator.
CPGN	Chronic proliferative glomerulonephritis.
CR1-CR6	Six distinct receptors for C3 fragments found on various cell types.
CREG	Cross-reactive group.
CRP	C-reactive protein.
CSA	Colony-stimulating activity.
CSF	Colony-stimulating factor.
CSIF	Cytokine synthesis inhibitory factor (see IL-10).
CTL	Cytotoxic lymphocytes.
CTLL	Cloned mouse cytotoxic T lymphocytic line.
DAT	Direct antiglobulin (Coombs test); also delay-accelerating factor.
DC	Dendritic cells.
DDS	Dapsone (diaminodiphenyl-sulfone).
DEAE	Diethylaminoethyl.
DGI	Disseminated gonococcal infection.
D_H	Diversity segment of immunoglobulin or T cell receptor gene.
DIC	Disseminated intravascular coagulation.
D-L	Donath-Landsteiner.
DLE	Dialyzable leukocyte extracts; disseminated lupus erythematosus.
DNCB	2,4-Dinitrochlorobenzene.
DNFB	Dinitrofluorobenzene.
DNP	Dinitrophenyl.
DP	Human class II MHC allele (formerly called SB).
DPO	Dimethoxyphenylpenicilloyl.
DPT	See DTP.
DQ	Human class II MHC allele (formerly called DC, MB, and DS).
DR	D-related HLA locus in humans.
DSCG	Disodium cromoglycate.
DST	Donor-specific transfusion.
DT	Diphtheria and tetanus toxoids.
DTH	Delayed-type hypersensitivity.
DTP	Diphtheria and tetanus toxoid combined with pertussis vaccine.
EA	Early antigens (of EBV).
EA	Erythrocyte amboceptor (sensitized erythrocytes).
EAC	Erythrocyte amboceptor complement.
EAE	Experimental allergic encephalitis or encephalomyelitis.
EAN	Experimental allergic neuritis.
EB	Epstein-Barr.
EBNA	Epstein-Barr nuclear antigen.
EBV	Epstein-Barr virus.
ECF	Eosinophil chemotactic factor.
ECF-A	Eosinophil chemotactic factor of anaphylaxis.
ECM	Erythema chronicum migrans (in Lyme disease).
ECP	Eosinophil cationic protein.
EDTA	Ethylenediaminetetraacetate.
EFA	Enhancing factor of allergy.

EIA	Enzyme immunoassay.
ELISA	Enzyme-linked immunosorbent assay.
EMIT	Enzyme multiple immunoassay technique; a homogeneous enzyme immunoassay.
ENA	Extractable nuclear antigen.
EP	Endogenous pyrogen.
Epo	Erythropoietin.
EPO	Eosinophilic peroxidase.
ER	Endoplasmic reticulum.
ESR	Erythrocyte sedimentation rate.
F_1	First generation.
F_2	Second generation.
FA	Fluorescent antibody.
FAB	French, American, British (system of leukemia classification).
Fab	Antigen-binding fragment.
FACS	Fluorescent-activated cell sorter.
Fc	Crystallizable fragment.
FCC	Follicular center cell.
FCM	Flow cytometry.
FCR	Fractional catabolic rate.
FcεR	Fc receptor specific for IgE.
FcγR	Fc receptor specific for IgG.
FcμR	Fc receptor specific for IgM.
FeLV	Feline leukemia virus.
FEV	Forced expiratory volume in 1 second.
FITC	Fluorescein isothiocyanate.
FSH	Follicle-stimulating hormone.
FTA-ABS	Fluorescent treponemal antibody absorption test.
FUDR	Fluorodeoxyuridine.
FVC	Forced vital capacity.
GALT	Gut-associated lymphoid tissue.
GBG	Glycine-rich beta-glyucoprotein.
GBM	Glomerular basement membrane.
G-CSF	Granulocyte colony-stimulating factor.
GEF	Glycosylation-enhancing factor.
GFR	Glomerular filtration rate.
GGG	Glycine-rich gamma-glycoprotein.
GIF	Glycosylation inhibition factor.
GLO	Glyoxylase.
GM-CSF	Granulocyte-macrophage colony-stimulating factor.
GMP	Guanosine monophosphate.
gp	Glycoprotein.
GPA	Guinea pig albumin.
GPC	Gastric parietal cell.
G6PD	Glucose-6-phosphate dehydrogenase.
GVH	Graft-versus-host (disease).
GVHR	Graft-versus-host reaction.
HAA	Hepatitis-associated antigen.
HAE, HANE	Hereditary angioneurotic edema.
HAT	Hypoxanthine, aminopterin, and thymidine.
HAV	Hepatitis A virus.
HbA	Adult hemoglobin.
HBcAg	Low-molecular-weight nucleocapsid antigen of hepatitis B virus.
HbF	Fetal hemoglobin.
HBeAG	Protein antigen of hepatitis B.
HBIG	Hepatitis B immune globulin.
HBsAg	Hepatitis B surface antigen.
HBV	Hepatitis B virus.
HCD	Heavy-chain disease.
hCG	Human chorionic gonadotropin.

HDL	High-density lipoproteins.
HDN	Hemolytic disease of newborn.
HDV	Hepatitis delta virus.
H&E	Hematoxylin and eosin (stain).
HETE	Hydroxyeicosatetraenoic acid.
HEV	High endothelial venules.
HI	Hemagglutination inhibition.
HIV	Human immunodeficiency virus.
HLA	Human leukocyte antigen.
HLA-B27	An HLA allele with several strong disease associations.
$(H_2L_2)n$	General formula for immunoglobulin molecule.
HMP	Hexose monophosphate (shunt).
HMW-NCF	High-molecular-weight neutrophil chemotactic factor.
HPETE	Hydroperoxyeicosatetraenoic acid.
HPLC	High-performance liquid chromatography.
HRF	Homologous restriction factor.
HPRT	Hypoxanthine phosphoribosyl transferase.
HSA	Human serum albumin.
HSF	Histamine-sensitizing factor, also hepatocyte-stimulating factor.
HSV	Herpes simplex virus.
5-HT	5-Hydroxytryptamine (serotonin).
HTC	Homozygous typing cells.
HTLV	Human T cell leukemia virus.
HuFcR	Human Fc receptor.
IBL	Immunoblastic lymphodenopathy.
ICA	Islet cell antibody.
ICAM	Intracellular adhesion molecule.
ICSA	Islet cell surface antibody.
IDAT	Indirect antiglobulin (Coombs) test.
ID	Idiotype.
IDDM	Insulin-dependent diabetes mellitus.
IDU	Idoxuridine.
IEF	Isoelectric focusing.
IEL	Intraepithelial lymphocyte.
IEP	Immunoelectrophoresis.
IF	Intrinsic factor (also initiating factor).
IFA	Indirect fluorescent antibody.
IFE	Immunofixation electrophoresis.
IFN	Interferon.
Ig	Immunoglobulin.
IGIM	Immune globulin for intramuscular use.
IGIV	Immune globulin for intravenous use.
Ii	Invariant chain.
IL	Interleukin.
INH	Isoniazid (isonicotinic acid hydrazide).
Ip_3	Inositol 1,4,5-triphosphate.
Ir	Immune response (genes).
ISG	Immune serum globulin.
ITP	Idiopathic thrombocytopenic purpura.
J	Joining segment of immunoglobulin or T cell receptor gene.
JRA	Juvenile rheumatoid arthritis.
K (cells)	Killer (cells).
K562	Erythroleukemic cell line.
KAF	Bovine conglutinin: conglutinin activating factor.
Kb	Kilobases or kilobase pairs.
KLH	Keyhole limpet hemocyanin.
La	See SS-B.
LAF	Leukocyte-activating factor (see IL-1).
LAK	Lymphokine-activated killer (cells).
LAV	Lymphadenopathy-associated virus.
LCMV	Lymphocytic choriomeningitis virus.
LCR	Ligase chain reaction.
LD	Lymphocyte-defined.
LDCC	Lectin-dependent cell-mediated cytotoxicity.
LDCF	Lymphocyte-derived chemotactic factors.
LDH	Lactate dehydrogenase.
LDL	Low-density lipoproteins.
LE	Lupus erythematosus.
Lf	Limit flocculation (unit) $1/1000 Lf = 0.0000003$ mg).
LFA	Lymphocyte functional antigen.
LGL	Large granular lymphocytes.
LH	Luteinizing hormone.
LIF	Leukocyte inhibitory factor.
LMI	Leukocyte migration inhibition.
LPL	Lamina propria lymphocyte.
LPS	Lipopolysaccharide.
LT	Leukotriene.
LT	Lymphotoxin or lymphocytotoxin (see TNF).
Lyb	Lymphocyte antigens on murine B cells.
LyNeF	Lytic nephritic factor.
Lyt	Lymphocyte antigens on murine T cells.
μm	Membrane-bound form of immunoglobulin μ heavy chain.
μs	Secretory form of immunoglobulin μ heavy chain.
MAC	(Complement) membrane attack complex.
$\beta_2 m$	β_2-Microglobulin.
MAC-1	Macrophage integrin 1.
Mac-1	Macrophage-1 glycoprotein.
MAF	Macrophage-activating (-arming) factor.
MALT	Mucosa-associated lymphoid tissue.
MBP	Major basic protein.
MC(DC)	Human MHC antigen of class II type.
MCA	Methylcholanthrene.
MCF	Macrophage chemotactic factor.
MCGN	Mesangiocapillary (membranoproliferative) glomerulonephritis.
MCP	Membrane cofactor protein.
M-CSF	Monocyte-macrophage colony-stimulating factor.
MCTD	Mixed connective tissue disease.
MDP	Muramyl dipeptide.
MeBSA	Methylated bovine serum albumin.
MER	Methanol extraction residue (of phenol-treated BCG).
MF	Mitogenic factor.
MHA	Major histocompatibility antigen.
MHA-TP	Microhemagglutination test for *Treponema pallidum*.
MHC	Major histocompatibility complex.
MHD	Minimum hemolytic dilution or dose.
MIF	Migration inhibitory factor.
ML	Malignant lymphoma.
MLC	Mixed lymphocyte (leukocyte) culture.
MLD	Minimum lethal dose.
MLR	Mixed lymphocyte (or leukocyte) response or reaction.
MMI	Macrophage migration inhibition.
MMR	Measles-mumps-rubella vaccine.
6-MP	Mercaptopurine.
MPG	Methyl green pyronin.
MPO	Myeloperoxidase.
MS	Multiple sclerosis.
MTX	Methotrexate.

MuLV	Murine leukemia virus.
MW	Molecular weight.
NADPH	Reduced form of nicotinamide adenine dinucleotide.
NBT	Nitroblue tetrazolium.
N-CAM	Neural cell adhesion molecule.
NCF	Neutrophil chemotactic factor.
NF	Nephritic factor.
NK	Natural killer (cells).
NSAID	Nonsteroidal anti-inflammatory drug.
NZB	New Zealand black (mice).
NZW	New Zealand white (mice or rabbits).
OAF	Osteoclast activating factor.
OPV	Oral poliovirus.
OS	Obese strain.
OSM	Oncostatin M.
OT	Old tuberculin.
PA	Pernicious anemia.
PAF	Platelet-activating factor.
PAIDS	AIDS in pediatric patients.
PAP	Peroxidase antiperoxidase.
PAS	*p*-Aminosalicylic acid; periodic acid-Schiff (reaction).
PBC	Primary biliary cirrhosis.
PCA	Passive cutaneous anaphylaxis.
PCM	Protein-calorie malnutrition.
PCP	*Pneumocystis carinii* pneumonia.
PCR	Polymerase chain reaction.
PDGF	Platelet-derived growth factor.
PE	Phycoerythrin.
PEC	Peritoneal exudate cells.
PFC	Plaque-forming cells.
PG	Prostaglandin.
Pg5	Urinary pepsinogen.
PGE	Prostaglandin E (PGE_1, PGE_2, $PGE_{2\alpha}$).
PGM_3	Phosphoglucomutase 3.
PGN	Proliferative glomerulonephritis.
PHA	Phytohemagglutinin.
PIE	Pulmonary infiltration with eosinophilia.
pIgA	Polymeric IgA.
PIP_2	Phosphatidyl inositol bisphosphate.
PK (P-K)	Prausnitz-Küstner (reaction).
PLCγ-1	Phospholipase Cγ isoform 1.
PLL	Poly-L-lysine.
PLT	Primed lymphocyte typing.
PMA	Phorbol myristate acetate; a tumor promotor that stimulates monocytes and lymphocytes nonspecifically.
PML	Progressive multifocal leukodystrophy.
PMN	Polymorphonuclear neutrophil.
PNA	Peanut agglutinin.
PNH	Paroxysmal nocturnal hemoglubulinuria.
PPD	Purified protein derivative (tuberculin).
PRP	Polysaccharide vaccine against *Haemophilus*.
PSS	Progressive systemic sclerosis.
PTH	Post transfusion hepatitis.
PTK	Protein tyrosine kinase.
PVP	Polyvinylpyrolidone.
PWM	Pokeweed mitogen.
-R	Receptor (eg, IL-R, IL-2R).
R	Roentgen (unit of radiation).
-RA	Receptor antagonist (eg, IL-1RA).
RA	Rheumatoid arthritis.
RAG	Recombination activating gene.
Ragg	Rheumatoid agglutinin.

RANA	Rheumatoid arthritis nuclear antigen.
RAST	Radioallergosorbent test.
RBC	Red blood cell (erythrocyte); red blood count.
RE	Reticuloendothelial.
RER	Rough endoplasmic reticulum.
RES	Reticuloendothelial system.
RF	Rheumatic fever; rheumatoid factor.
RFLP	Restriction fragment length polymorphism.
RLIg	Rh immune globulin.
RIA	Radioimmunoassay.
RIF	Receptor-inducing factor.
RIST	Radioimmunosorbent test.
RNP	Ribonucleoprotein.
Ro	See SS-A.
RPR	Rapid plasma reagin.
rRNA	Ribosomal RNA.
RSV	Respiratory syncytial virus.
S	S value or sedimentation coefficient.
SAA	Serum amyloid A.
SAC	Staphylococcal protein A of Cowan 1 strain.
SBE	Subacute bacterial endocarditis.
SC	Secretory component.
SCF	Stem cell factor.
SCID	Severe combined immmunodeficiency disease.
SCL-1	Antinuclear antibody found in scleroderma.
SD	Serologically defined.
SFA	Supressive factor of allergy.
SIDS	Sudden infant death syndrome.
sig	Surface immunoglobulin.
sigA	Secretory IgA.
SIRS	Soluble immune response suppressor.
SK-SD, SKSD	Streptokinase-streptodornase.
SLE	Systemic lupus erythematosus.
SMA	Smooth muscle antibody.
SMAF	Specific macrophage arming factor.
SNagg	Serum normal agglutinator.
SpA	Staphylococcal protein A.
SRBC	Sheep red blood cells.
SRF	Skin-reactive factor.
SRS-A	Slow-reacting substance of anaphylaxis.
SS	Systemic sclerosis.
SS-A	Sjögren's syndrome antibody to RNA.
SS-B	Sjögren's syndrome antibody to RNA.
SSPE	Subacute sclerosing panencephalitis.
STS	Serologic test for syphilis.
t(14,18)	Reciprocal translocation between chromosomes 14 and 18.
t(8,14)	Reciprocal translation between chromosomes 8 and 14.
TA	Transplantation antigens.
Tac	T cell activation receptor.
TAF	T cell-activating factor.
TATA	Tumor-associated transplantation antigen.
TBII	Thyroid-binding inhibitory immunoglobulin.
TBM	Tubular basement membrane.
Tc	Cytotoxic T cells.
TCGF	T cell growth factor (see IL-2).
TCR	T cell receptor.
TD	Thymus-dependent.
Td	Combined tetanus and diphtheria toxoid (adult type).
TdT	Terminal deoxynucleotidyl transferase.
TEBG	Testosterone-estrogen binding globulin.

TF	Transfer factor.	**TSI**	Thyroid-stimulating immunoglobulin.
TGF	Transforming growth factor.	**TSST-1**	Toxic shock syndrome toxin 1.
TGSI	Thyroid growth-stimulating immunoglobulin.	**TU**	Tuberculin units.
TH	Helper T cells.	**TX**	Thromboxane.
Thy	Thymus-derived.	**V**	Variable region.
TI	Thymus-independent.	**VCA**	Viral capsid antigen (of EBV).
TIL	Tumor-infiltrating lymphocyte.	**V-CAM**	Vascular cell adhesion molecule.
TL	Thymic lymphocyte (antigen) on pro-thymocytes.	**VDRL**	Venereal Disease Research Laboratory.
		VEA	Virus envelope antigen.
TLI	Total lymphoid irradiation.	**V**H	Variable domain of heavy chain.
TMP	Thymocyte mitogenic protein.	**VIG**	Vaccinia immune globulin.
TNF	Tumor necrosis factor.	**V**L	Variable domain of light chain.
TNP	Trinitrophenyl.	**VLDL**	Very low density lipoproteins.
Tp	Precursor T cells.	**VSG**	Variable surface glycoprotein (of trypano-somes).
TPH	Transplacental fetal hemorrhage.		
TPI	*Treponema pallidum* immobilization.	**VZIG**	Varicella-zoster immune globulin.
TRA	Thyrotropin receptor antibody.	**WBC**	White blood cell; white blood count.
Ts	Suppressor T cells.	**Z-DNA**	Methylated DNA coiled into a left-handed helix.
TSA	Tumor-specific antigen.		
TSab	Thyroid-stimulating antibody.	**ZIG**	Zoster immune globulin.
TSH	Thyroid-stimulating hormone.		

The CD Classification of Hematopoietic Cell Surface Markers*

Marker	Other Names	Cell Types/Lineages	Major Functions and Properties
CD1	T6	Cortical thymocytes, dendritic cells	Antigen presentation to γ/δ T cells
CD2	T11, sheep RBC receptor	T cells, NK cells	Binds LFA-3 (CD58); signaling
CD3	T3, Leu4	T lymphocytes	Transduces signals from T cell receptor; T lineage marker
CD4	T4, Leu3a	T lymphocytes, monocytes, macrophages, EBV-transformed B cells	Coreceptor for class II MHC; marker for helper T cells; signaling; receptor for human immunodeficiency virus (HIV)
CD5	T1	T lymphocytes, some B cells	Binds CD72; signaling; subset marker for B cells
CD6	T12	Some T and B cells	Unknown
CD7	Leu9	T cells, NK cells, some lymphoid and myeloid precursors	Signaling
CD8	T8, Leu2a	T lymphocytes	Coreceptor for class I MHC; marker for cytotoxic T cells; signaling
CD10	CALLA	B cell precursors	Endopeptidase; marker for acute lymphocytic leukemia
CD11a	LFA-1 α chain	T and B lymphocytes, monocytes, NK cells	Integrin; binds ICAM-1 (CD54) or ICAM-2; mediates leukocyte adhesion to other leukocytes or to endothelial cells
CD11b	MAC-1, CR3	NK cells, monocytes, neutrophils	Integrin; receptor for complement fragment C3bi, fibrinogen, or clotting factor X
CD11c	CR4	NK cells, monocytes, neutrophils	Integrin; receptor for complement fragment C3bi
CD14	LeuM3	Monocytes	LPS receptor
CD15	Sialyl Lewis X	Granulocytes; some cutaneous T cells	Oligosaccharide; bound by ELAM-1 protein on endothelial cells; T cell homing receptor for skin
CD16	FcγRIII	Macrophages, neutrophils, NK cells	Low-affinity Fc receptor for IgG; lineage marker for NK cells
CD18	LFA-1 β chain	T and B lymphocytes, monocytes, NK cells	Integrin; binds ICAM-1 (CD54) or ICAM-2; mediates leukocyte-endothelial cell binding
CD19	B4	B lymphocytes	Signaling
CD20	B1	B lymphocytes	Signaling
CD21	CR2, B2	B lymphocytes	Receptor for complement fragment C3d, CD23, and Epstein-Barr virus (EBV)
CD22		B lymphocytes	Binds CD45RO (on T cells) or CD75 (on B cells); signaling

(continued)

*Only selected markers are listed. Certain CD designations (such as CD3) refer to heteromeric complexes of multiple polypeptide chains. Some CD proteins (such as the integrins) must associate with other proteins to mediate the functions listed here.

Marker	Other Names	Cell Types/Lineages	Major Functions and Properties
CD23	FcεRII	Activated B cells, macrophages, eosinophils, thymic epithelium, platelets	Low-affinity Fc receptor for IgE; ligand for CD21
CD25	IL-2R α chain, Tac	Activated T and B lymphocytes, monocytes	Low-affinity IL-2 receptor; marker for lymphocyte activation
CD26		Activated T and B lymphocytes, monocytes	Serine exopeptidase; binds to collagen
CD28		Activated T lymphocytes (especially CD4 T cells), thymocytes	Mediates costimulation of T cells by binding B7 protein on activated APCs; signaling
CD29	Integrin β1	All hematopoietic and many other cell types	Integrin; binds to extracellular matrix components
CD32	FcγRII	B lymphocytes, macrophages, neutrophils, eosinophils	Medium-affinity Fc receptor for IgG complexes; signaling
CD34		Lymph node HEV, hematopoietic stem cells, endothelium	Sialomucin; ligand for L-selectin; vascular addressin in peripheral nodes
CD35	CR1	B lymphocytes, monocytes, neutrophils, some NK cells	Receptor for complement fragment C3b
CD38	T10	Activated lymphocytes	Unknown
CD39		Activated T, B, and NK cells	Intercellular adhesion
CD40		B lymphocytes	Mediates T cell help by binding inducible ligand (CD40L) on surface of activated T$_H$ cells; signaling
CD43	Leukosialin	T, B, and NK cells, monocytes	Sialomucin ligand for ICAM-1 (CD54); deficient in Wiskott-Aldrich syndrome
CD44	Hermes	T, B, and NK cells, monocytes	Hyaluronate receptor; mediates leukocyte binding to other leukocytes, to endothelium, or to extracellular matrix; signaling
CD45	Leukocyte common antigen; T200; B220 Isoforms: CD45R = 220 kDa CD45RA = 205–220 kDa CD45RO = 180 kDa	All leukocytes	Protein tyrosine phosphatase; multiple isoforms of extracellular domain owing to alternative RNA splicing; modulates signaling; CD45RO isoform (on T cells) binds CD22 (on B cells)
CD49b	VLA-2 α chain	Activated T cells	Integrin; binds collagen
CD49d	VLA-4 α chain	T and B lymphocytes, monocytes	Integrin; mediates leukocyte-endothelial cell interactions by binding VCAM-1
CD54	ICAM-1	Activated lymphocytes, endothelial cells	Binds LFA-1 or CD43; receptor for rhinoviruses and for *Plasmodium falciparum*
CD56	N-CAM	NK cells	NK cell adhesion; lineage marker for NK cells
CD58	LFA-3	Activated lymphocytes, many other cells	Ligand for CD2
CD64	FcγRI	Monocytes, macrophages	High-affinity Fc receptor for IgG
CD71	T9	Activated lymphocytes and macrophages, many proliferating cells	Transferrin receptor
CD72		B lymphocytes	Ligand for CD5
CD73	5′-Nucleotidase	Some B and T lymphocytes	Ecto-5′-nucleotidase; may regulate nucleotide uptake

Glossary of Symbols Used in Illustrations

▬▬▬▬▶	process of secretion (gray arrow, no outline)
⬢	virus
△ ⬡ ⬤ ▢	antigen epitopes
⏢	class I molecule
▢	class II molecule
▮	CD3
⊣	CD4
⊰	CD8
⋁	T cell receptor (TCR)
⋃	IL-2 receptor (IL-2R)
⊔	immunoglobulin Fc receptor (FcR)
⅄	immunoglobulin (Ig)

◎	stem cell
※	macrophage
◉	T cell or B cell
◉	pre-B cell
◉	activated B cell
⊗	plasma cell
◉	large granular lymphocyte (LGL) natural killer cell (NK)

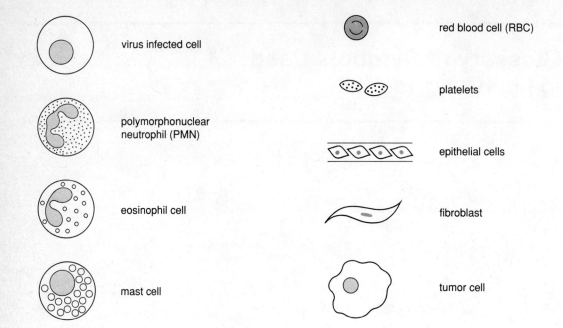

virus infected cell

polymorphonuclear
neutrophil (PMN)

eosinophil cell

mast cell

red blood cell (RBC)

platelets

epithelial cells

fibroblast

tumor cell

Index

Note: Page numbers followed by *t* or *f* indicate tables or figures, respectively.

ABO blood group system, 226–227, 227*t***
ABO incompatibility, 562–563
Abortion, spontaneous, recurrent, 562
ABO type, inheritance, 228*t*
Absidia, 662
Absorption spectrum, 178*f*
Acanthocheilonema persians, transfusion-transmitted, 232
Acarus siro, 331
Accessory receptor, 97–98
Accuracy, 176
ACE. *See* Angiotensin-converting enzyme
Acetaminophen, 791
  asthma and, 338
Achillobursitis, 398
Achillotendinitis, 398
Acquired hypogammaglobulinemia, 271–273
Acquired immunodeficiency syndrome (AIDS), 475–476, 689, 711
  cell-mediated immunity and, 147
  cellular immunodeficiency with abnormal immunoglobulin synthesis, 290
  clinical features, 693–694
  coccidioidomycosis and, 657
  cryptococcosis and, 661
  cytomegalovirus infection and, 701
  DR antigen-positive CD8 cells, 202, 203*f*
  drug allergy and, 373
  epidemiology, 692–693
  female genital tract mucosa and, 553
  focal glomerulosclerosis and, 489
  granulocyte colony-stimulating factor and, 783
  hairy leukoplakia and, 476*f*
  helper:suppressor T cell ratios and, 199
  hemophilia and, 439
  heterosexual transmission, 565–566
  histoplasmosis and, 658
  idiopathic thrombocytopenic purpura and, 436
  immunologic findings, 695–697
  immunopathogenesis, 583
  inosine pranobex and, 784
  interferon-gamma and, 783
  laboratory diagnosis, 694–695
  live vaccines and, 726
  lymphoma and, 619
  Mycobaterium avium complex and, 635
  ocular disorders and, 525–526
  opportunistic infection and, 694*t*
  pathogenesis, macrophages and, 697*t*
  Pneumocystis carinii pneumonia and, 663–664
  pseudomembranous candidiasis and, 475*f*
  Reiter's syndrome and, 407
  serum immunoglobulin levels, 157*t*
  subacute encephalitis and, 508
  syphilis and, 680
  toxoplasmosis and, 669
Acrodermatitis enteropathica, 288, 298
Acrosome reaction, 555
Actinobacillus actinomycetemcomitans, 471
Actinomycetes, 471
  thermophilic, hypersensitivity pneumonitis and, 366
Actinomycosis, serum immunoglobulin levels, 157*t*
Activation
  allergen-antibody, immunologic pathways and, 317*t*
  B cell, 45–46, 45*f*, 87–88
    bystander, 46
  complement, 47
    biologic consequences, 131–132
    inflammation and, 147–148
    pathways, 124
    periodontal disease and, 471–472
    regulatory molecules, 133
  kinin, 133
  lymphocyte, 203–209
    antigens and, 206–208, 207*f*, 207*t*, 208*f*
    biochemical and morphological events, 29*f*
    mitogens and, 205–206, 206*f*, 206*t*, 207*f*
  lymphocyte, 24, 25*f*, 29–30, 31*f*
  macrophage, 18–19
  phagocyte, 47
  platelet, 141
  T cell
    cytotoxic, 45–46, 46*f*
    helper, 44–45, 45*f*
    2-signal model, 99, 99*f*
Active immune suppression, 713
Active immunization, 712, 717–727
  materials available, 719–725*t*
Acute disseminated encephalomyelitis, 507–508
Acute inflammatory demyelinating polyneuropathy, 511–513
Acute lymphoblastic leukemia, bone marrow transplantation and, 759
Acute lymphocytic leukemia (ALL), 602–603
  T cell type, 610–612
Acute monocytic leukemia, 617
Acute myelogenous leukemia (AML), bone marrow transplantation and, 758–759
Acute myelomonocytic leukemia, 617
Acute-phase protein, 9
Acute-phase response, 110
  interleukin-6 and, 113, 114
  plasma proteins, 111*t*
Acyclovir, infectious mononucleosis and, 703
ADCC. *See* Antibody-dependent cell-mediated cytotoxicity
Addison's disease, 421

Adenohypophysitis, lymphocytic, 421
Adenosine, 794
  chemical structure, 144f
  inflammation and, 144
Adenosine deaminase, purine metabolic pathway and,
      296f
Adenosine deaminase deficiency, immunodeficiency and,
      295–297
Adenovirus, antigenic shift and, 734
Adhesion molecule, 98
Adjuvant, 51–52, 107, 712, 781
  desensitization therapy and, 743
  immune stimulation and, 714
Adoptive immunity, 712–713
Adoptive immunotherapy, cellular, 575–576
Adrenal cortex antibody, specificity and sensitivity, 414t
Adrenal insufficiency, 421
Adrenergic drugs, immediate hypersensitivity
      reactions and, 793
Adrenergic receptor, tissue distribution and effects, 793t
Adrenocorticotropic hormone (ACTH), multiple sclerosis
      and, 511
Adsorption of free ligand, 172
Adult respiratory distress syndrome (ARDS), 538–539
  C5a generation and, 131
  interleukin-1 receptor antagonist and, 784
Adult T cell leukemia (ATL), 112, 612
Aeroallergen, fungal, 332t
Afferent lymphatic vessel, 32
Affinity chromatography, 167
Affinity maturation, 33, 89
Aflatoxin A, 661
African river blindness, 678
African trypanosomiasis, 671–673
Agglutination, 184–186
  clinical tests involving, 185–186
  techniques, 184–185
Agglutination assay, sperm, 560
Agglutinin, 2
Agranulocytosis, 426
AHG. See Anti-human globulin
AIDS. See Acquired immunodeficiency syndrome
AIDS-related complex (ARC), 693
AIDS-related virus (ARV), 689
Airway disease, reversible obstructive, 335
Airway function testing, 318–320
Albuterol, 793
  asthma and, 340
Alcoholic cirrhosis, liver transplantation and, 750
Alcoholism, immunocompromised host and, 707
ALG. See Antilymphocyte globulin
Alkaline phosphatase deficiency, 306
Alkylating agents
  live vaccines and, 726
  rheumatoid arthritis and, 396
ALL. See Acute lymphocytic leukemia
Allele, 72
Allelic exclusion, 86
Allergen, 314
  allergic asthma and, 338
  anaphylaxis and, 350–351
  animal, 332
  arthropod, 330–331
  atopic, 329–332
  contact, 364, 364t
  environmental, atopy, atopic disease, IgE
      antibodies and, 328f
  food, 332
  hypersensitivity pneumonitis and, 366–367, 367t
  ingestant, urticaria and, 355
  mold, 329–330, 330f, 332t
  occupational, 339t, 366
  pollen, 329, 329t, 330f, 331f
  polymerized, desensitization therapy and, 743
Allergen-antibody activation, immunologic
      pathways and, 317t
Allergen bronchoprovocation testing, 324–325
Allergen extract, 332, 332t
Allergen injection therapy, 713
  allergic rhinitis and, 334–335
Allergen Unit (AU), 332
Allergic alveolitis, extrinsic, 366
Allergic angiitis, 449–450
Allergic asthma, 327, 338, 539
  desensitization, 740
  occupational allergens and, 339t
  serum IgE levels, 336f
Allergic bronchopulmonary aspergillosis (ABPA), 341,
      359–361, 369, 539, 661–662
  diagnostic criteria, 361t
  serum IgE levels, 336f
  stages of severity and chronicity, 361t
Allergic conjunctivitis, 334
  cromolyn sodium and, 792
Allergic contact dermatitis, 146–147, 363–365, 373, 375
  desensitization, 742
  patch test and, 320
Allergic disease
  active immunization and, 712
  airway function tests and, 318–320
  anatomic tests and, 320
  classification, 315–317, 315t
  effector T cell/lymphokine pathway, 317
  IgE and, 74
  IgE/mast cell/mediator pathway, 315–317
  IgE-mediated, treatment, 715
  IgG-IgM/complement/neutrophil pathway, 317
  immune complex, 357–361
  immune suppression and, 713
  interleukin-4 and, 116
  in vitro tests and, 322–324
  mechanisms, 315–317
  nonatopic, 327
  provocative tests and, 324–326
  skin tests and, 320–322
  tissue diagnosis and, 320
Allergic encephalomyelitis, experimental, 713
Allergic gastroenteropathy, 327, 343–344
Allergic granulomatosis of Churg and Strauss, 531
Allergic reaction
  eosinophils and, 138
  IgE-mediated, components, 323f
  T cell-mediated, components, 323f
  transfusion, 231–232
Allergic rhinitis, 327, 332–335, 338
  cromolyn sodium and, 792
  desensitization, 739, 740f, 742
  serum IgE levels, 336f
Allergic rhinoconjunctivitis, 327, 338
Allergoid, desensitization therapy and, 743
Allergy, 2, 137, 314
  atopic, 150
  atopic dermatitis and, 343
  clinical evaluation, 317–326

contact, eczematous, 363
desensitization, 739–743
  adverse effects, 741–742
  immunologic effects, 741, 741*f*
  indications, 742
  methods, 739–740
  modified allergens and, 743
  monitoring, 742–743
drug, 371–379
  diagnosis, 374–375
  hapten-carrier interaction, 373*f*
  immunologic basis, 371–374
  treatment, 375
factors determining expression of disease, 315*t*
food, 325
  cromolyn sodium and, 792
IgE-mediated, cromolyn sodium and, 792
immediate phase, 315
immune complex, desensitization therapy and, 742
insulin, 378–379
late phase, 317
latex, 351
occupational, 331
penicillin, 350, 375–377
prevalence, 314
role of immune system, 316*f*
selective IgA deficiency and, 274
serum IgE levels, 336*f*
skin testing, 320–322
  technique, 321*f*
sulfonamide, 372, 377–378
susceptibility, 314–315
T cell-mediated, 363–370
Alloantibody, platelet, 435
Alloantiserum, HLA, 242
Allograft rejection
  cyclosporin and, 776
  generation, 747*f*
  mechanisms, 747–749, 748*f*
Alloimmune thrombocytopenia, neonatal, 565
Alloimmunization, hemolytic disease of newborn
  and, 432
Allotype, 72
Alopecia, 388
Alpha chain, 59, 60
Alpha chain disease, 608–609
Alpha-fetoprotein, 572
Alpha heavy-chain disease, 462
Alport's syndrome, 479–480
ALS. *See* Amyotrophic lateral sclerosis
ALT. *See* Adult T cell leukemia
Aluminum acetate, allergic contact dermatitis and, 364
Alum precipitate, 52
Alveolitis, allergic, extrinsic, 366
Alzheimer's disease, 517
Amantadine, influenza A virus and, 639
Amebiasis, 533, 666
Amine, aromatic, 569
6-Aminopenicillanic acid, chemical structure, 372*t*
Aminophylline, 793
  asthma and, 340
  bronchial obstruction and, 353
  status asthmaticus and, 341
5-Aminosalicylic acid, Crohn's disease and, 460
Amiodarone pneumonitis, 530
AMIS. *See* Antibody-mediated immune suppression
AML. *See* Acute myelogenous leukemia

Amniocentesis, 432, 729
Amos wash step, 244
Amphotericin B
  aspergillosis and, 662
  blastomycosis and, 654
  bone marrow transplantation and, 759
  candidiasis and, 660
  chronic granulomatous disease and, 305
  coccidioidomycosis and, 657
  cryptococcosis and, 661
  histoplasmosis and, 658
  mucormycosis and, 663
Ampligen, human immunodeficiency virus and, 699
Amyloid, 608
Amyloidosis, 608
  classification, 609*t*
Amyloid protein, Alzheimer's disease and, 517
Amyotrophic lateral sclerosis (ALS), 516–517
ANA. *See* Antinuclear antibody
Anabolic steroids, hereditary angioedema and, 311–312
Analyte, 171, 176
Analyte concentration estimate, 176
Analytic method, 172, 176
  performance compared, 175–176
  types, 173–175
Analytic sensitivity, 175, 176
Analytic specificity, 176
Anamnestic immune response, 49
Anaphylactic reaction, 150
Anaphylactic shock, 347, 348, 352
  antibody-mediated, hydatid cyst and, 666
Anaphylactic shock syndrome, *Ascaris*-induced, 677
Anaphylactoid reaction, 347, 351–352
  cholinergic, 351
  drugs and additives causing, 352*t*
  ionic compounds and, 351
Anaphylatoxin, 131, 351
Anaphylaxis, 2, 327, 347–354, 373, 374
  aggregate, 351
  antivenin and, 733
  desensitization, 742
  drugs and diagnostic agents causing, 350*t*
  epinephrine and, 793
  exercise-induced, 351
  foods causing, 350*t*
  idiopathic, 352
  insect venom, desensitization, 740
  non-IgE, 351
  penicillin and, 376
Anaphylaxis kit, 353
ANCA. *See* Antineutrophil cytoplasmic antibody
Ancylostoma caninum, 676
Ancylostoma duodenale, 676
Androgen
  anti-DNA antibody formation and, 388
  hereditary angioedema and, 311–312
Anemia. *See also* Hemolytic anemia
  aplastic, 427, 434
    bone marrow transplantation and, 758
    granulocyte colony-stimulating factor and, 783
  erythropoietin and, 783
  hypoplastic, congenital, 434
  pernicious, 462–463
    selective IgA deficiency and, 274
  progressive systemic sclerosis and, 403
  sickle cell, immunocompromised host and, 707
  systemic lupus erythematosus and, 389

Anergy, 147, 195, 713
  clinical conditions and, 196t
  T cell, 99
    interleukin-2 and, 113
Anesthetic, pseudoallergic reactions and, 379
Angiitis
  allergic, 449–450
  central nervous system, 455
Angioedema, 354–356, 374. See also Urticaria-angioedema
  anaphylaxis and, 348, 353
  hereditary, 130, 311–312, 356, 380
    kinin-generating system and, 135
  idiopathic, 355
Angiofollicular hyperplasia, 618
Angioimmunoblastic lymphadenopathy, 618–619
Angioinvasion, 649
Angioneurotic edema, 354, 380
Angiotensin-converting enzyme (ACE), 377
Anhydride, hypersensitivity pneumonitis and, 366, 368
Animal allergen, 332
Animal serum, 729
Ankylosing spondylitis, 64–65, 398, 406–407, 521
  acute iridocyclitis, 521f
  HLA-B27 and, 384, 631
  immunosuppressives and, 792
Ann Arbor Staging System, 600, 615
Anogenital cancer, organ transplant recipients and, 581–582
Anthrax, 1, 629, 717
Anthroguinone, 784
Anti-acetylcholine receptor antibody, 514
Antiadhesin, 717
Antibiotics
  asthma and, 341
  beta-lactam, 375–376
    core structures, 376f
Antibody, 2, 25
  adrenal cortex, specificity and sensitivity, 414t
  anti-acetylcholine receptor, 514
  anticardiolipin, 440
  anticytoplasmic, systemic lupus erythematosus and, 391
  anti-DNA, systemic lupus erythematosus and, 390–391
  antierythrocyte, systemic lupus erythematosus and, 391
  antigliadin, 458
  anti-glomerular basement membrane, 479–481, 480f
  antigranulocyte, 426
  anti-hapten, epitope structure and, 54t
  anti-idiotype, 380
  anti-insulin, specificity and sensitivity, 414t
  anti-islet cell, specificity and sensitivity, 414t
  antilymphocyte, 778
  antimicrosomal, Hashimoto's thyroiditis and, 415
  antimyelin, plasmapheresis and, 512f
  antineuraminidase, 639
  antineutrophil cytoplasmic, 478
    ulcerative colitis and, 462
  antinuclear, 388t
    immunofluorescent staining, 390f
    polymyositis-dermatomyositis and, 404
    systemic lupus erythematosus and, 390
  anti-phospholipid, 562
  antiplatelet, systemic lupus erythematosus and, 391
  antisperm, 559–560
  antithyroglobulin, 416f
  antithyroid, 418f
  Donath-Landsteiner, 431
  enzyme-linked, 183
  erythrocyte, detection, 229–230
  ferritin-coupled, 183

HLA
  class I, 243t
  specificities, 242–243
immune hemolytic anemia and, 428
insulin receptor, specificity and sensitivity, 414t
monoclonal, 3, 67, 189–190, 711–712, 778–779, 784
  allograft rejection and, 749
  antiendotoxin, 784
  applications, 191t
  graft-versus-host disease and, 760
  HLA antigens, 242
  immune stimulation and, 714
  immune system neoplasms and, 601
  kidney transplantation and, 746–747
  liver transplantation and, 752
  technique of production, 190
  therapeutic activity, 576
neutralizing, 717
polyclonal, 778
reaginic, 683
Rh, hemolytic disease of newborn and, 432–433
serum, 229
treponemal, 683–684
tumor cell lysis and, 573
uptake by central nervous system neurons, 516f
Wassermann, 683
Antibody deficiency disease
  immune globulin and, 729
  passive antibody protection and, 712
Antibody-dependent cell-mediated cytotoxicity (ADCC), 47, 74, 103, 573, 618, 625, 748
Antibody-dependent killing, 573
Antibody-mediated anaphylactic shock, hydatid cyst and, 666
Antibody-mediated host defense, 624, 624t
Antibody-mediated immune suppression (AMIS), 564
Antibody-mediated immunity, evaluation, 267t
Anticardiolipin antibody, 440
Anticholinergic agents, anti-inflammatory effects, 715
Anticholinesterase agents, myasthenia gravis and, 514
Anticoagulants
  circulating
    endogenous, 439–440
    systemic lupus erythematosus and, 391
  lupus, 440
Anticonvulsants, selective IgA deficiency and, 275
Anticytoplasmic antibody, systemic lupus erythematosus and, 391
Antidiarrheal agents
  Crohn's disease and, 460
  ulcerative colitis and, 462
Anti-DNA antibody, systemic lupus erythematosus and, 390–391
Antierythrocyte antibody, systemic lupus erythematosus and, 391
Antigen, 25, 26, 30, 40, 42, 50, 51f. See also Human leukocyte antigen
  B cell, 52–53
  B cell tumor, immunophenotypes, 593t
  carcinoembryonic, 572
  cognate, 55
  common acute lymphocytic leukemia, 572
  cross-reactivity, autoimmunity and, 412
  detection, 184
  differentiation
    B cell, 201t
    T cell, 198t
  erythrocyte, 226–229
    detection, 229–230

hepatitis B, 465f
hepatitis B core, 465, 643
hepatitis B surface, 465, 643–645
Lewis, 227
lymphocyte activation and, 206–208, 207f, 207t, 208f
lymphocyte-determined membrane, 703
measles virus, subacute sclerosing panencephalitis and, 517
mechanisms of elimination, 46–47
processing and presentation, 42–44, 44f
Rh, 562
Sd, 227
self-
   autoimmune disease and, 380
   cross-reactivity and, 382
serum, detection, 164–165
Smith, 390
T cell, 55–56
T cell receptor recognition, 95, 96f
T cell tumor, immunophenotypes, 594t
thymus-dependent, 56
thymus-independent, 56
tumor-associated, 571–572
tumor cell, 570–572
tumor-specific, 571
Antigen-antibody complex, 147
   formation in agar, 152
Antigen-antibody glomerulonephritis, quartan malaria and, 666
Antigen-antibody precipitin curve, 152f
Antigen-binding site, 68
Antigenemia, hepatitis B, hepatitis B hyperimmune globulin and, 750
Antigenic, 50
Antigenic determinant, 2, 372, 380, 382. *See also* Epitope
Antigenic modulation, 574
Antigenic shift, 734
Antigenic variation, 734
Antigen-MHC complex, assembly and transport, 63f
Antigen-nonspecific therapy, 711, 713–715
Antigen-presenting cell (APC), 20, 26, 42–45, 55, 62–64, 381, 712
   B cells and, 88
   multiple sclerosis and, 509f
Antigen-receptor cell, interactions with T cells, 97–98
Antigen-receptor transmembrane signaling complex, 87f
Antigen-specific therapy, 711, 712–713
Antigliadin antibody, 458
Antiglobulin consumption test, 184
Antiglobulin test, 185–186, 229
Anti-glomerular basement membrane antibody, 479–481, 480f
Anti-glomerular basement membrane antibody disease, 479–481
Antigranulocyte antibody, 426
Anti-hapten antibody, epitope structure and, 54t
Antihistamines
   allergic contact dermatitis and, 364
   allergic disease and, 715
   allergic rhinitis and, 334
   anaphylaxis and, 353
   atopic dermatitis and, 343
   commonly used, 792t
   H1 receptors and, 142
   hypocomplementemic urticarial vasculitis and, 446
   immediate hypersensitivity reactions and, 792–793
   intradermal wheal-and-erythema skin test reactions and, 322
   serum sickness and, 359
   T cell sensitization and, 373
   urticaria and, 356

Anti-human globulin (AHG), 244–245
Anti-idiotype antibody, 380
Anti-idiotype antiserum, 77
Anti-idiotype autoantibody, 383
Anti-inflammatory drugs, 715, 786–794
   Crohn's disease and, 460
Anti-insulin antibody, specificity and sensitivity, 414t
Anti-insulin receptor antibody syndrome, 383
Anti-islet cell antibody, specificity and sensitivity, 414t
Antilymphocyte antibody, 778
Antilymphocyte globulin (ALG), 778
   allograft rejection and, 749
   aplastic anemia and, 434
   graft-versus-host disease and, 298
   kidney transplantation and, 746
   liver transplantation and, 752
   lung transplantation and, 538
Antilymphocyte serum (ALS), 778
Antimalarials, 791–792
   discoid lupus erythematosus and, 505
   relapsing panniculitis and, 409
   rheumatoid arthritis and, 396
   systemic lupus erythematosus and, 392
Antimicrosomal antibody, Hashimoto's thyroiditis and, 415
Antimyelin antibody, plasmapheresis and, 512f
Antineuraminidase antibody, 639
Anti-neutrophil cytoplasmic antibody (ANCA), 478
   ulcerative colitis and, 462
Antinuclear antibody (ANA), 388t
   immunofluorescent staining, 390f
   polymyositis-dermatomyositis and, 404
   systemic lupus erythematosus and, 390
Anti-oncogene, function and dysfunction, 579–580
Anti-phospholipid antibody syndrome, 562
Antiplatelet antibody, systemic lupus erythematosus and, 391
Antiretroviral therapy
   human immunodeficiency virus and, 698–699
   targets, 699t
Anti-Rh immunoglobulin prophylaxis, isoimmunization and, 563–564
Antiserum
   anti-idiotype, 77
   class II HLA typing, 243–244
   specific, 48
Antisperm antibody, 559–560
Anti-Tac, 112
Antithymocyte globulin (ATG), 778
   allograft rejection and, 749
   aplastic anemia and, 434, 758
   graft-versus-host disease and, 760
   kidney transplantation and, 746
Antithymocyte serum (ATS), 778
Antithyroglobulin antibody, 416f
Antithyroid antibody, 418f
Antitoxin, 2, 628, 717, 729
Antitrypsin deficiency, 158
   heart-lung transplantation and, 755
   liver transplantation and, 750
Antivenin, 733
APC. *See* Antigen-presenting cell
Aphthous stomatitis, 474–475
Aphthous ulceration, recurrent, 474–475, 474f
Aplastic anemia, 427, 434
   bone marrow transplantation and, 758
   granulocyte colony-stimulating factor and, 783
Apoptosis, 49, 100, 381, 383

Apronalide, immune thrombocytopenic purpura and, 438
Arachidonic acid, 715, 788
  chemical structure, 143*f*
  metabolic pathways, 142*f*
  metabolites, inflammation and, 143–144
ARC. *See* AIDS-related complex
ARDS. *See* Adult respiratory distress syndrome
Aromatic amine, 569
Aromatic hydrocarbon, polycyclic, 569
Arteriography, progressive systemic sclerosis and, 403
Arteritis
  giant cell, 451–453, 452*f*
    eyes and, 525
  Takayasu, 453–455
    angiographic findings, 454*f*
Arthritic joint, 111
Arthritis
  degenerative, 395
  gouty, 395
  hypogammaglobulinemia and, 409
  juvenile, 397–399
  Lyme, 685
  nonsteroidal anti-inflammatory drugs and, 790
  polymyositis-dermatomyositis and, 405
  psoriatic, 395, 408
    immunosuppressives and, 792
  Reiter's syndrome and, 407
  rheumatoid, 154, 383, 390, 392–397, 521
    chlorambucil and, 774
    cyclophosphamide and, 773
    experimental in swine, 384
    hydrocortisone and, 786
    immunopathogenesis, 393*f*
    immunosuppressives and, 791–792
    interleukin-1 receptor antagonist and, 784
    juvenile, 521
    plasma exchange and, 777
    prednisone and, 768
    scleral nodules, 522*f*
    scleral thinning, 522*f*
    serum immunoglobulin levels, 157*t*
    thymic hormones and, 782
  systemic lupus erythematosus and, 388, 392
Arthrodesis, rheumatoid arthritis and, 396
Arthroplasty, rheumatoid arthritis and, 396
Arthropod allergen, 330–331
Arthus reaction, 147, 148, 357, 366
  desensitization therapy and, 742
Arthus skin test, hypersensitivity pneumonitis and, 369
ARV. *See* AIDS-related virus
5-ASA. *See* 5-Aminosalicylic acid
Ascariasis, 677
Ascarid, 533
Ascaris, 676, 677
Aspergilloma, 361
Aspergillosis, 651*t*, 661–662
  allergic bronchopulmonary, 341, 359–361, 369, 539,
    661–662
    diagnostic criteria, 361*t*
    serum IgE levels, 336*f*
    stages of severity and chronicity, 361*t*
  immunologic abnormalities and, 653*t*
  immunologic diagnosis, 656*t*
  invasive, 361
  pathologic features, 652*t*
Aspergillus, 661–662, 709
  chronic granulomatous disease and, 303
Aspergillus flavus, 662

Aspergillus fumigatus, 359–360, 539, 662
  bone marrow transplantation and, 761
Aspergillus hypersensitivity pneumonitis, 361
Aspergillus niger, 662
Aspirin, 789–791
  anti-inflammatory effects, 790
  bronchospasm and, 528
  juvenile arthritis and, 399
  mechanism of action, 790–791
  prostaglandin synthesis and, 143
  pseudoallergic reactions and, 379
  rheumatoid arthritis and, 395–396
  rheumatoid eye disease and, 522
  sensitivity, asthma and, 337–338
  serum sickness and, 359
  systemic lupus erythematosus and, 392
  toxicity, 791
  urticaria and, 355
Asthma, 335–341
  allergic, 327, 338, 539
    desensitization, 740
    occupational allergens and, 339*t*
    serum IgE levels, 336*f*
  atopic, allergen bronchoprovocation and, 325
  drug-induced, 528
  extrinsic, 335
  intrinsic, 335–336
  kinins and, 135
  nonallergic, 327
  occupational, 338
Ataxia-telangiectasia, 154
  atopic dermatitis and, 343
  cancer and, 292*f*, 580
  immunodeficiency and, 290–292
  thymic hormones and, 782
Atelectasis, systemic lupus erythematosus and, 390
ATG. *See* Antithymocyte globulin
Atopic allergen, 329–332
Atopic allergy, 150
Atopic asthma, allergen bronchoprovocation and, 325
Atopic dermatitis, 327, 341–343
  desensitization, 740
  serum IgE levels, 336*f*
Atopic disease, 327–344
  environmental allergens and, 328*f*
  etiology, 328–329
  immunology, 327–328
Atopic eczema, 341
Atopic keratoconjunctivitis, 521
Atopy, 327
  asthma and, 335
  desensitization, 740, 742
  environmental allergens and, 328*f*
  IgE-mediated, allergen injection therapy, 713
Atropine
  rheumatoid eye disease and, 522
  sarcoid lesions of eye and, 524
Attenuated vaccine, 1, 56
Attenuated vaccine model, 675
AU. *See* Allergen Unit
Auranofin, rheumatoid arthritis and, 396
Autoantibody
  anti-idiotype, 383
  cross-matching, 245
  organ-specific, 412–413
  platelet, 435
    idiopathic thrombocytopenic purpura and, 436*t*
  specificity and sensitivity, 414*t*

systemic lupus erythematosus and, 387, 390–391
ulcerative colitis and, 461
Autocrine effect, 44, 105, 782
Autoimmune chronic active hepatitis, 467–468
Autoimmune disease, 64, 137, 380
animal models, etiologic factors, 384*t*
Arthus reaction and, 148
cancer and, 582
immune suppression and, 713
immunoblastic sarcoma of B cell type and, 606
immunoelectrophoresis and, 161
interleukin-10 and, 783
organ-specific, 384
polymyositis-dermatomyositis and, 404
selective IgA deficiency and, 274–275
testis and ovary, 560
thyroid, 413–419
Autoimmune endocrine disease
mechanism of development, 412
pathogenesis, 413*f*
Autoimmune hemolytic anemia
B cell neoplasms and, 591
cyclophosphamide and, 773
intravenous gamma globulin and, 778
prednisone and, 768
serologic findings, 429*t*
warm, 429–430
Autoimmune myocarditis, 442–443
Autoimmune neutropenia, 425
colony-stimulating factors and, 783
intravenous gamma globulin and, 778
Autoimmune oophoritis, 422, 560
Autoimmune orchitis, 560
Autoimmune-overlap syndrome, 413
Autoimmune polyglandular syndrome, 422–423
classification, 422*t*
Autoimmune thyroiditis, Arthus reaction and, 148
Autoimmunity
antigen cross-reactivity and, 412
complement deficiency and, 311
cross-reactivity and, 382
drug-induced, 372
idiotypy and, 382–383
immune system neoplasms and, 591
initiation through class II HLA expression, 413*f*
normal and disease-associated, 381*t*
oral unresponsiveness and, 549
Plasmodium malariae infection and, 668
Autonomic imbalance, 328
Autonomic reflex mechanism, bronchoconstriction and, 337
Autoradiography, 183–184
Autoreactivity, 49
disease-associated, 380–381, 381*t*
Avian leukosis virus, yellow fever vaccine and, 727
Avidin, immunofluorescence and, 183
Azathioprine, 768, 771–772
autoimmune hemolytic anemia and, 430
bone transplantation and, 762
bullous pemphigoid and, 495
corneal graft reactions and, 527
Crohn's disease and, 460
epidermolysis bullosa acquisita and, 500
graft-versus-host disease and, 760
heart transplantation and, 755
immune-complex glomerulonephritis and, 486–487
kidney transplantation and, 746
liver transplantation and, 752
lung transplantation and, 538, 757

lymphocytotoxic effects, 772
pemphigus vulgaris and, 503
polymyositis-dermatomyositis and, 406
primary biliary cirrhosis and, 469
properties and uses, 772*t*
Reiter's syndrome and, 407
systemic lupus erythematosus and, 392
ulcerative colitis and, 462
Azimexone, delayed hypersensitivity and, 784–785
Aziridine derivatives, 784–785
AZT. *See* Zidovudine
Aztreonam, 377
Azurophilic granule, 10
cytoplasmic, 612–613

B220, 88
B7, 44, 88, 99
Babesia microti, transfusion-transmitted, 232
Babesiosis, posttransfusion, 232
Bacillus, 629
Bacillus anthracis, 629
Bacillus Calmette-Guerin (BCG), 635, 718, 781
Bacillus cereus, 629
Bacteria
encapsulated, 627, 631–633, 632*f*
endogenous superantigens and, 383
immunomodulators derived, 781–782
intracellular, 627, 633–635, 634*f*
Bacterial disease, 627–635
endotoxins, 627–628
exotoxins, 627–628
serodiagnosis, 627
toxigenic, 627, 628–631, 628*f*
Bacterial infection, transfusion-transmitted, 232–233
Bacterial killing curve, 305*f*
Bacterial vaccine, 631, 633, 635
Bactericidal assay, 213*f*
Bactericidin, 2
Bacteriology, 1
Bacteriolysis, 717
Bacteriophage, live virus vaccines and, 727
Bacteroides fragilis, 633
Bacteroides gingivalis, 471
Bacteroides intermedius, 471
Bagassosis, 369
Balanitis circinata, 407
Band, 16
Bare lymphocyte syndrome, 299
Barnard, Christian, 757
Bartonellosis, serum immunoglobulin levels, 157*t*
Basophil, 74
atopic disease and, 327
electron micrograph, 141*f*
inflammation and, 141
properties, 140*t*
Basophil hypersensitivity, cutaneous, 150
Basophil kallikrein of anaphylaxis, 348
Batch, 176
Bayliascaris procynosis, 533
B cell, 3, 24–26, 63
acquired immunodeficiency syndrome and, 696–697
activated, progeny, 25*f*
activation, 30–31, 45–46, 45*f*, 87–88
bystander, 46
antigen, 52–53
antigen binding, 40
antigen presentation, 88*f*

B cell *(cont.)*
  as antigen-presenting cell, 88
  antigen-specific immune suppression and, 713
  assays, 200–202
    clinical applications, 209
    functional, 201–202, 260–261
  cancer, 49
  corticosteroids and, 766
  cross-matching, 245
  cyclophosphamide and, 773
  cytoplasmic immunoglobulins and, 201
  differentiation antigens, 201*t*
  DNA rearrangement, immunoglobulin genes and, 80–84
  early, 86
  enumeration, 259–260
  epitopes, 52–53, 52*f*, 53*f*
    complementarity, 55, 55*f*
    size and location, 52–53
  idiotypy, 382
  immune competence testing, 259–261, 260*t*
  interleukin-2 and, 113
  leukemias, 591*f*
    monoclonal surface immunoglobulins and, 591
  lymphocytic neoplasms, 601–607
  lymphomas, 591*f*
    DNA cell cycle, 597*f*
    immunophenotype, 597*f*
    monoclonal surface immunoglobulins and, 591
    pathogenesis, 585*f*
  malignancy, immunoglobulin gene rearrangements and, 91–92
  maturation, affinity, 33, 89
  mature, 86
    antigen-receptor transmembrane signaling complex, 87*f*
  memory, 26, 89
  monoclonal/polyclonal proliferation, 598*f*
  neoplasms, 590*f*
  ontogeny
    genetic events, 85*f*
    immunoglobulin gene rearrangements and, 84–86
    marker proteins, 85*f*
  proportion in normal tissues, 22, 24*t*
  self-tolerance and, 381
  subsets, 260
  surface immunoglobulins and, 200–201, 201*t*
  switch regions, 89
  systemic lupus erythematosus and, 385*t*
  tolerance, 91
  tumor antigens, immunophenotypes, 593*t*
  tumor cells and, 573
  virgin, maturation and release, 86–92
B cell growth factor I. *See* Interleukin-4
B cell immunodeficiency disorder, 266–278
  treatment, 265*t*
B cell-specific marker, 200
B cell stimulatory factor I. *See* Interleukin-4
BCG. *See* Bacillus Calmette-Guerin
BCGF-I. *See* Interleukin-4
Bcl-2, 49, 92
BCNU. *See* Bischloroethylnitrosourea
Beclomethasone, allergic rhinitis and, 334
Beclomethasone dipropionate, asthma and, 340
Beçhet's disease, 406, 446
  eyes and, 525
  recurrent aphthous ulceration and, 475
Bejel, 684

Benacerraf, Baruj, 5
Bence Jones myeloma, 158
  serum immunoglobulin levels, 157*t*
Bence Jones protein, 607
Bence Jones proteinuria, 608
Benign follicular hyperplasia, 618
Benign hypergammaglobulinemic purpura, 610
Benign monoclonal gammopathy, 609
Bentonite flocculation test, 186, 677
Besnier's prurigo, 341
Beta chain, 60
Between-batch random error, 176
Between-laboratory random error, 176
Bias, 176
Bible printer's lung, 369
Bile salts, liver transplantation and, 752
Biliary atresia, extrahepatic, liver transplantation and, 750
Biliary cirrhosis
  primary, 468–470
    percutaneous liver biopsy specimen, 468*f*
    serum immunoglobulin levels, 157*t*
Billingham, Rupert E., 3, 4
Binder, 171
Binder-ligand assay, 170–178
Binder-ligand reaction, 171–172, 172*f*
Biologic response modification, 713–714
Biotin, immunofluorescence and, 183
Biotin-avidin-enhanced immunoassay, 174–175, 175*f*
Biotin-dependent carboxylase deficiency, immunodeficiency and, 297
Bird breeder's disease, 366
Bird fancier's lung, 366
Bird handler's disease, 366, 369
Bischloroethylnitrosourea (BCNU), adverse pulmonary responses, 530
Black piedra, 650*t*
  immunologic abnormalities and, 653*t*
Blackwater fever, 667
Black widow spider bite
  passive immunization, 730*t*
  serum therapy, 733
Blastocyst, 555
Blastomyces dermatitidis, 654
Blastomycosis, 650*t*, 654
  immunologic abnormalities and, 653*t*
  immunologic diagnosis, 655*t*
  pathologic features, 652*t*
Blast transformation, 30
Bleomycin, adverse pulmonary responses, 530
Blood
  cross-matching, 229–230
  pretransfusion testing, 229
  screening, 229–230
  typing, 229–230
Blood-brain barrier, antihistamines and, 793
Blood cell, ontogeny, 9–10
Blood component therapy, 234–235
  guidelines, 234*t*
Blood dyscrasia, cyclophosphamide and, 773
Blood eosinophilia, 333
Blood group, 226
  ABO, 226–227, 227*t*, 227*t*
  H, 226–227
  Rh, 227–228, 228*t*
  structure, 227*f*
Blood transfusion, kidney transplantation and, 746

Bone
  avascular necrosis, systemic lupus erythematosus and, 388
  progressive systemic sclerosis and, 403
Bone marrow aplasia, 434
Bone marrow transplantation, 758–761
  aplastic anemia and, 434
  bare lymphocyte syndrome and, 299
  CML test and, 247
  complications, 760
  cytokines and, 427
  diseases treatable, 758*t*
  genetic diseases treatable, 758*t*
  graft-versus-host disease and, 760
  granulocyte-macrophage colony-stimulating factor and, 783
  immune system neoplasms and, 601
  indications, 758–759
  infection and, 761, 761*t*
  methotrexate and, 774
  procedure, 759
  venoocclusive disease of liver and, 760–761
Bone transplantation, 761–762
  immunosuppression and, 762
  rejection, 762
Bordet, Jules, 2, 3, 4, 8*f*
Bordetella pertussis, 629–630
Borrelia, 680, 686–687
Borrelia burgdorferi, 398, 685–686
Borrelia duttonii, 686
Borrelia hermsii, 686
Borrelia hispanica, 686
Borrelia parkeri, 686
Borrelia persica, 686
Borrelia recurrentis, 686
Borrelia turicatae, 686
Borreliosis, relapsing fever, 680, 686–687
Botulinum toxin, 628
Botulism, 628
  passive immunization, 730*t*
Bound fraction, 172
Bowel disease, inflammatory
  interleukin-1 receptor antagonist and, 784
  oral unresponsiveness and, 549
BP 180, 492, 495
BP 230, 492
Bradykinin, 133
  anaphylaxis and, 348
  hemolytic transfusion reactions and, 233
Breast milk immunology, 550
Breinl, Friedrich, 2, 4
Brent, Leslie, 3, 4
Bronchial obstruction, anaphylaxis and, 353
Bronchiectasis, 539
  heart-lung transplantation and, 755
Bronchiolitis, 640–641
  chest x-ray, 640*f*
Bronchiolitis obliterans, 367, 370
Bronchoconstriction, autonomic reflex mechanism and, 337
Bronchodilators, asthma and, 340
Bronchoprovocation testing, 318, 319*f*
  allergen, 324–325
  asthma and, 337
  hypersensitivity pneumonitis and, 369
Bronchopulmonary aspergillosis, allergic, 341, 359–361, 369, 539, 661–662
  diagnostic criteria, 361*t*
  serum IgE levels, 336*f*
  stages of severity and chronicity, 361*t*

Bronchospasm, drug-induced, 528
Brownian movement, 210
Brucella, 634
Brucella abortus, 634, 781
Brucella melitensis, 634
Brucella suis, 634
Brugia, 678
Brugia malayi, 533, 676
  transfusion-transmitted, 232
BSF-I. *See* Interleukin-4
Budd-Chiari syndrome, liver transplantation and, 750
Buerger's disease, 455
Bullous dermatosis, linear IgA, 503–504
Bullous pemphigoid, 492–495
  blisters, 494*f*
  histopathology, 494*f*
Burkitt's lymphoma, 91–92
  Epstein-Barr virus and, 570
  oncogenes and, 598
  t(8,14) chromosomal anomaly, 92*f*
Burnet, Frank Macfarlane, 2, 3, 4, 42, 578
Burns, thermal, serum immunoglobulin levels, 157*t*
Burow's solution, allergic contact dermatitis and, 364
Butterfly rash, 388
Bystander effect, 87

C1, 125–127
C1 esterase inhibitor deficiency, 312
C1INH deficiency, 311–312
C1 inhibitor (C1INH), complement system and, 129–130
C1q assay, 446
C1q binding assay, 127
C1q receptor, 132
C2, 127
C3, 127
C3a, 131
C3 convertase
  alternative pathway, 128
  classic pathway, 127
C3 deficiency, 310–311
C3 degradation pathway, 130*f*
C3 fragments, cellular receptors, 132*t*
C3 receptor, 127, 132–133
C4, 127
C4-binding protein (C4BP), complement system and, 130–131
C5a, 131, 145
C5 convertase
  alternative pathway, 128
  classic pathway, 127–128
C8-binding protein, 133
C9 deficiency, 311
Cachectin, 110
Cachexia, 111
Cadaveric transplantation, 745
Caddis fly, 331
Caffeine, 793
Calcification, subcutaneous, progressive systemic sclerosis and, 402
Calcineurin, 97
Calcinosis circumscripta, 402
Calcium channel blocker, progressive systemic sclerosis and, 403
Calcium ion, free, intracellular, 30
Calibration curve, 176
Calibrator, 171, 176
CALLA. *See* Common acute lymphocytic leukemia antigen
CAMPATH-1, 778

Cancer
  adoptive cellular immunotherapy and, 575
  ataxia-telangiectasia and, 292*f*
  autoimmune disease and, 582
  cerebellar degeneration and, 515
  colon, levamisole and, 784
  congenital immunodeficiency and, 580–581, 581*t*
  cyclophosphamide and, 773
  cytotoxic T cells and, 100
  human immunodeficiency virus and, 583–586
  immunocompromise and, 579–580
  interleukin-2 and, 113
  liver, hepatitis B virus and, 570
  lung, thymosin and, 782
  methotrexate and, 773–774
  organ transplant recipients and, 581–582
  patient, second tumors, 582
  polymyositis-dermatomyositis and, 405
  selective IgA deficiency and, 275
  skin
    organ transplant recipients and, 776
    ultraviolet radiation and, 570
Candida, 475, 476, 524, 526, 537, 649, 659–660
  hyper-IgE syndrome and, 307
  mucocutaneous candidiasis and, 283*f*
Candida albicans, 659
Candida krusei, 660
Candida tropicalis, 659–660
Candidemia, 660
Candidiasis, 651*t*, 659–660
  immunologic abnormalities and, 653*t*
  immunologic diagnosis, 656*t*
  mucocutaneous, chronic, 282–284, 659–660
    Candida infection and, 283*f*
    endocrinopathy and, 422
  oral, 476
    Sjögren's syndrome and, 401
  pathologic features, 652*t*
  pseudomembranous, 475*f*, 476
Candiduria, 660
Capillary tube method, 210
Caplan's syndrome, 394
Capnocytophaga, 471
Capping, 30
Caprine arthritis-encephalitis virus, 690
Captopril, 377
Carbohydrate, immunogenic, 42
Carboxylase deficiency, biotin-dependent, immunodeficiency
    and, 297
Carcinoembryonic antigen (CEA), 572
Carcinogen
  chemical, 569
  physical, 569–570
Carcinogenesis, radiation-induced, 569–570
Carcinoma
  cervical, human papilloma virus and, 570
  nasopharyngeal, Hodgkin's disease and, 570
  pyroglobulins and, 169
  renal cell, interleukin-2 and, 113, 783
  small cell, thymosin and, 782
Cardiac disease, 442–443
Cardiac transplantation, 754–756
Cardiomegaly, systemic lupus erythematosus and, 390
Cardiomyopathy, dilated, 443
Cardiopulmonary bypass, 755
Carpal tunnel syndrome, 394
Carrier, 54
Casoni skin test, 676

CD (cluster of differentiation), 26, 197
CD1, 817
CD2, 28, 98, 817
CD3, 26–28, 817
CD3 complex, 26, 44, 87
CD4, 28–29, 37, 42, 98, 583, 711, 714, 817
  acquired immunodeficiency syndrome and, 695–696
  cyclophosphamide and, 773
CD5, 87, 572, 714, 817
CD6, 817
CD7, 28, 817
CD8, 28–29, 37, 42, 98, 572, 583, 817
  cyclophosphamide and, 773
  DR antigen, 203*f*
CD10, 572, 817
CD11a, 817
CD11b, 617, 817
CD11c, 817
CD13, 617
CD14, 617, 817
CD15, 817
CD16, 103, 817
CD18, 817
CD19, 817
CD20, 817
CD21, 133, 817
CD22, 86, 817
CD23, 86, 818
CD25, 818
CD26, 818
CD27, 121
CD28, 44, 99, 714, 818
CD29, 39, 818
CD30, 121
CD32, 818
CD33, 617
CD35, 818
CD38, 818
CD39, 818
CD40, 86, 87, 818
CD40 ligand, 87–88, 121
CD43, 818
CD44, 818
CD45, 88, 98, 818
CD45RA, 98
CD45RO, 98
CD49b, 818
CD49d, 818
CD54, 818
CD56, 103, 818
CD58, 818
CD59, 133
CD64, 818
CD71, 818
CD72, 818
CD73, 86, 818
CDE blood group system, 562
CDR. *See* Complementarity-determining region
CEA. *See* Carcinoembryonic antigen
Ceftazidime, 377
Celiac disease
  lymphoma and, 582
  selective IgA deficiency and, 274
Celiac sprue, 457
Cell adhesion molecule, monoclonal antibodies and,
    779
Cell death, programmed, 49, 100, 381
Cell growth, polyclonal, nonmalignant regulated, 569

Cell-mediated cytotoxicity, antibody-dependent, 47, 74, 103, 573, 618, 625, 748
Cell-mediated hypersensitivity, 365
Cell-mediated hypersensitivity disease, 363–370
Cell-mediated immunity (CMI), 26, 146–147
    evaluation, 280t
    live vaccines and, 726
    periodontal disease and, 472
Cell-mediated lympholysis (CML), 208–209, 208f
Cell-mediated lympholysis (CML) test, 246f, 247–248
Cell membrane abnormality, immunodeficiency and, 298–300
Cell purification, flow sorting and, 204f
Cell sorter, fluorescence-activated, 202–203
Cell suicide, 49, 100, 381
Cell surface marker, hematopoietic, 817–818
Cellular adoptive immunotherapy, 575–576
Cellular assay, histocompatibility and, 246–248
Cellular immunity, 2
    cytomegalovirus and, 701
    immune system neoplasms and, 591
    influenza and, 638
    measles virus and, 642
    polymyositis-dermatomyositis and, 404
    recurrent aphthous ulceration and, 474–475
Cellular immunodeficiency with abnormal immunoglobulin synthesis, 289–290
Cellular immunology, 2–3
Cellular infiltrate, 137
Cellulose acetate zone electrophoresis, 158f
Central nervous system, isolated angiitis, 455
Central nervous system neuron, uptake of antibodies, 516f
Cephalosporin, 376f
    core structure, 376f
Cephamycin, 376f
    core structure, 376f
Cephapyrizone, 377
Cerebellar degeneration, paraneoplastic, 515
Cerebrospinal fluid, zone electrophoresis patterns, 160f
Cervical carcinoma, human papillomavirus and, 570
Cestode, 675–676
CFA. See Complete Freund's adjuvant
CGD. See Chronic granulomatous disease
Chagas' disease, posttransfusion, 232
Chancre immunity, 681
Charcot-Leyden crystal, 139, 336, 344
Charcot-Leyden crystal protein, 138
Chase, Merrill W., 2, 4
Chediak-Higashi syndrome, 306
    natural killer cells and, 261, 284
Chemical carcinogen, 569
Chemiluminescence, neutrophils and, 213
Chemoattraction, 118
Chemokine, 118–120, 119t
    inflammation and, 144–145
Chemoradiotherapy
    bone marrow transplantation and, 759
    venoocclusive disease of liver and, 760–761
Chemotactic factor
    asthmatic attack and, 337
    neutrophil, 12, 13t
Chemotaxin, 210, 478
Chemotaxis, 210, 479
    test, 210–211
Chemotherapeutic agents, adverse pulmonary responses, 530
Chemotherapy
    hairy cell leukemia and, 606
    immune system neoplasms and, 600–601
    multiple myeloma and, 608

Chest, progressive systemic sclerosis and, 403
Chest pain, systemic lupus erythematosus and, 389
Chitin, 649
Chlorambucil, 768, 774–775
    cold-agglutinin syndromes and, 430
    immune system neoplasms and, 600–601
    plasmacytoid lymphocytic lymphoma and, 606
    rheumatoid eye disease and, 522
    sympathetic ophthalmia and, 525
    systemic lupus erythematosus and, 392
    Vogt-Koyanagi-Harada syndrome and, 525
Chloramphenicol, chronic granulomatous disease and, 305
Chloroquine, systemic lupus erythematosus and, 392
Chlorpromazine
    chronic cholestasis and, 469
    lupuslike syndrome and, 389
Chlorpropamide, immune thrombocytopenic purpura and, 438
Cholangiocarcinoma
    liver transplantation and, 750
    primary sclerosing cholangitis and, 470
Cholangitis, sclerosing
    liver transplantation and, 750
    primary, 470
Choledochocholedochostomy, 751
Choledochojejunosotomy, 751
Cholera, 1, 629, 718
    active immunization, 719t, 735
    vaccination, 737
    vaccine, 736
Cholestasis, chronic, 469
Cholinergic anaphylactoid reaction, 351
Cholinergic urticaria, 355
Chorionic villus, trophoblast populations, 557f
Chorionic villus biopsy, 729
Chromatin, 26
Chromatography, 166–167
    affinity, 167
    gel filtration, 166–167, 167f
    ion exchange, 166, 166f
Chromoblastomycosis, 650t
    immunologic diagnosis, 655t
Chromomycosis
    immunologic abnormalities and, 653t
    pathologic features, 652t
Chromosomal translocation, neoplasms and, 599t
Chronic demyelinating polyneuropathy, 513
Chronic fatigue syndrome, natural killer cell deficiency and, 284
Chronic granulomatous disease (CGD), 303–305
    bacterial killing curves, 305f
    quantitative NBT test and, 212, 303
Chronic inflammatory infiltrate, 146
Chronic lymphocytic leukemia, 87
    serum immunoglobulin levels, 157t
Chronic mucocutaneous candidiasis (CMCC), 282–284, 659–660
    Candida infection and, 283f
Chronic myelogenous leukemia (CML)
    bone marrow transplantation and, 759
    interferon-alpha and, 782
Churg-Strauss syndrome, 449–450
Cicatricial pemphigoid, 494, 523
Ciliary neutrotropic factor (CNTF), 114
Cimetidine
    anaphylaxis and, 353
    H2 receptors and, 142
Circulation
    lymphatic, 32–35

Circulation *(cont.)*
  lymphocyte, 38–39
Cirrhosis
  hepatic, immunocompromised host and, 707
  liver transplantation and, 750
  primary biliary, 468–470
    liver transplantation and, 750
    percutaneous liver biopsy specimen, 468*f*
  serum immunoglobulin levels, 157*t*
Cladotanytarsus lewisi, 331
Claman, Henry N., 3, 4
Class switching, 89, 90*f*
  interleukin-2 and, 113
  interleukin-4 and, 116
Clindamycin-primaquine, *Pneumocystis carinii* and, 664
CLMF. *See* Interleukin-12
Clonal anergy, 91
Clonal deletion, 91
Clonality
  immune system neoplasms and, 592–596
  lymphocyte, gene rearrangement assay and, 220–221
Clonal restriction, 41–42, 86
Clonal selection, 3, 41–42, 41*f*
Clone, lymphocyte, 40
Clonorchis sinensis, 673
Clostridium, 628–629
Clostridium botinulum, 628–629
Clostridium perfringens, 629
Clostridium tetani, 625–626, 628
Clotting factor XI, 133
Cluster of differentiation. *See* CD
CMCC. *See* Chronic mucocutaneous candidiasis
CMI. *See* Cell-mediated immunity
CML. *See* Cell-mediated lympholysis; Chronic myelogenous
        leukemia
CMV. *See* Cytomegalovirus
c-myc oncogene, 570
c-myc proto-oncogene, 30, 92, 598
CNTF. *See* Ciliary neutrotropic factor
Coagulase, 630
Coagulation
  circulating inhibitors, 439–440
  disorders, 438–440
Coal tar, psoriatic arthritis and, 408
Coated particle reaction, 184
Cobra venom factor, 128
Coccidioidal meningitis, 657
Coccidioides immitis, 656–657
  phlyctenular disease and, 525
Coccidioidin, 657
Coccidioidomycosis, 650*t*, 654–657
  immunologic abnormalities and, 653*t*
  immunologic diagnosis, 655*t*
  pathologic features, 652*t*
  pregnancy and, 558
Cockroach allergen, 331
Cognate antigen, 55
Colchicine, 791
  Behcet's disease and, 446
  primary biliary cirrhosis and, 469
  progressive systemic sclerosis and, 403
  relapsing polychondritis and, 408
Cold-agglutin hemolytic anemia, chlorambucil and, 775
Cold-agglutinin syndrome, 430
Cold urticaria, 355
  familial, 355
Colitis, 459
  ulcerative, 461–462

rectal biopsy specimen, 461*f*
  selective IgA deficiency and, 274
Collagen disorder, serum immunoglobulin levels, 157*t*
Collagen vascular disease, 409, 537
  interferon-gamma and, 783
Colon cancer, levamisole and, 784
Colonic mucosa, normal flora, 623, 623*t*
Colony-stimulating factor (CSF), 10, 120–121, 783
Colony-stimulating factor-1 (CSF-1), clinical applications,
        427*t*
Combinatorial joining, 81, 94
Combined immunodeficiency, serum immunoglobulin levels,
        157*t*
Common acute lymphocytic leukemia antigen (CALLA),
        572
Common variable immunodeficiency, serum immunoglobulin
        levels, 157*t*
Competitive protein-binding assay, 170
Complement, 9
  activation, 47
    biologic consequences, 131–132
    inflammation and, 147–148
    pathways, 124
    periodontal disease and, 471–472
    regulatory molecules, 133
  allotype variants, 312–313
  assay, 186–189
  cascade, 125*f*, 126*f*
    late phase, 128–129, 129*f*
  components, 124
    deficiencies, 309–311
    functional assays, 188
    identification of defects, 261
    immunoassays, 188
    measurement, 188–189
    molecular weights and serum concentrations, 125*t*
  deficiencies, 309–313
    autoimmunity and, 311
    inherited, 310*t*, 409
    screening, 261
  fixation, 184, 190*f*
  fixation test, 189
    applications, 189*t*
    hypersensitivity pneumonitis and, 369
  functions, 124
  hemolytic transfusion reactions and, 233
  host defense and, 625
  immune competence testing, 261
  pathway, 47
    alternative, 124, 128
    classic, 124, 125–128
  receptors, 15, 132–133
    C1q, 132
    C3, 132–133
    deficiencies, 312
  regulatory factors, deficiencies, 311
  serum
    elevated, 189, 189*t*
    reduced activity, 188–189, 189*t*
  system, 124–133
    control mechanisms, 129–131
    systemic lupus erythematosus and, 390
Complementarity, 55, 55*f*, 216
Complementarity-determining region (CDR), 75
Complete Freund's adjuvant (CFA), 51, 781
Concentration estimate, 173
Concomitant immunity model, 675
Condom therapy, 560

Condyloma acuminatum, interferon-alpha and, 782
Confidence interval, 176
Confidence limit, 173, 176
Conformational epitope, 53, 53*f*
Congenital hypoplastic anemia, 434
Congenital immunodeficiency
  adoptive immunity and, 712
  immunoblastic sarcoma of B cell type and, 606
  neoplasia and, 580–581, 581*t*
Congenital thymic aplasia, 279–282
Conglutinating complement absorption test, 184
Conjunctiva, telangiectasis, 291*f*
Conjunctivitis
  allergic, 334
    cromolyn sodium and, 792
  giant papillary, 334
  Reiter's syndrome and, 407
  seasonal, antihistamines and, 792
  vernal, 520–521, 521*f*
Constant region, 68
Contact allergy, eczematous, 363
Contact dermatitis
  allergic, 146–147, 363–365, 373, 375
    desensitization, 742
    patch test and, 320
  eyes and, 525
  photoallergic, 365–366
Contact sensitivity, 196
Contagion, 1
Contingency table, two-by-two, 192*t*
Continuous-response assay, 176
Contrast media
  anaphylactoid reactions and, 351
  pseudoallergic reactions and, 379
Convoluted T cell lymphoma, 612
Coombs test, 185–186
  direct, 186
    hemolytic disease of newborn and, 432
    immune hemolytic anemia and, 428
    technique, 230*f*
  indirect, 186
    technique, 230*f*
Coons, Albert H., 2, 4
Copolymer I, multiple sclerosis and, 511
Coptic lung, 369
Coral snake bite, serum therapy, 733
Coreceptor, 98
Corneal graft reaction, 526–527, 526*f*
Corneal ulceration, systemic lupus erythematosus and,
  389
Cor pulmonale, 370, 402
Cortex, 33
Corticosteroid, 765–768, 786–789
  acute disseminated encephalomyelitis and, 508
  acute inflammatory demyelinating polyneuropathy and,
    513
  adrenal insufficiency and, 421
  allergic bronchopulmonary aspergillosis and, 361
  allergic contact dermatitis and, 364
  allergic gastroenteropathy and, 344
  allergic rhinitis and, 334
  allograft rejection and, 748–749
  anaphylaxis and, 353
  anti-inflammatory effects, 788–789
  asthma and, 340
  autoimmune hemolytic anemia and, 430
  autoimmune hepatitis and, 468
  autoimmune myocarditis and, 443

Beçhet's disease and, 406, 446
  bone transplantation and, 762
  cellular traffic and, 765–766, 766*f*
  clinical use, 767–768
  cold-agglutinin syndromes and, 430
  corneal graft reactions and, 527
  Crohn's disease and, 460
  epidermolysis bullosa acquisita and, 500
  giant cell arteritis and, 453
  gluten-sensitive enteropathy and, 458
  Goodpasture's syndrome and, 481, 536
  graft-versus-host disease and, 298
  heart transplantation and, 755
  hypersensitivity pneumonitis and, 369
  idiopathic pulmonary fibrosis and, 536
  idiopathic thrombocytopenic purpura and, 437–438
  immune-complex glomerulonephritis and, 486–487
  infertility and, 560
  juvenile arthritis and, 399
  live vaccines and, 726
  lung transplantation and, 538, 757
  mechanism of action, 787–788
  metabolic effects, 789
  minimal-change nephropathy and, 489
  myasthenia gravis and, 514
  nonspecific immunosuppression and, 715
  pancreas transplantation and, 754
  pemphigus vulgaris and, 503
  pharmacology, 786–787
  photoallergic contact dermatitis and, 365*t*
  Pneumocystis carinii and, 664
  polyarteritis nodosa and, 449
  polymyositis-dermatomyositis and, 406
  primary biliary cirrhosis and, 469
  progressive systemic sclerosis and, 403
  psoriatic arthritis and, 408
  recurrent aphthous ulceration and, 475
  relapsing panniculitis and, 409
  relapsing polychondritis and, 408
  rheumatoid arthritis and, 396
  rheumatoid eye disease and, 522
  sarcoid lesions of eye and, 524
  sarcoidosis and, 534
  Sjögren's syndrome and, 401
  small-vessel vasculitis and, 445
  status asthmaticus and, 341
  structures, 787*f*
  sympathetic ophthalmia and, 525
  systemic lupus erythematosus and, 388, 392
  Takayasu arteritis and, 453
  toxicity, 789
  tubulointerstitial nephritis and, 489
  ulcerative colitis and, 462
  urticaria and, 356
  Vogt-Koyanagi-Harada syndrome and, 525
  Wegener's granulomatosis and, 490
Cortisol, 786
  chemical structure, 787*f*
  half-life relative potency, 788*t*
Cortisone, 786
  chemical structure, 787*f*
  half-life relative potency, 788*t*
Corynebacterium diphtheriae, 629
Corynebacterium parvum, 781
Costimulation, 31, 113
Costimulatory signal, 44, 97, 105
Counterimmunoelectrophoresis, 165
Cowpox, 1

Cowpox virus, 717
Coxsackievirus, insulin-dependent diabetes mellitus and, 420
CR1, 132
CR2, 132–133
CR3, 132
CR4, 133
C-reactive protein, 9
Creatine, polymyositis-dermatomyositis and, 405
Creatinuria, polymyositis-dermatomyositis and, 406
CREST syndrome, 390
Creutzfeldt-Jakob disease, 515
Crevicular fluid, periodontal disease and, 471
Cricothyrotomy, 352
Crohn's disease, 459–461
    rectal biopsy specimen, 459f
    small-bowel barium contrast x-ray, 460f
Cromolyn
    allergic gastroenteropathy and, 344
    allergic rhinitis and, 334
    IgE-mediated allergic disease and, 715
Cromolyn sodium
    asthma and, 340
    immediate hypersensitivity reactions and, 792
Cross-linking, 30
Cross-matching, 229–230, 244–245
    autoantibodies, 245
    B cells, 245
    flow cytometry, 245, 245f
    kidney transplantation and, 745
    liver transplantation and, 752
    lymphocytotoxicity and, 244
    pancreas transplantation and, 753–754
    T cells, 244–245
Cross-reaction, 55, 176
Cross-reaction profile, 176
Cryoglobulin, 168–169, 607, 609
    classification of types, 169t
    clinical significance, 169
    IgG-IgM mixed, separation by gel filtration, 167f
    isolation and analysis, 168–169
Cryoglobulinemia, 154, 609
    essential, chlorambucil and, 775
    serum viscosity and, 168
Cryoprecipitate, 235
Cryptococcosis, 651t, 660–661
    immunologic abnormalities and, 653t
    immunologic diagnosis, 656t
    pathologic features, 652t
Cryptococcus, 526
Cryptococcus neoformans, 660–661
Cryptosporidium, 666
CSF. See Colony-stimulating factor
CTLS. See T cells, cytotoxic
Cuemulus oophorus, 555
Cumulative sum chart, 176
Cunninghamela, 662
Curare
    anaphylactoid reactions and, 352
    pseudoallergic reactions and, 379
Curschmann's spirals, 336
Cutaneous basophil hypersensitivity, 150
Cutaneous leishmaniasis, 670–671
Cutaneous T cell lymphoma, 613–614
Cutaneous test, 321
Cyclic neutropenia, 425–426
Cyclooxygenase, 788, 790–791
    asthma and, 337–338

    inhibitors, urticaria and, 355
    metabolites, 144
        chemical structures, 143f
Cyclophilin, 776
Cyclophosphamide, 768, 772–773
    autoimmune hemolytic anemia and, 430
    bone marrow transplantation and, 759
    bone transplantation and, 762
    bullous pemphigoid and, 495
    cold-agglutinin syndromes and, 430
    cytotoxic effects, 772–773
    effect on lymphocytes, 773f
    idiopathic thrombocytopenic purpura and, 437
    immune-complex glomerulonephritis and, 486–487
    immune system neoplasms and, 601
    kidney transplantation and, 746
    multiple myeloma and, 608
    multiple sclerosis and, 511
    pemphigus vulgaris and, 503
    polyarteritis nodosa and, 449
    properties and uses, 772t
    small noncleaved FCC lymphoma and, 605
    sympathetic ophthalmia and, 525
    systemic lupus erythematosus and, 392
    Takayasu arteritis and, 455
    Vogt-Koyanagi-Harada syndrome and, 525
    Wegener's granulomatosis and, 451, 490
Cyclosporin, 97, 775–776
    aplastic anemia and, 758
    autoimmune hemolytic anemia and, 430
    bone transplantation and, 762
    bullous pemphigoid and, 495
    chemical structure, 775f
    corneal graft reactions and, 527
    Crohn's disease and, 461
    graft-versus-host disease and, 298, 760
    heart transplantation and, 755
    kidney transplantation and, 746
    liver transplantation and, 752
    lung transplantation and, 538, 757
    multiple sclerosis and, 511
    nonspecific immunosuppression and, 714–715
    primary biliary cirrhosis and, 469
    properties and uses, 776t
Cyclosporin A, 113
    epidermolysis bullosa acquisita and, 500
    pemphigus vulgaris and, 503
Cysticercosis, 676
Cystic fibrosis, 539
    allergic bronchopulmonary aspergillosis and, 361
    heart-lung transplantation and, 755
    nasal polyposis and, 334
    serum immunoglobulin levels, 157t
Cystitis, cyclophosphamide and, 773
Cytogenetics, immune system neoplasms, 596–598
Cytokine, 19, 105–122, 782–784
    antagonists, 784
    atopic disease and, 328–329
    chemokine family, 118–120
    clinical applications, 427t
    defects, 288–289
    host defense and, 624
    immune stimulation and, 714
    immunoregulation and, 714
    immunoregulatory, 116
        properties, 106–107t
    implantation and, 555
    multiple sclerosis and, 509f

neutropenia and, 426–427
production, natural killer cells and, 103
receptor families, 121, 121*t*
tolerance and, 384
transplantation and, 427
Cytokine synthesis inhibitory factor. *See* Interleukin-10
Cytomegalovirus (CMV), 526, 700–701
  clinical manifestations, 700*t*
  insulin-dependent diabetes mellitus and, 420
  lung transplantation and, 757
  natural killer cells and, 104
  passive immunization, 730*t*
  transfusion-transmitted, 232
  vaccine, 738
Cytoplasmic azurophilic granules, 612–613
Cytotoxic drugs, 768–775
  clinical use, 771*t*
  combinations, 775
  cryoglobulinemia and, 609
  Goodpasture's syndrome and, 536
  idiopathic pulmonary fibrosis and, 536
  idiopathic thrombocytopenic purpura and, 437
  immunologic disorders and, 771*t*
  neutropenia and, 427
  nonspecific immunosuppression and, 714
  polymyositis-dermatomyositis and, 406
  relapsing polychondritis and, 408
Cytotoxicity, 28, 46
  cell-mediated, antibody-dependent, 47, 74, 103, 573, 618, 625, 748
Cytotoxic lymphocyte maturation factor (CLMF). *See* Interleukin-12
Cytotoxic T cells. *See* T cells, cytotoxic
Cytotrophoblast, 555
  invasive, 555
  noninvasive, 555

DAF. *See* **Decay-accelerating factor**
DAG. *See* Diacylglycerol
Dalen-Fuchs nodules, 524
Danazol, hereditary angioedema and, 312
Dapsone
  bullous pemphigoid and, 495
  dermatitis herpetiformis and, 458, 499
  epidermolysis bullosa acquisita and, 500
  herpes gestationis and, 497
  Pneumocystis carinii and, 664
  relapsing polychondritis and, 408
DAT. *See* Direct antiglobulin test
Dausset, Jean, 5
Davis, Mark, 3, 4
ddC. *See* Dideoxycytidine
ddI. *See* Dideoxyinosine
DEAE. *See* Diethylaminoethyl
Decay-accelerating factor (DAF), 133
Decidua, 552
Declining phase, 48
Decorin, transforming growth factor-beta and, 784
Defensin, 15
Degenerative arthritis, 395
Degranulation, 15, 74, 140
  assay, 212*f*
  extracellular, 16, 17*f*, 139
  tests, 211–212
Dehydration, status asthmaticus and, 341
Delay-accelerating factor (DAF), paroxysmal nocturnal hemoglobinuria and, 312

Delayed hypersensitivity, 2, 314, 363, 626
  azimexone and, 784–785
  lymphocyte activation and, 204
  skin testing, 195–197, 259
Delayed-type hypersensitivity (DTH), 100, 146
  acquired immunodeficiency syndrome and, 696
  corticosteroids and, 789
Delta agent, 466
Delta hepatitis, 466
Dementia
  presenile, 517
  senile, 517
Demyelinating disease, 507–513
Denaturation, 216
Dendritic cell, 63–64, 120
  blood, 63
  follicular, 33, 64
Dental caries, 473*f*
Dental plaque, 471
  normal flora, 623*t*
2'-Deoxycoformycin
  hairy cell leukemia and, 606
  immune system neoplasms and, 601
Deoxyribonuclease, 630
15-Deoxysporgualin, liver transplantation and, 752
de Quervain's thyroiditis, 416
Dermatitis
  atopic, 327, 341–343
    desensitization, 740
    serum IgE levels, 336*f*
  contact
    allergic, 146–147, 320, 363–365, 373, 375
    desensitization, 742
    eyes and, 525
    photoallergic, 365–366
  eczematoid, 374
    nonallergic, 327
  metal, 364
  Rhus, 364, 365, 739, 742
Dermatitis herpetiformis, 457–458, 494, 497–499, 498*f*
  IgA deposits, 499*f*
Dermatologic disease, 492–505
Dermatophagoides farinae, 330
Dermatophagoides pteronyssinus, 330
Dermatophyte, 649
Dermatophytosis, 342, 650*t*
  immunologic abnormalities and, 653*t*
Dermatosis
  bullous, linear IgA, 503–504
  vesiculobullous, 365
Dermographism, 355
Desensitization, 334–335, 365
  allergy, 739–743
    adverse effects, 741–742
    immunologic effects, 741, 741*f*
    indications, 742
    methods, 739–740
    modified allergens and, 743
    monitoring, 742–743
  anaphylaxis and, 353
  asthma and, 341
  penicillin, 377
  sulfonamide, 377
Desmoglein I, pemphigus foliaceus and, 501
Desmoplakin I, paraneoplastic pemphigus and, 503
Determinant selection, 64–65
Dexamethasone
  chemical structure, 787*f*

Dexamethasone *(cont.)*
  half-life relative potency, 788t
  rheumatoid eye disease and, 522
Diabetes mellitus
  immunocompromised host and, 707
  insulin-dependent, 419–421
    immunotherapy trials, 421t
  pancreas transplantation and, 753–754
Diacylglycerol (DAG), 30, 97
Diagnostic sensitivity, 176, 192
Diagnostic specificity, 176, 192
Dialysis, cadaveric kidney transplantation and, 746
Diaminodiphensylsulfone, dermatitis herpetiformis and, 458
Diamond-Blackfan syndrome, 434
DIC. *See* Disseminated intravascular coagulation
Dictyocaulus filaria, 676
Dictyocaulus viviparus, 676
Didanosine, human immunodeficiency virus and, 699
Dideoxycytidine (ddC, zalcitabine), human immunodeficiency virus and, 699
Dideoxyinosine (ddI, didanosine), human immunodeficiency virus and, 699
Dietary elimination testing, 325
Diethylaminoethyl (DEAE), 166
Diethyldithiocarbamate, human immunodeficiency virus infection and, 784
Differentiation, terminal, 10
Differentiation antigen
  B cell, 201t
  T cell, 198t
Differentiation factor, 783–784
Diffuse idiopathic skeletal hyperostosis (DISH), 407
DiGeorge's syndrome, 279–282, 280f
  thymic hormones and, 782
Digitalis glycoside, allergic reactions, 374
Dihydrofolate reductase, 773
Dilated cardiomyopathy, 443
Dimorphic fungus, 649
Dinitrochlorobenzene (DNCB), 196
Diphenhydramine, anaphylaxis and, 353
Diphenylhydantoin
  lupus syndrome and, 530
  pseudolymphoma and, 530
Diphtheria, 629, 717, 734, 736
  active immunization, 719t
  passive immunization, 730t
Diphtheria bacillus, 1–2
Diphtheria toxin, 2, 170, 629, 631, 712
Diphtheria toxoid, 2, 629
Diphyllobothrium latum, 675
Direct agglutination test, 184
Direct antiglobulin test (DAT), 229
Direct Coombs test, 186
  hemolytic disease of newborn and, 432
  immune hemolytic anemia and, 428
  technique, 230f
Direct immunofluorescence, 181, 181f
Discoid lupus erythematosus, 388, 391, 504–505, 504f, 505f
Disequilibrium assay, 171
DISH. *See* Diffuse idiopathic skeletal hyperostosis
Disodium cromoglycate, IgE-mediated allergic disease and, 715
Disseminated intravascular coagulation (DIC), 110, 233
Divalent, 68
DNA, 2, 3
  alkylation, 772–773
  amplification

ligase chain reaction and, 223f
    polymerase chain reaction and, 222f, 251f
  analysis, immune system neoplasms and, 592–596
  cell cycle, B cell lymphoma, 597f
  ligases, 223
  polymerases, 222
    thermostable, 223
  probes, methods for labeling and detecting, 218f
  rearrangement, 94
  rearrangement in B cells, immunoglobulin genes and, 80–84
  recombinant, 3, 216
  sequencing, HLA typing and, 254
  structure, 217f
  synthesis
    corticosteroids and, 789
    methotrexate and, 773
  transcription, steroid-receptor complex and, 787–788
  viral, detection by in situ hybridization, 222f
  viruses, oncogenic, 570
DNCB. *See* Dinitrochlorobenzene
Doherty, Peter C., 3, 4
Domain, 67
Dome area, 542
Dome cell, 542
Donath-Landsteiner antibody, 431
Dopamine, anaphylactic shock and, 352
Dose, 176
  minimum detectable, 177
Dot blot hybridization, 217, 219f
Double diffusion
  in agar, 152–54
  reactions, 152f
Double helix, 3
Double-negative lymphocyte, 29
Double-negative thymocyte, 102
Double-positive lymphocyte, 29
Double-positive thymocyte, 102
DPT combination vaccine, 629–630, 726
DR4 allele, oligonucleotide hybridization patterns, 252t
Dracunculus medinensis, 676
DR antigen, 203f
Drift, 176–177
Drug allergy, 371–379
  diagnosis, 374–375
  hapten-carrier interaction, 373f
  immunologic basis, 371–374
  treatment, 375
Drug fever, 374
Drug-induced eosinophilic pneumonia, 532, 532t
Drug-induced immune hemolytic anemia, 430–431
  clinical and laboratory features, 431t
Drug-induced immune neutropenia, 426
Drug-induced immune thrombocytopenia, 438
Drug-induced lupuslike syndrome, 389
Drug-induced respiratory disease, 528–530, 529t
Drugs
  anaphylaxis and, 350
  metabolic biotransformation, 372
  reactions, 618
  selective IgA deficiency and, 275
DTH. *See* Delayed-type hypersensitivity
DTP vaccine, 736–737
  reportable events, 728t
Duffy blood group antigen Fy(a-b-), 668
Duffy blood group system, 228–229
Duncan's syndrome, 277–278, 580, 619
Dwarfism, short-limbed, immunodeficiency and, 294–295, 294f

Dyscrasia
  blood, cyclophosphamide and, 773
  plasma cell, 607–610
    immunoelectrophoresis and, 161, 607
Dyshidrosis, 342

EBV. *See* **Epstein-Barr virus**
Echinococcosis, 676
Echinococcus granulosus, 676
Ectocervix, 552
Eczema, 341
  atopic, 341
  facial, Wiskott-Aldrich syndrome and, 293*f*
  hyper-IgE syndrome and, 307
  immunodeficiency and, 292–293
Eczema herpeticum, 343
Eczematization, 364
Eczematoid dermatitis, 374
Eczematous contact allergy, 363
Eczematous dermatitis, nonallergic, 327
Eczema vaccinatum, 343
Edelman, Gerald Maurice, 3, 4
Edema, 137
  angioneurotic, 354, 380
  laryngeal, anaphylaxis and, 352–353
  progressive systemic sclerosis and, 402
Effector cell, 24, 27*f*
Effector T cell/lymphokine pathway, 317
Efferent lymphatic vessel, 33
Eflornithine, *Pneumocystis carinii* and, 664
EGF. *See* Epidermal growth factor
Ehrlich, Paul, 2, 4, 8*f*
Eikenella corrodens, 471
Eisenmenger's syndrome, heart-lung transplantation and, 755
Electroimmunodiffusion, 164–165
  double
    clinical applications, 165*t*
    one-dimensional, 165, 165*f*
  single, one-dimensional, 165, 165*f*
Electromyography, polymyositis-dermatomyositis and, 405
Electrophoresis, 156–165
  immunofixation, 161–164, 164*f*
  zone
    cellulose acetate technique, 158*f*
    cerebrospinal fluid, 160*f*
    immunoelectrophoresis compared, 161*f*
    serum immunoglobulin abnormalities, 159*f*
    urine abnormalities, 160*f*
Elephantiasis, 678
Elimination diet testing, 325
ELISA. *See* Enzyme-linked immunosorbent assay
EM. *See* Erythema migrans
Emigration, 13*f*, 14
Emission spectrum, 178*f*
EMIT. *See* Enzyme-multiplied immunoassay
Emphysema, heart-lung transplantation and, 755
Encapsulated bacteria, 627, 631–633, 632*f*
Encephalitis
  influenza virus and, 639
  measles, 726
Encephalomyelitis
  allergic, experimental, 713
  disseminated, acute, 507–508
Endocarditis
  candidal, 660
  infective, 630
  subacute bacterial, serum immunoglobulin levels, 157*t*

Endocervix, 552
Endocrine disease, 412–423
  autoimmune
    mechanism of development, 412
    pathogenesis, 413*f*
Endocrine effect, 782
Endocrinopathy, candidiasis, mucocutaneous, 422
Endocytosis, receptor-mediated, 14*f*
Endogenous circulating anticoagulant, 439–440
Endogenous protein, 61
Endogenous pyrogen, 111
Endometrium, 552
Endomyocardial disease, Loffler's, 443
Endomyocardial fibrosis, tropical, 443
Endosalpinx, 552
Endothelial cell, inflammation and, 141–142
Endotoxin, 627–628, 631
  live virus vaccines and, 727
Endotoxin-mediated host injury, 626
Enprophylline, 794
Enteritis, regional, selective IgA deficiency and, 274
Enteropathy, gluten-sensitive, 457–458, 619
  jejunal biopsy specimen, 458*f*
  oral unresponsiveness and, 549
Enterotoxin, 629, 630, 631
Environmental lung disease, 533
Enzymatic label, 173–174
Enzyme deficiency, immunodeficiency and, 295–297
Enzyme-linked antibody, 183
Enzyme-linked immunosorbent assay (ELISA), 173–174, 174*f*
  anti-DNA antibodies and, 391
  Aspergillus precipitins and, 360
  drug allergy and, 375
  human immunodeficiency virus and, 694–695
  hypersensitivity pneumonitis and, 369
  Lyme disease and, 686
Enzyme-multiplied immunoassay (EMIT), 173, 173*f*
Eosinophil
  electron micrograph, 139*f*
  inflammation and, 138–139
  interleukin-5 and, 117
  peroxidase, 138
Eosinophilia, 100, 139
  blood, 333
  nasal, 333
  pulmonary
    simple idiopathic, 531
    tropical, 533
Eosinophilia-myalgia syndrome, 532
Eosinophilic gastroenteropathy, 343
Eosinophilic leukemia, 443
Eosinophilic pneumonia, 530–533, 531*t*
  acute, 531–532
  drug-induced, 532, 532*t*
  idiopathic, chronic, 531, 532*f*
  parasite-induced, 532–533, 532*t*
Epidermal growth factor (EGF), 783
Epidermal necrolysis, 630
Epidermolysis bullosa acquisita, 494, 499–500
Epinephrine
  anaphylaxis and, 352, 793
  asthma and, 340
  status asthmaticus and, 341
  urticaria and, 356
Epithelial basement membrane zone, 493*f*
Epithelial cell, IgA transport, 547*f*
Epithelial tumor, 580
Epithelioid cell, 19

Epitope, 50
  B cell, 52–53, 52f, 53f
    complementarity, 55, 55f
    size and location, 52–53
  conformational, 53, 53f
  linear, 53, 53f
  structure, anti-hapten antibody binding and, 54t
  T cell, 52, 55–56
Epo. See Erythropoietin
Epstein-Barr virus (EBV), 689, 701–703
  Burkitt-like non-Hodgkin lymphoma and, 580
  Burkitt's lymphoma and, 570
  CR2 and, 133
  diseases associated, 702t
  natural killer cells and, 104
  serologic response, 704f
  small noncleaved FCC lymphoma and, 605
  transfusion-transmitted, 232
Equilibrium assay, 171
E rosette-forming cell, 199, 200f
Erwinia, 631
Erythema, 137
Erythema migrans (EM), 686, 687
Erythema multiforme, 374, 502
Erythema nodosum, 374, 455, 455f
Erythroblastosis fetalis, 380, 432, 562
  antigen-specific therapy, 713
  passive immunization, 732t
Erythroblast, 562
Erythrocyte
  antibodies, detection, 229–230
  antigens, 226–229
    detection, 229–230
  disorders, 427–434
  substances adsorbing, 185t
  transfusion, 234–235
Erythrocyte aplasia, pure, 433–434
  cyclophosphamide and, 773
  intravenous gamma globulin and, 778
Erythroid pathway, 11f
Erythromycin, bullous pemphigoid and, 495
Erythropoietin (Epo), 120, 426, 783
  clinical applications, 427t
Escherichia, 631
Escherichia coli, 631, 718
Essential cryoglobulinemia, chlorambucil and, 775
Estrogen, anti-DNA antibody formation and, 388
Estrogen therapy, steroid clearance and, 786
Eukaryote, immunomodulator compounds derived, 782–784
Euroglyphus maynei, 331
Evan's syndrome, colony-stimulating factors and, 783
Excess-reagent method, 175
Exchange transfusion, hemolytic disease of newborn and, 433
Exercise-induced anaphylaxis, 351
Exogenous protein, 61
Exon, 80
Exotoxin, 627–628
Exotoxin A, 631, 712
Experimental allergic encephalomyelitis, 713
Experimental tolerance, 383–385
Exponential phase, 48
Extracellular degranulation, 16, 17f, 139
Extrahepatic biliary atresia, liver transplantation and, 750
Extrinsic allergic alveolitis, 366
Extrinsic asthma, 335
Eye, systemic lupus erythematosus and, 389
Eye disease, 520–527
  antibody-mediated, 520–523

  cell-mediated, 523–526
  rheumatoid, 521–523

Fab fragment, 68
Factor B, 128
Factor D, 128
Factor H, complement system and, 130–131
Factor I, complement system and, 130–131
Fagraeus, Astrid E., 2, 4
Falciparum malaria, 667–668
Familial cold urticaria, 355
Fanconi's syndrome, 488
Farmer's lung, 361, 366, 367, 369
  atypical, 369
Fas antigen, 121
Fascioliasis, 673
FCC lymphoma. See Follicular center cell (FCC) lymphoma
Fc fragment, 68
Fc receptor, 15, 47, 68, 74, 88
  inflammatory cell, 138t
  properties, 74t
Febrile reaction, transfusion, 231
Feline leukemia virus, 570
Felty's syndrome, 391, 394
  granulocyte colony-stimulating factor and, 783
Fenner, Frank, 2, 4
Ferritin-coupled antibody, 183
Fertilization, in vitro, 560
Fetal hydrops, 432
Fetal thymus transplantation, congenital thymic aplasia and, 282
Fetus, toxoplasmosis and, 669
FEV. See Forced expiratory volume
Fever, 111
  drug, 374
  host defense and, 624
  juvenile arthritis and, 398
  rheumatic, 398
    anti-cardiac immune responses, 380
FFP. See Fresh-frozen plasma
FGF. See Fibroblast growth factor
Fibroblast, interferons and, 115
Fibroblast growth factor (FGF), 783
Filariae, 676
Filariasis, lymphatic, 678
Filarid nematode, 678
FITC. See Fluorescein isothiocyanate
FK506, 97, 113, 776–777
  heart transplantation and, 755
  liver transplantation and, 752
  nonspecific immunosuppression and, 715
Flora, normal, 623, 623t
Flow cytometry, 202–203, 202f, 591–592
  cell analysis, 202
  clinical applications, 203, 205t
  cross-matching, 245, 245f
  neutrophils and, 213
Flow sorting, cell purification and, 204f
Fluconazole
  candidiasis and, 660
  coccidioidomycosis and, 657
Flucytosine
  candidiasis and, 660
  cryptococcosis and, 661
Fluke, 673
Flunisolide
  allergic rhinitis and, 334
  asthma and, 340

Fluocinonide, recurrent aphthous ulceration and, 475
Fluorescein, 178
Fluorescein isothiocyanate (FITC), 178–179
Fluorescence, 178
Fluorescence microscope
    epi-illumination and, 180*f*
    transmitted light and, 179*f*
Fluorescence polarization immunoassay (FPIA), 174, 174*f*
Fluorescent compound, absorption and emission spectra, 178*f*
Fluorochrome, 178
Fluorometric label, 174
5-Fluorouracil, 784
Focal glomerulonephritis, 484
Focal glomerulosclerosis, 489
Folic acid, 773
Folic acid cycle, 774*f*
Follicle
    lymphoid, transmission electron micrograph, 543*f*
    mucosal, 542
Follicular center cell (FCC) lymphoma, 604–605
Follicular dendritic cell (FDC), 33, 64
Follicular hyperplasia, benign, 618
Follicular lymphoma, 49, 92
Follicular zone, 542
Folliculitis, *Pityrosporum*, 650*t*
    immunologic abnormalities and, 653*t*
Food
    anaphylaxis and, 350
    allergen, 332
    allergy, 325
      cromolyn sodium and, 792
    poisoning, 629
Forced expiratory volume (FEV), 318, 337
Forced vital capacity (FCV), 325
N-Formylmethionine, 12
Foscarnet, cytomegalovirus and, 701
Fossa navicularis, 553
FPIA. *See* Fluorescence polarization immunoassay
Fracastoro, Girolamo, 1
Framework region, 75
Free fraction, 172
Fresh-frozen plasma (FFP), 235
Freund's adjuvant
    complete, 51, 781
    desensitization therapy and, 743
Frustrated phagocytosis, 211–212, 212*f*
FTA-ABS test, 683–684
Fulminant hepatic failure, liver transplantation and, 750
Fungal disease, 649–664
Fungus, dimorphic, 649
Fungus disease, serum immunoglobulin levels, 157*t*
Furosemide, 377
Fusobacterium nucleatum, 471
FVC. *See* Forced vital capacity

Gamete intrafallopian transfer, 560
Gamma chain disease, 609
Gamma globulin, 2, 3, 66
    acquired hypogammaglobulinemia and, 273
    anaphylaxis and, 351
    antibody deficiency disease and, 712
    hypogammaglobulinemia and, 269
    hypogammaglobulinemic arthritis and, 409
    idiopathic thrombocytopenic purpura and, 437–438
    intravenous, 777–778
    pure erythrocyte aplasia and, 434
    serum sickness and, 358
    severe combined immunodeficiency disease and, 288

Gammopathy, monoclonal, 607
    benign, 609
Ganciclovir
    bone marrow transplantation and, 759, 761
    cytomegalovirus and, 701
    hepatitis B virus and, 644–645
Gastroenteropathy
    allergic, 327, 343–344
    eosinophilic, 343
    protein-losing, serum immunoglobulin levels, 157*t*
Gastrointestinal disease, 457–463
    selective IgA deficiency and, 274
Gastrointestinal tract
    normal flora, 623, 623*t*
    progressive systemic sclerosis and, 402–403
    systemic lupus erythematosus and, 389
GBM. *See* Glomerular basement membrane
G-CSF. *See* Granulocyte colony-stimulating factor
Gel filtration chromatography, 166–167, 167*f*
Gene rearrangement assay, 220–221
Genetic engineering, 3, 714
Genetic identity determination, 254
Gentamicin, chronic granulomatous disease and, 305
Germinal center, 33, 33*f*
Germ theory of disease, 1
Giant cell arteritis, 451–453, 452*f*
    eyes and, 525
Giant papillary conjunctivitis, 334
Giardia lamblia, hypogammaglobulinemia and, 267
Giardiasis, 533, 666
Gingiva, healthy, 473*f*
Gingivitis, 471–473
Glands of Littre, 553
Gliadin, 457–458
Glioma, interferon-beta and, 782
Globulin
    antilymphocyte, 778
      allograft rejection and, 749
      kidney transplantation and, 746
      liver transplantation and, 752
      lung transplantation and, 538
    antithymocyte, 778
      allograft rejection and, 749
      aplastic anemia and, 758
      graft-versus-host disease and, 760
      kidney transplantation and, 746
    immune serum, measles virus and, 642
    Rh immune, 563–564
      incidence of Rh disease and, 564*f*
Glomerular basement membrane (GMB), 478
Glomerular cell, 479
Glomerulonephritis, 630
    antibody-induced, anti-glomerular basement membrane, 479–481
    antigen-antibody, quartan malaria and, 666
    focal, 484
    IgG deposits, 488*f*
    immune-complex, 481–487
      antigen-antibody systems and, 485*t*
      features, 483–484*t*
      histologic forms, 485*f*
      IgG deposits, 486*f*
    immune-induced
      cyclophosphamide and, 773
      prednisone and, 768
    interleukin-1 receptor antagonist and, 784
    membranoproliferative, 486
    mesangial, 484–485

Glomerulonephritis *(cont.)*
post-streptococcal, 485, 626
systemic lupus erythematosus and, 388–389
Glomerulonephrosis, transforming growth factor-beta and, 783–784
Glomerulosclerosis
focal, 489
transforming growth factor-beta and, 783–784
Glucocorticoid, 111
anti-inflammatory mechanisms, 715
asthma and, 340
cellular traffic and, 765–766, 766*f*
half-life relative potencies, 788*t*
metabolic effects, 789*t*
natural cytotoxic cells and, 573
side effects, 790*t*
Glucose-6-phosphate dehydrogenase, dermatitis herpetiformis and, 499
Glucose-6-phosphate dehydrogenase deficiency, 305–306
chronic granulomatous disease and, 305
plasmodial infection and, 668
Glucose tolerance test, 420
Glutamic acid decarboxylase, specificity and sensitivity, 414*t*
Glutaraldehyde, allergen polymerization and, 743
Gluten, dermatitis herpetiformis and, 499
Gluten-sensitive enteropathy, 457–458, 619
jejunal biopsy specimen, 458*f*
oral unresponsiveness and, 549
N-Glycolylneuraminic acid, 634
GM-CSF. *See* Granulocyte-monocyte colony-stimulating factor
Goiter, 413, 414, 415
thyrotoxicosis with diffuse, 417
Gold, 791–792
immune thrombocytopenic purpura and, 438
Gold salt
pneumonitis and, 530
rheumatoid arthritis and, 396
Goldstein, Gideon, 4
Gonococcus, 1, 633
vaccine, 738
Goodpasture's syndrome, 479–481, 480*f*, 536–537
Arthus reaction and, 148
chest x-ray, 536*f*
cyclophosphamide and, 773
influenza virus and, 639
plasma exchange and, 777
Gordon, Jon W., 3, 4
Gouty arthritis, 395
gpL-115 membrane glycoprotein deficiency, 300
Graft reaction, corneal, 526–527, 526*f*
Graft rejection, monoclonal antibodies and, 779
Graft-versus-host (GVH) disease, 233, 297–298, 469, 758
bone marrow transplantation and, 760
clinical staging, 760*t*
maculopapular rash and, 298*f*
Graft-versus-host (GVH) reaction, 712
cyclosporin and, 776
methotrexate and, 774
severe combined immunodeficiency disease and, 287
Graft-versus-leukemia (GVL) effect, 759
Gram-negative rod, 630–631
Granulocyte, 10
assays
bactericidal, 213*f*
functional, 262
degranulation, assay, 212*f*

Granulocyte colony-stimulating factor (G-CSF), 10, 120–121, 783
clinical applications, 427*t*
Granulocyte-monocyte colony-stimulating factor (GM-CSF), 10, 120–121, 783
clinical applications, 427*t*
macrophage-activating factor and, 573
Granulocytic leukemia, lymphocytic leukemia and, 617
Granuloma, 19–20, 20*f*
hepatic, schistosomiasis and, 666
Granulomatosis, 449–450
allergic of Churg and Strauss, 531
lymphomatoid, 537
Wegener's, 450–451, 490, 537
chlorambucil and, 774
saddle nose deformity, 450*f*
Granulomatous disease, chronic, 303–305
bacterial killing curves, 305*f*
quantitative NBT test and, 212, 303
Granulomatous ileitis, 459
Granulomatous inflammation, 146
Granulomatous vasculitis, 537*t*
Granzyme, 100
Graves' disease, 383, 417–419
antithyroid antibodies, 418*f*
Green nimitti midge, 331
Growth factor, 426, 783–784
interleukin-7 as, 117
Guillain-Barre syndrome, 511–513
plasma exchange and, 777
swine influenza virus and, 639
Guinea worm, 676
GVH disease. *See* Graft-versus-host (GVH) disease
GVH reaction. *See* Graft-versus-host (GVH) reaction

H1 receptor, 142, 142*t*
H2 receptor, 142, 142*t*
H3 receptor, 142, 142*t*
Haemophilus, 471
Haemophilus influenzae, 537, 615, 632–633, 718, 738
active immunization, 719*t*
hyper-IgE syndrome and, 307
hypogammaglobulinemia and, 267
splenectomized patient and, 707
type b, 735
vaccine, 737
Hageman factor, 133
anaphylaxis and, 348
hemolytic transfusion reactions and, 233
Hairy cell leukemia, 606
interferon-alpha and, 782
Hairy leukoplakia, 475, 476*f*
Hansen's disease, 635
H antigen, 631
Haplotype matching, 744–745
Hapten, 2, 54–55, 54*f*, 171
immune hemolytic anemia and, 431
Haptenation, 372
Hardy, James, 757
Hashimoto's thyroiditis, 413–415, 618
pathology, 415*f*
Haskins, Kathryn, 3, 4
Hassell's corpuscle, 37
Haurowitz, Felix, 2, 4
HAV. *See* Hepatitis A virus
Hay fever, 792
HBcAg. *See* Hepatitis B core antigen
HBIG. *See* Hepatitis B immune globulin

H blood group system, 226–227
HBLV. *See* Human B lymphotrophic virus
HBsAg. *See* Hepatitis B surface antigen
HBV. *See* Hepatitis B virus
HCV. *See* Hepatitis C virus
HDV. *See* Hepatitis delta virus
Heart
    progressive systemic sclerosis and, 402
    systemic lupus erythematosus and, 389
Heart-lung transplantation, 755–756
Heart transplantation, 754–756
Heat shock protein, 781
Heavy (H) chain, 25, 67–68
    allotypic forms, 72
    classes and subclasses, 69
    class switching, 89, 90*f*
        interleukin-2 and, 113
        interleukin-4 and, 116
    genes, 81–84
        rearrangement and expression, 83*f*
    properties, 69*t*
Heavy chain disease, 608–609
    alpha, 462
Helminthiasis, 329
Helminth infection
    eosinophils and, 138
    helper T cells and, 100
    immune response and, 673–678
    serum IgE and, 74
Helper factor, 31
Helper T cell. *See* T cell, helper
Hemagglutination, 184
    substances adsorbing to erythrocytes, 185*t*
Hemagglutination inhibition, 185, 186*f*
Hemagglutinin, 638, 639
Hematologic disease, 425–440
Hematopoiesis, 9
    cyclophosphamide and, 773
    schematic overview, 11*f*
Hematopoietic cell surface marker, 817–818
Hematopoietic colony-stimulating factor, 10, 120–121
Hematopoietic stem cell, 9–10, 22
Hematopoietic system, systemic lupus erythematosus and, 389
Hematopoietin receptor family, 121
Hematoxylin body, 388
Hemochromatosis, liver transplantation and, 750
Hemoglobin, sickle cell, *Plasmodium falciparum* and, 668
Hemoglobin A/S, 668
Hemoglobinuria
    nocturnal, paroxysmal, 133, 312, 433
    paroxysmal cold, 431–432
Hemolymphopoietic growth factor, clinical applications, 427*t*
Hemolysin, 2, 630
Hemolytic anemia, 626
    autoimmune
        B cell neoplasms and, 591
        cyclophosphamide and, 773
        intravenous gamma globulin and, 778
        prednisone and, 768
        serologic findings, 429*t*
        warm, 429–430
    cold-agglutin, chlorambucil and, 775
    immune
        classification, 428*t*
        drug-induced, 430–431, 431*t*
    systemic lupus erythematosus and, 387
Hemolytic assay, 187–188, 187*f*

Hemolytic disease, ABO, 562–563
Hemolytic disease of newborn, 233, 432–433
Hemolytic reaction, transfusion, 230–231
Hemophagocytic syndrome, 616
Hemophilia, 235, 438–439
Hemorrhagic Schwartzmann reaction, 110
Henoch-Schonlein purpura, 445–446, 490
Hepadnavirus, 643
Heparin
    immune thrombocytopenic purpura and, 438
    mast cell granules and, 139
Hepatic allograft rejection, 469
Hepatic cirrhosis, immunocompromised host and, 707
Hepatic failure, liver transplantation and, 750
Hepatic fibrosis, methotrexate and, 774
Hepatic granuloma, schistosomiasis and, 666
Hepatic sarcoidosis, 469
Hepatic transplantation
    primary biliary cirrhosis and, 469
    primary sclerosing cholangitis and, 470
Hepatitis
    chronic active, autoimmune, 467–468
    diagnosis, hepatitis B virus markers, 644*t*
    epidemic, live vaccines and, 727
    non-A, non-B, 466–467
    posttransfusion, 232
    serum immunoglobulin levels, 157*t*
    viral and serologic characteristics, 463*t*
Hepatitis A, 464
    passive immunization, 730*t*
    pregnancy and, 558
    vaccine, 738
Hepatitis A virus (HAV), 464, 645
Hepatitis B, 464–466, 737
    active immunization, 719–720*t*
    antigenemia, hepatitis B hyperimmune globulin and, 750
    antigens and antibody titers, 465*f*
    cirrhosis, liver transplantation and, 750
    liver biopsy specimen, 467*f*
    passive immunization, 730–731*t*
    polyarteritis nodosa and, 447–448
    pregnancy and, 558
    thymic hormones and, 782
    vaccination, 735
    vaccine, recombinant, 737
Hepatitis B core antigen (HBcAg), 465, 643
Hepatitis B hyperimmune globulin, hepatitis B antigenemia and, 750
Hepatitis B immune globulin (HBIG), 645
Hepatitis B surface antigen (HBsAg), 465
Hepatitis B virus (HBV), 464–466, 642–645, 718
    liver cancer and, 570
    markers and antibody responses, 644*f*
    markers for diagnosis of hepatitis, 644*t*
Hepatitis C, 466–467
    cirrhosis, liver transplantation and, 750
    kidney transplantation and, 746
    liver transplantation and, 750
Hepatitis C virus (HCV), 466–467
Hepatitis D, 466
Hepatitis delta virus (HDV), 643
Hepatitis E, 467
Hepatitis E virus (HEV), 467
Hepatobiliary disease, 463–470
Herd immunity, 734
Hereditary angioedema, 130, 311–312, 356, 380
    kinin-generating system and, 135
Hereditary complement deficiency, 409

Heroin addiction, immune thrombocytopenic purpura and, 438
Herpes gestationis, 495–497
  histopathology, 496*f*
Herpes labialis, thymic hormones and, 782
Herpes simplex virus
  eczema herpeticum and, 343
  type 1, recurrent aphthous ulceration and, 474
  vaccine, 738
Herpesvirus, 689
Herpes zoster, immunoblastic reactions, 618
Herpetic keratoconjunctivitis, interferon-alpha and, 782
Heteroduplex analysis, histocompatibility testing and, 254
HEV. *See* Hepatitis E virus
HHV-6. *See* Human herpesvirus type 6
High endothelial venule, 39, 116
High-molecular-weight kininogen, 133
High-zone tolerance, 51
Hinge region, 68
Histamine
  action at receptor sites, 792*t*
  anaphylaxis and, 348
  asthmatic attack and, 337
  bronchoprovocation testing and, 318
  chemical structure, 142*f*
  cholinergic anaphylactoid reaction and, 351
  inflammation and, 142
  inflammatory response and, 149
  mast cell granules and, 139
  receptors, 142*t*
Histiocyte, 18
Histiocytic medullary reticulosis, 616
Histiocytosis, malignant, 616
Histocompatibility
  cellular assays, 246–248
  molecular, techniques, 249*t*
Histocompatibility testing, 237–254
  flowchart for renal transplant patient, 239*t*
  heteroduplex analysis and, 254
  molecular-biologic methods, 248–254, 248*t*
  serologic methods, 240
  transplantation and, 237
Histology, 1
Histoplasma capsulatum, 657
Histoplasmosis, 651*t*, 657–658
  immunologic abnormalities and, 653*t*
  immunologic diagnosis, 655*t*
  pathologic features, 652*t*
History, allergic disease and, 317–318
HIV. *See* Human immunodeficiency virus
Hives, 150, 354, 355
HLA (human leukocyte antigen)
  alleles, class II, polymorphism, 249*t*
  alloantisera, 242
  antibodies
    class I, serum screening results, 243*t*
    specificities, 242–243
  antigens
    class II, tissue typing, 243–244
    inheritance, 298*f*
    microcytotoxicity testing, 241*f*
    monoclonal antibodies, 242
    sensitization, 240
    specificities, 238*t*
  class I, 58, 59–60
    diagrammatic structure, 60*f*
    peptide-binding site, 61*f*
    restricted, 58
    schematic representation, 59*f*

class II, 60–61
  autoimmunity and, 413*f*
  peptide-binding site, 62*f*
  restricted, 58
  schematic representation, 61*f*
complex, organization on human chromosome 6, 59*f*
gluten-sensitive enteropathy and, 458
Graves' disease and, 417
matching, renal allograft survival and, 239*t*
pemphigus vulgaris and, 501
sharing, spontaneous abortion and, 562
Sjogren's syndrome and, 400
system, 58
typing
  cadaveric transplantation and, 745
  class II, antisera, 243–244
  DNA sequencing and, 254
  oligonucleotide probes and sequence-specific, 252–253, 253*f*
  polymerase chain reaction and, 250–254
  restriction fragment length polymorphism and, 249–250, 250*f*
  sera, sources, 242
HLA-A, 58
HLA-A1, myasthenia gravis and, 513
HLA-A3, multiple sclerosis and, 508
HLA-B, 58
HLA-B7, multiple sclerosis and, 508
HLA-B8, myasthenia gravis and, 513
HLA-B8/DR3, autoimmune hepatitis and, 467
HLA-B27, 64–65
  ankylosing spondylitis and, 384, 631
  Reiter's syndrome and, 407
HLA-C, 58
HLA-DP, 58
HLA-DQ, 58
HLA-DQw1, multiple sclerosis and, 508
HLA-DR, 58
HLA-DR matching, pancreas transplantation and, 753
HLA-DR2, multiple sclerosis and, 508
HLA-DR3, myasthenia gravis and, 513
HLA-DR4 haplotype, rheumatoid arthritis and, 392
Hodgkin's disease, 614–616
  Ann Arbor Staging Classification, 600
  ataxia-telangiectasia and, 580
  human immunodeficiency virus and, 585
  live vaccines and, 726
  multiple-agent chemotherapy, 600*t*
  nasopharyngeal carcinoma and, 570
  radiation therapy and, 600
  Reed-Sternberg cell, 614, 614*f*, 615
  Rye classification, 614, 615*t*
  serum immunoglobulin levels, 157*t*
Hofbauer cell, 557
Homing receptor, 39
Homologous restriction factor (HRF), 133
  paroxysmal nocturnal hemoglobinuria and, 312
Homozygous typing cell (HTC) test, 247
Honeybee venom anaphylaxis, 351
Hookworm, 533, 676, 677
Hormone, nasal congestion and, 333
Horseradish peroxidase, 183
Host defense
  antibody-mediated, 624, 624*t*
  body surface, 622–623
  complement and, 625
  fever and, 624
  impaired, infectious complications, 707*t*

inflammation and, 623–624
macrophages and, 19–20
natural killer cells and, 103–104
neutrophils and, 16–17
nonimmunologic mechanisms, 623t
phagocytic cells and, 625, 625t
T cell-mediated, 624–625
House dust mite, 330
HPRT. *See* Hypoxanthine phosphoribosyl transferase
HPV. *See* Human papillomavirus
HRF. *See* Homologous restriction factor
HTC test. *See* Homozygous typing cell (HTC) test
HTLV. *See* Human T cell leukemia virus
HTLV-III. *See* Human T lymphotrophic virus type III
Human B lymphotrophic virus (HBLV), 705
Human chromosome 6
    HLA complex organization, 59f
    major histocompatibility complex, 239f
Human herpesvirus type 6 (HHV-6), 705
Human immune globulin, 728–729
Human immunodeficiency virus (HIV), 689–700, 711
    aplastic anemia and, 434
    cancer and, 583–586
    cells infected, 692t
    cellular immunodeficiency with abnormal immunoglobulin
        synthesis, 290
    epidemiology, 692–693
    etiology, 689–692
    genital transmission, 566f
    genomic organization, 691f
    hairy leukoplakia and, 476f
    heterosexual transmission, 565–566
    hypogammaglobulinemia and, 268
    idiopathic thrombocytopenic purpura and, 436, 437, 438
    infection
        antigenic variation and, 734
        CD4 lymphocyte numbers, 696f
        clinical features, 693–694, 693t
        diethyldithiocarbamate and, 784
        differential diagnosis, 697, 697t
        individuals at risk, 693t
        live measles vaccine and, 727
        recombinant DNA vaccine and, 738
        thymic humoral factor and, 782
        treatment, 697–700
    laboratory diagnosis, 694–695
    life cycle, 697–698
    malaria and, 668
    perinatal transmission, 566–567
    pseudomembranous candidiasis and, 475f
    recurrent aphthous ulceration and, 474
    replicative cycle, 698f
    serologic response, 694f
    vaccines, 700
        obstacles to development, 700t
    visceral leishmanisis and, 671
Human immunodeficiency virus-1 (HIV-1), transfusion-trans-
        mitted, 232
Human immunodeficiency virus-2 (HIV-2), 690
Human leukocyte antigen. *See* HLA
Human papillomavirus (HPV), cervical carcinoma and, 570
Human T cell leukemia virus (HTLV), T cell leukemia and,
        570
Human T cell leukemia virus type I (HTLV-I), 112,
        703–705
    multiple sclerosis and, 510
    transfusion-transmitted, 232
Human T cell leukemia virus type II (HTLV-II), 703–705

Human T lymphotrophic virus type III (HTLV-III), 689
Humidifier lung disease, 366
Humoral immunity, 2, 26
    drugs inducing, 373
    measles virus and, 642
Humoral response, primary and secondary, 90–91, 91t
Hyalohyphomycosis, 651t
    immunologic abnormalities and, 653t
Hyaluronidase, 630
Hybridization, 217
    dot blot, 217, 219f
    in situ, 221, 222f
Hybridization assay, 217–218, 219f
Hybridoma, formation, 191f
Hydatid cyst, 676
    antibody-mediated anaphylactic shock and, 666
Hydralazine
    lupuslike syndrome and, 389, 530
    systemic lupus erythematosus syndrome and, 372
Hydrocarbon, aromatic, polycyclic, 569
Hydrochlorothiazide, 377
Hydrocortisone, 786
    bronchial obstruction and, 353
    chemical structure, 787f
    status asthmaticus and, 341
Hydrocortisone sodium succinate, recurrent aphthous ulcer-
        ation and, 475
Hydrogen peroxide, generation, respiratory burst and, 304f
Hydrops fetalis, 562
Hydroxychloroquine, 791
    discoid lupus erythematosus and, 505
    rheumatoid arthritis and, 396
    rheumatoid eye disease and, 522
    systemic lupus erythematosus and, 392
21-Hydroxylase, specificity and sensitivity, 414t
Hymenolepis nana, 676
Hymenoptera venom anaphylaxis, 349, 350–351
    desensitization, 353, 740
Hypercoagulation, systemic lupus erythematosus and, 389
Hypereosinophilic syndrome, 443, 533
Hypergammaglobulinemia
    polyclonal
        polymyositis-dermatomyositis and, 404
        progressive systemic sclerosis and, 403
        rheumatoid arthritis and, 395
        serum immunoglobulin abnormalities, 159f
    Sjogren's syndrome and, 400
Hypergammaglobulinemic purpura, benign, 610
Hyper-IgE syndrome, 307
    serum IgE levels, 336f
Hyper-IgM syndrome, 88
Hypermutation, somatic, 89
Hypersensitivity, 2, 137
    basophil, cutaneous, 150
    cell-mediated, 365
    delayed, 2, 314, 363, 626
        azimexone and, 784–785
        lymphocyte activation and, 204
        skin testing, 195–197, 259
    delayed-type, 100, 146
        acquired immunodeficiency syndrome and, 696
        corticosteroids and, 789
    desensitization therapy and, 742
    immediate, 149, 314
        drugs suppressing, 792–794
    mechanisms, 314–326
    non-gluten, 459
    oral unresponsiveness and, 549

Hypersensitivity (cont.)
  pneumonia, allergen bronchoprovocation and, 325
  pneumonitis, 366–370, 539
    allergens causing, 367t
    Aspergillus, 361
  respiratory disease and, 528
  T cell, 363–370
  vasculitis, 444–445
    skin biopsy specimen, 445f
Hypersensitivity disease, cell-mediated, 363–370
Hypertension, lupus nephritis and, 389
Hypervariable region, 75, 75f, 84
Hyperviscosity, plasmacytoid lymphocytic lymphoma and, 606
Hyperviscosity syndrome, plasma exchange and, 777
Hypnozoite, 667
Hypoalbuminemia
  rheumatoid arthritis and, 395
  systemic lupus erythematosus and, 390
Hypochlorite, generation, respiratory burst and, 304f
Hypocomplementemia, splenectomized patient and, 707–708
Hypocomplementemic urticarial vasculitis, 446
Hypogammaglobulinemia
  acquired, 271–273
  arthritis and, 409
  immune system neoplasms and, 591
  passive immunization, 731t
  serum gamma-globulin concentrations, 158
  serum immunoglobulin abnormalities, 159f
  severe combined, 726
  transient of infancy, 270–271
  X-linked
    atopic dermatitis and, 343
    serum immunoglobulin levels, 157t
  X-linked infantile, 266–270
    periodontal disease and, 267f
Hypoparathyroidism
  idiopathic, 422
  immunodeficiency and, 279–282
Hypoplastic anemia, congenital, 434
Hypoproteinemia, 158
Hyposensitization, desensitization therapy and, 741
Hypothyroidism, primary, 419
Hypoxanthine phosphoribosyl transferase (HPRT), 190

IBL. See Immunoblastic lymphadenopathy
IBS-B. See Immunoblastic sarcoma of B cell type
Ibuprofen, 790
iC3b, 131
ICAM-1. See Intracellular adhesion molecule-1
IDAT. See Indirect antiglobulin test
IDDM. See Insulin-dependent diabetes mellitus
Idiopathic cold-agglutin hemolytic anemia, chlorambucil and, 775
Idiopathic pulmonary fibrosis, 534–536
  differential diagnosis, 535t
Idiopathic thrombocytopenic purpura (ITP), 435–438, 713
  children and adults, 436t
  cyclophosphamide and, 773
  immune globulin and, 729
  intravenous gamma globulin and, 777–778
  prednisone and, 768
  tests for platelet autoantibodies, 436t
Idiotype, 75–77
Idiotypy, 380, 382–383
IEL. See Intraepithelial lymphocyte

IFA. See Indirect fluorescent-antibody assay
IFN. See Interferon
IgA, 69
  biologic activities, 73
  breast milk and, 550
  deficiency, selective, 273–276
    serum immunoglobulin levels, 157t
  Fc domain, 545
  IgG polymerization and, 545
  immune exclusion, 545–547
  mucosal immune system and, 544–547
  myeloma, urine abnormalities, 160f
  properties, 71t
  secretory, 70f
  secretory component, 545
  secretory versus circulating, 547
  serum, 70f
    variation with age, 156f
  structural forms, 546f
  synthesis, regulation at mucosal sites, 548–549, 548f
  transport, 545
  transport across epithelial cell, 547f
Ig-alpha, 87
Ig-beta, 87
IgD, 69
  biologic activities, 73–74
  properties, 71t
  surface, 86
IgE, 69
  antibodies
    anaphylaxis and, 348
    drug allergy and, 374
    environmental allergens and, 328f
    molecule, 317f
    tests, 323
  biologic activities, 74
  elevated, diseases associated, 328t
  interleukin-4 and, 116
  myeloma, serum IgE levels, 336f
  properties, 71t
  serum, allergies and IgE disorders and, 336f
IgE/mast cell/mediator pathway, 315–317
IgE-mediated inflammation, 149–150
  immunologic events, 149f
IgG, 69
  antibodies
    hypersensitivity pneumonitis and, 366
    penicillin and, 371
    tests, 323
  biologic activities, 73
  deficiency, selective, 276–277
  development with age, 155f
  hypervariable regions, 75f
  myeloma, serum immunoglobulin abnormalities, 159f
  properties, 71t
  serum, variation with age, 156f
  subclasses, 261
    properties, 73t
IgG2 deficiency, 277
IgG2-IgG4 deficiency, 277
IgG3 deficiency, 277
IgG4 deficiency, 277
IgG/complement/neutrophil pathway, 317
IgG-IgM mixed cryoglobulin, separation by gel filtration, 167f
IgM, 69, 70f
  biologic activities, 73

deficiency, selective, 276
heavy chain disease, 609
properties, 71t
serologic test, toxoplasmosis and, 669
serum, variation with age, 156f
IgM/complement/neutrophil pathway, 317
Ileitis
granulomatous, 459
regional, 459
Iliojejunitis, ulcerative, 458
Imexone, 784
Imidizole, candidiasis and, 660
Immediate hypersensitivity, 149, 314
drugs suppressing, 792–794
Immediate phase, 315
Immobilization assay, sperm, 560
Immune adherence, 184
Immune competence, laboratory testing, 257–262, 258t
indications, 257t
Immune complex, 147
detection, 169–170
hypersensitivity pneumonitis and, 366
immune hemolytic anemia and, 431
systemic lupus erythematosus and, 390–391
Immune complex allergic disease, 357–361
desensitization therapy and, 742
Immune complex glomerulonephritis, 481–487
antigen-antibody systems and, 485t
features, 483–484t
histologic forms, 485f
IgG deposits, 486f
Immune complex-mediated inflammation, 147–149
clinical manifestations, 148–149
immunologic events, 148f
Immune disease, immunoblastic sarcoma of B cell type and, 606
Immune globulin, human, 728–729
Immune hemolytic anemia, 427–433
classification, 428t
drug-induced, 430–431
clinical and laboratory features, 431t
Immune interferon, 116
Immune neutropenia, drug-induced, 426
Immune reaction, abnormal, 618–619
Immune reactivity, normal, 380–381, 381t
Immune regulation, disordered, mechanisms, 380–385
Immune response, 9, 40–49
anamnestic, 49
antigen-nonspecific therapy, 711, 713–715
antigen-specific therapy, 711, 712–713
development, 769f
helminths and, 673–678
host, parasites and, 667f
localization, 47–48
major histocompatibility complex and, 64
modulation, 712–715
primary, 48, 48f
protozoa and, 666–673
quantitative and kinetic aspects, 48–49
secondary, 48f, 49
sequence of events, 43f
tumor cells escaping, 574–575
Immune serum globulin (ISG), measles virus and, 642
Immune stimulation, 713–714
Immune surveillance, 574, 578–579
Immune system
memory, 40

modulation, 713–714
mucosal, 541–551, 541–551
anatomy, 541–544
cell traffic, 550f
functions, 541
IgA and, 544–547
oral unresponsiveness, 549
sperm and, 554
neoplasms, 588–619
benign conditions mimicking, 618–619
classification, 588, 589t
cytogenetics, 596–598
DNA analysis, 592–596
immunologic features, 589–592
molecular genetics, 599–600
most common, 602t
therapy, 600–601
programmed cell death, 49
role in allergy, 316f
secretory, components, 553f
selection process and, 37
self and nonself discrimination, 40
specificity, 40
tumors, 580
virus infections, 689–705
Immune thrombocytopenia
B cell neoplasms and, 591
classification, 435t
drug-induced, 438
Immunity
adoptive, 712–713
antibody-mediated, evaluation, 267t
cell-mediated, 26, 146–147
evaluation, 280t
live vaccines and, 726
periodontal disease and, 472
cellular, 2
cytomegalovirus and, 701
immune system neoplasms and, 591
influenza and, 638
measles virus and, 642
polymyositis-dermatomyositis and, 404
recurrent aphthous ulceration and, 474–475
chancre, 681
herd, 734
humoral, 2, 26
drugs inducing, 373
measles virus and, 642
mucosal, 553–554
pregnancy and, 558–559
T cell
carcinoembryonic antigen and, 572
drugs inducing, 373
eye disease and, 523
Immunization, 717–738
active, 712, 717–727
materials available, 719–725t
adults and elderly, 736, 737t
adverse reactions, 726
age and, 735
childhood, recommendations, 735–736, 736t
clinical indications, 734–737
combined passive-active, 734
desensitization therapy and, 741
foreign travel, 737
hepatitis B virus, 645
historical milestones, 718t

Immunization *(cont.)*
  passive, 712, 727–734
    materials available, 730–733*t*
  risk:benefit ratio, 726
  simultaneous with multiple antigens, 736–737
  technique, 726
  vaginal, 553
Immunoassay. *See also* Radioimmunoassay
  biotin-avidin-enhanced, 174–175, 175*f*
  complement components and, 188
  enzyme-multiplied, 173, 173*f*
  fluorescence polarization, 174, 174*f*
  quantitative, comparative sensitivity, 191, 192*t*
Immunoblastic lymphadenopathy (ILB), 618–619
Immunoblastic reaction, 618
Immunoblastic sarcoma of B cell type (IBS-B), 605–606
Immunochemistry, 2
Immunocompromise, cancer and, 579–580
Immunocompromised host, opportunistic infection, 706–709
Immunocytochemistry, 591–592
Immunodeficiency
  ataxia-telangiectasia and, 290–292
  B cell, 266–278
    treatment, 265*t*
  causes, 263*t*
  cell membrane abnormalities and, 298–300
  cellular, abnormal immunoglobulin synthesis and, 289–290
  classification, 264*t*
  clinical features, 264*t*
  congenital
    adoptive immunity and, 712
    immunoblastic sarcoma of B cell type and, 606
    neoplasia and, 580–581, 581*f*
  enzyme deficiency and, 295–297
  hyper-IgM and, 273
  hypoparathyroidism and, 279–282
  initial screening evaluation, 264*t*
  mechanisms, 263–265
  natural killer cell deficiency and, 284
  pulmonary manifestations, 537
  respiratory disease and, 528
  serum immunoglobulin levels and, 157*t*
  severe combined, 279–282
    adoptive immunity and, 713
    bone marrow transplantation and, 758
    live vaccines and, 726
  short-limbed dwarfism and, 294–295, 294*f*
  T cell, 279–284
    treatment, 265*t*
  thrombocytopenia, eczema, recurrent infection and, 292–293
  thymoma and, 293–294
  treatment, 265*t*
Immunodiffusion, 152–156
  applications, 155–156
  double, 152–54
    analysis of antigen and antibody, 153*f*
    reaction patterns, 153*f*
  methods and interpretation, 152–155
  radial, 154–155
    in agar, 154*f*
    standard curve, 155*f*
Immunodominance, 54
Immunoelectrophoresis, 156–165, 607, 608
  serum patterns in disease, 162–163*f*
  technique, 161*f*
  zone electrophoresis compared, 161*f*
Immunofixation electrophoresis, 161–164, 164*f*

Immunofluorescence, 2, 178–183
  clinical applications, 183*t*
  direct, 181, 181*f*
  indirect, 181, 182*f*
  method and interpretation, 179–181
  quantitative, 183
  staining techniques, 181–183
  systemic lupus erythematosus and, 391
Immunogenetics, 3
Immunogenic, 50
Immunogenicity, 55–56
Immunogen, 42, 50–51, 51*f*
  adjuvants and, 51–52
Immunoglobulin, 15, 24–25. *See also* IgA; IgD; IgE; IgG; IgM
  abnormal synthesis, cellular immunodeficiency and, 289–290
  barrel, 67
  biologic activities, 73–74
  carbohydrate moieties, 72–73
  classes and subclasses, composition, 69–70
  classification, 68–72
  complementarity-determining regions, 75
  constant regions, 68
  cross-linking, 30
  cytoplasmic, B cells and, 201
  diversity, 66
  enzymatic digestion products, 68
  4-chain basic unit, 67–68, 67*f*
  framework regions, 75
  gene rearrangements
    B cell malignancy and, 91–92
    early B cell ontogeny and, 84–86
  genes, B cell DNA rearrangement and, 80–84
  gene superfamily, 78, 78*t*, 121
  heavy chains, 25
  hinge regions, 68
  hypervariable regions, 75, 75*f*, 84
  idiotypes, 75–77
  interchain disulfide bonds, 71*f*
  light chains, 25
  membranes, 70–72
  mucosal production, 548
  opsonizing effects, 15
  properties, 69*t*, 71*t*
  proteins
    membrane-bound and secreted forms, 25*f*
    organization and diversity, 66–68
  secreted, 70–72
  secretion, 88–89
  serum
    development with age, 270*f*
    disease and, 155–156, 157*t*
    immune system neoplasms and, 589–591
    normal distribution, 277*f*
    patterns of abnormalities, 159*f*
    single radial diffusion and, 154
  specificity, 66
  surface, B cells and, 200–201, 201*t*
  three-dimensional structure, 77–78, 77*f*
  transmembrane component, 72
  variable regions, 68, 74–77
    subgroups, 75
Immunohistochemistry, neonatal HIV infection and, 567
Immunologic reagent, tumor-reactive, 571
Immunologic screening test, 709*t*
Immunologic therapy, 711–715
Immunology
  cellular, 2–3

history, 1–5
molecular, 3
origin, 1–2
tumor, mechanisms, 569–576
Immunomodulator, 781–785
biochemical agents, 784–785
derived from bacteria, 781–782
derived from eukaryotic organisms, 782–784
Immunopathic effect, 637
Immunophenotype
B cell lymphomas, 597f
B cell tumor antigens, 593t
T cell tumor antigens, 594t
Immunophenotyping, 591–592
Immunopoietic cell neoplasm, 588
Immunoprecipitation, 152, 184
Immunoradiometric assay (IRMA), 173
Immunorestorative therapy, human immunodeficiency virus
and, 699–700
Immunoselection, 574
Immunostimulant, recurrent aphthous ulceration and,
475
Immunosuppression, 619, 714–715
active, 713
bone transplantation and, 762
cyclosporin and, 775–776
cytotoxic drugs and, 769–770
liver transplantation and, 752
lung transplantation and, 757
nonspecific, parasitic infection and, 666
pancreas transplantation and, 753–754
passive, 713
placenta and, 558–559
Immunosuppressive therapy, 765–779
acute disseminated encephalomyelitis and, 508
antibody-producing cells and, 770f
aplastic anemia and, 434, 758
autoimmune hemolytic anemia and, 430
corneal graft reactions and, 527
epidermolysis bullosa acquisita and, 500
Goodpasture's syndrome and, 536
graft-versus-host disease and, 760
herpes gestationis and, 497
hypocomplementemic urticarial vasculitis and, 446
idiopathic thrombocytopenic purpura and, 437
immune-complex glomerulonephritis and, 486–487
live vaccines and, 726
minimal-change nephropathy and, 489
myasthenia gravis and, 514
Reiter's syndrome and, 407
relapsing panniculitis and, 409
rheumatoid arthritis and, 396
rheumatoid eye disease and, 522
Sjögren's syndrome and, 401
sympathetic ophthalmia and, 525
systemic lupus erythematosus and, 392
Vogt-Koyanagi-Harada syndrome and, 525
Immunosurveillance, 100
Immunotherapy, 575–576
cellular, adoptive, 575–576
research, 578–579
type I diabetes mellitus and, 421t
Impetigo, 502
Implantation, 555
Imprecise joining, 84, 95
Imprecision profile, 175, 177
Inborn errors of metabolism, liver transplantation and,
750

Indirect agglutination test, 184–185
Indirect antiglobulin test (IDAT), 229
Indirect Coombs test, 186
technique, 230f
Indirect fluorescent-antibody assay (IFA), Lyme disease and,
686
Indirect immunofluorescence, 181, 182f
Indomethacin
asthma and, 338
Behcet's disease and, 446
hypocomplementemic urticarial vasculitis and, 446
Induration, 146
Infantile hypogammaglobulinemia, X-linked, 266–270
periodontal disease and, 267f
Infection
active immunization and, 712
bone marrow transplantation and, 761, 761t
immunologic defenses, 625–625
immunopathology, 625–626
nonimmunologic defenses, 622–624
opportunistic, 706–709
cyclosporin and, 776
parasitic, nonspecific immunosuppression and, 666
pregnancy and, 558
recurrent
hyper-IgE syndrome and, 307
immunodeficiency with, 292–293
serum immunoglobulin levels, 157t
splenectomized patient and, 708
transfusion-transmitted, 232, 232t
viral, 637–647, 689–705
immunologic sequelae, 638t
slow and latent, 517
Infectious hepatitis, serum immunoglobulin levels, 157t
Infectious mononucleosis, 430, 702–703
immunoblastic reactions, 618
pathogenesis, 703f
serum immunoglobulin levels, 157t
Infectious rhinitis, 333
Infectious syndrome, differential diagnosis, 708t
Infective endocarditis, 630
Infertility, 559–561
immune causes, 559–560
immune therapies, 560–561
Inflammation, 47, 137–150
acute, 16, 137
complement activation, 131–132
granulomatous, 146
host defense and, 623–624
IgE-mediated, 139, 149–150
immunologic events, 149f
immune complex-mediated, 147–149
clinical manifestations, 148–149
immunologic events, 148f
immunologically mediated, 145–150
classes, 145t
mediators, 142–145, 142t
Inflammatory bowel disease
interleukin-1 receptor antagonist and, 784
oral unresponsiveness and, 549
Inflammatory cell, 47, 138–142, 138t
immunoglobulin Fc receptors, 138t
Inflammatory infiltrate, chronic, 146
Inflammatory mediator, 47, 137, 142–145, 142t
chemotactic, 144–145
enzymatic, 145
smooth muscle-constricting, 142–144
vasoactive, 142–144

Inflammatory response, 137, 711
  cell-mediated, immunologic events, 146*f*
  corticosteroids and, 789
  immediate phase, 149–150
  immunologically mediated, 145–150
  late phase, 150
  modulation, 715
Influenza, 637–639
  active immunization, 719*t*, 720*t*
  pandemic, 637
Influenza A, pregnancy and, 558
Influenza A virus, 637–638
Influenza B virus, 638
Influenza virus, 637–639
  antigenic shift and, 734
  genetic reassortment, 638*f*
  insulin-dependent diabetes mellitus and, 420
  structural proteins, 638*t*
Initiation, 579
Innocent-bystander phenomenon, 426, 431, 435
Inosine pranobex, acquired immunodeficiency syndrome and,
    699–700, 784
Inositol 1,4,5-trisphosphate (IP3), 30, 97, 30, 97
Insect bite, wheal formation and, 355–356
Insect venom anaphylaxis, 350–351
  desensitization, 740
  prophylaxis, 322
Insemination, intrauterine, 560
In situ hybridization, 221, 222*f*
  neonatal HIV infection and, 567
Insulin
  allergy, 378–379
  covalent structure, 378*f*
  immunogenicity, 371
  receptor antibodies, specificity and sensitivity, 414*t*
Insulin-dependent diabetes mellitus (IDDM), 419–421
  immunotherapy trials, 421*t*
Integrin, 13, 132, 312
Intercellular adhesion molecule type-1 (ICAM-1), 13
Interdigitating cell, 35, 63
Interference, 175, 177
Interferon (IFN), 114–116, 782–783
  antiviral, 115–116
  host defense and, 624
  immune, 116
  influenza virus and, 639
  multiple sclerosis and, 384
  natural killer cells and, 573
  type I, 115
    induction and activity, 115*f*
Interferon-alpha, 115
  antitumor activity, 782
  hepatitis B virus and, 466, 644–645
  immune system neoplasms and, 601
  properties, 107*t*
Interferon-beta, 115
  antineoplastic activity, 782
  properties, 107*t*
Interferon beta-1b, multiple sclerosis and, 511
Interferon-gamma, 18, 39, 47, 100
  allograft rejection and, 748
  antitumor activity, 782–783
  leishmaniasis and, 671
  macrophage-activating factor and, 573
  multiple sclerosis and, 509
  properties, 107*t*
Interleukin, 3, 10, 711, 783
  properties, 106–107*t*

  receptors, 714
Interleukin-1 (IL-1), 45, 105–112, 478, 479
  actions on cells and tissues, 108*f*
  host defense and, 624
  inhibitors
    influenza and, 638
    as therapeutic agents, 111–112
  nonimmunologic effects, 110–111
  properties, 106*t*
  receptor, signal transduction and, 109–110
  receptor antagonist, 107, 784
  release, antigen stimulation and, 767*f*
  target cells and actions, 109*t*
  tolerance and, 383
Interleukin-2 (IL-2), 44, 100, 112–113
  allograft rejection and, 748
  clinical applications, 427*t*
  cyclosporin and, 776
  cytotoxic T cell activation and, 31
  effects on non-T cells, 113
  effects on T cells, 112–113
  human immunodeficiency virus and, 699
  lymphokine-activated killer cells and, 576
  malignancy and, 783
  natural killer cells and, 103, 573, 714
  properties, 106*t*
  receptor, 44, 714
    signal transduction and, 112
  related molecules as therapeutic agents, 113
Interleukin-3 (IL-3), 10
  clinical applications, 427*t*
  hematopoiesis and, 120
  lymphopoiesis and, 22
  natural cytotoxic cells and, 573
  properties, 106*t*
Interleukin-4 (IL-4), 100, 116–117
  antitumor activity, 783
  macrophage-activating factor and, 573
  properties, 106*t*
Interleukin-5 (IL-5), 100, 117
  eosinophils and, 139
  properties, 106*t*
Interleukin-6 (IL-6), 45, 88, 113–114, 114*t*
  clinical applications, 427*t*
  cytokine family, 114*t*
    activities, 114
  properties, 106*t*
  receptor, 114
Interleukin-7 (IL-7), 117
  properties, 106*t*
Interleukin-8 (IL-8), 118–120, 478, 479
  properties, 106*t*
Interleukin-9 (IL-9), 117
  properties, 106*t*
Interleukin-10 (IL-10), 117
  autoimmune disease and, 783
  properties, 106*t*
Interleukin-11 (IL-11), 114
  properties, 106*t*
Interleukin-12 (IL-12), 100, 117
  human immunodeficiency virus and, 699
  properties, 106*t*
Interleukin-13 (IL-13), 116–117
  properties, 106*t*
Interpolation, 173, 177
Interstitial fluid, 32
Interstitial pneumonitis, 366
Intracellular adhesion molecule-1 (ICAM-1), 479

Intracellular bacteria, 627, 633–635, 634*f*
Intracellular free calcium ion, 30
Intracellular killing
   myeloperoxidase deficiency and, 306
   tests, 212–214
Intradermal skin test, 321–322
Intraepithelial lymphocyte (IEL) compartment, 543
Intraepithelial lymphocyte (IEL), 543
Intraleukocytic killing test, 212
Intrauterine insemination, 560
Intrinsic asthma, 335–336
Intron, 80
Invariant chain (Ii), 62
Invasive aspergillosis, 361
In vitro fertilization, 560
In vitro testing
   allergic disease and, 322–324
   drug allergy and, 375
Ion exchange chromatography, 166, 166*f*
Ionic compound, anaphylactoid reactions and, 351
Ionizing radiation, carcinogenesis and, 570
Ipratropium bromide, asthma and, 341
Iridocyclitis, 523
   acute, 521*f*, 522*f*
   juvenile arthritis and, 398
IRMA. *See* Immunoradiometric assay
Ischemia-reperfusion injury, interleukin-1 receptor antagonist
     and, 784
ISG. *See* Immune serum globulin
Islet cell transplantation, 754
Isocyanate, hypersensitivity pneumonitis and, 366, 368
Isoetharine, 793
   asthma and, 340
Isoimmune hydrops, pathophysiology, 562
Isoimmunization, 562–565
   ABO incompatibility and, 562–563
   anti-Rh immunoglobulin prophylaxis, 563–564
   Rh, 233–234
     passive immunization, 732*t*
     prevention, 729–733
Isoimmunized pregnancy, management, 564–565
Isoniazid, lupuslike syndrome and, 389, 530
Isotype, 69
Isotype switching, 89
Isotypic exclusion, 86
ITP. *See* Idiopathic thrombocytopenic purpura
Itraconazole
   blastomycosis and, 654
   histoplasmosis and, 658
   paracoccidioidomycosis and, 659
Ixodes pacificus, 685
Ixodes ricinus, 685
Ixodes scapularis, 685

Japanese B encephalitis, formalin-inactivated vaccine, 737
Jarisch-Herxheimer reaction, 352, 684
Jaw claudication, giant cell arteritis and, 452
J chain, 69–70, 70*f*, 72
   properties, 69*t*
JC virus, 517–518
Jenner, Edward, 1, 3
Jenner, William, 711, 717
Jerne, Niels K., 3, 4, 5, 42
Job's syndrome, 306, 307*f*
Joint
   arthritic, 111
   juvenile arthritis and, 397–398

progressive systemic sclerosis and, 402
   rheumatoid arthritis and, 393–394
   systemic lupus erythematosus and, 388
Junctional diversity, 95
Juvenile arthritis, 397–399
Juvenile rheumatoid arthritis, 521

Kabat, Elvin A., 2, 4
Kallikrein
   basophil of anaphylaxis, 348
   tissue, 134–135
K antigen, 631
Kantrowitz, Adrian, 757
Kaposi's sarcoma, 694
   AIDS-associated, pathogenesis, 583, 584*f*
   interferon-gamma and, 782
   organ transplant recipients and, 582, 776
Kappa chain, 68–69
   genes, 81
     assembly and expression, 81*f*
     mechanism of rearrangement, 82*f*
Katayama fever, 675
Kawasaki disease, 713
   immune globulin and, 733–734
   intravenous gamma globulin and, 778
Kell blood group system, 228–229, 305
Keratin, 9
Keratoconjunctivitis
   atopic, 521
   herpetic, interferon-alpha and, 782
   phlyctenular, 525, 525*f*
   vernal, 334
Keratoconjunctivitis sicca, Sjogren's syndrome and, 400
Keratoderma blennorrhagicum, 407
Kernicterus, 562
Ketoconazole
   candidiasis and, 660
   coccidioidomycosis and, 657
   histoplasmosis and, 658
   paracoccidioidomycosis and, 659
   type I polyglandular syndrome and, 423
Kidd blood group system, 228–229
Kidney
   progressive systemic sclerosis and, 402
   systemic lupus erythematosus and, 388–389, 391
Kidney disease, multicystic with proteinuria, urine abnormali-
     ties, 160*f*
Kidney transplantation, 744–749
   blood transfusion and, 746
   cadaveric, 745
   CML test and, 247
   donor selection, evaluation, procedures, 745–746
   focal glomerulosclerosis and, 489
   Goodpasture's syndrome and, 537
   immunosuppression and, 746–747
   living related donor, 744–745
   patient, histocompatibility testing flowchart, 239*t*
   rejection, 747–749
   survival, 749
   technique, 746*f*
Kiel classification, 588, 589*t*
Killed vaccine, 56
Killing
   antibody-dependent, 573
   intracellular
     myeloperoxidase deficiency and, 306
     tests, 212–214

Kinin
  activation, 133
  asthmatic attack and, 337
  cascade, 133–135
    proteins, 133
  functions in disease, 135
  generation
    amplification and regulation, 134
    plasma inhibitors, 134
  hemolytic transfusion reactions and, 233
Kinin-generating pathway, 134*f*
Kininogen
  high-molecular-weight, 133
  low-molecular-weight, 134–135
Kitasato, Shibasaburo, 2, 3
Klebsiella, 631
Klebsiella pneumoniae, 631, 633
Koch, Robert, 1, 3, 4, 7*f*, 717
Koch's postulates, 1
Kohler, Georges J. F., 3, 4, 5, 189
Kraus, Rudolf, 2, 4
Kung, Patrick, 3, 4

Label, 171
  enzymatic, 173–174
  fluoremetric, 174
  radioisotopic, 173–174
Laboratory testing
  allergic disease and, 318
  immune competence, 257–262, 258*t*
    indications, 257*t*
  limitations, 257
  utility, 256
    clinical, 257
  variability, 256
Lactoferrin, 15
Laennec's cirrhosis, serum immunoglobulin levels, 157*t*
Lag phase, 48
LAK cell. *See* Lymphokine-activated killer (LAK) cell
Lambda chain, 68–69
  genes, assembly, 83*f*
  subtypes, 69
Lambert-Eaton syndrome, 515, 517
Lamina propria lymphocyte (LPL), 543–544
Lamina propria lymphocyte (LPL) compartment, 543
Lamina propria macrophage, 544
Lamina propria mast cell, 544
Lamina propria natural killer cell, 544
Landsteiner, Karl, 2, 4, 8*f*, 54
Landsteiner-Chase phenomenon, 364
Langerhans cell, 36, 63, 363
Large granular lymphocyte (LGL), 617
Large granular lymphocyte (LGL) leukemia, 617–618
Larva migrans, visceral, 533
Larygeal papillomatosis, interferon-alpha and, 782
Laryngeal edema, anaphylaxis and, 352–353
Latent phase, 48
Late phase, 317
Latex allergy, 351
Latex fixation test, 186, 395, 400
Laurell's rocket electrophoresis, 165
LAV. *See* Lymphadenopathy-associated virus
L chain disease, serum immunoglobulin levels, 157*t*
LCR. *See* Ligase chain reaction
Least squares method, 177
LE cell phenomenon, 387, 390
Legionella, 634

Legionella pneumophila, 634, 709
Leishmania, 669
Leishmania aethiopica, 670
Leishmania braziliensis, 670
Leishmania donovani, 671
Leishmania major, 670–671
  helper T cell response and, 100
Leishmania mexicana, 670
Leishmania mexicana subsp *pifanoi*, 670
Leishmaniasis, 533, 669–671
  cutaneous, 670–671
  lupoid, 670
  posttransfusion, 232
  recidiva, 670
  visceral, 671
Leishmania tropica, 670
Lennert's lymphoma, 613
Lens-induced uveitis, 523
Lentivirus, 690
Lepidoglyphus destructor, 331
Lepidoptera, 331
Lepromatous leprosy, interleukin-2 and, 113
Leprosy, 635
  interferon-gamma and, 783
  lepromatous, interleukin-2 and, 113
Leptospira, 680
Leptospira interrogans, 687
Leptospirosis, 680, 687
Letterer-Siwe disease, 298, 343
Leukemia
  acute lymphoblastic, bone marrow transplantation and, 759
  acute lymphocytic, 602–603, 610–612
  acute monocytic, 617
  acute myelogenous, bone marrow transplantation and, 758–759
  acute myelomonocytic, 617
  B cell, 591*f*
    monoclonal surface immunoglobulins and, 591
  chronic lymphocytic, 87, 157*t*
  chronic myelogenous
    bone marrow transplantation and, 759
    interferon-alpha and, 782
  eosinophilic, 443
  granulocytic, lymphocytic leukemia and, 617
  hairy cell, 606
    interferon-alpha and, 782
  immunocompromised host and, 707
  large granular lymphocyte, 617–618
  live vaccines and, 726
  lymphocytic
    granulocytic leukemia and, 617
    phenotypic markers, 595–596*t*
  monocytic, serum immunoglobulin levels, 157*t*
  natural killer cell, 617–618
  prolymphocytic, 604
    T cell type, 612
  small lymphocytic, 603–604
  T cell
    adult, 112, 612
    human T cell leukemia virus and, 570
Leukemic reticuloendotheliosis, 606
Leukocidin, nonhemolytic, 630
Leukocyte
  circulating, corticosteroids and, 765–766, 766*f*
  disorders, 425–427
  interferons and, 115
  polymorphonuclear, 10
Leukocyte adhesion deficiency, 299–300

Leukocyte adhesion glycoprotein, comparative structures, 300*f*
Leukocyte adhesion molecule deficiency, natural killer cell deficiency and, 284
Leukocyte functional antigen type-1 (LFA-1), 13, 98
Leukocyte functional antigen type-3 (LFA-3), 98
Leukocyte infiltration, 144
Leukocyte inhibitory factor (LIF), 114
Leukocyte movement disorder, 307
Leukoencephalopathy, multifocal, 727
  progressive, 517–518
Leukopenia, 425
  major causes, 426*t*
Leukoplakia, hairy, 475, 476*f*
Leukotriene, 144
  asthmatic attack and, 337
  rheumatoid arthritis and, 393
Levamisole
  Beçhet's disease and, 446
  colon cancer and, 784
Levey-Jennings chart, 177
Lewis antigen, 227
Lewis blood group system, 227
LFA-1. *See* Leukocyte functional antigen type-1
LGL. *See* Large granular lymphocyte
Lichen planopilaris, 505
Lichen simplex chronicus, 342
LIF. *See* Leukocyte inhibitory factor
Ligand, 171
  free, adsorption, 172
Ligand assay, 170
Ligase chain reaction (LCR), 223
  DNA amplification and, 223*f*
Light (L) chain, 25, 67–68
  allotypic forms, 72
  genes, 81
    assembly and expression, 81*f*
  properties, 69*t*
  surrogate, 86
  three-dimensional structure, 76*f*
  types and subtypes, 68–69
Limited-reagent method, 175
Linear epitope, 53, 53*f*
Linear IgA bullous dermatosis, 503–504
Lipid, immunogenic, 42
Lipomodulin, 715, 788
Lipopolysaccharide (LPS), 107, 782
Lipoxygenase, 788
5-Lipoxygenase metabolite, 144
  chemical structures, 143*f*
Liquid scintillation counter, 172
Lister, Joseph, 1
Listeria, 634
Listeria monocytogenes, 558, 634, 781
Listeriosis, postpartum, 558
Livedo reticularis, cold-agglutinin syndromes and, 430
Liver
  cancer, hepatitis B virus and, 570
  disease, serum immunoglobulin levels, 157*t*
  failure, liver transplantation and, 750
  venoocclusive disease, chemoradiotherapy and, 760–761
  transplantation, 749–752
    cross-matching and, 752
    immunosuppression and, 752
    indications, 750–751
    orthotopic, 751
    procedure, 751, 751*f*
    survival, 752

Loa loa, 676
  transfusion-transmitted, 232
Loeffler's endomyocardial disease, 443
Loeffler's syndrome, 531
Logit transformation, 172, 172*f*
Lou Gehrig's disease, 516–517
Louse-borne relapsing fever, 686
Lower detection limit, 175, 176, 177
Low-molecular-weight kininogen, 134–135
LPL. *See* Lamina propria lymphocyte
LPS. *See* Lipopolysaccharide
Lukes-Collins classification, 588, 589*t*
Lung
  cancer, thmyosin and, 782
  disease
    environmental, 533
    humidifier, 366
    obstructive, heart-lung transplantation and, 755
    occupational, 533
    rheumatoid, 398
  progressive systemic sclerosis and, 402
  systemic lupus erythematosus and, 389
  transplantation, 538, 755–756
Lungworm, 676
Lupoid leishmaniasis, 670
Lupus anticoagulant, 440
Lupus erythematosus (LE) cell phenomenon, 387, 390
Lupus nephritis, 389
  plasma exchange and, 777
Lupus syndrome, drug-induced, 530
Ly-49, 103
LYDMA. *See* Lymphocyte-determined membrane antigen
Lyme arthritis, 685
Lyme disease, 398, 680, 684–686
  multiple sclerosis and, 510
Lymph, 32
Lymphadenopathy, 35
  angioimmunoblastic, 618–619
  immunoblastic, 618–619
Lymphadenopathy-associated virus (LAV), 689
Lymphatic circulation, 32–35
Lymphatic filariasis, 678
Lymphatic vasculature system, 32*f*
Lymphatic vessel
  afferent, 32
  efferent, 33
  primary, 32
Lymph node, 32–35
  structure, 33*f*
Lymphoblast, 30
Lymphoblastic leukemia, acute, bone marrow transplantation and, 759
Lymphocyte, 9, 22–39. *See also* B cell; T cell
  activation, 24, 25*f*, 29–30, 31*f*, 203–209
    antigens and, 206–208, 207*f*, 207*t*, 208*f*
    biochemical and morphological events, 29*f*
    mitogens and, 205–206, 206*f*, 206*t*, 207*f*
  assays, 197–203
  circulation, 38–39
  clonality, gene rearrangement and, 220–221
  clonal organization and dynamics, 40–42
  clonal selection, 41, 41*f*
  clones, 40
  corticosteroids and, 766–767
  cyclophosphamide and, 773*f*
  cytotoxic, human immunodeficiency virus and, 696
  cytotoxic drugs and, 768–769
  double-negative, 29

Lymphocyte *(cont.)*
  double-positive, 29
  electron micrograph, 23*f*
  intraepithelial, 543
  lamina propria, 543–544
  large granular, 617
  memory, 24
  mixed culture, 208–209, 208*f*, 246–247
  primary repertoire, 41
  properties, 10*t*
  reactivity, pregnancy and, 559
  "resting" state, 22–23
  single-positive, 29
  suppressive factors in serum, 205*t*
  T-gamma, 617
  tumor-infiltrating, 714, 783
  "virgin", 23
Lymphocyte-determined membrane antigen (LYDMA), 703
Lymphocytic adenohypophysitis, 421
Lymphocytic leukemia
  acute, 602–603
    T cell type, 610–612
  granulocytic leukemia and, 617
  phenotypic markers, 595–596*t*
  small, 603–604
Lymphocytic lymphoma
  lymphoepithelioid, T cell type, 613
  plasmacytoid, 606–607
  small, 603–604
Lymphocytic neoplasm
  B cell, 601–607
  T cell, 610–614
Lymphocytotoxicity, cross-matching and, 244
Lymphocytotoxicity test
  complement-dependent, 240–241
  scoring, 241*t*
  tissue typing and, 240–242
Lymphoepithelioid lymphocytic lymphoma, T cell type, 613
Lymphoid aggregate, mucosal, 542
Lymphoid cancer, congenital immunodeficiency syndromes
    and, 581
Lymphoid cell, proportion in normal tissues, 24*t*
Lymphoid follicle, 33, 33*f*
  primary and secondary, 34*f*
  transmission electron micrograph, 543*f*
Lymphoid organ, 31–38
  peripheral, 23–24
  primary, 22
  secondary, 23–24
  subepithelial, 36
  tertiary, 39
Lymphoid pathway, 11*f*
Lymphoid stem cell, 22
Lymphoid tissue, mucosal, 36
  diffuse, 543–544
Lymphokine-activated killer (LAK) cell, 103, 544, 573, 576,
    714, 783
  interleukin-2 and, 113
  interleukin-7 and, 117
Lymphokine, 26, 105
  allograft rejection and, 748
  macrophage-activating factor and, 573
  natural killer cells and, 103, 573
Lympholysis, cell-mediated, 208–209, 208*f*, 246*f*, 247–248
Lymphoma
  AIDS-associated, 619
    pathogenesis, 584–585
  autoimmune disease and, 582

B cell, 591*f*
  DNA cell cycle, 597*f*
  immunophenotype, 597*f*
  monoclonal surface immunoglobulins and, 591
  pathogenesis, 585*f*
Burkitt's, 91–92
  Epstein-Barr virus and, 570
  oncogenes and, 598
  t(8,14) chromosomal anomaly, 92*f*
follicular, 49, 92
follicular center cell, 604–605
immunocompromised host and, 707
Lennert's, 613
live vaccines and, 726
lymphocytic
  lymphoepithelioid, 613
  plasmacytoid, 606–607
  small, 603–604
non-Hodgkin
  ataxia-telangiectasia and, 580
  human immunodeficiency virus and, 583–584
  interferon-alpha and, 782
  multiple-agent chemotherapy, 600*t*
  organ transplant recipients and, 582, 776
  radiation therapy and, 600
  phenotypic markers, 595–596*t*
  T cell, 611*t*
    convoluted, 612
    cutaneous, 613–614
    human immunodeficiency virus and, 584
    interferon-alpha and, 782
    peripheral, 613
Lymphomatoid granulomatosis, 537
Lymphoplasmapheresis, kidney transplantation and, 747
Lymphopoiesis, 22
  schematic overview, 24*f*
Lymphoproliferative disease
  pyroglobulins and, 169
  T-gamma, 617–618
Lymphoproliferative syndrome, X-linked, 277–278, 619
  cancer and, 580
  natural killer cell deficiency and, 284
Lymphotoxin, 110
  tumor cells and, 573
Lysin, 717
Lysosome, 10, 17
Lysozyme, 9, 15

MAC. *See* **Membrane attack complex;** *Mycobacterium*
    avium **complex**
Macroglobulinemia
  pyroglobulins and, 169
  Waldenstrom's, 154, 158
    monoclonal serum immunoglobulins and, 589
    plasmacytoid lymphocytic lymphoma and, 606
    plasma exchange and, 777
    serum immunoglobulin abnormalities, 159*f*
    serum viscosity and, 168
Macrophage, 9, 18, 63
  activation, 18–19
  corticosteroids and, 767
  enumeration, 262
  host defense and, 19–20, 624
  human immunodeficiency virus and, 697
  interferon-gamma and, 116
  interleukin-2 and, 113
  lamina propria, 544
  multiple sclerosis and, 509

phagocytic responses, 18–19
properties, 10t
secretory activity, 19
secretory products, 19t
splenic, 36
tumor cells and, 573–574
Macrophage-activating factor (MAF), 573
Maculopapular rash, graft-versus-host disease and, 298f
MAF. See Macrophage-activating factor
Major basic protein, 138
Major histocompatibility complex (MHC), 3, 26, 42, 52, 58
    antigen-specific immune suppression and, 713
    chromosome 6 and, 239f
    class I proteins, 42
        antigen presentation, 61–62
        interferon and, 115–116
        interferon-gamma and, 116
    class II proteins, 42, 86
        antigen presentation, 61–62
        interferon-gamma and, 116
        organ-specific disease and, 384
    disease and, 64–65, 64t
    genetic organization, 58–59
    immune responsiveness and, 64
    placental expression, 557
    T cell receptor, 713
    tumor-specific antigens and, 571
Malabsorption
    gluten-sensitive enteropathy and, 458
    hypogammaglobulinemia and, 269
Malaria, 533, 666–668
    antigen-antibody glomerulonephritis and, 666
    chemoprophylaxis, 737
    human immunodeficiency virus infection and, 668
    posttransfusion, 232
    pregnancy and, 558
Malignancy. See also Cancer; Neoplasia
    B cell, immunoglobulin gene rearrangements and, 91–92
    cyclophosphamide and, 773
    cyclosporin and, 776
    interleukin-2 and, 783
Malignant histiocytosis, 616
Malignant melanoma, interleukin-2 and, 783
Malignant transformation, molecular model, 580f
MALT. See Mucosa-associated lymphoid tissue
Mansonella ozzardi, transfusion-transmitted, 232
Margination, 12, 13f
Mast cell, 74
    atopic disease and, 327
    electron micrograph, 140f
    inflammation and, 139–141
    lamina propria, 544
    mediators, 140
    properties, 140t
Mast cell-associated mediator, asthmatic attack and, 337
Mastocytosis, systemic, cromolyn sodium and, 792
Maternal-fetal-placental complex, 556f
Maternal tissue, trophoblast, 555–557
Mayfly, 331
MC-1, 13
McDevitt, Hugh O., 3, 4
M cell, 542
McLeod phenotype, 229, 305
MCP. See Membrane cofactor protein
MCP-1. See Monocyte chemoattractant protein-1
M-CSF. See Monocyte colony-stimulating factor
Measles, 641–642, 717, 736
    encephalitis, 726

immunization, 718
    active, 720t
    passive, 731t
    vaccine, age recommendations, 735
    vaccinination, reportable events, 728t
Measles virus, 641–642, 718
    antigens, subacute sclerosing panencephalitis and, 517
Mechlorethamine, Hodgkin's disease and, 616
Medawar, Peter Brian, 3, 4
Mediastinum, drug-induced inflammation, 530
Medulla, 33, 35
Medullary reticulosis, histiocytic, 616
Melanoma
    interleukin-2 and, 113
    malignant, interleukin-2 and, 783
Melphalan, multiple myeloma and, 608
Membrane attack complex (MAC), 128–129, 129f, 478
Membrane cofactor protein (MCP), 133
Memory
    immune system, 40
    lymphocytes, 24
    thymus-independent antigens and, 56
Meniere's disease, antihistamines and, 793
Meningitis
    coccidioidal, 657
    cryptococcal, 661
    neonatal, 632
Meningococcus, 633
    active immunization, 720–721t
    splenectomized patient and, 707
6-Mercaptopurine, 771
    Crohn's disease and, 460
    ulcerative colitis and, 462
Mercuric chloride, anti-glomerular basement membrane antibody response and, 480
Merozoite, 667
Metabolic burst, 16
Metacholine, bronchoprovocation testing and, 318, 319f
Metacholine challenge test, 324
Metachromatic, 139
Metal dermatitis, 364
Metaproterenol, 793
    asthma and, 340
Metchnikoff, Elie I. I., 2, 3, 4, 7f
Methimazole, Graves' disease and, 418
Methotrexate, 768, 773–774
    adverse pulmonary responses, 530
    graft-versus-host disease and, 760
    pemphigus vulgaris and, 503
    polymyositis-dermatomyositis and, 406
    properties and uses, 774t
    Reiter's syndrome and, 407
    rheumatoid arthritis and, 396
    Takayasu arteritis and, 455
    Wegener's granulomatosis and, 451
Methyldopa
    immune hemolytic anemia and, 431
    lupuslike syndrome and, 389
Methylprednisolone
    allergic contact dermatitis and, 364
    allograft rejection and, 748–749
    bronchial obstruction and, 353
    liver transplantation and, 752
    multiple sclerosis and, 511
    status asthmaticus and, 341
Methylxanthine, immediate hypersensitivity reactions and, 793–794
Metronidazole, Crohn's disease and, 460

MHA-TP test, 684
MHC. *See* Major histocompatibility complex
Microbicidal assay, 213–214
Microcytotoxicity testing, 241*f*
Microfilaria, 678
Microglobulin, 59
Microsomal antigen, specificity and sensitivity, 414*t*
Milk protein
  hypersensitivity, oral unresponsiveness and, 549
  immune response and, 382
Milstein, Cesar, 3, 4, 5, 189
Mineralocorticoid
  adrenal insufficiency and, 421
  mechanism of action, 787–788
Minimal-change nephropathy, 489
Minimum detectable dose, 177
Minimum detection limit, 177
Mite, allergenic, 330–331
Mitogen, 30, 30*t*
  B cell activation and, 201
  lymphocyte activation and, 205–206, 206*f*, 206*t*, 207*f*
Mitogenesis, 29
Mitotic cycle, 768*f*, 769
Mixed connective tissue disease, progressive systemic sclerosis and, 403
Mixed hemadsorption, 184
Mixed lymphocyte culture (MLC), 208–209, 208*f*
Mixed lymphocyte culture (MLC) test, 246–247, 246*f*
Mixed-lymphocyte reaction (MLR), 246
MLC. *See* Mixed lymphocyte culture
MLR. *See* Mixed-lymphocyte reaction
MMR vaccine, 726, 736
Mold allergen, 329–330, 330*f*, 332*t*
Molecular genetics, immune system neoplasms and, 599–600
Molecular histocompatibility, techniques, 249*t*
Molecular immunology, 3
Molecular mimicry, 382, 413*f*
Monobactam, 376*f*
  core structure, 376*f*
Monoclonal antibody, 3, 67, 189–190, 711–712, 778–779, 784
  allograft rejection and, 749
  antiendotoxin, 784
  applications, 191*t*
  graft-versus-host disease and, 760
  HLA antigens, 242
  immune stimulation and, 714
  immune system neoplasms and, 601
  kidney transplantation and, 746–747
  liver transplantation and, 752
  technique of production, 190
  therapeutic activity, 576
Monoclonal gammopathy, 607
  benign, 609
  serum immunoglobulin levels, 157*t*
Monoclonal paraproteinemia, cryoglobulins and, 169
Monocyte, 9, 17–18
  assays, 197–203
  corticosteroids and, 766–767
  electron micrograph, 18*f*
  enumeration, 262
  host defense and, 624
  human immunodeficiency virus and, 697
  interleukin-1 release, antigen stimulation and, 767*f*
  interleukin-2 and, 113
  multiple sclerosis and, 509
  properties, 10*t*
Monocyte chemoattractant protein-1 (MCP-1), 478

Monocyte colony-stimulating factor (M-CSF), 10, 120
Monocyte-macrophage assay, 209
Monocyte-macrophage system, 17–20
  cells, 17*t*
Monocytic leukemia
  acute, 617
  serum immunoglobulin levels, 157*t*
Monocytopenia, corticosteroids and, 765–766
Monokine, 105
Mononeuritis multiplex, 451
Mononuclear phagocyte system, 17
  neoplasms, 616–617
Mononucleosis
  human immunodeficiency virus and, 693
  immunoblastic reactions and, 618
  infectious, 430, 702–703
    pathogenesis, 703*f*
  posttransfusion, 232
  serum immunoglobulin levels, 157*t*
Monovalent, 68
Montenegro test, 670
Mortierella, 662
Motility, neutrophil, tests, 210–211
Motion sickness, antihistamines and, 793
MS. *See* Multiple sclerosis
Mu chain disease, 609
Mucocutaneous candidiasis, chronic, 282–284, 659–660
  Candida infection and, 283*f*
  endocrinopathy and, 422
Mucormycosis, 649, 651*t*, 662–663
  immunologic abnormalities and, 653*t*
  immunologic diagnosis, 656*t*
  pathologic features, 652*t*
Mucor stalonifer, 369
Mucosa
  host defense and, 622–623
  immunoglobulin production, 548
  normal flora, 623*t*
Mucosa-associated lymphoid tissue (MALT), 36
Mucosal follicle, 542
Mucosal homing, 549–550
Mucosal immune system
  anatomy, 541–544
  cell traffic, 550*f*
  functions, 541
  IgA and, 544–547
  oral unresponsiveness, 549
  sperm and, 554
Mucosal immunity, 553–554
Mucosal lymphoid aggregate, 542
Mucosal lymphoid tissue, diffuse, 543–544
Multicystic kidney disease with proteinuria, urine abnormalities, 160*f*
Multifocal leukoencephalopathy, 727
Multinucleated giant cell, 20
Multiple myeloma, 66, 154, 158, 607–608
  interferon-alpha and, 782
  monoclonal serum immunoglobulins and, 589
  serum viscosity and, 168
Multiple sclerosis (MS), 158, 508–511, 713
  cell interactions, 509*f*
  cerebrospinal fluid patterns, 160*f*
  cerebrospinal fluid specimen, 510*f*
  interferon and, 384
  magnetic resonance image of brain, 510*f*
  plasma exchange and, 777
Mumps, 524, 736
  active immunization, 721*t*

vaccine, age recommendations, 735
vaccinination, reportable events, 728*t*
Mumps virus, insulin-dependent diabetes mellitus and, 420
Mu protein, 86
Muramyl dipeptide, 52
Murray, Joseph E., 5
Muscle
  polymyositis-dermatomyositis and, 405
  progressive systemic sclerosis and, 402
  systemic lupus erythematosus and, 388
Mutation, 570
Myalgia, systemic lupus erythematosus and, 388
Myasthenia gravis, 383, 513–515
  intravenous gamma globulin and, 778
  plasma exchange and, 777
Myasthenic syndrome, 515, 517
Mycetoma, 650*t*
  immunologic abnormalities and, 653*t*
  immunologic diagnosis, 655*t*
  pathologic features, 652*t*
Mycobacterium, 634–635
Mycobacterium avium complex (MAC), 634–635, 694, 695
Mycobacterium leprae, 635
Mycobacterium paratuberculosis, 459
Mycobacterium tuberculosis, 366, 524, 634–635, 695
Mycoplasma, 624
Mycoplasma pneumoniae, 430, 626
Mycoplasma tuberculosis, 626
Mycosis, 649–664
  cutaneous, 650*t*
  immunologic abnormalities and, 653*t*
  subcutaneous, 650*t*
    immunologic diagnosis, 655*t*
    pathologic features, 652*t*
  superficial, 650*t*
  systemic
    immunologic diagnosis, 655–656*t*
    pathologic features, 652*t*
  systemic invasive, 650–651*t*
    opportunistic pathogens, 659–664
    primary pathogens, 654–659
Mycosis fungoides, 615
Mycotoxicosis, pulmonary, 369
Mydriatics, rheumatoid eye disease and, 522
Myelin basic protein, 384, 508, 510, 713
Myelodysplasia, granulocyte colony-stimulating factor and, 783
Myelogenous leukemia
  acute, bone marrow transplantation and, 758–759
  chronic
    bone marrow transplantation and, 759
    interferon-alpha and, 782
Myeloid pathway, 11*f*
Myeloma
  Bence Jones, 158
    serum immunoglobulin levels, 157*t*
  IgA, urine abnormalities, 160*f*
  IgE, serum IgE levels, 336*f*
  IgG, serum immunoglobulin abnormalities, 159*f*
  multiple, 66, 154, 158, 607–608
    interferon-alpha and, 782
    monoclonal serum immunoglobulins and, 589
    serum viscosity and, 168
  proteins, 66, 74
Myelomonocytic leukemia, acute, 617
Myeloperoxidase, 15–16
  deficiency, 306
    chronic granulomatous disease and, 305

Myeloproliferative disorder, granulocyte colony-stimulating factor and, 783
Myocardial disease, 442–443
Myocardial fibrosis, progressive systemic sclerosis and, 402
Myocarditis
  autoimmune, 442–443
  systemic lupus erythematosus and, 389
Myopericarditis, influenza virus and, 639
Myxedema, nasal congestion and, 333

NADPH-dependent oxidase, 15
NAPDH oxidase, respiratory burst and, 304
Nasal congestion, drugs causing, 333*t*
Nasal decongestants, allergic rhinitis and, 334
Nasal eosinophilia, 333
Nasal polyposis, 334
  allergic rhinitis and, 335
  aspirin sensitivity and, 338
Nasal provocation testing, 325
Nasopharyngeal carcinoma, Hodgkin's disease and, 570
National Childhood Vaccine Injury Act (1986), 727
National Marrow Donor Program (NMDP), 759
Natural cytotoxic (NC) cell, 573
Natural killer (NK) cell, 22, 102–104
  assays, 209
    functional, 261
  cytokine production, 103
  deficiency, immunodeficiency and, 284
  development and tissue distribution, 102–103
  enumeration, 261
  host defense and, 103–104
  immune competence testing, 261
  interleukin-2 and, 113
  lamina propria, 544
  leukemia, 617–618
  nonspecific immune stimulation and, 714
  OK432 and, 781
  proportion in normal tissues, 24*t*
  T cells compared, 103
  tumor cells and, 573
Natural killer cell stimulatory factor. *See* Interleukin-12
Natural killing, 103
Natural selection, 1
  theory, 3
NBT test. *See* Nitro Blue Tetrazolium (NBT) test
NC cell. *See* Natural cytotoxic (NC) cell
Necator americanus, 676
Necrolysis, epidermal, 630
Necrotizing vasculitis, systemic, 447–450
Nedocromil, IgE-mediated allergic disease and, 715
Nedocromil sodium, 792
Negative predictive value, 192
Negative selection, 49, 102
Neisseria, 633
Neisseria gonorrhoeae, 407, 565, 633
Neisseria meningitidis, 633, 718, 735
Nematode, 676–678
  filarid, 678
Neonatal alloimmune thrombocytopenia, 565
Neonatal meningitis, 632
Neoplasia
  congenital immunodeficiency and, 580–581, 581*t*
  immune surveillance and, 578–579
  interferon-alpha and, 782
  intrinsic defense and, 578
  pathogenesis, 579*f*
Neoplasm
  B cell, 590*f*

Neoplasm *(cont.)*
  chromosomal translocation and, 599*t*
  human immunodeficiency virus and, 585
  immune system, 588–619
    benign conditions mimicking, 618–619
    classification, 588, 589*t*
    cytogenetics, 596–598
    DNA analysis, 592–596
    immunologic features, 589–592
    molecular genetics, 599–600
    most common, 602*t*
    therapy, 600–601
  lymphocytic of B cell origin, 601–607
  lymphocytic of T cell origin, 610–614
  mononuclear phagocyte system, 616–617
  plasma cell, 607–610
  T cell, small, 612–613
  urticaria-angioedema and, 355
Neostigmine, myasthenia gravis and, 514
Nephelometry, 170, 171*f*
  rate, 170
Nephritic factor, membranoproliferative glomerulonephritis
    and, 486
Nephritis
  lupus, 389
    plasma exchange and, 777
  tubulointerstitial, 487–489
Nephropathy, minimal-change, 489
Nephrotic syndrome, 158
  focal glomerulosclerosis and, 489
  immune-complex glomerulonephritis and, 482
  serum immunoglobulin levels, 157*t*
Nerve growth factor (NGF), 121
Nervous system
  slow and latent virus infections, 517
  systemic lupus erythematosus and, 389
Neuraminidase, 638, 639
Neurodermatitis, 341, 364
  localized, 342
Neurofibrillary tangle, 517
Neurologic disease, 507–518
  immunologic abnormalities, 515–518
Neuromuscular junction, normal and myasthenic, 514*f*
Neuromuscular transmission, disorders, 513–515
Neuron, central nervous system, uptake of antibodies, 516*f*
Neurosyphilis, multiple sclerosis and, 510
Neutralizing antibody, 717
Neutropenia
  autoimmune, 425
    intravenous gamma globulin and, 778
  cyclic, 425–426
  granulocyte colony-stimulating factor and, 783
  immune, drug-induced, 426
  management, 426–427
Neutrophil, 9, 10–17
  adhesion, 479
  antimicrobial systems, 212*t*
  bands, 16
  chemiluminescence and, 213
  chemotactic factors, 12, 13*t*
  degranulation, tests, 211–212
  electron micrograph, 12*f*
  emigration, 13*f*, 14
  engulfment and digestion of target, 15*f*
  enumeration, 262
  flow cytometry and, 213
  functions, 209–214
    disorders, 214*t*

  granules, 10
    contents, 12*t*
    release of contents, 17*f*
  host defense and, 16–17
  ingestion, tests, 211
  interleukin-2 and, 113
  intracellular killing, tests, 212–214
  margination, 12, 13*f*
  metabolic burst, 16
  microbicidal activity, 14–16
  microbicidal assay, 213–214
  motility, tests, 210–211
  oxidative microbicidal pathway, 16*f*
  polymorphonuclear, 209
  properties, 10*t*
  recognition and adhesion, tests, 211
  respiratory burst, 16
  segmented, 10
  tissue invasion, 10–14
Neutrophilia, corticosteroids and, 765
New Guinea thatched roof lung, 369
Nezelof's syndrome, 289–290
NGF. *See* Nerve growth factor
Niacinamide, bullous pemphigoid and, 495
Nickel
  allergic contact dermatitis and, 147
  sensitivity, 364, 365
Nicolle, Charles Jules Henri, 4
Nikolsky's sign, 502
Nippostrongylus brasiliensis, 677
Nitro Blue Tetrazolium (NBT) test, 212
  quantitative, 212–213, 303
Nitrofurantoin, pulmonary disease and, 529–530
Nitroglycerin, allergic reactions, 374
NK cell. *See* Natural killer (NK) cell
NKSF. *See* Interleukin-12
NMDP. *See* National Marrow Donor Program
Nocardia, 537, 781
Non-gluten hypersensitivity, 459
Nonsteroidal anti-inflammatory drugs (NSAIDs), 789–791
  anti-inflammatory effects, 790
  anti-inflammatory mechanisms, 715
  asthma and, 337–338
  available in USA, 790*t*
  bronchospasm and, 528
  mechanism of action, 790–791
  prostaglandin synthesis and, 143
  pseudoallergic reactions and, 379
  relapsing polychondritis and, 408
  rheumatoid arthritis and, 396
  side effects, 791*t*
  Sjögren's syndrome and, 401
  systemic lupus erythematosus and, 392
  toxicity, 791
  urticaria and, 355
Nontropical sprue, 457
Normal flora, 623, 623*t*
Northern blot technique, 224
N region, 83, 95
NSAIDs. *See* Nonsteroidal anti-inflammatory drugs
Nuclease protection assay, 217, 219*f*
Nucleic acid, immunogenic, 42
Nucleic acid probe, 216–217
  hybridization assays using, 219*f*
  methods for labeling and detecting, 218*f*
Nucleoside analog
  hepatitis B virus and, 644–645
  human immunodeficiency virus and, 699

Nucleoside phosphorylase
deficiency, immunodeficiency and, 295–297
purine metabolic pathway and, 296*f*
Nucleotidase, 86
deficiency, immunodeficiency and, 297
Nuttall, George H. F., 2, 3
Nystatin, candidiasis and, 660

O antigen, 631
Obstructive airway disease, reversible, 335
Obstructive lung disease, heart-lung transplantation and, 755
Occupational allergen, 339*t*, 366
Occupational allergy, 331
Occupational asthma, 338
Occupational lung disease, 533
Ocular sarcoidosis, 523–524
Ocular toxoplasmosis, 669
Ocular vasculitis, systemic lupus erythematosus and, 389
OK432, 781
Oligoadenylate synthetase, 116
Oligonucleotide probe, sequence-specific, HLA typing and, 252–253, 253*f*
Onchocerca volvulus, 676, 678
Onchocerciasis, 678
Oncogene, 570
Burkitt's lymphoma and, 598
Oncogenesis, 579
viral, 570
Oncostatin M (OSM), 114
Onion skin lesion, 388
Oophoritis, autoimmune, 422, 560
Ophthalmia, sympathetic, 524–525
Opiates
anaphylactoid reactions and, 352
pseudoallergic reactions and, 379
Opportunistic infection, 706–709
cyclosporin and, 776
Opsonin, 2, 15, 25, 47, 717
Opsonization, 15*f*, 47, 74, 124, 127
Oral candidiasis, 476
Sjögren's syndrome and, 401
Oral contraceptive
nasal congestion and, 333
steroid clearance and, 786
Oral disease, local, immunologic mechanisms, 471–474
Oral mucosa, normal flora, 623*t*
Oral provocation testing, 325–326
Oral ulceration, 474–475
Oral unresponsiveness, 549
Orchitis, autoimmune, 560
Organ transplantation. *See* Transplantation
Organ transplant recipient, cancer and, 581–582
Ornithodorus, 686
Orodental disease, 470–476
Orthopedic surgery, rheumatoid arthritis and, 396
OSM. *See* Oncostatin M
Osteoarthritis, spinal, 407
Osteoporosis, interleukin-1 receptor antagonist and, 784
Ostwald viscosimeter, 168
Otitis media, allergic rhinitis and, 335
Ouchterlony, O., 152
Ouchterlony analysis, 152–54
Ovarian failure, premature, 422
Ovary, 554
autoimmune disease, 560
Overlap syndrome, 450
Owen, Ray D., 2, 4

Oxytriphylline, 793
Oxyuriasis, 532

p56, 97
p59, 97
PAF. *See* Platelet-activating factor
Pancreas
disorders, 419–423
transplantation, 752–754
cross-matching and, 753–754
immunosuppression and, 753–754
indications, 753
procedure, 753
survival, 753
Pancreatitis, tissue kallikreins and, 135
Pancytopenia, 434
Pandemic influenza, 637
Panencephalitis, sclerosing, subacute, 517, 641–642, 726
Panniculitis, relapsing, 408–409
Panuveitis, 523
Papain, 68
Papillomatosis, laryngeal, interferon-alpha and, 782
PAP method. *See* Peroxidase-antiperoxidase (PAP) method
Paprika slicer's lung, 369
Paracoccidioides brasiliensis, 658
Paracoccidioidomycosis, 651*t*, 658–659
immunologic abnormalities and, 653*t*
immunologic diagnosis, 655*t*
pathologic features, 652*t*
Paracortex, 35
Paracrine effect, 44, 105, 583, 782
Paragonimus, 673
Parallelism testing, 177
Paraneoplastic cerebellar degeneration, 515
Paraneoplastic pemphigus, 503
Paraproteinemia, 160–161
monoclonal, cryoglobulins and, 169
Paraprotein, 607
Parasite-induced eosinophilic pneumonia, 532–533, 532*t*
Parasite
disease, 666–678
transfusion-transmitted, 232
host immune response and, 667*f*
infection
eosinophils and, 138
nonspecific immunosuppression and, 666
serum IgE and, 74
Parasitemia, trypanosomiasis and, 672*f*
Parasitism, 666
Parathyroid gland, embryologic development, 281*f*
Paroxysmal cold hemoglobinuria, 431–432
Paroxysmal nocturnal hemoglobinuria (PNH), 133, 312, 433
Pars cavernosa, 553
Partitioning step, 172
Passive hemagglutination assay, 185*t*
Passive immune suppression, 713
Passive immunization, 712, 727–734
materials available, 730–733*t*
Pasteur, Louis, 1–2, 3, 7*f*, 629, 646
Patch testing, 196, 320–321, 364
allergic drug reactions and, 375
contact allergens used, 364*t*
interpretation, 364*t*
Pauciarticular disease, 398
Pauling, Linus, 2
PCR. *See* Polymerase chain reaction

PDGF. *See* Platelet-derived growth factor
Pediculus humanus, 686
Pemphigoid, cicatricial, 523
Pemphigus, paraneoplastic, 503
Pemphigus erythematosus, 502
Pemphigus foliaceus, 500–503
   characteristic features, 501*t*
Pemphigus vulgaris, 494, 500–503
   characteristic features, 501*t*
   conjunctival bullae and, 523
   histopathology, 501*f*
   IgG deposition, 503*f*
   lesions, 502*f*
Penciclovir, hepatitis B virus and, 644–645
Penem, 376*f*
   core structure, 376*f*
Penicillamine, 791–792
   lupus syndrome and, 530
   pemphigus and, 501
   primary biliary cirrhosis and, 469
   progressive systemic sclerosis and, 403
   rheumatoid arthritis and, 396
Penicillin
   allergy, 350, 375–377
   biotransformation products, 372*t*
   chemical structure, 372*t*
   chronic granulomatous disease and, 305
   core structure, 376*f*
   cross-reactions, 377
   desensitization, 377
   IgG antibodies and, 371
   Lyme disease and, 686
   skin test, 376
   syphilis and, 684
Penicillin G, 372, 376
Penicillium marneffei, 658
Penicilloic acid, 376
   chemical structure, 372*t*
Penicilloyl-polylysine, 350, 376
Pentadecylcatechol, 363, 365
Pentamidine, *Pneumocystis carinii* and, 288
Pentamidine isethionate, *Pneumocystis carinii* and, 664
Pentapeptide, 382
Pentostatin, immune system neoplasms and, 601
Peptide-binding site, 60
   class I HLA molecule, 61*f*
   class II HLA molecule, 62*f*
Peptide-MHC complex, assembly and transport, 62
Peptide-prolyl *cis-trans* isomerase (PPIase), 776
Peptide-transporter protein, 62
Peptidomannan, 649
Perforin, 100
Periarteriolar lymphoid sheath, 35
Pericardial disease, 442
Pericarditis
   nonsteroidal anti-inflammatory drugs and, 790
   relapsing, 442
   systemic lupus erythematosus and, 388
Periodontal disease, 630
   inflammatory, 471–473
   pathogenesis, 472*f*
   X-linked infantile hypogammaglobulinemia and, 267*f*
Periodontitis, 471–473
   advanced, 473*f*
Periodontium, normal, 473*f*
Peripheral lymphoid organ, 23–24
Peripheral T cell lymphoma, 613
Peritonitis, systemic lupus erythematosus and, 388

Pernicious anemia, 462–463
   selective IgA deficiency and, 274
Peroxidase-antiperoxidase (PAP) method, 183
Pertussis, 629, 717, 736
   vaccination, 735
     active, 721*t*
   vaccine, 629, 726
Peyer's patch, 36
   antigen-specific suppressor T cells, 549
   histologic section, 542*f*
   microscopic anatomy, 36*f*
   transmission electron micrograph, 543*f*
P glycoprotein, 776
Phaeohyphomycosis, 651*t*
   immunologic abnormalities and, 653*t*
Phagocyte, 9–20
   activation, 47
   dysfunction disease, 303–307
     treatment, 265*t*
   mononuclear, 17
     neoplasms, 616–617
Phagocytic cell, 623*t*
   corticosteroids and, 767
   enumeration, 262
   host defense and, 623–624, 625, 625*t*
   immune competence testing, 261–262
   microbicidal proteins, 625*t*
Phagocytosis, 2, 14–16, 14*f*, 717
   corticosteroids and, 789
   evaluation, 304*t*
   frustrated, 211–212, 212*f*
   steps in progression, 210*f*
   tests, 211
Phagolysosome, 211
Phagosome, 15, 211
Pharyngitis, 630
Phenobarbital, steroid clearance and, 786
Phenotypic marker, lymphoma and lymphocytic leukemia, 595–596*t*
Phenylbutazone, pemphigus and, 501
Phenylephrine, 793
   rheumatoid eye disease and, 522
   sarcoid lesions of eye and, 524
Phenylketonuria, eczema and, 343
Phenylpropanolamine, 793
Phenytoin
   lupuslike syndrome and, 389
   selective IgA deficiency and, 275
   steroid clearance and, 786
Phlyctenular keratoconjunctivitis, 525, 525*f*
Phosphatidylinositol bisphosphate (PIP2), 97
Phosphodiesterase, 793
Phosphoinositide glycosidic linkage, 133
Phospholipase A2, 715
Phospholipase C, 97
Phosphorylation, 29–30
Photoallergic contact dermatitis, 365–366
Photoallergic reaction, topical causes, 365*t*
Photopatch testing, 320–321, 365
Photosensitivity, 365
Phototoxic reaction, topical causes, 365*t*
Physical carcinogen, 569–570
Physical examination, allergic disease and, 318
Physical therapy
   juvenile arthritis and, 399
   rheumatoid arthritis and, 395
Picornavirus, 645, 646
PIE syndrome, 361

Pigeon breeder's disease, 366
Pigmentation, progressive systemic sclerosis and, 402
Pinocytosis, 14*f*
Pinta, 684
Pinworm, 532
Piperacillin, 377
Pirbuterol, 793
 asthma and, 340
Pituitary snuff, immunogenicity, 371
Pit viper bite, serum therapy, 733
Pityriasis versicolor, 650*t*
 immunologic abnormalities and, 653*t*
Pityrosporum folliculitis, 650*t*
 immunologic abnormalities and, 653*t*
Placenta
 as immune organ, 557
 local immunosuppression and, 558–559
Placental bed, trophoblast populations, 557*f*
Placental protein, secretion, 559
Placental steroid hormone, secretion, 559
Plague, 737
 active immunization, 722*t*
Plaquenil, rheumatoid eye disease and, 523
Plasma
 exchange, 777
  bullous pemphigoid and, 495
 fresh-frozen, 235
 products, transfusion, 235
 proteins, acute-phase response, 111*t*
Plasma cell, 25, 26, 88
 dyscrasia, 607–610
  immunoelectrophoresis and, 161
 electron micrograph, 27*f*
 neoplasms, 607–610
Plasmacytoid lymphocytic lymphoma, 606–607
Plasmacytoma, solitary, 608
Plasmapheresis, 713, 777
 acute inflammatory demyelinating polyneuropathy and, 512*f*
 antimyelin antibody and, 512*f*
 cryoglobulinemia and, 609
 Goodpasture's syndrome and, 481
 myasthenia gravis and, 514
 pemphigus vulgaris and, 503
 renal vasculitis and, 490
Plasmin inhibitor, hereditary angioedema and, 311
Plasmodium, 667, 738
Plasmodium falciparum, 667–668
Plasmodium ovale, 667
Plasmodium vivax, 667–668
Plateau phase, 48
Platelet
 activation, 141
 disorders, 434–438
  immunologic mechanisms, 435
 inflammation and, 141
 transfusion, 235
  bone marrow transplantation and, 759
Platelet-activating factor (PAF), 141, 479
 asthmatic attack and, 337
 chemical structure, 144*f*
 inflammation and, 144
Platelet-derived growth factor (PDGF), 479, 783
Plateletpheresis, 235
Pleura, drug-induced inflammation, 530
Pleural effusion
 rheumatoid, 394
 systemic lupus erythematosus and, 390
Pleurisy, systemic lupus erythematosus and, 388

Pleuritic chest pain, systemic lupus erythematosus and, 389
Pleuritis, juvenile arthritis and, 398
PLT test, 274
PMN. *See* Polymorphonuclear neutrophil
Pneumococcus, 615, 631–632
 active immunization, 722*t*
Pneumoconiosis, 366
Pneumocystis, 709
Pneumocystis carinii, 537, 649, 663–664, 706
 pneumonia, 475, 663
  bone marrow transplantation and, 759
 pneumonitis, 694
 severe combined immunodeficiency disease and, 287, 288
Pneumocystosis, 651*t*, 663–664
 immunologic abnormalities and, 653*t*
 pathologic features, 652*t*
Pneumonconiosis, 369
Pneumonia
 eosinophilic, 530–533, 531*t*
  acute, 531–532
  chronic idiopathic, 531, 532*f*
  drug-induced, 532, 532*t*
  parasite-induced, 532–533, 532*t*
 hypersensitivity, allergen bronchoprovocation and, 325
 mycoplasmal, 430
 Pneumocystis carinii, 475, 663
  bone marrow transplantation and, 759
Pneumonitis
 amiodarone, 530
 hypersensitivity, 366–370, 539
  allergens causing, 367*t*
  Aspergillus, 361
 interstitial, 366
 juvenile arthritis and, 398
 Pneumocystis carinii, 694
PNH. *See* Paroxysmal nocturnal hemoglobinuria
POHS. *See* Progressive ocular histoplasmosis syndrome
Poisoning, food, 629
Poison ivy, 147, 363, 364, 739, 742
Poison oak, 363, 364, 739, 742
Poisonous bite, serum therapy, 733
Pokeweed mitogen (PWM), B cell activation and, 201
Poliomyelitis, 646–647, 717, 734
 active immunization, 722*t*
 live vaccines and, 727
 pregnancy and, 558
 vaccination, 735
  reportable events, 728*t*
Poliosis, 524
Poliovirus, 646–647
 vaccine, oral attenuated, paralytic illness and, 726–727
Pollen allergen, 329, 329*t*, 330*f*, 331*f*
Poly(I:C), 115
Polyarteritis nodosa, 447–449, 490, 626
 eyes and, 525
 hepatic angiogram, 448*f*
 interleukin-1 receptor antagonist and, 784
 muscle biopsy, 447*f*
Polyarthralgia, systemic lupus erythematosus and, 388
Polyarthritis, hypogammaglobulinemia and, 269
Polychondritis, relapsing, 408
Polyclonal antibody, 778
Polyclonal hypergammaglobulinemia
 polymyositis-dermatomyositis and, 404
 progressive systemic sclerosis and, 403
 rheumatoid arthritis and, 395
 serum immunoglobulin abnormalities, 159*f*
Polycyclic aromatic hydrocarbon, 569

Polyglandular syndrome
  autoimmune, 422–423
    classification, 422*t*
  type I, 422
  type II, 422
  type III, 422–423
Polymerase chain reaction (PCR), 221–223
  amplification
    allele-specific, 251–252
    DNA, 222*f*, 251*f*
    types, 250–251
  hepatitis C viremia and, 466
  HLA typing and, 250–254
  Leishmania and, 670
  method, 250
  neonatal HIV infection and, 566–567
Polymorphonuclear leukocyte, 10
Polymorphonuclear neutrophil (PMN), 209
Polymyalgia rheumatica, 452
Polymyositis, 380
  defection "recognition", 404*f*
  methotrexate and, 774
Polymyositis-dermatomyositis, 390, 391, 404–406
  autoimmune myocarditis and, 443
Polymyxin, immunogenicity, 371
Polymyxin B, anaphylactoid reactions and, 351
Polyneuropathy, demyelinating
  acute inflammatory, 511–513
  chronic, 513
Polyposis, nasal, 334
  allergic rhinitis and, 335
Polyribosinic agents, 784
Polysaccharide, anaphylactoid reactions and, 352
Polyserositis, systemic lupus erythematosus and, 388
Polyvalent, 69
Pompholyx, 342
Pooled response-error relationship, 177
Porphyria cutanea tarda, 494
Porter, Rodney Robert, 3, 4, 5
Portier, Paul, 2, 4
Positive predictive value, 192
Positive selection, 49, 95, 102
Postinfarction syndrome, 442
Postpartum thyroiditis, 416
Postpericardiotomy syndrome, 442
Posttransfusion purpura, 438
  plasma exchange and, 777
Power function, 177
PPIase. *See* Peptide-prolyl *cis-trans* isomerase
Prausnitz-Kustner reaction, 322, 372
Prausnitz-Kustner skin test, 741
Pre-B cell, 86
Precipitation, 172
  reaction, 152
Precipitin, 2
  curve, antigen-antibody, 152*f*
  reaction, 147
  test, hypersensitivity pneumonitis and, 369
Precision, 177
Precision profile, 177
Predictive value
  effect of prevalence, 192*t*
  negative, 192
  positive, 192
  theory, 191–193
Prednisolone
  chemical structure, 787*f*

half-life relative potency, 788*t*
  sarcoid lesions of eye and, 524
Prednisolone acetate, corneal graft reactions and, 527
Prednisone, 786
  allergic bronchopulmonary aspergillosis and, 361
  allergic contact dermatitis and, 364
  allergic rhinitis and, 334
  allograft rejection and, 748–749
  asthma and, 340
  autoimmune hemolytic anemia and, 430
  bullous pemphigoid and, 495
  chemical structure, 787*f*
  cryoglobulinemia and, 609
  epidermolysis bullosa acquisita and, 500
  giant cell arteritis and, 453
  graft-versus-host disease and, 760
  half-life relative potency, 788*t*
  herpes gestationis and, 497
  Hodgkin's disease and, 616
  idiopathic thrombocytopenic purpura and, 437
  liver transplantation and, 752
  multiple myeloma and, 608
  multiple sclerosis and, 511
  pancreas transplantation and, 754
  pemphigus vulgaris and, 503
  plasmacytoid lymphocytic lymphoma and, 606
  polyarteritis nodosa and, 449
  polymyositis-dermatomyositis and, 406
  recurrent aphthous ulceration and, 475
  rheumatoid arthritis and, 396, 768
  status asthmaticus and, 341
  systemic lupus erythematosus and, 392
  Takayasu arteritis and, 455
  Wegener's granulomatosis and, 451
Pregnancy
  immunity and, 558–559
  infection and, 558
  isoimmunized, management, 564–565
  lymphocyte reactivity and, 559
  toxoplasmosis and, 669
  yellow fever immunization and, 726
Prekallikrein, 133
Premature ovarian failure, 422
Premunition, 668
Presenile dementia, 517
Presensitization, kidney transplantation and, 745
Pressure urticaria, 355
Pretransfusion testing, 229
Prevalence, effect on predictive value, 192*t*
Prick testing, 349
Primary biliary cirrhosis, 468–470
  liver transplantation and, 750
  percutaneous liver biopsy specimen, 468*f*
Primary follicle, 33, 33*f*, 34*f*
Primary humoral response, 90–91, 91*t*
Primary hypothyroidism, 419
Primary immune response, 48, 48*f*
Primary immunodeficiency, respiratory disease and, 528
Primary lymphatic vessel, 32
Primary lymphocyte repertoire, 41
Primary lymphoid organ, 22
Primary sclerosing cholangitis, 470
Primer, 222
Priming event, 48
Pro-B cell, 84
Probe, 216
  nucleic acid, 216–217

hybridization assays using, 219*f*
methods for labeling and detecting, 218*f*
Procainamide, lupuslike syndrome and, 389, 530
Procarbazine, Hodgkin's disease and, 616
Procaterol, 793
Programmed cell death, 49, 100, 381
Progression, 579
Progressive multifocal leukoencephalopathy, 517–518
Progressive ocular histoplasmosis syndrome (POSH), 658
Progressive systemic sclerosis, 380, 391, 401–404
Proinflammatory, 47
Prolymphocytic leukemia, 604
T cell type, 612
Promastigote, 669, 670
Promotion, 579
Properdin, 128
Propylthiouracil, Graves' disease and, 418
Prostaglandin, 144, 791
anti-inflammatory agents and, 715
asthmatic attack and, 337
inhibitors, relapsing panniculitis and, 409
nonsteroidal anti-inflammatory drugs and, 790
rheumatoid arthritis and, 393
Protein
deficiency, complement-related, inherited, 310*t*
denaturation/precipitation, 172
peptide-transporter, 62
placental, secretion, 559
Protein A, 167
Protein kinase C, 97
Protein-losing gastroenteropathy, serum immunoglobulin levels, 157*t*
Protein tyrosine kinase (PTK), 29–30, 87, 97
Proteinuria
Bence Jones, 608
immune-complex glomerulonephritis and, 482
Proteoglycan, inflammation and, 145
Proteus, 631
Proto-oncogene, function and dysfunction, 579–580
Protozoa, immune response and, 666–673
Provocation testing, 324–326
allergic drug reactions and, 375
nasal, 325
oral, 325–326
Provocative-dose challenge, 375
Prozone phenomenon, 152
Pruritus, 150
Pseudoallergic reaction, 379
Pseudo-Goodpasture's syndrome, 530
Pseudomembranous candidiasis, 475*f*, 476
Pseudomonas, lung transplantation and, 757
Pseudomonas aeruginosa, 631, 660, 738, 781
Pseudomonas exotoxin A, 712
Pseudopelade, 505
Psoriatic arthritis, 395, 408
immunosuppressives and, 792
Psyllium, asthma and, 528
PTK. *See* Protein tyrosine kinase
Pulmonary eosinophilia
simple idiopathic, 531
tropical, 533
Pulmonary fibrosis, idiopathic, 366, 534–536
differential diagnosis, 535*t*
Pulmonary function testing, 318–320
asthma and, 336–337
Pulmonary hypertension, heart-lung transplantation and, 755
Pulmonary mycotoxicosis, 369

Pulmonary-renal syndrome, 481
Pulmonary vascular disease, heart-lung transplantation and, 755
Pulmonary vasculitis syndrome, 537
Pure erythrocyte aplasia, 433–434
cyclophosphamide and, 773
intravenous gamma globulin and, 778
Purine analog, rheumatoid arthritis and, 396
Purine metabolic pathway, 296*f*
Pus, 16
PWN. *See* Pokeweed mitogen
Pyridostigmine, myasthenia gravis and, 514
Pyrimethamine-sulfadoxine, *Pneumocystis carinii* and, 664
Pyrimidinolone, 784
Pyrogen, endogenous, 111
Pyroglobulin, 169

Quality control chart, 177
Quality control pool, 177
Quantal-response assay, 177
Quantitative immunoassay, comparative sensitivity, 191, 192*t*
Quantitative immunofluorescence, 183
Quantitative Nitro Blue Tetrazolium (NBT) test, 212–213, 303
Quartan malaria, 667–668
antigen-antibody glomerulonephritis and, 666
Quinidine
immune thrombocytopenic purpura and, 438
lupuslike syndrome and, 389
Quinine, 790
blackwater fever and, 667
immune hemolytic anemia and, 431
thrombocytopenia and, 372

Rabies, 1
immunization, 735
active, 723–724*t*
passive, 731–732*t*
vaccine, adverse reactions, 726
Rabies virus, 646
Radiation, live vaccines and, 726
Radiation-induced carcinogenesis, 569–570
Radiation therapy, immune system neoplasms and, 600
Radioactive counting, 172
Radioallergosorbent test (RAST), 323, 324*f*, 332
Aspergillus precipitins and, 360
drug allergy and, 375
hypersensitivity pneumonitis and, 369
Radiocontrast media, pseudoallergic reactions and, 379
Radioimmunoassay (RIA), 170, 171–173. *See also* Immunoassay
anti-DNA antibodies and, 391
binder-ligand reactions, 172*f*
hypersensitivity pneumonitis and, 369
logit transformation, 172, 172*f*
ultrasensitive enzymatic, 174, 175*f*
Radioiodine, Graves' disease and, 418–419
Radioisotopic label, 173
RAG-1, 84
RAG-2, 84
Raji cell assay, 446
Random error, 177
between-batch, 176
between-laboratory, 176
within-assay, 178

Ranitidine
anaphylaxis and, 353
H2 receptors and, 142
Rapamycin, nonspecific immunosuppression and, 715
Rappaport classification, 588
RAST. *See* Radioallergosorbent test
Rate nephelometry, 170
Rattlesnake bite, serum therapy, 733
RAU. *See* Recurrent aphthous ulceration
Raynaud's phenomenon
cold-agglutinin syndromes and, 430
polymyositis-dermatomyositis and, 405
progressive systemic sclerosis and, 402
Sjögren's syndrome and, 400
systemic lupus erythematosus and, 389, 391
Raynaud's syndrome, 455
Reaginic antibody, 683
Receptor-mediated endocytosis, 14*f*
Recidiva leishmaniasis, 670
Recombinant DNA, 3, 216
Recombinant vaccine, 56
Recombination signal sequence, 82*f*, 84
Recovery, 177
Recurrent aphthous ulceration (RAU), 474–475, 474*f*
Recurrent spontaneous abortion, 562
Red pulp, 36
Reed-Sternberg cell, 614, 614*f*, 615
Regional enteritis, selective IgA deficiency and, 274
Regional ileitis, 459
Reinherz, Ellis, 4
Reiter's disease, 521
acute iridocyclitis, 522*f*
Reiter's syndrome, 395, 407
methotrexate and, 774
Relapsing fever borreliosis, 680, 686–687
Relapsing panniculitis, 408–409
Relapsing pericarditis, 442
Relapsing polychondritis, 408
Relative response (RR), 246–247
Remittive agents, juvenile arthritis and, 399
Renal allograft survival
HLA-A, -B, -DR mismatches and, 240*t*
HLA matching and, 239*t*
Renal arteriography, progressive systemic sclerosis and, 403
Renal cell carcinoma, interleukin-2 and, 113, 783
Renal dialysis, alternative complement pathway and, 131
Renal disease, 478–490
humorally mediated, immunopathogenesis, 479*t*
Renal transplantation. *See* Kidney transplantation
Reovirus, insulin-dependent diabetes mellitus and, 420
Replicate, 177
Reproductive system
anatomy
female, 552
male, 553
human immunodeficiency virus and, 565–567
mucosal immunity, 553–554
RER. *See* Rough endoplasmic reticulum
Residual, 177
studentized, 177
Respiratory burst, 16, 304*f*
chronic granulomatous disease and, 303
NAPDH oxidase and, 304
Respiratory disease, 528–539
drug-induced, 528–530, 529*t*
environmental, 533
occupational, 533
Respiratory failure, treatment, 341

Respiratory obstruction, lower, anaphylaxis and, 348
Respiratory syncytial virus, 639–641, 738
bronchiolitis, chest x-ray, 640*f*
Response, 172, 177
Response-error relationship, 178
"Resting" state, 22–23
Restriction, 95
Restriction enzyme, 218–219
Restriction fragment length polymorphism (RFLP)
HLA typing and, 249–250, 250*f*
tissue typing and, 250*f*
Restriction fragment, 219
Reticular cell, 32
Reticulin fiber, 32
Reticuloendothelial cell, corticosteroids and, 767
Reticuloendotheliosis, leukemic, 606
Reticulosis, medullary, histiocytic, 616
Retina, cotton-wool spots, 523, 523*f*
Retrovirus, 570, 571, 689
classification, 690*t*
endogenous superantigens and, 383
evolutionary relationships, 691*f*
Reverse transcriptase, 570
Reverse transcriptase PCR (RT-PCR), 224
Reversible obstructive airway disease, 335
RFLP. *See* Restriction fragment length polymorphism
Rh antibody, hemolytic disease of newborn and, 432–433
Rh antigen, 562
Rh blood group system, 227–228, 228*t*, 562
Rh disease, incidence, Rh immune globulin and, 564*f*
Rheumatic disease, 387–409
cytotoxic drugs and, 771, 771*t*
immunocompromised host and, 707
methotrexate and, 774
Rheumatic fever, 398, 630
anti-cardiac immune responses, 380
Rheumatoid arthritis, 154, 383, 390, 392–397, 521
chlorambucil and, 774
cyclophosphamide and, 773
experimental in swine, 384
hydrocortisone and, 786
immunopathogenesis, 393*f*
immunosuppressives and, 791–792
interleukin-1 receptor antagonist and, 784
juvenile, 521
plasma exchange and, 777
prednisone and, 768
scleral nodules, 522*f*
scleral thinning, 522*f*
serum immunoglobulin levels, 157*t*
thymic hormones and, 782
Rheumatoid arthritis-like disease, multifactorial etiology, 384*t*
Rheumatoid disease, B cell neoplasms and, 591
Rheumatoid eye disease, 521–523
Rheumatoid factor
juvenile arthritis and, 397
polymyositis-dermatomyositis and, 404
rheumatoid arthritis and, 393, 521
Sjögren's syndrome and, 400
systemic lupus erythematosus and, 391
Rheumatoid vasculitis, 394, 395
plasma exchange and, 777
Rh haplotype, frequencies, 228*t*
Rh immune globulin, 563–564
incidence of Rh disease and, 564*f*
Rh incompatibility, 127
Rhinitis
allergic, 327, 332–335, 338

cromolyn sodium and, 792
   desensitization, 739, 740f, 742
   serum IgE levels, 336f
  infectious, 333
  kinins and, 135
  nonallergic, 327
   chronic, 333
  seasonal, antihistamines and, 792
Rhinitis medicamentosa, 333
Rhinoconjunctivitis, allergic, 327, 338
Rhinoscopy, 333
Rhinovirus infection, interferon-alpha and, 782
Rh isoimmunization, 233–234
  passive immunization, 732t
  prevention, 729–733
Rhizopus arrhizus, 649, 662
Rhodamine, 178
Rhodopsin receptor, interleukin-8 receptor and, 119
Rh prophylaxis, 233–234
Rhus dermatitis, 364, 365, 739, 742
RIA. *See* Radioimmunoassay
Ribavirin, respiratory syncytial virus and, 641
Richet, Charles Robert, 2, 4
Ricin, 712
Rifampin, steroid clearance and, 786
Rimantadine, influenza A virus and, 639
RNA
  methods of analyzing, 223–224
  probes, methods for labeling and detecting, 218f
RNA virus, oncogenic, 570
Rose-Waaler test, 186, 395
Rotavirus, 738
Rough endoplasmic reticulum (RER), MHC molecules and, 62
Roundworm, 676, 677
Roux, P. P. Emile, 2, 3
RR. *See* Relative response
RS-61443, liver transplantation and, 752
RT-PCR. *See* Reverse transcriptase PCR
Rubella, 717, 736
  immunization
   active, 724–725t
   hazards, 726
  vaccine, age recommendations, 735
  vaccinination, reportable events, 728t
Rubella virus, insulin-dependent diabetes mellitus and, 420
Run, 178
Rye classification, 614, 615t

Sabin-Feldman test, 669
Sabin vaccine, 647, 727, 735
Saksenaea, 662
Salicylate, 790
  juvenile arthritis and, 399
  rheumatoid arthritis and, 395–396
  ulcerative colitis and, 462
Salk vaccine, 647, 727, 735
Salmonella, 623, 633–634
Salmonella choleraesuis, 633
Salmonella enteritidis, 633
Salmonella typhi, 633
Salmonella typhimurium, 781
Salting out, 172
Sandwich assay, 173, 173f
Sarcoidosis, 366, 533–534
  chest radiography, 534f, 534t
  hepatic, 469
  multiple sclerosis and, 510

ocular, 523–524
  serum immunoglobulin levels, 157t
Sarcoma
  immunoblastic of B cell type, 605–606
  Kaposi's, 694
   AIDS-associated, 583, 584f
   interferon-gamma and, 782
   organ transplant recipients and, 582, 776
Saturation analysis, 170
Scarlet fever, 630
SCF. *See* Stem cell factor
Schick, Bela, 4
Schick test, 629
Schistosoma haematobium, 674
Schistosoma japonicum, 674
Schistosoma mansoni, 673, 674–675
Schistosoma mekongi, 674
Schistosome, 674
Schistosomiasis, 674–675
  hepatic granuloma and, 666
Schlossman, Stuart, 4
Schmidt's syndrome, 422
SCID. *See* Severe combined immunodeficiency disease
Scleral nodule, 522f
Scleral thinning, 522f
Scleritis, systemic lupus erythematosus and, 389
Scleroderma, 390
Scleromalacia, 394
Scleromalacia perforans, 394
Scleronodular disease, rheumatoid arthritis and, 394
Sclerosing cholangitis
  liver transplantation and, 750
  primary, 470
Sclerosing panencephalitis, subacute, 517
  measles vaccine and, 726
Scorpion sting, antisera, 733
Sd antigen, 227
Seasonal conjunctivitis, antihistamines and, 792
Seasonal rhinitis, antihistamines and, 792
Seborrhea, 342
Secondary follicle, 33, 33f, 34f
Secondary humoral response, 90–91, 91t
Secondary immune response, 48f, 49
Secondary immunodeficiency, respiratory disease and, 528
Secondary lymphoid organ, 23–24
Secretor blood group system, 227
Secretory component, 70, 70f, 72
  properties, 69t
Secretory immune system, components, 553f
Sedormid, immune thrombocytopenic purpura and, 438
Segmented neutrophil, 10
Selectin, 12
E-Selectin, 12
L-Selectin, 12, 39, 86
P-Selectin, 12
Selection, 37
Self-antigen
  autoimmune disease and, 380
  cross-reactivity and, 382
Self-nonself discrimination, suppressor T cells and, 387
Self-tolerance, 2, 102
  loss, 381–382
Senile dementia, 517
Sensitivity
  analytic, 175, 176
  contact, 196
  diagnostic, 176, 192
Sepsis syndrome, 626

Septic shock, 110, 626
   interleukin-1 receptor antagonist and, 784
Sequential epitope, 53
Seroconversion, 694
Serodiagnosis, 627
Serology, 2, 48
Serratia marescens, chronic granulomatous disease and, 303
Serum
   antibodies, 229
   disease, 358
   lymphocyte suppressor factors, 205t
   proteins, single radial diffusion and, 154
   therapy, 733
   viscosity, 168, 168
      increased, disorders associated, 168t
Serum sickness, 147, 148–149, 358–359, 734
   antivenin and, 733
   desensitization therapy and, 742
   immunologic events, 358f
   latency period, 374
   penicillin and, 376
Serum sickness-like syndrome, 465
Severe combined immunodeficiency disease (SCID), 286–288
   adoptive immunity and, 713
   bone marrow transplantation and, 758
   live vaccines and, 726
   maculopapular rash and, 298f
Sex hormone, mechanism of action, 787–788
Sexually transmitted disease (STD), female genital tract mucosa and, 553
Sezary syndrome, 615
Sheehan's syndrome, 421
Sheep erythrocyte test, 395
Shewhart chart, 177
Shigella, 623, 738
Shigella flexneri, 631
Shock
   anaphylactic, 347, 348, 352
      hydatid cyst and, 666
   septic, 110, 626
      interleukin-1 receptor antagonist and, 784
Short-limbed dwarfism, immunodeficiency with, 294–295, 294f
SI. *See* Stimulation index
Sialic acid, 632
Sicca complex, 389
Sicca syndrome, progressive systemic sclerosis and, 403
Sick building syndrome, 533
Sickle cell anemia, immunocompromised host and, 707
Sickle cell hemoglobin, *Plasmodium falciparum* and, 668
Sickle cell trait, 668
Side chain theory, 2
Signal transduction
   interleukin-1 receptors and, 109–110
   interleukin-2 receptors and, 112
   T cell receptors and, 96–97
   tumor necrosis factor receptors and, 110
Simian immunodeficiency virus (SIV), 690
   genital transmission, 566f
Similarity testing, 177
Single-positive lymphocyte, 29
Single-positive thymocyte, 102
Single radial diffusion, 154–155
Sinopulmonary infection, recurrent, selective IgA deficiency and, 274
Sinusitis, allergic rhinitis and, 335
SIV. *See* Simian immunodeficiency virus
Sjögren's syndrome, 383, 390, 399–401, 618

   lymphoma and, 582
   multiple sclerosis and, 510
   polymyositis-dermatomyositis and, 405
   progressive systemic sclerosis and, 403
   rheumatoid arthritis and, 394
   serum immunoglobulin levels, 157t
   systemic lupus erythematosus and, 389
Skin
   cancer
      organ transplant recipients and, 581, 776
      ultraviolet radiation and, 570
   host defense and, 622–623
   normal flora, 623, 623t
   polymyositis-dermatomyositis and, 405
   progressive systemic sclerosis and, 402
   systemic lupus erythematosus and, 388, 391
Skin testing, 145
   adverse reactions, 197
   allergic drug reactions and, 375
   allergy, 320–322
      technique, 321f
   anaphylaxis and, 349–350, 349t
   cutaneous, 321
   delayed hypersensitivity, 195–197, 259
   interpretation, 196–197
   intracutaneous concentrations, 349t
   intradermal, 321–322
   passive transfer, 322
   penicillin allergy and, 375–377
   technique, 195–196
   wheal-and-erythema, 322t
SLE. *See* Systemic lupus erythematosus
Sleeping sickness, 671
Small cell carcinoma, thymosin and, 782
Small lymphocytic leukemia, 603–604
Small lymphocytic lymphoma, 603–604
Smallpox, 1, 711, 717
   active immunization, 725t
   vaccination, risk:benefit ratio, 726
Small-vessel vasculitis, 444–445, 537
   syndromes associated, 445–447
   systemic diseases associated, 447t
Smith antigen, 390
Snakebite
   passive immunization, 732t
   serum therapy, 733
Snell, George Davis, 5
Sodium benzoate, hives and, 355
Solid crystal gamma counter, 172
Solitary plasmactyoma, 608
Somatic hypermutation, 89
Southern blot technique, 218–220, 220f
Specific antiserum, 48
Specific granule, 10
Specificity
   analytic, 176
   diagnostic, 176, 192
   immune system, 40
   immunoglobulin, 66
   tests, 182f
Sperm, mucosal immune system and, 554
Sperm agglutination assay, 560
Sperm-egg fusion, 554–555
Sperm immobilization assay, 560
Spirochetal disease, 680–687
Spirochete, 680, 685
Spleen, 35–36
   microscopic anatomy, 35f

Splenectomy
  autoimmune hemolytic anemia and, 430
  cold-agglutinin syndromes and, 430
  hairy cell leukemia and, 606
  idiopathic thrombocytopenic purpura and, 437–438
  immunocompromised host and, 707
  thymus-independent antigens and, 726
Spondylitis
  ankylosing, 64–65, 398, 406–407, 521
    acute iridocyclitis, 521*f*
    HLA-B27 and, 384, 631
    immunosuppressives and, 792
    rheumatoid arthritis and, 394
Spondyloarthropathy, immunopathogenesis, 631
Spontaneous abortion, recurrent, 562
Sporotrichosis, 650*t*
  immunologic abnormalities and, 653*t*
  immunologic diagnosis, 655*t*
  pathologic features, 652*t*
Sporozoite, 667
S protein, complement system and, 131
Sprue, 457
SSPE. *See* Subacute sclerosing panencephalitis
Standard, 171, 176
Standard deviation, 178
Staphylococcus
  atopic dermatitis and, 343
  splenectomized patient and, 707
Staphylococcus aureus, 630, 660, 781
  hyper-IgE syndrome and, 307
  phlyctenular disease and, 525
  protein A, 167
  toxin, 383
  toxin TSST-1, 96
Staphylococcus epidermidis, 630
  bone marrow transplantation and, 761
  chronic granulomatous disease and, 303
Status asthmaticus, treatment, 341
STD. *See* Sexually transmitted disease
Steady-state phase, 48
Stem cell
  hematopoietic, 9–10, 22
  lymphoid, 22
Stem cell factor (SCF), lymphopoiesis and, 22
Steroid
  anabolic, hereditary angioedema and, 311–312
  anti-inflammatory mechanisms, 715
  bullous pemphigoid and, 494–495
  discoid lupus erythematosus and, 505
  herpes gestationis and, 497
  mechanism of action, 788*f*
  placental, secretion, 559
Stevens-Johnson syndrome, 373, 374, 377
Stichocyte, 673
Still's disease, 398
Stimulation index (SI), 246
Stomatitis, aphthous, 474–475
Storage mite, 331
Stratum functionale, 552
Streptococcus, 630
Streptococcus agalactiae, 632
Streptococcus pneumoniae, 537, 631–632, 735
  hyper-IgE syndrome and, 307
  hypogammaglobulinemia and, 267
  splenectomized patient and, 707
Streptococcus pyogenes, 630, 781
Streptococcus sanguis, recurrent aphthous ulceration and, 474

Streptokinase, 630
Streptolysin, 630
Streptozyme test, 630
Strongyloides stercoralis, 533, 537, 666, 676
Studentized residual, 177
Subacute sclerosing panencephalitis (SSPE), 517, 641–642
  measles vaccine and, 726
Subcapsular sinus, 32
Sulfamethoxazole, 377
Sulfasalazine
  adverse pulmonary responses, 530
  Crohn's disease and, 460
  ulcerative colitis and, 462
Sulfisoxazole, 377
  chronic granulomatous disease and, 305
Sulfonamide
  allergy, 372, 377–378
  immune thrombocytopenic purpura and, 438
Superantigen, 95–96, 383, 781
  interaction with T cell receptor, 96*f*
Superoxide, generation, respiratory burst and, 304*f*
Suppressor T cell. *See* T cell, suppressor
Surrogate light chain, 86
Swine influenza virus, 639
Switch region, 89
Sympathectomy, progressive systemic sclerosis and, 403
Sympathetic ophthalmia, 524–525
Sympathomimetic drugs
  anti-inflammatory effects, 715
  asthma and, 340
  immediate hypersensitivity reactions and, 793
Syncytiotrophoblast, 557
Synovectomy
  juvenile arthritis and, 399
  rheumatoid arthritis and, 396
Synovial fluid, rheumatoid arthritis and, 394
Synthetic vaccine, 56
Syphilis, 680–684
  course of untreated, 681*f*
  posttransfusion, 232
  primary, 682
  secondary, 682
  serologic tests, 683*f*
    false-positive, systemic lupus erythematosus and, 391
  tertiary, 682–683
Systemic lupus erythematosus (SLE), 50, 154, 374, 380, 383, 385, 387–392, 618
  autoimmune myocarditis and, 443
  chlorambucil and, 774
  cyclophosphamide and, 773
  drug-induced, 530
  immune-complex deposits, 485–486
  immunosuppressives and, 792
  impaired tolerance, B cells, T cells and, 385*t*
  multiple sclerosis and, 510
  pyroglobulins and, 169
  retinal cotton-wool spots, 523, 523*f*
  serum immunoglobulin levels, 157*t*
Systemic lupus erythematosus syndrome, hydralazine and, 372
Systemic mastocytosis, cromolyn sodium and, 792
Systemic necrotizing vasculitis, 447–450
Systemic sclerosis, transforming growth factor-beta and, 784

t(8,14), 91, 92*f*
t(14,18), 92
Tachyzoite, 669

Taenia saginata, 675
Taenia solium, 676
Tail piece, 72
Takayasu arteritis, 391, 453–455
  angiographic findings, 454*f*
Talmage, David W., 3, 4
Tapeworm, 675–676
Target amplification technique, 221–223
Tartrazine yellow dye, hives and, 355
TBII. *See* Thyrotropin binding-inhibitory immunoglobulin
Tc cell. *See* T cell, cytotoxic
T cell, 3, 26–30
  acquired immunodeficiency syndrome and, 696
  activated, progeny, 28*f*
  activation, 30–31
    2-signal model, 99, 99*f*
  allograft rejection and, 748
  anergic, 99, 113
  antigen, 55–56
    differentiation, 198*t*
    tumor, immunophenotypes, 594*t*
  antigen binding, 40
  antigen-presenting cells and, 97–98
  antigen-specific immune suppression and, 713
  assays, 198–199
    clinical applications, 209
    functional, 258–259
  azathioprine and, 771
  corticosteroids and, 766
  cross-matching, 244–245
  cyclophosphamide and, 773
  cytotoxic, 28, 100
    activation, 31, 45–46, 46*f*
    influenza virus and, 639
    interleukin-4 and, 116
  enumeration, 258
  epitopes, 52, 55–56
  E rosette-forming, 199, 200*f*
  helper, 100
    activation, 44–45, 45*f*
    heterogeneity, 100
  helper:suppressor ratios, 199, 199*t*
  host defense and, 624–625
  idiotypy, 382
  immune competence testing, 258–259, 259*t*
  immunity
    carcinoembryonic antigen and, 572
    drugs inducing, 373
    eye disease and, 523
  immunodeficiency disorders, 279–284
    abnormal cytokine production and, 289
    treatment, 265*t*
  interleukin-2 and, 112–113
  leukemias
    adult, 112, 612
    human T cell leukemia virus and, 570
  lymphomas, 611*t*
    convoluted, 612
    cutaneous, 613–614
    human immunodeficiency virus and, 584
    interferon-alpha and, 782
    peripheral, 613
  maturation, intrathymic, 38*f*
  membrane defects, 289
  membrane molecules, 714
  memory, 98
  monoclonal antibodies and, 779
  multiple sclerosis and, 509*f*
  natural killer cells compared, 103
  neoplasms
    lymphocytic, 610–614
    small, 612–613
  ontogeny, 101–102, 101*f*
  proportion in normal tissues, 22, 24*t*
  self-tolerance and, 381
  subsets, 28, 28*t*, 99–101, 199, 258
  suppressor, 101
    antigen-nonspecific, 549
    antigen-specific, 549
    immunologic tolerance and, 387
    nonsteroidal anti-inflammatory drugs and, 791
    tumor-specific, 574–575
  surface molecules, 28*t*
  systemic lupus erythematosus and, 385*t*
  tumor cells and, 572–573
  tumor-specific antigens and, 571
T cell growth factor. *See* Interleukin-2
T cell receptor (TCR), 3, 26, 94–97
  accessory molecules, 97–99
  alpha and beta genes, 94–95
    rearrangement, 96*f*
  coreceptors, 97–99
  epitope recognition, 55
  interaction with superantigens, 95–96, 96*f*
  recognition of antigen, 95, 96*f*
  signal transduction, 96–97
  structure, 94, 95*f*
  transmembrane signaling, 97*f*
T cell receptor-CD3 complex, 714
T cell receptor-major histocompatibility complex (TCR-MHC), 713
T cell-specific marker, 198–199
TCR. *See* T cell receptor
TCR-MHC. *See* T cell receptor-major histocompatibility complex
TdT. *See* Terminal deoxynucleotidyltransferase
Telangiectasis, conjunctival, 291*f*
Template, 222
Tendinitis, nonsteroidal anti-inflammatory drugs and, 790
Teratogenesis, cyclophosphamide and, 773
Terbutaline, 793
  status asthmaticus and, 341
Terminal deoxynucleotidyltransferase (TdT), 84, 95
Terminal differentiation, 10
Tertiary lymphoid organ, 39
Testis, 554
  autoimmune disease, 560
Test specimen, 178
Test specimen "unknowns", 173
Tetanospasmin, 628
Tetanus, 628, 717, 734, 736
  active immunization, 725*t*
  passive immunization, 732*t*
Tetanus toxin, 625, 628
Tetanus toxoid, 2, 628, 718, 726
  reportable events, 728*t*
Tetracycline
  bullous pemphigoid and, 495
  Lyme disease and, 686
  recurrent aphthous ulceration and, 475
Tetrahydrofolate, 773
Tetramethylrhodamine isothiocyanate, 179
TGSI. *See* Thyroid growth-stimulating immunoglobulin
Th cell. *See* T cell, helper

Theophylline, 793
  anti-inflammatory effects, 715
  asthma and, 340
  bronchial obstruction and, 353
  status asthmaticus and, 341
Thermal burn, acute, serum immunoglobulin levels, 157t
Thiazide, immune thrombocytopenic purpura and, 438
Thmyic hormone, 782
Thomas, E. Donnall, 5
Thomas, Lewis, 578
Thromboangiitis obliterans, 455
Thrombocytopenia
  alloimmune, neonatal, 565
  immune
    B cell neoplasms and, 591
    classification, 435t
    drug-induced, 438
  immunodeficiency and, 292–293
  quinine and, 372
  systemic lupus erythematosus and, 387
Thrombocytopenic purpura
  differential diagnosis, 437t
  idiopathic, 435–438, 713
    children and adults, 436t
    cyclophosphamide and, 773
    immune globulin and, 729
    intravenous gamma globulin and, 777–778
    platelet autoantibodies and, 436t
    prednisone and, 768
  immune globulin and, 734
Thrush, 476, 659–660
Thymectomy, myasthenia gravis and, 514
Thymic aplasia, congenital, 279–282
Thymic humoral factor, 37, 782
Thymocyte, 37
  development, stages, 101–102, 101f
  double-negative, 102
  double-positive, 102
  negative selection, 102
  positive selection, 102
  single-positive, 102
Thymoma, immunodeficiency and, 293–294
Thymopentin, 782
Thymopoietin, 37
Thymosin, 37, 782
Thymostimulin, 782
Thymulin, 37, 782
Thymus, 36–38
  embryologic development, 281f
  microscopic anatomy, 37f
  transplantation, fetal, congenital thymic aplasia and, 282
Thymus-dependent antigen, 56
Thymus-independent antigen, 56
Thyroglobulin, specificity and sensitivity, 414t
Thyroid atrophy, 419
Thyroid autoimmune disease, 413–419
Thyroid cell, immunofluorescent staining, 416f
Thyroid growth-stimulating immunoglobulin (TGSI), 418, 418f
  specificity and sensitivity, 414t
Thyroiditis
  autoimmune, Arthus reaction and, 148
  chronic, 413–415
  de Quervain's, 416
  Hashimoto's, 413–415, 618
    pathology, 415f
  postpartum, 416

Thyroiditis syndrome, transient, 415–417
Thyroid peroxidase, specificity and sensitivity, 414t
Thyroid-stimulating immunoglobulin (TSI), 418, 418f
  specificity and sensitivity, 414t
Thyrotoxicosis with diffuse goiter, 417
Thyrotropin binding-inhibitory immunoglobulin (TBII), 418, 418f
  specificity and sensitivity, 414t
Tick-borne relapsing fever, 686
TIL. *See* Tumor-infiltrating lymphocyte
Tinea, 505
Tinea nigra, 650t
  immunologic abnormalities and, 653t
Tinea versicolor, 650t
  immunologic abnormalities and, 653t
Tinnitus, 396
Tiselius, Arne Wilhelm, 2, 4, 156
Tissue immunofluorescence, systemic lupus erythematosus and, 391
Tissue kallikrein, 134–135
Tissue typing, 237
  class II HLA antigens, 243–244
  lymphocytotoxicity test and, 240–242
  reagents, 242
  restriction fragment length polymorphism and, 250f
  test, interpretation, 241–242, 242t
  transplantation and, 237–240
  variability in results, 244
TMP-SMZ. *See* Trimethoprim-sulfamethoxazole
TNF. *See* Tumor necrosis factor
Tolerance, 51
  B cell, 91
  experimental, 383–385
  high-zone, 51
  self-, 2, 102
    loss, 381–382
  suppressor T cells and, 387
  systemic lupus erythematosus and, 385t
Tonegawa, Susumu, 3, 4, 5
Tonsil, 36
Torulopsis glabrata, 659–660
Toxic disease, active immunization and, 712
Toxic epidermal necrolysis, 373, 374
Toxic shock syndrome, 96, 383, 630
Toxigenic bacterial infection, 627, 628–631, 628f
Toxin, neutralization, 46
Toxocara canis, 533
Toxocara cati, 533
Toxoplasma, 526, 666, 669
Toxoplasma gondii, 537
  transfusion-transmitted, 232
Toxoplasmosis, 508, 533, 666, 668–669
  ocular, 669
Tracer, 171
Tracheostomy, 353
Transcobalamin II deficiency, immunodeficiency and, 297
Transformation, 570
  malignant, molecular model, 580f
Transforming growth factor-beta, 117–118, 783–784
  cell sources and target cells, 118f
  properties, 107t
Transfusion reaction, 230–233, 231t
  allergic, 231–232
  febrile, 231
  hemolytic, 230–231
  immunologic mechanisms, 233
  selective IgA deficiency and, 276

Transfusion-transmitted infection, 232, 232*t*
Transient thyroiditis syndrome, 415–417
Transitional zone, 552
Transmembrane signaling
    complex, antigen-receptor, 87*f*
    T cell receptor, 97*f*
Transplantation, 744–763
    ABO testing and, 744–746
    adoptive immunity and, 712
    bone, 761–762
        immunosuppression and, 762
        rejection, 762
    bone marrow. *See* Bone marrow transplantation
    heart, 754–756
    heart-lung, 755–756
    histocompatibility testing and, 237
    kidney. *See* Kidney transplantation
    liver. *See* Liver transplantation
    lung, 755–756
    pancreas. *See* Pancreas transplantation
    tissue typing and, 237–240
Trematode, 673–675
Treponema carateum, 684
Treponemal antibody, 683–684
Treponema pallidum, 487, 680–684
Treponema subsp *endemicum*, 684
Treponema subsp *pertenue*, 684
Treponematosis, nonvenereal, 684
Treponeme, 681–682
Triamcinolone
    allergic contact dermatitis and, 364
    chemical structure, 787*f*
    half-life relative potency, 788*t*
    recurrent aphthous ulceration and, 475
Triamcinolone acetonide, asthma and, 340
Trichinella spiralis, 677
Trichinosis, 677
Trichophyton, 502, 524
Trichophyton tonsurans, 505
Trichopyton rubrum infection, thymic hormones and,
        782
Trichosporon beigelii, 649
Trichuriasis, 532
Trichuris trichiura, 673
Trimethoprim-dapsone, *Pneumocystis carinii* and, 664
Trimethoprim-sulfamethoxazole (TMP-SMZ), 373
    bone marrow transplantation and, 759
    Pneumocystis carinii and, 288, 664
Trimetrexate, *Pneumocystis carinii* and, 664
Tropheryma whippelii, 463
Trophoblast, 557
    invasion of maternal tissue, 555–557
Tropical endomyocardial fibrosis, 443
Tropical pulmonary eosinophilia, 533
Tropical sore, 670
Tropical spastic paraparesis, multiple sclerosis and, 510
Trypanosoma brucei, 671
Trypanosoma cruzi, transfusion-transmitted, 232
Trypanosoma rhodesiense, 671, 673
Trypanosome, 671–672
Trypanosomiasis
    African, 671–673
    antigenic diversity, molecular mechanism, 673*f*
    antigenic variation and parasitemia, 672*f*
TSI. *See* Thyroid-stimulating immunoglobulin
Tuberculin, 2
    skin testing, live virus vaccines and, 727
    test, 322

Tuberculosis, 2, 626, 635
    active immunization, 725*t*
    pregnancy and, 558
    serum immunoglobulin levels, 157*t*
d-Tubocurarine, anaphylactoid reactions and, 352
Tubulointerstitial nephritis, 487–489
Tuftsin deficiency, 306–307
Tumor
    development, 569–570
    epithelial, 580
    immune system, 580
    immunology, mechanisms, 569–576
    interferon-alpha and, 782
    interferon-gamma and, 782–783
    interleukin-4 and, 783
Tumor-associated antigen, 571–572
Tumor-associated determinant, 571
Tumor cell
    antigens, 570–572
    escape from immune response, 574–575
    immunization and, 575
    immunologic effector mechanisms and, 572–574
    macrophages and, 573–574
    natural killer cells and, 103–104, 573
    T cells and, 572–573
Tumor-infiltrating lymphocyte (TIL), 714, 783
Tumor necrosis factor (TNF), 45, 105–112, 478, 783
    actions on cells and tissues, 108*f*
    host defense and, 624
    inhibitors as therapeutic agents, 111–112
    macrophage-activating factor and, 573
    nonimmunologic effects, 110–111
    receptors, signal transduction and, 110
    target cells and actions, 109*t*
    tumor cells and, 573
Tumor necrosis factor-alpha, 88, 110
    mast cell granules and, 139
    properties, 106*t*
Tumor necrosis factor-beta, 110
    properties, 106*t*
Tumor-reactive immunologic reagents, 571
Tumor-specific antigen, 571
Tyan, Marvin L., 3, 4
Tympanometry, 318
Typhoid, 633
    active immunization, 725*t*
Tyrosinemia, liver transplantation and, 750
Tyrosine phosphatase, 88, 98
Tyrpanosomiasis, 533

Ulceration, aphthous, recurrent, 474–475, 474*f*
Ulcerative colitis, 461–462
    rectal biopsy specimen, 461*f*
    selective IgA deficiency and, 274
Ulcerative iliojejunitis, 458
Ultrasensitive enzymatic radioimmunoassay (USERIA), 174,
        175*f*
Ultraviolet light, psoriatic arthritis and, 408
Ultraviolet radiation
    photoallergic contact dermatitis and, 365
    skin cancer and, 570
Unknown, 178
Upper detection limit, 178
Urethritis, Reiter's syndrome and, 407
Urinary creatine, polymyositis-dermatomyositis and, 405
Urine, abnormalities, zone electrophoresis patterns, 160*f*
Ursodeoxycholic acid, primary biliary cirrhosis and, 469

Urticaria, 150, 354–356, 374
  anaphylaxis and, 348, 353
  cholinergic, 355
  cold, 355
    familial, 355
  desensitization therapy and, 742
  idiopathic, 355
  pressure, 355
Urticaria-angioedema, 327
Urticarial vasculitis, hypocomplementemic, 446
Urticaria pigmentosa, 356
USERIA. *See* Ultrasensitive enzymatic radioimmunoassay
Uteroplacental circulation, 555
Uveitis, lens-induced, 523

Vaccination
  immunoblastic reactions, 618
  reportable events, 728*t*
Vaccine, 56
  attenuated, 1, 56
  bacterial, 631, 633, 635
  currently in development, 737–738
  human immunodeficiency virus, 700, 738
    obstacles to development, 700*t*
  influenza virus, 639
  killed, 56
  live, hazards, 726–727
  Lyme disease, 686
  measles virus, 642
  poliovirus, 647
  recombinant, 56
  respiratory syncytial virus, 641
  special populations and, 737
  synthetic, 56
  types, 718
  vaccinia, contaminated, epidemic hepatitis and, 727
Vaccine Adverse Event Reporting System, 727
Vaccinia
  passive immunization, 732*t*
  vaccine, contaminated, epidemic hepatitis and, 727
Vaccinia virus, 639, 726
  eczema vaccinatum and, 343
Vagina, normal flora, 623*t*
Vaginal immunization, 553
Vaginitis, candidal, 659–660
Valid analytic range, 178
Vancomycin, bone marrow transplantation and, 761
Variable-folding theory, 2
Variable region, 68, 74–77
  subgroups, 75
Variance, 178
Varicella
  passive immunization, 732–733*t*
  vaccine, 738
Varicella-zoster virus, natural killer cells and, 104
Variolation, 1, 717, 726
Vascular addressing, 39
Vascular disease, 443–455
  classification, 445*t*
  pulmonary, heart-lung transplantation and, 755
Vascular purpura, cold-agglutinin syndromes and, 430
Vascular system, systemic lupus erythematosus and, 389
Vasculitides, 443–455
  classification, 445*t*
Vasculitis, 147
  Beçhet's, 406
  granulomatous affecting lung, 537*t*
  hypersensitivity, 444–445

    skin biopsy specimen, 445*f*
  necrotizing, systemic, 447–450
  nongranulomatous affecting lung, 537*t*
  polymyositis-dermatomyositis and, 405
  pulmonary, 537
  renal, 489–490
  rheumatoid, 394, 395
    plasma exchange and, 777
  small-vessel, 444–445, 537
    syndromes associated, 445–447
    systemic diseases associated, 447*t*
  systemic lupus erythematosus and, 389
  urticarial, 355
    hypocomplementemic, 446
Vasodilating agents, progressive systemic sclerosis and, 403
V/D/J joining, 83
  molecular basis, 84
V/D/J recombinase, 84
VDRL test, 683, 684
  false-positive, systemic lupus erythematosus and, 391
Venom desensitization, 740
Vernal conjunctivitis, 520–521, 521*f*
Vernal keratoconjunctivitis, 334
Vesicle, dermatologic disease and, 499
Vesiculobullous dermatosis, 365
Vibrio cholerae, 629, 718
Villus
  atrophy, 458, 459
  intermediate, cross-fractured immature, 563*f*
Vincristine
  Hodgkin's disease and, 616
  idiopathic thrombocytopenic purpura and, 437
Virus
  antigenic shift and, 734
  DNA, detection by in situ hybridization, 222*f*
  endogenous superantigens and, 383
  infection, 637–647
    immune system, 689–705
    immunologic sequelae, 638*t*
    natural killer cells and, 104
  insulin-dependent diabetes mellitus and, 420
  neutralization, 46–47
  oncogenesis, 570
  slow and latent infections, 517
  vaccines, adverse effects, 727
Visceral larva migrans, 533
Visceral leishmaniasis, 671
Viscosity, serum, 168
  disorders associated with increased, 168*t*
Visna virus, 690
Vitamin B12 deficiency, 462–463
  multiple sclerosis and, 510
Vitamin D, mechanism of action, 787–788
Vitiligo, 524
Vitronectin, complement system and, 131
V/J joining, 81
v-*myc* proto-oncogene, 598
VNTR typing, 254
Vogt-Koyanagi-Haradi syndrome, 524–525
von Behring, Emil, 2, 3, 4, 8*f*
von Krogh equation, 172, 187–188
von Pirquet, Clemens P., 2, 4
von Willebrand's disease, 438–439

Waldenstrom's macroglobulinemia, 154, 158
  monoclonal serum immunoglobulins and, 589
  plasmacytoid lymphocytic lymphoma and, 606
  plasma exchange and, 777

Waldenstrom's macroglobulinemia *(cont.)*
 serum immunoglobulin abnormalities, 159f
 serum viscosity and, 168
Wassermann antibody, 683
Weber-Christian disease, 408–409
Wegener's granulomatosis, 450–451, 490, 537
 chlorambucil and, 774
 cyclophosphamide and, 773
 saddle nose deformity, 450f
Weighting, 178
Weil's disease, 687
Western blot analysis, human immunodeficiency virus and, 695f
Wheal-and-erythema skin test, 322t, 375
Wheal-and-flare reaction, 144
 drugs causing, 350t
Whipple's disease, 463
Whipworm, 532
White piedra, 650t
 immunologic abnormalities and, 653t
White pulp, 35
Whooping cough, 629
Wilson's disease, liver transplantation and, 750
Wiskott-Aldrich syndrome, 292–293
 atopic dermatitis and, 343
 cancer and, 580
 facial eczema, 293f
Within-assay random error, 178
Wright, Almoth E., 2, 4
Wuchereria, 678
Wuchereria bancrofti, 533, 676
 transfusion-transmitted, 232

Xanthine, asthma and, 340
X-linked hypogammaglobulinemia
 atopic dermatitis and, 343

serum immunoglobulin levels, 157t
X-linked infantile hypogammaglobulinemia, 266–270
 periodontal disease and, 267f
X-linked lymphoproliferative syndrome, 277–278, 619
 cancer and, 580
 natural killer cell deficiency and, 284

Yalow, Rosalyn, 5
Yaws, 684
Yellow fever
 immunization, 726
  active, 725t
 vaccination, 737
 vaccine, 736
  contaminated, 727
Yersin, A. E. J., 2, 3
Yersinia, 631

Zalcitabine, human immunodeficiency virus and, 699
ZAP70, 97
Zidovudine (AZT), 689
 human immunodeficiency virus and, 698–699
 idiopathic thrombocytopenic purpura and, 438
Zinkernagel, Rolf M., 3, 4
Zona pellucida, 555
Zone electrophoresis, 157–158
 cellulose acetate technique, 158f
 cerebrospinal fluid, 160f
 immunoelectrophoresis compared, 161f
 serum immunoglobulin abnormalities, 159f
 urine abnormalities, 160f
Zoster, thymic hormones and, 782
Zygomycosis, 649, 651t, 662–663
 immunologic abnormalities and, 653t
 immunologic diagnosis, 656t
 pathologic features, 652t